Proceedings of the
XXIII International Congress of the
History of Medicine

Volume 1

Proceedings of the XXIII International Congress of the History of Medicine

LONDON 2–9 SEPTEMBER 1972

Organized by the
British Society for the History of Medicine
and
The International Society of the History of Medicine

Patron:
HER MAJESTY QUEEN ELIZABETH II

Honorary President:
THE RT. HON. THE LORD COHEN OF BIRKENHEAD

President:
DR. F. N. L. POYNTER

Volume 1

London
Wellcome Institute of the History of Medicine
1974

PRINTED IN GREAT BRITAIN AT
THE UNIVERSITY PRESS
ABERDEEN

Council of Honour

The Lord Mayor of London, *Vice-Patron*
The Vice-Chancellor, University of London, *Vice-President*
The President, The Royal Society of London, *Vice-President*
The President, Royal College of Physicians of London, *Vice-President*
The President, Royal College of Surgeons of England, *Vice-President*
The President, Royal College of Obstetricians and Gynaecologists, *Vice-President*
The President, Royal College of General Practitioners, *Vice-President*
The President, Royal College of Pathologists, *Vice-President*
Chief Medical Officer, Department of Health and Social Security
The President, British Medical Association
The President, Royal Historical Society
The President, British Society for the History of Pharmacy
The President, British Society for the History of Science
The Master, Worshipful Society of Apothecaries of London
The President, Medical Society of London
The President, Pharmaceutical Society of Great Britain
The President, Royal Society of Medicine
The President, The Harveian Society
The President, The Hunterian Society
The President, Osler Club of London
The President, Scottish Society of the History of Medicine
The President, Society for the Social History of Medicine
The Director, Institute of Historical Research
The Director, The Warburg Institute
The Regius Professor of Physic, University of Cambridge
The Regius Professor of Medicine, University of Oxford
Rt. Hon. Lord Brock
Sir Zachary Cope
Dr. Douglas Guthrie
Professor Rupert Hall, Professor of History of Science, Imperial College, London
Sir Geoffrey Keynes
Sir John McMichael, Deputy Chairman, The Wellcome Trust
Dr. Joseph Needham
Dr. Walter Pagel
Professor Hugh Trevor-Roper
Dr. P. O. Williams, Director, The Wellcome Trust
Mr. A. Dickson Wright

Organizing Committee

Dr. F. N. L. Poynter, *Chairman*
Dr. D. Geraint James, *Secretary*
Dr. A. White Franklin, *Treasurer*

Mr. R. A. Cohen
Dr. J. K. Crellin
Miss Jessie Dobson
Dr. Ruth G. Hodgkinson
Dr. K. D. Keele
Dr. A. H. T. Robb-Smith
Dr. A. J. Rook
Dr. Hugh Sinclair
Dr. K. Bryn Thomas
Mr. G. Wilson
Dr. G. E. W. Wolstenholme

Secretariat
Wellcome Institute of the History of Medicine
183 Euston Road
London, NW1 2BP

International Society of the History of Medicine Council 1972

F. N. L. Poynter, Great Britain, *President*
A. Pazzini, Italy, *Honorary President*
F. A. Sondervorst, Belgium, *Honorary Vice-President*
F. Guerra, Spain, *Vice-President*
C. Martinez-Duran, Guatemala, *Vice-President*
M. Nadjmabadi, Iran, *Vice-President*
C. Coury, France, *Vice-President*
L. Dulieu, France, *Secretary-General*
E. Reti, Hungary, *Assistant Secretary-General*
I. Simon, Israel, *Treasurer*

CONTENTS

VI. Congress Theme: Relations between British Medicine and Medicine in Other Countries

Special note: the following papers delivered at the Congress are being published elsewhere:

BRODNY, L. M. (U.S.A.). Clinical and cultural history of connotative medical pewter. (This paper is to be expanded and published in book form.)

COWEN, D. L. (U.S.A.). The spread and influence of British pharmacopoeial literature.

DA SILVA ARAUJO, C. (Brazil). The immortalized cow: smallpox vaccine and Wright's vaccines in Brazil. Rio de Janeiro, Grafico Olimpica Editora, 1972, pp. 69, illus.

I INAUGURAL ADDRESS AND INTRODUCTION

1. Presidential Address

Dr. F. N. L. Poynter
(*Great Britain*)

My Lords, Ladies and Gentlemen,

It is a great honour and a rare privilege to welcome to London the delegates and associates of this 23rd International Congress of the History of Medicine.

As you will see when you look around this hall, it is a very well-attended meeting. In fact, it has proved to be the largest of the whole series, with 637 members representing no less than forty-eight countries. Its importance is acknowledged by the high level of support which it has received in Britain, and the seal was set upon this official support by the patronage graciously accorded to it by Her Majesty, Queen Elizabeth II.

Her Majesty is at present in Scotland, enjoying a well-earned rest from her official duties, and is unable to be with us today. However, on your behalf and in your name I have sent Her Majesty the following message:

The delegates and associates of the XXIII International Congress of the History of Medicine send Greetings to Her Majesty and express their gratitude for Her Majesty's patronage of their Jubilee meeting.

Representing medical and academic bodies in nearly fifty countries, delegates will present more than 350 formal papers. Many of these will analyse the influence which British Medicine has exerted throughout the world, and in a special Symposium the rise of the British National Health Service will be discussed in the light of developments in many other countries.

We hope to ensure that, by contributing to a deeper understanding of medical and scientific and social problems in many parts of the world, and by extending the spirit of friendliness and mutual cooperation which is so notable a feature of the relations between doctors of every nationality, this Congress will prove worthy of the recognition which Your Majesty has graciously accorded it.

Her Majesty has sent the following reply to this message:

Please convey to all the delegates and associates of the XXIII International Congress of the History of Medicine the sincere thanks of The Queen for their kind and loyal message of greetings which Her Majesty, as Patron, much appreciated. The Queen wishes the Congress every success in its aims for extending the knowledge and application of medical and scientific discoveries in this country and throughout the world, and hopes that all delegates will take away a new inspiration for their professional labours.

The Minister of Health and Social Security, Sir Keith Joseph, has other duties which prevent him from being here this morning, but he has sent us the following message:

It is a pleasure to welcome more than 500 participants from so many countries to this twenty-third International Congress of the History of Medicine. That history is the inheritance of the world and to it all have contributed. In an age when advance in medical science in any country immediately becomes the concern of all, it is of great importance that we should understand the way in which our present practices have evolved. I am sure that this Congress will help that process and I wish it all success.

It usually falls to the lot of a Congress President, as one of the first duties of his office, to extend a formal welcome to the President of the International Society which founded this series of congresses more than fifty years ago.

I was looking forward to having at my side today in that capacity my old friend Professor Maurice Bariéty, whose wisdom and inspiring eloquence created such a profound impression at the 22nd Congress in Bucharest. He has left his own mark on this meeting, for it was his idea to introduce into the usual Congress programme the special symposia which are a novel feature of this London meeting, and it was he who suggested the discussion on the development of concepts in clinical medicine.

His sudden death last year, half-way through his term of office, has been a great loss to our Society and to this Congress. How great a loss was expressed in moving terms in the formal Éloge by his great friend and closest associate at the Hôtel Dieu in Paris, Professor Charles Coury, now himself a Vice-President, which he delivered at the meeting of the Society's Permanent Committee last May.

When, at that meeting, I was elected to succeed our late President, I was deeply conscious of the difficulty of proving a worthy successor to such a man and I take this first opportunity of repeating publicly my assurance to your Permanent Committee that I shall do my best to justify the trust you have placed in me.

However, it is a great pleasure to have with us today a former President and now the Honorary President of the International Society, Professor Pazzini, of Rome. To him, and to all the officers and council of the Society, I give cordial greetings and a warm welcome from the British Society for the History of Medicine. We hope that by the end of the week you will all feel that *our* efforts and *your* journeys have been abundantly justified and that this 23rd Congress will prove a truly memorable one.

It is also a great pleasure to have with us Members of the Congress Council of Honour. Between them, they represent the most important medical and scientific bodies in Britain and it has been a very great encouragement to the Organizing Committee to have their warm support at all times.

They have sent messages of welcome and good wishes to the Congress and I now call upon the Congress Secretary, Dr. James, to read these to you.

Dr. D. Geraint James then read the following messages:

Our Vice-Patron, the Lord Mayor of London, is abroad at this time, but he has sent us greetings and wishes us a happy and successful meeting.

Our President of Honour, Lord Cohen of Birkenhead, is today opening another International Medical Congress as its President, but he has sent the following message to Dr. Poynter.

It is particularly apt that at a time when there is in the United Kingdom a vigorous resurgence of interest in the history of medicine the International Congress should be held in London under your Presidency for you have played so notable a role in stimulating this interest. May I as Honorary President send to you and to all participants in the Congress my best wishes to the certain knowledge that under your guidance and leadership the 1972 Congress will prove an outstanding success.

The Vice-Chancellor of the University of London reminds us that it is now fifty years since the International Congress last met in London. On behalf of the University, which is one of the great centres of medical education in this country, he sends his felicitations and expresses the wish that this meeting will be as successful as its predecessors have been.

The President of the Royal Society sends greetings and good wishes to all participants and is delighted that so many different countries are represented.

Sending his best wishes for a very successful Congress, the President of the Royal College of Physicians looks forward to welcoming you to the Reception at the College tomorrow evening 'where you will see 450 years of medical history in the setting of very attractive modern surroundings'.

The President and Council of the Royal College of Surgeons of England has sent us the following message:

As the inheritors of so much, both tangible and intangible, from our predecessors in this Royal College and its forebears, and as the guardians of a heritage valued by all students of the History of Medicine, we have a special interest in your meeting and are confident that it will prove successful in every way.

The President and Council of the Royal College of Obstetricians and Gynaecologists welcome you to London and look forward to receiving a party of delegates on Wednesday afternoon when they will be shown the College's fine historic collections of books and instruments, among which are the original Chamberlen forceps.

A message of welcome and good wishes has also come from the President of the Royal College of General Practitioners, who will also be receiving a party of delegates.

The Regius Professor of Physic at Cambridge sends greetings and good wishes, and adds:

May I express the hope that in its consideration of medical education, the Congress will be able to encourage the study of the History and Philosophy of Medicine in the medical schools of universities throughout the world.

Sir George Godber, the Chief Medical Officer of the Department of Health and Social Security, sends his personal greetings and best wishes for a successful Congress, adding that the Programme cannot fail to be of the greatest interest to all.

Dr. Douglas Guthrie of Edinburgh, for long a familiar figure at many of these International Congresses and an old friend of many delegates visiting us from abroad, is unable to attend this one and sends greetings to all. On Friday next, when we shall be enjoying the Congress Banquet, Dr. Guthrie will be celebrating his 87th birthday and in your name we shall send him a telegram of greetings on his anniversary.

Another old friend of many of us here, Sir Zachary Cope, now in his 92nd year, sends a warm personal letter from his retirement in Oxford and remarks that this Congress would have given the greatest pleasure to Sir Henry Wellcome.

Special messages of greeting have also come from Professor Sir Eric Gombrich, Director of the Warburg Institute, from Dr. Rupert Hall, Professor of the History of Science at Imperial College, and other members of the Council of Honour. Among them is a personal telegram from Dr. Joseph Needham in Pekin, where he is pursuing his researches for the continuation of his great work on the History of Science and Civilization in China. Dr. Needham is also President of the important International Union of the History and Philosophy of Science, and its Secretary-General writes to Dr. Poynter associating the full Council of the Union with their President's message and adds:

We recognise no dividing line between your field of interest and our own, and we know that the results of your work will be of great value far beyond the field of the History of Medicine itself. To our good wishes for the success of the Congress we add our expression of respect and admiration for your own personal contribution to historical scholarship, to which the world-wide study of the history, not only of medicine but of science at large, is so much in debt.

2. Messages from the Five Continents

Europe Professor A. Pazzini

(*Rome*)

For me it is a matter of pride and satisfaction to deliver to this distinguished gathering a message on behalf of the European states. As a European, and as honorary President of the International Society of the History of Medicine, I am especially proud to pay homage to Her Majesty the Queen, who is the gracious Patron of this Congress.

To Lord Cohen of Birkenhead, honorary President; to you Dr. Poynter, President of the Congress and of the International Society; and to all the members of the Secretariat, I extend my sincere thanks for the work you have done and I express my admiration for the splendid organization which you have achieved. I offer my best wishes for the success of this meeting and for the future.

To you all, my dear colleagues and friends, you who have made this meeting possible, I should like to express my most sincere greetings and feelings of friendship.

You who are gathered here are in a privileged and enviable position. You have come together, without heed to social position or whatever else, in the hope and expectation of seeing truth emerge from your studies and investigations. Together we shall rejoice in that supreme experience.

There was once a time when I arrived at another congress, flying in above the clouds and the storms, above the seas and the mountains, and I remember then saying: 'I have arrived here like a pilgrim who travels in the light of the sun and over the earth's clouds.'

The truth is, we are all pilgrims passing out of this earthly life, passionately seeking to extract some truth from our studies and researches: above the clouds, whilst below us tragedy unrolls across the surface of a planet called Earth.

After paying tribute to the memory of those devoted colleagues who have passed away and after acknowledging their great contributions to our discipline, I should like now to present greetings to this Congress: from myself as the longest-standing member of the International Society; from the University of Rome to which I have the honour of belonging; from the Italian National Academy for the History of the

Healing Arts, of which I am President; from the Italian Society of the History of Medicine, of which I am honorary President; and from all our colleagues throughout Europe, from that spiritual brotherhood to which I feel proud and honoured to belong.

Africa Dr. T. R. Lambo
(Nigeria)

On the occasion of the XXIII International Congress of the History of Medicine, it is with great pleasure that I send this short message on behalf of Africa. First of all, allow me to congratulate you for the many achievements in this field, especially in your efforts to preserve and utilize historical material and evidence to stimulate further scientific work for the ultimate good of the individuals and of our societies.

The whole framework of medical thinking is changing: we now have at our disposal a corpus of organized concepts and scientific knowledge, and we are also facing a Copernican revolution parallel to the Age of Enlightenment. We still remember with inspiration great names and events which have conditioned our perceptions and motivations, occasionally providing world images of medicine which may determine the tracks along which action may be pushed by the dynamic of interests. Such events and names that were connected with Hippocratic medicine, with Pasteur, Descartes, Galen, Harvey, Andreas Vesalius, Pavlov or even Claude Bernard, who has been termed the apostle of physiological determinism, still linger in our memory to provide the ethos and an orientation.

Future discoveries and creativity may put us in yet another place, with even greater respect for our environment, for human potentialities and, possibly even for each other as well. The history of medicine has aptly demonstrated that medicine as a science and as an art is inextricably connected with the structure and evolution of our civilizations. Galdston (1963) has observed that 'individual man, the infinite being, is an "accident" in time. But he is also the issue of a long past, that is of historic and collective man. To understand the individual, the finite person, we need to know a great deal about the extended past of the collective historical man. . . .'

Life in the tropics today has altered considerably: mortality and morbidity rates have decreased significantly, human energy and quality of life have improved considerably, man is now able to release his energy for creativity. There is no doubt that the present health conditions in Africa testify to the fact that scientific medicine, during the past few decades, has to its credit a remarkable development of insight into many medical problems, for example, communicable diseases and nutritional disorders. The control of many endemic diseases has paved the way to exponential growth and socio-economic development almost unparalleled in the history of many nations.

At this point, I would like to refer to the exotic and exciting historical material waiting to be explored in Africa. Tropical medicine has gone through many revolutions and has achieved a great deal within the last decade. For the medical historian, these and other cultures still constitute a virgin soil. The relative isolation of some of these cultures has led paradoxically to the evolution of some ideas and practices that form the basis of the indigenous forms of medicine. There is no doubt that this aspect of human culture should be reflected in our medical history.

America Dr. C. Martínez Durán

(*Guatemala*)

Au nom de l'Amérique, continent d'utopies et d'espoirs, je présente mes salutations aux distingués collègues, historiens de la Médecine, participants à ce 23e Congrès International, et je remercie les organisateurs britanniques de leur aimable hospitalité, de leur efficacité dans la coopération et de l'excellente organisation de ce Congrès.

Ici, à Londres, au XVIIe siècle, William Harvey, dans son œuvre fondamentale en Physiologie, De Motu Cordis, disait en latin: «Philosophi enim veri, qui amori veritatis et sapientiae flagrant, nunquam se tam sapientia plenos reperiunt, aut suo sensu abundant, quin veritate, a quocunque et quandocunque venerit, locum dent.»

Merveilleuses paroles toujours en vigueur pour l'esprit humain. L'amour de la vérité, de ce que nous croyons notre vérité, doit laisser passer tout ce qui est nouveau sans tenir compte de qui et d'où proviennent ces vérités.

Peu de temps avant cela, Bacon dans son aphorisme Livre 1,124 avait également dit dans la langue universelle et œcuménique: «Itaque ipsissimae res sunt (in hoc genere) veritas et utilitas: atque opera ipsa pluris facienda sunt, quatenus sunt veritatis pignora, quam propter vitae commoda.»

La vérité et l'utilité peuvent se confondre, mais, pour agir, il faut être fidèle à cette vérité même si l'on doit renoncer aux commodités de la vie.

Face au monde qui nous entoure, il nous faut la liberté de pensée et d'expression la plus complète: le dialogue entre les hommes est un enrichissement mutuel. Comme tout est sujet à discussion on a donc besoin de la raison, de l'observation juste, sans préjugés et de l'expérimentation qui confirme. Médecine d'hier et d'aujourd'hui a valeur pédagogique et éthique dans le noble enseignement de l'Histoire de la Médecine. Cette discipline philosophique et scientifique constitue un pont solide entre la Technique et les Humanités, entre l'utile, le pragmatique et les intérêts sacrés de l'esprit.

La politique de la santé est la plus grande des politiques selon Virchow et la politique de l'esprit chère à Paul Valéry.

L'Histoire de la Médecine offre aux jeunes une culture authentique leur permettant de comprendre l'exercice de leur profession et le sommet de la vie humaine.

L'Histoire de la Médecine, nous devons le dire avec clarté et vérité, a presque cessé d'être une question controversée, mais si n'avait été la passion qui encore enflamme quelques vieux maîtres dans certaines nations, elle aurait disparu totalement des plans d'études des écoles de Médecine.

Si son enseignment s'ajustait à la rigueur scientifique et à la philosophie la plus élevée, nous serions fidèles à Bertrand Russell, respectant la relation étroite entre ces nobles disciplines créatrices, signe de l'homme de tout les temps.

Dans la Société Internationale d'Histoire de la Médecine, dans chacune des Sociétés Nationales, dans le présent Congrès, nous devons agir sans hésitations, avec la volonté souveraine de Don Santiago Ramón y Cajal, avec la dévise de Ruskin, l'esthète, *To Day*, pour que l'enseignment de l'Histoire de la Médecine soit maintenu et amélioré en faveur de la culture médicale.

Pour conclure ces mots de remerciement je voudrais rappeler Sydenham dans sa réponse au Dr. Blackmore: «Lisez Don Quichotte, c'est un excellent livre que je lis encore.» En tant qu'hispanoamericain, ce conseil me plaît, mais peut être a-t-il été donné, comme l'affirment quelques historiens, pour indiquer le manque de bonnes publications médicales en cette époque. Mais à mon avis ce conseil va plus loin: il sert à signaler la multiple et merveilleuse aventure de l'homme dans la realité et l'enchantement, la valeur de la justice, la valeur de la culture au service de la vie.

Chers collègues: en 1728, l'Histoire de la Médecine du Dr. Freind, citoyen anglais, était publiée en français. Dans la préface nous trouvons ces paroles que je vous laisse comme guide de nos sessions et discussions: «On trouve en lui (l'auteur Freind) des charmes auxquels il est difficile de résister. Il répand dans ses écrits une force et une douceur qui le rend maître des esprits. On admire dans ses conversations les agréments de l'esprit, la justesse du raisonnement et l'étendue de ses lumières.» Qu'il en soit ainsi pour le Congrès.

Asia Dr. M. Nadjmabadi
(*Tehran*)

C'est pour moi un grand honneur de me trouver encore une fois parmi vous, mes chers collègues et la grande famille de l'histoire de la médecine. Je suis certain que je serai enrichi de vos sciences. Pour moi qui suis un des anciens membres de la Société Internationale d'Histoire de la Médecine, il est la plus grande réussite de pouvoir assister chaque deux ans à cette réunion, afin de faire des échanges de nos connaissances sur les questions historiques médicales.

Il me semble qu'il faut reconnaître que nos anciens confrères et savants ont rendu de grands services à l'humanité. Cette reconnaissance est en réalité le condiment de notre vie. A mon avis, s'il n'y avait pas ce condiment dans notre vie, certainement l'aliment de la vie serait fade. Il faut toujours rappeler et dire des dévouements des anciens médecins que la jeune génération sache qu'on remercie toujours les serviteurs de l'humanité.

Pour l'Asie, ce grand continent qui était le berceau de la civilisation, il y a des milliers de siècles que les peuples ont travaillé pour l'humanité et la médecine. Il est bien clair que les tâches des hindous, chinois, japonais, arabes, indochinois, philippiniens, indonésiens, pakistaniens, afghans, libanais, syriens, turcs, des habitants de l'Asie centrale, de l'Iraq d'aujourd'hui ou des anciens mésopotamiens, de l'Arabie, de Palestine et enfin des perses sont bien importantes et que les peuples mentionnés ont rendu des grands services à la médecine. Maintenant nous avons en Asie quelques Instituts d'Histoire de la Médecine: à l'Inde, au Pakistan, au Japon, en Chine, en Turquie, en Iran ainsi que dans d'autres pays du continent de l'Asie qui ont tous une part bien importante pour les recherches historiques. Comme exemple je peux vous signaler la nouvelle Société d'Histoire de la Médecine et l'Institut de Recherches

Historiques Médicales de New Delhi, qui est fondé sous les bons soins du Professeur Hakim Abdul-Hameed, du Professeur Subba Reddy et de leurs confrères.

En ma qualité de Délégué pour toute l'Asie et ses peuples, je remercie le Dr. N. Poynter ainsi que le Dr. Geraint James, Secrétaire Général du Congrès, et notre Secrétaire Général de la S.I.H.M., le Docteur L. Dulieu, et tous les autres membres qui ont déjà rendu des services pour le progrès de cette réunion.

Merci à vous tous.

Australia Professor K. F. Russell

(*Melbourne*) (read by Professor de Gruchy)

I send you cordial greetings and best wishes for the success of the Congress, not only from myself but also from all those in Australia who are inspired by the study of medical history.

With the many papers to be presented by the delegates, I do not doubt that the meeting will be an unqualified success. It is the getting together of historians from around the world that enhances the importance of such a gathering which to my sorrow I cannot attend in person.

As the International Society of the History of Medicine and the International Academy of the History of Medicine so well demonstrate, medical history knows no geographical or political boundaries. One hopes that the co-operation fostered by these bodies will always be present and that they will continue to flourish.

Although isolated from the great centres of culture, we in Australia are very conscious of our medical heritage and while much of this has been reported, a lot still remains to be done for there is no lack of material for the medical historian. I sincerely hope that the deliberations of 2 to 9 September fulfil all the expectations of those responsible for the organization and that the London Congress will be long remembered by the delegates. To you, as its President, I send my warmest regards and congratulations.

3. Message from the International Academy of the History of Medicine

L. Belloni, Honorary President

(*Bologna, Italy*)

J'ai l'honneur de saluer ce XXIIIe Congrès de la Société Internationale d'Histoire de la Médecine au nom de l'Académie Internationale d'Histoire de la Médecine. Je suis heureux de cette occasion pour souligner les liens étroits qui existent entre ces deux associations: une véritable fraternité de buts qui, souvent, est plus d'une fraternité, lorsqu'elle se fonde sur l'identité des personnes.

Un cas typique est celui d'Ernest Wickersheimer, le vénérable Président de la Société Internationale d'Histoire de la Médecine, qui fut en même temps l'un des fondateurs de notre Académie, née il y a juste dix ans, au cours d'un déjeuner de travail à la Cornell University d'Ithaca.

La série des symposium – qui font partie des buts institutionnels de l'Académie – fut ouverte elle aussi au cours d'un Congrès international: le symposium sur la *Matière médicale au XVIe siècle* qui eut lieu à Bâle en 1964.

Depuis lors, les symposium se sont succédés régulièrement tous les trois ans:

en 1967, à Liège, sur le thème *Théories sur la structure de la matière vivante et leur influence sur la médecine*, suggéré par le Président Florkin;
en 1970, ici à Londres, à la Wellcome Foundation, sur le thème *Influence des sciences de base sur le développement de la médecine*, thème suggéré par le Président Charles Donald O'Malley, que la mort a précocement arraché à la présidence du symposium et à notre amitié.

Le symposium de 1973 aura lieu à Vienne et aura pour sujet l'histoire de la glorieuse Wiener medizinische Schule.

D'autres symposium ont été patronnés par l'Académie et, en particulier, celui sur Stenon, tenu à Copenhagen en 1965, sous la présidence du regretté Père Scherz, et dont les actes constituent un volume de *Analecta.*

En effet, parmi les buts institutionnels de l'Académie il y a aussi l'édition et notamment la publication de *Clio Medica* qui – grâce surtout au travail intelligent et passionné de Madame Lesky – a désormais atteint le 7e volume.

C'est ainsi que les publications de l'Académie sont placées dans nos librairies à côté des volumes des comptes-rendus des Congrès de la Société Internationale: et ils en complètent, bien que sous une physionomie différente, la valeur comme instruments de travail.

C'est justement cette intégration que j'estime important de souligner en cette occasion: une intégration qui nait de l'amour commun pour l'histoire de la médecine et qui se propose de stimuler l'étude sérieuse et engagée, dans le cadre de l'histoire de la science et du développement du contexte social.

Il s'agit du reste de la même empreinte donnée par Noël Poynter à ce XXIIIe Congrès, qu'il a organisé d'une façon si magistrale. Grâce à son activité et à celle de ses collaborateurs, ce Congrès qui se tient dans la ville de Pott, de Paget, de Bright, de Hodgkin, de Addison – pour ne mentionner que des noms connus par tous les médecins et non pas seulement par les historiens – passera certainement à l'histoire de l'historiographie médicale comme l'un des plus réussis.

4. Presidential Address Conclusion

To the Organizing Committee I should like to express my gratitude for all their labours. The Congress Secretary, Dr. Geraint James, has carried out his task with verve and imagination and has given to all his work his own pronounced individual character. The Congress treasury has been firmly and tactfully handled by Dr. White Franklin. For arranging the visits to Oxford and Cambridge, which have proved attractive features of this Congress for our guests from other countries, we are indebted to Dr. Robb-Smith of Oxford and Dr. Arthur Rook of Cambridge. Many of the practical and sometimes tedious chores which form a large part of the preparations for any Congress have been most competently dealt with by Mr. Gordon Wilson, of the Wellcome Institute.

To them and to all the other helpers, including the members of my own staff who have worked so diligently behind the scenes, I give my thanks.

I must also express my gratitude to the Secretary-General of the International Society, Dr. Louis Dulieu, for his timely advice throughout the preparation of the Congress. Dr. Dulieu has the interests of the Society very much at heart and his labours over many years, quietly and modestly given, have been a great contribution to its continuing success.

At the Bucharest Congress in 1970 the International Society was celebrating the completion of its first half-century and our Honorary Vice-President, Dr. Sondervorst, told us of the growth and achievements of this body which owed so much to the energy and inspiration of its founders, Professor Tricot-Royer and Professor Laignel-Lavastine.

Its Third International Congress was held in London in 1922, just fifty years ago, so once again we are celebrating a jubilee. I do not propose to take up your time with a detailed account of how the history of medicine has fared in this country since that date, but it seems worth recalling some of the salient features in the development of interest in the subject here to the point where it has become strong enough to support a great international meeting of this kind.

And if the name WELLCOME occurs more than once or twice in my remarks I hope that you will not put it down to 'local pride' but accept it as part of the historical record.

To give you a clear picture I have to go back a little beyond the date of the Third Congress of 1922 to that very large 17th International Medical Congress held in London in 1913 and attended by 7,000 delegates. It had an important section devoted to the History of Medicine which reflected the dynamic influence of Sir William Osler, then Regius Professor of Medicine at Oxford and the President of the recently founded Section of the History of Medicine of the Royal Society of Medicine.

The Congress Committee persuaded Henry Wellcome, whose avid collecting of everything to do with the history of medicine was already well known, to prepare a special Historical Exhibition for that meeting. This made such a great impression on all the delegates that Wellcome was urged to establish it as a permanent institution and in the following year it was opened as the Wellcome Historical Medical Museum. At the opening ceremony, Wellcome declared: 'The value of history to research workers is beyond estimation. . . . This collection is intended to be useful to students and to all those engaged in research. I have found that the study of the roots and foundations of things greatly assists research and facilitates discovery and invention.'

When the International Congress met in London in 1922 Osler was no longer with us. Charles Singer was the Congress President and Wellcome was a Member of the Executive Committee, giving a memorable Reception to all Congress Delegates in his Museum at its former home in Wigmore Street.

Apart from the Royal College of Physicians, which sponsored the annual Fitzpatrick Lectures on the history of some medical topic, the Royal Society of Medicine was still the only medical institution that had a special concern for the History of Medicine.

Six years later, in 1928, still under the influence of William Osler, two young medical students at St. Bartholomew's Hospital, Walter Bett and Alfred White Franklin, founded the Osler Club of London, a small and intimate group of medical students and their teachers that met regularly to discuss special topics in the history of medicine. One of those founders is still with us and is indeed the Treasurer of this Congress, while the Club which he founded has prospered exceedingly and now has over 300 members.

If I now have to mention the name of Wellcome again it is to recall the fact that at his death, at the age of 82, in 1936, he left everything which he owned, including the world-wide pharmaceutical company trading under his name, to a body of Trustees who were charged with the responsibility of distributing all the revenues which they received from the property to advance medical research anywhere in the world. Among the beneficiaries of this generous will was the history of medicine and the museum and library which Wellcome had founded, now joined together as the Wellcome Institute.

The world-wide disruption caused by war delayed the full impact of this gift to posterity, but in 1949 the Wellcome Library first opened its doors freely to scholars from all countries.

In the following decade many attempts were made to introduce the history of medicine as a regular subject into the curriculum of the medical schools. There was still no university department anywhere in Britain which could provide teachers or who could help to train them.

At its close, however, in 1959, a group led by the late Dr. W. S. C. Copeman, with the support and encouragement of the Royal Colleges, established what they called the Faculty of the History of Medicine and Pharmacy in one of our most ancient medical corporations. This was the Society of Apothecaries of London. It had a royal charter dating from the year 1617 and had done great work in the nineteenth century in the training and examining of general medical practitioners, a role now passing almost entirely to the universities.

The aims of the Faculty were to foster and extend more general interest in medical history by enlisting the support of all medical corporations, schools, societies, clubs and individuals in a co-ordinated effort to this end. The Faculty also welcomed the interest and support of general historians in forging closer links between medical history and general, social and economic history. The support came promptly and willingly from every medical institution in the country. Series of annual lectures were founded and honorary lecturerships were established at a number of medical schools.

At the end of its first decade, in 1969, the efforts of the Faculty were crowned by the establishment of a postgraduate Diploma in the History of Medicine, an officially recognized qualification granted after examination by the Society of Apothecaries as one of our medical licensing bodies. A one-year course of study and instruction given by teachers recruited from members of the Faculty was begun immediately and has already attracted more than fifty candidates, most of them being themselves teachers in the medical schools. So far, fifteen successful candidates have been awarded this Diploma.

Yet another activity of the Faculty was to initiate a series of biennial national congresses beginning in 1960. These were so successful that by 1965 the Faculty thought the time had come to establish the first British Society for the History of Medicine, bringing together with it for this purpose the History Section of the Royal Society of Medicine, the Osler Club of London and the flourishing Scottish Society of the History of Medicine, with Dr. Douglas Guthrie as its first President. To this new federated Society was entrusted the organization of the British Congresses of the History of Medicine and the national representation on the International Society.

In recent years, the number of affiliated societies has increased from four to six with the accession of the British Society for the History of Pharmacy and the new and successful Society for the Social History of Medicine.

At about the same time, the Wellcome Trust, which had for many years been awarding Wellcome Research Fellowships in the History of Medicine to individual researchers, began to re-examine its policy for supporting the subject. It soon became apparent to the committee studying this matter that young scholars could not look forward to a secure career in the history of medicine unless there were more academic openings for them in the universities. As a result, new departments financed by the Trust have been set up at University College, London, and at both Oxford and Cambridge. A second department in the University of London has been founded independently at King's College Hospital Medical School, staffed by teachers and successful candidates of the Apothecaries Diploma Course. A lecturer has been appointed to the Welsh National School of Medicine and a new Welsh Society of the History of Medicine is becoming appended to the British Society.

It is against this historical background, and assured of the benevolent support of the Wellcome Trust, that we felt confident in inviting medical historians from all countries of the world to meet together in our capital city in this 23rd International Congress.

A great many of you are university teachers, and Britain is not the only country where there are difficulties in integrating the study of the history of medicine with the ordinary medical subjects. You will be interested therefore in seeing how we in Britain have brought together academic and professional bodies to advance our common cause. It is my firm belief that without the informed interest and support of the medical profession our subject would become a minor branch of general history and its practitioners the inhabitants of a number of isolated ivory towers. On the other hand, without the guidance that is given by research and without the example and the standards set by rigorous scholarship, the subject could indeed become a fitting pursuit for elderly and retired doctors.

Our field is a very large one and there is plenty of room for all. No one man can match the desiderata required by the late Henry Sigerist for a medical historian and be physician, archaeologist, anthropologist, philologist, sociologist, philosopher and historian all rolled into one. Such skills can only be brought together by co-operative endeavour, and at its best, such endeavour produces the kind of medical history which can earn the respect of the professional historian as well as the physician, which can attract the young and give them a secure base in the humanistic tradition even while it gives them a deeper understanding of the special medical and scientific skills which go to make a good doctor.

I am sure that it is in this spirit that we embark on our discussions and I am sure that by next Friday evening there will not be one of us who will not carry away from this meeting new ideas, new aspirations and new enthusiasm to speed his own individual labours.

II SYMPOSIUM

Some Concepts of Clinical Medicine

Charles Coury
Paris (France)

Introduction

Honoured Chairmen;
You will no doubt permit me to follow the tradition prevailing in all international Congresses and to speak in my own native language, it being French, forgetting how strongly attracted I have always been by that of Shakespeare, Byron and Shelley. I also wish to call up the memory of my regretted countryman and beloved master, our late President Professor Bariéty, who passed since we last met in Bucarest. He would have been one of today's prominent speakers on a subject which he had personally suggested in view of this meeting. He belongs to those of whom the great American poet Longfellow has written: departing, they leave behind them 'Footprints on the sands of time'.

Monsieur le Président,

En me confiant la coordination de cette première séance du XXIIIe Congrès International d'Histoire de la Médecine et le soin d'ouvrir ce Symposium sur l'histoire de la médecine clinique, vous m'avez, certes, fait un grand honneur et donné une marque touchante de votre amitié. Mais vous m'avez par là même placé dans un grand embarras. Dans une ville telle que Londres et dans un haut-lieu de l'histoire de la médecine comme le Wellcome Institute, on se sent en effet mal à l'aise pour définir – ne fut-ce que sommairement – les grandes étapes du raisonnement médical et du développement de la clinique. La civilisation britannique a produit au cours des âges trop de génies médicaux d'une – exceptionnelle qualité – pour qu'on puisse songer à confiner leur oeuvre dans le cadre artificiel et étroit de concepts abstraits. Aussi me limiterai-je à quelques considérations cursives sur les débuts de la clinique et sur leur place épistémologique, heureux si elles peuvent servir de prélude aux exposés érudits qui vont suivre et à une discussion que je souhaite animée.

Mes chers Collègues, Mesdames, Mesdemoiselles, Messieurs,
L'idée de soigner – donc de connaître et d'inventorier les maladies – est une des modalités de l'instinct de conservation. Elle est aussi vieille que le mal physique lui-même. Elle résulte d'une impulsion naturelle à laquelle obéissent tous les êtres vivants. L'observation zoonomique courante donne à penser que ce besoin est instinctif dans les espèces animales les plus évoluées. Chez l'homme, il est devenu très tôt intuitif.

Une des premières démarches du raisonnement médical a consisté à établir une distinction entre les maux dont l'origine était évidente ou apparente, et les autres. La logique qui poussait l'homme primitif à éloigner la cause flagrante du mal chaque fois qu'il en avait l'occasion et la possibilité, s'inscrit dans l'affirmation classique de Kurt Sprengel (1792) selon laquelle la chirurgie serait la plus ancienne des thérapeutiques. A une date précoce, les hommes des temps archaïques comprirent que tous les désordres du corps humain ne s'expliquent pas seulement par l'effet d'agents extérieurs immédiatement appréhensibles; une place croissante fut accordée à des facteurs moins directs, notamment à certaines forces de la nature. Un pas de plus dans ce domaine fit naître la médecine magique dont le principe est de maintenir l'équilibre entre celles de ces influences indiscernables qui étaient réputées maléfiques ou bénéfiques.

Dès lors, la médecine – ou ce qui en était la lointaine anticipation – s'est engagée simultanément sur deux voies distinctes, le plus souvent divergentes mais parfois aussi confondues: celle de l'empirisme et celle de la foi, au sens le plus large du terme. Les connaissances médicales empiriques se sont initialement inspirées d'une logique élémentaire appuyée sur des constatations occasionnelles mais répétées, enregistrées par la mémoire; elles sont une sorte de préfiguration lointaine de la médecine clinique d'observation. De son côté, la médecine magique est devenue religieuse, puis sacerdotale, dès que l'esprit humain, mûri par les débuts de la vie en société, s'est élevé jusqu'à la conception du métaphysique. Décisif sur le plan spirituel, cet élan vers les divinités n'a été, à l'origine, qu'un cas particulier du recours au surnaturel.

Ces deux courants primitifs ont longtemps coexisté; l'un et l'autre ne s'adressaient le plus souvent ni aux mêmes cas, ni aux mêmes maladies. La médecine magique ou théurgique a d'ailleurs fait à la médecine empirique des emprunts de plus en plus larges; elle n'en représente pas moins l'aspect le plus répandu et le plus général des médecines archaïques.

La médecine magique résume en effet la plupart des caractères initiaux de l'art de soigner. Elle s'adresse aux affections dites internes, tant que leur siège demeure inconnu et leur cause indiscernable. Par analogie avec l'action des corps étrangers, la plupart de celles-ci ont été attribuées à l'action de forces invisibles, immatérielles et mystérieuses. La maladie est considérée comme une présence indépendante, incorporée temporairement à l'homme, mais étrangère à lui. Les symptômes cliniques ne sont que les manifestations secondes de cette présence occulte qui «possède» physiquement le malade. La maladie résulte en définitive d'une imposition.

La médecine religieuse n'en est qu'une variété plus tardive qui substitue à cette présence magique invisible celle d'une déité ou d'un démon qui peut aussi bien – selon ses intentions – exercer une action néfaste et punitive s'il est irrité, offensé, vengeur, justicier, ou, à l'inverse, une action bienfaisante et curative, s'il est bienveillant, satisfait, ou indulgent. L'effet divin peut être individuel ou collectif sans que les victimes soient nécessairement conscientes de la faute commise. Face à cette conception supranaturelle de la maladie, la reconnaissance de son siège et de sa nature perd tout intérêt devant l'identification de la puissance responsable. Suivant les cas, ce rôle est dévolu au prêtre-devin ou au sorcier-magicien. La nosologie clinique n'est encore que mythologie et divination. Au demeurant, la mentalité primitive n'attribue pas seulement la maladie à l'intervention de dieux ou de démons dont chacun a, pour ainsi dire, sa spécialité pathologique: le mal physique ou moral peut être également le fait d'un être humain malveillant agissant à distance, d'un défunt haineux, voire d'un ennemi vivant exerçant un sortilège.

Le diagnostic clinique et le pronostic appartiennent donc à ceux – sorciers ou prêtres – qui savent pénétrer les mystères de l'inconnu et qui utilisent à cet effet des moyens très variés, inspirés par les événements astronomiques, les phénomènes météorologiques, certaines analogies morphologiques. Le jeûne, l'ivresse ou la transe divinatoire, l'exploitation des rêves spontanés ou orientés des malades, l'invocation verbale accompagnée ou non de danses rituelles, jouent un rôle favorisant. L'action propre des mots et des gestes occupe en effet une grande place dans le diagnostic clinique, c'est-à-dire dans l'identification de la puissance malfaisante. Elle est encore plus importante dans les différentes mesures thérapeutiques dont il serait hors de propos de parler ici et qui associent aux procédés de conjuration, d'oraison, d'expulsion, d'évacuation, de propitiation sacrificielle ou de confession médicale, certains rites de transfert ou de substitution par exemple, sur lesquels nous aimerions pouvoir nous étendre plus longuement.

Entre-temps, l'empirisme médical, exploité avec intelligence, relevait de nombreuses corrélations cliniques. Les papyrus égyptiens et les tablettes mésopotamiennes en donnent une illustration particulièrement éloquente sous forme de propositions à trois panneaux reliant entre eux des symptômes, des diagnostics élémentaires et des pronostics. La pharmacopée s'enrichissait en outre de possibilités thérapeutiques dont l'efficacité, reconnue au cours des siècles, surclassait celle des procédés magiques ou religieux.

Dès la fin de la période homérique – du moins dans le monde méditerranéen – le bon plaisir des dieux, les fabulations mythologiques, les conjonctions astrologiques et autres phénomènes surnaturels ont progressivement cessé d'expliquer le fonctionnement pathologique de l'organisme humain. La maladie, en tout cas, n'est plus considérée comme une manifestation étrangère à l'homme, mais comme une partie intégrante de son comportement déréglé. Ce progrès fondamental qui a rayonné sur l'ère hippocratique et sur les siècles qui l'ont suivie, a cependant eu une contrepartie fâcheuse dont l'effet a été aussi durable que celui des croyances primitives. La pensée médicale ne s'est en effet libérée de l'emprise religieuse que pour tomber sous celle des constructions de l'esprit et des systèmes philosophiques successifs qui l'ont emporté pendant plus de deux mille cinq cents ans sur la réalité des faits. Celle-ci était inéluctablement soumise à des *a priori* intellectuels. On peut se demander si le spéculatif et l'abstrait n'ont pas autant ralenti le développement de la médecine clinique que ne l'avaient fait, avant eux, le divin et le fabuleux.

A de rares exceptions près, la médecine clinique est demeurée telle jusqu'à la Renaissance. Les méthodes d'examen et les connaissances sémiologiques se sont à peine enrichies – même en Orient – durant toute la fin de l'Antiquité et la plus grande partie du Moyen Age. Certes l'interprétation des faits élémentaires constatés a varié quelque peu selon les tendances individuelles; mais les ressources de la médecine sont restées très limitées, faute de pouvoir s'appuyer sur des données anatomiques ou physiologiques valables. La médecine clinique se réduisait à une énumération topographique de symptômes ou de signes pour la plupart évidents, dépourvus de lien entre eux et grossièrement classés de la tête aux pieds. Rares sont les auteurs médicaux qui se sont aventurés à ébaucher certains regroupements sommaires. Chaque trouble était considéré en soi comme une maladie autonome: la nosologie était purement symptomatique ou, au mieux, syndromique. Les maux de tête, les hémoptysies, les douleurs de ventre, les fièvres, les hydropisies, les catarrhes, les esquinancies, les cachexies, les jaunisses, les paralysies, les grosseurs contre nature, pour ne donner que quelques exemples, constituaient autant de maladies; on en dissociait à peine les différentes composantes, et on en distinguait mal les variétés, en dépit des tentatives de quelques médecins inspirés ou en avance sur leur temps.

Chacun sait qu'un changement radical, bien que lent et progressif, s'est opéré en Europe entre la fin du XVe et le milieu du XVIIe siècle. Il a surtout été marqué par la rénovation de l'anatomie et par la naissance de la physiologie marquée par une découverte décisive: celle de la circulation du sang. Et cependant la médecine clinique n'en a pas bénéficié de façon immédiate: la plupart des livres de clinique médicale parus jusqu'au début du XIXe siècle sont en grande partie calqués sur ceux des époques précédentes.

La première expression de la clinique moderne est issue de la confrontation, devenue progressivement systématique, entre les troubles ou symptômes observés sur le vivant et les lésions anatomiques observées à l'autopsie. Avec Bonet, Morgagni et leurs émules d'Italie, de Leyde, d'Edimbourg, de Vienne, puis de Paris, le souci séculaire d'attribuer une cause aux diverses maladies a enfin pris une orientation scientifique. Dans le même temps ou presque – aux très vieux procédés empiriques d'interrogatoire, d'inspection et de palpation, se sont ajoutés de nouveaux moyens d'exploration clinique, plus précis, plus objectifs, plus permanents, notamment tactiles et auditifs comme la percussion d'Auenbrugger propagée par Corvisart, et l'auscultation de Laennec. La modification qualitative des humeurs élémentaires a enfin perdu l'importance imaginaire que lui avaient accordée les Anciens. Désormais, la maladie va se définir par un couple formé de son expression clinique et de la lésion anatomique tenue pour en être responsable. L'exploitation et la diffusion de ce principe a fait le rayonnement principal de l'Ecole française du XIXe siècle. Dans l'ensemble, il a régi la médecine depuis 150 ans.

Et pourtant cette méthode anatomo-clinique portait en elle-même le germe de ses quelques insuffisances et de ses rares échecs. Elle impliquait en effet le postulat d'une corrélation étroite, significative et constante entre le trouble et la lésion, ce qui n'est pas toujours vérifié. Certes, l'épanouissement de l'histologie pathologique, sous l'impulsion de Virchow et de l'Ecole allemande, lui a donné des assises plus solides et plus précises, mais qui ne répondent cependant pas à tous les cas. Elle confondait trop exclusivement l'anomalie lésionnelle avec le facteur étiologique et lui conférait un caractère de spécificité qui est loin d'être absolu. Or, le dogme de la spécificité, proclamé notamment en France par Bretonneau, a été une des lignes de force de la médecine au XIXe siècle: l'anatomie pathologique – même reflétée sur le plan humoral – n'était pas seule à pouvoir le satisfaire. La perturbation fonctionnelle prédomine souvent sur la lésion, quand même elle ne joue pas un rôle exclusif. Du temps des Broussais et des Bouillaud, l'inflammation – préfiguration lointaine du «stress» de Selye – se voyait attribuer toute la responsabilité du désordre clinique, sans qu'intervienne la nature ou le siège de la lésion. Vers le milieu du XIXe siècle, les progrès prodigieux accomplis par la biochimie et la physiologie ont éclairé la médecine clinique d'un jour nouveau: à la clinique appartient en effet en propre la particularité – souvent signalée – de ne ressembler à aucune des autres sciences, d'en être à peine une et de les utiliser toutes. Elle-même s'est enrichie de moyens d'investigation nouveaux parmi lesquels je me bornerai à rappeler les enregistrements graphiques ou électriques, la radiologie dont les applications actuelles appartiennent à l'examen clinique, les méthodes isotopiques et combien d'autres qui ont transformé profondément les descriptions sémiologiques et les conceptions nosologiques traditionnelles. En attendant que l'immunologie contemporaine en affaiblisse le principe lui-même, la spécificité des maladies a pris de plus en plus une tonalité physio-pathologique. Une véritable explosion de procédés d'exploration physiques, chimiques – ou, pour employer un qualificatif plus général, biologiques – a caractérisé la médecine des cent dernières années au point de s'imposer à la clinique traditionnelle et, souvent, de se substituer à elle. La spécificité microbiologique née des découvertes de Pasteur et de Koch a dû elle-même céder du terrain devant les les explications infracellulaires, métaboliques, génotypiques ou moléculaires: la médecine a pris une dimension ultrastructurale.

C'est dire à quel point la médecine clinique a fait désormais place à la médecine biologique et à ses antennes les plus avancées et les plus perçantes. Vers 1900, les acquisitions médicales faites au cours du XIXe siècle faisaient l'admiration de ceux qui s'attardaient un moment à porter leur regard en arrière. Quelque soixante quinze années plus tard, combien plus prodigieux encore apparait le pas franchi à l'époque contemporaine, si tant est qu'on ait même le loisir de s'attarder à le mesurer!

Dans toute science et principalement en médecine, les appréciations de l'historien n'ont en effet qu'une valeur «actuelle», donc toute relative.

Mais j'aurais scrupule à m'étendre plus longuement sur ce thème qui risquerait de pécher par manque d'originalité. Je m'en voudrais de différer plus longtemps l'intérêt et le plaisir que nous prendrons tous à écouter les éminents orateurs qui vont animer ce Symposium.

L. J. Rather
Stanford, California (U.S.A.)

Some aspects of the theory and therapy of inflammation: from William Harvey to Clemens von Pirquet

'Theory of inflammation' as used here comprises (*a*) causal and physiopathological explanations of clinically and experimentally observed phenomena grouped together under the heading of inflammation by medical writers of past and present times and (*b*) interpretations of the clinical or biological significance of inflammation, together with the corresponding explanations of its beneficial or baneful effects. Whether any given phenomenon should be included under the heading of inflammation is itself a prior conceptual or theoretical issue, but it will be skirted in the present paper.

Repeated revisions of a theory of inflammation deriving largely from Galen have accompanied, more or less *pari passu*, advances in our understanding of anatomy, physiology and pathology since the time of Harvey. The therapy of inflammation, on the contrary, has changed significantly only in the past three or four decades. Since physicians have usually asked for some degree of consonance between theory and therapy, it follows that during the past three and a half centuries different rationales must have been put forward for the same therapeutic procedures. Blood-letting is a case in point. But ought the physician to treat inflammation, as such, at all? Making use of the analogy developed at length by Thomas Campanella at the beginning of the seventeenth century, does inflammation represent disease or a war *against* disease?[1] Campanella was dealing with the interpretation of fever. With respect to inflammation the question was first clearly formulated by Georg Ernst Stahl a century later. As he put it, is inflammation a *passio*, i.e. something suffered by the body? Or is it an *actio*, an active or reactive response to disease or injury? Stahl held that inflammation was an active and essentially beneficial response, hence the physician should attempt to check it only under special circumstances. The same conclusion was reached by John Hunter, later in the eighteenth century, and again by Ilya Mechnikov toward the end of the nineteenth century, although each of these men had quite different ideas regarding the causes and physiopathological mechanisms of the inflammatory process.

Turning now to the beginning of the period to be spanned in this paper, it might seem obvious to the modern reader that Harvey's account of the circulation should have had repercussions in respect to the theory and therapy of inflammation. What is called the Galenic 'circulation' of the blood is in a limited sense, if at all, circulatory – it is the slow outward movement, by way of venous channels, of a fluid thought to be used up in the tissues. In Galenic physiopathology corrupt or superfluous humours are sometimes shifted to the periphery, where they form inflammatory tumours. The incompatibility, in respect to the theory and therapy of inflammation, of Harvey and Galen was recognized by Jean Riolan, the eminent champion of Galenism at Paris. Harvey's circulation would invalidate the whole Galenic theory of 'fluxions', said Riolan, and was incompatible as well with the accepted rationales of revulsive, derivative and evacuative bleeding.[2] Certain other physicians were less acute, or more tolerant of contradiction, than Riolan. V. F. Plemp, for example, left his account of the physiopathology of inflammation and the rationale of blood-letting unchanged after he accepted the Harveian circulation in 1654.[3] And the same may be said of the younger Horst, a few years later.[4] It is perhaps unnecessary to add here that physicians continued to bleed their patients as before. In time new rationales were developed.

Georg Ernst Stahl, whose medical career dates from the latter half of the seventeenth century, long after the Harveian circulation had been generally accepted, is notable less for his views on the mechanism of the inflammatory process than for those on its significance. As he put it, inflammation has a 'final' as well as a 'physicomechanical' explanation. That the small blood vessels become blocked in zones of inflammation had been a Galenic tenet. In Stahl's opinion it sufficed as an explanation of the mechanics of the situation. In the face of complete blockage extensive death of tissue could result. But the body was not a mere machine; it was watched over and controlled by an *anima* (more or less corresponding to the idea of the Hippocratic *physis*, according to Stahl). In order to prevent massive death of tissue the *anima* saw to it that fresh blood was pumped at higher intensity through the obstructed vessels of the inflamed zone, breaking up the log jam, so to speak, and under favourable conditions producing complete resolution. Thus the inflammatory process, in Stahl's view, is itself a therapeutic act on part of the body under control of the *anima*, one designed to overcome the mechanical proximate cause of the disturbance. It followed that the process should be allowed to run its beneficial course, within limits, and that the patient should be advised that the associated disability or discomfort was preferable to what would happen in the absence of this response.[5] Inflammation was, as Stahl's successor at the University of Halle wrote, an *actus salutarius*, a salutary act or reaction.[6] It appears that Stahl's interpretation encountered some opposition. In a short poem appended to a dissertation of 1705 he writes,

Quae tanta invidia est, ut quod Natura saluti
Consulit, hoc medicus damnet et aeger idem.[7]

How odious it is that both physician and patient condemn Nature's healing measure!

In John Hunter's often quoted statement that inflammation is 'not to be considered as a disease, but as a salutary operation consequent either to some violence or some disease' Stahlian influence is evident. The same may be said of his remark that 'if a part under the influence of such irritation as should naturally excite inflammation, had either no powers or disposition to exert them, the consequences would be much worse, for mortification would probably take place'. But the salutary operation of Hunter does not consist in the overcoming of vascular obstruction. It is a tissue-reparative process. The activated small blood vessels in inflamed zones throw off a 'coagulable lymph' that subsequently undergoes organization and so replaces tissue destroyed by violence or disease. (It should also be noted that

Hunter's inflammation is in no sense a defensive process.) Not all tissue repair requires the participation of the inflammatory process. Cleanly incised wounds heal without it when their edges are approximated. But where greater violence has been done to the tissues 'an action . . . called inflammation', whereby the activated small blood vessels throw off the larger amounts of coagulable lymph required, takes place. The complexity of Hunter's views on the subject of inflammation can only be touched on lightly here. He held that the inflammatory process could, under special circumstances, become 'depraved' or 'unnatural', hence harmful. The physician often found himself facing a therapeutic dilemma. For example, when suppurative inflammation follows on obvious violence to the tissues it is a restorative process, Hunter believes – but what, he asks, of 'those suppurations which appear to arise spontaneously?' At times, then, 'it is almost impossible to determine whether the inflammation itself be the real disease . . . or whether it may not be a salutary process of nature to restore parts whose functions, and perhaps texture, have been destroyed by some previous, and almost imperceptible cause'. It seems plain to him that where inflammation 'cannot accomplish its salutary purpose, as in cancer, scrofula, venereal disease, etc., it does mischief'.[8]

The therapeutic effects of blood-letting depend, in Hunter's opinion, on its ability to 'lower the constitution', i.e. to lower the general state of reactivity of the body, including the salutary act of inflammation. For this reason blood-letting 'should in all cases be performed with great caution', he warns. Hunter denied that the beneficial effects of bleeding in cases of inflammatory disease resulted from diminution of the amount of blood in the affected part or in the body as a whole. Reading his remarks on the proper site for withdrawal of blood we learn that the debate that had flared up in the sixteenth century around Pierre Brissot was still alive. Hunter suggests that the efficacy of 'bleeding on the left side for an inflammation in the right, upon the sole principle of derivation' may actually depend on 'remote sympathy'. For the most part, however, he holds that 'the site from which the blood is withdrawn is unimportant', and 'repulsion, derivation, revulsion and translation' have been accorded exaggerated importance.[9] The interested reader will find these topics treated fully by one of Hunter's contemporaries, Borsieri di Kanilfeld (Burserius), professor of materia medica at Pavia. Burserius states that the proponents of revulsive bleeding prefer to open veins remote from the inflamed part, so as to direct blood away from that part, whereas the proponents of derivative bleeding open veins near the affected part, so as to increase the impetus of the blood entering that part and thus contribute to the relief of inflammatory stasis (Borsieri's 'revulsive' is Hunter's 'derivative'). Borsieri himself denied that vascular obstruction was the proximate cause of inflammation.[10]

At the end of the eighteenth century a new period in the study of the inflammatory process was inaugurated by the use of the microscope. Examining blood vessels in the exposed mesenteries of rabbits and in the swimming webs of frogs with microscope lenses uncorrected for spherical and chromatic aberration, investigators – beginning with Wilson Philip in 1799 – described the initial acceleration and subsequent retardation of flow within irritated small blood vessels, the phenomenon of axial flow, even the clustering of blood corpuscles on the margins of vessels in inflamed areas. In the earlier accounts red and white corpuscles were not as a rule distinguished from each other. Corrected lenses came into general use in the 1830s.

In 1842 Wharton Jones observed white corpuscles drifting along the walls of small vessels in inflamed areas and compared them to round pebbles moving along the bottom of a stream. He noted also that at times they could be seen to 'line the walls of small veins like epithelium'.[11] In 1844 William Addison half-observed and half-hypothesized that the white corpuscles passed out into the tissues, and two years later Waller described their passage through intact walls, albeit faultily. Addison thought that the white cells were embryonal forms, contributing to the growth and maintenance of the tissues; Waller expressed no opinion as to the significance of the phenomenon.[12]

It was not until nearly forty years later that the white cells of the blood were accorded a central place in the theory of inflammation, in the new form given it by Ilya Mechnikov. The way was prepared by Julius Cohnheim's more accurate description of the passage of leucocytes from the blood stream to the tissues, made in 1867, and the rapid development of bacteriology in the latter nineteenth century. Cohnheim had been unable to account satisfactorily for the phenomenon he had described, but in 1883 Mechnikov did so in a manner eminently suited to the needs of the new era. Impressed by Cohnheim's findings, and aware that bacteria had been found within leucocytes, Mechnikov argued that the complex phenomena of inflammation in higher animals had the biological purpose of bringing leucocytes into action where they were needed. Inflammation was, he wrote, in essence a 'defence of the organism against microorganisms, the leucocytes in this struggle devouring and destroying the parasites'. To critics offended by his teleology Mechnikov replied that his theory was compatible with Darwin's principle of natural selection, i.e. the apparently purposeful character of the inflammatory reaction was merely a reflection of its real survival value.[13] As in the case of Stahl and Hunter, Mechnikov's theory of inflammation implied that the physician should allow the process to run its course. The goal of the 'salutary process' has changed, of course. It is neither the overcoming of vascular obstruction, as with Stahl, nor the repair of tissue damage, as with Hunter, but the elimination of disease-producing microorganisms from the body.

It was to become evident shortly that not all inflammatory processes could be interpreted in this way. Physicians had long been familiar with the observation that some individuals were immune to certain diseases. Mechnikov attempted to relate immunity to phagocytic activity on part of the leucocytes. A rival theory made immunity dependent on protective humoral substances of proteinaceous character, present in the blood. The point to be made here is that only a short time after it had been shown that on exposure to *harmful* agencies the body generated protective humoral substances capable of preventing, containing or suppressing inflammatory responses in some instances, it was found also that under certain circumstances exposure to initially *harmless* agencies could elicit destructive inflammation. A general response of this kind – not involving the inflammatory process – was first described by Portier and Richet. In 1902 they found that repeated small doses of a toxin derived from the tentacles of *Actinia*, although at first innocuous, would after a time elicit a fatal generalized response. 'We term *anaphylactic* (the contrary of phylaxis)', they wrote, 'the property of a toxin to diminish instead of reinforcing immunity, when it is injected in non-fatal doses'.[14] In 1903 Maurice Arthus showed that repeated injections of horse serum into rabbits, at first harmless, eventually caused a severe, localized inflammatory lesion.[15] Three years later Clemens von

Pirquet noted the apparent paradox involved and suggested that the term allergy be applied to instances in which the 'immune' response was harmful, retaining the term immunity for the protective response.[16] And so a new aspect of the Janus-faced process of inflammation began to reveal itself.

References

1 RATHER, L. J. and FRERICHS, J. B., 'On the use of military metaphor in western medical literature. The *bellum contra morbum* of Thomas Campanella (1568–1639)', *Clio Medica*, 1972, **7/3**, 201-8.

2 RIOLAN, JEAN, *Opuscula anatomica nova*, London, 1649, pp. 543–45.

3 PLEMP, V. F. *Fundamenta medicina*, 3rd ed., Louvain, 1654, pp. 128–32.

4 HORST, GREGOR, *Opera*, Gouda, 1661, vol. 1, p. 439b.

5 STAHL, GEORG ERNST, *Theoria medica vera*, ed. Choulant, Leipzig, 1831–33, vol. II, pp. 219–23.

6 ALBERTI, MICHAEL, *Introductio in universam medicinam*, Halle, 1718–21, 257–59.

7 STAHL, GEORG ERNST, *Disputatio medica inauguralis de inflammationis vera pathologia . . .*, Halle, 1705.

8 HUNTER, JOHN, *A Treatise on the Blood, Inflammation and Gun-shot Wounds*, London, 1794, pp. 206, 248, 249, 250, 260.

9 Ibid., pp. 345, 353, 375.

10 BURSERIUS, J. B., *The Institutions of the Practice of Medicine*, Edinburgh, 1800, vol. 1, pp. 86, 87.

11 WHARTON JONES, THOMAS, 'Observations on some points in the anatomy, physiology, and pathology of the blood', *Brit. for. med. Rev.*, 1842, **14**, 585–600.

12 RATHER, L. J., *Addison and the White Corpuscles*, London and Los Angeles, 1972, ch. II.

13 Ibid., chs. III, IV.

14 PORTIER and RICHET, CH., 'De l'action anaphylactique de certains venins', *C. r. Soc. Biol. Paris*, 1902, **54**, 170–72.

15 ARTHUS, MAURICE, 'Injections répétées de serum de cheval chez le lapin', *C. r. Soc. Biol.*, 1903, **55**, 817–20; ARTHUS, MAURICE and BRETON, MAURICE, ibid., 1903, **55**, 1478–80.

16 PIRQUET, C. V., 'Allergie', *Muench. med. Woch.*, 1906, **53/2**, 1457–58.

L. Belloni
Milan (Italy)

La conception de la maladie selon l'École Galiléienne

Cet exposé se rattache à quatre autres que j'ai développé aux Symposia de Liège (1967)[1] et de Londres (1970)[2] de l'Académie Internationale d'Histoire de la Médecine, au Symposium Boerhaave à Leyde (1968)[3] et au Symposium van Swieten à Vienne (1972)[4]; et, comme les précédents, il tend à présenter sous son vrai jour l'importance qu'il faut attribuer à l'Ecole Galiléienne dans le développement de la biologie et de la médecine.

En effet, cette école est souvent laissée dans l'ombre dans les traités d'histoire de la médecine, où elle apparait plutôt émargée en tant qu'école douée d'une continuité bien précise. Eloquente est au contraire la succession de savants qui la composèrent et qui répondent aux noms de: Galilée, B. Castelli, Borelli, Malpighi, Valsalva, Morgagni, pour ne pas citer Redi et Vallisneri: tous des maillons d'une chaine qui dépasse un siècle et demi: de 1610 à 1761, dates de la parution, respectivement, du *Sidereus nuncius* de Galilée et du *De sedibus* de Morgagni.

L'élévation du grossissement optique à instrument de la science, pronée dans le premier de ces ouvrages, contribua puissamment à la relance de l'atomisme qui se vérifia au XVIIe siècle, et détermina le dévoloppement de l'anatomie microscopique, laquelle, attribuant une structuration mécanique à notre organisme, contribua largement à l'application de la nouvelle mécanique galiléienne du monde inorganique au monde organique. Fruit de cette application est le *De motu animalium*, paru en 1680/1, auquel Giovanni Alfonso Borelli (1608–79) travailla pendant plusieurs dizaines d'années, après avoir publié en 1649 ce qui peut être considéré comme son manifeste iatromécaniste: le livre *Delle cagioni delle febbri maligne della Sicilia negli anni 1647 e 1648.*[5]

Deux influences sont facilement reconnaissables à la lecture de cet ouvrage:
(*a*) la doctrine de la circulation du sang, pour laquelle les galiléiens romains, réunis autour de B. Castelli, furent parmi les premiers à montrer de l'intérêt: un intérêt que l'on peut documenter dès 1636, en coïncidence avec le voyage de Harvey à Rome et à Naples.[6]
(*b*) le *De statica medicina* (1614), qui enseignait à évaluer quantitativement la *perspiratio insensibilis* et qui fut écrit par Santorio Santorio (1561–1636), celui-là même qui proposa le thermomètre et l'hygromètre pour quantifier les qualités élémentaires du système quaternaire traditionnel (chaud-froid-sec-humide).

Dans le livre *Delle cagioni delle febbri maligne della Sicilia* . . . que nous venons de citer, Borelli renversa la conception de la maladie, en repoussant la doctrine quaternaire traditionnelle, et proposa au contraire une interprétation atomistico-mécaniste. Le système quaternaire, fondé sur les correspondance entre le macrocosme et notre microcosme, admettait que, d'une intempérie ou déséquilibre entre les quatre qualités élémentaires (chaud, froid, sec, humide) du premier, dérivât une noxa avec un effet morbigène sur le second. Dans ce dernier s'établissait, en effet, une intempérie ou déséquilibre analogue entre les quatre humeurs (sang, bile jaune, bile noire, flegme) qui constituent notre organisme et dans la juste proportion desquelles consiste la santé.

Ayant démoli, à l'aide de simples expériences, la thèse suivant laquelle «des premières qualités élémentaires l'air peut s'altérer et se corrompre de manière à devenir apte à causer l'épidémie courante» (p. 7), Borelli attribue la corruption de l'air à des exhalaisons toxiques d'origine terrestre qui rappellent les «semences d'épidémie» chantées par l'atomiste Titus Lucrèce Caro (Ier siècle avant J.C.) dans le *De rerum natura*. C'est-à-dire qu'on peut penser que «le soleil appliqué par la nature, soulève en l'air par un artifice chimique, . . . des exhalaisons extrêmement perverses et venimeuses, corrosives et destructives: ainsi que nous en avons un exemple tout prêt dans les éclairs» (p. 107) que la science n'avaient pas encore interprêtés comme des phénomènes électriques. Les éclairs, au contraire, offrent un modèle approprié pour expliquer comment des «noeuds» de semences d'épidémie peuvent frapper une certaine localité, à un certain moment. Condensées par des forces d'ordre physique, et ainsi atterries à nouveau, ces semences pénètrent dans notre organisme et provoquent la maladie, agissant directement sur les organes, au lieu que sur les humeurs: dans le cas spécifique de l'épidémie sicilienne de 1647/8, en agissant sur les poumons, que les sections cadavériques montrent «putrides et pourris», d'une couleur noire et livide, et parfois parsemés de petites taches semblables à celles de Palerme, où, en effet, le médecin Giuseppe Galeano les avait trouvé «enflammés et parsemés de certaines petites taches livides ressemblant à des pétéchies» (p. 127).

L'indication thérapeutique n'a donc pas pour but de purger l'organisme de l'humeur peccante, mais «de procurer un antidote approprié, qui ait la faculté spécifique de résister et d'enlever sa force à la cause venimeuse» (p. 133), c'est-à-dire aux semences d'épidémie: et Borelli croit avoir trouvé cet antidote dans le soufre, dont il conseille l'emploi, également d'après les résultats de l'expérience thérapeutique, et non pas pour le tempérament «chaud» qui lui est attribué par le système quaternaire.

Borelli, lui aussi, conçoit la fièvre comme un facteur de guérison: mais, à l'encontre de la doctrine traditionnelle, il n'attribue pas cet effet à la coction de l'humeur peccante, mais à une accélération du *mouvement* en quoi son iatromécanique fait consister la vie: le mouvement *interne* de l'organisme vivant, que Borelli continuera à étudier – de même que le mouvement *externe* et *local* – pendant les trente années restantes de sa vie, construisant son grand ouvrage qui s'intitule justement *De motu animalium*.

Le mouvement organique de Borelli a effectivement comme centre la pulsation cardiaque, mais se répand largement au delà du lit circulatoire: «il faut que, par l'impulsion conférée au sang par le débat des artères, s'échappent par les *pores* et par leurs extrémités d'innombrables *particules* qui étaient contenues dans le sang, lesquelles, avec l'impulsion reçue en s'insinuant dans les espaces restés vides après la transpiration d'autres particules, viennent, par un merveilleux artifice, à conserver ce flux et reflux de particules, ou ce *mouvement*, en quoi consiste la conservation et la vie de l'animal» (p. 159).

On configure ainsi une physiologie fondée sur le mouvement, sur les particules, sur les pores; et avec elle, une pathologie basée sur des altérations du mouvement corpusculaire normal: «Finalement je peux considérer que les parties qui sont actuellement contenues dans l'animal peuvent se mouvoir de deux façons: certaines fois, par les voies normales, avec l'ordre et la vitesse habituelle et ordonnée par la nature: d'autres fois, toutes ces choses peuvent se confondre et se perturber. Il me semble manifeste que, dans le premier cas, l'on doive conserver la localisation, la structure, la composition et la disposition habituelle de toutes ces parties ordonnées par la nature et, en conséquence, l'état de santé; et que, dans le second cas, ceci ne se vérifie pas» (pp. 159–60).

L'apparition d'une tuméfaction dans un point de l'organisme n'est plus un rassemblement de *materia peccans* dérivant du trouble humoral, mais une accumulation de particules dérivant d'une altération de leur mouvement physiologique: «De cet exemple sensé on peut affirmer que, chaque fois que les parties d'un animal ne conservent pas cet ordre et cette disposition de mouvement, et qu'il ne se fait pas par les voies et avec la vitesse ordonnées par la nature, il s'en suit nécessairement une disposition et un arrangement pervers, et donc une infirmité dans les parties de cet animal» (p. 161).

C'est justement pour débloquer et mobiliser ces particules placées et disposées d'une façon perverse, et «pour ôter l'obstruction des pores, qui est la compagne assidue des infirmités» que s'accentue le mouvement cardiaque et, par conséquent, le mouvement de l'organisme en entier, de sorte que la fièvre est essentiellement un mouvement fébrile au lieu qu'une augmentation de chaleur servant à cuire l'humeur peccante. En effet: «Les opérations naturelles telles que la digestion, la maturation, la nutrition et la séparation des excréments s'exercent généralement chez l'animal au moyen du mouvement des esprits et des humeurs, et des parties solides réduites en toutes petites particules» (pp. 157–58).

Ces particules doivent être en mesure de se séparer et, aussi, de se mélanger. Il est bien sûr facile d'admettre a priori qu'une séparation – telle que celle, par exemple, du suc gastrique qui «se sépare» dans l'estomac – s'effectue à travers les pores; mais l'hypothèse atomistico-mécaniste resterait plus ou moins à l'état où elle était dans l'antiquité classique si on ne démontrait pas, dans notre organisme, sinon tous ces pores, du moins les mécanismes minuscules qui en constituent le support ou qui sont, de toutes façons, nécessaires au déroulement des mouvements corpusculaires.[7]

Pour construire une iatromécanique pas purement théorique et aprioristique comme celle de René Descartes (1596–1650), Borelli sollicita l'anatomie à découvrir les «machines» minuscules cachées dans les différentes parties de notre organisme: et il eut la chance singulière d'orienter sur cette voie un chercheur de la trempe de Marcello Malpighi (1628–94), qui, à l'habileté manuelle pour l'anatomie dont il était doué d'une façon extraordinaire, sut associer l'observation au microscope. Ce fut ainsi que Malpighi[8] fonda l'anatomie microscopique et se servit de celle-ci pour donner à l'organisme une structure mécanique minuscule: ses découvertes vont des alvéoles pulmonaires au capillaires sanguins, du récepteur tactile à la machine de la sécrétion et à celle de la diurèse avec son glomérule de capillaires et son tubule en partie droit et en partie tordu.

La structuration minuscule de l'organisme représenta un apport essentiel à la conception mécaniste de la maladie exposée par Borelli.

Notre organisme est un complexe mécanique: et sa vie est le fonctionnement des machines, certaines desquelles particulièrement délicates et petites, qui le constituent. De même que celles inorganiques, les machines organiques sont elles aussi sujettes à des détériorations, à des avaries, à des pannes qui en altèrent le fonctionnement. Ces pannes ont une incidence aux niveaux les plus petits des machines organiques; mais, étant donné l'état actuel des instruments dont on dispose, il est possible d'effectuer une étude valable seulement au niveau macroscopique, à travers l'examen des lésions d'organes à la table anatomique. Les altérations fonctionnelles qui dérivent de ces pannes produisent des troubles dans l'économie de l'organisme, qui se traduisent par des manifestations cliniques proportionnées au siège et à la nature des pannes mêmes.

C'est le programme implicite dans le titre même de l'ouvrage de G. B. Morgagni (1682–1771) *De sedibus et causis morborum per anatomen indagatis* (1761),[9] lequel, s'étant mis à suivre systématiquement une voie que Malpighi avait déjà commencé à tracer, est aujourd' hui indiqué comme le fondateur de l'anatomie pathologique.

La pathologie par «contagium vivum seu animatum»[10] apporta elle aussi des développements à la conception de la maladie formulée par Borelli. Dans son interprétation des fièvres malignes, l'intempérie entre les quatre humeurs disparait par rapport à la lésion locale: la lésion précisément des poumons, constamment démontrée à la table anatomique et provoquée par les semences d'épidémie introduites par voie respiratoire. Au lieu de purger l'organisme de l'humeur peccante, l'indication thérapeutique vise à l'anéantissement de ces semences.

La première acquisition pratique de cette conception est l'étiologie acarienne de la gale, démontrée en 1687 par Giovan Cosimo Bonomo et qui est un produit de la structuration microscopique des insectes et de la négation de la théorie de leur génération spontanée dérivée des expériences de Redi. Au lieu d'une intempérie entre les quatre humeurs, comme on l'admettait auparavant, la gale dépend d'une noxa externe, et précisément de l'acare, qui explique localement, sur la peau, son action nocive. L'indication thérapeutique ne vise donc pas à libérer l'organisme de l'humeur peccante, mais à tuer l'acare qui est la cause de la maladie: et Bonomo obtint ce résultat d'une façon brillante grâce à la médication topique appliquée sur la peau atteinte. Les récentes victoires sur certaines maladies bactériennes, grâce aux antibiotiques et aux chimiothérapiques, ne sont, ni plus ni moins, que l'équivalent actuel de la victoire sur la gale grâce aux onctions tendant à tuer l'acare.

Je viens d'indiquer seulement quelques uns des points les plus saillants du bouleversement de la notion de maladie apporté par l' Ecole Galiléienne; et je renvoie ceux qui voudraient approfondir la question au *De recentiorum medicorum studio*[11] qui constitue l'oeuvre méthodologique de Malpighi, son testament scientifique paru posthume, ici à Londres, en 1697.

References

1 'De la théorie atomistico-mécaniste à l'anatomie subtile (de Borelli à Malpighi) et de l'anatomie subtile à l'anatomie pathologique (de Malpighi à Morgagni)', *Clio Medica*, 1971, **6**, 99–107.

2 'L'influence exercée sur la médecine clinique par les sciences de base développées par l'école Galiléienne (Génération spontanée et "contagium vivum" de la gale)', *Clio Medica*, 1973, **8**, No. 2.
3 'Boerhaave et la doctrine de la glande', dans G. A. LINDEBOOM (ed.), *Boerhaave and his Time*, Leiden, 1970, pp. 69–82.
4 'G. B. Morgagni und die Bedeutung seines "De sedibus et causis morborum per anatomen indagatis', dans E. LESKY et A. WANDRUSZKA (ed.), *Gerard van Swieten und seine Zeit* (B. VIII der 'Etudien zur Geschichte der Universität Wein'), Wein (H. Böhlaus), 1973, pp. 133–42.
5 'J'ai donné une première analyse de ce livre dans mon travail "Dal Borelli al Malpighi" ', *Atti della Società Italiana di Patologia*, 1967, **10**, 381–94; *Simposi Clinici*, 1967, **4**, pp. xvii–xxiv. Voir aussi l'introduction (pp. 15–20) du livre cité à la note 8.
6 BELLONI, L., 'La dottrina della circolazione del sangue e la Scuola Galileiana 1636–61', *Gesnerus*, 1971, **28**, 7–34.
7 Voir le travail cité à la note 3.
8 MALPIGHI, M., *Opere scelte* a cura di L. Belloni, Torino (Utet), 1967.
9 Voir le travail cité à la note 4.
10 Voir le travail cité à la note 2.
11 Voir les pp. 491–631 du livre cité à la note 8.

A. H. T. Robb-Smith
Oxford (Great Britain)

Morgagni and English medicine

Just over two hundred years ago, in December 1771, there was buried in the little Paduan Church of St. Massimo, Giovanni Baptista Morgagni, who had held with distinction the chair of Anatomy in the University of Padua for some fifty-six years, a worthy successor to his illustrious predecessors – Vesalius, Fallopius, Fabricius, Casserius and Spigelius.

It seemed appropriate for two reasons to discuss the impact on English medicine of Morgagni's most famous work *De Sedibus et Causis Morborum per anatomen indigatis*, a work which he had been preparing for twenty years and completed in 1761 when he was almost eighty.

In accordance with the Congressional themes I will hope to show how Morgagni was influenced by English medical thought and his impact on English medicine, but my second reason is that Professor Bariéty, whose tragic death last June has robbed this Congress and the world of a notable medical historian and clinician, had proposed that one of our themes should be 'L'évolution du Concept de Nosologie au cours des Ages', and there is little doubt that Morgagni's masterwork was a major factor in the development of nineteenth-century nosology.

If we turn to any book on the history of medicine we will find Morgagni described as the 'Father of Modern Pathology', but by his contemporaries he was hailed as 'His Anatomic Majesty', 'Anatomicorum totius Europae princeps'. Is this difference in attitude of importance? I think it is. Nowadays by Pathology, we can mean three things – the study of disease causation, its aetiology and pathogenesis, or we may mean morbid or pathological anatomy and histology, the recognition of morphological changes in the organs, and lastly there is clinical pathology, the application of laboratory methods to assist in the diagnosis and treatment of disease.

In the eighteenth century, pathology had only the first meaning and we find Hieronymus Gaub, Boerhaave's successor at Leyden, in his *Institutiones Pathologiae Medicinalis* of 1758 which remained the standard text for several generations of medical students, defining Pathology as that which it is useful to know of the nature, differences, cause and progress of disease; he mentions that there is also pathological semiotics or symptomatology, the knowledge of the signs which reveal all that is obscure in a disease, and which it should be known whether they are present, have occurred or may appear during the course of a disease. Even in this sense it is quite a modern word; it is occasionally found in Galen, but it was Jean Fernel who really introduced the word 'pathology' in his *Medicina* of 1554, though twelve years earlier he had used the galenic term aetiology for the same concept. Fernel still accepted as a basis the humoral concept of disease and we must confess that we have not in this day and age entirely shaken ourselves free from this metaphysical approach, yet he stressed that much disease has a specialized and localized seat in this or that organ and he made this the basis of his classification of disease.

In the succeeding two hundred years, remarkably little progress had been made in the knowledge of the nature of disease. There had been considerable advances in physiology, and gross anatomy had almost reached its zenith. The application of the microscope and vascular injection by Leeuwenhoek and Malpighi had uncovered the marvels of micro-anatomy and by revealing the capillary circulation had converted Harvey's logical necessity into a histological certainty, and yet as Richard Davies, a Cambridge scientist whose achievements have not been fully appreciated, wrote to Stephen Hales in 1759, 'The discovery of the circulation has not been followed by so great an advancement in the science of medicine as was naturally to be expected from it. The reason for which is that our theory has not advanced much in the knowledge which is naturally founded upon this grand principle.' This disparity remained until the purpose of respiration was revealed.

So the eighteenth-century physician devoted himself to the classification of disease either by symptoms or on the basis of a system of pathology which was largely theoretical. I need not bore you with an account of these theories but it should be recognized that the majority of their originators were good clinical observers, who contributed very considerably to our knowledge of the natural history of disease, and are illustrative of the paradox, so often to be seen in medicine, even today, of the sound clinician who insists on propounding a fantastic philosophical theory to support his excellent observations. One of the difficulties was that they had no idea of how the tissues of the body were composed, for their microscopes could not resolve the cells that lay between the fibres and blood vessels, and so they had to imagine that these fibres and capillaries consisted of globules of lymph or other substances which were built up from chemical elements and that disease arose from some disturbance of this process.

But, as I have said, Morgagni was not regarded by his contemporaries as a great pathologist, nor was he, but as an anatomist and so we must look in a different direction.

Until the last hundred years, the way of an anatomist seeking to dissect the human body and display its structure to students has always been difficult and dangerous, whereas from the thirteenth century post-mortem examinations were being performed in Italy, at the behest of the judiciary, to determine whether a death was natural or due to poisoning or witchcraft and sometimes, during an epidemic, to try and ascertain the cause.

By the fifteenth century it had become a regular practice for physicians to make post-mortem examinations on their patients in order to confirm or correct their diagnosis; we find Leonardo da Vinci writing 'And so there being an old man sitting on a bed in the hospital of Santa Maria Nuova in Florence, without another movement or any sign of accident, he passed away from his life and I did an autopsy on him to see the cause of such a sweet death'. Unhappily, as Kenneth Keele has told us, Leonardo left no account of his findings other than his observations on the old man's blood vessels. (See *Med. Hist.*, **17**, July 1973.)

A contemporary Florentine physician, Antonio Benivieni, kept notes of everything – his clothes, his fees, his debts and his clinical records, which were published in 1507, five years after his death, 'On some hidden and remarkable causes of disease and recovery'. It consists of some hundred and eleven case histories and in fifteen a post-mortem examination was made and Benivieni remarks casually that only on one occasion in all his practice was permission not granted. One would not pretend that the observations either clinical or anatomical in *De Abditis causis* were of major importance, but it was a beginning and for the next two hundred years many of these collections of completed cases with anatomical observations were published in Italy, Germany and Switzerland. England did not contribute much in this field. As Morgagni pointed out, there were scattered post-mortem reports in the clinical writings of Willis, Highmore, Glisson and Lower and in particular in Harvey's writings; indeed in Harvey's first letter to Jean Riolan he spoke of a projected Medical Anatomy which was never written and Morgagni adopted this term to designate what we would call clinico-pathological correlation, though Harvey's proposal was a book on morbid anatomy, such as Matthew Baillie was to compile, for he wrote 'I might undertake to relate from the many dissections of sick bodies and the most grievous and wonderful diseases of dead persons, in what manner and how the inward parts of them are changed in place, bigness, condition, figure, substance and other sensible accidents from their natural form and appearance which all anatomists commonly described'. Harvey makes no suggestion of relating the visceral changes to symptoms or clinical manifestations.

It is remarkable how many of these volumes of medical anatomy were never written, for in addition to Harvey's book, Vesalius was compiling a collection of post-mortem findings in puzzling and chronic diseases; Pietro Castelli died before his 'Sepulchretum' of two hundred cases was completed, while Thomas Bartholin's book on which he had spent twenty years was burnt and it might well be but for his remarkable longevity that Morgagni's book would also have been lost.

Probably the earliest English book of this type was John Browne's *Compleat Treatise of Preternatural Tumours* which appeared in 1678; Browne, who had practised at Norwich, was nominated Surgeon to St. Thomas's Hospital by Charles II, against the wishes of the Governors, who discharged him eight years later for misdemeanours and neglect of duty. It was during this period that he reported to the Royal Society an account of a soldier who contracted ascites by drinking much water when he could not stir from his duties. The post-mortem revealed an enormous glandular liver and the excellent engraving by William Faithorne is the earliest representation of a cirrhotic liver. Joseph Payne discovered a manuscript volume of 'Anatomical Practical Observations in St. Thomas Hospital' written by one James Molins in 1677, and both these books give good accounts of cirrhosis, aneurysms and growths. However for the most part these sixteenth- and seventeenth-century morbid-anatomical observations were not very illuminating to their contemporaries, partly because they chiefly record the more remarkable masses and the like, partly because there was no clear distinction between ante-mortem and post-mortem changes – it was not until 1673 that Kerckring pointed out that the cardiac polyp so frequently recorded was a post-mortem clot – and partly because a humoral hypothesis of disease causation did not in most instances require a local lesion as an explanation; so there was little interest in attempts at correlation of clinical history and post-mortem findings. This is of course not completely true; obstructive lesions and visceral rupture could be identified and there was a growing understanding of a relationship between paralysis and cerebral abnormality, but it was not a large achievement for all the labour.

How little had been achieved became apparent when Théophile Bonet, a Genevese physician who abandoned practice owing to defective hearing, devoted the rest of his life to gathering together all these reports, some 3,000 of them, which were published in 1679 in two massive volumes of some 1,700 pages under the title of *Sepulchretum Anatomicum sive Anatomica Practica*. The cases are arranged in anatomical order from the head downwards and though Haller praised the book as worth an entire pathological library, yet it is impossible to learn what the author claimed that it revealed – the hidden causes of disease. However it was the gadfly that inspired Morgagni.

Probably Malpighi was the first to adopt a rational approach to morbid anatomy, when he said that it advances medicine by demonstrating the seat, the origin and the cause of disease as well as the mechanisms by which it is produced. Malpighi had a stroke in July 1694 at the age of sixty-six and a second fatal one five months later. The post-mortem was performed by his young pupil, Giorgio Baglivi, and he found a large heart with an abnormally thick left ventricle; the right kidney was small with a dilated pelvis and there was a stone in the bladder. The right ventricle of the brain contained two ounces of extravasated blood and the left an ounce of yellow phlegm. Giovanni Lancisi, the epidemiologist, reported the post-mortem findings to the Royal Society and explained that 'they proved that the conglobated glands in the whole body had thrown into the mass of blood an acid lymph and that the conglomerated glands of the hypochondria, especially those of the liver, had thrown into it a melancholy humour and that these two sorts of humours being carried into the vessels of the brain had disposed the blood to coagulate there, and that these having corroded and broken through the tunics which served for a stop to them, they had run into the ventricles where they caused death without a remedy.'

Thus we see the contrasting voices of the anatomist and pathologist of the late seventeenth century, but before we deplore the obscurantism of the theoretical pathologist, remember that once or twice a week we make post-mortem examinations on patients dying from cardiac failure in whom we find fibrosis and ischaemic changes in the myocardium and a variable degree of narrowing of the coronary blood vessels and then read the remarkable statements as to the causation of a mystical condition called coronary heart disease; a few years ago 'Stress' was the cause of all the more obscure diseases, then they were collagen disease, next it was auto-immunity. Are we really so much wiser than our predecessors?

The achievements of medicine in the first half of the eighteenth century are negligible when compared with the century before and what was to come later. On the continent the Age of Reason provided the popular teaching and textbooks of Boerhaave, Hoffman and Stahl, and the symptomatic nosology of de Sauvages which was to inspire Linnaeus, but these, for the most part, were creations of the library rather than the laboratory or the bedside.

In England the situation was slightly different; there was not the urge to write textbooks to attract students, as university remuneration was unlike that on the continent, while something of the sceptical empiricism of Sydenham may have had a restraining influence. So we find the English physicians of this period were men of culture and highly successful in their practice; it was Alexander Pope who said that physicians were in general the most amiable companions and the best friends as well as the most learned men he knew and the names come tripping off the tongue – Mead, Freind, Arbuthnot, Akenside, Garth, Askew, Sloane, Lawrence, William Hunter, but what did English medicine of this period contribute? Some good clinical descriptions by Fothergill, Huxham and Heberden, improvements in midwifery by Smellie and in surgery by Cheselden and Pott, Floyer's pulse watch and Pringle's work on military sanitation. The only epoch-making contributions I can think of are Robert Whytt's work on experimental neurology and James Lind's study of scurvy. But just as physicians could be able poets, connoisseurs of the arts or expert botanists, so it was that the amateur could advance medical knowledge, the physiological studies of the curate of Teddington, the Reverend Stephen Hales, Lady Mary Wortley Montague's advocacy of smallpox inoculation and the discovery of the value of salicylates in rheumatism by the Rector of Chipping Norton. The Age of Reason also provided the economical humanitarianism that was to create the voluntary hospitals, the dispensaries and charity schools – all part of the desire to advance mankind by conquering ignorance – and the resultant was the industrial revolution.

It may seem that I have strayed from my main theme, yet is is only possible to measure progress against the background of the climate of thought. These accounts of individual diseases by Fothergill, Huxham and Heberden, following in the Sydenham tradition that disease entities are characterized by their symptoms and natural history, were very different from the encyclopaedic approach of the pathological or symptomatic nosologies; furthermore the *Philosophical Transactions of the Royal Society* are rich in individual case histories with post-mortem changes, such as James Douglas' (1715) account of aortic regurgitation, and observations resulted in a gradual recognition that it was possible to correlate clinical manifestations and visceral lesions.

Morgagni was elected a fellow of the Royal Society in 1722. At that time he had been Professor of Anatomy at Padua for seven years and his publications had consisted for the most part of detailed anatomical studies while his sole contribution to the *Philosophical Transactions* was an account of a lunar eclipse. Nevertheless in 1704 when Morgagni was only twenty-two, he had been elected President of the Bologna Academy of Sciences and had selected as the theme of his address, Bonetus' *Sepulchretum*, in which he praised the industry of its preparation, yet deplored its shortcomings, which had not been overcome in Manget's new edition. What was required was an adequate index both of symptoms and morbid appearances, and this germinal idea was to provide one of the most valuable features of *De Sedibus*.

It was not until 1741, when Morgagni was fifty-nine, that he decided to write his own book on the localization of disease and there is the well-known story of the young medical student – unfortunately as nameless as the importunate visitor from Porlock – who asked him to gather together his and others' observations, and so the seventy letters began to be written; he followed the masterly system of indexing which he had adopted in his anatomical epistles, and which enormously simplified preparation of the text for the printer. The letters had roman numbers while the individual cases and their commentaries had arabic numbers and so in the four indices – the first a table of contents, the second an index of symptoms and nominal details of the cases, the third dealing with morbid lesions and the fourth referring to authors' names, historical facts, observations and controversies – the references are to the letter and its section and there is no need for pagination as each page is headed by the number of the letter.

Of course the design of Morgagni's book was Baconian in concept, of which he was well aware, for in a letter to Monsignor Celendiss he quotes the passage from the *Advancement of Learning* pleading for post-mortem examinations on the victims of illness 'because in the differences of the internal parts are often found the immediate causes of many diseases'.

Morbid anatomy and its clinical correlation had not stood still in the twenty years that were to elapse while Morgagni was polishing his letters and commentaries and there was increasing awareness that in many instances it was possible to relate symptoms and disease to visceral abnormalities. It would take too long to recount all these observations, and so I shall only instance a few of which, perhaps, the most significant was that of Morgagni's other Bolognian anatomical teacher, Albertini. An essay of his on dyspnoea associated with heart disease, published posthumously in 1748, gives a clear account of pulmonary oedema and passive venous congestion consequent on heart disease, and shows that the dyspnoea is a resultant of the retarded pulmonary circulation, often arising from valvular heart disease; in other words mechanical factors are responsible rather than a serous constitution of the blood.

Picchione in 1741, anticipated Haller's famous aphorism 'Pathologia docet physiologiam' by quoting Malpighi as having said 'Since in Anatomy the morbid state reflects the idea of the healthy, why should not disease indicate the function of an organ especially when experiments cannot assist us.'

However, it must be confessed that Haller's contributions to morphological pathology are in no way comparable to his physiological researches and are more in the Bonetian tradition – random observations discovered at autopsy with little clinical correlation, though he does provide excellent accounts of aneurysms and congenital malformations. Jean Baptiste de Sénac's *Traité des Maladies du Coeur* (1749) was far more important as Morgagni later acknowledged in the third of his dedicatory prefaces.

In England some interesting advances were made. I mentioned briefly John Fothergill's excellent clinical descriptions of disease, but as a catalyst in the new approach of clinico-pathological correlation he was even more important. Fothergill had been trained at Edinburgh and so indirectly had absorbed the Boerhaavian approach, and when a friend and contemporary, George Cleghorn was stationed in Minorca as an Army Surgeon, Fothergill encouraged him to publish in 1751 his observations on more than 120 post-mortem examinations, correlating these with the clinical symptoms; it contains a number of valuable observations particularly the modification of acute and chronic disease by intercurrent malaria. In 1753 Cleghorn was appointed Anatomist to Trinity College, Dublin, where he met a twenty-nine-year-old medical student, Samuel Clossy, who had started keeping notes on the post-mortem examinations of cases he had been clerking, which covered the period from 1752 to 1756 and were published in 1763, *Observations on some of the Diseases of the Parts of the Human Body Chiefly taken from Dissections of Morbid Bodies* and it is a remarkable achievement. Although published shortly after

Morgagni's book, it makes no reference to *De Sedibus* as the text was probably completed before a copy arrived in England, but it shows a wide knowledge of medical literature both English and continental. Clossy explains that 'our knowledge of the affections of the Human System is acquired by seeing symptoms and dissecting bodies and both are improved by reason and reflection, which will allow me to explain the phenomena of the symptoms and prove the explanations and this is the method I have endeavoured to follow in these observations'. It is based on a study of fifty-three cases arranged in relation to symptoms and each case history is given with post-mortem findings and a commentary; in fact on a small scale it corresponds to the pattern of Morgagni's book, although it is clear that Clossy had arrived at a similar concept independently. It would take too long to discuss his significant observations, but one might mention Jacksonian epilepsy associated with a meningioma, the distinction between spinal and cerebral paralysis, oedema of renal origin, intestinal obstruction due to impaction of worms and many more. Just before his work was published, Clossy left for New York and gave private lectures on anatomy, though he had difficulty in obtaining bodies. In 1765 he was appointed Professor of Natural Philosophy at King's College, afterwards Columbia University and two years later became Professor of Anatomy. In his inaugural address he spoke of Morgagni's latest book as a work 'never enough to be admired as well for its utility as elegance of style' and mentioned that copies had been imported to America from Naples. As a Loyalist, Clossy suffered during the American war of independence and returned to England in 1780 having lost both his possessions and his professorial chair, for which he received meagre compensation from the British Government, and he died in 1784 at the age of sixty.

In the late summer of 1760 Morgagni completed his great work, writing the preface and the five important dedicatory letters and a year later the two noble folio volumes were issued from the Venetian press of Remonini. It was an immediate success for it fulfilled a need and as I have shown, the medical world was ready to receive its approach; but a different fate met a little pamphlet of ninety-six pages that was published in Vienna in the same year, Leopold Auenbrugger's *Inventum Novum*, the account of mediate percussion, the first step in the development of clinical examination. Like Morgagni, he had verified his observations by post-mortem examinations, but Auenbrugger, content in the elegant society of Vienna, had no desire for fame and notoriety, though it must have been gratifying for him when, in his eighty-eighth year, Corvisart acclaimed his achievements.

But to return to Morgagni's *De Sedibus*. The seventy letters, each dealing with a particular symptom and illustrated by case histories, post-mortem findings and commentaries, were preceded by the indices on which he had rightly set so much store, a preface explaining how the book came to be written and five letters of dedication addressed to members of the learned societies to which Morgagni had been elected. It was unfortunate that these letters were omitted from the original English translation, but they do appear in the reprint which the late Dr. Paul Klemperer, a devoted Morgagnian, both in his scientific and historical work, edited for the New York Academy of Medicine. The first dedicatory epistle is addressed to Christopher Trew, a member of the Academia Naturae Curiosorum, and in this Morgagni argues against those who have claimed that morbid anatomy is of no value in elucidating the nature of disease. He explains that both the dogmatists and their opponents, the empiricists, accept the value of morbid anatomy as the illuminator of medicine, although the latter group are not in sympathy with microscopic anatomy, and with this viewpoint Morgagni would disagree, as he feels that it is often only by the application of detailed anatomy that the cause of a disease may be found. However, there are those who are totally opposed to dissections, little presumptive men, sceptics, who perhaps are frightened lest their diagnostic errors may be revealed; they argue that the lesions that can be found may be artefacts or they may not be the result of the disease but of poor treatment, or they may not be the cause, but the effects of the disease and it is these effects which are the cause of death.

Morgagni at once admits that one must distinguish post-mortem from ante-mortem changes and that this can only be achieved by great experience.

With regard to the other objection, he suggests that if one compares the detailed clinical history with the morbid anatomical findings, it is usually possible to recognize the lesions that have caused the illness, as against those that have resulted therefrom. He then quotes Glisson who pointed out that if post-mortem examinations are carried out on a large number of patients suffering from the same disease, and the findings compared, that abnormality which is common to all of them should be the cause; although Morgagni would not be prepared to go as far as this, yet he would agree with the principle and it is for this reason that he has often given a number of case histories of the same disease to illustrate its variations.

The second preface is addressed to William Bromfield, Surgeon to St. George's Hospital, as a representative of the Royal Society. He had selected Bromfield, as his son, William Heriot Bromfield, had been a student at Padua and lived in Morgagni's house, but died in 1762. In this he traces the history of morbid anatomy from the Ancient Egyptians to Benivieni, and then to modern times and naturally gives a pæn of praise to William Harvey.

The third preface is addressed to Jean Baptiste de Sénac (though he calls him Pierre), Physician to the King and the Académie Royale des Sciences and is the most interesting of the five as in it Morgagni opposes the view of those who hold that because post-mortem examinations are unable to detect the first and most hidden causes of disease, which are inaccessible to the senses, therefore they are of no value.

Morgagni specifically mentions a physician who lived at the end of the last century who was a careful observer of diseases but was biased against anatomy. It has been assumed that Morgagni was referring to Thomas Sydenham, but this is unlikely, particularly as he says that the criticism had been made in Italy not many years ago. It seems much more probable that Morgagni is referring to the attacks which Malpighi suffered from his colleagues, in particular Giovanni Gerolamo Sbaraglia (1641–1709) whose *De Recentiorum Medicorum Studio dissertatio epistolaris ad amicum* (Naples 1689) was full of satirical invective to which Malpighi replied in his *Risposta*, published in 1697, three years after his death.

It is true that Sydenham in his concern to characterize the natural history of disease had little enthusiasm for experimental inquiries, but his scepticism as to the possibility of determining the aetiology of disease was on religious rather than scientific grounds. His attitude to morbid anatomy is revealed in a passage in the essay *On Dropsy* (1683) in which he comments on a statement in the Hippocratic

On Ancient Medicine '. . . it is very necessary for a physician to know well and thoroughly the structure of the human body; so that he form true ideas concerning nature and concerning the causes of certain diseases. How can one who knows not the structure of the kidneys and the ducts that lead from them to the bladder, see his way to those symptoms which arise from a calculus; . . . So necessary is this knowledge, that he who wants it is like a man fighting blindfold. . . . It may be learned well and thoroughly by dissection . . . and that easily and by men whose wit and judgment are limited' and then he goes on to say 'Nevertheless in all acute diseases – and two thirds are acute – we must fairly own that there is in their nature some specific property which no speculations deduced from the contemplation of the human frame will ever be enabled to discover and exhibit. Hence I think that all which was meant by Hippocrates was this – that men should not spend their labour in dissections only but that they should rather promote the art of medicine by the dutiful observations of natural phenomena.' But in the *Schedula Monitoria* he reveals his puritanical scruples. . . . 'Man, indeed, may so have his intellectual faculties shaped by Nature, as to be enabled to perceive not what is absolute truth, but only that which is necessary for him to know, and fitted to his nature' and elsewhere he expresses the same idea: 'However much, by seriously inclining our minds, we may discover what Nature does, and by what organs she does it, the way in which she does it will always be unknown to man.' On the other hand one finds both in the essay on Dropsy and the Epistle dedicatory to Dr. Cole, references to post-mortem findings in explanation of the progress of disease and in the *Medical Observations* he postulates morphological changes to explain clinical manifestations.

It was Locke rather than Sydenham who took the extreme view, as a consequence of his physical hypothesis of perception, that knowledge could not be gained beyond the realm accessible to the unaided eye and therefore that detailed anatomy and microscopy were useless and what could not be observed, would never be observed – 'Nature performs all her operations on the body by parts so minute and insensible that I think noe body will ever hope or pretend even by the assistance of glasses or any other invention to come to a sight of them'. . . . But Locke's views remained unknown until Fox Bourne revealed them in 1876 as a result of his studies of the Shaftesbury papers in the Public Records Office. It is clear that the pragmatic view-points of Sydenham and Morgagni were not dissimilar. Morgagni, like Sydenham, was not concerned 'with these hidden reasons which man can under no circumstances attain' but 'it does not follow that the effects of those causes necessarily also escape our senses; for they affect perceptible parts and the abnormal alterations which we discern in them are the manifest internal causes of very many diseases'. While Sydenham wrote 'By diligent research during dissection and by careful scrutiny we may attain to the knowledge of those larger organs by which Nature conducts her more visible operations. . . . By diligently examining and comparing all those points – the exact observations of the natural phenomena of the diseases themselves, I learn the nature of the disease . . . hypotheses directly derived from the facts themselves and arising from those observations only which are suggested by practical and natural phenomena are stable and permanent.' This digression seemed desirable as it is often maintained that Sydenham was opposed to pathological enquiries and therefore to the Morgagnian approach, and that Morgagni was replying to Sydenham's criticisms in the letter to de Sénac, but this is a confusion of thought. Sydenham, like Morgagni, had no enthusiasm for theoretical pathology, speculations on the cause of disease based on theories unrelated to clinical and morbid anatomical observations, but Sydenham, no doubt influenced by Locke, was not prepared to accept the idea that micro-anatomy might illuminate our knowledge of disease, whereas Morgagni, though his studies were based on gross morbid anatomy, admired the achievements of the microanatomists.

The fourth and fifth prefaces addressed to Johann Schreiber of the Russian Imperial Academy of Sciences and Johann Meckel of the Berlin Royal Academy are less important, the one showing that the study of morbid changes in the commoner diseases is more valuable than in rare ones, and the fifth that it is more valuable from the point of view of medical research to examine diseased bodies than healthy ones.

I do not need to remind you of the quality of Morgagni's letters and observations and the vast body of clinicopathological correlation which he presents, but it is interesting to notice the large number of English authors from whom he quotes. They embrace Harvey, Willis, Lower, Highmore, Glisson, Frank Nicholls, Freind, Mead, James Young, Cheselden, John Hunter, John Rutherford and Robert Whytt, revealing the breadth of his knowledge and reading. The first reference to *De Sedibus* that I have found in an English book occurs in Richard Browne Cheston's *Pathological Inquiries and Observations in Surgery from the Dissections of Morbid Bodies* which was published in 1766, a book written by an apprentice surgeon in a small county town.

Browne Cheston, who was born in Gloucester in 1738, was apprenticed to his father, an apothecary, and in 1762 he was appointed to the staff of the Gloucester Infirmary. He became a full surgeon in 1784 and three years later received an M.D. from the Archbishop of Canterbury, that curious survival of Henry VIII's act of 1511, which persisted for more than three centuries. With his M.D., Browne Cheston became physician to the Infirmary until his death in 1815. The *Pathological Inquiries* were written when he was aged twenty-eight and are dedicated to Henry Watson, Surgeon to the Middlesex and Westminster Hospitals.

It is in the preface that he refers to Morgagni's influence and justifies his book by saying 'In the course of such enquiries many diseases will occur, which from their particular nature, situation and connections must have been absolutely incurable, yet even for such we may reap advantage, since by being made acquainted with the original cause, we may collect sufficient hints how to attack the disease with more propriety in an earlier state, and in an advanced one, may be better able to form our prognostics in a certain and satisfactory manner.'

One cannot pretend that Browne Cheston made any epoch-making observations. There are good accounts of surgical emphysema, of psoas abscess from spinal tuberculosis, which Percival Pott would describe thirteen years later, and of renal and liver disease, but it was the attitude, not the achievements, that was significant for he was concerned with the correlation of morphological changes with disease states rather than symptoms.

While Browne Cheston was working in Gloucester, another young man, only twenty-five, was making even more important studies at St. George's Hospital. William Stark had started his medical training in Scotland, but dissatisfied with the teaching, came to London to work with John Hunter, obtained a Leyden degree and continued at St. George's when Hunter came on to the staff. Unhappily Stark turned from clinical medicine to experimental dietetics and as you probably recall, succumbed on 23 February 1770, to self-induced scurvy. His writings were published by his friend Carmichael Smyth in 1788 and except in one particular disease – tuberculosis – it was the attitude rather than the achievements that are significant, for he divided his cases into two groups, in one of which he analysed the effects of treatment on the progress of the disease. I would not pretend that this resulted in a controlled clinical trial – of which I think one of the first was carried out by William Cobbett as British political propaganda against Benjamin Rush, but it illustrated the increasing awareness of the value of clinico-pathological correlation. Apart from his tragic self-experimentation, which unhappily did not add much to our knowledge of the nutritive value of foodstuffs, Stark's major contribution was his study of tuberculosis, in which he traced the progress from the tubercle to the caseous cavity using both the microscope and injection methods; in fact, he was the first to prove, by morphological evidence, the unity of tuberculous disease, observations which were confirmed by Matthew Baillie and in greater detail by Laënnec. This view was reversed by Virchow who regarded tubercles and caseous metamorphosis as distinct entities and this dualistic approach was adopted by the German clinicians led by Felix von Niemeyer with his dictum that 'the greatest evil which can happen to a consumptive is that he should become tuberculous'. They ignored the beautiful experiments of Villemin and it was only with the work of Robert Koch that the Germans were convinced of the specificity of tuberculosis.

There are other instances of the recognition of Morgagni's work in England. At Oxford, John Parsons, one of the first teachers in the Radcliffe Clinical School, discussed the importance of Morgagni in his inaugural lecture as Lee's Reader in Anatomy in 1767, and in the following year there was a visitor to the city who was also aware of the great Paduan Anatomist. Dr. Samuel Johnson spent the spring with his friend, Dr. Chambers, Principal of New Inn Hall and Boswell, arriving fresh from his adventures in Italy, told Johnson that he had seen an experiment in which a ring of burning coals was placed around a scorpion which forthwith retired to the centre and committed suicide by piercing its head with its sting. Johnson was sceptical suggesting that it was killed by the heat and suffered a convulsion, but he would be satisfied if the great anatomist Morgagni, after dissecting the scorpion on which the experiment had been tried, should certify that its sting had penetrated into its head.

Of course England was not the only country to welcome Morgagni's clinico-pathological approach to nosology. In Vienna under Van Swieten it was readily accepted, for in 1749 he had made a regulation that post-mortem examinations should be made on all patients dying in hospital and the value of the Morgagnian approach is reflected in the fifteen volumes of de Haen's *Ratio Medendi*, and the four beautifully illustrated volumes of Sandifort's *Observationes*. In France although de Sénac was entirely in accord with the Morgagnian viewpoint, its general acceptance was delayed, and Joseph Lieutaud's vast *Historia Anatomica Medica* which appeared in 1767 is still in the Bonetian style.

Nor did the theoretical systems of medicine vanish overnight. In Scotland, William Cullen, a great teacher and wise clinician, gained his greatest fame by his nosology, published in 1769, which was based on the theories of Frederick Hoffman, and had the great merit, so it seemed, that once one had determined the theoretical nature of a condition, one knew what type of drug to use, while soon the Brunonian theory caught the fancy of half Europe.

Morgagni enjoyed a very different fame. Books were dedicated to him, students from all over Europe and indeed from as far as America, came to visit him, amongst them John Morgan of Philadelphia, who was to play such an important part in American medical education and found Morgagni, at the age of eighty-two, reading without spectacles and as alert as a man of fifty. It was about this time that the well-known drawing was made by the English artist, Nathaniel Dance, and engraved by his then girl friend, Angelica Kauffman.

Morgagni continued to teach until a few weeks before his death, in his eighty-ninth year, on 6 December 1771. Two years earlier he had been gratified to learn that *De Sedibus* had been translated into English, and an excellent translation it is, by Dr. Benjamin Alexander about whom all too little is known.

Alexander qualified from Leyden in 1761, was admitted as a licentiate of the College of Physicians in 1765 and in the same year was appointed Physician to the London Hospital at the age of twenty-nine, the only applicant for the post. He used to say that he had undertaken the translation as a consequence of a taunt from Sir George Baker, the President of the College of Physicians, but Wadd suggests that he was more interested in the guinea a sheet that the publishers paid him. He died in 1768 before the work was published and was said to have been so great a devotee of the Brunonian System that he drank thirteen pints of porter on the day of his death.

Unfortunately Alexander omitted Morgagni's dedicatory letters and substituted three of his own addressed to John Fothergill, Alexander Russell of St. Thomas's and William Hunter who once wrote 'Were I to guess at the most probable future improvement in physic, I should say that this would arise from a more general and more accurate examination of diseases after death and were I to place a man of proper talents in the most direct road of becoming truly great in this profession, I would choose a good practical anatomist and put him into a large hospital to attend the sick and dissect the dead.' It was a prognostication which his nephew fulfilled. Naturally Alexander's translation made Morgagni's work more accessible to English-speaking countries, for there is no doubt that by the second half of the eighteenth century, an intimate knowledge of latin was on the wane save for those who had gone to a university and few English medical books were written in latin.

There are many references to Morgagni in that great storehouse of late eighteenth-century clinico-pathological observations, the *Medical Transactions of the Royal College of Physicians*; it is there that one finds the papers by Heberden, Fothergill and others on Angina Pectoris, and you will recall that John Hunter carried out two of the post-mortem examinations, failing to look at the coronaries in one, but in Fothergill's case where there was extensive myocardial scarring, both coronaries showed severe calcification.

I think it would not be unfair to say that John Hunter had little enthusiasm for the Morgagnian clinico-pathological approach. He was an experimental pathologist who wished to study function by experiment and observation and his collections were directed to reveal pathogenetic rather than morphogenetic principles.

It was John Hunter's nephew, Matthew Baillie, about whom Professor Rodin spoke at our conference, who concerned himself with morphological pathology and his 'Morbid Anatomy of some of the most important parts of the Human Body' which was published in 1793 was quite distinct in approach from that of Morgagni, upon whom, as he said 'it would be difficult to bestow too high praise'. By Baillie's time, morbid anatomy had progressed to the stage in which visceral lesions could be described in their own right and his clinical comments, which first appeared in the second edition, were cursory in the extreme. Later he published an atlas of engravings, drawn for the most part by William Clift, of specimens either from the Hunterian museum or his own collection which he presented to the Royal College of Physicians and was later transferred to the College of Surgeons and was utterly destroyed during the bombing of London.

Baillie's atlas was soon to be surpassed by that of Robert Carswell, who, before he became Professor of Morbid Anatomy at University College, had been assistant to John Thompson, John Hunter's pupil, whom the University of Edinburgh appointed to the first Chair of Pathology in Great Britain. Matthew Baillie's *Morbid Anatomy* was an immediate success, going through five editions in England as well as being translated into German, French, Italian and Russian, while Baillie, as William Hunter had foretold, was equally successful as a consulting physician and it was remarked, as unusual at that time, that it was his custom to examine his patients very carefully.

To continue to trace the progress of the Morgagnian approach we must cross the Channel, where 'le flambeau de la Nosolgie' as Corvisart put it, burnt most brightly at the beginning of the nineteenth century. Stimulated by Bichat's concept of the pathology of tissues rather than organs and enlightened by the work of the Viennese school, it was Corvisart who initiated the concept of diagnostic methods which he revealed in his great book on cardiology; there he suggested that someone should write a new version of Morgagni entitled 'De Sedibus et causis morborum per signa diagnostica investigatis et per anatomen confirmatis' and though the book was never written, it was his pupils – Bayle, Bretonneau and Laënnec who fulfilled his ideals. Nor was Morgagni's original work forgotten, for a French translation appeared in 1820 and two years later William Cooke, a London practitioner and founder of the Hunterian Society, issued an abridgement of Alexander's translation which was reprinted in America. Dr. Cooke almost equalled Morgagni in longevity, for he died at the age of eighty-eight, having performed a paracentesis on a hydrocoele the year before he died, while he started practising obstetrics before the age of sixteen.

While the French school of clinical medicine flourished, interest in the new attitude developed in Guy's Hospital under the influence of Bright, Addison and Hodgkin and it was Bright who made the next major advance for in 1842, in order to pursue his studies on renal disease, he established one of the first clinical research units with a laboratory attached to the wards where his students, Golding Bird and George Rees examined the patients' urine and blood, while another student, George Robinson, published a paper on 'Granular Disease of the Kidney' before his twenty-first birthday. In this great triumvirate of clinicians, who illuminated their clinical observations by morbid anatomy, we see the ultimate flowering of the Morgagnian concept but it is a concept which in the future will continue to yield rich rewards as it does today, and we have only to think of Dorothy Anderson's work on mucoviscidosis or the recognition of the carcinoid syndrome to realize how short-sighted was Sir James Goodhart when he delivered the Harveian Oration sixty years ago entitled 'The Passing of Morbid Anatomy'.

In conclusion I would like to mention briefly a curious association between England and Morgagni's writings. A week before Morgagni died he wrote to his favourite pupil, Michele Girardi that there were four boxes of manuscripts in his study which he wished to give him, but when Girardi arrived from Parma, Morgagni had died, alone in his home but for his servants and a medical student, Luigi Calza, and the manuscripts were nowhere to be found; subsequent Morgagnian scholars sought them all over Italy but they had vanished and their rediscovery twenty years ago is due to the detective skill of Professor Pazzini. In December 1952, one of the professor's associates, Dr. Borri, went to Florence to see what medieval medical manuscripts there might be in the Laurentian Library. Passing through the old library with its magnificent display of manuscripts on the reading desks, he went down to consult the catalogue, printed in 1896, of which there are copies in most of the principal libraries in the world. Naturally Dr. Borri found a rich treasure trove of medieval medical works but then was amazed to find the name of Morgagni in the manuscript index; when Professor Pazzini examined these manuscripts he realized that he had discovered the volumes which had been sought for nearly two centuries; not only were there the manuscript drafts of *De Sedibus*, the *Adversaria* and the *Epistolae*, but also an autobiography and over two hundred lectures which Morgagni had delivered when he first came to Padua as Professor of Theoretical Medicine. But where had the manuscripts been and how did they come to the Laurentian Library? It would seem that on Morgagni's death, his servants were anxious to burn as rubbish all the papers their old master had accumulated but the medical student, Luigi Calza, removed the manuscripts and in due course sold them to a book-loving Paduan surgeon, Dr. Dainose, from whom they went to the private library of Marchese Paolini Gianfilippi of Verona. In 1842 the family sold most of the library to a Paris book collector and dealer, Guglielmo Libri, who was not over-scrupulous as to how he acquired his books, indeed he stole large numbers from French public libraries. In 1844 Lord Ashburnham decided to form a library and bought a large collection from Libri for £8,000. The Earl continued to enlarge his library until his death in 1878, but in 1853 had printed a catalogue of part of his collection which mentions the Morgagni items as did the 1883 report of the Historical Manuscript Commission. The fifth Earl wished to sell his father's collection, but by now it was known that it contained the books that Libri had stolen from France and no library would touch it, while the French Government were demanding their books back. There was a considerable scandal, but in the end the British Museum bought the Stowe manuscripts for £45,000, the Italian Government paid £23,000 for the Libri collection, apart from the books claimed by France for which their Government paid £24,000 and some of the other books were sold privately. The Italian Government gave the Libri manuscripts to the Laurentian Library and so they returned to Italy after their forty years in England, catalogued but unknown until Professor Pazzini discovered this new Morgagni which he and his students are revealing; perhaps we shall learn the name of the medical student who inspired Morgagni to write one of the great books in medicine, a book which by concept and example has had a profound influence on English medicine.

L. S. King
Chicago, Illinois (U.S.A.)

Rationalism and empiricism in early eighteenth-century medicine

The desire to label the great thinkers had produced some peculiar distortions. We call Francis Bacon or John Locke or Thomas Sydenham empiricists, and we call Leibniz or Boerhaave or Hoffmann rationalists. How basic is the distinction between them? Actually, there is only a difference of degree. The rationalist lays particular stress on something called reason and the empiricist on something called observation or sense data or facts. But both terms, rationalism and empiricism, are indissolubly connected and neither can exist without the other, any more than we can have 'up' without 'down', or an 'inside' without an 'outside'.

The difference between a rationalist and an empiricist, a difference that loomed so large in eighteenth-century thought, is best illustrated by familiar detective stories. The great Hercule Poirot, for example, is the prototype of the rationalist. He solves problems not by rushing around in search of facts (or clues), as do the lesser detectives. Instead, Poirot uses his little grey cells and reflects. He meditates. He seeks the inner connexions among events. A suitable term is 'the eye of reason', that indicates a rational activity that 'sees' more deeply and perceives truth hidden from those with lesser vision.

In what we call rationalism the philosopher could safely go far beyond the immediate experience, if only he used right reason. Reason would be a reliable guide to penetrating the secrets of the universe, for the universe was rational and amenable to analysis through reason. Experience was merely the starting point.

The empiricist, however, distrusted the conclusions attained principally through the exercise of reason, and wanted to stay relatively close to concrete experience. In the empirical viewpoint the physician could safely go only a very short distance beyond actual observation. He might make low level generalizations, but not sweeping abstractions.

Let me give two examples that illustrate the 'rational' process in science. Galileo, in one of his writings, was discussing what happens when a stone is dropped from the top of a mast of a moving ship. In the dialogue the character Salviata says, 'Without making the experiment I am sure that the result will be as I am telling you, because it must necessarily come out this way.' Necessity holds sway and the power of reason can perceive and identify the necessity without any further sense perception, such as making the actual experiment. Thought, by penetrating into the underlying reality, is superior to mere observation which then becomes unnecessary.

A further and somewhat different example comes from the writings of Christian

Wolf, the disciple of Leibniz. Wolf, believing that the planets were inhabited, proved that the inhabitants of Jupiter were much larger than those on earth. His reasoning was quite logical. The pupil of the eye, he declared, contracts or dilates according to the intensity of the light. But the light on Jupiter is much more dim than on earth because Jupiter was further away from the sun. Hence the inhabitants of Jupiter had pupils much larger than the men on earth. Now, the size of the pupil is proportional to the size of the eye, and the size of the eye proportional to that of the body. Therefore, the inhabitants of Jupiter, with their large pupils, would necessarily be much larger in size than the inhabitants of earth. This is a delicate bit of reasoning that achieves a logical solution worthy of Sherlock Holmes.

The rationalists held very explicitly that medicine rested on a twin base. As Hoffmann declared, 'In medicine there are two supports – experience, which is the first parent of truth; and reason, which is the key to medical science. Experience comes first in order, and reason follows. Hence in medical affairs reasons which are not founded on experience have no value.'

The problem is perfectly clear. We start with some facts or sense data which are accepted as true. Then by the exercise of reason we reach conclusions that are also accepted as true. The great question is, How much fact, how much data, do you need to warrant any given exercise of reason? Rationalists claim that with a small amount of fact you could achieve a great deal of truth through reasoning. The empiricists held that you must have a great deal of fact in order to support a very small amount of reasoning. The issue between the two groups is quantitative only – how much fact to support how much reasoning? At what point does reasoning become speculation? What is the dividing line between inference and imagination? What are the criteria for valid reasoning?

Each rationalist physician felt that his own reasoning was sound and valid and his own logic quite impeccable. But he might have considerable doubt about his colleague or his rival. Indeed, different writers, starting with the same facts, might come out with quite different conclusions, infer quite different causal factors, assert a quite different character to Reality. Each protagonist, confident that his own reasoning was just, would conclude that his opponent's was not. The opponent, clearly, was indulging not in sound reasoning but in *hypothesis*.

This is a key word in eighteenth-century medicine and almost always a word of opprobrium, to express disapproval of the methods and conclusions of those with whom you disagree. 'Hypothesis' implied speculation and imagination rather than reason, and in the 'Age of Reason' speculation and imagination were not to be encouraged.

When we speak of hypothesis we immediately think of Newton who said, 'Whatever is not deduced from the phenomena is to be called an hypothesis.' To apply to eighteenth-century medicine, Newton's dictum needs only a single emendation, to read, 'Whatever is not *properly* deduced from the phenomena is to be called an hypothesis.' In this sense, 'hypothesis' is a distinctly pejorative term, as any acquaintance with eighteenth-century medical writings makes immediately apparent.

We are, therefore, left with a critical but undefined word, 'properly'. If we examine the two examples that I gave, we can readily say that Galileo's assertion regarding the fall of the cannon ball from a moving ship is a proper deduction from the phenomena, and Wolf's assertion regarding the size of men on Jupiter is not a proper deduction from the known facts.

How can we decide what is *proper*? Let us study two medical writers at the turn of the eighteenth century.

George Baglivi, born in 1668, the same year as Boerhaave, died at the early age of thirty-nine, but he exerted an important influence over his contemporaries. In his writings he devoted a great deal of attention to the problem of empiricism and rationalism, and he expressed some interesting points of view.

Reason, he emphasized, is not in any way to be opposed to experience, and those who try to make such an opposition, one to the other, are wrong. The two are co-ordinate and correlative. Baglivi expressed well (p. 8) the particular function of reason – it is the activity 'by which a physician perceives consequences, brings together the principles and causes of diseases, foretells their progress and outcome, and by understanding the present looks forward to the future'. Or again, disease is so complex – 'the innumerable causes of diseases, the various temperaments . . ., age, sex, way of living, diverse climate . . . and an infinity of other things that concur toward the production or removal of disease' – these he said, are so perplexing 'that it is a hard matter to trace the truth, unless the totality [*complexus*] of them all be weighed and illustrated by a discrete use of reason'. Reason seems to have a practical function throughout, to sort out the complexity of observation.

However – and this is a matter of great significance – while Baglivi denies any opposition between reason and experience, he does make a sharp distinction between theory and practice. It is the function of theory 'to give the causes [*rationem*] of the phenomena that accompany diseases; to make a proper comparison between what went before and what is present; to trace the hidden causes of diseases, and the true origins of these causes; and to explain other things of that nature; by which means the physician may be enabled to proceed more openly in determining indications . . .'.

This description of theory is remarkably similar to that of reason just quoted. Theory seems to be merely the elaboration and systematization of what reason does. But again, the goal seems to be practical, directed toward the improvement of medical practice.

Baglivi has many pointed criticisms of theory, and these criticisms illustrate very well some of the conflicts of the early eighteenth century.

In the period we are discussing there was great interest in the relative merits of the so-called Ancients and the Moderns. This opposition between the old and the new became prominent first in literary circles and then spread over to the scientific world. It has been known as the Battle of the Ancients and the Moderns, a topic admirably studied by many fine scholars. In medicine Baglivi straddled the issues in an interesting fashion. He claimed that in matters of theory the Moderns are far superior to the Ancients, but in the matters of practice the Ancients – especially Galen and Hippocrates – were superior.

Baglivi had no difficulty in establishing the superiority of the Moderns in regard to theory, which derived from physics and experimental philosophy. The theory of the Moderns, said Baglivi, is much more certain than that of the Galenists, for it is 'grounded upon experiments made with diligence and repetition and drawn from the storehouse of natural philosophy, and demonstrates causes and symptoms of diseases, not by uncertain conjectures but by mathematical truths, that shine as clear as the sun'. The Galenic theory, on the other hand, 'does not only seduce weak minds from the true road of practice . . . but by . . . a barrenness of invention, and an ostentation of logical quibbles in refuting and retorting arguments, covers its practice with the greatest obscurity'.

If modern theory is so much superior to that of the Ancients, why does modern practice not enjoy an equal degree of superiority? In his answer Baglivi indicates, by indirection, the difficulties of eighteenth-century medical rationalism.

The great defect lies not in the theory itself but in its application to practice. Theory can indicate the causes of diseases but difficulty arises if any one 'promiscuously forms his notions of practice from the rules of theory'. Successful practice requires not merely theoretical justification but concrete experience. Among the Ancients, said Baglivi, the medical practice – the concrete problems of what to do for the patient in particular circumstances – rested upon proven and well-established experience. The Aphorisms of Hippocrates, for example, represent careful observation and accumulated wisdom, and rejection of this experience is wrong unless the innovation has equally convincing experience in support.

Theory does not offer enough justification for innovations, unless these are backed up by concrete experience. We should not reject the old approved methods merely because the new philosophical theories suggest a different course. Theory is always to be subservient to observation and theory alone can give rise to error. The Moderns, he said, '. . . by virtue of dissections and experiments made upon natural things, attained some certainty in the way of theory', but they thought that this certainty of theory would also apply to the natural history of diseases and procedures for cure. The Moderns 'formed conclusions of practice from the rules of theory, and, by confounding the one with the other . . . gave occasion to the pernicious errors that physick groans under at this day'. Progress can only come from carefully noting what does in fact take place. And this is the way of observation, not of theory.

Surely, it would seem to us that if theory – rational analysis – does not permit direct practical application to the cure of disease, it is not very good theory. If we try to work our way out of this impasse we see several logical possibilities. For example, we can say that any failure of theory to improve the practice of medicine means that the theory is wrong and should be discarded in favour of something better. This view, however, did not have any adherents. No one would admit that therapeutic failures indicated the falsity of his own basic theory.

A second view, to which Boerhaave adhered (and Baglivi inclined towards, to some degree), holds that if theory did not seem to be helpful in practice, the theory might be partly wrong. Although basically sound it may have jumped to hasty conclusions or indulged in improper inferences. We will analyse this viewpoint further when we discuss Boerhaave.

A third view, and one which carried a lot of weight with Baglivi, was a basic scepticism – science could never know enough to affect practice. Baglivi's reasoning on this point is quite interesting.

He strongly supported the school of iatromechanists. They held 'that a human body, as to its natural actions, is truly nothing else but a complex of chemico-mechanical motions, depending on such principles as are purely mathematical'. He compared different organs to shears, wedges, bellows, levers, pulleys, tubes, springs. These data were drawn from experiment and experience. Baglivi indicated that these 'mathematical-experimental principles' are best suited to explain both normal and pathological conditions. Now, if diseases arose only from defects of the solid parts – the organs – then these principles would clearly apply. However, most diseases arose not from disorders of the solids but from disorders of the fluids. And the nature of the fluids escapes human comprehension. 'The ablest philosopher . . . will be forced to acknowledge . . . in tracing the constituent parts of any humors, that the *minima* or least particles . . . lie beyond the reach of all art and speculation' (p. 121). In other words, theory can never reach the true understanding of the fluids, and consequently we must rely on empirical and observational methods. 'The art of curing human bodies is acquired only by use and exercise' and consequently he said, 'practice is of more importance than the theory, to the cure of diseases' (p. 121). He would deny that the art of curing could be derived from following out the dictates and inferences of theory. In line with this view he went on to say, 'I would not have you to take all your conception of physick to be truths, til they have stood the test of practice. What repeated experience recommends to you for a truth, that you may always depend upon as such' (p. 122).

We have here indeed a rather confused picture. Baglivi seems to be saying something like this: the human body is a machine governed by the laws of mechanics but this does not help medical practice much, because the real seat of disease, the humours, is not amenable to analysis through the mechanical philosophy. So, instead of trying to improve our science and get to understand the humours, we should pay little attention to theory. Rather, we should make continued observations on the natural history and description of diseases. Baglivi held that such observations should be recorded in aphoristic form, for the guidance of others, rather than in a rationalistic or systematic form. Baglivi seems to be entering on a schizoid course, with a fairly sharp separation between theory and practice.

Perhaps we can divide physicians into two groups – those who are more interested in knowledge, in theory, in system formation and conceptual analysis. Such physicians start with data but, like good Platonists, try to achieve the universals behind the phenomena. They do this by reason, which is the tool for achieving truth. And it is reason which constructs theory. Then we have the second group, more interested in activity than in reflection, in practice rather than in theory, who want to stay close to the phenomena rather than find conceptual formulations. For them reason is merely a tool to enable them to achieve better practical results. Baglivi belongs, I believe, to the latter group, and Boerhaave to the former. While both were influenced by the intellectual turmoil of the era, they reacted in different ways. The mode of the action is, I believe, a personality response, rather than a carefully reasoned position.

Baglivi was really a pessimist regarding man's ability to penetrate into the secrets of nature. He adopted mechanistic explanations and scorned the Aristotelians and the chemists, but nevertheless he had a highly ambiguous attitude in regard to theory and practice. Theory, good in its way, would not go very far in helping practice. This must develop from observation and not rational analysis. It must proceed *a posteriori*, and any *a priori* projections of theory he condemned.

Hermann Boerhaave, on the other hand, had great faith in the power of reason. As a systematist he organized all concepts into a hierarchal and highly rational form. While he expressed great respect for observation and the primacy of facts, he had no doubts regarding the power of theory to embrace all the phenomena of medicine.

In an early lecture of 1703 Boerhaave firmly expressed the importance of observation and the data provided by sense experience; yet he emphasized that the inferences we draw from the data, through the mathematical method – i.e. the process of reasoning – would uncover far more than the senses alone could achieve. And, he stressed, these conclusions of reason are no less precise nor certain nor useful than the data of sense. Observation and reason are the twin methods of discovering truth. On this all eighteenth-century writers were agreed but they had different degrees of esteem for each. Boerhaave held reason in particularly high esteem.

Boerhaave denied any sharp distinction between theory and practice. His medical theory, based on the science of mechanics, had the utmost value for both understanding (*noscendis*) diseases as well as curing them. Anyone who understands the causes of perfect health will understand the sources and causes (*rationem*) of disease. And physicians who see most clearly the proximal causes of disease are the very ones most suitable for combating these causes. Theory, thus, has the utmost importance for practice, and theory is a function of reason.

The science of mechanics can explain many normal and disturbed bodily functions – e.g. the defects of vision that are corrected by the use of spectacles – but this is only a small part of medicine. Boerhaave realized that the defects of the fluids and the causes of internal disease were not yet known, nor could cure of such diseases as yet be referable to mechanics. He asked whether this reference was something intrinsically impossible to attain, or merely a result that had not yet been achieved. His answer, simple and clear, seems directed specifically against the objections of Baglivi. Said Boerhaave, we must not expect a science so new and only so recently turning its attention to medicine to achieve in a short time what everyone else had been unable to achieve in three thousand years (p. 176). Boerhaave thus had the *faith* that the various pathological states *will* be explained by mechanics. He had faith that the secrets of the body *are* amenable to the investigations of the mechanistic physicians.

In his *Institutes of Medicine*, first published in 1708, Boerhaave declared that medicine arose first from the faithful collection of observations. Then the causes of experience (*experimentum*) were investigated by the exercise of reason (*disputationem rationis*). The former aspect – the data of experience – always remains constant in clarity, use, and necessity. Experience does not deceive. On the other hand, the assertions of reason and causation are doubtful, for every sect offers a different schema.

Many sects have offered many different medical theories, but all these explanations have merely some degree of probability. 'Probable opinion' (par. 19) is something not so self-evident that it would compel acceptance by every competent person. We must distinguish the kernel of fact, the data of observation, from the inferences to which they may give rise. Experience is beyond doubt – and here I must emphasize the double meaning attached to the Latin *experimentum*, which connotes both experience and experiment. Experiments in physics, mechanics, anatomy, and chemistry, as well as the experiences of medical practice, must all be accepted as given. But when we try to extend the data from one setting to another, then we can fall into error. For example, chemistry describes changes produced in certain bodies under the influence of fire, and these experiments are indubitable and correct. But trying to apply these data to the human body and to draw conclusions from this transfer can lead to error. Experience cannot be doubted but inference is subject to error, and he repeats this concept in many different aspects and modalities.

However, reason was just as important as sense observation. While we must have very accurate observation of phenomena of both health and disease, we must also have knowledge of what is hidden from the senses. And this can be acquired by sound reasoning. The data are sacrosanct, yet they can be extended through reason. We must add nothing to the data, said Boerhaave, except what follows so manifestly therefrom that no competent person – the Latin is *nemine gnaro et cordato* – can refuse assent. We can add to the data whatever can be inferred therefrom *by strict principles of reasoning* (*deducuntur severa lege ratiocinii*).

What is it that reason actually does? In reasoning, he said, we examine the data, carefully compare them with each other, so that agreements or differences become clear. Then all those things are inferred which are clearly seen to be contained therein. And these inferences, he went on to say, are no less assured or dependable (*minus firma vel fida*) than the data. In a note he expounds this further (note 7). We speak of reasoning when we compare among themselves the ideas that arise from experience, and perceive distinctly all those concepts (*notiones*) of which the ideas are composed, and thence are able to judge what the ideas have in common and wherein they differ. Nor is anything required for science other than this comparison carefully undertaken. The physician needs this process of reasoning (i.e. sound reasoning) since many things in the human body lie far beyond the limits of senses.

The inferences achieved by reason are no less certain than the data furnished by the senses – provided the inferences are correct. The criterion of correctness seems to be the assent of those who are competent to have an opinion on the subject – a refinement of Descartes' doctrine that the clarity and distinctness of an idea is the guarantee of its truth. Similarly for Boerhaave. If an inference is clear and distinct to all competent persons, then that reasoning is sound. Boerhaave used various descriptive terms to describe proper reasoning – *severa, vera, exacta, justa* – but the import is the same. Reasoning of this type is just as reliable as sense perception or experiment.

But Boerhaave had nagging doubts. Experiments in mechanics are valid, as are the rules derived from such experiments; but 'great care must be taken never to apply those rules to bodies upon which the like experiments have never been tried' (1742). A law may apply in a thousand cases and yet yield an exception on the very next case. Thus he is emphasizing that experience and experiments are valid but inference may be fallacious.

The caution – that the inference from one experiment cannot be applied to a different set of circumstances – in a sense negates the entire concept of inductive reasoning, whose essence is the transference of things which are already known to things which are not yet known. Lurking behind his discussion, as was also the case with Baglivi, is the poorly organized thought that inferences can never be absolutely assured until the implied prediction has been verified, and the rational projection established in concrete sense experience.

Boerhaave was indeed in the grip of a dilemma. On the one hand he believed that reasoning can give knowledge which is just as certain as sense experience. On the other hand, he also realized that rational inference can never be absolutely certain until it has been verified by sense experience. This dilemma he did not resolve. He tended to regard his own reasoning as certain, the reasoning of others as at best probabilistic.

Boerhaave's views represent not scepticism but caution. What we confidently believe has universal application nevertheless can be found to have exceptions. Our errors arise, however, not from impossibility of attaining truth nor from weakness of reasoning, but from impatience and haste. We reach conclusions before the matter has been sufficiently examined. To prove his point he gave an example that is most instructive. What, he asked, is the cause of bodily heat? The Ancients considered the source of heat in the body to reside in the heart, but they came to this conclusion when the nature of heat and the action of the heart were not yet known. This knowledge had to wait until the time of Harvey. Had the Ancients waited until Harvey's time they could have correctly placed the cause of heat in the motion of the blood, determined by the heart (i.e. bodily heat is induced by the passage of blood through the vessels).

Then, in a gesture toward realism, Boerhaave asked, 'But who would suspend judgment for the 2,200 years that elapsed between Hippocrates and Harvey?' And he answered this question, *Sed oportebat tamen*. 'Nevertheless, they should have done so!' Only by such patience can the art of medicine be purged of its errors and become conscious of its strength. Where there are doubts that can be resolved only through hypothesis, we must go cautiously [*pes figendus est*] and leave it to our descendants to solve the doubts – after experiments, which we have not yet made, have kindled the light for them. He recommended this caution, this deliberate withholding of judgment, this refusal to indulge in speculative hypothesis. And he declared that for certain problems still current – e.g. the use of the spleen, the properties of many plants, or the causes of plague or smallpox – for problems such as these we should remain without any opinion until time has brought forth the truth. In this way, he said, the art of medicine would be made true and reliable. If, however, from inadequate [*mutilis*] experiments we fall into speculations and conjectures [*concludimus ad theoremata & opiniones*] then our art will be merely fables, more suitable for the dreams of the learned than for directing the practice of physicians.

Two features here call for specific comment. Boerhaave clearly shows the limitations of early eighteenth-century thought. In regard to bodily heat he believed that, after having waited for 2,200 years, he at last had the true explanation. This, for him, was a variant of the friction theory – that heat is produced by the friction of the blood in the vessels. This he accepted as the definitive truth, based upon the knowledge of mechanics and of cardiac physiology as expounded by Harvey. But if anyone had suggested to him that maybe this was not true, and that he should wait for several hundred years more before he came to a conclusion, he would have brushed aside any such suggestion. In the early eighteenth century the idea that an explanation is inadequate or wrong is a judgment that applied to your predecessors but not to yourself.

Boerhaave had two classes of reasoning (or concepts or theories). In the one class he was entirely sure that he had the right answer and would have completely rejected any intimation to the contrary. Then, there was a further group to which he was willing to admit some uncertainty. Yet, when we read Boerhaave we realize that his recommendations to avoid hasty conclusions in unsolved problems was nothing more than a gesture. Rarely would he admit ignorance, but for the most part he went boldly ahead, offering theoretical elaborations and rational inferences, to produce a well-rounded rational system. His system, indeed, is riddled with speculation and unproven assumptions, with false analogies and fallacious inferences, but all this he could not perceive. He was making a gesture toward sound methodology, but it was a wan and feeble gesture. It is as if the ideas of Francis Bacon had wafted into his mind and were slowly germinating, but they had not yet produced any real roots.

As we study these two men – and limitations of time prevent the inclusion of others – we realize that the terms empiricism and rationalism are so intimately intermingled that there is no sound way to disentangle them. Perhaps the terms themselves are bad and should be discarded, although they are so firmly entrenched in historical usage that they would be sorely missed. However, I suggest that as labels they have little significance. We should, rather, when we study individual physicians, consider not whether they were empiricists or rationalists, but rather whether they were critical of their observations and their inferences. Both Baglivi and Boerhaave were beginning to show some critical awareness in regard to inference. But Baglivi floundered badly and was unable to work his way out of the morass in which he found himself. Boerhaave had much greater critical ability, but still his critical judgment was quite vague. And while both of these men paid attention to the problems of inference, they quite ignored the equally pressing problem, What constitutes a 'fact'? Is any given observation 'really' true?

These problems began to receive significant attention during the middle and latter part of the eighteenth century. The earlier writers were making the problems vivid, and – at least to retrospective analysis – dimly indicating the course which critical thinking had to take.

I suggest that when we study the history of medical ideas in the eighteenth century – and this is a part of intellectual history – that the terms empiricism and rationalism have relatively little meaning. A deeper understanding of the era will emerge if we study instead the growth of critical thinking.

J. Poulet
Paris (*France*)

Naissance de la méthode anatomo-clinique

L'histoire universelle de la médecine peut être divisée en deux périodes: avant le XIXe siècle et depuis celui-ci.

Après vingt-cinq siècles de stagnation, d'Hippocrate à Laennec, la médecine va connaître, en quelques décennies, un essor prodigieux grâce à la méthode anatomo-clinique.

Jusqu'à la fin du XVIIIe siècle, à quelques exceptions près, les médecins ne savaient pas examiner les malades et ignoraient les lésions provoquées par les maladies. Ils ne pouvaient s'en tenir qu'à des idées vagues qu'ils essayaient de compenser par des systèmes *a priori* et des doctrines toutes faites, relevant de suppositions arbitraires. La plupart de ces systèmes étaient de conception étiopathogénique et s'efforçaient de réduire toutes les causes des maladies à un principe unique.

Après la perpétuation des conceptions de Galien et leur déformation dans l'esprit scolastique, la médecine s'était refugiée dans des doctrines telles que l'iatro-chimie, l'iatro-mécanicisme, le vitalisme, qui prétendaient pouvoir tout expliquer à partir de postulats.

Il s'agissait là, d'ingénieuses constructions de l'esprit qui dirigeaient la pensée dans l'interprétation des faits et qui avaient l'avantage de faciliter la pratique de la médecine.

La faiblesse des connaissances rendait la pratique médicale incertaine, et aléatoire. Par ailleurs, le niveau des études était médiocre dans des Facultés restées longtemps marquées de scolastique et plus attachées à défendre le passé, qu'à préparer l'avenir.

La conscience d'un certain charlatanisme décourageait les vocations et le nombre des médecins allait décroissant. De 1786 à 1789, la Faculté de Paris ne décerna pas un seul diplome.

En août 1792, la Législative supprima toutes les Facultés de France.

Un an plus tard, sur l'initiative de Fourcroy, la médecine allait se dégager de ce chaos et en décembre 1793, furent créées des Ecoles de Médecine à Paris, à Montpellier, à Strasbourg. Avec ces nouvelles Ecoles est apparu un esprit médical nouveau. L'enseignement ne reposait plus sur l'exégèse des classiques, mais était centré sur l'étude du malade. Il n'y avait plus de discussions philosophiques et métaphysiques, ni d'assertions dogmatiques, mais un retour à une conception de la médecine essentiellement hippocratique, libérée des superstructures galéniques et scolastiques.

Si la tendance systématique et particulière d'un esprit médical doctrinaire s'est encore perpétuée au XIXe siècle, avec Pinel et sa «Nosographie Philosophique», puis avec la médecine physiologique de Broussais et l'homépathie d'Hahnemann, à l'opposé dès le XVIIIe siècle, certains esprits allaient annoncer la révolution médicale qui se préparait.

L'apport du XVIIIe siècle, en effet, a été considérable. Siècle rationnel, il a débarrassé la médecine du fardeau accablant des anciens. Siècle cultivé, il a commencé d'intégrer à la médecine, les progrès de la chimie et de la physique.

C'est ainsi que s'est amorcée la substitution de la recherche des systèmes et des doctrines à l'utilisation des méthodes.

Littré désigne sous ce terme, «L'ensemble des procédés rationnels employés à la recherche de la vérité», alors que la doctrine est «Un ensemble de dogmes qui dirigent l'esprit dans une voie particulière».

La méthode anatomo-clinique réside dans la confrontation des maladies et des lésions anatomiques.

Encore faut-il pour la concevoir et la réaliser connaître les unes et les autres. Si Paracelse avait émis dès le XVIe siècle l'idée d'une spécificité morbide, on n'avait identifié par la suite que bien peu d'entités pathologiques et pratiquement pas de maladies individualisées. On ignorait tout de l'anatomie pathologique. L'anatomie elle-même, était restée purement descriptive.

On voit tout de suite les exigences que comporte la méthode anatomo-clinique et pourquoi elle était restée si longtemps inconcevable. Il faut d'abord connaître, de la maladie, des signes suffisamment nombreux et assez précis pour lui donner une véritable individualité. En effet, la seule connaissance de quelques symptômes isolés risque de réunir dans une description commune, des affections parfois profondément différentes.

La méthode anatomo-clinique exige d'autre part, une connaissance détaillée des lésions tant microscopiques que macroscopiques, puisque c'est de leur confrontation aux signes que l'on peut déduire l'individualité d'une maladie. Ceci suppose une connaissance anatomique et histologique de l'organisme sain et une longue pratique des autopsies.

Laennec est souvent considéré comme le père de la méthode anatomo-clinique. En fait, il n'en fut que le plus brillant utilisateur par son extraordinaire génie de clinicien et par sa rigueur d'anatomo-pathologiste.

La méthode anatomo-clinique n'est pas le fait d'un seul. Elle résulte des conceptions et des efforts de nombreux médecins et n'a été possible qu'à partir du moment où les autopsies sont devenues de pratique courante.

Galien s'était déjà inquiété du «lieu» des maladies, mais les localisations qu'il a pu établir relevaient davantage de l'intuition que de constatations anatomiques.

La pratique des autopsies, déjà prônée par Harvey chez lequel on trouve des apports importants à l'étude de l'anatomie pathologique, s'est développée au cours du XVIIe siècle et surtout du XVIIIe. Peyer, Hoffmann, von Haller et quelques autres avaient entrevu l'utilité probable de disséquer davantage.

Un premier pas considérable fut franchi par Théophile Bonet, de Genève, qui dans son «Sepulchrum anatomicum» (1679) a réuni les observations correspondant à plus de 3.000 autopsies, dont les lésions constatées avaient été notées. Il a édifié à l'anatomie pathologique un monument véritablement digne d'elle. Dans son oeuvre gigantesque, il a présenté de nombreuses compilations qui avaient occupé une bonne partie de sa vie. Malheureusement, les signes décrits étaient de peu d'importance et les principaux d'entre eux avaient été négligés.

Le véritable créateur de l'anatomie pathologique fut Morgagni. C'était un anatomiste, élève de Malpighi et de Valsalva, mais aussi un observateur de génie. Dans la dédicace de son premier livre, il précise que les autopsies ne peuvent être utiles que faites par un clinicien expérimenté, ayant une connaissance profonde de l'anatomie normale, «le flambeau de l'anatomie pathologique», selon son expression, et comparées à une étude précise et détaillée de l'histoire de la maladie.

Il dit ailleurs qu' «Il faut recueillir et comparer entre elles, le plus possible d'histoire de maladies et de dissections» (Lettre XLIX à l'illustre J. Fred. Schreiber). C'est de lui que découle toute l'école anatomo-pathologique macro et microscopique qui allait jeter un si vif éclat pendant le XIXe siècle.

Morgagni eut une influence énorme sur l'évolution de la médecine. Ce ne fut qu'à l'âge de 79 ans, en 1761, qu'il publia le livre qui devait immortaliser son nom: «Le siège et les causes des maladies démontrés par l'anatomie.»

L'oeuvre de Morgagni est capitale. Il pose nettement son principe. «Il n'est pas de meilleur moyen de s'instruire que de réunir le plus grand nombre possible d'observations et de dissections, aussi bien personnelles qu'étrangères.»

Ainsi Morgagni s'attache dans chaque cas à décrire l'histoire de la vie de chaque patient, celle de sa maladie, le contexte de sa mort, et les lésions anatomiques découvertes à l'autopsie. Il tente d'expliquer comment les symptômes peuvent résulter des lésions.

C'est lui qui a introduit le concept anatomique dans la pratique de la médecine. Jusqu'à lui, les maladies étaient des entités vagues. Il va essayer de préciser les lésions qu'elles provoquent. Créant une discipline anatomo-pathologique, il recherche sur le cadavre les lésions correspondant aux troubles observés pendant la vie, ce qui lui permet de dresser un premier tableau, des lésions qui accompagnent les principaux états morbides.

Morgagni décrit entre autres, l'origine vasculaire de l'apoplexie, les gommes du cerveau, la tuberculose rénale; Il établit la contro-latéralité lésionnelle dans les hémiplégies, l'origine cérébrale des épilepsies, la mort subite par rupture d'anévrysme, la condensation du poumon dans la pneumonie, enfin, il entrevit les différentes causes des hydropisies. C'est à cette date que la méthode anatomo-clinique s'est dessinée, mais ses possibilités étaient encore faibles parce qu'elle n'avait pas acquis une somme suffisante de connaissance. En effet, Morgagni, s'il avait soigneusement étudié les lésions observées à l'autopsie des malades, ignorait les signes objectifs recueillis durant la vie et n'avait guère la possibilité de faire de confrontations valables.

Simultanément, le Montpellierain Lieutaud, devenu à la mort de Sénac médecin de Louis XV, puis de Louis XVI, disséqua plus de douze-cents cadavres en s'intéressant plus particulièrement aux désordres découverts après la mort. Certains l'ont considéré comme le fondateur en France de l'anatomie pathologique.

Peu après, Bichat s'illustra par l'originalité et l'ampleur de ses vues aussi bien que par sa prodigieuse puissance de travail. Schopenhauer disait de lui «Sur 50 millions de bipèdes, on aurait peine à rencontrer une tête pensante telle que celle de Bichat» et lors de sa mort prématurée, survenue à l'âge de 31 ans, Corvisart déclarait à Bonaparte: «Personne, en si peu de temps, n'a fait autant de choses, et si bien.» En effet, de 1799 à 1802, il publie un «Traité des membranes en général», des «Recherches physiologiques sur la vie et la mort», une «Anatomie générale appliquée à la physiologie et à la médecine», et une «Anatomie descriptive», sans compter plusieurs mémoires.

En quelques mois, il ouvre plus de six cents cadavres et rédige le plan d'un cours d'anatomie pathologique.

Il fut à la fois et simultanément anatomiste, anatomo-pathologiste, physiologiste et médecin, mais son grand souci résidait dans sa formule: «Qu'est-ce qu'une maladie, si l'on n'en connait pas le siège?»

En dehors de bien d'autres conceptions originales, qui attestent de son génie et auraient suffi à sa gloire, ne seront retenus ici que ses apports à la méthode anatomo-clinique. Il anima d'un souffle nouveau l'anatomie pathologique et créa l' «Anatomie générale».

Jusqu'à lui, l'anatomie n'avait distingué que des viscères et des organes. Le grand mérite de Bichat est d'avoir montré que ceux-ci n'étaient pas homogènes, mais que les éléments qui les composent et qu'il appelle «les tissus» peuvent se retrouver dans chacun d'entre eux: «La chimie a ses corps simples qui forment par les combinaisons diverses dont ils sont susceptibles les corps composés. De même l'anatomie a ses tissus simples qui par leurs combinaisons forment les organes.» . . . «Dans les appareils différents, il y a des tissus qui eux sont identiques.»

Les notions fondamentales que Bichat a introduites sont à la base du développement de l'histologie normale et pathologique. Il a d'ailleurs dressé lui-même un programme d'avenir.

La classification de Bichat, claire et simple, partage l'anatomie pathologique en deux catégories. D'une part, l'étude des altérations communes à chaque système anatomique, c'est à dire à chaque tissu (cellulaire, artériel, veineux, nerveux, osseux, musculaire, etc. . . .) D'autre part, l'examen des maladies propres à chaque région. Cette seconde partie découle en droite ligne de Morgagni qui avait mis au point la pathologie des organes, mais tandis que celui-ci n'était pas sorti des faits particuliers qu'il avait observés, Bichat s'élève vers la loi générale par la pathologie tissulaire et tente de tout expliquer par elle.

Bichat s'affirme comme l'un des fondateurs les plus importants de la méthode anatomo-clinique lorsqu'il écrit dans l«Anatomie Descriptive»: «Disséquer en anatomie, faire des expériences en physiologie, suivre les malades et ouvrir les cadavres en médecine, c'est là une triple voie, hors laquelle il ne peut y avoir d'anatomiste, de physiologiste, ni de médecin.»

Bichat avait d'ailleurs fait établir dans son service des feuilles imprimées où devaient être consignés dans le même ordre, les renseignements recueillis sur l'âge, le sexe, le tempérament, l'histoire du malade et de sa maladie, le compte-rendu de l'autopsie, le traitement, le régime.

Lorsque Flaubert écrit: «La grande école médicale française est sortie du tablier de Bichat», il exagère, ne serait-ce qu'en oubliant Laennec, mais cette assertion contient certainement une grande part de vérité.

Morgagni et Bichat, ces deux grands créateurs de l'anatomie pathologique, ne produisirent leurs oeuvres qu'à la fin du XVIIIe siècle. Si par leur vie, ils lui appartiennent, par leurs doctrines, ils font partie du XIXe siècle.

Simultanément à l'occasion de la Révolution Française, l'enseignement de la médecine change considérablement et l'esprit médical s'en trouve modifié d'autant. Dès 1766, Desault, qui devait former Bichat, entreprit un cours de clinique chirurgicale qui fut bientôt suivi par plus de deux cents auditeurs, parmi lesquels, son ainé, le grand chirurgien Louis. Il va d'ailleurs plus loin que l'enseignement de la clinique, lorsqu'il écrit: «En cas de mort prévue ou imprévue, le Professeur, après la récapitulation de l'histoire de la maladie et du traitement mis en usage, fera l'ouverture du cadavre, examinera chaque partie en détail et en tirera des conséquences utiles à l'instruction et au progrès de l'art. L'enseignement clinique apparait et l'emporte rapidement sur l'enseignement dogmatique. Cessant de lutter férocement contre les nouveautés, les médecins les adoptent avec enthousiasme. Les hôpitaux se multiplient, surtout en France, après le rapport de Tenon qui montre l'encombrement et ses dangers. Après l'incendie de l'Hôtel Dieu en 1773, quatre nouveaux hôpitaux sont crées à Paris entre 1778 et 1788.

La vieille Faculté vermoulue de Gui Patin, jetée bas par le nouveau régime est bien morte. Elle a été remplacée par des Ecoles de Médecine où enseignent des Professeurs, nommés jeunes à des postes importants. Ainsi après avoir détruit, la Révolution a-t-elle reconstruit. Sous l'influence de Vicq d'Azyr, de Cabanis et de Fourcroy, la réforme allait se préciser. On restreint les cours théoriques et les exercices purement dialectiques, au profit d'une instruction plus objective. Enfin, deux événements vont donner tout son essor à la médecine française. La création en 1802 de l'Internat des Hôpitaux de Paris, pépinière de cliniciens et la fondation en 1805, par Dupuytren de la Société Anatomique qui groupera des cliniciens et des anatomo-pathologistes.

Ces conditions associées à la découverte de nouveaux moyens d'investigation, allaient enfin permettre la naissance de l'exploration clinique.

Corvisart est généralement considéré comme le chef de l'école clinique française au XIXe siècle. C'est lui qui créa l'enseignement de la sémiologie.

Enthousiasmé par la découverte de la percussion, due à Auenbrugger, il se sert de cette méthode pour le diagnostic des maladies organiques du coeur et il écrit: «Une maladie organique existe, selon moi, quand un organe solide vivant quelconque est, dans son tout ou dans une de ses parties, assez dégénéré de sa condition naturelle, pour que son action facile, régulière et constante en soit lasse ou dérangée, d'une manière sensible et permanente.»

Par ailleurs, Corvisart contrôlait ses diagnostics par l'autopsie. Ce fut un vrai clinicien. Il ne fit pas de théories. Son but était de donner au praticien une ligne de conduite qui empêchât la médecine de devenir de moins en moins «un art conjectural» et celà par les moyens qu'il expose lui-même:

«J'ai voulu prouver que si les maladies organiques dans leur nombre et leur histoire ne sont pas encore bien connues, que si l'on s'est souvent mépris à cet égard, la faute en est là, depuis la Renaissance des lettres, aux médecins qui ont négligé l'anatomie jointe à la physiologie, telle que je l'ai définie; que cette faute a conduit nécessairement dans une autre, celle de négliger l'ouverture des cadavres; que de là dérivent des méprises fréquentes, j'ose dire grossières, en substituant souvent des effets à leur cause; en prenant les maladies, les unes pour les autres.»

Professeur au Collège de France, il fit ses cours de clinique d'abord à l'hôpital Necker, puis à la Charité, où il enseignait devant plus de trois cents élèves. Excellent organisateur, il donna à l'enseignement médical un essor inconnu jusque là. Il a conçu une école dite empirique dans laquelle il substitue le diagnostic à la prognose et distingue les symptômes des signes reconnus par les sens.

Corvisart fut donc le créateur de la médecine française avec ses traditions: examen complet du malade et contrôle des diagnostics par l'autopsie des sujets qui succombent.

Il eut pour élèves Bayle, Laennec et Dupuytren.

Bayle fut surtout un anatomo-pathologiste, mais aussi un très grand praticien. Il fut le premier à proclamer l'unité de la tuberculose dans toutes ses formes.

Le plus grand médecin du XIXe siècle et, peut-être, de tous les temps, fut René-Théophile Laennec. La percussion avait été découverte par Auenbrugger, utilisée et développée par Corvisart. Laennec découvrit et utilisa l'auscultation médiate et sut d'emblée l'amener à sa perfection. D'ailleurs, le stéthoscope allait «devenir le symbole du médecin comme autrefois au Moyen-Age, l'urinal».

Outre les découvertes que lui a permis l'auscultation, Laennec a su utiliser une méthode qui découlait de son principe. «Rassembler des faits, et, de leur rapprochement, déduire les conséquences les plus immédiates, tel est le seul moyen que nous ayons, dans les sciences naturelles, pour parvenir à la connaissance de la vérité.»

Il s'est ainsi situé entre, d'une part, les doctrinaires dont les systèmes exclusivement basés sur l'imagination de leur auteur conduisirent à l'incompréhension de la réalité et, d'autre part, les empiristes qui réunissent des faits, mais qui, par leur refus de tout raisonnement, sont amenés à les laisser dans l'incohérence.

Laennec, restant dans la ligne hippocratique joint le raisonnement à l'observation; c'est ainsi qu'il a su créer et exploiter la méthode anatomo-clinique. Dès 1804, il formule une classification anatomo-pathologique fondée sur: 1⁰ les altérations de structure; 2⁰ les lésions dues à des corps étrangers animés; 3⁰ les altérations de la nutrition; 4⁰ les vices de forme et de position.

Les maladies n'étant pas individualisées de son temps, Morgagni ne pouvait que comparer les signes présentés par les malades et les lésions trouvées à l'autopsie. Par ailleurs, il avait tendance à partir de la lésion découverte pour expliquer les symptômes.

Laennec ayant découvert un nouveau procédé d'examen, compare les résultats de son investigation aux lésions du cadavre. Il y cherche l'explication et la cause des manifestations cliniques.

En effet, il ne s'est pas contenté de préciser la nature et les caractères des bruits respiratoires; il a établi à quelles lésions ils correspondaient. Avant lui, toutes les maladies du poumon et de la plèvre étaient réunies dans un chaos confus.

Laennec a apporté partout la lumière. Il isole la pleurésie de la pneumonie. Il décrit tous les aspects de la tuberculose pulmonaire et la sépare du cancer. Il reconnait par leurs signes cliniques et par leurs lésions anatomiques, des affections jusqu'alors ignorées, comme l'emphysème, l'infarctus, l'oedème pulmonaire, la dilatation des bronches, le catarrhe suffocant, les cirrhoses.

Laennec a décrit lui-même les principes de sa méthode: «Le but que je me suis constamment proposé dans mes études et recherches a été la solution des trois problèmes suivants: 1⁰ distinguer sur le cadavre un cas pathologique aux caractères physiques que présente l'altération des organes; 2⁰ le reconnaître sur le vivant à des signes certains, indépendants des symptômes; 3⁰ combattre la maladie par les moyens que l'expérience a montré être les plus efficaces.»

Partout, il précise la nécessité et la valeur de la méthode anatomo-clinique: «Je crois que cette étude est la seule base de connaissance positive en médecine et qu'on ne doit jamais perdre de vue, dans la recherche étiologique, sous peine de poursuivre des chimères et de se créer des fantômes pour les combattre.»

Simultanément, Dupuytren fait pour la chirurgie ce que Laënnec avait fait pour la médecine. Bon clinicien, habile opérateur, et excellent anatomiste, il superpose les signes observés aux lésions qui les provoquent. En collaboration avec Bayle et Cruveilhier. Dupuytren fonde la Chaire d'Anatomie Pathologique de la Faculté de Médecine de Paris.

Par la suite, d'autres médecins français ont continué d'illustrer la méthode anatomo-clinique de Bichat et de Laennec, bien qu'après ceux-ci, il restât peu à découvrir. Bretonneau décrit la diphtérie et le croup et reconnait la fièvre typhoïde. Louis observe et identifie les tuberculoses laryngées, intestinales et hépatiques. Il complète admirablement le tableau clinique et anatomique de la fièvre typhoïde. Andral écrit un traité d'anatomie pathologique.

Cruveilhier publie entre 1828 et 1842, un magnifique atlas où sont minutieusement reproduites presque toutes les lésions qu'on peut retrouver dans le corps humain, et où il affirme qu'à chaque maladie correspond une lésion «sui generis». Bouillaud en 1835 est le premier à établir les signes de l'endocardite rhumatismale et ses lésions.

Si, à la suite de Morgani, la méthode anatomo-clinique est vraiment l'oeuvre des médecins français, d'autres médecins étrangers en ont ébauché les prémisses ou développé les possibilités, en particulier, en Grande Bretagne. Dans un document inédit de la Faculté de Médecine de Paris, on trouve une liste des élèves de Laennec, parmi lesquels figure une très grande majorité de britanniques et son appréciation: «M. Hodgkin, D. M. anglais, quaker, assez bien.»

Déjà Harvey, dans son «De Motu Cordis» avait-il ébauché une méthodologie comparative et affirmé que la base du diagnostic doit être cherchée dans l'autopsie. Il faut citer l'oeuvre de clinicien de ce remarquable observateur que fut Sydenham. Malheureusement, il considère l'anatomie comme une «baliverne». John Hunter a fondé l'école anatomo-pathologique anglaise. Les plus illustres médecins britanniques furent à Londres Bright, Hodgkin, Addison, à Dublin Graves, Adams et Stokes, à Edimbourg Corrigan et Fraser.

La médecine allemande eut beaucoup de difficultés à se dégager du transcendantalisme romantique du début du siècle. C'est Schönlein de Bamberg qui fit connaître en Allemagne les nouveaux moyens d'investigations et la méthode anatomo-clinique. Celle-ci devait être brillamment représentée par Rokitansky et Von Hebra à Vienne, puis plus tard par Virchow à Berlin qui devait fonder la pathologie cellulaire.

Il n'est pas de pays dont les médecins n'aient pas épousé la méthode anatomo-clinique et ne l'aient fait progresser. Néanmoins, née des conceptions de Morgagni, cette méthode est une réalisation française par Bichat, par Laennec et par les autres grands cliniciens français de la première moitié du XIXe siècle. C'est elle qui fut à l'origine du développement de toute la médecine moderne et elle demeure, aujourd' hui tout aussi valable car loin d'avoir l'exclusive des doctrines, elle n'est pas incompatible avec d'autres méthodes par exemple physiologiques ou humorales.

A. Pecker
Paris (France)

Discussion

N'ayant malheureusement pas eu la possibilité d'assister à la réunion d'hier et ignorant donc si cela a déjà été mentionné, je voudrais, à la suite du passionnant exposé général du Pr. Poulet et des très remarquables communications que nous venons d'entendre, rappeler simplement que parmi les précurseurs de Morgagni on relève le nom d'un anglais Robert Morton; il vécut de 1637 à 1698 et localisa avec précision les ganglions hilaires des phtisiques ainsi que l'ont noté les Professeurs Bariéty et Coury dans leur histoire de la Médecine.

Mais nous voudrions surtout souligner qu'une opposition du type de celle qui se manifesta entre les opinions de Morgagni et de Boerhaave reste d'actualité; il en e de même des idées judicieuses de Baglivi évoquées si opportunément par le Dr. Lester King. Si Morgagni opérait ses déductions à partir d'autopsies et Boerhaave partir d'examens cliniques, l'un comme l'autre n'avait qu'une approche limitée du malade. Certes depuis le XVIIème siècle cette approche s'est considérablement perfectionnée; elle n'en reste pas moins encore très imparfaite et entraîne de ce fait d'importantes différences d'interprétation.

Nous tirerons argument de la variabilité dans le temps – temps parfois très court ou même nul – de l'opinion des savants de toutes les époques pour insister sur l'intérêt des études médico-historiques qui étudiant cette variabilité incitent forcément le médecin à une utile modestie. Somme toute l'historique d'une question médicale est un peu comme l'étude d'une erreur diagnostique ou thérapeutique, laquelle ne saurait être exceptionnelle. Nous ne devons pas oublier en effet qu'il est impossible d'observer deux faits cliniques rigoureusement identiques et que contrairement aux physiciens nous ne pouvons jamais faire de comparaisons «toutes choses égales d'ailleurs». Aussi malgré la somme des données que peuvent enregistrer le cerveau humain ou les ordinateurs devrons-nous toujours, comme au temps de Boerhaave et de Morgagni, admettre que certaines inconnues peuvent fausser des déductions apparemment logiques et garder comme Baglivi un certain scepticisme.

III CONGRESS THEME

Clinical Medicine

R. E. Siegel
Buffalo, New York (U.S.A.)

Galen's concept of reflex and functional co-ordination

The use of the term reflex in the title of this paper is actually a misrepresentation, since it does not correctly correspond to the concepts of biological reactions used in Galen's time, the second century A.D. Originally the word reflex or reflexion referred to the rebound of an optical ray. It is the Latin translation of the Greek word *anaklasis*, the bending back.

Galen mentioned in his treatise *Commentaries on the Doctrines of Hippocrates and Plato*[1] that the *pneuma psychikon* (*spiritus animals*, from *anima*, the soul), activates brain and nerves by spreading diffusely into all neural structures, like light expands through space.[2] With this comparison Galen only wanted to indicate the uniform penetration of space by a visually sensitive pneumatic emanation issuing from the eye but was not thinking of distinct light rays.

Later authors thought that they took up Galen's idea, when they wrote that the animal spirit propagates like light rays through the nervous system and that sensory impressions were reflected in the brain like light rays before turning into a motor response.[3] Thus, a misinterpretation of Galen's doctrine of nerve action was introduced into neurophysiology even before the anatomical basis of reflex action could be discussed. The discovery of the nerve fibre by Fontana (1720–1805) hardly justified the further use of this originally optical term.

When we employ, for convenience, the term reflex in the following discussion of Galen's doctrine of human and animal responses, we should remain aware that Galen only described the behaviour of the organism as a whole but did not think of isolated stimuli passing through preset reflex arcs.

Furthermore, he did not consider that circumscript areas of the brain or spinal cord were endowed with specialized functions. The only exception was that he attributed conscious perception of smell to the olfactory bulb, because it is distinctly separated from the larger mass of the brain in those domestic animals which he dissected.[4] Galen generally presumed that the brain acted as a single functional unit. Since inadequate observation suggested further to him that each peripheral nerve could conduct sensory and motor impulses between brain and effective organ, he postulated that every stimulus proceeded (especially in larger nerves) by pneumatic activation along a single hollow central canal, but in the smaller nerves through the solid nerve matter itself in absence of a visible pathway.[5] He never raised the question of possible interference between the centripetal and centrifugal countercurrents of pneumatic movement in the same nerve. In view of these differences it appears difficult to us to decide: (1) whether the modern concepts of reflex and instinct correspond to Galen's terminology; and (2) whether he already distinguished reflex and instinct as separate responses.

Galen employed mainly two terms to indicate the whole range of spontaneous reaction. The word *horme* (from *hormao*, to rush, to be eager) is best translated as impulse, because it stressed the motor response. The other Greek term, *orexis* (from *orego*, yearning; also to reach out) indicated more the psychological aspect of the reaction and its motive; it should be translated as desire or instinct. A third word was *ephesis* (from *ephiemi*, to aim at, to desire), which more closely approached the meaning of *orexis*. Evidently a word-by-word translation of these terms as instinct or reflex appears not possible, because exact synonyma in the two languages do not exist. Thus the second question whether Galen distinguished reflex from instinct could not occur to Galen in this form.

The following analysis will approach the problems of reflex and instinct from three angles: We will see that Galen considered only the level of awareness of an individual during the response to a stimulus; that he regarded these responses as inherited or as learned, and finally that he discussed at great length the biological purpose of these reactions. The answer to the third question depended mainly on his philosophical outlook. In view of the unquestionable influence of Aristotelian ideas on Galen the concepts of this philosopher shall first be briefly examined.[6]

Aristotle spoke of three types of awareness and thus of three forms of responses: (*a*) he thought that voluntary, i.e. active and conscious movements of the skeletal muscles, required the participation of the so-called rational part of the soul, which supposedly entered the organism of man at the time of birth. (*b*) He believed that *non*-voluntary movements resulted as response to stimuli perceived during sleep or waking; he included in this class such involved activities as walking and speaking. Voluntary and *non*-voluntary movements require the participation of the cerebral pneuma. This did not apply to *in*voluntary movements. (*c*) He considered the activity of the viscera as *in*voluntary movements (for instance heartbeat or peristalsis). Normally we do not become aware of these activities.

When Galen attributed the tonus of the circular sphinctor muscles to different states of awareness, indicating the need of evacuation of bowel or bladder, he could not yet know that this was due to a combined action of striated and smooth muscles (anus) or to the co-ordination of spinal (voluntary) and autonomous (involuntary) innervation (urinary bladder).[7] We should, therefore, exclude the response of these muscular organs from the following discussion.

Galen stressed more than Aristotle the transition between voluntary and non-voluntary movements. Non-voluntary responses included, besides walking and speech, more complicated reactions, such as the blinking of an eye on close approach of a finger, or retraction of a limb in response to painful stimulation. Acquired and more complex performances during sport or speech had to be learned step by step, but could become non-voluntary. He did not include in this description the artificial reflexes which we invented for clinical diagnostic purposes.

Only the voluntary and non-voluntary responses involved in Galen's doctrine the participation of the *cerebral pneuma* (*animal spirit*), because they were mediated through the cranial and spinal nerves. Of the responses thus transmitted we define, in our own terms, the simpler responses as reflex, but the more involved reactions as instinct. Galen's terminology did not lend itself to this distinction. A modern author[8] (Fearing) pointed out that even the current usage of the term reflex still lacks unanimity as to what shall be included. And the neurophysiologist Sherrington[9] wrote that it is impossible to draw a line between motor acts performed 'by will and by non-will'. His opinion makes it plausible that Galen already did not want to draw a sharp line between non-voluntary and voluntary movements.

When Galen defined all voluntary and non-voluntary responses performed by the skeletal muscles as *kineseis psychikas* (*kinesis*, movement), he simply wanted to indicate that only the *pneuma psychikon* was the motive force. By the use of this term Galen did, however, not suggest the activity of a separate soul. He only wanted to distinguish the voluntary and the non-voluntary movements from the involuntary motions of intestinal or cardiac contractile fibres, the *kineseis physikas*. The usual translation of the latter term as 'natural movement' fails to convey the correct sense of Galen's expression, since he often defined even consciously performed movements as natural (*kata physin*). The Greek term *physikos* is derived from *phyo*, to grow, and *phyton*, the plant. Its Latin translation as vegetative, plant-like, gives the correct meaning of the Greek word, because it suggests that these activities are not connected with conscious endeavour. When modern physicians speak of vegetative functions, they still use the time-honoured Galenic term.

Galen did not relate these natural or involuntary motions to participation of any form of pneuma, since he did not believe in a *pneuma physikon*, as later postulated by his successors.[10] But Galen assumed that the contractile fibres of the viscera reacted to local stimulation by a natural irritability. He defined the response of each organ as specific function (*dynamis*),[11] but he did not employ the more abstract concept of irritability for which a corresponding term did not exist in ancient medical nomenclature.

Other authors of antiquity defined the spontaneous reaction of skeletal and visceral (smooth) muscles as subject to biological laws (*hypo heimarmene*, Alexander of Aphrodiseas),[12] or as ruled by necessity (*anangke*).[13] But they were not aware of the structural differences of these tissues. However, Galen avoided these rather philosophical terms and preferred describing the facts. He was especially interested in the spontaneous, automatic relaxation of a skeletal muscle during contraction to the opposite antagonistic muscle.[14] Since he did not suspect the participation of spinal or higher nerve structures, he assumed an inborn mechanism.

He also found it remarkable that many types of movement could be started with deliberate intention, but that in the further course the same action was conducted on a lower level of awareness: Galen recalled that, when he was actually sleeping during a prolonged night-march, he only awoke when he stumbled. In other instances, when the earlier intention was forgotten, the action continued subconsciously even though sleep might not supervene. Thus, awareness of certain activities frequently sinks to a lower level.

Galen particularly mentioned that respiratory movements could be performed either at a conscious or at a subconscious level, since they were always mediated by peripheral nerves and (striated) voluntary muscles. This mechanism seemed to be susceptible to an act of will, and it was thought only to depend on the degree of awareness. He referred to the story of a greatly angered slave who allegedly committed suicide solely by wilful arrest of respiration.[15] The modern concept of sudden cardiac arrest as an alternative diagnosis was unknown to the ancient physicians. However, this story proves that Galen failed to understand that respiratory movements can result from chemical stimulation of the nerve centres by the blood passing through the brain. The basis for this concept was lacking in the absence of chemical science, and because Galen's concept of a very slow blood flow to the periphery of the body would not even let him consider such mechanism. Nevertheless, Galen understood that respiration normally occurred under the urgent (*epeigon*) and overwhelming need of the body, which was entirely depending on certain functions, which must be performed in absence or against our will. Galen used here the term *doulos*, slave, in regard to our body to indicate the overruling demand of biological processes.[16]

Galen further mentioned that acquired habits can ultimately result in instinctive or reflex-like responses of which we are not aware. Only during the time of learning the action is performed consciously, but then becomes 'second nature' (*physis epikteton*). He wrote: 'Habit (*ethos*) becomes an attribute of the physical constitution and should preferably be defined as acquired constitution.'[17]

Many habits which had not to be taught appeared to him characteristic for each species of animals. A baby duck, hatched in separation, will take to the water, while a young eagle will start to fly even if it never saw the example of its parents. Galen also observed that young animals try to fight playfully with horns not yet grown or with claws still too soft to be used.[18] He put in the same category the feeding habits of young animals which accept suitable but refuse noxious products.

Galen regarded such reactions as natural (*kata physin*) since they arise from a specific organization of the body. A creative thought appeared to provide the co-ordination of all parts of the body and to guarantee its adaptation to the environment. The Greeks called the harmony of the interacting parts of the body and their adaptation to their surroundings *sympatheia* (sympathy). Galen referred this idea to Hippocrates: 'Hippocrates said that all parts are in unison by sympathy; each part in relation to the activity of each other'. He thus taught us that all constituents of the body, so to say, are combined in one purpose of action, and that each [part] operates in this manner, that all may live and perform a balanced activity of the body and each part its own particular function.[19]

Hippocrates and Aristotle also expressed this principle by the term *oulomenlia* (*oulos*, whole, *melos*; limb), which also indicated a musical harmony, and they applied it even to the co-ordinated courses of stars and planets, because this term expressed the permanent co-ordination of the movement of all parts. In biology this expression introduced a teleological definition. Galen stressed that the co-ordination of all parts and the responses of the organism to stimuli served mainly for the self-preservation of the individual and of the species.[20] It was Galen's conviction that the multitude of such intricate mechanisms could not have arisen by chance. He quoted the philosopher Zeno: 'Self-preservation is the principal drive of every living organism.'[21]

Since reflex and instinctive responses served this purpose admirably, they seemed to result from an original plan (*logos*),[22] which produced the predestined harmony between the *milieu interne* and the *milieu externe*, to use Claude Bernard's expressions. Galen also suggested this idea by the term sympathy.[23]

In contrast to the Galenic idea, the modern concept of survival of the fittest favours the selection of random-variations among many individuals of the same species. Galen's system suggested a static concept of all species. Only minor and temporary changes of individuals seemed possible, although the influence of external factors could lead to adaptive modifications, as Hippocrates so impressively described in the treatise *On air, waters and places*. In this famous book Hippocrates explained the distinct mental and somatic features of the various races by the influence of soil, climate, food and customs. But the recognition of occasional changes did not contradict the traditional philosophical concept of stability and permanency of biological forms. In this sense we have to understand the words of Hippocrates quoted by Galen: 'Nature does not require an education.'[24]

Every inherited somatic and mental constitution and all the learned and acquired responses of the organism seemed to be perfectly co-ordinated and in harmony with the environment. Therefore Galen wrote, especially in regard to sexual propagation: 'Did thus nature not give us both the ability to trust [our body] and use our organs without instruction.'[25]

The preceding analysis showed that the scientists of a bygone period observed the same phenomena as we do but described these in different terms according to their basic philosophical concepts of nature.

ACKNOWLEDGEMENTS

Research for this study was supported by the National Library of Medicine and The National Institute of Health, Education and Welfare. Grant No. 1 R01–LM–984–01.

Bibliography

1 GALEN, *Opera omnia*, ed. by D. C. G. Kuehn, Leipzig, 1821–33; reprint by Olms, Hildesheim, vol. 5, pp. 181–805.
2 SIEGEL, R. E., *Galen's System of Physiology and Medicine; An Analysis of his Doctrines and Observations on Bloodflow, Respiration, Humors and Internal Diseases*, Basle, Karger, 1968, pp. 113 ff.
3 WILLIS, T., *Scientia brutorum*, ch. 6.
4 SIEGEL, R. E., *Galen on Sense Perception; His Doctrines, Observations and Experiments on Vision, Hearing, Smell, Taste, Touch and Pain and Their Historical Sources*, Basle, Karger, 1970, p. 140.
5 SIEGEL, R. E., op. cit., 1968, pp. 192 ff.; 1970, pp. 46, 71 ff.
6 ARISTOTLE, *Movement of Animals*, 703 b 4–20.
7 KUEHN, op. cit., vol. 4, p. 439.
8 FEARING, F., *Reflex action*, New York, Hafner, 1964.
9 SHERRINGTON, C. S., *The Integrative Action of the Nervous System*, New Haven, Yale University Press, 1906.
10 SIEGEL, op. cit., 1968, p. 186; TEMKIN, O., 'Galen's pneumatology', *Gesnerus*, 1951, 8, 180–89.
11 SIEGEL, op. cit., 1968, pp. 183 ff.
12 VON ARNIM, J., *Stoicorum veterum fragmenta*, 4 vols, Stuttgart, 1902, vol. 2, p. 285, line 8.
13 ARISTOTLE, *Parts of animals*, 639 b 25.
14 KUEHN, op. cit., vol. 4, pp. 384–87.
15 Ibid., pp. 448–50.
16 Ibid., p. 449.
17 Ibid., p. 452.
18 GALEN, *De usu partium*, book 1, ch. 3; KUEHN, op. cit., vol. 4, p. 6.
19 KUEHN, op. cit., vol. 15, p. 359.
20 Ibid., vol. 3, pp. 17 ff.
21 DIOGENES LAERTIUS, book 7, ch. 85, referring to Zeno.
22 KUEHN, op. cit., vol. 4, pp. 643, 693.
23 Ibid., vol. 3, p. 18.
24 Ibid., vol. 8, p. 443.
25 Ibid., p. 446.

S. H. Greenblatt
Hanover, New Hampshire (U.S.A.)

Some philosophical and clinical background to Sherrington's concept of integrative action*

Sir Charles Sherrington (1857–1952) published his ten Silliman lectures on *The Integrative Action of the Nervous System* in 1906.[1] From that time forward he has been recognized as one of the most important figures in the history of modern physiology. In the two decades since his death in 1952, the importance of his work has been emphasized by the appearance of four scholarly monographs and numerous shorter essays in which he is the central subject.[2] This growing body of secondary historical sources has clarified Sherrington's debt to his nineteenth-century predecessors in experimental physiology. It has also provided some analysis of the philosophical views which he expressed so eloquently in the final few decades of his ninety-five years. At least in part, the origin of his later interest in the philosophical implications of his own work has been traced to his early grounding in the classics. But it is obvious that the young Sherrington must have been influenced by other currents in his intellectual milieu besides experimental biology and the study of the classics.

For several years I have been vaguely aware of this historiographical weak spot in our understanding of Sherrington. The contrast between two recent historical monographs has emphasized the importance of this problem, while also suggesting an approach to its solution. In his study of *Mind, Brain and Adaptation in the Nineteenth Century*, Robert Young has traced the history of 'Cerebral localization and its biological context from Gall to Ferrier'.[3] According to his Preface he has presented his work as a contribution to the historical background of modern experimental psychology. In the process of his analysis, Young has shown how the introspective associationist psychology of the eighteenth-century philosophers was transformed into the working theoretical basis of much of modern neurophysiology during the nineteenth century. Among the important figures in this transformation were Alexander Bain (1818–1903), Herbert Spencer (1820–1903), John Hughlings Jackson (1835–1911), and Sir David Ferrier (1843–1928). All of this is quite intriguing with regard to Sherrington, because *The Integrative Action* is dedicated 'To David Ferrier in token of recognition of his many services to the experimental physiology of the central nervous system'. Young mentions this fact, but his historical study is not taken beyond Ferrier.

In the most recent monographic treatment of Sherrington's work, Judith Swazey

* This essay was written during the author's tenure as Tiffany Blake Fellow on the Hitchcock Foundation.

has specifically analysed the historical foundations of *The Integrative Action.*[4] Ferrier's scientific contributions are noted, of course, along with the vast array of other data which Sherrington assimilated in creating his synthesis. But the non-scientific aspects of Sherrington's background are not systematically explored. If one reads first Young's book, and then Swazey's, one gets the feeling of passing through the same forest while observing different trees. Surely the philosophical psychology that so strongly influenced Ferrier and his contemporaries could not have been of so little import for Sherrington. It is true that in his later years Sherrington provided his own philosophical analysis of the mind-body problem. He expressed a definite preference for Cartesian dualism.[5] But it does not necessarily follow that the explicitly stated philosophical positions of his later years were actually his operating assumptions when he was younger. The intellectual climate of the 1870s and 1880s was quite different from that of the 1930s and 1940s. If we wish to understand the extra-scientific background of *The Integrative Action*, we must look to the intellectual milieu in which it was conceived.

At this juncture some biographical details may be helpful. Sherrington received his formal education and scientific training in the period from 1870 to 1887.[6] Although there is no evidence that he made any extensive study of contemporary philosophical trends, there were some rather strong currents of thought in late Victorian England which he could hardly have missed. More specifically, the analytical philosophy of John Stuart Mill, and its conjunctive associationist psychology, were well entrenched in the philosophical atmosphere at Cambridge when Sherrington was a student there.[7] Furthermore, we must not forget that he was a qualified physician, well trained in the English clinical school of the late nineteenth century. This was the very heyday of clinical neurology. Ferrier, after all, was a practising neurologist and a staff member at Queen Square. The leading neurological theorist of the day was Hughlings Jackson, whose work had been a direct inspiration to Ferrier. Jackson's place in the associationist tradition was well established.[8] It would seem extremely unlikely that such a keen mind as Sherrington's would have been unaware of all this excitement in a field directly contiguous to his own.

These historical suspicions can be at least partially substantiated by an appropriate analysis of *The Integrative Action.* The first six lectures are concerned with reflex phenomena, progressing from the simplest paradigm examples to the complexities of compound reflexes, facilitation, and inhibition. But it is in the final four lectures that Sherrington first reveals himself in print as a theorist beyond the bounds of experimental physiology. In Lecture VII he discusses 'Reflexes as Adapted Reactions'. The first paragraph introduces the difficulties of the mind–body problem and teleology. Sherrington immediately adopts a Darwinian position with regard to the 'purpose' of reflexes. Toward the end of the lecture he draws heavily on the work of William James and, to a lesser extent, Herbert Spencer, in his discussion of the 'Bodily resonance of emotions'.[9]

Lecture VIII explores 'Some Aspects of the Reactions of the Motor Cortex'. In addition to the experimental studies of Fritsch and Hitzig, and Ferrier, Sherrington acknowledges the clinical contributions of Broca, Jackson, and Bastian. The bulk of his discussion is concerned with the results of contemporary experimental work on the functions of the cortex. But in several facets of his work he finds useful analogies in clinically derived concepts, especially those of Jackson. The 'march' of a unilateral seizure is compared to the 'spreading' phenomenon of a 'spinal reaction'. In his consideration of decerebrate rigidity, Sherrington notes that: 'Hughlings Jackson with characteristic penetration of thought argued nearly thirty years ago that rigidity ensuing in hemiplegia (hemiplegic contracture) is not owing to the cerebral lesion nor to the lateral sclerosis', but rather to the release phenomenon caused by a disruption of the normal co-operative 'antagonism' between the cerebrum and the cerebellum.[10]

In quoting Sherrington's references to Jackson and others outside of the experimental tradition, I am not claiming that Sherrington took his direct inspiration from them. Rather, he found that his own experimental results were remarkably congruent with functional concepts which had been derived from other sources. Similar correlations are also found in Lecture IX, 'The Physiological Position and Dominance of the Brain'. Again, the general point of view is evolutionary. Within any given organism, the integrative complexity of each neural segment increases with increasing proximity to the 'leading segment', the brain. In this regard, Sherrington notes that, 'The "three levels" of Hughlings Jackson is an expressive figure of this grading of rank in nerve-centres.'[11] Further on, he continues in the same vein: '. . . it is in the integration of long series, or of the *whole* series, of segments one with another, that, apart from psychical phenomena, the nervous system seems to reach its acme of achievement. Here it is that we see eminently what Herbert Spencer has insisted on, namely, that integration keeps pace with differentiation.'[12]

I would be saying nothing new if I were simply to remind everyone that Charles Sherrington was much influenced by the theories of Charles Darwin. This has been remarked upon many times. The Honorary President of this Congress, Lord Cohen, has stated that Sherrington was introduced to Darwin's evolutionary concepts while still a young boy in the household of his stepfather, Dr. Caleb Rose, Jr.[13] But Darwin's writings contain more than just evolutionary theories. In fact, Sherrington does not refer to *The Origin of Species* in *The Integrative Action*. Rather, his only direct citation of Darwin's writings is to *The Expression of the Emotions in Man and Animals*.[14] It was in this latter work that Darwin presented his rather incomplete ideas about the evolutionary relationship between the nervous system and the psychical functions of the organism. The evolutionary concepts, of course, were largely Darwin's own original creations, but the psychological ideas were borrowed.

Darwin's views on psychological function were largely associationist. In the first chapter of *The Expression of the Emotions* ('General Principles of Expression'), he states quite bluntly at one point: 'The power of Association is admitted by everyone.'[15] He also makes copious references to Bain and Spencer. We have already seen that Sherrington knew Spencer's work and utilized his broad conceptualizations in *The Integrative Action*. Where Darwin had made a cautious foray into the straits between biology and psychology, Spencer sailed in full sheets to the wind. Though Spencer's results were less well founded, they were decidedly more comprehensive. In their aspect of comprehensiveness Spencer's theories were frequently useful in the more solidly based applications of other thinkers (e.g. Hughlings Jackson). There is no direct evidence that Sherrington became acquainted with Spencer's ideas through his interest in Darwin, but this kind of intellectual progression was a common phenomenon in late nineteenth-century England.

In the foregoing analysis I have tried to show that the associationist psychology was an integral part of Sherrington's intellectual milieu during the first several decades of his life. In fact, at several points in Lecture IX he specifically uses the terms 'associative memory' or 'associative recall'.[16] By the time Sherrington began his own work in the 1880s the fields of psychology and physiology were somewhat separate in Great Britain. But they shared certain basic assumptions. Among these were the sensory-motor reflex paradigm, cerebral localization, and the association of ideas. Spencer had brought the principles of evolutionary adaptation to psychology, and Jackson had applied Spencer's concepts to clinical neurology.[17] Where Darwin had left the theory of biological evolution largely at the morphological level, Sherrington demonstrated its importance for physiology. In Sherrington's hands the pervasive themes of neurophysiology came to include: reflex action, cerebral localization, and the role of the nervous system in the organism's adaptation to its environment.

Sherrington's concepts of integrative action were solidly based on the rock of exhaustive experimental study. But it is not mere coincidence that at many points they bear a striking resemblance to the clinically derived theories of Hughlings Jackson and the philosophical notions of Herbert Spencer. In the intellectual sense, Sherrington was a strong and independent man, but he was not an island. In the first few decades of his life he absorbed the fundamental assumptions of the times. The mark of his genius was his ability to give those assumptions greater clarity and stronger scientific expression.

References

1 New York, Scribner's.

2 COHEN OF BIRKENHEAD, LORD, *Sherrington. Physiologist, Philosopher and Poet*, Liverpool University Press, 1958; LIDDELL, E. G. T., *The Discovery of Reflexes*, Oxford, Clarendon Press, 1960; GRANIT, RAGNAR, *Charles Scott Sherrington. An Appraisal*, London, Nelson 1966; SWAZEY, JUDITH P., *Reflexes and Motor Integration: Sherrington's Concept of Integrative Action*, Cambridge, Mass., Harvard University Press, 1969.

3 Oxford, Clarendon Press, 1970.

4 Op. cit. Lest my criticisms of Young's and Swazey's scholarly works be misconstrued, it should be pointed out that neither intended to explore the area which is the subject of this paper.

5 COHEN, op. cit., pp. 51–64; GRANIT, op. cit., pp. 165–76. Swazey's bibliography of secondary sources, op. cit., pp. 262–68, contains references to several other studies of Sherrington's philosophical writings.

6 SWAZEY, op. cit., pp. 4–14.

7 SIDGWICK, HENRY, 'Philosophy at Cambridge', *Mind*, 1876, **1**, 235–46. I am indebted to Mr. James Hughes of the Dartmouth Medical School and St. John's College, Cambridge, for bringing this article to my attention.

8 YOUNG, op. cit., pp. 197–210 and *passim*. See also GREENBLATT, SAMUEL H., 'The major influences on the early life and work of John Hughlings Jackson', *Bull. Hist. Med.*, 1965, **39**, 346–76; and 'Hughlings Jackson's first encounter with the work of Paul Broca: the physiological and philosophical background', *Bull. Hist. Med.*, 1970, **44**, 555–70.

9 For a discussion of James' relationship to Spencer and the associationist psychology, see YOUNG, op. cit., pp. 194–95 and 251.

10 *Integrative Action*, pp. 303–4.

11 Ibid., p. 314.

12 Ibid., p. 344.

13 COHEN, op. cit., pp. 1–2.

14 London, Murray, 1872. Sherrington's citation is found in *Integrative Action*, p. 396.

15 DARWIN, op. cit., p. 31.

16 *Integrative Action*, pp. 331–32 and 352.

17 Part of the historical analysis in the preceding few sentences is based on YOUNG, op. cit., pp. viii–x and *passim*.

L. Morgenstern
Los Angeles, California (U.S.A.)

The surgical inviolability of the spleen: historical evolution of a concept

Smooth muscle is absent in the capsule and trabeculae of the spleen in lower vertebrates, appearing first in reptiles and reaching highest development in certain mammals, such as the horse, cow, pig and dog; the fragile organ in man, however, is devoid of well-developed smooth muscle and elastic fibres and is thus highly vulnerable, once its capsule is breached, to exsanguinating haemorrhage. Therein lies the core of this historical survey of surgical procedures on the spleen.

Modern textbooks of surgery invariably recommend splenectomy for splenic trauma, whether the latter is trivial or major. Moreover, no modern surgical text recommends less than total splenectomy for any disorder for which splenectomy is indicated. Today any operation on the spleen short of total splenectomy is looked upon not only with surprise, but also (and more likely) with chagrin and utter disfavour.

Yet it was not always so. Incision of the spleen (splenotomy), suture of the spleen (splenorrhaphy), fixation of the spleen (splenopexy) and partial resection of the spleen have been described in many authenticated reports from the sixteenth century onwards. At some point in the historical evolution of modern surgery, however, it became axiomatic that the spleen was surgically inviolable, and non-resective splenic operations disappeared from the surgical scene.

It is not the purpose of this paper to recount the fascinating history of surgery on this organ. This has been excellently done in many other reviews.[1, 2, 3, 4] This account will stress conservative operations on the spleen (less than total splenectomy), their fall into disrepute, and the first faint glimmer of a possible modern revival of such operations.

Ancient and even medieval references to surgical procedures on the spleen are probably apocryphal. The Babylonian Talmud (second to sixth century A.D.) makes reference to splenectomy performed on horses and men, in Biblical times, to increase their running ability and Pliny (A.D. 23–79), in his *Natural History*, relates that 'professed runners in the race that may be troubled with the splene have a devise to burne and waste it with a hot yron'. Sir Richard Blackmore, in his *Critical Dissertation Upon the Spleen*[5] written in 1725, quotes Paul of Aegina's description (seventh century A.D.) of the burning of the spleen by 'an oblong, red-hot Iron, that Two Crusts or Escars may be made by one Impression only'. He also quote Trallianus' (Greek, sixth century A.D.) account of a soldier who had the 'Region of the

Spleen burnt with red hot Barbarian Instruments of Iron' and survived. In the fifth century A.D., Caelius Aurelianus, the last of the medical writers of the Western Roman Empire, is said to have applied a red hot iron to destroy the spleen. Yet these and other accounts of early splenic surgery are impossible to authenticate and scarcely to be believed.

Nevertheless, observations on the spleen probably began very early, since most ancient cultures regarded it as a principal or cardinal organ. The Talmud (Tractate Chullin 55 a) states that a piercing wound to the animal spleen is lethal, although animals in which the spleen is removed may live normally.[6] The earliest authenticated experiments on extirpation of the spleen are to be found in the late seventeenth century in the writings of Clarke (1676) and Zambeccari (1680). Sir Christopher Wren (1632–1723), while serving as Professor of Anatomy, is also said to have demonstrated that the spleen could be removed from a dog without affecting the animal's health. Similar experiments are ascribed to Johann Konrad Brunner (1653–1727).

The earliest experiments on more conservative surgery of the spleen were recorded in the nineteenth century. Assolant (1802)[7] first demonstrated the segmental blood supply of the dog spleen by selective ligation of terminal arterial divisions. Philipeaux (1869)[8] divided the rat spleen transversely and replaced it in the abdominal cavity, with survival of the rat. Jordan (1898)[9] described partial splenectomy in three dogs, one of which died of shock and the other two of which made excellent recoveries.

The clinical literature of the seventeenth, eighteenth and nineteenth centuries abounds with cases of successful conservative procedures on the spleen. The first successful total splenectomy has been ascribed to Andriano Zaccarello of Palermo, in 1549. Thereafter partial resections of the spleen were reported chiefly as a consequence of stab wounds or gunshot wounds. Among the first of these was the case of Nicolaus Matthias,[10] surgeon of Colberg, who in 1678 treated a stab wound victim whose spleen was partially protruding, first by ligature of the protruding portion, then three days later by removal of all the remaining spleen except for a portion the size of a hazel nut. The patient recovered. In 1732, John Ferguson,[11] a London surgeon, treated Thomas Conway, 'who received a Wound with a Skane or great Knife . . . into the Left Hypochondrium'. The spleen was 'out at the Wound', whereupon Mr. Ferguson 'made a Ligature with a strong wax'd Thread' about the 'unsound Part' of the spleen and cut off 'three Ounces and a half of the Spleen'. The remaining part of the spleen was replaced and the patient recovered without incident. Larrey, surgeon extraordinaire of the Napoleonic wars, reported three wounds of the spleen which he managed without splenectomy during the Napoleonic campaigns. In 1867 B. N. Hyatt,[12] an English civil servant serving in India, successfully resected a hand-sized ($3\frac{1}{2}$ oz.) portion of spleen protruding from a knife wound in a thirty-year-old Rajpoot, after preliminary ligature. In the United States, H. C. Markham[13] in 1874 reported the case of a Winnebago Indian, all of whose multiple stab wounds had been successfully treated by the 'Indian doctor' except for one in the left upper quadrant, where three-quarters of the spleen protruded. The wound was then thirty-six hours old. Markham resected the protruding portion of spleen with a 'common bistoury'. Although the 'hemorrhage was appalling', he succeeded in controlling it with ligatures. 'Whiskey was given freely', and a year later the Indian presented himself healed and well, with his only statement being: 'Indian heap no run'. Similar reports are those of Faris[14] (U.S.A., 1874), of a stab wound and excision of a large portion of protruded spleen; Deeble[15] (U.S.A., 1889), of a gunshot wound in a young Indian, in which he 'relieved him of at least three-fourths of the spleen'; James[16] (U.S.A., 1892), of a gunshot wound of the spleen and diaphragm, in which he sutured both spleen and diaphragm with No. 8 silk; and Zikoff[17] (Russia, 1895), of the successful suture of a lacerated spleen. These, among other reports, kept alive the notion prevalent before the twentieth century that splenic trauma was not necessarily lethal and was indeed amenable to surgical repair. This was reflected in the medical texts of the times, as will be discussed later.

Other surgical procedures of the spleen were also quite frequently reported. Cysts and abscesses were apparently much more common before this century, although it is quite possible that most of the splenic abscesses previously reported were in reality subphrenic abscesses. Péan[18] in 1867 performed a splenic resection of a huge cyst of the spleen in a young woman. Although he eventually resected the entire spleen, he first excised the cyst and was the first surgeon to put forth the concept of controlled segmental resection of the spleen. ('Considering the arrangement of the arterial system of the spleen, which divides it in departments independent of each other, I proceeded with the ligature in succession of the different branches of the splenic artery in a manner which would enclose and isolate the portion of the spleen which had the cyst.') Cysts were also aspirated (Garcia,[19] 1884), abscesses drained (Lauenstein,[20] 1887; Fountain,[21] 1891) or aspirated (Trafton,[22] 1874), and the spleen injected with arsenicals and other medications (Mosler,[23] 1867).

Yet somewhere between the late nineteenth and mid-twentieth centuries, lesser procedures on the spleen seemed to fall into disrepute and total splenectomy became the procedure of choice in any surgical condition involving the spleen. The exact transition point in surgical thought and practice in this area is difficult to document precisely. Presumably there were an increasing number of complications of conservative procedures accumulating at the same time as the operation of splenectomy became increasingly safe. However, there are scarcely any detailed reports of such adverse results, perhaps because surgeons are generally loth to report complications. It is interesting to follow this gradual change in surgical practice as reflected in the surgical textbooks of the last 100 years.

Textbooks of a century ago barely mentioned the spleen. Thus Druitt[24] in 1867, in his entire text had only one sentence: 'Wounds of the spleen, if deep, are also fatal, from the great haemorrhage that follows, although the whole organ has been removed from animals, and from man, without much consequent evil.' Billroth,[25] in his *Clinical Surgery* (1881), gives only brief mention to the spleen, describing one case of rupture of the spleen found incidentally at post-mortem: 'On the upper surface the capsule was torn, and the parenchyma of the organ traversed in its whole thickness by a rent, full of loose blood-clot. From the appearance of the rent and the small quantity of blood effused, we concluded that this injury might have healed up completely.' Samuel Gross' *System of Surgery*[26] in 1882 still stressed that treatment of splenic wounds 'should be conducted upon general antiphlogistic principles, of which rest and light diet are among the most important. If copious haemorrhage exist, acetate of lead, ergot, and opium should be administered in large and sustained doses, aided by the internal and local use of ice. . . .' Gross, however, does recommend removal of a protruding portion of spleen which has become inflamed, citing examples in which this had successfully been done. In Gross's time the mortality following splenectomy for even benign conditions averaged 50 per cent.

By the turn of the century a change is discernible, inasmuch as splenectomy is mentioned much more freely for both injury and disease, but conservative procedures are still described and advocated. Von Esmarch's *Textbook on Operative Surgery*[27] (1901) relates that: 'Under some circumstances – for instance, in cysts or a partial crushing – only a portion of the spleen should be removed; the haemorrhage from the surface of the incision is arrested by tamponade, by indirect ligature or with thermo-cautery; also by elastic constriction with a rubber tube, portions of the spleen can be ligated . . .'. Although not in a textbook, W. J. Mayo's *Principles Underlying Surgery of the Spleen,*[28] presented to the American Medical Association in 1910, is appropriate to review at this point. Mayo reported on ten total splenectomies with one operative death, and three 'conservative' operations with no deaths. 'One case was a gunshot injury in which haemorrhage from the lacerated spleen was readily controlled by buttonhole catgut suturing and gauze packing. In the second case a movable spleen . . . was cured by fixation by means of suture and gauze packing. The third case consisted of evacuation and drainage of a typhoid splenic abscess.' Further: 'If partial resection is to be done, temporary compression of the pedicle seems to be harmless . . . and after the application of the clamp, the desired amount can be resected and the haemorrhage controlled by buttonhole catgut suturing with a round needle. . . .' By 1911, Theodor Kocher[29] writes that: 'Injuries of the spleen demand excision of the gland.' But he also mentions that the spleen may be incised to open an abscess and for the purpose of transplanting the thyroid. DaCosta's eighth edition of *Modern Surgery*[30] (1919) still mentions in the description of treatment of wounds and rupture of the spleen that: 'If the spleen is damaged we may do splenectomy, total or partial, may use the suture, the cautery or the tampon.' At this time, the mortality from splenectomy due to wounds or rupture was still 34 per cent.

By the fourth decade of the twentieth century, conservative operations on the spleen had all but disappeared. Max Thorek, in *Modern Surgical Techniques*[31] (1938), mentioned that 'suture of the spleen is indicated where the rent is small and the condition appears remediable'. By 1949, Orr[32] states that: 'Splenectomy is usually the operation of choice when surgery of the spleen is indicated.' Yet C. Grey Turner[33] in 1955 still states: 'In all forms of injury haemorrhage is the main cause of death and as the structure of the spleen makes suture almost impossible, splenectomy is the operation of choice except in some stab wounds, in which it may be justifiable to attempt conservative surgery.' By 1968 and 1969, the surgeon's choice is clear and unequivocal: 'It is imperative to remove the spleen when it is injured, whether haemorrhage occurs immediately or after an interval . . .' (*Operative Surgery*, Rob and Smith);[34] and: 'The only acceptable treatment of any splenic injury is splenectomy. Even a slight non-bleeding tear of the splenic capsule may lead to recurrent fatal bleeding' (Schwartz, 1969).[35]

Contemporary surgical theory and craft having reached such a conclusion, there would seem to be little reason to pursue any further the concept of more conservative approaches to surgical procedures on the spleen. Yet there has remained a lingering doubt that the spleen is truly as completely expendable an organ as now believed. And there has persisted the technical challenge of a surgical 'Everest', that of overcoming the great difficulties which splenic surgery imposes. For these reasons, experimental and clinical studies on conservative surgery of the spleen have continued to the present day.

In a little-known paper,[36] published in Rome in 1901, Dr. Gaetano Funaioli described partial splenectomy and splenic hemostasis in dogs using segmental arterial ligation and an elastic ligature about the cut end of the spleen. He was the first to suggest the application of these techniques to man. In 1923, Volkmann independently suggested the feasibility of partial splenectomy in humans, based on his anatomical studies of the splenic vasculature in man. Similar experimental and anatomical studies have followed in papers by Henschen (1928),[37] Huu (1956),[38] Finochietto (1961),[39] Campos Christo (1961),[40] Bourgeon (1966),[41] and Upadhyaha (1971),[42] among others. All of these studies not only described the anatomic basis for conservative surgery on the spleen, but suggested the feasibility of applying these principles to man. Henschen,[37] Campos Christo[40] and Bourgeon[41] have been especially eloquent in their plea for surgeons to spare the healthy, albeit injured, spleen, citing experimental as well as clinical evidence that this is possible.

There have been a few new techniques of haemostasis described, in addition to the experimental and anatomical studies cited above. Topalov[43] (1960) described a new haemostatic suture of the cut end of spleen tied over a pedicled omental graft, successfully used in dogs and suggested for humans. Cooper (1966)[44] described the use of a freezing clamp (liquid nitrogen) and metallic staples, also successfully used in dogs for subtotal splenectomy. Parenthetically it should be stated, however, that the lower animals tolerate splenic injury relatively well because of the contractility of their spleens. Injuries which most certainly would be lethal in man without treatment can be overcome in the dog, rabbit, pig and monkey without any treatment. Thus application of principles which seem valid for splenic surgery in the lower mammals must be done with great caution in man.

Conservative splenic surgery performed on human subjects in the modern era is limited to a relatively few instances. Campos Christo (1962)[45] reported on eight cases in which he had performed subtotal splenectomy for trauma, utilizing the concept of 'controlled' resection. Two were stab wounds, four, bullet wounds, and the remaining two, rupture due to blunt trauma. The extent of resection ranged from polar segments (15–20 per cent) to more than half the splenic parenchyma. Seven of the eight survived. The fatal case (bullet wound) succumbed to a subphrenic abscess and mesenteric vascular occlusion. In no instance was there a complication due to postoperative bleeding.

Bourgeon and Mouiel (1966)[41] reported five partial splenic resections performed for the purpose of transposing the spleen transthoracically in cases of cirrhosis and splenoportal thrombosis. They reported excellent and complete haemostasis using a special technique of sectioning and suturing the spleen. They have also performed open splenic biopsies without incident during operative procedures such as portacaval shunt.

Morgenstern (1966)[46] reported the use of cyanoacrylate monomer (physiologic adhesive) as an adjunct to subtotal splenectomy for massive splenomegaly due to myeloid metaplasia in a middle-aged woman. He also successfully used the monomer, combined with gold leaf and a collagen patch, for the control of bleeding due to capsular tears in six human subjects.[47]

Bodon and Verzosa[48] challenged the necessity for splenectomy in all cases of incidental splenic injury, reporting on three cases of splenic injury occurring during operation successfully managed with the application of a gelfoam patch.

In a recent paper entitled 'The conservative management of splenic trauma',[49] Douglas and Simpson outlined a scheme for observation and non-operative treatment in children suspected of having splenic trauma. They suggested that not all traumatized spleens in children warrant removal and that minor lacerations may heal. Only six of thirty-two cases of suspected splenic rupture over a seven-year period required splenectomy.

Finally, splenic puncture for the purpose of splenoportography is still performed in some centres, although recent developments in angiography and umbilical vein catheterization have lessened the need for such studies.

CONCLUSION

There are reasons to continue exploring means of salvaging all or part of the spleen in cases of trauma and even in some pathological states, as pointed out by a number of students of this subject. Certainly in infants below the age of two the effects of total splenectomy are known to be hazardous. In older children and adults the complete immunologic consequences of splenectomy are still imperfectly known, and reports of the infectious and thrombotic consequences of splenectomy continue to appear in the literature. Moreover, the surgical complications of splenectomy are not inconsequential. These sequelae of total splenectomy, both questionable and proven, have given a small group of surgeons pause in totally accepting the modern dictum of the surgical inviolability of the spleen. It remains to be seen whether today's challenge of this concept will mature into tomorrow's practice. If so, another meaningful chapter will have been added to the history of surgery on the 'organ of mystery', the spleen.

References

1 HERRLINGER, R., *Die Milz. C. Z.*, 1958, **90**, 2982–3012.

2 RICKETTS, B. M., 'Surgery of the spleen', in *Surgery of the Prostrate, Pancreas, Diaphragm, Spleen, Thyroid and Hydrocephalus, a Historical Review*, Cincinnati, 1904, pp. 92–137.

3 PEARCE, R. M., KRUMBHAAR, E. B. and FRAZIER, C. H., 'The history of extirpation of the spleen', in *The Spleen and Anemia*, Philadelphia, J. B. Lippincott, 1918, pp. 3–57.

4 PUGH, H. L., 'Splenectomy with special reference to its historical background', *Int. Ab. Surg.*, 1946, **43**, 209–24.

5 BLACKMORE, R., *A Critical Dissertation upon the Spleen*, London, J. Pemberton, 1725.

6 ROSNER, F., 'The spleen in the Talmud and other early Jewish writings', *Bull. Hist. Med.*, 1972, **46**, 82–85.

7 CAMPOS CHRISTO, M., 'Dados experimentais', in *Esplenectomias parciais sistematizadas ('reglees')*, Brazil, Belo Horizonte, 1961, pp. 69–70.

8 PHILIPEAUX, J. M., 'Section transverale complète de la rate en deux parties sur un rat albinos; guérison; état de l'organe splénique au moment de la mort six mois après l'opération', *C. r. Soc. Biol., Paris*, 1870, **22**, 40–41.

9 JORDAN, H. M., 'Conservative surgery of the spleen', *Lancet*, 1898, i, 208–17.

10 MATTHIAS, N., *De exciso liene ex homine, sine noxa. Ephem. Med. Physicar*, Dec. II, ann. III, 1684, 378.

11 FERGUSON, J., 'An account of the extirpation of part of the spleen of a man', *Phil. Trans. R. Soc. Lond.*, 1737–38, **40**, 425–27.

12 HYATT, B. N., 'Wound of the spleen; removal of portion; recovery', *Ind. med. Gaz.*, 1868, **3**, 85.

13 MARKHAM, H. C., 'Excision of a portion of the spleen – recovery', *Med. Rec.*, 1874, **9**, 482–83.

14 FARIS, A. A., 'Wound of the spleen with partial excision – recovery', *Amer. Pract.*, 1878, **42**, 299–300.
15 DEEBLE, H. M., 'On a case of the partial removal of the spleen', *J. Amer. med. Ass.*, 1897, **29**, 277–78.
16 JAMES, R. L., 'A case of gunshot wound of the spleen: suturing of the diaphragm: recovery', *N. Amer. Pract.*, 1892, **4**, 232–33.
17 ZIKOFF, V., 'Suturing of the spleen', *Vrach*, 1895, **16**, 995–1000; (Rus.).
18 PÉAN, J., *Ovariotomie et Splénotomie*, 2nd ed., Paris, Germer-Baillière, 1869, pp. 129–38.
19 GARCIA, M. V., 'Quiste del bazo', *La Cronica Medica*, 1884, **1**, 253–54.
20 LAUENSTEIN, C., 'Ueber einen Fall von operativ geheilten Milzabscess nebst Bemerkungen', *Dt. med. Woch.*, 1887, **13**, 1098–99.
21 FOUNTAIN, H. L., 'Two cases of abscess of the liver and one of abscess of the spleen – operation – recovery', *Courier Rec. Med.*, 1890–91, **8**, 194–95.
22 TRAFTON, A., 'Case of splenic disease. Tapping with pneumatic aspirator', *Trans. med. Soc. State Calif.*, 1874–75, **5**, 116–19.
23 MOSLER, F., 'Zur localen Behandlung chronischer Milztumoren', *Dt. Arch. klin. Med.*, 1874–75, **15**, 117–22.
24 DRUITT, R., *The Principles and Practice of Modern Surgery*, Philadelphia, Henry C. Lea, 1864, p. 464.
25 BILLROTH, T., *Clinical surgery*, London, The New Sydenham Society, 1881, p. 229.
26 GROSS, S., *A System of Surgery*, Philadelphia, Henry C. Lea., 1882, vol. II, p. 636.
27 VON ESMARCH, F., and KOWALZIG, E., *Surgical Technic. A Textbook on Operative Surgery*, ed. by N. Sena, New York, MacMillan, 1901, p. 739.
28 MAYO, W. J., 'Principles underlying surgery of the spleen', *J. Amer. med. Ass.*, 1910, **54**, 14–18.
29 KOCHER, T., *Text-book of Operative Surgery*, ed. by H. J. Stiles and C. B. Paul, 3rd Eng. ed., London, Adam & Charles Black, 1911, p. 565.
30 DACOSTA, J. C., *Modern surgery*, Philadelphia, W. B. Saunders, 8th ed., 1919, p. 1203.
31 THOREK, M., *Modern Surgical Techniques*, Philadelphia, J. B. Lippincott, 1938, vol. 3, p. 648.
32 ORR, T. G., *Operations of General Surgery*, Philadelphia, W. B. Saunders, 1949, p. 682.
33 TURNER, C. G., 'Operations on the spleen', in *Modern Operative Surgery*, ed. by C. G. Turner and L. C. Rogers, London, Cassell, 4th ed., 1955, p. 1003.
34 HUNT, A. H., 'Splenectomy', in *Operative surgery*, ed. by C. Rob, R. Smith and C. N. Morgan, Philadelphia, J. B. Lippincott, vol. 4, 2nd ed., 1968, p. 254.
35 SHIRES, G. T., 'Trauma', in *Principles of Surgery*, ed. by S. I. Schwartz, New York, McGraw-Hill, 1969, p. 195.
36 FUNAIOLI, G., 'Splenectomia parziale ed emostasi splenica', *Giornale Medico del Rel Esercito Roma*, 1901, **49**, 1160–66.
37 HENSCHEN, C., 'Die chirurgische Anatomie der Milzgefässe', *Scweiz med. Woch.*, 1928, **58**, 164–77.
38 HUU, N., 'Territoires artériels de la rate. II études experimentales. Possibilités de résection partielle réglée de la rate', *Presse méd.*, 1956, **64**, 1749–50.
39 FINOCHIETTO, R., 'Esplenectomias parciales', *Piensa Medica Argentina*, 1960, **47**, 2861–62.
40 CAMPOS CHRISTO, M., 'Bases anatomicas e esperimentais das esplenectomias parciales', *Rev Brasil. Cirugia*, 1963, **46**, 80–90.
41 BOURGEON, R. and MOUIEL, J., 'La chirurgie conservatrice de la rate: splénorraphie, splénectomie partielle', *Presse méd.*, 1966, **74**, 303–6.
42 UPADHYAHA, P., NAYAK, N. C. and MOITRA, S., 'Experimental study of splenic trauma in monkeys', *J. ped. Surg.*, 1971, **6**, 767–73.
43 TOPALOV, I. B., 'A new hemostatic suture in partial splenectomy', *Khirurgiia (Mosk)*, 1960, **36**, 126–27; (Rus.).
44 COOPER, I. and HIROSE, T., 'Application of cryogenic surgery to resection of parenchymal organs', *New Engl. J. Med.*, 1966, **274**, 13–18.
45 CAMPOS CHRISTO, M., 'Segmental resection of the spleen', *O Hospital*, 1962, **62**, 187–204.
46 MORGENSTERN, L., KAHN, F. and WEINSTEIN, I., 'Subtotal splenectomy in myelofibrosis', *Surgery*, 1966, **60**, 336–39.
47 MORGENSTERN, L., DICKMAN, J. and SHORE, J. M., 'Splenic hemostasis', in *A Symposium on Physiological Adhesives*, ed. by J. E. Healey, Jr., Houston, University of Texas, 1966, pp. 121–29.
48 DOUGLAS, G. and SIMPSON, J., 'The conservative management of splenic trauma', *J. ped. Surg.*, 1971, **6**, 565–70.
49 BODON, G. and VERZOSA, E., 'Incidental splenic injury', *Amer. J. Surg.*, 1967, **113**, 303–4.

A. E. Rodin
Galveston, Texas (U.S.A.)

The influence of Matthew Baillie on disease concepts

The influence of Matthew Baillie's book, *The Morbid Anatomy* was predetermined, in part, by the circumstance of his birth. Born in 1761 to the sister of William Hunter and John Hunter, he came under their influence during his formative years. Baillie received his medical education largely at their Anatomical Theatre and Museum on Windmill Street in London. He rapidly became an expert dissector and, in 1783 on William's death, assumed the yearly series of anatomy lectures. His fame as a lecturer grew, and he published his *Morbid Anatomy* in 1793. However, Baillie gave up the lectureship to enter the full-time practice of medicine in 1799. By the time of his death in 1823, he had become one of the most renowned physicians of his time in London. He remains honoured today as the last recipient of the Gold-Headed Cane, and by busts in the Royal College of Surgeons of England, the Royal College of Physicians of London and St. James's Chapel of Westminister Abbey.

Matthew Baillie's activities in anatomy extended over a period of twenty years and were quite varied. He collected 1,281 museum specimens, of which he had personally prepared over 900. Forty per cent of these preparations were of diseased states. In 1818, five years before his death, he presented the entire collection to the Royal College of Physicians of London, along with £400 for their upkeep. In 1938 the specimens were transferred to the Royal College of Surgeons of England. There they were all destroyed during the 1941 bombing raids over London which also damaged the Hunterian collection. All that remains is the handwritten catalogue listing the labels for each specimen. From this Baillie's interest and industry in morbid anatomy is evident, but it is not possible to judge his expertise.

Baillie published many articles on the morbid anatomy of various diseases. Twenty-four of these were collected by Wardrop in 1825. The most significant one is on diabetes. Baillie rejected the then current theories of etiology. It is not due to retrograde flow of chyle from lacteals into kidney lymphatics because chyle is not very sweet. Baillie also killed two dogs, one that had been on a normal diet and one fed only on bread and butter. Chyle from the former was not sweet and from the latter only slightly sweet, again contrary to the chyle hypothesis of diabetes. This was one of the first recorded animal experiments on diabetes, Minkowski's dog experiments not being performed until 1889. This analysis and experimental study by Baillie is indicative of a rejection of supposition and a reliance on logic based on direct observations, also characteristic of his book.

Baillie's *Morbid Anatomy of Some of the Most Important Parts of the Human Body* was published at the age of thirty-two in 1793, the same year as John Hunter's death. It was more widely read than his papers, as evidenced by the publication of many editions, eight English, three American, two French, one German and one Italian. Baillie's *Morbid Anatomy* had an active period of publication of almost half a century, from 1793 to 1838, the last one being fifteen years after his death in 1823. Not only the relative brevity of the *Morbid Anatomy*, but also its clearness, conciseness and freedom from long pathogenetic dissertations contributed to its popularity. These attributes were in direct contrast to Morgagni's weighty tome of 1761 and Rokitansky's of 1842.

Baillie's *Morbid Anatomy* differs from Morgagni's *De Sedibus* in not being based on specific cases, but being structured according to each system with concise descriptions of the various disease changes that can occur therein. There are twenty-four chapters, beginning with the pericardium and ending with the brain. A comparison of all editions reveals relatively few changes from the first except for the second edition in which a section on symptoms was appended at the end of each chapter. His comments on clinical-pathological correlations in the preface are surprisingly advanced for the eighteenth century. For example, some symptoms may be associated with different morbid changes, some morbid changes may have different symptoms, and morbid changes may have no corresponding symptoms. Such comments are indicative of a wide experience and careful study of patients both before and after death.

Baillie's *Morbid Anatomy* was considerably enhanced by the publication of an atlas titled *A Series of Engravings Accompanied with Explanations, which are Intended to Illustrate the Morbid Anatomy of Some of the Most Important Parts of the Human Body*. The drawings were executed by William Clift, later to become Conservator of the Royal College of Surgeons. They were printed as ten separate fascicles between 1798 and 1802 and collated as a first edition in 1803. A total of eighty-one diseases are represented in the figures. The sequence corresponds to that of the *Morbid Anatomy*. Krumbaar has labelled this atlas as the first of its kind. Taken together with his textbook, they represent an innovative presentation of disease changes, at least for his time.

In addition to providing a readable account of anatomical changes in disease, Baillie made significant contributions to the delineation of several diseases, in particular cirrhosis and emphysema. Garrison has given Baillie credit for the first accurate description of cirrhosis. Morgagni did not specifically mention this entity and Rokitansky's description adds little. Baillie's description of cirrhosis is quite detailed, including small and large tubercles, and increased firmness and decreased size of the liver. Even more significant is Baillie's association of cirrhosis to alcoholism. 'This disease is hardly met with in a very young person, but it is likewise more common in men than in women. This seems to depend upon the habit of drinking being more common in one sex than in the other; for this disease is most frequently found in hard drinkers.' Baillie's avoidance of unfounded theorizing is apparent in his statement that, although no connexion is apparent between cirrhosis and alcoholism 'very commonly we can see little connexion between cause and effect'.

In addition to cirrhosis, Baillie provided the first definitive gross delineation of emphysema. He specifically referred to the basic abnormality of dilated alveoli. 'The lungs are sometimes, although I believe, rarely formed into pretty large cells. The enlargement of the cells cannot well be supposed to arise from any other cause, than the air being not allowed the common egress from the lungs. It is not improbable also, that this accumulation may sometimes break down two or three contiguous cells into one, and thereby form a cell of a very large size.' Although Morgagni had described lungs filled with a great quantity of air, he did not appreciate the enlargement of alveoli. Rokitansky's microscopic studies of the next century added little further to the basic anatomy and pathogenesis of emphysema.

Baillie's descriptions of cirrhosis and emphysema are examples of his detailed and accurate descriptions of disease changes, uncluttered by supposition. His *Morbid Anatomy* and his *Atlas* made available a straightforward account of pathologic abnormalities and related symptoms in an attractive format suitable for practitioners. The multiple editions attest to the extent of his audience. It was the combination of experience in both anatomy and medical practice in an individual gifted with clarity of vision, thought and statement, that resulted in this first practical textbook and atlas of pathology and clinical pathologic relationships.

E. Borlone
Rome (*Italy*)

Il concetto di malattia dall'antichità ai nostri giorni

Se noi avessimo chiara l'idea di quello che è la malattia 'in sé', nei testi di patologia speciale dovremmo leggere come intestazione dei vari capitoli: 'la malattia, quando è provocata dal tale agente e si sviluppa con il tal processo patogenetico, dando luogo ai sintomi tali e tali, prende il tal nome.' Purtroppo, però, ciò oggi non è realizzabile: la nosografia è ordinata, quando è possibile, secondo la eziologia e, quando essa è sconosciuta, secondo il quadro anatomopatologico od il quadro sintomatologico. Infatti esistono delle definizioni della malattia come cosa in sé, ma un concetto unitario scientificamente definito, sperimentalmente comprovato e praticamente utilizzabile in clinica, manca nella scienza medica contemporanea, che dell'argomento, a quanto almeno mi risulta, si disinteressa, preferendo la ricerca dei fattori exiologici e di una terapia eziologicamente orientata. Eppure, malgrado i trionfi della moderna terapia, pur dopo la distruzione o la rimozione dei fattori eziologici vediamo, non di rado, purtroppo, l'organismo morire in preda ad un irreversibile decadimento di tutte le sue attività metaboliche, vittima di quel fatto tuttora misterioso nella sua intima essenza, che è la malattia.

Nell'antichità greco-romana troviamo un primo cenno esplicito del concetto di malattia nel 'De Natura hominis' nel Corpus ippocratico. Leggesi nel 4⁰ capitolo di detto libro: 'Il corpo dell'uomo ha in sé sangue, flemma, bile gialla e nera: questi elementi costituiscono la natura del corpo e per essi soffre ed è sano. E' sano precisamente quando questi elementi stanno in armonia fra di loro rispetto alla mescolanza, alla forza, alla quantità e alla perfetta fusione; è malato invece quando uno di questi elementi è in difetto o in eccesso o se è isolato nel corpo e non è mescolato con tutti gli altri.'

In seguito l'autore attribuisce anche agli umori le 4 qualità temperamentali, il caldo, il freddo, il secco e l'umido, e da questa concezione derivano i temperamenti dell'uomo ed il variare dei medesimi e delle malattie con essi connesse col variare delle stagioni ed il fondamentale precetto igienico e terapeutico consistente nel cercare di mantenere l'equilibrio dell'appositio con l'ablatio, che in termini moderni possiamo tradurre con l'equilibrio tra anabolismo e catabolismo. In sintesi possiamo dire che il concetto di salute per gli ippocratici risiede nell'armonia dei componenti elementari del corpo, e quello di malattia nella rottura di questa armonia. In altri libri del Corpus, come ci rammenta il Pazzini, compare anche il pneuma come fattore e regolatore dell'armonia organica; ma ciò non cambia sostanzialmente il concetto sopra esposto.

Galeno riprende il pensiero ippocratico, sviluppandolo razionalisticamente, con perfetto rigore logico, senza perdere, però, il contatto con la realtà clinica e con lo scopo didattico dei suoi scritti, rivolti a favorire un corretto esercizio dell'arte medica. Nel capitolo 1º del 'De morborum differentiis liber' Galeno si propone esplicitamente il quesito 'Primum dicendum est, quid morbum vocemus' e nei successivi 13 capitoli esaurisce diligentemente il proposito. La prima ovvia definizione della malattia, così come appare evidente all'uomo malato, è la lesione di una funzione (energeia), onde esso ne deduce la lesione della struttura che a quella funzione è deputata. Di quì la prima definizione galenica di salute e malattia: salute è la naturale struttura di tutte le parti, né il discorso cambia dicendo 'causa delle funzioni' invece di struttura; e se questa è la salute il contrario sarà la malattia, o una qualche struttura in condizione non naturale o una qualche causa non naturale di lesa funzione. E siccome è proporzionato (symmetros) ciò che è secondo natura e sproporzionato (ametros) ciò che non è secondo natura, potremo dire anche che salute è proporzione e malattia sproporzione. Tale discorso è valido sia per la teoria quantitativa dei pori (poros) che per quella qualitativa dei temperamenti: sicché malattia sarà la sproporzione dei pori, ma anche la intemperie (discrasia) dei 4 elementi (prota stoikeia), caldo, freddo, secco ed umido. Successivamente Galeno precisa che nelle sproporzioni delle parti e nella discrasia dei 4 elementi vi sono dei limiti entro i quali si ha una salute più o meno buona ed oltre i quali si ha la malattia vera e propria fino alla dissoluzione (dialysis ftorà).

Questi concetti ippocratico-galenici sono rimasti più o meno alla base della dottrina medica, ed ancor oggi, leggendo le definizioni di salute e di malattia nelle enciclopedie e nei dizionari, vediamo che il principio di armonia-disarmonia è tuttora valido. Nuovi indirizzi patogenetici sono stati introdotti dagli animisti, da Paracelso a Stahl e Hahnemann, e dai sistematici del XVIII e XIX secolo con la dottrina dell'irritabilità della materia vivente. La 'cellular patologie' di Virchow e la microbiologia di Pasteur hanno portato ad un grande progresso nella sistematizzazione nosologica, ma la loro influenza sulla formulazione di una dottrina unitaria della malattia è stata piuttosto negativa.

Su questo argomento è tornato con una nuova dottrina basata su una valida ed ampia sperimentazione Aleksej D. Speranskij, direttore dello Istituto di Patologia Generale e Sperimentale dell'Accademia delle Scienze mediche dell'URSS, ed allievo di Pavlov, i metodi fisiologici del quale, egli transporta nella patologia.

Questa dottrina è esposta nel suo libro, che nella traduzione inglese si intitola 'A basis for the theory of Medicine', edito a Mosca nel 1935, quando l'A. aveva 47 anni. Essa parte, come abbiamo detto, da una vasta sperimentazione e si basa su alcune deduzioni fondamentali, che in sintesi Vi espongo:

– l'azione trofica non è limitata a settori distinti del Sistema Nervoso, ma è implicita in qualsiasi attività del S.N. su organi e tessuti;

– il S.N. deve esser concepito come una *rete nervosa*, sicché una qualche struttura nervosa, che esercita una qualche azione trofica su un qualche organo o tessuto, è collegata con tutte le altre, che a loro volta sono collegate alla periferia con organi e tessuti; pertanto tutte le strutture e tutti i tessuti possono interferire in un processo trofico che si manifesti in un qualche distretto, e rappresentano come l'anello di una catena di riflessi;

– di conseguenza qualsiasi punto del S.N., comprese le strutture nervose periferiche, può diventare d'origine di processi neurodistrofici, fungendo da centro nervoso temporaneo o permanente per tali processi.

Nel campo, poi, più specificamente patologico, col lavoro sperimentale suo e dei suoi collaboratori, Speranskij ha ritenuto di aver dimostrato che:

– molti processi patologici la cui causa veniva considerata come assolutamente estranea ad influenze nervose, originano in realtà interamente da queste ultime;

– in qualsiasi processo patologico la componente nervosa è dall'inizio alla fine il fattore che regola il suo stato generale;

– le modificazioni indotte dall'irritazione di un punto qualsiasi della 'rete nervosa' consistono in trasformazioni delle condizioni nervose interne, in *combinazioni nervose nuove*, che si sviluppano e si estinguono; le combinazioni nervose fisiologiche sono caratterizzate da una maggiore stabilità; una combinazione nervosa nuova è sempre patolologica e può con maggior facilità esser rimossa;

– se l'irritazione locale produce alterazioni irreversibili in qualche punto, il processo non si esaurisce nel punto leso, in quanto questo a sua volta diventa un centro irritativo, un focolaio di nuove irritazioni patologiche: per tal modo una combinazione nervosa patologica può acquistare la stabilità di una combinazione fisiologica;

– una combinazione nervosa patologica può essere eliminata solo indirettamente, creando nuove combinazioni che portino alla sua disintegrazione;

– anche ogni intervento terapeutico che agisce sul S.N. rappresenta un trauma, il cui effetto è imprevedibile, perché dipende da come è combinato il S.N. su cui si agisce: *la predisposizione, pertanto, non è un indebolimento delle difese organiche verso un determinato agente patogeno, ma il modo come sono combinate le correlazioni interne del S.N. dell'individuo*;

– se l'irritazione supera una certa intensità limite, indipendentemente dal luogo di inizio e dalla qualità dell'agente, *essa si generalizza a tutto il S.N.*, *assumendo una forma standard di sviluppo: allora il suo decorso è inarrestabile e cessa con distrofia generale e morte.*

Sulla base di quanto sopra ho molto succintamente esposto, Speranskij ritenne di poter concludere che lo studio 'della componente nervosa' in patologia realizza le premesse necessarie per una 'dottrina della Medicina'. Infatti dà un'idea concreta dello *anello fondamentale* di ogni processo patologico e stabilisce l'inquadramento di tutte le forme patologiche in un unico sistema. *Occorre pertanto abbandonare la credenza erronea che la malattia sia l'irruzione di qualcosa di estraneo che può e deve essere espulso.* Questo punto di vista è legato al 'concetto causale', che vede i fenomeni patologici come una collusione di due fattori, l'agente patogeno e l'organismo; ma questi due fattori rapidamente si fondono in uno solo, diventando un centro di alterazione nella catena nervosa, a sua volta punto di partenza di un processo a catena: di conseguenza noi *non avremo una malattia dell'organismo, ma un nuovo organismo.*

Con questo Speranskij ritiene di aver risolto il problema del concetto di malattia: le condizioni patologiche sono caratterizzate da reazioni nervose; la presenza di queste dimostra che si ha a che fare con un processo patologico. Non si tratta né di disarmonia di fenomeni che esistono normalmente né di disorganizzazione delle correlazioni di funzionamento delle singole parti dell'organismo, ma della comparsa di processi nuovi, qualitativamente distinti. La disorganizzazione delle correlazioni, la disarmonia sono solo conseguenze. Certo la base per lo sviluppo di processi nervosi distrofici risiede nelle peculiarità strutturali e funzionali del S.N., cioé nelle sue proprietà fisiologiche; ma la loro alterazione crea una nuova attività nervosa, nuove reazioni nervose, non necessarie e dannose per la vita. Ne segue che la Medicina può finalmente esser considerata come una Scienza indipendente, perché studia fenomeni nuovi, estranei agli altri campi della biologia.

La nuova dottrina elaborata da Speranskij, come lui stesso riconosceva ancora nel 1953, ha incontrato e continuerà ad incontrare, accanto ai consensi anche resistenze ed avversioni, ma è tempo, insiste Speranskij, che anche i difensori del passato abbandonino la protezione delle pure e semplici espressioni verbali e rivelino la vera sostanza delle loro dottrine. Speranskij attacca a fondo il vecchio edificio della Medicina, ma accanto alla distruzione del vecchio presume, ed a nostro avviso con buone ragioni, di aver presentato un valido indirizzo per una nuova teoria della Medicina, basato su un concetto di malattia assolutamente originale e ricco di promesse e non solo per la teoria, ma anche per la clinica. Infatti in appendice al suo libro sono riportati numerosi interventi terapeutici sul S.N. che, rispettando la integrità anatomica di esso, hanno dato inaspettati risultati positivi nelle più svariate malattie. Ma il tempo concessomi mi impone di fermarmi a questi brevi cenni; rimango con la speranza di aver destato l'interesse dei colleghi su problemi di sempre, che meritano tutta la nostra attenzione.

Riferimenti bibliografici

ARIAM, E., 'Una recente discussione sulla teoria di Speranskij', in appendice di *Fondamenti per una teoria della Medicina*, di A. D. Speranskij, trad. italiana di F. Ormea, Torino, Einaudi, 1956.

Dizionario Enciclopedico Italiano, s.v. malattia e salute, Roma, Treccani, 1970.

Dictionnaire de la philosophie, Paris, Larousse, 1964.

Enciclopedia Italiana, s.v. malattia, Roma, Treccani.

IPPOCRATE, *Opere*, Torino, Boringhieri, 1961.

IPPOCRATE, *Della natura dell'uomo*, trad. di A. Capparoni, Roma, Istituto di Storia della Medicina, 1960.

KRUEGER, H. C., *Avicenna's Poem on Medicine*, U.S.A., Springfields, 1963.

KÜHN, C. G., *Cl. Galeni Opera Omnia*, reprint la edizione di Leipzig, 1821, G. Holms-Hidelsheim, 1959.

PAZZINI, A., *La medicina nella storia nell'arte nel costume*, Milano, Selvi, 1968–70.

PREMUDA, L., *Storia della fisiologia*, Udine, Del Bianco, 1966.

SPERANSKIJ, A. D., *A Basis for the Theory of Medicine*, International Publisher, New York, 1935.

L. L. Langley
Bethesda, Md. (U.S.A.)

Homeostasis – origin of the concept

If the word homeostasis is analysed it is found to consist of *homeo*, which means like or similar, and *stasis*, a standing. A better idea of stasis can be obtained by considering how it is used in medicine. One speaks of stasis in reference to the circulation to indicate a stoppage of circulation. Likewise, it is used to connote retarded movement of the intestinal contents. Homeostasis, then, conveys the impression that something is stopped, unchanging. If we look in the dictionary, we find homeostasis defined as 'the tendency of a system, especially the physiological system of higher animals, to maintain internal stability, owing to the co-ordinated response of its parts to any situation or stimulus tending to disturb its normal condition or function'. There are thus two essential ideas therein: (1) internal stability, and (2) the co-ordinated response responsible for the maintenance of that internal stability.

One's body temperature, blood pressure, heart rate, respiratory rate, urine output, body weight, blood composition, total body composition, to name but a few, day after day, year after year are static. A whole battery of clinical tests have been developed which measure something. In each instance, the results are meaningful because we know that certain values are always obtained in a state of health and that those values may vary in sickness. We expect these values to be static. We have come to understand many of the physiological mechanisms that maintain this internal stability. When abnormal values are detected that fact alone tells us something about the responsible physiological mechanism. Thus, the importance of the concept of homeostasis to physiology and to medicine. Without an appreciation of homeostasis and comprehension of homeostatic mechanisms, medicine is empirical, not rational. Such was the state of the art prior to the landmark papers that established this concept.

First, the means had to be developed for accurate measurement. The early physician depended upon his own senses. He could estimate body heat by virtue of his own temperature receptors, he could count the pulse, he could smell the breath, he could detect sugar in the urine by his sense of taste, he could gain much knowledge by using his eyes. But to measure specific body temperature, blood pressure, blood and urine sugar, the chemical makeup of the whole body and its components all awaited appropriate instrumentation. Just as our current knowledge of the biochemistry of inheritance could not have developed without radioisotope detectors and the amino acid analyser, our understanding of body temperature required the thermometer. It is with the thermometer and the measurement of body temperature that I have elected to begin this survey.

Early man, by means of his own senses, detected that certain living things are warm and others are not. He was also able to ascertain that the former maintained about the same warmness despite the ambient temperature whereas the latter varied with the ambient temperature. Obviously, however, progress depended upon the development of instrumentation; in this case, a means of actually measuring temperature. The first thermometer is said to have been produced in 1592 by Galileo. Early instruments contained water, then wine, and finally, in 1670, mercury. But the inquiring mind could not wait for these refinements. An Italian physician with the marvellous name of Sanctorio Sanctorius, made his own clinical thermometer, determined body temperature with it, and concluded that man's temperature remains remarkably constant except during illness when it rises. He published his findings in 1614 in *De Statica Medicina*. In 1714, Gabriel Fahrenheit, a German physicist, constructed a thermometer with mercury but took a rather arbitrary reference point for zero. That happened to be the lowest temperature observed in his hometown during a particular winter. And, it was not the air temperature but rather the temperature of a mixture of snow and sal ammoniac! The boiling point of water he set at 212 degrees. Why, I do not know. At any rate, he did measure body temperature with this instrument and found it to be constant at 96 degrees. About the same time, a Swedish astronomer by the name of Anders Celsius constructed a thermometer too. He decided to use the freezing point of water as zero and the boiling point as 100° thereby producing a very logical instrument. Why the Fahrenheit thermometer became more popular than the Celsius one in some countries would be interesting to know. And, why Antoine Reaumur, in 1731 decided to make still another thermometer with only 80 degrees between freezing and boiling, could be made part of that investigation. But whatever the scale, there was now a means of measuring temperature of the air as well as of the living body. Just where the instrument should be placed on, or in, the body has still to be resolved. At first, investigators pressed it against the skin, or in the armpit, or between the thighs. Dr. George Fordyce was the first to suggest that the bulb of the thermometer be placed under the tongue.

Charles Blagden (1748–1820) was born in Edinburgh. He obtained his M.D. in 1768 and, at age twenty-four, became a Fellow of the Royal Society. His contributions were such that he later became Sir Charles Blagden. His publications illustrate beautifully the depths of his inquiring mind. The origins of much of our knowledge of the physiology of temperature regulation are to be found therein. He states, for example, in an atmosphere of high temperature, that 'The external circulation was greatly increased; the veins had become very large, and a universal redness had diffused itself over the body.'

In another paper, he says that '. . . it appears beyond all doubt, that the living powers were very much assisted by the perspiration, that cooling evaporation is a further provision of nature for enabling animals to support great heats'. And, 'Perhaps no experiments hitherto made furnish more remarkable instances of the cooling effect of evaporation than these last facts; a power which appears to be much greater than hath commonly been suspected.'

John Hunter (1728–93), another Englishman, in this case a surgeon, was born twenty years before Charles Blagden. His main work was done at St. George's Hospital in London, both as a surgeon and as an anatomist. But he was also a physiologist much concerned with body temperature. Hunter appeared to be unaware of the work of Blagden; at least he never mentions his name. Still, this was not unusual in those days as the citing of previous work by others was not generally practised. They both belonged to the Royal Society of London, and read their papers at about the same time; thus they more than likely were acquainted. John Hunter was not content with putting the thermometer on the skin, or in the armpit, or under the tongue. He wanted to know what the body temperature was in a variety of places. So he had relatively small thermometers made and inserted them everywhere; in the male urethra, the rectum, and in experimental animals in the body cavities and a variety of organs. He carried out hundreds of experiments. His curiosity was obviously insatiable. Most importantly, he confirmed that body temperature remains constant despite broad variations of the external environmental temperature.

Blagden concentrated on high temperatures and was impressed with 'the power of the body to destroy heat'. Hunter found that the body could generate heat as well. The ability of the body to generate heat in a cold environment, and to dissipate heat when the ambient temperature rises are, of course, fundamental homeostatic mechanisms.

In 1853, Charles Robin published a book, *Treatise on Anatomical and Physiological Chemistry, Normal and Pathologic*. On page 14, he discusses the relationship of the living organism and its environment. He then refers to 'the humours (this milieu de l'intérieur). . .'. But he goes no further with the concept. A year later, in 1854, Bernard presented his first lecture as the occupant of the newly-created chair of physiology of the University of Paris. This lecture was promptly published in *Le Moniteur des Hôpitaux*. In this opening lecture, Bernard discusses broad, general principles. He defines the field of physiology and then states that 'There are two general conditions necessary for the understanding of the mechanism of life: 1. the environment (le milieu); 2. the organism.' This environment is the external one. In his second lecture he speaks of the internal environment without actually using the expression 'le milieu interieur'. He says, '. . . mais si l'on arrive a l'individu, ou existent un grand nombre de molecules, il est impossible qu'elles soient toutes en rapport avec l'exterieur; il faut donc, pour qu'elles soient en rapport avec le milieu, un artifice. . . . Cet artifice, c'est la circulation; le sang est ce milieu.' So the blood is the internal environment, or at least an important component of it and, at least in this early lecture, 'interieur' was merely implied. In later writings, 'interieur' was added and, more importantly, the concept was steadily developed to embrace physiological mechanisms responsible for the maintenance of the constancy of the internal environment which is, after all, the very definition of homeostasis. Robin did nothing to develop this idea. Yet Robin later claimed that he had been overlooked as the originator of the concept. Clearly, he should be given credit for the first use of the term; but little for its development.

Charles Philippe Robin (1821–85) was a prominent histologist of the Faculty of Medicine. He organized biology into four fields, one of which was entitled 'The science which studies the influence of the environment, or, if one prefers, of external agents, on living organisms'. He helped found the Society of Biology, as did Claude Bernard. They were thus contemporaries, both noted biologists, and Bernard may well have first heard Robin use the expression 'milieu de l'interieur'.

Claude Bernard (1813–78) studied French, Latin, history, and elementary mathematics. During this period, corresponding to our high school, he had no contact with science. He had little idea what he wanted to do. To make a living, he took a job in a pharmacy. Somehow he came to fancy himself as an author, a playwright, and even enjoyed limited success in this endeavour. Flushed with success in a small town, he went to Paris to win fame and fortune, but there the best thing he won was the sound advice to abandon any thought of making a career in the theatre. He took that advice, gave up the theatre, began the study of medicine, and came under the influence of the leading French physiologist, François Magendie. He graduated from medical school in 1843 and turned immediately to physiology. Beyond doubt, although his contributions were many, his greatest was the development, introduction, and urging of the experimental method. A life of thought and work on this subject is expressed magnificently in his *Introduction to the Study of Experimental Medicine* published in 1865.

Eduard Pfluger (1829–1910) was born in Germany, in Hanau. He studied under J. P. Muller and Du Bois-Reymond in Bonn. In 1868, he founded the *Archiv für die gesamte Physiologie*, and ten years later, the new Institute of Physiology at Bonn. His range in physiology was broad. He worked and published in the fields of metabolism, embryology, and respiration. In embryology, he carried out experiments with cross-fertilization of the eggs of different species of frogs; in respiration he established that the respiratory centre (seat of respiration) lies not in the blood or the lungs, but rather in the nervous system. All of this would seem to establish him as a solid investigator, as dedicated to the experimental method as Bernard, but the publication cited by Walter Cannon, *Die teleologische Mechanik der lebendigen Natur* published a year before Bernard's death would seem to predate Bernard by years, even centuries, for it is a bewildering mixture of philosophy, theology, and pure speculation with but a sprinkling of what could today be called physiology. The statement in this article that Cannon quotes is 'The cause of every need of a living being is also the cause of the satisfaction of that need.' This is what Pfluger calls the 'law of teleologic causality'. He then goes on to cite numerous examples. For example, in his most noted field, namely respiration, he states 'The respiratory motions are primarily regulated by need and demand.' No argument there, but there is also no discussion of mechanism, merely the conclusion that if there is a greater need for oxygen, breathing increases to satisfy that need. Teleology, so proudly championed by Pfluger in this very long and rambling article, is the despair of every teacher of physiology because it is so dearly depended upon by so many inadequately prepared students. One is hard pressed to believe that Cannon really read this article, or read it in its entirety.

Leon Fredericq (1852–1935) was a very distinguished Belgian physiologist. He was a modern experimentalist who made important contributions in many fields, but particularly in circulation and respiration. He was among the first to recognize the role of the atrial-ventricular node, he studied the relationship between respiration and blood pressure oscillations. He established much of our basic understanding of the regulation of breathing by the nervous system using sophisticated and pioneering techniques. He was also well known for his work on the mechanism of temperature regulation, on the protein content of blood, the mechanism of coagulation, and the respiratory exchange of gases. Fredericq worked with a variety of animals and was greatly interested in comparative physiology. He attained world stature and in 1952, the centennial of his birth was commemorated at the University of Liège. Fredericq clearly understood the importance of regulatory mechanisms that served to maintain the internal environment despite variations in the external environment. His work is obviously of primary importance in the development of the concept of homeostasis.

The concept of the constancy of the internal environment did not spread rapidly. Leon Fredericq in Belgium certainly understood it and contributed to its development. Sir Michael Foster, in his *A Textbook of Physiology* published in 1877, made mention of it but one really has to wait until the twentieth century to pick up the trail once again. A considerable number of physiologists, particularly in England, Germany, France, and the United States were making major contributions in various façets of physiology in the early years of the new century. The experimental method, urged so consistently by Bernard, was now the rule. Paper after paper was published which added to the sum total of our knowledge of regulatory mechanisms and could be included in this survey. Certainly those of Bayliss, Starling, Haldane, Henderson, and Cannon, to name a few, are significant to the development of this concept.

Walter Bradford Cannon (1871–1945) was born in Wisconsin but received his A.B., A.M., M.D., and Sc.D. degrees all from Harvard. Not surprisingly, he stayed at Harvard where in 1906, only six years after receiving his M.D. degree, he succeeded his mentor, the noted H. P. Bowditch. Cannon first directed his attention to movements of the gastrointestinal tract. This led him to an investigation of the autonomic nervous system. During his long career at Harvard, he published not only voluminously, but each publication was an entity rather than a fragment, and in each he furthered our knowledge of basic physiologic mechanisms. As Cannon's work on the autonomic nervous system progressed, he came to recognize it as an important factor contributing to the ability of the organism to maintain the internal environment relatively constant. Finally, in 1926, he first used the term 'homeostasis', a term he coined. In this respect, mention should be made of the fact that although, as John Fulton states, Cannon outlined for the first time his classic concept of homeostasis in 1926 in an article included in a very obscure volume, a year earlier he had published almost the identical material in the now defunct and little known *Transactions of the Congress of American Physicians and Surgeons*. A close comparison proves revealing. Finally, in 1929, in an article in *Physiological Reviews*, entitled *Organization for Physiological Homeostasis*, Cannon develops completely the concept of homeostasis. Here we see that he first mentions Pfluger, Fredericq and Richet, but he does give credit to Claude Bernard using the date 1878 which, as previously documented, is much too late. Nonetheless, Cannon's 1929 publication is a true landmark. Walter Cannon took Bernard's basic concept of 'La fixité du milieu intérieur' a giant step forward both by virtue of his own research, and by his ability of conceptual synthesis. He coined the term 'homeostasis' to designate stability of the organism; 'homeostatic conditions', to indicate details of the stability; and 'homeostatic reactions', to signify means for maintaining stability. Since then the concept has been broadened, additional knowledge of intricate homeostatic mechanisms gained, and a host of new terms introduced. 'Feedback', 'loops', 'servomechanisms', 'transfer functions', 'cybernetics', and many other expressions are used. In addition, the basic principle is applied by engineers, sociologists, economists, ecologists, and mathematicians as well as all types of biologists.

Any paper published today, at least in physiology, which is worth the paper it is printed on, should further clarify a homeostatic mechanism. Happily, the good ones do.

Bibliography

BERNARD, CLAUDE, *Le Moniteur des Hopitaux*, 1854, **2**, 409–10, 450.

BERNARD, CLAUDE, *Leçons sur les Propriétes physiologiques et les Alterations pathologiques des Liquides de l'Organisme*, vol. 1, pp. 1–27, 1859.

Ibid., pp. 41–62.

BERNARD, CLAUDE, 'Experimental considerations common to living things and inorganic bodies', *An Introduction to the Study of Experimental Medicine*, 1865, pp. 59–86.

BERNARD, CLAUDE, *Leçons sur les Phenomènes de la Vie, communs aux Animaux et aux Vegetaux*, 1878–79, pp. 66–124.

BLAGDEN, CHARLES, 'Experiments and observations in a heated room', *Phil. Trans. R. Soc. Lond.*, 1775, **65**, 111–23.

BLAGDEN, CHARLES, 'Further experiments and observations in a heated room', ibid., pp. 484–94.

CANNON, WALTER B., 'The physiological basis of thirst', *Proc. R. Soc. Lond.*, 1917–19, **90**, 283–301.

CANNON, W. B., MCIVER, M. A. and BLISS, S. W., 'Studies on the conditions of activity in endocrine glands', *Amer. J. Physiol*, 1924, **69**, 44–66.

CANNON, W. B., 'Some general features of endocrine influence on metabolism', *Trans. Cong. Amer. Phys. Surg.*, 1925, **13**, 31–53.

CANNON, W. B., 'Physiological regulation of normal states: some tentative postulates concerning biological homeostasis', *Selected Readings in the History of Physiology.*, 1926, pp. 329–32.

CANNON, W. B., 'Organization for physiological homeostasis', *Physiol. Rev.*, 1929, **9**, 399–431.

FREDERICQ, LEON, 'Influence of the environment on the composition of blood of aquatic animals', *Notes Rev. Arch. Zool. exper. gen.*, 1885, **3**, 34–38.

HUNTER, JOHN, 'Of the heat, etc., of animals and vegetables', *Phil. Trans. R. Soc. Lond.*, 1778, **68**, 7–49.

PFLUGER, E., 'The teleologic mechanisms of living nature', *Pfluger's Arch.*, 1877, **15**, 57–103.

ROBIN, CHARLES and VERDEIL, F., *Traité de Chimie anatomique et physiologique normale et pathologique*, vol. 1, pp. 11–15.

H. D. Isaacs
Hyde, Cheshire (Great Britain)

Some clinical methods used by the Arabs in the Middle Ages

Arab physicians in the Middle Ages, although needing 'aid to diagnosis', were skilled observers and founded their clinical methods along the same lines as their Greek predecessors. They highly respected Galen and Hippocrates from whose works they drew most of their theoretical knowledge and through their own experience they became adept in the interpretation of signs and symptoms – relying mainly upon their instinct and senses.

Of the main clinical methods that we still use, even in our modern age, history, inspection and palpation were the main items upon which they laid greater emphasis. The fourth clinical method, namely percussion, was to come later to us through the *Inventum Novum* of Leopold Auenbrugger (1722–1809) which was published in Latin in 1761. Auscultation of the immediate variety, i.e. placing of the examiner's ear directly in contact with the chest, was not new when Laennec (1781–1826) made his epoch-making discovery.

If one reads through the works of Isaac Israeli, Rhazes and Avicenna one finds that great emphasis is placed upon their critical observations at the patient's bedside and upon their physical findings. They studied their patients very closely and recorded all their findings accurately; no detail, however trivial, would escape them. Even before the period of translations, i.e. the latter part of the ninth century and the first part of the tenth when Ḥunayn and his co-workers rendered most of the Greek works into Syriac and Arabic, a few Arab physicians at the dawn of Islam had shown a keen interest in their profession. Their methods, however primitive and crude, were quite sufficient to aid them in their diagnosis. To illustrate, we may give the case of the death of the Caliph ʿUmar b. al-Khaṭṭab. After the Caliph had been stabbed by Abu-Lu'lu'ah who had struck him with a sharp instrument in the abdomen a physician was called in. I quote from al-Muqaddisī the following: 'The physician made him [the Caliph] drink some date-water, which oozed through the wound unchanged. And because of its reddish colour it was impossible to decide whether the liquid which came out of the wound was date-water or blood. And so another physician was called in, who gave ʿUmar milk to drink. The milk oozed through the wound and could be seen to be milk. Upon seeing this the physician said: I perceive that the wound is mortal; make now O! Commander of the faithful your last will and testament.'

Among the famous clinicians of the period following the age of translation were three well-known physicians who not only relied on what had been transmitted to them from the Greeks through the translators Ḥunayn and Ḥubaysh but also added their own observations. These were Isḥāq b. Sulaymān al-Isrā'īlī (855–950) the author of a celebrated *Book of Fevers*, Rhazes (865–925) and Avicenna (980–1037), all of whom were instrumental in immortalizing the period known as the 'Golden Age'.

In his *Book of Fevers* which was later translated into Latin by Constantinus Africanus of Monte Casino (1010–87) Israeli draws on Ḥunayn's translation of Galen's treatise *Liber Febribus*. Despite a quantity of false reasoning which follows from his dependence on his ancient predecessors' concepts of physiology and pathology Israeli does communicate to us a great deal of clinical truth as he assembles all that could be said at that time about the various stages of pulmonary tuberculosis. Its signs and symptoms are accurately described and the important relationship between loss of weight and the persistent low-grade pyrexia is clearly recognized by him as diagnostically significant. He actually starts his chapter on the hectic fever generated by tuberculosis with an introductory note on the subject of 'wasting' which he calls 'al-Dhubūl'. This is a commendable observation for we still consider that loss of weight is one of the early clinical signs of tuberculosis. Israeli defines wasting as the dispersal of the essential bodily moistures and the degeneration of the organs from a state of growth and development to a state of wasting and atrophy.

Israeli goes on to describe T.B. facies. Like Galen and Hippocrates before him, he was familiar with the type of person who has a predisposition to the disease, namely, persons with a smooth and ruddy complexion, thin elongated thorax and winged scapulae. He regarded the years eighteen to thirty-five as the dangerous years and noticed that diarrhoea supervening in the course of the disease was an ominous sign.

Pyrometry was primitive then and the only 'thermometer' a physician had was his own hand. A sense of touch will indicate the presence of a temperature above the normal. Yet Israeli says 'If you palpate the patient suffering from hectic fever you will find the body dry and rather cold because there is not enough heat to reach the skin. If you keep your hand long enough on the surface of the body you will notice the heat creep slowly beneath it.' This account fits well with Galen's clinical observations.

Another sign which is the result of extreme wasting and which does not augur well is described by Israeli. 'If you uncover the abdomen it will appear as though it is devoid of viscera. If you then touch it you will find the skin flat and as hard as a board and similar in texture to parchment. When the skin of the abdominal wall is pinched and pulled upwards it stretches outwards and remains in an upright position for lack of the moisture which would normally keep it malleable and allow it to return to its normal position.'

Israeli, like his predecessors Galen and Hippocrates describes the urine of the emaciated tuberculous patients as copious, thin and oily; 'it appears to be plated with casts (*Ṣafā'iḥ*)'. It is not uncommon to find amyloid or lardaceous changes in the kidneys of patients with chronic tuberculosis. Hippocrates noticed that fatty substances settling on the surface of the urine were alarming as being signs of severe wasting (Jones II, 27). Rhazes, on the other hand who was a very careful clinician with a critical mind, says: 'I have never seen any such thing in the urine of phthisic patients. To my mind this is wrong; it can never happen.' (Iskandar, *Majallat-al-Mashriq*, April 1962, p. 233).

On the subject of 'Causus' Fever Israeli describes this fever as being ardent and continued with serious consequences. 'At first', he says, 'the pulse is broad and slow, occasionally the fever declines and then rises vehemently until it reaches its fastigium (*Sawra*). One of its worst complications is diarrhoea with sanguinous stools.' This records well with Sydenham's description of continued fever or what he also calls 'dysenteric fever'. It may well be that both were referring to enteric fever or typhoid fever described by Thomas Willis.

Certainly Rhazes was the observer, the recorder and bedside physician par excellence. For differential diagnosis was a subject to which he attached the importance it merits. His treatise on this subject *Kitāb Al-Furūq* is still in manuscript form. The Wellcome Institute of the History of Medicine is fortunate enough to possess a copy of it but it has never been yet studied.

In diagnosis the Arabs stress examination of the pulse, then a close inspection of urine. Rhazes was no exception to the general run of physicians since he also took careful note of the pulse and urine. But he did differ from his predecessors and colleagues in that not only did he take detailed case histories, but he also realized the futility of relying on 'modified factors' of the pulse alone as a means of diagnosis. In the last chapter of his book '*al-Furūq*' (Differential Diagnosis) he discusses the pulse, its character, frequency, rhythm and size. He, like Israeli, does not elaborate on the fantastic kinds of pulse which Avicenna enumerated (Browne, p. 79). He restricts them to six and points out that there are two types of irregularities: the regularly irregular and the irregularly irregular. In fevers, he states, pulse goes hand in hand with respiration which may be deep, rapid, short, slow, infrequent or hurried.

In another part of his same book 'Al-Furūq' he discusses the differential diagnosis between chronic inflammatory swellings and cancer. 'Cancer', he says, 'disseminates around its site and grows in time, whereas other swellings remain stationary in size and growth.' He is also familiar with palpation of the spleen and differentiates between the hard and soft spleen, ascribing the former to black bile and the latter to a preponderance of yellow bile.

The next greatest name in the field of systematization is that of Ibn-Sīna or Avicenna as he was called in Latin. His prodigious memory, his command of language and logic, his profound knowledge of the subject matter and his unflagging energy enabled this great muslim to classify and arrange all the medical knowledge of his time. This knowledge, which he augmented with his own observations is assembled in a work known as al-Qanūn fi-Ṭibb or better known to Europeans as 'The Canon of Medicine'. Avicenna may well have been indebted to his great predecessor Rhazes for some proportion of his clinical knowledge, and if a provisional judgment may be made on the capabilities of the two men, we might say that the originality of Avicenna probably lay in the theory of medicine, while that of Rhazes lay rather in its practice. Avicenna was also a keen and a perceptive diagnostician, though how much of his knowledge in this field he owed to observations of Rhazes who had been born 115 years previously in A.D. 865 is still not entirely clear. So far as we know he was the first to write a careful description of meningitis: 'Most of these patients die from Asphyxia. I say this is probably (that the cause of death here) is due to the involvement of some important organ (other than the brain) such as respiratory muscles.' In other words he is speaking of respiratory failure probably in a case of polio when the muscles of the diaphragm are paralysed. He also observes

(I, p. 73) that one of the signs of pneumonia is malar flush and that clubbing of the fingers occurs in tuberculous patients and ulceration of the lung (I, p. 113).

So much for these famous physicians. It should be noted, however, that interesting clinical observations, made by others, may be gleaned from other sources. For instance, one finds in the book *The Creation of the Foetus* by ʿArīb b. Saʿīd Al-Qurṭubi the following: 'If a woman suffers from pain in her hip or head or in any other parts of her body and then becomes pregnant, these pains will disappear.' We also find the following clinical observations: 'If the breasts of a pregnant woman suddenly get smaller she is certain to miscarry.' The author also notes the signs of toxaemia of pregnancy and its consequences: 'If a woman becomes pregnant and her eyes are sunk, her face and feet swollen, her ears pale and her lips greenish then she will either go into confinement which ends in a still birth or she might give birth to a sick baby that dies soon after parturition or to a live infant that does not last long.'

Many historians believe that, with the fall of the Arab Muslim Empire in the East and later the eclipse of Muslim Spain in the West, Arabic medicine receded into obscurity. This is not quite so, as Elgood has shown that the traditions of Arabic medicine were carried on by other Muslim legatees, mainly Persians and Turks. Bahā'-ul-Dawla, a Persian savant, whose date of birth is not known, lived in the latter part of the fifteenth century and died, according to Haji Khalifa, in Rayy in A.D. 1507. This man Bahā'-ul-Dawla who wrote: *The Quintessence of Experience* must have been a keen clinical observer. According to Elgood he was the first to record the spontaneous cure of cutaneous Leishmaniasis after twelve months of ulceration. He also describes three varieties of rash: measles (*Ḥuṣba*), smallpox (*jadrī*) and chickenpox (*Ḥumayqa*). I quote here Elgood's translation 'Know that the chickenpox is a condition midway between measles and smallpox. The signs and symptoms of this disease are like the signs and symptoms of these diseases but in all respects it is less dangerous.' Here again we have a translation from his work concerning what he calls a disease of the eye which is known to us nowadays as an ophthalmic manifestation of the allergic disease – hay-fever: 'I have seen many patients whose brain has become heated in the spring by the smell of red roses. They get a catarrh and a running nose. They have also had irritation of the eyelids, which, when this season passed, subsided together with the catarrh and nasal discharge. These people benefited very little by treatment.' No doubt this is a description of hay-fever and one may ask whether Bahā'-ul-Dawla had access to a previous work attributed to Rhazes, *A Book on Catarrh* which is mentioned by Ibn-abī-ʾUṣaybiʿa on Rhazes and which is also mentioned by Al-Birūnī in his treatise on the works of Rhazes. (See Paul Kraus's *Epître de Birūnī.*) Bahā'-ul-Dawla's description of syphilis is the earliest known account of this disease to be written outside Europe. He referred to it as the 'Armenian Sore', a condition which he believes arose in Europe and from there spread to Constantinople and Arabia. The symptoms, he says, are similar to smallpox. Hence it is also known as '*Abileh-i-faranq*' – 'Frankish pox'. The latter should be differentiated from *atishak* 'little fire'.

I now come to another interesting manuscript written about the middle of the seventeenth century or probably later, copies of which are scattered in different libraries. Its title is 'Thoroughness in the management of the human body', and it was written by Saliḥ b. Naṣr Allah al-Ḥalabī, known as ʾIbn Sallūm who was the head of the medical fraternity in Constantinople and court-physician to the Sultan

Muḥammad b. Ibrahīm Khan. The author must have been well trained in the tradition of Graeco-Arabic medicine as well as having had access to the works of his earlier and contemporary European physicians. For his son Yaḥya who collected his father's work writes of him: 'He [his father] collected it from these famous physicians – Greek and Latin.' Saliḥ Effendi, the author himself, was a keen observer and a good compiler. He leaves an impression of modesty, claims very little honour and tries to cover himself by quoting his predecessors and, as usual, gives frequent praise to God. He writes a special chapter on what he calls 'The New Chemical Medicine' attributed to Paracelsus of whom he thought highly and some of his methods of treatment he recommends. He devotes a chapter to Dyspnoea and Bronchospasm, the Arabic title of which is *Faṣl fi Ḍīq Majārī al-Ri'ah* and quotes a European doctor whose name he gives – doubtless in corrupt form as 'Aranbus' or probably he meant Heurnius (1543–1601): 'I saw a chemist who suffered from this disease. He lost weight and became dyspnoeic. He then died. Postmortum examination revealed that his lung was desiccated and dry like a dried apple.' He cites this physician on what is clearly a case of fibrosis of the lung. He also mentions Daniel Sennert (1572–1637), Luiz de Mercado (1520–1606), Jean Fernel (1497–1558), Matthew Platerius (*c.* 1130–50) and John of Gaddesden (*c.* 1280–1361). In a special chapter dedicated to what he calls 'The sweating fever or the English sweat' he mentions: 'This fever appeared first in the English Island in A.H. 897. It affected many people and after 40 years it spread to the whole continent of Europe and the Islamic countries at a later date. Now we see many cases in Constantinople. The Franks believed it a new disease which was not mentioned before by the previous doctors yet Sennert claims that Galen refers to this fever as Synochos. It differs from Hecticus in that it attacks the humours whereas Hecticus attacks the organs of the body.'

He also speaks of the disease scurvy, which is described 'as not having been mentioned by the muslim doctors but by the Franks'. He refutes this statement by referring to Daniel Sennert who claimed that Avicenna mentioned a clinical syndrome which fits in with this disease. Another disease, namely chlorosis, is described by Ṣaliḥ Effendi. The same author also described a certain syndrome on which he quotes Avicenna in support of his own observations on the subject: 'On the subject of amenorrhoea, we may note that any woman, whose menstrual flow is incarcerated within her, may in consequence of the residue develop like a man. Bodily hair will grow in profusion and she will develop a beard. Her voice will grow gruff and hoarse and she may even die.' One may ask whether he was in fact describing a 'Cushing Syndrome'.

He also describes certain autopsies carried out by European doctors. One case was that of a patient who died from ascites, but was found on post-mortem examination to have multiple cysts in her abdominal cavity. The other case was that of a man who could not be diagnosed when alive, yet on autopsy he was found to have multiple cysts in his kidneys.

We also find yet another reference to Sennert, this time on the subject of anorexia. His observations concern the story of a young woman, aged eighteen, whose appetite for food was lost. This went on for three years without food or drink. Her menstruation stopped, her urine and stools increasingly diminished, her hair and finger-nails grew longer and then she lost her voice and she continued to lose weight until in the end she died.

When one reads the manuscript one soon notes that this doctor has not only drawn on European sources but also adopted European terminology; for example, cremotartar, mercuriale, aqua Teriacalis, Diarosen, Cardo Santo or Carduus Benedictus, Dia Prunus, Aromaticum Rosatum and Guiaco.

I have chosen these two muslim physicians, Bahā' ul-Dawla and Saliḥ Effendi b. Naṣrallah, for although the gap between the two was a century, the former represents a different era from that of the latter. Bahā' ul-Dawla was the last of what Elgood describes as 'Persian Isolation'. The latter was at the beginning of a new epoch. During these hundred years there was a new approach to the West by the Muslim East. Papal envoys, Venetian merchants and ambassadors from various European countries started to appear on the scene of the Middle East. East India company was active, travellers, missionaries and probably doctors brought with them their culture. The impact of western civilization on the Ottoman Empire was tremendous. After a succession of victories the Ottoman Muslim stopped at the gates of Vienna. This was followed by decisive and unmistakable defeats in battles and loss of territory which ended in the treaty of Carlowitz (1699). This was a very painful experience. Then the younger generation of the Ottomans started to look westward for science including medicine, technology and military knowhow.

Bibliography

ISRAELI, ISAAC, *De Febribus* (*Kitab al-Hummayat*), MS. Bodleian, Hatton 35.
HUNAYN b., ISHAQ, *Liber Febribus* (*Kitāb fi Aṣnāf al-Hummayāt*), MS. Escorial 797.
JONES, W. H. S., *Hippocrates*, Loeb series, 4 vols. Cambridge, Mass., 1949.
SYDENHAM, THOMAS, *The Whole Works of . . .*, 8th ed., London, 1722.
BROWNE, E., *Chahar Maqala*, Gibbs memorial series, Oxford University Press, 1921.
ELGOOD, C., 'Baha'-ul-Douleh and the Quintessence of Experience', *Science, Medicine and History*, vol. 1, Oxford University Press, 1953.
'ARIB b. SA'ID al-QURTUBI, *Kitāb Khalq al-Janin*, Algiers, Librairie Ferraris, 1956.
RHAZES, *Kitāb al-Furūq*, Wellcome Institute of the History of Medicine, MS. WMS. Or. 145.
AVICENNA, *Kitab al-Qanūn fi al-Tibb*, Bulāq Press, Cairo, 3 vols.
SHAH, M. H., *The General Principles of Avicenna*, Karachi, 1966.
LLAMAS, J., *Ishaq Israeli, Tratado de leas Fiebres*, Madrid–Barcelona, 1945.
KÜHN, W. (ed), *Claudii Galeni opera omnia*, Leipzig, 1821–33.
MORATA, N., 'Un catalogo de fondos arabes prinitivos de el Escorial', *al-Andalus*, 1934, II
MAJOR, R., *Classic Descriptions of Disease*, Springfield, Illinois, 1963.
IBN ABI-Usaybi'a, *Kitab Tabaqāt al-Attiba'*, 2 vols., Cairo, Bulaq Press.
IBN SALLUM, Ṣalih b. Nasrallah al-Halabi, *Thoroughness in the Management of the Human Body*, Wellcome Institute of the History of Medicine, WMS. Or. 131.

F. Guido
Rome (Italy)

Luci ed ombre nel sistema dottrinario di Thomas Sydenham

La necessità di dare un metodo alla scienza, e alla medicina in particolare, fu sentita, nel mondo culturale inglese del '600, da Francesco Bacone (1561–1626) e da colui che è stato considerato il suo erede spirituale, John Locke (1632–1704). Ambedue questi filosofi condividono almeno l'avversità contro l'astrattismo delle scuole, contro le dispute pompose quanto sterili, contro il dogmatismo, l'erudizione libresca, le affermazioni arbitrarie, le ipotesi fantasiose che minano l'obbiettività della ricerca scientifica.

La stessa avversione fu sentita da un amico del Locke, anch'egli medico, cioè da Thomas Sydenham (1624–1689), il quale credette di superare questa difficoltà richiamandosi, in una fase di vivo e ribelle fermento rinnovatore, alla fonte ippocratica. L'opera e il pensiero di Thomas Sydenham costituirono quindi una reazione costruttiva all'esasperato sperimentalismo del secolo, che era a sua volta espressione di una ribellione alla mentalità dogmatica che aveva imperato per tutto il Medioevo sulla scia della cultura classica. Il pensiero di Thomas Sydenham è quindi un ammonimento a non dimenticare quanto di positivo e di duraturo e di perennemente valido era contenuto nei principi ippocratici, e quindi un richiamo al passato. Diciamo un richiamo, non un ritorno al passato, giacchè il Sydenham era cosciente del fatto che il progresso è generato da idee nuove e rivoluzionarie, ma era convinto che queste idee, appunto perchè nuove e rivoluzionarie, dovevano essere incanalate secondo un orientamento realistico e costruttivo, e quindi non dovevano perdere di vista il fine supremo del medico, e cioè l'osservazione, lo studio la cura del malato.

Lo studio della malattia, secondo il Sydenham, doveva quindi essere condotto sull'osservazione minuziosa e continua dei fenomeni morbosi e del loro andamento evolutivo.

Il rifiuto, che egli fa, dell'indagine delle cause nascoste delle malattie – indagine che era uno dei cardini della medicina razionale – non è dettato dalla coscienza della loro inutilità ai fini della cura, ma della impossibilità della mente umana di penetrare nei misteri della natura. E' impossibile, per lui, una scienza della natura intesa nel senso moderno, e questo suo scetticismo appare anche nel frammento sull'Anatomia, in cui, pur riconoscendo l'utilità dell'anatomia macroscopica, il Sydenham per voce del Locke ritiene inutile indagare sulla struttura microscopica degli organismi. In ogni caso, l'anatomia, pur utile al chirurgo, non può illuminare sulle cause dei fenomeni morbosi. La conoscenza dei fenomeni biologici è impedita dalla loro stessa complessità e la sola via per appressarsi alla loro conoscenza è l'osservazione minuziosa dei fenomeni morbosi.

Diciamo: osservazione minuziosa. Tanto minuziosa da costituire, di per se, una nuova via di ricerca, un nuovo sistema. E' questo il lato positivo del dottrinale del Sydenham, che altrimenti si potrebbe identificare col puro empirismo.

La metodologia del Sydenham è basata su tre cardini. Il primo è rappresentato dalla necessità di una 'storia' o descrizione della malattia, per quanto possibile esatta e completa; il secondo dal ripudio di ogni ipotesi filosofica; il terzo dalla necessità di separare i fenomeni costanti e particolari da quelli accidentali ed estranei. L'espressione 'notitia clara ac distinta', da lui impiegata, indica il suo personale modo di intendere l'insegnamento ippocratico. Come giustamente osserva Lain Entralgo, il Corpo ippocratico è la culla della medicina scientifica europea. Da essa possono derivare però creature storiche ben diverse. Galeno, Van Helmont e Sydenham, tutti e tre ippocratici, danno però una differente impronta alle loro particolari dottrine. Più che parlare di medicina neo-ippocratica, bisognerebbe parlare di medicina sydenhamiana.

Galenismo, iatromeccanica e iatrochimica costituiscono gran parte del mondo intellettuale in cui si è formato il Sydenham. E' superfluo sottolineare la profonda insoddisfazione del Sydenham per le teorie iatromeccaniche e iatrochimiche, così lontane dalla sua dottrina. Più interessante è notare le differenze tra il suo pensiero e quello galenico, che certamente gli è più congeniale. Alla classificazione galenica delle cause dei morbi – cause nascoste, cause antecedenti, cause contingenti – il Sydenham oppone la sua classificazione, per cui le cause morbose sono divise in tre categorie: particelle miasmatiche occasionalmente pervenute nel sangue e non convenienti agli umori; perturbazioni atmosferiche; fermentazione e putrefazione degli umori.

Anche l'essenza del processo morboso è differente. Per Galeno, si tratta di una diatesi contro natura; per Sydenham, è uno sforzo della natura, è un movimento reattivo alla 'causa morbi', indirizzata alla cura dell'infermo.

Per conseguenza, i sintomi della malattia sono, per Galeno, 'accidentia morbi'; per Sydenham sono tentativi concatenati della natura per espellare la materia peccante, e sono quindi 'utili' per la eliminazione della 'causa morbi'. Il che non esclude la esistenza di sintomi nocivi a proposito del reumatismo.

Il medico deve – secondo il Sydenham – ordinare i casi della sua esperienza clinica come i botanici ordinano le piante. Primo scopo del medico deve essere quello di condurre i processi morbosi individuati a 'specie', le 'species morbose'. In ciò, egli deve non tenere alcun conto delle 'ipotesi fisiologiche', intendono con questo termine le varie disquisizioni iatromeccaniche e iatrochimiche del suo tempo. Ma deve separare i sintomi costanti e particolari da quelli accidentali e avventizi. In fine, è necessario osservare la possibile relazione dell'infermità con la stagione. Con il termine di 'costituzione dell'anno' il Sydenham indica l'influenza dei vari periodi dell'anno sull'incidenza, sull'andamento evolutivo e sulla gravità delle forme morbose. Il Sydenham parla anche di una 'costituzione epidemica', denominazione assai usata nei tempi antichi, ma che, per il Sydenham, vuole indicare l'influenza che una epidemia esercita sulle malattie comuni di un paese, la frequenza insolita di malattie simili fra loro ma non contagiose nè sistematiche, o il grado analogo di malignità che esse presentano, o il predominio di alcuni sintomi. Così egli parla di una costituzione epidemica nervosa, infiammatoria, anemica-gastrica, putrida, catarrale, reumatica ecc.

Questa metodologia sydenhamiana apre la strada a un 'sicuro metodo' di terapia, a una terapia specifica, che egli però confessa di non conoscere ancora – all'infuori dell'uso della china e dell'oppio – ma di cui si augura il ritrovamento. Egli preconizza cioè, per ogni forma morbosa, l'uso di un medicamento specifico, che agisca in modo diverso da quello comunemente accettato di derivazione di umori peccanti. Con questi concetti, erroneamente si rifiuta di considerare specifico il mercurio, a causa della salivazione che il suo uso produce.

Per quel che riguarda il salasso, in alcune circostanze il Sydenham ritiene di averne ottenuti ottimi risultati, quando si trattava di controllare o diminuire l'ebollizione del sangue, quando il sangue era cioè troppo attivo nella sua lotta contro le cause patogene. Così, riteneva utile il salasso nella peste, specialmente se praticato presto e in abbondanza. E se un malato pur salassato, veniva a morte, egli cercava di spiegare il caso dicendo che sarebbe stata necessaria una ulteriore sottrazione di sangue, perchè quella già praticata non era stata sufficiente ad espellare tutta la materia peccante; meglio sarebbe stato, in questo caso non salassare affatto, perchè allora vi sarebbe stata la possibilità della formazione di un'accesso salutare, possibilità che un salasso insufficiente aveva compromesso.

Questo tipo di ragionamento è assai simile a quello che fa il Molière, pure a proposito del salasso, in una scena de *l'Amour médecin* (commedia rappresentata per la prima volta nel Settembre del 1665). Esso è indicativo di un insufficiente spirito critico, che è stato bene messo in luce da Lester S. King, e dimostra che il Sydenham non era privo di quei difetti che egli rimproverava ai razionalisti.

Luci ed ombre, quindi sono evidenti nel dottrinale sydenhamiano; del quale però dobbiamo riconoscere l'originale impostazione e l'influsso notevole che eserciterà nel progresso scientifico. Le 'species plantarum' di John Ray sono, ad esempio, parallele alle 'species morborum' di Thomas Sydenham. I due inglesi coetanei danno inizio, nei campi di specifica loro competenza, a quello che sarà l'orientamento della scienza moderna. Indubbio l'influsso, su questo indirizzo scientifico, del pensiero baconiano e della interpretazione della natura che Bacone aveva proposto. Indubbio l'influsso che questo indirizzo scientifico ha, a sua volta, sul pensiero di Locke, il quale nega la realtà delle specie che sarebbero solo 'i modelli umani' delle cose. Osserva quindi Lain Entralgo: le 'species' botaniche di John Ray e le 'species morbosae' di Sydenham si collocano, cronologicamente e concettualmente, tra le 'forme' di Bacone e le 'essenze nominali' di Locke. Esse sono le espressioni – rispettivamente fitologica e nosologica – della scienza naturale del XVII secolo e di cui troviamo un'eco anche in autori italiani, come il Baglivi nel 1696. Frutti di questa attitudine intellettuale saranno le numerose nosografie del secolo XVIII. La storia clinica alla maniera di Sydenham si continuerà con la patografia anatomo-clinica di G. B. Morgagni.

Bibliografia

BAGLIVI, G. *De praxi medica*, lib. II, cap. III (*Opera omnia medico – practica et anatomica*), Venet 1738, p. 106.

CARLINI, A., *La filosofia di Giovanni Locke*, Firenze Vallecchi, 1928, pp. 26–28.

DEWHURST, K., *Dr. Thomas Sydenham (1624–1689) – His life and original Writings*, London, The Wellcome Historical Medical Library, 1966.

KING, L., 5, 'Empiricism and Rationalism in the Works of Thomas Sydenham', *Bull. Hist. Med.*, **44**, no. 1, January-February, 1970.

LAIN ENTRALGO, P., *La Historia Clìnica*, Madrid, 1950.

PAYNE, J. F., *Thomas Sydenham*, Londra, T. Fischer Unwin, 1900.
PAZZINI, A., *Storia della Medicina*, Milano, S.B.L., 1946.
PREMUDA, L., 'Ritorno alla Scuola di Coo. Tommaso Sydenham L'Ippocrate inglese, rinnovatore della Clinica moderna (1624–1689)', in *Rassegna Giuliana di Medicina*, **1**, p. xxxvii.
SYDENHAM, T., *Opera Medica*, Genevae, Fr. De Tournes, 1749.
TEMKIN, O., 'Die Krankheitauffassung von Hippokrates und Sydenham in ihren Epidemien' *Arch. J. Gesch. Med.*, 1928, **4**, 327–52.
VITALI, E. D., 'Thomas Sydenham, il suo tempo, il suo metodo, le sue opere con particolare riguardo al "De podagra" ', in *Collana di Pagine di Storia della Medicina, Miscellanea*, no. 5, Roma, 1961, pp. 75–99.
VITALI, E. D., 'Thomas Sydenham il suo tempo, il suo metodo', *Atti, e Memorie dell'Accademia di Storia dell'Arte Sanitaria*, S. II, A. XXVIII, no. 4, Ottobre-Dicembre 1962, pp. 176–84.

C. Hodel
Basle, Switzerland

An early definition of myocardial infarction by E. Ziegler

Myocardial infarction is a common and well defined disease today. It belongs to the most important diseases of the century with an annual toll of hundreds of thousands of victims. Single cases of typical myocardial infarction have been described and illustrated (under various names) from the times of the ancient Egyptians until the middle of the last century. However, a clear etiology was never mentioned. The most famous descriptions are those of Harvey (1649), Heberden and Cruveilhier. Towards the end of the nineteenth century various pathologists in different countries realized the causal connexion between disturbed blood flow in the coronary arteries and necrosis of the heart wall. They defined it as a distinct entity and a common cause of death. Clinicians accepted the theory only at the beginning of this century (Obrastzow). Leibowitz treated recently, in brilliant fashion, the evolution of the notion and concept of this important disease. From an anatomico-pathological viewpoint it is fascinating to observe how different scientists discovered within a few years the causal relationship between a soft necrotic heart wall, sometimes ruptured, fatty degeneration and concomitant degeneration of the coronaries (e.g. arteriosclerosis, thrombosis and inflammation). Besides the intellectual effort of logical combination of cause and effect, it was of extreme importance to prove the observation in many cases. Therefore the merit of confirming this view and making it widely accepted was as important as the first description. Ziegler played an important part to further this end.

During his ambulant career which led him from Bern to Freiburg, Würzburg, Zürich and Tübingen back to Freiburg, Ziegler must have seen quite often the signs of myocardial infarction. In his first years at Freiburg he published a paper on causes of renal sclerosis in which he also described a necrosis and fibrosis of the heart wall combined with occlusion of the left coronary artery (1879). He called this condition myomalacia cordis and compared it to arteriosclerotic encephalomalacia. Fibrosis was compared with renal shrinkage. Three years later another paper appeared on myomalacia cordis. In these same years Ziegler included a paragraph on this disease in the first edition of his textbook. The time spent in Freiburg was quite important for Ziegler. The Institute (with its chairman R. Maier who was a student of Rokitansky) had a marked effect on Ziegler, who in later years influenced its development. A complete collection of Ziegler's reference papers is still available. All dissection protocols of his from 1880 were mainly handwritten and can be studied to this day in the present pathology institute. Careful examination of these allows recognition of what influenced Ziegler in following up the thought of causal relationship between coronary disease and myocardial infarction. This is of the utmost importance since Ziegler had a wide influence on many generations of doctors through his international gathering of students and through his textbook. This was widely used and translated into many languages.

The dissection protocols in Freiburg around 1880 reveal that tuberculosis was the eading cause of death which came to the attention of the pathologist. Other infectious diseases were also frequent, e.g. typhoid fever. The average age of 145 corpses dissected in 1882 was forty years. Older people died at home and were not dissected. In addition, it is interesting to note that wealthy people, those prone to heart disease because of their way of life, did not enter hospital. Heart infarction was therefore not a very common finding in the autopsy room. Hearts were often described as fatty, degenerated or inflamed. One has to keep in mind that both conditions are also frequent in myocardial infarction and can easily obscure diagnosis. In preparing his textbook Ziegler was certainly consulting previous textbooks. Rokitansky had already mentioned in his textbook of 1844 that fat infiltration of the heart wall was often accompanied by sclerosis of the coronaries. In addition, Ziegler was well informed on recent papers. He added accurately all references in his textbook after each paragraph. These references coincide with his paper collection. Including references in a textbook was very uncommon at that time. One of his students evaluated all known references in 1886 in his thesis (Beck). Blood vessel damage in the kidneys and brain was also often observed. Single cases of similar damage in the heart were occasionally dissected. For these reasons Ziegler concluded that there was a definite correlation between disease of the coronary arteries and myomalacia cordis. When he was convinced he stated it clearly. His description of myomalacia cordis remained almost unchanged throughout all eleven editions of his textbook.

Als Myomalacia cordis bezeichnet man passend eine Erweichung des Herzmuskels, wie sie sich nach arterieller Anämie einstellt. Die häufigste Ursache dieser Anämie bilden Erkrankungen (Sklerose und Atherom) der arteriellen Ernährungsgefässe des Herzens, der Kranzarterien und ihrer Aeste, seltener embolische Verstopfung derselben. Die Erweichungsherde sehen je nach ihrem Alter und ihrem Gehalt an Blut verschieden aus. Ist die Erweichung noch frisch, so sehen sie meist weiss-gelb aus, die Muskelsubstanz ist zugleich weiss und zerreisslich; zuweilen sinkt die Schnittfläche etwas ein, idem die Substanz sehr weich ist. Mit unter kommt es zufolge der Obliteration und Verstopfung der Arterien zu Blutaustritt aus den Kapillaren, zu Infarktbildung. Dann sieht der Herd dunkelrot-hämorrhagisch aus, oder er ist dunkelrot, braun und gelb gefleckt. Aeltere Herde sehen nicht selten grau-gelb oder grau-braun, oder wohl mehr rostfarben aus. Noch ältere gewinnen eine grau durch scheinende Beschaffenheit und sinken etwas unter das Niveau der Schnittfläche zurück. Solche Herde findet man am häufigsten im linken Ventrikel, namentlich in der Umgebung der Spitze der Vorder – und Hinterwand. Hat der Erweichungsherd eine erhebliche Ausdehnung und greift er durch die ganze oder nahezu die ganze Muscularis hindurch, so kommt es zur Ruptur der Herzwand. Bei der Sektion findet man alsdann den Herzbeutel durch ausgetretenes Blut stark ausgedehnt. Der Riss hat meist einen unregelmässig zackigen Verlauf, ist im übrigen meist nicht breit.

A description of histological changes with a picture follows the macroscopic explanation. Ziegler shows clearly that muscle cells degenerate first, showing swelling and pyknosis. Haemorrhages might occur at the same time. Later on, pigmentation is found and fatty degeneration develops. At the end fibrosis is the result. Discussing the results Ziegler writes critically: myomalacia has until now not received much attention, i.e. the disease runs under different names. Clinicians commonly call this form of heart disease myocarditis or fatty heart. Neither opinion is correct. The affection is an anaemic necrosis. Fat infiltration and inflammation can accompany it, but never as the main and primary change. Myomalacia is a process which can be compared with encephalomalacia. The affection is not rare and leads in severe cases to death by heart insufficiency or rupture and bleeding. Only for dissections performed in Freiburg after 1880 are complete protocols available. The collection of cases from Tübingen (1882–89) are reviewed in the thesis of Beck. He described eight patients with heavy sclerosis of the coronary arteries, aneurysms of the heart and partial ruptures of the left ventricular wall. Only in one case is a detailed clinical description given.

After Ziegler's return to Freiburg in 1890 quite a number of cases of myomalacia cordis with sclerosis of the coronaries appear in the dissection protocols.

Autopsy 2, 1890*:* describes a 57-year-old man.
Die Spitze des linken Ventrikels ist in eine schwielige Masse verwandelt, von Muskulatur ist nichts zu erkennen. Hier sitzt der Intima ein alter Thrombus an. Die Koronargefässe sind stark verkalkt.

Autopsy 30, 1890*:* deals with a 72-year-old woman.
Das Herz ist stark vergrössert, und zwar sowohl in der Breite als auch in der Höhe. Die Spitze wird vom linken Ventrikel gebildet. Der linke Ventrikel fühlt sich sehr fest an, ebenso der ausgedehnte rechte Ventrikel. Der rechte Ventrikel ist erweitert, die Muskulatur hypertrophisch, blass-grau. An der Spitze des rechten Ventrikels findet sich ein fast 3 cm, im Zentrum bereits erweichter, gemischter rot- und weissgefleckter polypöser Thrombus, welcher die Spitze des Ventrikels einnimmt. Die Spitze der Papillarmuskeln sind gelb gefärbt. In der Herzspitze und an der Vorderwand sitzt auch im linken Ventrikel ein grosser polypöser Thrombus. Die Muskalutur des linken Ventrikels ist sehr stark hypertrophisch, etwas gelb gefärbt. Kleinere Thromben sitzen auch da und dort zwischen den Trabekeln. Die Arteriae coronariae zeigen in den Innenwänden zahlreiche weisse Flecken, sind etwas verdickt, zeigen Verkalkungen.

About five to six cases out of 250 autopsies showed sclerosis of the coronary artery and myomalacia cordis. In the textbook Ziegler did not change much of his first description. He added only a macroscopic picture to the histological one.

Myocardial infarction does not seem to be a new disease. Certainly many people have died of it previously. A clear definition of the disease became possible only through the evolution and perfection of pathology in the nineteenth century. The history of evolution of the notion of myocardial infarction reveals the immense value of anatomico-pathological observation. Of course some basic notions had to be created. Sclerotic coronaries were first described in Egyptian mummies. Fatty degeneration and softness of the heart were not uncommon findings since the first autopsies were performed. Cases of rupture of the heart wall were published before the second half of the nineteenth century. It is interesting to note here that Heberden and his school preceded the pathologists with their notion of angina pectoris.

A clear notion of arteriosclerosis was defined by Scarpa in the 1830s. Ten years later the genial Virchow introduced the concept of thrombosis with subsequent infarction, e.g. in the kidneys. Another twenty years later histological techniques were much more refined. All these developments allowed the pathologists of the second half of the nineteenth century to conceive a causal relationship between vessel damage and heart infarction. Many single observations were published (Malmsten 1861, Boettger 1863, Tautin 1866 to mention a few). At the same time as Ziegler, Weigert reported on anaemic necrosis of the heart in a paper on pathological clotting mechanisms. Ziegler therefore, was only one of many, to observe the condition. His invaluable contribution, however, is the extension of the thought through his famous and much re-edited and translated textbook.

Literature

BECK, H., 'Zur Kenntnis der Entstehung der Herzruptur und des chronischen, partiellen Herzaneurysmas', Thesis, Tübingen, 1886.

BOETTGER, H., 'Ueber die spontanen Rupturen des Herzens', *Archiv der Heilkunde*, 1863, **4**, 502–21.

CRUVEILHIER, J., *Anatomie pathologique du Coeur humain*, vol. III, Paris, Baillière, 1829–42.

HODEL, C. und BUESS, H., 'E. Ziegler (1849–1905): Ein grosser Forscher und Lehrer', *Clio Med.*, 1966, **1**, 303–18.

LEIBOWITZ, J. O., *The History of Coronary Heart Disease*, London, Wellcome Institute of the History of Medicine, 1970.

LEYDEN, E., 'Ueber die Sklerose der Coronararterien und die davon abhängigen Krankheitszustände, *Z. klin. Med.*, 1884, **7**, 459–86.

MORTON, L. T., *A Medical Bibliography*, 3rd ed., London, Deutsch, 1970.

OBRASTZOW, W. P. und STRASCHESKO, N. D., 'Zur Kenntnis der Thrombose der Coronararterien des Herzens', *Z. klin. Med.*, 1910, **71**, 116–32.

ROKITANSKY, C., *Handbuch der speziellen pathologischen Anatomie*, Band 1, Vienna, Traumüller und Seidel, 1844.

WEIGERT, K., 'Ueber die pathologischen Gerinnungsvorgänge', *Virchows Arch. path. Anat.*, 1880, **79**, 87–123.

ZIEGLER, E., 'Ueber Myomalacia cordis', *Virchows Arch. path. Anat.*, 1882, **90**, 211.

ZIEGLER, E., *Lehrbuch der allgemeinen und speziellen pathologischen Anatomie*, 1st ed., Jena, G. Fischer, 1881–85; 11th ed., 1911.

ZIEGLER, E., 'Ueber die Ursachen der Nierenschrumpfung nebst Bemerkungen über die Unterscheidung verschiedener Formen von Nephritis', *Dtsch. Arch. klin. Med.*, 1879, **25**, 586–623.

W. Baroni
Bologna (Italy)

Arrigo Montanari e il sondaggio cardiovasale

Se Werner Forssmann ha il merito indiscutibile di aver compreso appieno l'importanza del cateterismo del cuore e di averlo coraggiosamente attuato su se stesso, fu un medico italiano, il ravennate Arrigo Montanari, che per primo ne prospettò le varie possibilità di utilizzazione pratica nella metodologia clinica, pubblicando nel gennaio del 1928 sulla rivista 'Lo Sperimentale' i risultati di una serie di ricerche sul sondaggio dei vasi sanguigni e del cuore da lui eseguite con successo su animali vivi e nel cadavere. Ma pochi, forse anche in campo medico, conoscono le benemerenze di questo nostro studioso. Anche le informazioni biografiche che abbiamo su di lui sono scarse e questa carenza di notizie é dovuta alla profonda modestia che sempre pervase il Montanari in tutti i suoi atteggiamenti. Nacque a S. Alberto di Ravenna il 1^{0} agosto 1892 da antica famiglia romagnola. Trascorse i primi anni della sua vita nel paese d'origine poi andò a Faenza dove il padre era segretario comunale. Dal 1915 al 1919 fu soldato. Ottenuto il congedo entrò come allievo interno all'Istituto di Fisiologia della Università di Bologna e vi restò fino alla laurea, conseguita a pieni voti nel 1921, discutendo una tesi sperimentale di fisiologia col prof. P. Albertoni. Dopo tre anni di attività all'Ospedale Civile di Faenza entrò come assistente nella Clinica Medica di Firenze diretta dal prof. Schupfer. Nel 1925 ottenne col massimo punteggio i diplomi di specializzazione in Clinica Medica e Otorinolaringoiatria; l'anno dopo quello in Anatomia Patologica. Nel 1930 conseguì l'abilitazione alla libera docenza in Patologia Speciale Medica e nel 1933 assunse la direzione dell'Ospedale Civile di Lecce. Nel 1958, quando per raggiunti limiti di età fu collocato a riposo, si trasferì a Bologna sua città prediletta, ma di tanto in tanto amava trascorrere brevi soggiorni a Faenza, sede in passato della sua famiglia. Qui morì nel settembre del 1971.

La sua vita di studioso é documentata da oltre 100 pubblicazioni scientifiche. Ha compiuto ricerche importanti sulla coagulazione del sangue e sulla autoemoagglutinazione, sul midollo, sull'equilibrio calcio-potassio in alcune disfunzioni endocrine e nel carcinoma, sulla genesi extra epatica della bilirubina, sulla bile, sull'urea, sulla reazione xantoproteica nel siero di sangue e sulla distribuzione del glucosio nel sangue nei diversi distretti circolatori. Originali sono i suoi contributi in alcune malattie neurologiche e pregevoli le pubblicazioni a carattere monografico sui carcinomi primitivi del fegato, sugli ascessi sottodiaframmatici e sulla encefalite epidemica. Si é occupato delle meningopatie tubercolari, del tifo e di altre malattie infettive quali il tetano, di cui aveva una indiscutibile competenza avendo per oltre un anno, dal 1927 al 1928, retto l'incarico di assistente straordinario presso l'Istituto Antirabbico di Firenze. Ma certamente i suoi lavori più noti e che costituiscono un vanto per la scienza italiana sono quelli che riguardano il sondaggio dei vasi sanguigni e del cuore. Arrigo Montanari fu il primo a intuire la possibilità di introdurre una lunga sonda flessibile in una vena del braccio per farla risalire fino al cuore destro e a concretizzare l'idea realizzando con successo l'esperimento nell'animale vivo e nel cadavere, e fu anche il primo a proporre l'esplorazione dei vasi sanguigni e del cuore per la soluzione di problemi di fisiopatologia.

Prima del nostro Montanari i fisiologi e i chirurghi erano intervenuti sui vasi ma per tratti brevissimi e con intendimenti diversi. Chauveau, Marey e Faivre nel 1861 avevano introdotto cannule rigide attraverso i grossi vasi del collo nel cavallo per registrare su tamburi scriventi le contrazioni delle orecchiette e dei ventricoli. Questi autori erano stati preceduti nelle manovre di intubazione vasale dal rev. inglese Stephen Hales che nel 1733 aveva congiunto l'arteria di un vecchio cavallo con un lungo tubo di vetro per misurare la pressione arteriosa. Nel 1912 Bleichröder, Unger e Loeb avevano compiuto manovre più ardite per far giungere medicamenti in modo più diretto e in maggior concentrazione a determinati organi, ma non si erano proposti di raggiungere il cuore o di servirsi del sondaggio come mezzo di indagine.

Il Carrel aveva tentato una intubazione permanente dell'aorta toracica con un tubo rigido e il Mattioli aveva introdotto nella carotide primitiva un sottile zaffo di garza iodoformica contenendolo con sutura applicata sui margini della ferita.

Anche il Caucci aveva praticato tentativi di zaffamento intravasale e il Baccelli aveva introdotto, attraverso un ago-cannula, una piccola molla nel sacco degli aneurismi di forma ampollare e a collo ristretto per provocare la formazione di coaguli compatti e occludenti. Il Montanari intraprese i suoi esperimenti sul sondaggio, quando era assistente alla Clinica di Firenze, col preciso intento di raggiungere il cuore e per la soluzione di questi problemi:
(1°) dimostrare la possibilità e l'innocuità del sondaggio negli animali,
(2°) ricercare l'utilità di questo mezzo di indagine nella patologia del cuore,
(3°) dimostrare la possibilità meccanica del cateterismo cardiaco prima nel cadavere poi nell'uomo vivo.
Iniziò i suoi esperimenti sui cani servendosi di una sonda flessibile e lunga tanto da poter seguire agevolmente le tortuosità vasali e raggiungere i vasi più interni. Sistemato l'animale su di un apparecchio di contenzione metteva allo scoperto una delle vene dell'arto anteriore, applicava al vaso due pinze emostatiche leggermente distanziate, praticava una piccola incisione nel tratto compreso fra le due pinze e vi introduceva il capo della sonda che poi spingeva nell'interno del vaso in senso centrale dopo aver tolta la pinza emostatica prossimale. In queste manovre cercava di evitare infezioni operando con tecnica perfettamente asettica; di evitare il pericolo di emorragie agendo celermente e introducendo la sonda a vaso reso esangue; di non provocare embolie servendosi di sonde o prive di lume o piene di liquido isotonico.

In un primo tempo fu indispensabile sacrificare gli animali ma in seguito lo si poté evitare ricorrendo all'aiuto radiologico. La sonda una volta entrata nell'atrio lo attraversava e penetrava infallibilmente nella cava inferiore fino alle vene iliache. Questo fu il risultato di quattro esperimenti su cinque condotti nel cane. Ma poiché nel quinto animale di maggior mole rispetto ai precedenti, in un secondo tentativo di sondaggio, il tratto di sonda introdotta risultò sensibilmente più corta (aveva infatti seguito una via diversa da quella solita, era penetrata nel ventricolo e, attraversatolo in tutta la sua lunghezza, aveva imboccato l'arteria polmonare raggiungendo il punto della sua biforcazione), il Montanari compì ulteriori esperimenti per scoprire la ragione di questo diverso risultato. Constatò che il fatto si registrava prevalentemente nei cani più grandi e mai in quelli più piccoli e che la deviazione verso la polmonare avveniva quando il catetere era spinto lentamente in quel tratto in cui il capo esplorante passava dallo sbocco della cava superiore a quello della cava inferiore.

Il medico revennate praticò poi nel cane il sondaggio dalle vene dell'arto posteriore e notò che nella quasi totalità dei casi il sondino oltrepassata la cavità auricolare penetrava nella cava superiore e in una delle vene succlavie, più di rado nella giugulare interna.

Poi dal cane spostò sul coniglio i suoi esperimenti servendosi di sonde di calibro inferiore e utilizzando la stessa metodica. Ottenne risultati sovrapponibili a quelli riscontrati nel cane, però nel coniglio, come del resto si era verificato nei cani di piccola taglia, non riuscì a far penetrare la sonda nel ventricolo destro per farle imbucare l'arteria polmonare.

Sulla base di questi dati il Montanari poté concludere che:

(1°) il sondaggio venoso nell'animale vivo é possibile,

(2°) é innocuo se si prendono alcune precauzioni,

(3°) non é doloroso se non nella sua prima parte (incisione della cute e delle parti molli),

(4°) La sonda può essere spinta attraverso il torace e l'addome fino all'origine di una delle vene iliache interne e negli animali di grossa taglia può raggiungere la biforcazione dell'arteria polmonare se il sondaggio verrà praticato con estrema lentezza nel tratto intra-auricolare,

(5°) quando non é possibile ricorrere all'esame radiologico la diversa via seguita dalla sonda può essere intuita senza sacrificare l'animale dalla diversa lunghezza del tratto esploratore (più lungo per la cava inferiore, più breve per la polmonare).

Per la conferma della possibilità meccanica del sondaggio nel cadavere si servì di sonde di gomma flessibilissime, lunghe più di un metro ma con calibro di pochi millimetri e come porta di entrata utilizzò le vene della piega del gomito. Seguì la metodica già sperimentata sugli animali: praticata l'incisione introduceva la sonda e la spingeva centralmente poi aperto il torace controllava la sede del capo esplorante.

Negli esperimenti più riusciti la sonda si fermò a pochi centimetri dall'orecchietta destra a causa dei coaguli sanguigni che si opponevano al suo progresso.

Create le premesse indispensabili per l'applicazione del sondaggio alla patologia umana il Montanari ne prospettò anche e chiaramente l'utilità proponendolo:

(1°) per la ricerca di stenosi vasali,

(2°) per rilevare variazioni del decorso dei vasi, spesso indizio di spostamenti anomali dei visceri,

(3°) per il prelevamento isolato del sangue refluo da quell'organo di cui si vuole saggiare la funzionalità,

(4°) per l'immissione di medicamenti in un determinato distretto,

(5°) per l'infusione diretta intracardiaca di generosi quantitativi di soluzione fisiologica dimostratasi di più pronta efficacia rispetto alle fleboclisi.
Gli studi e le proposte di questo nostro studioso ottennero ben presto il consenso di scienziati illustri.

Il tedesco Werner Forssmann nel 1929, col procedimento identico a quello descritto dal Montanari, fu il primo a praticare il cateterismo cardiaco nell'uomo vivo, attuandolo coraggiosamente su se stesso. Il primo in Italia fu Silvestrini di Perugia che nel 1930 introdusse direttamente digitale nell'orecchietta destra in un cardiopatico scompensato. Nel 1941 il metodo assunse la fisionomia e l'importanza che oggi gli competono grazie agli studi di Cournand e Richards che resero possibile la sua applicazione su vasta scala. Successive e ulteriori applicazioni sono state proposte allo scopo di rendere il metodo più innocuo e più fecondo di risultati.

Al cateterismo cardiaco, realizzato dal Montanari negli animali vivi e nel cadavere e da lui proposto per la soluzione di problemi di patologia umana, attuato per la prima volta nell'uomo vivo da Forssmann e valorizzato da Richards e Cournand, spetta un ruolo preminente nelle conoscenze attuali della fisiologia circolatoria e delle sue variazioni nelle cardiopatie congenite, conoscenze che sono state anche l'indispensabile presupposto al rapido ed entusiasmante progresso della cardiochirurgia.

Bibliografia

BACCELLI, Citato da Caucci, *Policlinico*, Roma, 1918, Sez. Prat. 509.
BLEICHRODER, 'Introarterielle Therapie', *Berl. klim. Wschr.*, 1912, no. 32.
CAUCCI, *Policlinico*, Roma, 1919, Sez. Prat. 509.
CHAUVEAU, cit dai Trattati di Fisiologia, 1861.
COURNAND, *Proc. Soc. Exp. Biol. Med.*, 1941, **46**, 462; *Fed. Proc.*, 1945, **4**, 207; *J. clin. Invest.*, 1945, **24**, 106.
CRAINZ, *Riv. Osped. Roma*, 1915, **5**, 734–42.
DONEGAN, *J. Physiol. Lond.*, 1921-22, **55**, 226–45.
FORSSMANN, W., 'Sondierung des rechten Herzens', *Klin. Wchr.*, 1929, nos. 45 and 49.
GATELLIER, *Bull. et mém. Soc. de chir. de Par.*, 1918, **44**, 1175.
GIORGI, *Policlinico*, Roma, 1921, XXVIII, Sez. Prat., 1361–63.
LOEB, 'Introarterielle Therapie', *Berl. klin. Wschr.*, 1912, no. 32.
LUBICH, T., FOSCARINI, M., MANZINI, E., DE NOVELLIS, M., 'La posizione attuale del cateterismo cardiaco nella diagnostica clinica', *Collezioni di monografie e memorie scientifiche*, serie II°, vol. IX, Bologna, Soc. Tip. Mareggiani, 1960.
LUCIANI, *Fisiologia dell'uomo*, 5, a. ed., Milano, Soc. Ed. Lib., 1921.
MAREY, Citato dal Luciani.
MONTANARI, A., 'Il sondaggio dei vasi sanguigni', *Lo Sperimentale*, 1928, no. 82, I–II, p. 93.
PALADINI, P., *Rivista di Storia della Medicina*, anno 1°, vol. 1°, ed., Universo, Roma, 1957.
ROBERT, *Dt. med. Wschr.*, 1921, **47**, 333.
RONCATO, *Arch. di fisiologia*, Firenze, 1922, **20**, 159–64.
RUHL, *Dt. med. Wschr.*, 1915, **41**, 710.
SILVESTRINI, R. and GUARDABASSI, M., *Boll. Acc. med. chir. di Perugia*, 21 giugno 1930.
TUFFIER, *Bull. Acad. de méd.*, Par. 3 s., **74**, 455–60.
UNGER, 'Introarterielle Therapie', *Berl. klin. Wschr.*, 1912, no. 32.

G. Keil
Freiburg i. Br. (*West Germany*)

Makroskopische Hämatoskopie

Caesar der Feldherr – so berichtet die Legende – kam zu Hippokrates' Grab, und weil er glaubte, daß ein Schatz darin verborgen sei, ließ er es öffnen. Und in der Tat findet er eine Elfenbeinkapsel unter dem Haupt des Toten: Hippokrates hatte nämlich sein Lesepult mit sich begraben lassen, in dem er ein Buch verwahrte: εἶχε γὰρ ἐν ἑαυτῷ ἐγκεκρυμένα θεῖα μυστήρια – „darin hielt er verborgen heilige Geheimnisse".

Welches sind nun die Geheimnisse, die Hippokrates der Arzt mit sich begraben ließ? Ein Wunderheilmittel? Eine durchschlagende therapeutische Methode? Nichts dergleichen. Das, was Caesar der Kapsel entnimmt und seinem Leibarzt anvertraut, ist ein simples Diagnose-Schema, das anhand weniger Paragraphen prognostisch-diagnostische Schlüsse zieht.

Das Geheimnis ärztlichen Erfolges für Hippokrates – ein Diagnose-Schema. Gewiß, nur eine Legende, aber nichts zeigt besser als eben diese Legende, welche Wertschätzung der Diagnose in der mittelalterlichen Medizin entgegengebracht wurde und welche Hoffnungen mittelalterliche Praktiker auf einfache Diagnose-Schemata setzten.

Verhältnismäßig selten sind ärztliche Taschenbücher überliefert. Es genügt festzuhalten, daß sie seit dem 14. Jh. bezeugt sind und daß sie den spätmittelalterlichen Praktiker auf seinen Krankenbesuchen begleiteten. In keinem dieser ärztlichen Taschenbücher der Frühzeit fehlen Diagnose-Schemata, oft stellen sie sogar den inhaltlichen Hauptteil, und dieselbe Gewichtung zeigen praxisbezogene Arzneibücher, die mitunter den Diagnose-Abschnitt an den Anfang stellen: Der hundertfach überlieferte „Bartholomäus" beginnt mit einem Harntraktat, und das „Boec van medicinen in Dietsche" leitet sich mit einer ganzen Reihe von Diagnose-Schemata ein.

Diagnose-Schemata gehören zu den gängigen Gattungen medizinischer Kleinliteratur. Im Spätmittelalter und der frühen Neuzeit ist ihrer Legion. Sie verraten mit einiger Deutlichkeit, welche diagnostischen Verfahren angewandt wurden und welche Methoden der Praktiker beim Diagnose- und Prognosestellen bevorzugte.

Für die systematisierte Diagnose standen zwei Gruppen von Verfahren zur Verfügung. Die erste Gruppe, die sich aus einer einzigen Methode rekrutiert, stammt aus der Pneumalehre und bietet die Pulsdiagnostik.

Die zweite Gruppe, die mehrere Verfahren aufweist, fußt auf der Humoralpathologie; sie umfaßt diejenigen Methoden, die aus den Körperausscheidungen die

Säftemischung abzulesen versuchen und auf diese Weise eine Prognose oder Diagnose anstreben.

Am bekanntesten von diesen humoralpathologisch ausgerichteten Methoden ist die Uroskopie. Vom Frühmittelalter bis ins 19. Jh. belegt hat sie durch ihre vieltausend Überlieferungen für ausreichende Repräsentanz in der Medizinhistorie gesorgt. Mehrere Monographien befassen sich mit ihrer Geschichte. Andere humoralpathologische Diagnose-Praktiken haben demgegenüber sich historischem Scharfblick teilweise entzogen. In der Regel spielten sie im ärztlichen Alltag kaum eine Rolle – wie beispielsweise die Koproskopie, die Paulos von Nikaia nach Ruphos noch empfiehlt, die anschließend aber weitgehend aufgegeben wurde. Jedenfalls ist mir bislang kein mittelalterliches Kot-Schema begegnet. Einige Verfahren wurden dagegen ernster genommen und in ihrer Semiotik durch katalogartige Schemata aufgeschlüsselt. Hierher gehören die Hautausschläge, von denen das ebengenannte Buch aus Hippokratens Grabe berichtet; hierher gehört die Sputumdiagnostik, von der schematisierend das „Boec van medicinen" handelt, und hierher gehört ein Abschnitt über den Schweiß, der den Leser des „Boec van medicinen" über das Schwitzen und seine Zeichen diagnostisch-prognostisch aufklärt.

Das „Boec van medicinen in Dietsche" ist für den Physicus, nicht für Chirurgen geschrieben. Das zeigt bereits die Anordnung des Stoffes, die von der Pädiatrie über Frauenheilkunde bis zur Pharmakologie und materia medica reicht, und das zeigt die Auswahl der behandelten Diagnoseschemata, die mit der Uroskopie einsetzen und anschließend die Semiotik von Schweiß, Auswurf und Hautausschlägen bringen. Eines der grade für den Wundarzt aufschlußreichen Verfahren fehlt: die Haematoskopie.

Der Aderlaß als therapeutisches Verfahren ist alt, und ebenso alt wie die Phlebotomie ist die diagnostische Wertung des gelassenen Blutes. Als festgefügtes diagnostisches Verfahren begegnet die Blutschau jedoch erst später: ebenso wie die Uroskopie wurde auch die Haematoskopie nicht vor Beginn des Mittelalters systematisiert und zum Diagnoseschema ausgebaut.

Die erste Stufe dieses Ausbaus ist eng mit der Aderlaßtechnik gekoppelt. Frühe systematische Hinweise zur diagnostischen Wertung des Aderlaßblutes begegnen in der pseudohippokratischen „Phlebotomie". Und ebenso unselbständig wie bei der „Phlebotomia Hippocratis" sind die Blutschau-Regeln, die als Unterabschnitt in Ortolfs „Arzneibuch" begegnen.

Die zweite Stufe systematischen Ausbaus ist mit der textlichen Selbständigkeit erreicht. Ebenso wie die Harnschau im Frühmittelalter eigenständige Traktate aufweist, läßt sich für die Blutschau literarische Selbständigkeit bereits für vorsalernitanische Zeit bezeugen. Belegt für diese frühe Zeit ist ein zwei Quartblätter umfassender Traktat, der in Katalogform aufgebaut ist und den Stil des Briefes lediglich im Titel nachahmt: „Es beginnt" – so lautet die Überschrift – die „epistula Hippocratis de sanguine cognoscendo a medico qualis sit".

Dieser Titel, der erst im Zuge der Überlieferung sich herausgebildet hat und nicht der Urfassung eignet, läßt bereits erkennen, daß der Text in frühmittelalterlicher Tradition pseudoepigraphischer Hippokrates-Zuweisungen steht. Auf frühmittelalterliche Entstehung deutet auch die Sprache, die – am Sprechlatein orientiert – die Merkmale langobardischer Übersetzungen erkennen läßt. Und frühmittelalterliche Genese läßt schließlich sich an strukturellen Eigenheiten ablesen: Wie schon gesagt, ist der Text in Katalogform aufgebaut, wobei – wie den colores urinarum – jeder Blutfarbe ein eigener Text-Paragraph entspricht. Und wie bei urognostischen Traktaten ist jeder Farbe eine bestimmte Diagnose zugeordnet. Diese Diagnose indessen wird – wiederum parallel zu den frühen Harntraktaten – keineswegs allein aus dem Aussehen des Leibessafts gewonnen, sondern polysymptomatisch auch aus anderen Zeichen sowie der Krankengeschichte abgeleitet. Daneben finden sich – und auch das korrespondiert mit frühen Harntraktaten – verstreut über die Paragraphen vereinzelte therapeutische Winke.

Die Blutschau in der zweiten Ausbaustufe korreliert also weitgehend mit der gleichzeitigen Uroskopie, und es ist anzunehmen, daß die ersten Blutschautexte parallel zu den frühmittelalterlichen Harntraktaten entstanden. Zwar setzt die Überlieferung später ein – die Hämatoskopie wird erst zu Beginn des neunten und nicht schon im achten Jh. greifbar – ,doch ist die Überlieferungsdichte im ganzen gesehn bei der Blutschau geringer – fürs Frühmittelalter beträgt sie nur 8 Prozent, gemessen an den Textzeugen der Uroskopie – ,und bei dieser geringen Dichte bedeuten zwei Abschriften aus dem neunten Jh. lediglich einen terminus ante quem: beide Textzeugen der pseudohippokratischen ,,Epistula de sanguine cognoscendo'' sind durch mindestens ein Zwischenglied vom Urtext getrennt, und beim jetzigen Stand der Untersuchungen ist es nicht ausgeschlossen, daß die Textentstehung ins 7., wenn nicht ins 6. Jh. zurückreicht.

Wie weit die frühmittelalterliche Hämatoskopie ausgestrahlt hat, läßt sich noch nicht sagen. Belegt ist sie nur in zwei Handschriften, deren Provenienz auf Deutschland oder Frankreich weist, aber nicht eindeuting bestimmt ist. Ob landessprachige Übersetzungen sich nachweisen lassen, steht offen, ist aber nicht wahrscheinlich: Bei den frühmittelalterlichen Harntraktaten sind derartige volkssprachige Reflexe bisher nicht aufgezeigt, obwohl die Texte die salernitanische Periode überdauerten und in praxisnahen Sammelhandschriften sich bis an die Schwelle der Neuzeit behauptet haben. Vermutlich gilt für die pseudohippokratische ,,Epistula de sanguine cognoscendo'' ähnliches, wenngleich Spuren einer hoch- oder spätmittelalterlichen Texttradition noch fehlen.

Aus dem 10. bis 13. Jh. sind keine Blutschau-Traktate bezeugt; die Überlieferung setzt erst wieder ein mit der dritten Ausbaustufe der Hämatoskopie. Diese dritte Stufe systematischer Blutschau hat mit der zweiten die textliche Selbständigkeit gemein – nach wie vor sind es Kurztraktate, die vom iudicium sanguinis handeln – im Gegensatz zur zweiten Stufe ist die Hämatoskopie jedoch weiter systematisiert worden, so daß sie nicht mehr unterschiedliche Zeichen zur Krankheitsfindung benutzt, sondern die Diagnose allein aus dem Blut ohne Wertung irgendwelcher anderer Symptome vornimmt.

Dieser Schritt zur monosymptomatischen Diagnose wird in Byzanz vollzogen, wobei Salerno in Anlehnung an Isaak wie Theophilus die Entwicklung nachvollzieht und weiter vorantreibt. Auslösend ist eine Vervollständigung der Farbenskala, der ein fester Humoralbezug beigeordnet wird; weiterführend wirken Beobachtungen der Beimengungen, und ihre Krönung findet die Systematisierung in der Regionenlehre, die eine Organrepräsentanz mit einschließt.

All dies sind wohlbekannte Tendenzen aus der Geschichte hochmittelalterlicher Uroskopie, wobei die Entwicklung wiederum zweigleisig verläuft: die Systematisierung der Blutschau ist offensichtlich nicht eigenständig abgelaufen, sondern in enger Anlehnung an den Ausbau der Uroskopie erfolgt. Das geht so weit, daß die Blutschau in Ansätzen die nur für den Urognosten sinnvolle Regionenlehre übernimmt. Im übrigen zeigt sie Abhängigkeit von den Harnfarben, wobei gelbes Blut die Leber und Galle, weißliches das Phlegma und dunkles Blut die schwarze Galle repräsentiert.

Mit dieser humoralpathologischen Farbenskala indessen nicht genug: Die mittelalterliche Hämatoskopie zeigt Ansätze, auf dem Wege der Signaturenlehre die Harnschau zu überholen. Charakteristisch für hochmittelalterliche Blutschau-Regeln sind Diagnosen, die weniger von der Farbe als der Gestalt des makroskopischen Blutbildes ausgehn: Ein geklumpter Blutkuchen beispielsweise, umgeben von Serum, wird als Indiz für Harnsteine gewertet; häutige Koagula deuten, wenn sie von Serum unterlagert sind, auf die *intercutanea pestis*, die Wassersucht, während kleine, im Serum schwimmende Blutkuchenpartikeln im Sinne der Apostasenlehre als Absonderungen innerer Geschwüre angesehen werden. Besonders sinnfällig wird dieser Signaturbezug in der Prognose eines bairischen Textes vom Jahr 1427, wo es heißt: *Sind denn pläterl ob dem pluet als dy auf dem wasser werdent, wenn es regent, der prich ains auf, vnd vindestu ain grüebel dar ůnder, das beczaichent den tod.*

Die Texte der dritten Ausbaustufe sind in zahllosen Handschriften überliefert, doch lassen sich die Textzeugen – von wenigen Ausnahmen abgesehn – auf zwei Grundschemata zurückführen, die trotz allen Ergänzungen und Umstellungen im Kern nur wenig variieren. Diese geringe Zahl an Ausgangstexten kontrastiert deutlich mit der Uroskopie, die im Mittelalter über ein ganzes Arsenal von Texten verfügt, wobei die Textlänge – je nach inhaltlicher Ausrichtung – zwischen wenigen Sätzen eines Kurztraktats und zahlreichen Kapiteln eines Lehrbuchs schwankt. Eine entsprechende Variationsbreite fehlt der Haematoskopie, deren vielen Überlieferungen – soweit bekannt – immer nur der eine oder andere von zwei Kurztraktaten zugrundeliegt. Diese Monotonie mag damit zusammenhängen, daß die Blutschau außerhalb der Universitäten blieb und von der Schulmedizin nur wenig beachtet wurde. In der Praxis spielte sie jedoch eine ungleich größere Rolle, und zumindest gebietsweise scheint sie Ende des Mittelalters der Pulskontrolle den zweiten Platz in der Diagnostik streitig gemacht zu haben. Allein aus dem deutschen Sprachgebiet sind zehn mittelalterliche Übersetzungen belegt, von denen etliche in mehreren Überlieferungen vorkommen. Diese Übersetzungen wurden bis weit in die Neuzeit benutzt, und über Drucke – beispielsweise das „Feldbuch" Gersdorffs – sicherten sie sich ihre Verbreitung bis an die Schwelle des 18. Jhs.

Blutschau-Schemata sind Kurztraktate, doch haben sie ungeachtet textlicher Eigenständigkeit innerhalb medizinischer Sammelhandschriften einen bestimmten Stellenwert: In der Regel sind sie dem Aderlaß-Abschnitt eingeordnet, und als Bestandteil des Aderlasses haben wir uns die Blutschau vorzustellen. Die Phlebotomie ist ein therapeutischer Eingriff; daß er eigens zu diagnostischen Zwecken vorgenommen wurde, ist nicht belegt.[1] Indessen wissen wir, daß er häufig gefordert wurde, und diese Häufigkeit des Aderlassens erlaubt Rückschlüsse auf die Häufigkeit der Hämatoskopie.

Blutschau ist im Gegensatz zur Harn- und Pulskontrolle ein abhängiges diagnostisches Verfahren; damit ist gesagt, daß ihr Substrat nicht beliebig zur Verfügung steht und daß ihre Durchführbarkeit äußeren Faktoren – hier der Indikationsstellung zu einem therapeutischen Eingriff – unterworten ist. Da diese therapeutische

Maßnahme aber häufig indiziert war, können wir mit einer relativen Häufigkeit auch mit der Blutschau rechnen. Die überlieferten Texte bestätigen diese Überlegung.

Neuere Darstellungen mittelalterlicher Diagnose-Techniken beschränken sich in der Regel auf Uroskopie und Pulskontrolle. In der Tat sind damit die beiden wichtigsten Verfahren erfaßt. Die historische Darstellung mittelalterlicher Diagnostik wird jedoch erst dann vollständig, wenn sie ein drittes Verfahren mitberücksichtigt. Und diese dritte wichtige Technik ist die makroskopische Hämatoskopie.

Note

1 Eine Ausnahme macht lediglich die Lepraschau, vgl. beispielsweise Carlowitz, S. 12, 17, 19.

Benutztes Schrifttum

[BLEKER-] BERGER, JOHANNA, *Die Entwicklung der Harndiagnostik aus der Harnschau zur Harnuntersuchung*, med. Diss. Münster/Wf., 1965.

BLANKE, DIETRICH, *Die pseudohippokratische „Epistula de sanguine cognoscendo“* [Arbeitstitel], med. Diss. Bonn, 1973.

BRAEKMAN, WILLY und GUNDOLF KEIL, „Die ‚Vlaamsche leringe van orinen‘ in einer niederfränkischen Fassung des 14. Jahrhunderts. Randbemerkungen zur Gliederung des mittelalterlichen Harntraktats“, *Niederdtsch. Mitt.*, 1968, **24**, 75–125.

CARLOWITZ, HANS, *Der Lepraabschnitt aus Bernhard von Gordons „Lilium medicinae“ in mittelalterlicher deutscher Übersetzung*, med. Diss. Leipzig, 1913.

CHRISTOFFEL, HANS, „Grundzüge der Uroskopie“, *Gesnerus*, 1953, **10**, 89–122.

CZARNECKI, ROMUALD, *Ein Aderlaßtraktat angeblich des Roger von Salerno samt einem lateinischen und einem griechischen Texte zur „Phlebotomia Hippocratis“*, med. Diss. Leipzig, 1919.

DAEMS, WILLEM FRANS, *Boec van medicinen in Dietsche. Een Middelnederlandse compilatie van medisch-farmaceutische literatuur*, Leiden, 1967 (=Janus, Beiheft 7).

EIS, GERHARD und KEIL, GUNDOLF, „Nachträge zum Verfasserlexikon“, *Studia neophilol*, 1971, **43**, 377–429 (ärztliche Taschenbücher: S. 377 ff.).

KEIL, GUNDOLF, *Der „kurze Harntrakat“ des Breslauer „Codex Salernitanus“ und seine Sippe* (med. Diss. Bonn), Feuchtwangen: C.-E. Kohlhauer, 1969.

ders., „Acht Parallelen zu den Blutschau-Texten des Bremer Arzneibuchs. Untersuchungen zur spätmittelalterlichen Hämatoskopie“, *Niederdtsch. Mitt.*, 1969, **25**, 117–35.

ders., „Zur mittelniederdeutschen Blutschau“, *Niederdtsch. Mitt.*, 1970, **26**, 125–28.

KOELBING, HULDRYCH M., *Der Urin im medizinischen Denken*, I–VII, Basel, 1967.

LEISINGER, HERMANN, *Die lateinischen Harnschriften Pseudo-Galens*, med. Diss. Zürich, 1925 (=Beitr. z. Gesch. d. Med., 2).

MUSCHEL, JESAJA, „Die pseudohippokratische Todesprognostik und die Capsula eburnea in hebräischer Überlieferung“, *Sudhoffs Arch.*, 1932, **25**, 43–60.

ORTOLF, *Das Arzneibuch Ortolfs von Baierland*, hrsg. von James Follan, Stuttgart, 1963 (=Veröffentl. Internat. Ges. Gesch. Pharmazie, N.F. 23).

SCHRÄPLER, KARIN und KEIL, GUNDOLF, „Die Blutschau-Texte des Kasseler Kodex 4° med. 10“, *Niederdeutsch. Mitt.*, 1973, **29**.

SCHUBRING, KONRAD, „Wieder einmal Vorläufiges zu Paulos von Nikaia“, *Verh. XIX. Int. Kongr. Gesch. Med.*, Basel, 1966, S. 214–22.

STEUDEL, JOHANNES [Hrsg.], VON GERSDORFF, HANS, *Feldbuch der Wundarznei*, Straßburg, 1517, Neudruck Darmstadt, 1967.

SUDHOFF, KARL, „Die pseudohippokratische Krankheitsprognostik nach dem Auftreten von Hautausschlägen, ‚Secreta Hippocratis‘ oder ‚Capsula eburnea‘ benannt“, *Sudhoffs Arch.*, 1916, **9**, 79–116.

ders., „Ein deutscher diagnostischer Leitfaden zur Aderlaßblutschau“, *Sudhoffs Arch.*, 1917, **10**, 318 f.

ders., „Ein deutsch Aderlaßschau-Vorschrift“, *Sudhoffs Arch.*, 1920, **12**, 192.

TALBOT, CHARLES, ‘A mediaeval physician's Vade mecum’, *J. Hist. Med.*, 1961, **16**, 213–33.

L. Lauridsen
Svendborg (Denmark)

Laterna magica in corpore humano (from the early history of cystoscopy)

Diseases of the lower urinary tract was one of the most important fields of surgery for many centuries. The operative treatment was mainly confined to lithotomy, which was usually performed via the perineal route. Lithotripsy of small bladder stones was added in the 1820s. Palliative treatment dominated, however, with the catheter and bougie as the sovereign instruments. Diseases of the upper urinary tract were not treated surgically at all.

The introduction of antiseptic wound treatment in 1867 by Joseph Lister (1827–1912) laid the foundation for a tremendous expansion within many branches of surgery, but this did not apply to operations on the urinary tract. The main reason was above all a lack of adequate diagnostic procedures. Progress was not really made until the invention of the electric cystoscope, followed a few years later by the introduction of X-ray examination of the urinary tract. These two events form the basis of modern urinary tract surgery and of the development of urology as a specialty.

As yet the history of cystoscopy has been given rather modest attention, and we do not have any complete and comprehensive description of it. Smaller sections have been discussed in some detail, for example the first attempts at endoscopy in 1805–7 by Philip Bozzini (1773–1809), which form the prelude to the history of cystoscopy. His invention was of no practical use, but he put forward some of the principles which later should make endoscopy so valuable. Bozzini was aware that the ideal solution would be to use a source of light, which could be introduced into the hollow organ itself. He would use lenses to enlarge the picture, and he suggested a system of mirrors in order to change the course of the beam of light.

A few names should be mentioned as the most important shortly after Bozzini, i.e. Pierre Segalas (1792–1875) (Paris, 1827), John Fisher (1797–1850) (Philadelphia, 1827), and John Avery (1807–55) (London, 1840s). They all used candles as the source of light in their endoscopes. The experiments of these men were made in a period that in many ways was marked by attempts at converting physical theories into practical methods of clinical examination. The most successful results were the introduction of stethoscopy in 1816 and opthalmoscopy in 1851. The urological endoscopes from that period were, however, of little practical value.

In 1853 Antonin Jean Desormeaux (1815–82) from Paris constructed a universal endoscope, which for a time created great expectations. He used a gazogen lamp as the source of light. Several surgeons improved the instrument, in particular Francis

Cruise of Dublin, and it then became of some diagnostic and therapeutic value in patients with diseases of the urethra. It could also be used to confirm the diagnosis of stones in the bladder. The examination was not in actual fact a cystoscopy, as it was far from possible to inspect the whole of the inside of the bladder. The instrument was, however, only used by specially enthusiastic surgeons.

In 1841 the Finnish physician Gustav Samuel Crusell (1810–58) got the idea of using a glowing platinum thread (electrocauter, galvanocauter) for surgical burning, and the method was further developed in 1854 by the German Albrecht Theodor Middeldorf (1824–68). In 1866 Julius Bruck the younger (1840–1902) from Breslau demonstrated that it was possible to obtain light from a platinum thread, which was brought to glow by an electric current. A cooling system was used in order to prevent the thread burning through. Bruck first invented a stomatoscope for illuminating the oral cavity and the throat, and then a large lamp which he misleadingly called a urethroscope. The lamp was to be placed in the rectum or vagina, and in the opinion of Bruck it would then be possible to inspect the inside of the bladder wall through a catheter in indirect illumination. The lamp consisted of two glass tubes with the platinum thread in the inner one, and between the tubes water circulated to cool the wire.

The suggestion of Bruck was of no practical importance, but the idea was taken into use in another way: for a sort of examination of the internal female genitals. When the lamp was introduced into the vagina, it was just possible to discern the outlines of the uterus and ovaries through the abdominal wall. The method was called diaphanoscopy and was introduced in 1875 at the Stadtkrankenhause in Dresden by Julius Schramm.

Two years later a young doctor in Dresden, Maximilian Nitze (1848–1906), presented an instrument which he called 'kystoscope with device for enlargement of the field of vision'. The event took place at a meeting in the old Institute of Pathology, where he had carried out his experiments. Nitze demonstrated the instrument on a cadaver in which he had previously placed some stones in the bladder. Success was ensured, when one of the professors present could state that what he saw through the cystoscope was gall stones and not bladder stones. This was true, as Nitze had no other stones available at the time.

Nitze had participated in the diaphanoscopic experiments as an assistant to Dr. Schramm and was thus aquainted with Bruck's platinum thread lamp with cooling system. He found out that he would obtain a far better illumination if the source of light was introduced into the bladder 'in a similar way to bringing a candle with you when entering a dark room'. Nitze was also aware that it was necessary to enlarge the field of vision and considered that it could be done with a system of lenses. He thus thought that he had found the two principles which could really utilize the method of endoscopic examination. He allied himself with the university optician Bénèche from Berlin and with a local instrumentmaker Wilhelm Deicke, and the result of their work was the first experimental cystoscope, which was presented in Dresden in 1877. At the same time experiments were carried out with other endoscopes, among these the gastroscope and rectoscope.

The trial instrument was found to be useless. Mr. Deicke did not think that he had enough professional expertise to improve it – neither did he have means to pay for further experiments – and he therefore sent word to his colleague Josef Leiter

(1830–92) in Vienna. Nitze sent the construction plans to Leiter and made him an offer of co-operation, and negotiations were started when Leiter had decided that he could improve Nitze's inventions. In November 1878 he visited Nitze in Dresden, and the final result was that Leiter bought the patent rights; it was also agreed that Nitze should move to Vienna so they could work together in developing the instruments further. The two men co-operated there from the beginning of 1879, and they received permission to try out the endoscopes at the 3. University Clinic of Surgery under Professor Leopold von Dittel (1815–98). The public presentation took place at a meeting in Königliche Kaiserliche Gesellschaft der Aerzte in Wien on 9 May 1879.

Professor Dittel opened by demonstrating cystoscopy on a cadaver, and then together with Nitze on an eighteen-year-old man. Nitze demonstrated the various endoscopes for cystoscopy, urethroscopy and rectoscopy and gave a survey of the principal improvements that he had invented. Finally Leiter gave a detailed account of the technical construction of the instruments.

Reports of the new discovery created great expectations all over Europe. It was arranged that Nitze should procure and publish clinical material in order to judge the method, and he was offered patients from the three University Clinics of Surgery. Leiter was to publish a technical description of the endoscopes. So the future prospects looked bright.

For unknown reasons Nitze did not set to work, much to the dissatisfaction of Leiter. A dispute was brewing, and Nitze claimed that his absolute priority to the invention of the cystoscope was being challenged. It ended with a complete break and Nitze moved to Berlin, where he joined forces with the instrumentmaker Paul Hartwig (1846–1928), who started production of platinum thread cystoscopes.

Leiter published his technical description as a monograph in 1880, and then left on a business trip to present the cystoscope to the leading surgeons of the time. Theodor Billroth (1829–94) took care that Leiter was well received all over Europe.

The prominent surgeons were interested and bought cystoscopes – but to nearly all of them it proved a disappointment and they gave up further trials. Nitze continued his experiments in Berlin, but, judging from the literature, von Dittel's department in Vienna was the only one that employed cystoscopy and considered that some benefit was obtained from it.

In 1880 Thomas Alva Edison (1847–1931) invented the electric incandescent lamp, where the source of light was a carbon thread built into a glass-globe from which the air had been evacuated. The invention was rapidly taken into use in medical examination techniques, particularly within oto-rhino-laryngology. A cystoscope with an Edison lamp, however, was not forthcoming until 1887, when two models appeared almost at the same time, from Leiter and von Dittel in Vienna, and from Nitze and Hartwig in Berlin. Both were an improvement of the original platinum thread cystoscope.

Von Dittel started clinical trials in January 1887 with an incandescent lamp cystoscope constructed by Leiter, and the instrument was presented at a meeting on 11 March. At a meeting in January 1887 Nitze stated that he had experimented with the incandescent lamp but had returned to the platinum thread which he found to be better. Nevertheless he published two months later an article on a cystoscope with Edison lamp, which had been constructed together with Hartwig. Argument started again as to who had the priority. Leiter's instrument had certain advantages for instance the electric bulb was placed in a closed house, while it was unprotected in Nitze's model and could therefore break within the bladder.

A reliable and really serviceable cystoscope was now available since the troublesome cooling mechanism had become superfluous, and the method of cystoscopic examination was taken into daily use by the leading surgical departments. A large number of technical improvements soon followed. In 1887 Alexander Brenner (1859–1936) designed a cystoscope for ureteral catheterization in women, but this procedure first became routine in men after Joaquin Albarran (1860–1912) in 1897 invented a small device to move the ureteral catheter up and down.

At the presentation of the platinum thread cystoscope in 1879 Nitze only very briefly referred to Bénèche and Deicke, while he mentioned Leiter in an extremely commendatory manner and emphasized that some important constructive improvements were Leiter's own intellectual property. As mentioned, a complete break between them occurred within a short time, for reasons unknown. When Leiter published his monographic description of the instruments he wrote in the introduction, that he only sought priority for the construction and completion of the serviceable instruments, carried out after he had been inspired by the ideas of Nitze. This was interpreted by Nitze as an attempt to deprive him of the priority for the invention of the cystoscope, and when in 1889 he published the first textbook of cystoscopy it was provided with a postscript which is unique because of its exceedingly controversial character. In vehement phrases Leiter was stamped as being mendacious, his conduct as morally degrading and his means as base.

It is difficult from the literature to estimate the dispute between Nitze and Leiter. Professor Erna Lesky has given me permission to study a collection of letters in the manuscript archives in the Institut für Geschichte der Medizin in Vienna. It consists of twenty-three letters from Nitze to Leiter from the years 1878 to 1880 (collection numbers 1 to 23), two drafts of a letter from Leiter to Nitze (coll. nos. 24 and 25), three letters from Bénèche to Leiter (coll. nos. 27, 28, 29), four from Deicke to Leiter (coll. nos. 30, 31, 32, 33), and one from Billroth to Leiter (coll. no. 35).

The examination of these letters did not give enough information to clear up the matter, but contributed somewhat to an understanding of why the two men parted ways.

In the first letter dated 29 June 1878 Nitze writes to Leiter and tells of his invention and asks if he would consider taking over the practical work with application for patents in Austria and Hungary, together with production and distribution of the endoscopes. From the following letters it can be seen that Leiter showed his interest and soon started to improve the instruments. A visit to Nitze in Dresden also seems to have been planned. In a letter dated 6 October 1878 Nitze apologizes for not having answered letters and admits that Leiter has reason for being angry. Nitze also has to confess that he lacks money and he asks Leiter to pay the expenses connected with the patents. In several letters Nitze presses Leiter to arrange a meeting in Dresden, and on one occasion he begs most humbly for it.

It can be established that the meeting took place in the period between 12 and 26 November 1878 in Dresden, and that a draft of an agreement for future co-operation was discussed. Nitze demanded as his part 20 per cent of the retail price of the endoscopes, and considered that he got a verbal agreement to this at the meeting.

Nitze mentions with regret, that there was some bad feeling at the end, but does not give any details. On 30 November 1878 Nitze writes to say that he will not accept the final offer of Leiter of 15 per cent of the retail price. Nitze expresses his anxiety with regard to the business side of the matter; he would rather continue to co-operate without any financial connexion, and for this reason he offers Leiter to buy all the rights for a lump sum.

The next letter is dated 6 January 1879 and is written in Vienna, where Nitze now resides. It is very cool in its tone, and it is obvious that there has been some disagreement as Nitze 'for the last time' requests that his experimental models be returned, and he threatens to approach his lawyer. The time for Nitze's arrival to Vienna can be fixed to the latter half of December 1878, as is evident from two letters from Deicke to Leiter dated 11 and 12 December 1878. It can also be seen that Deicke has payed Nitze 600 guilders on behalf of Leiter.

The disagreement which finds expression in the letter of 6 January seems to have been of short duration, as they sign a contract on 20 February 1879 to the effect that Leiter takes over all rights for a sum of 5,000 guilders. The co-operation appears to have otherwise been harmonious as is reflected in the only letter written during the following months. Nitze left Vienna for a few days in March and wrote from Eisenach, that many colleagues had admired the instruments produced by Leiter, similarly they congratulated Nitze on having found such a man to complete his invention.

As mentioned Nitze praised Leiter greatly in May 1879, when the cystoscope was presented publicly. It was agreed that Leiter should write a monograph on the technical side of the matter, while Nitze should carry out the clinical trials and publish his results. This, however, he did not accomplish. In a very formal letter dated 1 July 1879 Nitze writes that the arrangement was that he should have the necessary aids and instruments for the clinical work. Obviously he has not received them as he now asks if he can buy them. He got an answer the same day and writes again on 2 July. From this letter it appears that Leiter has refused to sell him any instruments, and possibly has threatened to do everything in his power to harm Nitze in the future. Nitze will not submit to such treatment and suggests that they meet alone. On 9 July he again asks permission to buy instruments, just as he inquires about an instalment which is due according to the contract on the sale of the rights. On 4 October and again on the 5th Nitze writes, begging that he might buy instruments as he has still not obtained any.

Finally on 2 November 1879 he has received a cystoscope, but with very poor lenses which he wants to have exchanged.

A draft of a letter from Leiter to Nitze dated 7 January 1880 puts a stop to the row of letters from Nitze. Leiter offers to sell back all the rights for 10,000 guilders. At the same time he returns the original experimental instruments (model Nitze/Deicke) – as mentioned Nitze had asked to get them back already in January 1879.

Unfortunately we lack the second half of the correspondence, all the letters (but one) from Leiter to Nitze. They were possibly amongst the personal papers left behind by Nitze and deposited in Berlin. However, these disappeared in the hectic months of 1945 after the fall of Berlin.

It will probably never be possible to give a complete explanation of the relationship between Nitze and Leiter. Maybe the cause of the break should be sought in the personality of the two men. Leiter was a self-educated man, who won a position for himself as the leading instrumentmaker of Central Europe. He was industrious and valued work higher than everything, and his only ambition was to prove his professional skill and win recognition for his achievements. Nitze was introvert by nature, and was difficult to get on with; he did not fit into an ordinary environment. The dispute placed them in the wrong light in the eyes of their contemporaries – as Edwin Hurry Fenwick (1856–1944) wrote: 'Neither space, inclination, nor accurate knowledge permit me to enter into the details of the quarrel between Dr. Nitze and Mr. Leiter, which is now distracting somewhat from the real credit of the invention'.

The history of cystoscopy begins with Bozzini, who in 1805–7 put forward important principles for a method of examination of body cavities. Desormeaux constructed in 1853 the first usable endoscope and is therefore called the father of endoscopy. Nitze deserves the honour of having invented the method of cystoscopy, based on his platinum thread kystoscope from 1877. The new and most important feature was the system of lenses permitting enlargement of the field of vision, and the placing of the source of light in such a manner that it could be introduced into the bladder. It is, however, reasonable that Leiter is given a place in this history since he added many technical improvements to the instrument and manufactured the first specimen which was of real practical use. The history of the invention and development of cystoscopic instruments shows that a new era was on the way: with growing demands for a more refined technique, the demarcation between the contributions of the physician and the technician is becoming obliterated.

F. Schultze-Seemann
Berlin (West Germany)

Verbesserungen der Cystoskope nach Nitze's Erfindung
(Vorwiegend im deutschsprachigen Raum)

Bis in die achtziger Jahre des vorigen Jahrhunderts war in der vorcystoskopischen Zeit die Urologie nur ein Gebiet von engbegrenztem Umfang. Dittel in Wien, Sir Henry Thompson in London und Guyon in Paris führten durch ihre bewundernswürdige klinische Beobachtungsgabe und ihre operative Kunst – Nitze in Berlin durch die epochemachende Erfindung der Cystoskopie- eine wesentliche Erweiterung des Fachgebietes herbei. Seinem ersten Instrument hafteten aber noch viele technische Mängel an, die dringend der Verbesserung bedurften. Sicher lag auch hierin mit ein Grund, daß sich die Methode der Blasenspiegelung zunächst so schwer durchsetzen konnte.

Während der Physiker Helmholtz 1851 mit seinem Augenspiegel sofort ein technisch perfektes Instrument schuf und v. Graefe damit das Fach Augenheilkunde unter Abspaltung von der Chirurgie relativ schnell auf eigene Füße stellen konnte, ging diese Entwicklung in der Urologie, speziell in Deutschland, wesentlich langsamer vor sich.

Dies konnte erst ab 1886 nach Einführung der Mignonlampe geschehen: Damit wurde das ursprünglich starkkalibrige und unhandliche Cystoskop Nitze's für die Praxis anwendbar, die Grundvoraussetzung für die Möglichkeit seiner technischen Weiterentwicklung.

Zunächst wurden, da sich bei kranken Blasen leicht Eiter, Schleim oder Blut auf das Prisma legte, die *sog. Irrigationscystoskope* konstruiert, bei denen nach Einführung des Instrumentes das Prisma durch einen darüber hingehenden Wasserstrahl gereinigt wurde. 1895 führte Güterbock in Berlin ein anderes Prinzip des Irrigationscystoskops ein. Zum Unterschied gegenüber dem Nitze'schen waren hier Lampe, Prisma und Fernrohr in einem Mandrin eingearbeitet, der in einen in die Blase eingeführten Metallkatheter eingeschoben wurde, nachdem diese zuvor durch einen in dem Metallkatheter befindlichen Mandrin klargespült worden war.

Eine weitere technische Verbesserung führte Schlagintweit ein. Seine Modifikation bestand darin, daß eine Spülvorrichtung angebracht wurde, die durch einfache Hahnregulierung zu betätigen war. Dieses Instrument – sinnreich konstruiert – wurde der Vorläufer des seit 1907 allgemein gebräuchlichen Ringleb'schen Irrigationscystoskops. Der dabei angegebene Ventilklappenverschluß hat sich so bewährt, daß er bis heute noch im Gebrauch ist.

Als ein besonderer Nachteil wurde empfunden, daß mit allen diesen Cystoskopen einzelne Partien der Blase – speziell in der Umgebung des Sphincters und an der

Blasenhinterwand – nicht ausreichend eingesehen werden konnten. Schon Nitze hatte mehrere Versuche unternommen, um diesem Übelstand Abhilfe zu schaffen. Die entscheidende Lösung zur Sphincterbesichtigung gelang jedoch erst 1903 dem Münchener Urologen Schlagintweit mit seinem retrograden Cystoskop: Führte man dessen Optik ganz in den Schaft ein, so wurde ein besonderes Klapprisma am Okular herausgeschoben, womit der Blaseneingang besichtigt werden konnte.

1927 griff der jüngste Nitze-Schüler Jahr die Idee eines Rückblick-Cystoskopes in seinem sog. Proretro-Spiegelcystoskop wieder auf. Solange jedoch die 90°-Optik beibehalten wurde, gehörte auch die hintere Blasenwand trotz aller Variationsversuche noch zum toten Winkel der Cystoskopie. Bereits 1926 hatte deshalb Jahr die 90°-Optik durch eine 110°-Stumpfwinkeloptik ersetzt, wodurch jetzt die Besichtigung der Blasenrückwand und damit die lückenlose Cystoskopie möglich war.

Ein ganz wesentliches Problem der alten Urologen lag in dem unzulänglichen optischen System, das der Berliner Optiker Bénèche für Nitze konstruiert hatte und das seitdem unverändert geblieben war. Dadurch waren die Blasenbilder nicht in ihrer natürlichen Lage, sondern spiegelverkehrt zu sehen. Der erste, dem endlich im März 1907 eine Aufhebung der Bildumkehrung gelang, war der Berliner Optiker Kollmorgen. Zuvor hatte noch 1904 der Nitze-Schüler Jacoby mit seinem Stereocystoskop eine merkliche Erhöhung der Tiefenwahrnehmung in der Blase versucht. Auch diese Bilder waren jedoch noch seitenverkehrt und relativ lichtschwach. Dieses Stereocystoskop hat sich daher innerhalb des urologischen Instrumentariums nicht weiter durchgesetzt.

Zur Verbesserung des optischen Systems ging Ringleb – ein weiterer Nitze-Schüler – ab 1909 den einzigen folgerichtigen Weg, indem er sich mit der Fa. Zeiss-Jena in Verbindung setzte. In enger Zusammenarbeit mit dem dortigen Abteilungsleiter Professor v. Rohr wurde ein neues optisches System entwickelt, mit dem aufrechte und seitengleiche Bilder und durch doppelte Umkehr eine weitaus größere Lichtstärke erreicht wurden. Ringleb liess 1923 außerdem Farbfilter zum Vorsatz vor das Okular des einfachen Untersuchungscystoskops konstruieren, um die Tiefenwahrnehmung in der Blase zu steigern. – Seit Anfang 1925 führte der schon oben erwähnte Jahr in Zusammenarbeit mit der Fa. Heynemann kürzere Lampen für Cystoskope unter gleichzeitiger Verkürzung ihrer sogenannten „schädlichen" Länge ein, was besonders für Blasen kleinen Fassungsvermögens von größter Wichtigkeit war. Jahr's Prioritätsrechte wurden aber später bestritten. So soll schon zwei Jahrzehnte zuvor Israel in Berlin ein Instrument mit sehr verkürzter Schnabel – form konstruiert haben, desgleichen unabhängig von ihm Pilcher in den U.S.A., 1909.

1933 gab Usadel die Konstruktion eines Dauer-Irrigationscystoskops bekannt, mit dem bereits Klarspülung und Auffüllung der Blase während der Cystoskopie möglich waren. Der endgültige Übergang von der sog. statischen zur dynamischen Cystoskopie gelang dann durch die Strahlcystoskope nach May und Heynemann 1952.

Die in den letzten Jahren neu berechneten optischen Systeme haben zu einer kaum noch zu überbietenden Bildqualität geführt. Aber auch hier ist durch Einführung der Glasfiber-Optik noch eine weitere Vereinfachung durch Fortfall der endovesicalen Lampe am Cystoskop eingetreten. Die Lichtquelle befindet sich jetzt wieder außerhalb des Cystokops wie beim Erfinder des Lichtleiters Philipp Bozzini

1806. So hat sich über einen Zeitraum von 160 Jahren der Kreis zur ursprünglichen Idee wieder geschlossen.

Neben dieser Entwicklung der einfachen Übersichtscystoskopie mußten für die nun notwendigen und möglichen diagnostischen und therapeutischen Eingriffe noch besondere Cystoskopmodelle konstruiert werden. Denn der Ausbau dieser Methode fiel gleichzeitig zusammen mit der sich stürmisch entwickelnden Nierenchirurgie. Sie verlangte nach einer möglichst exakten praeoperativen Seitenlokalisierung der Nierenerkrankung. Das 1894 von Nitze geschaffene Uretercystoskop zur Sondierung des einzelnen Harnleiters hatte sich infolge seiner feststehenden Krümmung in der Praxis nicht bewährt. –

Das erste wirklich brauchbare Uretercystoskop legte im Januar 1895 der Berliner Urologe Casper vor. Durch eine auf der Oberseite des Instrumentes einzusetzende Rinne mit Schiebedeckel konnte Casper dem Ureterkatheter die für die Einführung in den Harnleiter notwendige Winkelung geben. Außerdem konnten die Katheter im Harnleiter liegenbleiben, während das Cystoskop herausgenommen wurde. Der Harn jeder einzelnen Niere konnte nun gesondert aufgefangen und untersucht werden. Casper wurde dadurch zusammen mit dem Berliner Richter einer der Begründer der funktionellen Nierendiagnostik.

Nach Entdeckung der Röntgenstrahlen und Einführung der retrograden Kontrastdarstellung des Nierenbeckens durch Voelcker und v. Lichtenberg im Jahre 1905 erfuhr die urologische Diagnostik zusätzlich einen ungeahnten Aufschwung.

Inzwischen hatte 1897 der Pariser Urologe Albarran das retrograde Cystoskop mit dem Schiebedeckel durch die Einführung, des sog. Katheterhebels wesentlich vervollkommnet, den Jahr 1925 noch durch Fensterung verbesserte. In dieser Form ist er bis heute noch in Gebrauch.

Das alte Casper'sche Uretercystoskop wurde von ihm selbst 1908 auch zu operativen Zwecken ausgebaut. Nitze's erste Veröffentlichung eines Operationscystoskopes stammte schon aus dem Jahre 1891, während die eingehende Beschreibung erst 1895 erfolgte: Es bestand aus einer Drahtschlinge zum Abschnüren größerer und einer Platiniridium-Elektrode zum Koagulieren kleinerer Tumoren.

Das Verdienst, die Entfernung von Blasentumoren mit der Drahtschlinge häufiger ausgeführt zu haben, gebührt besonders Schlagintweit. Er benutzte dazu seit 1900 ein Uretercystoskop als Operationsinstrument und legte damit eine Nickeldrahtschlinge um den Tumor, die nach Entfernung des Cystoskopes alle zwei Stunden weiter zugeschnürt wurde, so daß der Tumor meist nach 24 Stunden spontan abging. Blieb der Erfolg bei dieser Behandlung aus, mußte die Schlinge zur Tumorzerstörung glühend gemacht werden.

Die gutartigen Papillome der Harnblase wurden nun mit zunehmender cystoskopischer Beobachtung viel häufiger festgestellt, als man früher angenommen hatte. Die entscheidende Wendung in ihrer Bekämpfung brachte im Februar 1910 Edwin Beer [vom Mount Sinai-Hospital] aus New York, der erstmals gutartige Papillome mit dem (Oudin'schen) Hochfrequenzstrom zerstörte. Ein sehr wichtiger Schritt in der Bekämpfung der Blasentumoren war damit getan.

Eine andere Anwendungsmöglichkeit bot der weitere Ausbau der Operationscystoskope zur Bekämpfung der Blasensteine. Hier hatte 1824 Civiale in Paris den bis dahin geübten Steinschnitt durch Einführung der blinden Lithotrypsie abgelöst, die durch ihn und die folgenden Urologen zu großer Vollkommenheit gebracht wurde.

Bigelow in Boston gelang 1875 ein weiterer Fortschritt durch Einführung der Litholapaxie. In einer Sitzung wurden nun die Steine zertrümmert und vollständig aus der Blase abgesaugt. Die postoperative Mortalität und Infektionsgefahr konnte entschieden gesenkt werden. Während die Diagnose „Blasenstein" vor Nitze's Erfindung nur durch Fühlen und Ausmessen mit der Steinsonde gestellt werden konnte, erfolgte diese seit Nitze mit dem Cystoskop.

Der Übergang von der blinden zur optischen Lithotrypsie ging jedoch nicht schnell vonstatten. Dies hatte zwei Gründe: Um eine Bruchfestigkeit des Instrumentes zu erzielen, mußte sein Querschnitt vergrößert werden, da die Optik noch zusätzlich eingefügt werden mußte. Die Instrumente konnten daher nur sehr starkkalibrig oder sehr wenig bruchsicher sein.

Der Urologe Kneise in Halle konnte nun seit 1908 beginnend in Zusammenarbeit mit Heynemann-Leipzig eine Fremdkörperzange entwickeln, die die Lithotrypsie kleiner Steine unter Leitung des Auges ermöglichte. Nach Verbesserung der Zangenbacken durch Einführung besseren und härteren Stahles war diese Kneise-Heywalt-Blasensteinzange lange Jahre in Gebrauch.

Ähnlich Kneise hatte schon der Berliner Urologe Schwenk 1910 einen cystoskopischen Lithotryptor, der eine Kombination eines Lithotryptors mit einem Spülcystoskop darstellte, publiziert. Eine ähnliche Kombination gab auch Young aus Baltimore im Jahre 1911 an. Beide gingen von dem Prinzip der Fremdkörperzange aus. Nur waren die Zangenbacken erstmalig nicht wie beim blinden Lithotryptor in der Längsrichtung sondern quer, also zangenartig, beweglich. Durch eine seitliche Anbringung der Optik zu den Backen des Instrumentes durch den Engländer Canny-Ryall konnten diese Zangenbacken nun auch bei weiter Öffnung übersehen werden. Alle diese Instrumente wurden seit 1931 durch die Einführung der v. Lichtenberg-Heywalt-Blasensteinzange wesentlich verbessert. In Ergänzung dazu wurde im gleichen Jahre das Morgenstern-Dauerspülcystoskop geschaffen, mit dem die Steintrümmer wesentlich schmerzloser abgesaugt werden konnten.

Früh tauchte schon der Gedanke auf, das in der Blase Gesehene zu Lehrzwecken und zur Dokumentation photographisch festzuhalten. Erste Versuche unternahm 1889 v. Antal in Budapest. Die ersten, wenn auch noch sehr unscharfen Bilder gelangen Kutner 1891 in Berlin. Nitze's Photocystoskop wies dagegen wesentliche Verbesserungen durch stärkeres Kaliber, wirksamere Lampen und eine praktischere Suchereinrichtung auf. In seinem 1894 veröffentlichten „Kystophotographischen Atlas" waren die Bilder jedoch noch recht unscharf bedingt durch die Grobkörnigkeit der photographischen Platte, die sich bei der notwendigen Vergößerung für den Atlas sehr störend bemerkbar machte.

Seit 1905 hatte der Nitze-Schüler Jacoby die stereophotographische Methode ausgearbeitet. Er wandte dabei gemeinsame Winkelsysteme an, die eine größere Lichtstärke gestatteten. Seine Arbeitsergebnisse legte er 1911 in seinem „Lehrbuch der Kystoskopie und Stereophotographischen Atlas" vor. Diese Methode konnte sich nicht durchsetzen, da die Bilder keine Verbesserungen gegenüber denen von Nitze und Casper aufwiesen und Einzelheiten z. T. nicht erkennbar waren.

Einen wirklich brauchbaren kystophotographischen Atlas schufen erst 1913 Fromme und Ringleb unter Verwendung der inzwischen von Zeiss-Jena wesentlich verbesserten optischen Systeme. Das Buch galt zwei Jahrzehnte lang als unübertroffenes Standardwerk auf diesem Gebiet. Fromme hatte auch 1908 die ersten

Versuche zu Farbaufnahmen in der Blase unternommen. Die Ergebnisse waren jedoch bei dem sehr groben Korn der damaligen Farbfilme recht unbefriedigend. Erst nach Schaffung feinkörnigerer Farbfilme konnte Ringleb Mitte der dreißiger Jahre brauchbare Farbdiapositive der Harnblase vorlegen.

Immer schon hatte die vergrößerte Prostata ein besonderes Problem dargestellt. Um dieses Hindernis auf transurethralem Wege zu beseitigen, wurden zunächst katheterförmige Messer angegeben, bei deren Anwendung aber starke Nachblutungen aufgetreten waren. Daher empfahl Bottini 1874 in Padua die galvanokaustische Methode mit Platinplättchen zur Einkerbung der Prostata. 1887 wurde diese Methode in Deutschland durch Freudenberg eingeführt, der 1897 eine eigene Modifikation des Bottini'schen Prostataincisors vorlegen konnte. Die 1913 von Luys konstruierte „Forage" zur Verschorfung des vorstehenden Prostatagewebes und das von Young 1913 geschaffene Cold-Punch-Gerät, sowie das von Thompson, waren noch z. T. blind arbeitende Instrumente oder zur direkten Sicht wie beim Rektoskop ohne Linsensystem konstruiert. Der Vorteil dieser Punch-Geräte lag in der glatten Schnittfläche ohne Nekrosen; ihr Nachteil wiederum in der z.T. recht starken Nachblutung. Aus diesem Grunde empfahlen Bumpus die vorherige Koagulation der Prostata und Caulk 1920 statt der kalten Stanze einen elektrischen Kauter. Von Kirwin wurde ein sog. Rotary-Resektoskop zur Resektion speziell der Prostataseitenlappen konstruiert.

Das erste brauchbare Elektroresektoskop zur transurethralen Beseitigung der Prostatahypertrophie veröffentlichte 1926 Stern in den U.S.A. Unter Benutzung des Hochfrequenzstromes. Von Beer demonstrierte seine Methode 1930 an der Chirurgischen Universitätsklinik Berlin bei dem Urologen Joseph. Der unglückliche Ausgang zweier Operationen verzögerte zunächst die Einführung dieser Methode in Deutschland, für die besonders v. Lichtenberg eintrat. Bis dahin wurde in Deutschland vorwiegend die Elektrokoagulation der Prostata angewandt, während die Bottini'sche Incision zunehmend in den Hintergrund trat. Bei den nun folgenden heftigen Diskussionen um die richtige Methode äußerte u.a.der Hamburger Kropeit 1931, daß er schon seit 1909 – ähnlich den Amerikanern – mit der Hochfrequenztechnik gearbeitet hätte. 1911 hätte er mit der Fa. Reiniger, Gebbert und Schall ein Instrument entwickelt, bei dem es sich technisch „um die endoskopisch ausgeführte modifizierte Bottini'sche Operation, der aber die früheren Gefahren genommen sind", handelte. 1924 demonstrierte er auf dem 6. Deutschen Urologen-Kongreß in Berlin seinen flexiblen Unterwasser-Kaltkauter als Einsatz zum Irrigationsurethroskop nach Goldschmidt. Damit konnte unter Leitung des Auges, Vermeidung von Nebenverletzungen und weitgehender Ausschaltung der Blutungen durch den kaustischen Schnitt operiert werden.

Das ursprüngliche Stern'sche Instrument wurde 1932 durch MacCarthy und den amerikanischen Instrumentenbauer Whappler als Stern-MacCarthy-Instrument herausgebracht. In Deutschland hatte v. Lichtenberg zusammen mit der Fa. Heynemann 1932 das v. Lichtenberg-Heywalt'sche Blasenhalsinstrumentarium konstruiert und damit die breitere Anwendung der Prostataresektionen ermöglicht.

Die fehlende Lichtquelle am Elektrotom, die zu kleine Schlinge und der noch zu enge Spülkanal, der oft verstopft war, liess im Höchstfall nur die Resektion bis zu 15g Prostatagewebe zu. Diese Mängel beseitigte das seit 1937 in Gebrauch befindliche Staehler-Heywalt-Blasenhals-Elektroschneidgerät. Durch Anbringung zweier

Lampen war bessere Sicht und damit auch leichtere Blutstillung möglich; mit größerer Schlinge und stärkerer Spülung konnte mehr Gewebe reseziert werden. –

Betrachtet man die Entwicklung all dieser Cystoskopmodifikationen, dann ist abschließend zu sagen, daß Nitze außer einem Prostata-Operationsgerät alle anderen Entwicklungen richtig vorausgesehen und dafür z.T. schon grundsätzliche Modelle geschaffen hatte. Die nachfolgenden Urologen und ihre Instrumentenbauer haben in langer Entwicklungsarbeit diese Grundtypen dann zu dem reichhaltigen Cystoskop- und transurethralen Operationsinstrumentarium ausgebaut, das uns heute zur Verfügung steht.

B. Lieberman
Oakland, California (U.S.A.)

Morgagni's syndrome – the evolution of an eponym

Medicine and the medical sciences abound in eponyms – proper names applied to anatomic parts, physiological phenomena, micro-organisms, laboratory or clinical tests, surgical procedures, syndromes, signs, and innumerable diseases. A recent compilation by Jablonski refers to 10,000 eponyms.[1] Stedman's *Medical Dictionary* lists 265 syndromes.[2] The names are usually those of physicians whose subsequent fame depends on the tissue, test or treatment by which the student knows them.

In 1935 a woman, aged forty-one years, came to a hospital clinic in a mid-western state. She complained of chronic headache, dizziness, ringing in the ears, weakness and numbness in the hands, all of which bothered her for about two years. Her family history was not significant. Examination disclosed only mild hypertension and obesity of moderate degree. The usual laboratory tests and spinal fluid examination yielded normal findings. Roentgen examination of the skull showed marked thickening of the frontal bone with some increased thickening of the calvarium as a whole. She was observed in the clinic over the years as an example of hyperostosis frontalis interna (HFI), or Morgagni's Syndrome.

Twenty-six years later, in 1961, she developed diabetes mellitus. Periodic roentgen examinations did now show progression of the skull thickening. She died in July 1963 of diabetic vascular complications at age sixty-nine.

She was the proposita of a family kindred of three generations with HFI, consisting of four daughters and a granddaughter. Two of the daughters were obese and also developed diabetes. One of these developed hypo-thyroidism and a psychiatric disorder unrelated to the thyroid condition. A third daughter developed rheumatoid arthritis. The two diabetic patients died in March 1970 and November 1971 of diabetic vascular complications, age fifty-one and fifty-five years respectively. Unfortunately, periodic skull roentgen examinations on the daughters were not possible, but at a three-year follow-up on three of the four daughters there was no progression in the skull thickening.

The granddaughter was found to have no signs of HFI at age fourteen, early signs at seventeen, with considerable increase at age twenty-two. A growth hormone assay done in December 1966 was found to be within the normal range. This conforms with the findings in nine patients with the Morgagni syndrome reported in 1966 in the German literature by Weinheimer and Bruhl.[3] Comparing the growth hormone levels in obese patients without the syndrome, they concluded that a distinct relationship could not be proven.

In 1935, the same year when the index case was first seen in the clinic, Dr. Sherwood Moore of St. Louis presented a radiological exhibit at the annual convention of the American Medical Association. It was entitled '. . . a new metabolic disorder and its pathognomonic signs in the skull'. Surveys of several thousand films showed 3.5 per cent of them with HFI. He also presented a paper on 'A clinical syndrome with radiologic lesions in the frontal bone'. In 1936 he proposed the term 'metabolic craniopathy' to encompass all the features of the syndrome, with emphasis on the conspicuous skull changes.[4] His interest and extensive research in this field culminated in the publication of his monograph in 1955, entitled *Hyperostosis cranii*.[5]

Although workers in palaeopathology have discovered skulls of many centuries ago showing HFI,[6] all writers on the subject credit the first medical report in an autopsy examination by Giovanni Battista Morgagni. This is recorded in his historic treatise, *De Sedibus et Causis Morborum per anatomen indagatis libri quinque*, or 'The seats and causes of diseases investigated by anatomy'. The work was published in 1761, when Morgagni was seventy-nine years old. The eponymic case report deserves extended quotation from the 1769 English translation of Dr. Benjamin Alexander (1736–68).[7] 'A woman of seventy-five years of age, of manly aspect, and very fat, having been quite slender to her five-and-fortieth year, was in the latter years of her life, become a valetudinarian; yet in such a manner as never to complain of a pain in her head, much less of any violent indisposition that could be referr'd thereto; but she rather complain'd of other things, among which her acquaintance, though but little accustom'd to attend minutely to these lamentations of a querulous old woman, particularly mention'd a kind of swoonings, as it were, and other disorders of that kind.'

The autopsy revealed as the likely cause of her death a ruptured left ventricular aneurysm. He continues, '. . . at length having open'd the cranium, we found the dura mater to be so much more closely affix'd to the sutures . . . than it generally is that it could not be pull'd away without laceration . . . the os frontis was prominent in that part, in the form of very frequent tuberosities: and the same kind of appearances were also in the basis of the cranium, especially on the petrose processes . . . all these tuberosities were made up of a more white substance than the bones in any other part of the cranium were; so that they seemed to consist of a new accession and, as it were, an effusion of bony matter'.

Morgagni offers an explanation of possible symptoms from the new bone within the cranial cavity by saying, '. . . and though the surface of each of these prominences was very smooth, and shining, yet the very great inequality and exhuberating state of them all, could not but extremely compress the brain, wherein there appear'd to be, in other respects, no kind of injury, in what part soever it corresponded with these tuberosities. The dura mater show'd no mark of injury in itself where it cover'd these tuberosities; nor did it adhere to them very closely as it did to some other certain parts of the cranium'.

More knowledge about Morgagni's original finding came slowly. There were isolated case reports of 'osteo-phytes' on the inner surface of the calvarium and considerable speculation as to their nature. In the latter part of the nineteenth century British reports associating the skull findings at autopsy with psychiatric symptoms during life in women proposed a possibly significant etiologic relationship. With the recent availability of roentgenologic examinations on a large scale, surveys among apparently normal populations, homes for the aged, and persons in general and psychiatric hospitals yielded evidence to warrant a clinical association between the radiologic findings and symptoms in some instances, but a negative association in others. Ferdinand Morel in 1930,[8] is credited with the first diagnosis during life; he emphasized the psychiatric symptoms. Folke Henschen suggested in 1936, that the condition be called Morgagni's syndrome in a paper so titled.[9]

Two reference sources, *Index Medicus* and *Current Medical Information and Terminology* of the American Medical Association[10] give primary listing under the anatomic feature of 'hyperostosis, frontal, internal'. *Index Medicus* also carries the eponyms of Morgagni and Morel while the American Medical Association publication also carries the sub-eponyms of Stewart–Morel and Morel–Moore syndromes. Recognition is accorded the priority of Morgagni's report, and his eponym should be used when the anatomic feature occurs in women in association with symptoms of obesity, headache, vertigo, diabetes, or psychiatric disorders suggesting an organic brain syndrome.

Familial occurrence of the condition has attracted considerable interest, with such reports as that by Knies and LeFever[11] in a mother and three daughters. In the present state of our incomplete knowledge the medical geneticist Dr. Victor McKusick considers 'the condition may be dominant, but whether autosomal or X-linked is not known'.[12] It is probable that hereditary cases with asymptomatic skull findings only may be more prevalent than reports would indicate. Because of its predominance in females it must be considered as X-controlled if not X-linked.

Who is the man behind this eponym as well as the twenty-nine other eponyms that carry his name?[13, 14, 15] Morgagni was born in the town of Forli, province of Romanga, in northern Italy in 1682. At sixteen, in 1698, he became a medical student at the University of Bologna and worked with Antonio Valsalva, also of eponymic fame, in his research on the anatomy of the ear, published in 1704. After six years of study, Morgagni was graduated in 1704 with degrees in medicine and philosophy. Biographers refer to his election as president of a student group known as 'Academia Inquietorum'. Literally translated, it was the 'Academy of the Restless', not concerned with socio-political issues as might be expected today, but devoted to search for scientific truth.

From 1706 to 1719 Dr. Morgagni issued a series of publications entitled *Adversaria Anatomica* or anatomical notebooks based on his early investigations in this field. In 1715, at thirty-three, he was appointed Professor of Anatomy at Padua. But the crowning accomplishment of his fifty-six years at Padua, to the time of his death in 1771 at eighty-nine, was the publication in 1761 of one of the great works in medicine, *De Sedibus et Causis Morborum*. This was issued in Latin in the form of seventy letters to a young friend. The letters were revised for publication of the books in Venice. The material in the letters carries some homely information about the patients, as well as the detailed findings in almost 700 autopsies, arranged mainly by bodily regions – diseases of head, thorax, abdomen, surgical diseases, those of the whole body. The work contains an extensive index. The patient identified with the HFI syndrome is described in Book 2, Epistle 27.[6] Excerpts from his writings in English translation[16] as well as the entire *De Sedibus* are available for the English-language reader in a new edition published in 1960 under the editorship of the late Dr. Paul Klemperer (1887–1964).[16] Though his biographers attribute about thirty eponyms, mostly anatomical, to Morgagni, he is undoubtedly best known and most frequently referred to by the hyperostosis syndrome. But his name is also identified, because of his original descriptions, with several common clinical conditions met with by physicians in daily practice – lung changes in pneumonia, cirrhosis of the liver, heart-block, coronary sclerosis, rupture of aortic aneurysm, mitral stenosis and the familial occurrence of apoplexy, suggesting the familial or genetic factor in hypertension.[14]

In the two centuries since his death Morgagni has come to be recognized as the founder of pathological anatomy, the study of grossly visible organ changes resulting from disease, or the 'seat' of disease.[19] Today he is accorded the distinction of being at the head of a lineage that includes Marie Xavier Bichat (1771–1802), who emphasized the changes in tissues resulting from disease; Dr. Rudolf Virchow (1821–1902), and his theory of the cell in disease mechanisms, and Sir Archibold Garrod (1857–1936), in relation to molecular abnormalities[18] and the numerous biochemical disorders that have been discovered in the past sixty years as a result of rapidly expanding knowledge in genetics. In the words of Dr. Klemperer, 'Morgagni's great work gave strength to and confidence in the reliability of the perceived facts established by pathologic anatomic investigation and in the importance of their correlation with observation at the bedside.'[19]

Since 1930 single and collected case reports, especially in the European medical literature, have broadened the spectrum of the manifestations of the condition and offered clues to the understanding of its causation and treatment. In addition to the classical triad of obesity, virilism and hyperostosis, associated endocrine disorders have been noted, namely diabetes mellitus, diabetes insipidus, acromegaly, hyper- and hypo-thyroidism, vertigo and various psychiatric manifestations, all determinable by present-day tests.[20, 21]

Whether or not HFI is a clinical entity depends on the presence of clinical features in association with the skull changes, and nosological concepts applied to 'disease' criteria. Studies of 'normal' populations have the shortcoming of lacking long-term follow-up. While the condition remains etiologically unexplained, its cardinal features of its occurrence in women, familial incidence and the triad described by Morgagni led early observers to postulate pituitary dysfunction. In light of modern neuro-physiology one may invoke some aberrant function of the hypothalamus and its releasing factors as causative, as proposed in a recent experimental study. With the use of oestrogenic materials Dr. G. Rudale has succeeded in producing frontal hyperostosis in mice which he believes may be mediated through the hypothalamus.[22] A similar explanation with respect to the Albright syndrome has been advanced just this year.[23]

Though eponyms have become part of the physician's vocabulary, the tags on our verbal baggage, there is not unanimous agreement on their use. The American medical historian Fielding Garrison (1870–1935), was especially outspoken in his opposition. Writing in 1909, he labelled the eponym as 'Conceptual shorthand', but reluctantly conceded we should retain some eponyms, 'to awaken and stimulate a lively interest in the great names of medicine among ambitious, inquiring students whose minds are still in the plastic stage.'[24] With respect to Morgagni himself, Sir William Osler (1849–1919) was more specific in his advice in saying, 'I cannot too warmly commend to young clinicians the reading of Morgagni.'[25]

Two physicians deserve particular mention on the subject of eponyms. In writing on neurological tests, the late Dr. Robert Wartenberg of San Francisco (1887–1956) bemoans the profusion of proper names in his specialty and warns against the trend toward 'eponymania' by saying that 'we need more physiology and fewer eponyms'.[26] Having himself described a sign in cortico-spinal disease, he had an eponym thrust upon him.[27]

In 1937 Dr. Fuller Albright of Boston (1900–69) described an interesting endocrine condition with a title of seventeen words.[28] It was captioned 'Syndrome characterized by osteitis fibrose disseminate, areas of pigmentation and endocrine dysfunction with precocious puberty in females'. After four years another writer adopted the eponymic designation of Albright's syndrome, as it is still known today, despite Dr. Albright's protestation in 1947.[29] That is what happens when the discoverer is at a loss for words – succinct ones – to name his discovery.

Recent comments on eponyms are more tolerant. An editorial writer in the *Journal of the American Medical Association* on the 'Half life of eponyms' states that 'an important threat to the longevity of an eponym resides in the expanding knowledge of the disease which it designates. We like eponyms because they are convenient and commemorative, easy to remember and comfortingly familiar.'[30]

Eponyms in medicine are here to stay. Some may be consigned to the archives of medical literature, medical dictionaries and histories. When the ultimate 'causes of diseases' are as clearly definable as the 'seats' are presently, we shall be justified in replacing them with scientific terms. Until then eponyms deserve to be retained and used, so we may assign a measure of immortality to our professional forebears.

References

1 JABLONSKI, S., *Illustrated Dictionary of Eponymic Syndromes and Diseases and their Synonyms*, Philadelphia, W. B. Saunders, 1969.

2 *Stedman's Medical Dictionary*, 22nd ed., Baltimore, Williams & Wilkins, 1972.

3 WEINHEIMER, B. and BRUHL, P., 'Growth hormone concentration in the Morgagni syndrome', *Med. Welt.*, 1966, **34**, 1746–48.

4 MOORE, S., 'Metabolic craniopathy', *Amer. J. Roentgenol. Radium Ther.*, 1936, **35**, 30–39.

5 *Hyperostosis cranii*, Springfield, Illinois, C. C. Thomas, 1955.

6 ARMELAGOS, G. J., 'Disease in ancient Nubia', *Science*, 1969, **163**, 255–59.

7 MORGAGNI, G. B., *The Seats and Causes of Diseases*, trans. from the Latin by Benjamin Alexander, M.D., London, 1769.

8 MOREL, F., *Hyperostosis frontalis interna*, Paris, Gaston Doin, 1930.

9 HENSCHEN, F., 'Morgagni syndrome', *Hygeia*, 1936, **98**, 65–85.

10 *Current Medical Information and Terminology*, 4th ed., Chicago, American Medical Association, 1971, p. 193.

11 KNIES, P. T. and LEFEVER, H. E., 'Metabolic craniopathy: Hyperostosis Frontalis Interna', *Ann. int. Med.*, 1941, **14**, 1858–92.

12 MCKUSICK, V., *Mendelian Inheritance in Man*, 3rd ed., Baltimore, Johns Hopkins Press, 1971, p. 160.

13 TEDESCHI, C. G., 'Giovanni Battista Morgagni, the founder of pathologic anatomy', *Boston med. Quart.*, 1961, **12**, 112–25.

14 Editorial: 'Morgagni (1682–1771)', *J. Amer. med. Ass.*, 1964, **187**, 948–50.

15 CREIGHTON, C., 'Morgagni, Giovanni Battista (1682–1771)', *Encyclopedia Britannica*, 11th ed., New York, 1911, vol. 18, pp. 831–33.

16 KELLY, E. C., *Medical Classics*, 1940, **4**, 628–839.

17 *The Seats and Causes of Diseases investigated by Anatomy*; with a preface, introduction and a new translation of five letters, by Paul Klemperer, M.D., Sc.D., New York, Hafner, 1960.

18 GARROD, SIR ARCHIBALD E., *Inborn Errors of Metabolism*, London, H. Frowde, 1909.

19 KLEMPERER, P., 'Pathologic anatomy at the end of the eighteenth century', *J. Mt. Sinai Hosp.*, 1957, **24**, 589–603.

20 HARPMAN, J. A., 'Vestibulometry in a case of Morgagni-Stewart-Morel syndrome', *J. Laryngol, Otol.*, 1972, **8**, 43–62.
21 MOORE, M. T., 'The Morgagni-Stewart-Morel Syndrome. Report of a case with pneumoencephalographic findings', *Arch. int. Med.*, 1944, **73**, 7–12. (The findings showed 'pronounced cortical atrophy over the frontal and parietal lobes, atrophy of islands of Reil and moderately advanced internal hydrocephalus with assymetry and irregularity of the lateral ventricles.')
22 RUDALI, G., 'Experimental production of hyperostosis frontalis interna in mice', *Israel J. med. Sci.*, 1968, **4**, 1230–35.
23 HALL, R. and WARRICK, C., 'Hypersecretion of hypothalamic releasing hormones: a possible explanation of the endocrine manifestations of polyostotic fibrous dysplasia (Albright's syndrome)', *Lancet*, 1972, **i**, 1313–16.
24 GARRISON, F. H., 'Eponymic expressions in medical literature', *Boston med. surg. J.*, 1909, **161**, 618–22.
25 OSLER, SIR W., *The Evolution of Modern Medicine*, New Haven, Conn., Yale University Press, 1922, p. 188, footnote.
26 WARTENBERG, R., *Diagnostic Tests in Neurology*, Chicago, Year Book Publishers, 1953, p. 33.
27 BRAIN, LORD and WALTON, J. N., *Brain's Diseases of the Nervous System*, 17th ed., London, Oxford University Press, 1968, p. 22.
28 ALBRIGHT, F., BUTLER, A. M., HAMPTON, A. O., *et al.*, 'Syndrome characterized by osteitis fibrosa disseminata, areas of pigmentation and endocrine dysfunction, with precocious puberty in females, report of five cases', *New Engl. J. Med.*, 1937, **216**, 727–46.
29 ALBRIGHT, F., 'Polyostotic fibrous dysplasia: a defence of the entity', *J. clin. Endocrin.*, 1947, **17**, 307–24, p. 320.
30 SV, Editorial: 'Half life of eponyms', *J. Amer. med. Ass.*, 1970, **213**, 456.

D. Novak
Hamburg (West Germany)

Radiological diagnosis of brain tumours – a historical review

In the history of radiological evaluation of intracranial tumours, the following three periods of development might be distinguished: (1) diagnosis of brain tumours by means of plain X-ray films; (2) demonstration of intracranial masses by ventriculography, encephalography and cerebral angiography; (3) localization and diagnosis of intracranial lesions with the aid of brain scanning.

The X-ray study of the skull in early days of roentgenology was unsatisfactory. There was the difficult problem of differentiating tissue changes within superimposed structure of the same density. The roentgenological diagnosis and localization of intracranial tumours was mainly restricted to the cases in which the neoplasm had affected the skull. It was only the calcified area of the tumour that could be differentiated from normal cerebral tissue by X-rays.

Probably the first attempt to diagnose an intracranial tumour roentgenologically is to be attributed to Obici and Bollici.[20] Obici and Bollici experimented post-mortem with a large tumour of the temporal region. Oppenheim found experimentally that tumour mass put into the skull could be differentiated within the brain tissue. It was also Oppenheim who confirmed roentgenologically the diagnosis of a pituitary tumour as far back as 1897.[11, 21] The case of a calcified brain tumour demonstrated on the plain X-ray film was described in 1899 by Lichtheim.[15] The first attempt to demonstrate a cerebellar tumour was described by Church in 1899.[7] In 1902 Fittig[10] published the case of a calcified glioma in a nine-year-old child. The roentgenological findings were confirmed by operation and autopsy. Also Benedikt published two cases of intracerebral masses demonstrated with X-ray film.[3] Mills and Pfahler reported in 1902 on a tumour of the brain diagnosed clinically and roentgenologically.[16] Schüller was the first to recognize the importance of the displaced calcified pineal gland as a valuable sign of an intracranial lesion. Further cases of roentgenologically diagnosed pituitary tumours were published by Albers-Schönberg.[1] Henschen found that acoustic neuromas widened the internal auditory meatus. He described the first case in which the radiographic findings were confirmed at autopsy.[13] Holzknecht[14] as well as Henschen[13] gave a classical account of the value and limitations of plain film roentgenology in the diagnosis of brain tumours.

The important roentgenographic procedures of ventriculography were initiated in 1918 by Dandy.[8] In 1919 Dandy[9] described the method of encephalography and at the same time predicted the procedure of air myelography for the localization of spinal tumours. Obviously independent of Dandy's discovery, also Bingel introduced in 1921 pneumo-encephalography for the diagnosis of intracranial lesions.[4]

Since X-rays penetrate normal brain tissue, cerebrospinal fluid and non-calcified tumour tissue almost equally, and because most of all intracranial tumours either directly or indirectly modify the size or shape of the ventricles, Dandy considered the possibility of filling the cerebral ventricles with a medium that would produce a shadow in the roentgenogram. To achieve this, Dandy injected various solutions and suspensions (thorium, potassium, iodine, collargol, argyrol, bismuth subnitrate and subcarbonate) in various concentrations into the ventricles of dogs but with fatal results. Dandy states: 'Any substance injected into the ventricles must satisfy two very rigid exactions. (1) it must be abolutely non-irritating and non-toxic; and (2) it must be readily absorbed and excreted. . . . Ventriculography, therefore, seems possible only by the substitution of gas for cerebrospinal fluid.[8] It means that . . . the cerebral ventricles can be sharply outlined in a roentgenogram if the ventricular fluid be withdrawn and replaced by an equal quantity of air.'[9]

At first Dandy performed ventriculography in the diagnosis of internal hydrocephalus in infants. Dandy did not apply ventriculography to adults, but he defined the value of ventriculography in the diagnosis of intracranial masses as follows: 'Tumours in either cerebral hemisphere may dislocate or compress the ventricle and in this way localize the neoplasm. Tumours growing into the ventricles may show a corresponding defect in the ventricular shadow.'[6] The important step made by Dandy still left too many problems unsolved in the diagnosis and localization of brain tumours.

Early in 1925, Moniz and Lima[17, 18] began to review the possibilities of making visible the cerebral vessels. They put rubber tubes of the diameter of medium-sized cerebral arteries, containing sodium bromide solutions, into the macerated skull. These 'intracerebral vessels' were radiographed successfully. Further experiments were carried out on mongrel dogs and the results confirmed the harmlessness of contrast media. They continued their experiments on animals and obtained the first cerebral angiogram in a dog. In order to study normal radiographic anatomy of intracranial vessels, further injections of contrast media were performed on cadavers. After improving the roentgenologic technique, the roentgenographic visualization of cerebral arteries in a hopeless case with a massive brain tumour was attempted. The experiment failed. The further seven attempts failed too. Only owing to the tremendous determination of Moniz was the work continued. He succeeded with the ninth case, in which the carotid artery was surgically exposed and 5 ml of 25 per cent sodium iodide was injected. Moniz states with deliberation: 'Nous avions réalisé notre desideratum. On pouvait tirer, chez le vivant, la radioartériographie du cerveau et il semblait, par ce premier cas, que cette visibilité des artéres pourrait fournir des éléments pour la localisation des tumeurs.'[18]

The work and intellectual attitude of Moniz to accomplish his own idea is characterized very much to the point by Babinski:[2]

'L'idée neuve, que personne ne semble avoir envisagée avant M. Moniz et qui surgit un jour dans son esprit en quète de moyens capables de perfectionner la sémiologie des tumeurs intracraniennes, de facilite leur localisation, . . . est le fruit d'une méditation soutenue et de nombreuses expériences conduites avec une méthode rigoureuse . . . il se décide à mettre son projet à exécution et se lance courageusement dans cette entreprise comme autrefois ses compatriotes Dias et Vasco de Gama s'élançaient à travers l'Océan à la recherche de la route des Indes.'

On 7 July 1927 Moniz presented his epoch-making discoveries before the Société de Neurologie de Paris in a paper entitled: 'L'encephalographie artérielle: son importance dans la localisation des tumeurs cérébrales'.[18] For his work Moniz was awarded the Nobel Prize in 1949.

The neuroradiological evidence of an intracranial tumour by means of encephalography and angiography is mainly indirect. Both methods have a definite incidence of morbidity and mortality. The use of isotopes for the detection of brain tumours makes possible a direct demonstration of the intracranial lesion without risk for the patient.

The pioneer work in the brain scanning was done by Moore,[19] who tagged diiodofluorescein, a substance taken selectively by brain tumours, with ^{131}J. After intravenous injection of radioactive diiodofluorescein, Moore detected gamma radiation of ^{131}J from the tumour using Geiger–Müller counter. Moore localized twelve out of fifteen brain tumours successfully. Subsequently Moore studied a series of 500 patients, showing that brain scanning is a simple, safe and accurate method that makes possible direct demonstration of intracranial lesions. Progress in nuclear medicine and brain tumour diagnosis has been the result of improved radiopharmaceuticals and better detection instruments. Blau and Bender[5] introduced in 1959 ^{203}Hg-labelled chlormerodrin. Further significant improvement was achieved through introduction of ^{99m}Tc-Pertechnetate as a scanning agent by Harper in 1964.[12] Improvements have been made in detection instruments through replacement of Geiger–Müller detector by crystal scintillation counters in 1950 by Cassen.[6] At the beginning of scanning era heavily shielded detectors were used. They were moved manually from point to point over the skull. These were replaced by motor-driven detectors. The recent development is the scintillation camera which has the ability to produce an image of the distribution of radioactivity in the region of interest, and which obviates the necessity to move the detector mechanically from point to point.

The introduction of radioisotope technique in the diagnosis of brain tumours has been of great importance. Brain scanning can be performed also in outpatients without need for hospitalization, and without discomfort or danger to patients. These are obvious advantages compared to pneumo-encephalography and cerebral angiography. Brain scanning has become a universally accepted method in the diagnosis and localization of brain tumour.

References

1 ALBERS-SCHÖNBERG, H. E., 'Zwei Fälle von Hypophysentumoren', *Aerztlicher Verein in Hamburg*, 9 Februar 1904.

2 BABINSKI, J., Préface in: MONIZ, E., *Diagnostic des tumeurs cérébrales et épreuve de l'encéphalographie artérielle.* Paris, Masson, 1931.

3 BENEDIKT, M., 'Das Röntgenlicht im Dienste der Krankheiten des Schädels und des Gehirns, und der gerichtlichen Medizin', *Dtsch. med. Wschr.*, 1902, **28**, 405.

4 BINGEL, 'Encephalographie, eine Methode zur roentgenographischen Darstellung des Gehirns', *Fortschr. Rôntgenstr.*, 1921/22, **28**, 205.

5 BLAU, M. and BENDER, M. A., 'Radiomercury (Hg-203) labelled Neohydrin: A new agent for brain tumor localization', *J. nucl. Med.* (Convention Issue), 1959, p. 35.

6 CASSEN, B., CURTIS, L. and REED, C., 'Sensitive directional gamma-ray detector', *Nucleonics*, 1950, **6**, 78.

7 CHURCH, 'Pituitary tumor in its surgical relations', *J. Amer. med. Ass.*, 1909, **53**.

8 DANDY, W. E., 'Ventriculography following the injection of air into the cerebral ventricles', *Ann. Surg.*, 1918, **68**, 5.

9 DANDY, W. E., 'Roentgenography of the brain after the injection of air into the spinal canal', *Ann. Surg.*, 1919, **70**, 397.

10 FITTIG, O., 'Ueber einen roentgenographisch lokalisierten Fall von Hirntumor. Nach einem Vortrag, gehalten in der medizin' (Sektion der Schles. Gesellsch. fuervaterlaend. Kultur am 28. Nov. 1902), *Fortschr. Roentgenstr.*, 1903, **6**, 258.

11 FUERNROHR, W., *Die Roentgenstrahlen im Dienste der Neurologie*, Berlin, S. Karger, 1906.

12 HARPER, P. V., BECK, R., CHARLESTON, D. and LATHROP, K. A., 'Optimization of a scanning method using Tc-99m', *Nucleonics*, 1964, **22**, 50.

13 HENSCHEN, F., 'Die Akustikustumoren, eine neue Gruppe radiographisch darstellbarer Hirntumoren', *Fortschr. Roentgenstr.*, 1912, **18**, 207.

14 HOLZKNECHT, G., Bemerken zu der vorläufigen Mittheilung von M. Benedikt 'Das Röntgenlicht im Dienste der Krankheiten des Schädels und des Gehirns und der gerichtlichen Medizin', *Dtsch. med. Wschr.*, 1903, **28**, 619.

15 LICHTHEIM, 'Gehirntumor' (Discussion zu dem Vortrag von Ludloff), *Dtsch. Med. Wschr.*, 1899, **25** (Vereinsbeilage no. 40, p. 240, 1899).

16 MILLS, PFAHLER, 'Tumor of the brain localized clinically and by the Roentgen rays. With some observations and investigations relating to the use of the Roentgen rays in the diagnosis of lesions of the brain', *Phila. med. J.*, 1902, **9**.

17 MONIZ, E., *Diagnostic des Tumeurs cérébrales et épreuve de l'encéphalographie artérielle*, Paris, Masson, 1931.

18 MONIZ, E., 'L'encéphalographie artérielle; son importance dans la localisation des tumeurs cérébrales', *Rev. neurol.*, 1927, **34**, 72.

19 MOORE, G. E., *Diagnosis and Localization of Brain Tumors. A clinical and experimental study employing fluorescent and radioactive tracer methods*, Springfield, Ill., C. C. Thomas, 1953.

20 OBICI, BOLLICI, 'Applicazioni dei raggi "X" alla diagnosi di sede dei corpi estranei della testa e dei tumori intracranici' (Ferrara, 18 November 1897). *Riv. pathol. nerv. ment.*, 1898, **2**, no. 10; *Münch. Med. Wschr.*, 1898, **45**, 227.

21 OPPENHEIM, H., 'Hypophysentumor' (Discussion zu dem Vortrag von Cassirer), Berl. Ges. f. Psych. u. Nervenheilkunde 13 November 1899.

22 SCHUELLER, A., *Roentgen-Diagnostik der Erkrankungen des Kopfes*, Vienna and Leipzig, Alfred Hoelder, 1912.

E. Vaubel and D. Dünschel
Berlin (West Germany)

Ernst Jeger, ein Beitrag zur Geschichte der Gefässchirurgie

Die Herz- und Gefäßchirurgie hat sich in den letzten Jahren stürmisch entwickelt. Die 1929 von Dos Santos angegebene Angiographie ermöglicht heute eine klare Indikation zur Gefäßoperation, rekonstruktive Eingriffe an großen Gefäßen gehören zur Routine, das Risiko der Operation am offenen Herzen ist wesentlich gesenkt und die Mikrochirurgie ermöglicht jetzt durch Anastomose kleinster Gefäße selbst die Reimplantation, z.B. eines Fingers. Die Grundlagen für diese Entwicklung wurden bereits um die Jahrhundertwende gelegt in den Laboratorien der Physiologie und experimentellen Chirurgie, heute vor allem verbunden mit den Namen Carrel und Guthrie. Etwa zur gleichen Zeit (1913) erschien ein jetzt im Handel kaum erhältliches Buch über Gefäß- und Herzchirurgie von Ernst Jeger. Dieses Buch ist in seiner Konzeption so modern und enthält eine derartige Fülle experimenteller Untersuchungen, die kriegsbedingt erst Jahrzehnte später Eingang in die Klinik fanden, daß man sich entschlossen hat, dieses Buch als Reprint neu herauszugeben. Gestatten Sie mir, wenn ich den Versuch unternehme, an Hand der wenigen uns zugänglichen Dokumente den Lebensweg und die Arbeit Ernst Jeger's aufzuzeichnen.

Jeger wurde am 9. November 1884 in Wien geboren. Seine Familie, sicher jüdischen Ursprungs, wanderte um die Jahrhundertwende der Labourbewegung Englands folgend, nach London aus. Einen ersten Hinweis über die wissenschaftliche Tätigkeit Ernst Jeger's finden wir im Jahre 1908. Er arbeitete damals an der Experimentellen Biologischen Abteilung der Universitätsklinik in Berlin als Mitarbeiter Adolf Bickels über Stoffwechseluntersuchungen nach portocavaler Anastomose (ECK'sche Fistel), wahrscheinlich im Rahmen seiner Dissertation. Zwei Jahre später finden wir ihn als Assistenten am Allgemeinen Krankenhaus in Wien. Dort hatte er Gelegenheit, seine in Berlin konstruierte dreibranchige Gefäßklemme zur Durchführung von Seit-zu-Seit-Anastomosen bei der damals sehr bekannten Firma Josef Leiter herstellen zu lassen. Bevor Jeger im Jahre 1912 wieder nach Berlin übersiedelte, unternahm er eine Studienreise nach Amerika. Er suchte im Sinai-Hospital in New York den Thoraxchirurgen Charles Elsberg auf und es ist anzunehmen, daß er auch Alexis Carrel und die Physiologen Melzer und Auer vom Rockefeller-Institut persönlich kennenlernte. Die Eindrücke dieser Reise gaben ihm Anregungen, vor allem zur Weiterentwicklung des gefäßchirurgischen Instrumentariums.

So veröffentlichte er 1913 ein Gerät, um die Dreipunkt-Naht von Carrel zu erleichtern, modifizierte die ursprünglich für die Bluttransfusion gedachte Gefäßklemme von Elsberg als Doppelklemme für Anastomosen und versah den

Melzer-Auer'schen Narkoseapparat mit einem doppelläufigen Trachealtubus und einem Gummiballon zur Abdichtung. Nach dieser Reise setzte er seine experimentellen Untersuchungen am Jüdischen Krankenhaus in Berlin unter James Israel fort, zunächst mit Arbeiten über Aortenersatz mit gedoppelter Carotis, die portocavale Anastomose nach der von ihm entwickelten Technik und dann – auf eine Anregung von James Israel hin – die Neuimplantation der Nierenvenen nach hoher Unterbindung der V. cava.

Am 27. März 1913 konnte er zwei Hunde neun und zehn Monate nach diesem Eingriff vorstellen. Im gleichen Jahre empfahl der amerikanische Chirurg Matas auf dem Internationalen Medizinkongress in London das von Jeger angegebene Verfahren auch als Operationsmethode zur Behandlung von Aortenaneurysmen.

An diesem Arbeiten waren beteiligt Wilhelm Israel, später nach London emigriert, Helmuth Joseph, der 1913 mit Jeger nach Breslau übersiedelte und Ernst Unger, von 1919 an Chef des Rudolf-Virchow-Krankenhauses Berlin, bis er 1934 aus politischen Gründen entlassen wurde und möglicherweise gewollt bei einem Unfall tragisch ums Leben kam. 1912 erhielt Alexis Carrel für seine gefäßchirurgischen Arbeiten den Nobelpreis und in diesem Jahre muß auch Jeger sein 1913 im Hirschwald Verlag erschienenes Buch: „Die Chirurgie der Blutgefäße und des Herzens" abgeschlossen haben. Dieses mit 231 Abbildungen reich illustrierte Buch gibt an Hand der Literatur eine eindrucksvolle Übersicht des Standes der Gefäßchirurgie um die Jahrhundertwende. Doch hat sich Jeger nicht damit begnügt, die damals z.B. von Carrel entwickelten und heute noch gültigen Prinzipien der Nahttechnik aufzuzeigen. Seine große gefäßchirurgische Erfahrung ermöglichte es ihm, selbstentwickelte Instrumente anzugeben und die Technik auch mit eigenen Operationspräparaten zu erläutern.

Die Aktualität seiner Versuche ist überraschend. Jeger beschreibt Experimente mit resorbierbaren Gefäßprothesen aus formolgehärtetem Parakasein, damals als erster Kunststoff unter dem Namen Galalith im Handel, ähnlich den Payr'schen Ringen aus Magnesium, die Jahrzehnte später in ähnlicher Form in Nakajamas Gefäßnahtapparat Verwendung fanden.

Er gibt den inneren und äußeren Shunt bei Eingriffen an großen Gefäßen an und beschreibt die Bypasstechnik mit autologen Venentransplantaten. Interessant sind seine Versuche zusammen mit Julius Wohlgemuth, zur Blutstillung eine mechanische aus tierischen Membranen hergestellte resorbierbare Gaze zu verwenden. Weit über alle bisherigen Experimente hinaus gehen jedoch seine Versuche, aus invaginierten Venen widerstandsfähige Klappen herzustellen und diese Transplantate bei Aorten- und Mitralstenosen in ventriculo-pulmonale oder-aortale Shunts einzusetzen. Es gelang ihm, Hunde nach diesen Eingriffen mit suffizienten Venenklappen bis zu elf Tagen am Leben zu halten. 1913 wird Jeger Mitglied der Deutschen Gesellschaft für Chirurgie und verläßt im gleichen Jahre Berlin, um an der Königl. Chirurgischen Universitätsklinik in Breslau unter Hermann Küttner seine experimentellen Arbeiten zusammen mit seinem Berliner Kollegen Helmuth Joseph fortzusetzen. Neben einer Reihe technischer Anregungen, z.B. einer Pleura-Aspirationsdrainage, widmete er sich den Problemen der operativen Behandlung von Aortenaneurysmen. Es gelang ihm im Experiment, resezierte Aortenanteile durch End-zu-Seit anastomosierte Venentransplantate zu überbrücken. Ein Verfahren, das erst 1949 – also 30 Jahre später – Kunlin als Saphena-Umkehrplastik in die Klinik einführen konnte.

Zur Behandlung der portalen Hypertension gab er bei ungünstigen anatomischen Verhältnissen die mesentericocavale Anastomose an. Zwei der so operierten Hunde lebten bei Kriegsausbruch noch. Am 8. August 1914 wurde Jeger als landsturmpflichtiger Zivilarzt eingezogen und im Oktober in die freigekämpfte Festung Przemysl versetzt. Dort arbeitete er als Mitarbeiter Barany's im Festungs-Spital Nr. 8. Am 11. November 1914 wurde die Festung erneut von den Russen eingeschlossen. Die große Zahl schwerster Verletzungen in diesen Kämpfen ermöglichten es Jeger, seine gefäßchirurgischen Kenntnisse voll einzusetzen. Bereits im November gelingt es ihm, Manuskripte über seine Erfahrungen einem in der Festung gelandeten Piloten mitzugeben. Die Arbeiten erscheinen im Dezember 1914 in der Berliner Klinischen Wochenschrift und im Januar 1915 in Brun's Beiträgen.

So berichtet er über acht Gefäßverletzungen durch Schuß, Schrapnell oder Stich der A. femoralis, poplitea und brachialis, in fünf Fällen hatte die primäre Gefäßnaht Erfolg, in drei Fällen mußte wegen nachfolgender Infektion eine Amputation vorgenommen werden. Die damals übliche Unterbindung der Gefäße hätte jeweils mit Sicherheit eine Gangrän der betroffenen Extremität zur Folge gehabt. In einem Fall gelang es ihm, einen durch einen Gewehrnahschuß fast völlig abgetrennten Arm durch Naht der A. und V. brachialis, der N. ulnaris und medianus nach Stabilisierung der Humerusfraktur zu erhalten. Aufgrund dieser Erfahrungen forderte Jeger, eine primäre Gefäßrekonstruktion selbst unter ungünstigsten Bedingungen zu versuchen. Die gefäßchirurgischen Erfolge der Amerikaner anläßlich des Koreakrieges 1953/54 haben diese Erfahrung Jeger's voll bestätigt. Die Amputationsrate betrug damals nur noch einen Bruchteil im Vergleich zu den Zahlen des letzten Weltkrieges.

Jeger konstruierte während der Belagerung ein einfaches Narkoseüberdruckgerät, beschreibt ein Verfahren zur intravenösen Dauerinfusion und gibt Apparate zur Stabilisierung von Schußbrüchen an. Die große Zahl von Toten gibt ihm die Möglichkeit, auch seine experimentellen Studien voranzutreiben. So führt er an 20 Leichen mesenterico-cavale Anastomosen, teils unter Zwischenschaltung eines Jugularis-transplantates durch.

Das Verhältnis zu seinem Lehrer Barany war ausgezeichnet. Barany erwähnt in einer Arbeit über die Behandlung von Hirnabszessen, daß er die Idee der Drainage mit Guttaperchastreifen seinem Mitarbeiter Jeger verdanke. Jeger selbst führt auf Anregung Barany's bei Kopfschußverletzungen die primäre Duraplastik mit freitransplantierter Fascie durch. Der Versuch, einen traumatisch bedingten Hydrocephalus durch ein Venentransplatat in die Vena jugularis abzuleiten, bleibt ohne Erfolg. Am 9. März 1915 gerät Jeger in Gefangenschaft, zwei Wochen später ergibt sich General von Kusmanek mit 40 000 Mann. 1915 erhält Barany in Gefangenschaft den Nobelpreis zugesprochen. Durch Vermittlung von Prinz Carl von Schweden wird er gegen einen russischen Gefangenen ausgetauscht. Den Österreichern gelingt es jedoch nicht, den geforderten – einen Tänzer – in ihren Lagern ausfindig zu machen. Sie liefern deswegen einen Mann gleichen Namens aus. Aber ehe diese Täuschung bemerkt wird, ist Barany in Sicherheit. Am 30. August wird Jeger, schwer an Typhus erkrankt, in das Spital von Kainsk im Bezirk Tomsk eingeliefert und verstirbt am folgenden Tag im Alter von 30 Jahren. 1916 erscheint posthum noch eine Arbeit über tierexperimentelle Untersuchungen in Breslau. 1920 tritt nach sechsjähriger Pause die Deutsche Gesellschaft für Chirurgie wieder zusammen. Bei der Totenehrung der im Krieg Gefallenen und Vermißten werden die Nahmen von 160 Kollegen verlesen, darunter auch Ernst Jeger.

Es ist ein beliebtes Bonmot, den Krieg als den großen Lehrmeister der Chirurgie anzusprechen. Bedenkt man aber, daß mehr als 40 Jahre nach den ersten klinischen und experimentellen Arbeiten von Rehn, Carrel, Guthrie, Stich, Doyen, Jeger u.a. vergingen, ehe sich die Gefäß- und Herzchirurgie zum heutigen Stand entwickeln konnte, daß durch die Weltkriege bekannte chirurgische Schulen wie die des Jüdischen Krankenhauses in Berlin zerstreut wurden, daß die kriegsbedingten Grenzen den unerläßlichen wissenschaftlichen Austausch unmöglich machten oder daß durch Tod – wie im Falle Jeger's – eine impulsgebende Lebensarbeit jäh unterbrochen wurde, dann kann der Gedanke eines positiven Einflusses des Krieges auf die Entwicklung der Wissenschaft eigentlich nur als Blasphemie erscheinen.

K. E. Rothschuh and J. Bleker
Münster (West Germany)

Die Einführung naturwissenschaftlich-messender Methoden in die klinische Diagnostik in der deutschen Medizin des 19. Jahrhunderts

Veranlaßt durch die neue naturwissenschaftliche Denkweise hat die Physiologie im 19. Jahrhundert von etwa 1840 an eine außerordentliche Anzahl neuer Apparate, Geräte und Meßverfahren entwickelt, um Lebensvorgänge zu analysieren, zu objektivieren und zu quantifizieren. Darüber liegen 2 Arbeiten aus Münster aus jüngster Zeit vor.[1, 2] Diese Einstellung zum analytisch messenden Vorgehen ist nicht selbstverständlich. Sie setzte sich seit etwa 1840 in Deutschland durch, geleitet von der Überzeugung, daß erstens auch Lebensvorgänge gesetzlich, d.h. unter gleichen Bedingungen gleichartig ablaufen, daß sie zweitens den Prinzipien der Physik und Chemie folgen ohne dem Einfluß irgend welcher vitaler Sonderkräfte zu unterliegen, und drittens, daß physikalische und andere Meßverfahren die untersuchten biologischen Größen zutreffend erfassen, z.B. die tierische Wärme und die Größe der Herzkraft. Wie verhielt sich die Klinik gegenüber dieser Entwicklung?

Wir gewannen bei der Durchsicht viel gebrauchter Lehrbücher der klinischen Diagnostik den Eindruck, daß zwischen der Verwendung von objektivierenden oder messenden Verfahren in der Forschung und ihrer Anwendung in der klinischen Diagnostik nicht selten mehrere Jahrzehnte vergangen sind.[3] Wir haben versucht, diesen Eindruck durch eine genauere Untersuchung zu sichern oder zu widerlegen. Anschließend wollen wir versuchen, unsere Ergebnisse zu interpretieren.

Die Generation der deutschen Physiologen nach Johannes Müller, z.B. Ernst Brücke (+1892), H. Helmholtz (+1894), E. du Bois-Reymond (+1896), Carl Ludwig (+1895), K. v. Vierordt (+1884), G. G. Valentin (+1883), hat der objektivierenden, quantifizierenden Methode in der Physiologie zum Siege verholfen. Das beginnt im Zeitraum zwischen 1840 und 1850. Auch einzelne Kliniker und Pathologen nahmen damals diese Art des Denkens und Forschens auf, so z.B. Ludwig Traube (1818–76), Theodor Frerichs (1819–85), Carl Aug. Wunderlich (1815–77), Rudolf Virchow (1821–1902) und Jakob Henle (1809–85).

Man folgte dabei aber weniger dem pathologisch-anatomischen Konzept der Pariser oder Wiener Schule auf der Suche nach dem Sitz der Krankheiten. Man wollte vielmehr die Ursache der pathologisch veränderten Lebensvorgänge enträtseln. C. A. Wunderlich verlangte 1842 eine Medizin, die ,,die Gesetze lehren muß, nach denen der Organismus lebt und erkrankt, genest und stirbt".[4] In der jungen naturwissenschaftlich exakten Physiologie sucht man die Wege zur Erforschung dieser Gesetze. Auf diese Physiologie sollte die neue Krankheitslehre aufgebaut werden. Jakob Henle (1809–85) schreibt: ,,die Physiologie des gesunden und des kranken Menschen sind nicht verschieden, Physiologie und Pathologie sind Eins".[5] Die Reformer erklären weiter, daß die Krankheiten nur ,,den Ablauf der Lebenserscheinungen unter veränderten Bedingungen darstellen"[6] und daß daher die Krankheitserscheinungen nichts anderes seien ,,als die abgeänderten Funktionen des erkrankten Organismus".[7]

Die Aufgaben dieser neuen physiologischen Medizin definiert der junge Rudolf Virchow (1821–1902) im Jahre 1846 als ,,die Erforschung der veränderten Bedingungen, unter denen sich der erkrankte Körper oder das einzelne leidende Organ befinden, die Feststellung der Abweichungen, welche die Lebenserscheinungen unter bestimmten Bedingungen erfahren, endlich die Auffindung der Mittel, durch welche diese abnormen Bedingungen aufzuheben sind".[8] Die physiologische Medizin, die nicht mehr die lokale Läsion, sondern die Functio laesa in den Mittelpunkt stellt, verlangt somit diagnostische Methoden, die es erlauben, die Abweichung von der Normalfunktion objektiv festzustellen und, wenn möglich, quantitativ zu erfassen. Man sollte meinen, daß bei solchem Programm die physiologisch entwickelten Verfahren bald in der Klinik ausprobiert wurden. Dem ist aber nicht so.

Welches waren die gebräuchlichen diagnostischen Verfahren um 1840? Bei Lukas Schönlein (1793–1864) in Berlin gehören die folgenden Verfahren zum ständigen klinischen Rüstzeug (1842, Klinische Vorträge): nämlich Auskultation, Perkussion und Palpation, die chemische und mikroskopische Untersuchung von Harn, Stuhl, Sputum und Erbrochenem, sowie die chemische und mikroskopische Blutuntersuchung.[9]

Vergleichen wir nun, welche Untersuchungsmethoden etwa 30 Jahre später in der deutschen Klinik gebräuchlich waren, so müssen wir feststellen, daß sich seit Schönleins Zeit kaum etwas geändert hat. In Niemeyers vielbenutztem ,,Lehrbuch der speziellen Pathologie und Therapie", das in den Jahren 1874 bis 1877 seine 9. verbesserte Auflage erfuhr, finden wir, daß von einer Bereicherung der diagnostischen Verfahren fast nicht die Rede sein kann.[10] Zwar erscheinen die chemischen und mikroskopischen Untersuchungsverfahren in manchen Gebieten erweitert, aber es fehlt das wesentlich Neue. Die messenden Verfahren der Physiologie finden bis auf eine Ausnahme keine Verwendung in der klinischen Diagnostik, weder das Thermometer, noch der Sphygmograph, noch Respirationsapparate, Pneumographen, Atemdruckmesser, oder Aerometer, Blutkörperchenzählung usw. Das einzige neue Hilfsmittel, das aus dem Bereich der physiologischen Forschung stammt, ist das 1847 von Hutchinson entwickelte Spirometer, dem zur Kapazitätsbestimmung bei tuberkulösen Lungen eine gewisse Bedeutung zugestanden wird.

Das ist auffallend. Die Pulsregistrierung mit Sphygmographen wurde durch Vierordt 1853 angegeben, von Marey (1860) klinisch anwendbar gemacht, aber erst James Mackenzie[11] macht seit 1880 von dem Verfahren zur Analyse des menschlichen Pulses bei der unregelmäßigen Herztätigkeit Gebrauch. Im ,,Taschenbuch der Medizinisch-Klinischen Diagnostik" von Müller-Seifert[12] wird die Methode der Pulsregistrierung erstmals im Jahre 1886 angegeben. Die Blutdruckmessung mit dem Sphygmomanometer von v. Basch, entwickelt 1880, brauchte 15 Jahre, um in der Klinik Fuß zu fassen. ,,Einige liebenswürdige Kollegen, von Patienten diesbezüglich interpelliert" – so schreibt v. Basch 1896 – ,,äußerten sich in überaus wohlwollender Weise dahin, das was ich thue, sei purer Schwindel. Zum Pulsfühlen brauche man die Finger und die Uhr, sonst nichts".[13] Mit dem Thermometer ging es ähnlich; seit etwa 1850 weiß man, daß die fieberhafte Körperwärme chemische Quellen hat und weder vom Herzen noch von den Nerven ihren Ursprung nimmt. Die Thermometerkonstruktionen wurden allmählich handlicher und zuverlässiger. Ludwig Traube[14] beginnt 1850/51 mit der systematischen Temperaturmessung am Krankenbette. C. A. Wunderlichs Monographie[15] über die Eigenwärme des menschlichen Körpers erschien 1868, aber bei Niemeyer[16] wird die klinische Thermometrie 1874/77 noch nicht erwähnt. Erst Müller-Seifert besprechen 1886 das Verfahren ausführlich. Die Methode der Blutkörperchenzählung, 1852 von Vierordt angegeben, braucht ca. 30 Jahre, um in der Klinik Fuß zu fassen.

Im Einklang mit der Armut an messenden Methoden steht auch das Angebot an medizinischen Instrumenten auf den Ausstellungen des 19. Jahrhunderts. Auf der Pariser Weltausstellung von 1867 wurden offenbar überhaupt keine diagnostischen Geräte vorgestellt.[17] Die deutsche Ausstellung auf dem Gebiete der Hygiene und des Rettungswesens von 1882/83 zeigte dagegen schon Auskultations- und Perkussionsinstrumente, Spekula für Nase, Ohr, Schlund und Kehlkopf, Thermometer und Laryngoskope. Vorgestellt werden auch ein Cardio-Sphygmo-Chronograph, das Spirometer, Aesthesiometer zur Prüfung der Sensibilität, Dynamometer und Galvanometer. Nicht im Einklang mit den allgemeinen diagnostischen Lehrbüchern steht die Fülle von ophthalmologischen Instrumenten. Beschrieben werden Augenspiegel, Refraktometer, Optometer, Perimeter und so weiter.[18] Die Augenheilkunde, der die physiologischen Kenntnisse den größten direkten Nutzen gebracht hatten, war um diese Zeit schon eine Spezialdisziplin.

Danach zeichnet sich folgendes Bild ab: Erst seit den 80er Jahren wurde den apparativen und quantitativen Hilfsmitteln der Diagnostik mehr Aufmerksamkeit zugewandt. Es liegen also für viele Verfahren Jahrzehnte zwischen dem Zeitpunkt ihrer ersten Konstruktion und ihrem Eingang in die klinische Anwendung.

Welches mögen wohl die Gründe dafür sein?

Einige dieser Gründe beruhen auf der historischen Situation der Medizin im 19. Jahrhundert, andere berühren auch die Probleme des diagnostischen Vorgehens im Allgemeinen. Es soll versucht werden, dies in einigen Punkten zu präzisieren:

1. Man wußte lange Zeit nicht recht, ob das Messen biologischer Größen überhaupt dem Lebendigen adäquat ist. Ich erinnere an die Bedenken von Bichat und Claude Bernard.[19]

2. Neben diesen grundsätzlichen Bedenken empfanden viele der älteren Ärzte eine deutliche Abneigung dagegen, ihre subjektive Erfahrung der objektiven Messung unterzuordnen. So berichtet Helmholtz, er habe noch um 1850 behaupten hören, Auskultation und Perkussion seien „grob mechanische Untersuchungsmittel, deren ein Arzt von hellem Geistesauge nicht bedürfe". Selbst das Pulszählen mit der Sekundenuhr habe „bei den alten Herren als ein Verfahren von nicht ganz gutem Geschmack" gegolten.[20]

3. Das pathophysiologische Denken von Wunderlich, Traube und anderen wurde seit 1850 durch die Entwicklung der pathologischen Anatomie in den Hintergrund gedrängt. Man fragte mehr nach dem Sitz und der Erscheinungsweise als nach Art und Ursachen krankhafter Störungen. Die Fortschritte der Morphologie förderten zwar die pathologischen Erkenntnisse, brachten aber dem Kliniker für Diagnose und Therapie wenig Anregungen. Aus diesem Unbehagen erwächst wieder eine stärkere Tendenz, die physiologischen Kenntnisse in den Dienst der Klinik zu

stellen. 1878 erklärt Ottomar Rosenbach (1851–1907) in seiner Arbeit über Mageninsuffizienz: „Uns muß es, da wir heilen wollen, darauf ankommen, nicht einen irreparablen pathologischen Zustand zu diagnostizieren, sondern die Entstehung des Leidens, den Beginn des Prozesses, die Functio laesa des Organs frühzeitig zu erkennen, und darum müssen wir auf die Funktionsprüfung unser Augenmerk legen."[21] Während es den Reformern der 40er Jahre zunächst darum ging, „die Abweichungen, welche die Lebenserscheinungen erfahren", zu erforschen, verlangte Rosenbach nun die Feststellung der gestörten Funktion zum Zwecke der Diagnostik.

So ändert sich in den 80er Jahren langsam die Szene.

4. Der Kliniker benötigt Verfahren, die dem Patienten nützen, ihm sicher nicht schaden und möglichst nicht belästigen. Der Praktiker fürchtete, seine Patienten zu verlieren, wenn er sie mit dem Licht des Augenspiegels blendete,[22] ihm zur Temperaturmessung für eine halbe Stunde ein Thermometer anlegen mußte,[23] wenn er ihm Blut abnehmen mußte und dgl. Auch der Patient mußte also in Funktionen denken lernen, und das brauchte Zeit.

5. Die Pathophysiologie der Hauptkörperfunktionen, z.B. für Kreislauf, Atmung, Stoffwechsel, Verdauung, Nierenfunktion usw., stand noch in den Anfängen. Man mußte erst lernen, sinnvolle und klinisch wichtige Fragen zu formulieren, bevor Meßgeräte zu praxisnahen Ergebnissen führen konnten.

6. Die Praxisnähe eines klinisch diagnostischen Verfahrens liegt vor allem darin, daß ein Krankheitsbild durch dieses Verfahren gesichert werden kann. Die Abgrenzung von Krankheitsbildern muß also eine gewisse Reife erreicht haben. Alles das ist um 1870 noch in vollem Gange. Ein deutliches Beispiel dafür, in wie starkem Maße die Anwendung eines diagnostischen Verfahrens von der Präzisierung eines bestimmten Krankheitsbildes abhängen kann, kennen wir aus der Geschichte der Harndiagnostik. Die chemische Harnuntersuchung blieb fast 200 Jahre klinisch ungenutzt, bis die Entdeckung der Bright'schen Krankheit im Jahre 1827 die Anwendung dieser Methode unumgänglich machte. Dagegen war es nicht unbedingt notwendig, ein Ophthalmoskop zu benutzen, wenn bei einem bekannten Nierenleiden Sehstörungen auftraten. Ebenso verhielt es sich um 1900 mit der Blutdruckmessung. Man wußte zwar um den Zusammenhang, der zwischen Nierenleiden, Herzvergrößerung und einer Erhöhung des arteriellen Drucks besteht. Doch nach dem Stand der Krankheitslehre schien es unwichtig für die Diagnose und Prognose, das Ausmaß dieser Druckveränderung festzustellen. Die wissenschaftliche Medizin hatte bis zum Ende des 19. Jahrhunderts die Pathogenese mancher Krankheiten eingehend erforscht, dabei kam es jedoch nur in wenigen Fällen zur funktionellen Abgrenzung von neuen Krankheitsbildern, zu deren Diagnose neue messende Verfahren benötigt wurden.

Aus allen diesen Gründen mag sich die immerhin merkwürdige Tatsache erklären, daß die Medizin – vor allem die innere Medizin – die messenden Verfahren der Physiologie erst mit Jahrzehnten Verspätung in ihre diagnostischen Routineverfahren aufgenommen hat.

Anmerkungen

1 ROTHSCHUH, K. E., „Die Bedeutung apparativer Hilfsmittel für die Entwicklung der biologischen Wissenschaften im 19. Jahrhundert", in *Geschichte der Naturwissenschaften und der*

Technik im 19. *Jahrhundert,* 7. Gespräch der G. Agricola-Gesellschaft, Hrsg. v. Verein Deutscher Ingenieure, Düsseldorf, 1971.

2 RAPP, DIETMAR, „Die Entwicklung der physiologischen Methodik von 1784–1911. Eine quantitative Untersuchung", *Münstersche Beiträge zur Geschichte und Theorie der Medizin,* nr. 2, Münster, 1970.

3 Neben zahlreichen Einzeldarstellungen vgl. besonders: KEELE, KENNETH, *The Evolution of Clinical Methods in Medicine,* London, 1963.

4 WUNDERLICH, CARL AUGUST, „Uber die Mängel der heutigen deutschen Medicin und und über die Nothwendigkeit einer entschieden wissenschaftlichen Richtung in derselben", *Archiv für physiologische Heilkunde,* 1842, **1**, I–XXX, S. iii.

5 HENLE, JAKOB, *Handbuch der rationellen Pathologie,* bd. I, Braunschweig, 1846, S. 25.

6 VIRCHOW, RUDOLF, „Uber die Standpunkte in der wissenschaftlichen Medicin", *Archiv für pathologische Anatomie und Physiologie und für klinische Medicin,* 1847, **1**, 3–19, S. 3.

7 HENLE, JAKOB, *Handbuch der rationellen Pathologie,* bd. I, Braunschweig, 1846, S. 25.

8 VIRCHOW, RUDOLF, „Uber die Standpunkte in der wissenschaftlichen Medicin", *Archiv für pathologische Anatomie und Physiologie und für klinische Medicin,* 1847, **1**, 3–19, S. 4.

9 Vgl. SCHOENLEIN, JOHANN LUKAS, *Schönlein's klinische Vorträge,* Redigiert und herausgegeben von Dr. L. Güterbock, 2. Aufl. Berlin, 1842.

10 Vgl. NIEMEYER, FELIX VON, *Lehrbuch der speziellen Pathologie und Therapie mit besonderer Rücksicht auf Physiologie und pathologische Anatomie,* Neu bearbeitet von Eugen Seitz, 9. Aufl. bd. I, Berlin, 1874, bd. II, Berlin, 1877.

11 MACKENZIE, JAMES, *The study of the pulse arterial, venous, and hepatic and the movements of the heart,* Edinburgh and London, 1902.

12 Vgl. SEIFERT, OTTO und MÜLLER, FRIEDRICH, *Taschenbuch der medicinisch-klinischen Diagnostik,* 2. Aufl. Wiesbaden, 1886 (1. Aufl. April 1886, 3. Aufl. ebenfalls 1886).

13 BASCH, S. V., „Fünfzehn Jahre Blutdruckmessung", *Wiener Klin. Wschr.,* 1896, **46**, 617–20.

14 TRAUBE, LUDWIG, „Über die Wirkungen der Digitalis, insbesondere über den Einfluß derselben auf die Körper-Temperatur in fieberhaften Krankheiten, mit einem Anhang über Temperaturmessungen bei Kranken", *Charité-Annalen, Jg.* 1850, **1**, 622; Abgedruckt in Ludwig Traube, *Gesammelte Beiträge zur Pathologie und Physiologie,* bd. II, Berlin, 1871, S. 97 ff.

15 WUNDERLICH, C. A., *Das Verhalten der Eigenwärme in Krankheiten,* Leipzig, 1868. Vgl. auch ders. „Die Thermometrie", *Arch. physiol. Heilkunde,* N.F., 1857, **1**, 15–16.

16 NIEMEYER, FELIX VON, vgl. 10.

17 Vgl. *Études sur l'Exposition de* 1867 *ou les Archives de l'industrie au XIXe siècle,* 8 Bde, Hrsg. Eug. Lacroix, Paris, 1868/69, bd. 8, *Appareils et Instruments de l'Art Medical.*

18 Vgl. *Bericht über deutsche Ausstellung auf dem Gebiete der Hygiene und des Rettungswesens . . .,* Berlin, 1882–83, Hrsg. P. Boerner, bd. II, Breslau, 1885.

19 BICHAT, XAVIER, *Recherches physiologiques sur la vie et la mort,* Sec. Ed., Paris, 1802, p. 81; BERNARD, CLAUDE, *Cahier de notes* 1850–60, ed. M. D. Grmek, Paris, 1965, pp. 173–74.

20 HELMHOLTZ, HERMANN V., „Das Denken in der Medizin" (Rede, Berlin, 1877), in *Vorträge und Reden,* 2. bd., Braunschweig, 1896, S. 179.

21 ROSENBACH, OTTOMAR, „Der Mechanismus und die Diagnose der Mageninsuffizienz", *Sammlung klinischer Vorträge,* von Volkmann, nr. 51 (1878); Abgedruckt in *Ausgewählte Abhandlungen von Ottomar Rosenbach*", Hrsg. Walter Guttmann, Leipzig, 1909, bd. II, S. 59.

22 HELMHOLTZ, HERMANN V., vgl. 20.

23 EBSTEIN, ERICH, „Die Entwicklung der klinischen Thermometrie", *Ergebnisse der inneren Medizin und Kinderheilkunde,* 1928, **33**, 407–503, S. 482.

V. Martinelli and G. Viviano
Rome (Italy)

Malformazioni congenite: casistica, storia, osservazioni

La storia delle malformazioni congenite è strettamente legata alla storia dell'uomo. Tutto ciò che è stato considerato come una deviazione del normale sviluppo non è mai passato inosservato ed ha sempre preoccupato l'uomo forse più della malattia che ben presto ha trovato una logica spiegazione ed è proprio questa impotenza nel trovare un nesso causale che ha fatto la storia di queste aberrazioni somatiche, storia che si è spesso identificata in una paura reverenziale della collera divina. Ne fanno fede le rappresentazioni degli antichi eroi e degli dei, personificati spesso in corpi irrazionali, fantasiosi che trovano posto soltanto nel loro olimpo soprannaturale.

Naturalmente questa premessa non esclude un interesse scientifico da parte di alcuni sull'argomento, perciò, prima di illustrare i dati da noi raccolti sulle malformazioni congenite, faremo una brevissima sintesi storica, anche se siamo consapevoli di omettere, in così breve spazio, molti nomi che andrebbero ricordati.

Il primo vero tentativo di ricerca causale di questa patologia si fa risalire ad Empedocle, è perciò appannaggio della scuola italica. Questi tentò di spiegare le mostruosità come aberrazioni non logiche del seme.

Con Ippocrate si affaccia la possibilità che una causa meccanica possa alterare il seme e dare origine alla malformazione.

In epoca romana i pregiudizi su questa patologia vennero alimentati sia da naturalisti che da letterati: Tito Livio, Cicerone, Tacito non riuscirono a scrollarsi di dosso l'elemento magico e soprannaturale e ad eccezione di Galeno che aveva ripreso quanto già affermato da Empedocle, in questo periodo non troviamo idee nuove sull'argomento.

Nel periodo di decadenza e nel medio evo le interpretazioni magiche ebbero largo consenso, anzi furono confermate dal pensiero astrologico che sembrò aver trovato la soluzione per spiegare ogni capriccio della natura. Claudio Tolomeo, S. Alberto Magno e S. Tommaso d'Aquino furono le voci più autorevoli e, per la diffusione dei loro scritti, condizionarono senza speranza il pensiero del loro tempo. Le teorie aristoteliche ed empedoclee vennero rielaborate con nozioni astrologiche e sopratutto Alberto Magno pensò di aver trovato una soluzione a problemi che lo stesso Aristotele aveva lasciati insoluti. Il seme, esso afferma, ha la possibilità di somigliare al genitore, alla specie, al genere. Quando questa somiglianza si limita al genere, soltanto allora si hanno in natura i mostri; fu anche assertore della possibilità di fecondazione tra uomo e animale. La sola voce originale di questo periodo fu quella di Guglielmo da Saliceto che, parlando dell'idrocefalo del neonato, lo fa derivare esclusivamente da una causa naturale, rinnegando coraggiosamente le idee correnti.

In periodo umanistico è ancora il pensiero empedocleo che domina incontrastato, ma non sono molti che si occupano dell'argomento, mentre nel Rinascimento la schiera s'infittisce, ma le congetture eziologiche rimangono nel campo della pura fantasia e lo confermano voci autorevoli come lo svizzero Giacomo Rueff e Ambrogio Parè che, nel fare un elenco delle cause che possono influire nel generare i mostri, inserisce come moventi determinanti anche l'immaginazione della madre, l'opera dei demoni, la gloria di Dio. Ma è proprio in questo periodo storico che, nell'appendice ad un trattato anatomico di Realdo Colombo, troviamo il primo abbozzo di scienza teratologica, con una discussione logica sulle cause che hanno portato a generare le malformazioni da lui descritte.

Il primo a smitizzare le leggendarie figure degli Ippogrifi, delle Chimere e delle Arpie fu Ulisse Aldovrandi che le considerò soltanto parto dell'umana fantasia e ad un suo allievo Bartolomeo Ambrosini è attribuito il primo vero trattato di teratologia comparata.

A Fabrizio d'Acquapendente si fanno risalire i primi studi embriologici. Comunque la scienza teratologica non è appannaggio dei soli italiani: Cornelio Gemma fiammingo, Levinus Lemmens zelandese, Giovanni Schenk di Friburgo sono soltanto alcuni degli stranieri che si occuparono delle deviazioni dello sviluppo. Tutti furono però dominati dalle fantasiose credenze che imperavano, come del resto avvenne per il nostro Fortunato Liceti che, pur avendo scritto il più ponderoso trattato di teratologia dell'epoca (De monstrorum causis, natura et differentiis – Padova, 1616), subì l'influenza dei suoi predecessori. Comunque nel suo libro va notato come, tra le molte cose ovvie, per la prima volta si parla di malattia come causa diretta di malformazione ed anche l'impianto anomalo di placenta viene indicato come possibile fattore di alterazione fetale.

Di vero rapporto di causalità tra malattie e malformazioni ereditarie si cominciò a parlare soltanto nel XVII° secolo quando Ingrassia, Sthal e Boerhàave si occuparono dell'argomento. Fodéré per primo attribuì al matrimonio tra consanguinei la possibilità di dare con più incidenza malformazioni.

Haller nel suo libro 'De monstribus' raccolse tutto lo scibile del suo tempo ed anche se, da un punto di vista eziologico, dalla sua grandiosa opera non nasce nulla di nuovo, egli, avendo collegato lo studio delle malformazioni con l'anatomia e l'embriologia, fu il primo a dare alla teratologia un abito scientifico.

Con Giovanni Battista Bianchi si comincia a parlare di malattie fetali, mentre con lo Zacchia si fa una distinzione netta tra embriopatie e fetopatie. Gli esperimenti di teratogenesi iniziano invece nel XVIII° secolo con Stefano Geoffroy, Dareste e Meckel e fu proprio quest'ultimo che dedusse dai suoi studi una delle leggi fondamentali della teratologia che cioè la malformazione non è altro che un arresto di sviluppo.

Un veterinario italiano, il Lombardini, si servì dell'elettricità per provocare delle alterazioni sull'embrione di pollo e corredò un suo libro di una appendice con disegni delle malformazioni così ottenute.

Siamo arrivati così, anche se con uno sguardo estremamente panoramico al nostro secolo: la microchirurgia, l'irradiazione, la chimica sono i mezzi di cui si serve l'embriologia teratologica ed i lavori si susseguono con un crescendo impressionante; le fantasiose descrizioni di ciclopi e di sirene si riducono ad una rigida affermazione di Wolff: irradiando nel blastoderma, intorno alla ventesima ora, zone diverse si possono ottenere, sperimentalmente, tutta quella genia di mostri che avevano turbato i nostri avi.

Con le esperienze molti punti oscuri sembrano chiarirsi, ma una branca nuova, eredità di una società che si evolve, viene a svilupparsi: la chemioteratogenesi cioè lo studio delle malformazioni derivanti dall'azione lesiva di sostanze tossiche. Gli studi su questo specifico argomento sono iniziati all'inizio del secolo: Stockard, Leplat, Cotronei, Lehmann, Müller, Ancel sono soltanto alcuni della fittissima schiera di medici che si sono applicati a questi studi sino ad arrivare a Fraser e Fainstat che nel 1951 dimostrarono l'azione teratogena del cortisone, specie per la formazione del palato, e nel 1954 l'azione dimile dell'ACTH. Ricordiamo gli studi di Giroud e De Rotschild che affermarono che la tiroxina può essere causa di cataratta, le esperienze di Gerarde nel 1964 sui danni da chemioterapici antitumorali, quelle di Harley e di Done sugli antibiotici, quelle di Chassagne sugli iperdosaggi da Vit. A. Naturalmente è impossibile, in questa sede, fare una disamina completa degli studi sulle malformazioni congenite anche perchè la moderna teratologia, ormai, si confonde ed è parte integrante della genetica. Comunque l'incidenza delle malformazioni è senz'altro andata aumentando negli ultimi anni.

Nella casistica da noi effettuata presso l'Ospedale Pediatrico del Bambino Gesù in Roma abbiamo preso in considerazione i ricoveri dal 1954 al 1971 compreso. Questi sono risultati 158.742 di bambini compresi tra 0 e 12 anni, le malformazioni ospedalizzate sono state 3614, quindi il 2,27 per cento dei ricoveri, incidenza questa ben lungo dalla realtà, sia perchè, naturalmente, solo un modesto numero di questi malati viene ospedalizzato, sia perchè l'esito in aborto o nato morto non ci permette di fare un censimento reale di esse. La prevalenza dei maschi è stata notevole: 66,02 per cento. I decessi, avvenuti quasi sempre per complicazioni sopraggiunte, sono stati l'8,24 per cento dei malformati.

Tipo di malformazione	*Maschi*	*Femmine*	*Totale*
Cardiopatie congenite	242	174	416
Cardiopatie congenite e mongolismo	20	19	39
Malformazioni congenite dell'encefalo	60	16	76
Spina bifida (meningocele e mielomeningocele)	141	174	315
Labbro leporino e palatoschisi	482	274	756
Stenois ipertrofica del piloro	142	29	171
Anomalie congenite dell'esofago, malformazioni, malrotazioni stomaco e intestino	124	80	204
Malformazioni ano-rettali	46	10	56
Malformazioni delle vie biliari	14	4	18
Reni policistici congeniti	11	7	18
Estrofia della vescica	16	5	21
Malformazioni dell'uretra	130		130
Criptorchidismo	187		187
Lussazione congenita dell'anca	28	93	121
Piede torto congenito	250	150	400
Altre malformazioni ossee e dell'estremità	366	133	499
Malformazioni multiple	127	60	187
Totale casi	2386	1228	3614

Tipo di malformazione	*No. casi*	*Mesi* 1	2	3	4	5	6	7	8	9	10	11	12	*Deceduti*	*% decessi*
Cardiopatie congenite	416	37	12	8			2	5	7		4	3	4	88	21,17
Cardiopatie congenite e mongolismo	39	6	3	1	1									11	28,25
Malformazioni congenite dell'encefalo	76	2		3		1	2						1	8	10,52
Spina bifida (meningocele e mielomeningocele)	315	49	2	3			2							58	18,40
Labbro leporino e palatoschisi	756	4		3		2	1		1		4		4	21	2,77
Stenosi ipertrofica del piloro	171	4												4	2,34
Anomalie congenite dell'esofago															
Malformazioni, Malrotazioni stomaco e intestino	204	67												67	32,84
Malformazioni ano-rettali	56	9	1				2							12	21,40
Malformazioni delle vie biliari	18	3												3	16,60
Reni policistici congeniti	18		1					1						3	16,60
Estrofia della vescica	21	1			1	1								3	14,20
Malformazioni dell'uretra	130													—	—
Criptorchidismo	187													—	—
Lussazione congenita dell'anca	121													—	—
Piede torto congenito	400				1									1	0,25
Altre malformazioni ossee e delle estremità	499	2												2	0,40
Malformazioni multiple	187	15						1				1		17	9,09
Totale casi	3614	199	19	18	3	4	9	7	8		8	4	9	298	8,24
							Anni								
Cardiopatie congenite	416		3	1			2							88	21,17
Cardiopatie congenite e mongolismo	39													11	28,25
Malformazioni congenite dell'encefalo	76													8	10,52
Spina bifida (meningocele e mielomeningocele)	315		1	1										58	18,40
Labbro leporino e palatoschisi	756		1		1									21	2,77
Stenosi ipertrofica del piloro	171													4	2,34
Anomalie congenite dell'esofago															
Malformazioni, Malrotazioni stomaco e intestino	204													67	32,84
Malformazioni ano-rettali	56													12	21,40
Malformazioni delle vie biliari	18													3	16,60
Reni policistici congeniti	18		1											3	16,60
Estrofia della vescica	21													3	14,20
Malformazioni dell'uretra	130													—	—
Criptorchidismo	187													—	—
Lussazione congenita dell'anca	121													—	—
Piede torto congenito	400													1	0,25
Altre malformazioni ossee e delle estremità	499													2	0,40
Malformazioni multiple	187													17	9,09
Totale casi	3614		6	2	1		2							298	8,24

Per quanto riguarda il tipo le malformazioni ossee risultano le più numerose, seguite dalle cardiopatie congenite che però sono tra quelle che incidono di più sulla mortalità, precedute soltanto dalle malformazioni dell'intestino, delle quali ben il 32,84 per cento è venuto a morte. Per ciò che concerne l'epoca di morte è evidente che è massima nel primo mese di vita e va decrescendo per ogni tipo di malformazione ad eccezione delle cardiopatie che mantengono una certa costante per tutto il primo anno.

Da questa statistica, che abbraccia un arco di 17 anni, non vogliamo quì trarre delle conclusioni, ma è indubbio che le malformazioni congenite sono andate aumentando nel nostro secolo. Pensiamo. Perciò, di essere nel giusto se i nostri sforzi saranno dedicati ad una medicina preventiva più efficace. Attualmente noi possiamo, già all'inizio del IV^0 mese di sviluppo intrauterino, mediante amniocentesi, conoscere il probabile difetto enzimatico alla base della malformazione e se consideriamo che, sino ad ora, le malattie metaboliche ereditarie, dovute ad una mutazione genetica, sono più di cento, viene con sè che la prevenzione non è più una cosa astratta ed anche se, attualmente, questa si risolve spesso in una indicazione all'aborto eugenico, essa può indirizzare, se non altro, ad una tempestiva terapia subito dopo la nascita e, nei casi più fortunati, ad una terapia farmacologica sul feto ed anche dietetica, attraverso la madre, nei casi accertati di malattia metabolica.

Bibliografia

BICKEL, H., *Prospettive in pediatria*, 1971, **3**, 219.
CAFFARATO, T. M., *Vitalità*, **26**, ottobre, 1964.
DE CARLI, L. e NUZZO, F., *Rassegna clinico-scientifica*, 1971, XLVII, 12, 396.
GOMIRATO-SANDRUCCI, M., *Minerva Pediatrica*, 1960, XII, 160.
FRASER, F. C. e FAINSTATT, T. D., *Pediatrics*, 1951, **8**, 527.
LA CAVA, A. F., Castalia, 1947, **3**, 6.
MARTINELLI, V., *Rivista di Storia della Medicina*, 1970, XIV, 1.
PAZZINI, A., *Storia della Medicina*, Soc. Editrice Libraria, Milano, 1947.
RUSSO, A., MARTINELLI, V. e ROMANI, L., *Aggiornamento pediatrico*, 1961, XII, 12, 791.
TESTA, I., *Infanzia*, **37**, settembre, 1960.
VALENTI, O., *Prospettive in pediatria*, 1971, **3**, 209.
VIGNOTTI, F. e FERRANTE, E., *Le malattie da aberrazioni cromosomiche*, ed. Minerva Medica Torino, 1971.

T. G. Benedek
Pittsburgh, Pa. (U.S.A.)

Recognition of the relationship of sex to disease susceptibility

Answers to the question of 'why do certain diseases occur more frequently in one sex than the other' reveal not only an aspect of medical thinking, but also provide insight into the attitudes of educated men toward women in a given period. The first systematic attempt to evaluate the influences that the sex of a patient may exert on disease was published in 1829 by Carl L. Klose (1791–1863), a professor of pathology, legal medicine and medical history at the University of Breslau. His work was entitled *On the Influence of the Sexual Difference on the Development and Cure of Diseases.* Prior to the nineteenth century the only presumedly systemic diseases that were usually considered to have a sex-related predilection were gout, a disease of men, hysteria, the disease most generally associated with women, chlorosis, which was usually thought to be a variant of hysteria confined almost exclusively to young women, and hypochondriasis, the male analogue of hysteria. A female predisposition to tuberculosis was suggested in the seventeenth century, but became a topic of scientific discussion only in the nineteenth.

Interest in factors which influence susceptibility to diseases grew during the nineteenth century. The monograph on the effect of sex on predisposition published by W. R. Williams in London in 1885 listed thirty-seven 'diseases' with a female and forty-eight having a male preponderance. Some of the diagnoses are categories, such as 'malignant growths' and 'insanity', both said to predominate in women; others are symptoms of various diseases, such as 'ileus' and 'coxalgia' in men, and 'ascites' and 'erythema' predominant in women; several, such as 'febricula' are not recognized today at all.

I have chosen three examples to demonstrate the interrelationships between explanations of sex-related susceptibility to diseases and what these explanations reveal about the relationship between the sexes. Gout, the venerable disease of men, will be presented first, then tuberculosis, about which the question of sex-related predisposition engendered much debate, and finally chlorosis, which is a diagnosis that is no longer made, but was believed to be a disease of women.

Gout differs from the other diseases to be cited not only because it occurs principally in men, but because its pathogenesis since ancient times has had moral connotations. Gout was popularly considered to occur as punishment for, or at least as a consequence of excessive eating, drinking and venery. Pathophysiologic explanations of how such behaviour causes the disease centred about the symptom of 'plethora'. Seventeenth-century hypotheses chiefly pertained to specific humours which were created and/or activated by overindulgence and revealed themselves in part by a plethoric appearance. The symptoms of acute gout depended on the localization of these humours. Gradually the emphasis on blood-born humours diminished in favour of excess of blood volume, usually considered to be associated with an abnormal state of the blood vessels.

A less well-known hypothesis, which had been advanced by Aretaeus in the second century, was that excessive mental strain may also precipitate gout. This was a convenient explanation for gouty authors, such as Sydenham, for whom it certainly was more desirable to offer their intellectual labours as the cause of their ailment than debauchery. However, this idea had greater implications. For instance, Friedrich Hoffmann, early in the eighteenth century, wrote that 'Whoever would live free from gouty pains ought to refrain from weighty cares, the labours of the mind, much thought, anxiety and solicitude. All immoderate passions of the mind eminently and speedily disturb the regular healthful functions of the body . . .'. A century later Charles Scudamore stated that 'Severe study comprises not only want of exercise, lateness and irregularity in the hours of rest and sleep, but also its consequences, weakness of stomach, and inactive bowels; by its effects on the nervous system, from the over-action of the brain, produces that form of irritative debility, which increases the susceptibility of the frame to disease, and consequently to gout, if such be the predisposition of the individual.' The opinion of Charcot, after another half century, was that 'We may not longer deny the influence exercised by cerebral causes; and intellectual labour, moral emotion, and intensity of thought have always occupied an important position in the etiology of gout . . .'.

We must consider three explanations for the occurrence of gout in women: menstrual abnormalities, licentiousness, and inheritance. The Hippocratic aphorism that 'A woman does not take the gout unless her menses be stopped,' was the foundation of the ideas about the relationship of gout to amenorrhea, as well as the first recorded recognition of the rarity of this disease in women. Women were considered less susceptible to plethora, and therefore to gout, because in the eyes of most authors their behaviour did not tend to generate it; furthermore, their structure, being more delicate than that of men inherently restrained the development of plethora; and finally, the menses act as a safety valve and counteract tendencies toward plethora. Thus, cessation of menses, whether due to age or disease, permits gouty humours to accumulate.

To Seneca, the tutor of Nero, may be attributed the first statement that gout occurs in women for the same reason as in men, that is, as a consequence of licentiousness. He believed that the prevalence of gout had risen markedly in women since the time of Hippocrates, four centuries before, and that the increase in gouty women resulted from the circumstance that in his generation as many women as men engaged in debauchery. Until the seventeenth century only lay authors used this explanation. Then, well into the nineteenth century, both laity and physicians employed Seneca's statement, frequently emphasizing the licentiousness of the women who were their contemporaries in comparison to the propriety of the women of their mothers' and grandmothers' generations.

Authors differed about the prevalence of heritably transmitted gout and in ideas about just what was transmitted. According to Gerard van Swieten (1776): '. . . several of the fair sex have been attacked by this disease, notwithstanding they had these discharges in great abundance and regularity: but this, indeed, is more frequently the case with those in whose family it has been hereditary . . .'. William Cullen (1792) stated unequivocally that 'The Gout is generally a hereditary disease.' Charles Scudamore, who made a great effort to study familial occurrence of gout, concluded that some degree of predisposition may be inherited, but that 'body conformation, constitution, temperament, and particular habits of living' are far more important factors. However, A. B. Garrod and some other authorities agreed with van Swieten. Garrod was of the opinion that inheritance was important in two aspects of gout: it results in onset at an early age, and it is responsible for 'most female cases'.

The other way to explain the occurrence of gout in decorous women was to modify the diagnosis with terms such as retrocedent gout, or rheumatism. For example, Benjamin Rush (1805) cited the following case: 'In the year 1794 I attended Mrs. Lloyd Jones, who had a swelling of the same kind in her foot and leg. Her constitution, habits, and the sober manners of her ancestors, gave me no reason to suspect it to arise from the usual remote causes of gout. . . . I mention these facts as an additional proof of the sameness of the gout and rheumatism. . . .'

Now let us proceed to tuberculosis. At one time there had been an hypothesis that amenorrhea may actually cause tuberculosis, and even for some time after 1882, when its bacterial cause was discovered, conjectures about the significance of menstrual abnormalities persisted. According to Richard Morton (1689): 'This is most commonly the original of women's consumptions and I have very seldom seen any woman that was capable of the monthly purgations . . . who ever fell into a consumption without an obstruction of these purgations coming upon it. . . . 'Tis true, indeed, this obstruction may arise in the progress of a consumption from the impoverished state of the blood . . . and therefore is to be accounted an effect rather than a cause of this disease. But many times it is the occasion of the consumption.'

As long ago as Aretaeus and Paul of Aegina haemoptysis was often considered a vicarious and beneficial mechanism for the discharge of the noxious humours that were retained due to amenorrhea. However, in contradistinction to other diseases in which menstruation or its lack was deemed to play an important role, this was not used as an explanation by the advocates of increased female susceptibility to tuberculosis. The question of susceptibility, together with conjectures about its mode of transmission began to receive increasing attention in the latter part of the eighteenth century. The problem of susceptibility was mainly approached in three ways, two of which were analogous to approaches to the other diseases which concern us, namely inheritance and emotional disturbance, and one different, that is biostatistics.

Data which indicated that certain manifestations of tuberculosis were observed more frequently in one sex or the other, as well as regional differences presented difficulties to the theorizers. For instance, in England in the early nineteenth century scrofula and abdominal tuberculosis were more common in men and pulmonary and nervous system tuberculosis in women. Ancell (1852) analysed the statistical data exhaustively and could only conclude that in England 'there is presumptive evidence of the female sex operating in a slight degree as a predisposing cause of tuberculosis.' He considered the most likely explanation for this to be 'that the female sex transmits tuberculosis hereditarily more frequently than the male sex; it probably transmits it more frequently to the female than to the male offspring'.

The following quotation from an 1835 treatise on tuberculosis remarkably resembles a quotation I have given from Scudamore about gout, and also applies to beliefs about chlorosis.

Intense application to study is a powerful cause of tuberculous diseases. This operates in several ways: it necessarily implies sedentary habits, and, consequently, liability to all the evils which arise from them, such as imperfect digestion, constipated bowels, etc. The sensorial power, moreover, is so much exhausted as to weaken the nervous system, and to deprive the various organs, the functions of which are essential to health, of their due proportions of nervous influence. Mental depression also holds a very conspicuous place among those circumstances which diminish the powers of the system generally, and it often proves one of the most effectual determining causes of consumption. Disappointment of long-cherished hopes, slighted affections, loss of dear relations, and reverse of fortune, often exert a powerful influence on persons predisposed to consumption, more particularly in the female sex (James Clark).

Theophilus Thompson carried this thesis forward. He wrote:

. . . although in the country at large many more women than men fall victims to consumption, yet in London the mortality of women from this disease is much less than that for men, and their comparitive immunity is especially observable in married life. . . . The physical circumstances of the two sexes in a great city being for the most part similar, we must seek in mental causes for the explanation of this remarkable circumstance; and such are easily assigned. On the one hand, we see man struggling in this crowded metropolis for the support of his family, beset with the wasting influences of anxious care; whilst, on the other hand, we find woman, endowed with more faith and patience (provided she receive her just share of consideration and tenderness), fulfilling cheerfully the duties of the day, and not so anxiously regarding the morrow. . . .

Thompson correlated the prevalence of illegitimate births and adult deaths attributed to tuberculosis in various localities and did not, as we might expect, conclude that consumption is a retribution for vice. Rather: '. . . in any district most notorious for the number of children born out of wedlock, the women must be assumed to be least happy in condition, most exposed to hope deferred, unrequited affection, bitter ingratitude, and all the causes which tend to wither the heart of those whose life may be said to ebb and flow with their emotions.'

The last disease we shall consider is chlorosis, or 'morbus virgineus'. This now is recognized to have been iron deficiency anaemia due to various causes. As recently as fifty years ago, shortly before the diagnosis ceased to be made, some writers restricted this term exclusively to women. In the original description by Johannes Lange (1554) the typical patient was described to appear 'as if exsanguinated'. However, the disease was not attributed to a deficiency of a component of blood until methods for haematologic examinations were developed in the nineteenth century. Lange believed the ailment to be caused by intoxication from retained menstrual blood, and therefore treatment was directed toward relieving the obstruction. The most effective relief was deemed to result from pregnancy, and thus marriage was recommended as therapy.

We may be tempted to smile about such naivité, but must pause to consider why such ideas continued to have prominent adherents into the twentieth century, when the role of iron deficiency in this disease was already well established. There appear to have been two main reasons for this persistence: the slow development of scientific knowledge about menstruation, and the belief in the inferiority of women. Robert Thomas wrote in 1822: 'The cause of this disease seems to be a want of power in the system arising from weakness to propel the blood into the uterine vessels with a force sufficient to open their extremities, so as to allow a discharge of blood from them. . . . To procure a flow of the menses proves in some cases a very difficult matter. . . . By marriage, and a change in the mode of life, the disorder has in several instances been removed. . . .'

The French clinician, Armand Trousseau, half a century later shifted from biologic to moral conjecturing about the role of catamenia in chlorosis: 'Marriage is one of the hygienical measures recommended to chlorotic girls. . . . The strange idea, after germinating in the heads of some physicians, has become popularized, that the erotic instincts are more developed in chlorotic than in other women. I willingly admit that puberty indicates a woman's fitness to conceive; but I deny that this fitness arouses in her instincts similar to those which it arouses in a man. In our order of society, young girls are as remarkable for chastity in thoughts as in actions. . . .'

Carl von Noorden, a German professor of medicine at the turn of this century, expressed in regard to chlorosis a concern that had become widespread since education of women became more prevalent, namely, that the stresses of obtaining an education would lead to diseases. '. . . No one will deny that the physical and mental growth of many girls is quite sufficient to stand the fatigue and exertion which the higher education and the learned professions have always been accustomed to place upon the growing youths of the male sex. In the enormous majority of young girls this is not so. . . . In view of the frequency of chlorosis in girls who are subjected to physical or mental overexertion, and in view of the significance which the normal maturing of the female organism has for the coming generations, the physician must at least require the great majority of girls to postpone that rigid training of the mind. . . .'

I have sought to show that concern with the question of the predisposition to diseases due to sex was largely a nineteenth-century development and that two schools of thought can be discerned therein. C. L. Klose and nearly a century later P. J. Möbius exemplify ideas that were predominantly sociological; the other, of which W. R. Williams and von Noorden are representatives, emphasizes biological differences. Klose summarized his ideas as follows:

> If the woman shows a greater tendency to diseases than the man it in no way follows that this relationship is based in the nature of the sexes themselves. . . . When her upbringing has not coddled the woman, but rather has aimed to strengthen her body, to restrict the sensitivity of the nerves, and to set the intellect and emotion into the necessary equilibrium so far as possible, we do not see that the man has a lesser predisposition to diseases than the woman. . . . If the female sex is more susceptible to diseases than the masculine, the mode of life which has been assigned to women, and the upbringing which is designed for this mode of life and prepares them for all of its unfortunate consequences. Even if Nature originally gave disease susceptibility equally to both sexes, . . . (this) has been changed to the detriment of women by the influence of civilisation, which has placed them on a higher plane, more befitting them. . . .

Möbius, a German neuropsychiatrist, while he took the greater longevity of women into account, arrived at a more simplistic conclusion: '(1) Men fall ill and die as a result of their activities more frequently than women, and the main causes for the greater mortality in men than women are consumption of alcohol and venereal diseases. (2) There is no logical reason to believe that longevity or resistance against diseases is inherent in the feminine sex.'

The belief in the biologic inferiority of women that is implicit in the opinion of von Noorden about the potentially disastrous consequences of subjecting girls to education was stated even more bluntly by W. R. Williams. According to this English physician the two sexes are susceptible to different diseases because 'There are in women two constitutional peculiarities not immediately attributable to sex, . . . defective sanguinification and a highly nervous organisation. . . . Men are stronger, more passionate, more violent and intemperate than women, yet withal possessed of superior mental powers. They are also more exposed to climatic influences and to the wear and tear of life.'

The various formulations I have related, of course, shed more light on the authors' attitudes toward women than on disease processes. Contemporarily the question of sex-related predisposition to diseases has slipped from polemics into the realm of the biostatistician. Whether the advice of St. Peter to husbands to 'Give honour onto the wife, as onto the weaker vessel' has not only moral, but also biologic meaning remains unresolved.

J. Cule
Llandysul, Wales (Great Britain)

The use of the tobacco enema in the treatment of strangulated inguinal hernia

'The direction given by writers on this subject [of strangulated hernia] is hardly to be trusted; the symptoms which are generally mentioned by them as indications that the time for the operation is come, are most frequently signs that the proper time is just elapsed.'[1]

Ambroise Paré (1510–90) knew what came 'lastly, a vomitting and evacuation of the excrements by the mouth being hindered from the other passage of the fundament. They vulgarly call this affect *Miserere mei*. That you may helpe this symptome, you must rather assay extreame remedies, than suffer the Patient to die by so filthy and loathsome a death. And we must cure it by Chirurgery. . .'[2]

But recourse to surgery, even by the time of Percivall Pott (1714–88), who wrote the warning in the opening paragraph, was not to be undertaken if any other remedy held out a hope of cure. In 1970, there came into my possession, by the kindness of Miss Rosemary Leach, a manuscript written by her forebear Robert Jones of Denbigh (?1807–43), which will eventually be deposited at the Wellcome Institute of the History of Medicine. This apothecary and secretary of the Denbighshire Infirmary (1826–36) recorded some case notes of interest there between 1826 and 1828. Most of the rest of the manuscript is taken up with an account of his education as a pupil in medical and surgical practice in Dublin, where he went for about six months in 1836/7 before his return to Denbigh.

Two of the case notes concern the treatment of Strangulated Scrotal Hernia.

Case 1

William Jones aet. 31, a game keeper & a strong athletic man was admitted 26th May [1826] with a strangulated scrotal rupture on the right side. The tumor was distended & painful – He had been bled – had taken nauseating doses of Antimony & the taxis had been employed, before his admission & all without effect. As soon as he was brought into the House he was put into a Warm Bath & kept there untill syncope came on. The taxis was now tryed but with the same result as before – he was next administered a Tobacco Glyster which produced after the lapse of a few minutes the most distressing effects. The powers of life appeared to be completely overcome, this favorable opportunity was again taken in indeavouring to return the Bowel to its natural situation – not succeeding after giving it every chance, the operation was deemed necessary & was immediately resorted to.[3]

Case 2

Robert Hughes aet. 65 Admitted 21 Sept. [1826] – The Bowel had been strangulated about 60 hours tho' several attempts had been made to reduce it – The tumor was very large & painful – great tenderness over the abdomen – hiccup – cold clammy sweats – pulse small and quick – He was put into the warm Bath & had a Tobacco Glyster which produced great distress The taxis was applied for about 20 minutes but without effect – as there was no time now to be lost the operation was resorted to without further delay. . . .[4]

These patients were treated by a recognized series of therapeutic steps; taxis, then bleeding, taxis, a warm bath, another attempt at taxis, the tobacco enema, taxis again and operation only if all that had failed.

The Enema Nicotianae of the 1807 Pharmacopoeia of the Denbighshire Infirmary consisted of:

Tabacci dr 1
Aquae ferventis oz 8
Infuse.

After such a dose of nicotine,[5] it was small wonder that it 'produced after the lapse of a few minutes the most distressing effects'. But it will not have escaped attention that though 'the powers of life appeared to be completely overcome' the *favourable opportunity* of another attempt at taxis was the aim.

The London Pharmacopoeia of 1836 gives a strength for the Tobacco Enema of 1 drachm of Tobacco to a Pint of Boiling Water, to be macerated for an hour and strained. Professor Redwood commented in 1847 that it had 'been sometimes given in cases of hernia. It is a dangerous application'.[6]

Reduction by taxis was recommended as the initial line of therapy by Astley Cooper (1768–1841) in his *Anatomy and Surgical Treatment of Inguinal and Congenital Hernia*, London, 1804. His instructions were detailed and clear. Empty the bladder, lay the patient on his back, with a pillow under his pelvis and another under his shoulders, the loins then becoming dependent. The thighs were to be flexed to a right angle, with the knees sufficiently together to allow space only for an arm between them, so that the operator could maintain pressure for quarter to half an hour. If this failed, bleeding of 14 to 20 ounces, sufficient to bring on 'a degree of faintness' was recommended. It was hoped the patient would faint and thus produce one of the 'favourable opportunities' for renewed attempts at taxis. The student was advised not to worry about a thready pulse before bleeding, because this was usual in strangulated hernia and would become larger after 'this evacuation'. Next in order came the warm bath at 100 degrees, raising the temperature until once again the patient fainted, 'or feels inclined to do so'. This usually took place in 15 to 20 minutes, after which taxis was again to be tried. Astley Cooper found both bleeding and baths disappointing as they usually failed. 'The two remedies on which, as far as my observation goes, the firmest reliance is to be placed, are, the tobacco glyster, and the application of cold; and if these fail I should be little inclined to await the trial of any other remedy.'

The tobacco glyster could be given in either smoke or liquid form. Sir Astley preferred the liquid enema and liked it prepared by infusing 1 drachm of tobacco in 12 ounces of boiling water for 10 minutes. 'But as the effect of this potent remedy varies very much in different constitutions, and perhaps according to the quality of the tobacco', half only was to be injected at first, and the remainder half an hour later if necessary. He advised against the practice of using two drachms. If effective, he expected to find the patient in a state of extreme languor, with a quick, weak pulse, a cold sweat and no power to exert his voluntary muscles. This seems to be the description of a severely collapsed patient. And one is not surprised to learn that only slight pressure is required for taxis. Possible pre-operative manoeuvres were not yet exhausted for there was still the cold treatment, produced by locally applied brandy and vinegar, vinegar and sal ammoniac, 'or simply dashing cold water upon the naked abdomen'; best of all broken ice, though he warns against the dangers of frost bite! Leeches and fomentations also played a part in his thinking on alternative methods of reducing strangulated hernia. He gave opium during his efforts at reduction, advising against strong purgatives, although permitting opium with calomel and cathartic extract as an aperient. Despite these exhausting and time consuming preliminaries, he claimed to be fully aware of the dangers of delay. If the above trials failed, he operated.[7]

In the notes made by Richard Parton for his certificate of attendance on two courses of Anatomy and Operations signed by Henry Cline and Astley Cooper in April 1803, is recorded Mr. Cline's views on the use of tobacco.

Clysters may be useful as tending to sooth and foment the large intestines, and for this purpose a considerable quantity of tepid water should be thrown up either alone or united with some mild ingredient; but of all injections Mr. Cline prefers the Tobacco and he says all others should give way to it. He makes it by infusing dr 1 of the herb in a pint of boiling water and which he recommends to be injected at once – it produces a Sedative effect – faintness – weak pulse – cold perspiration – looses the power of Speech frequently – lying nearly in an insensible state, so that people round him suppose him Dead – and Mr. Cline says it is common for him to remain so for one hour – after which Mr. Cline has repeatedly succeeded in returning the Hernia and that when many other means had been ineffectually tried. . . .[8]

Lawrence in *A Treatise on Ruptures* (1838) discusses the finer points of the techniques of reduction. Mr. Wilmer of Coventry used a common smoothing iron, which he left on an irreduceable hernia for several hours.[9] A Mr. Macleod believed in prolonged and steady taxis with the right hand, whilst compressing the neck of the tumour with the left. He was present when Mr. Hood, 'after the tobacco-glyster had been administered . . . with the assistance of two carters, applied compression to the tumour' whilst he applied pressure to its neck. 'A full hour was expended under the most unremitting exertions of the four individuals already mentioned, before the displacement was overcome, and yet our patient recovered without a bad symptom.'[10] Lawrence comments that it sounded more like a simple irreduceable hernia, which was not a strangulated one, and that in any case its return was more likely to have been attributable to the tobacco glyster than to the taxis.

The great Jean Amussat (1796–1856) recommended prolonged taxis and went 'to work without previous bleeding or use of the bath'. And should the hand of the operator tire, he was to be assisted by another person who should place his fingers on those of the operator and act in concert with him. Monsieur Amussat was said to persist for several hours, and never to quit before complete reduction of prolapsed parts and the sac! Lawrence found his technique objectionable and dangerous, due to the possibility of reduction 'en masse'.[11] The British methods do not seem to have been entirely free of this danger.

Thomas Sydenham (1624–89) had used the tobacco smoke enema in the treatment of the Iliac Passion, the symptoms of which are those of intestinal obstruction. Once 'the *Peristaltick* Motion (by which, according to the Law of Nature, all things should be conveyed downwards) begins to be inverted, and all things tend upwards, and the Patient is grievously tormented, and provoked to Vomit, the Disease now ending in an *Iliac Passion*. In this Case the Physician can proceed no further in the method of Cure; which the Fever, the Antecedent cause of this Symptom, required, than to order bleeding in the Arm for once: For how many, and whatsoever *Cathar-ticks* you prescribe, will presently become *Emetick*, and so the more promote the inverted Motion of the Bowels; for as much as the strongest purging Medicines, or indeed the least part of them, can scarce pass the Guts, and cause a Stool. In this Case I think it most advisable first to bleed in the Arm, and an hour or two after, to inject a strong Glister. I reckon the smoak of Tobacco, strongly blown up through a large Bladder into the Intestines by a Pipe inverted, to be the best, and most effectual Glister I know, which may be repeated a little while after, unless the former, by giving a Stool, open the passage downwards. But this Symptom being not totally conquered by this Remedy, it is necessary, that a *Cathartick* somewhat stronger, be used, how difficult so ever it be to make way.'[12]

John Woodall (?1556–1643) also used the tobacco smoke enema in the treatment of the Iliac Passion and describes it in the passage on 'Enema Fumosum or a Fumous Glister' of his *Surgeon's Mate*.[13] Despite his enthusiasm for the 'Glister of smoake, . . . very convenient in many occasions, experimented, to bee not onely safe; but also most comfortable, pleasant, profitable, and easie to be perceived in', he makes no reference to it as a restorative. Yet by the eighteenth century, it had achieved a transient popularity in resuscitation of the apparently drowned. Its use in the navy coming to an end in 1812, when that 'portion of the Apparatus for the Use of the Smoke of Tobacco in the Case of Suspended Animation' was banned, 'Because, Tobacco in such Case, howsoever employed, so far from animating must always have a deadly tendency. And consequently, that the Instructions for the Use of Tobacco should be expunged from the printed Directions accompanying the Apparatus.'[14]

This apparatus, as supplied by Messrs. Simpson and Smith, Surgical Instrument Makers to the Navy, consisted of a common bellows connected to a brass box with a wooden casing, which contained the tobacco and supplied the smoke. From this emerged a long brass nozzle, leading into a flexible tube ending in an ivory rectal cannula. For fluid injections such as the tobacco infusion, the bellows and brass box were replaced by a simple syringe.[15]

The pharmacological action of nicotine is complex. It stimulates and then de-presses all autonomic ganglia. At the neuromuscular junction after an initial acetyl-choline-like action depolarizing the end plate and stimulating skeletal muscle, there follows a curare-like effect with a neuromuscular block. The relaxing effect on skeletal muscle is weak. Centrally, it stimulates the respiratory centre before de-pressing it, which does not justify its use in resuscitation as it is so likely to be followed by death. Benjamin Brodie (1783–1862), who had experimented with rectal injections of tobacco on cats and dogs had found a uniformly fatal result. In the *Philosophical Transactions of the Royal Society* for 1811, he describes the vomiting, the syncope, the spasm of the voluntary muscles, cardiac arrest and then on his opening the thorax the considerable cardiac dilatation. He concluded 'from these experiments, that the effect of the infusion of tobacco, when injected into the intestine of a living animal, is to destroy the action of the heart, stopping the circulation and producing syncope'.[16] Dobson believes it was this report which induced the Court of Examiners, who inspected all Naval Surgeons' instruments on behalf of the Royal College of Surgeons, to condemn the use of tobacco 'howsoever employed' in the treatment of 'suspended animation'.[14]

Dr. Daniel Legare of the University of Pennsylvania had already condemned the practice in the United States of America in his inaugural dissertation of 1805, and his was by no means the first warning voice.[17] Tobacco, which had received wide acclamation as a panacea since its introduction into Europe, had also received much general criticism as early as the royal condemnation of James I in his *Counterblast to Tobacco* of 1604.

The continued use of the tobacco enema in nineteenth-century surgical practice was an heroic measure for a desperate situation. Strangulated hernia was a painfully unpleasant and fatal condition, but surgery without either anaesthesia or antisepsis was to be avoided if at all possible. Even toxic doses of nicotine, sufficient to cause severe collapse was regarded by leading surgeons as a justifiable alternative. Whilst its rationale was to reduce the inflammation in the swollen area by decongesting the blood vessels, the ease of the reduction afterward was mainly achieved by the loss of muscle tone and general collapse of the patient. It appears to have been effective enough to have become an accepted part of British surgical practice.

Both of the Denbighshire patients recovered after operation. The young Mr. William Jones was discharged cured after twenty-one days and the elderly Mr. Robert Hughes after thirty-three.

References

1 POTT, PERCIVALL, *A Treatise on Ruptures*, London, 1756, p. 106.
2 PARÉ, AMBROISE, *The Apologie and Treatise of Ambroise Paré* [1585], ed. Geoffrey Keynes, London, 1951, p. 107.
3 Robert Jones of Denbigh MS., p. 14.
4 Ibid., p. 23.
5 Ibid., p. 11 of *Pharmacopoeia*.
6 *Gray's Supplement to the Pharmacopoeia*, re-written by Theophilus Redwood, London, 1847, p. 757.
7 COOPER, ASTLEY, *The Anatomy and Surgical Treatment of Inguinal and Congenital Hernia*, London, 1804, pp. 23–26.
8 Royal Society of Medicine MS. Cline (Henry) Lecture on Surgery: MS. notes taken by Rd. Parton (with Certificate of Attendance on two Courses of Anatomy and Operations, signed Henry Cline and Astley Cooper, 7 April 1803), p. 80. Shelf mark 52 c. 1.
9 LAWRENCE, W., *A Treatise on Ruptures*, 5th ed., London, 1838, p. 143.
10 Ibid., p. 145, citing *London med. Gaz.*, **7**, 264.
11 Ibid., p. 146.
12 SYDENHAM, THOMAS, *The Whole Works of that Excellent Practical Physician Dr. Thomas Sydenham*, 3rd ed., corrected by John Pechey, London, 1701, p. 428.
13 WOODALL, JOHN, *The Surgeons Mate or Military and Domestique Surgery*, London, 1639.
14 DOBSON, J., *J. Roy. Navy Med. Service*, 1957, **43**, 23–28.
15 A Description of the Apparatus for Restoring Suspended Animation from Messrs. Simpson and Smith, Surgical Instrument Makers to the Navy.
16 *Phil. Trans. R. Soc. Lond.*, 1811, pt. I, 186–90.
17 STEWART, G. G., 'A history of the medicinal uses of tobacco 1492–1860', *Med. Hist.*, 1967, **11**, 228–68.

M. Gourevitch
Paris (*France*)

Un psychothérapeute à Bicêtre sous Louis-Philippe, François Leuret

La maladie mentale exprime toujours une lésion du cerveau, au moins hypothétique; le rôle du médecin consiste donc en principe à agir sur cette pathologie lésionnelle en recourant aux thérapeutiques médicamenteuses habituelles et, faute d'y parvenir, il doit observer envers son malade une attitude de compassion, qui s'appelait charité et qui se nomme désormais philanthropie. Tels étaient les caractères essentiels par lesquels la psychiatrie du XIXe siècle apporte une amélioration radicale au sort des malades mentaux, mais s'oppose non moins essentiellement à l'attitude des psychiatres d'aujourd'hui. Dans la première moitié du XIXe siècle, les conceptions modernes ont un seul précurseur direct, qui de son temps a eu très mauvaise presse et qui aujourd'hui a sombré dans l'oubli, François Leuret (1797–1851), médecin de Bicêtre. Il n'a fait aucune concession à la philanthropie. «N'employez pas les consolations, dit-il dès 1834, car elles sont inutiles; n'ayez pas recours aux raisonnements, ils ne persuadent pas; ne soyez pas tristes avec les mélancoliques, votre tristesse entretiendrait la leur; ne prenez pas avec eux un air de gaîté, ils en seraient blessés. Que votre raison soit leur règle de conduite. Une seule corde vibre encore chez eux, celle de la douleur, ayez assez de courage pour la toucher.»

Cette corde douloureuse, c'est la douche qui était chargée de la faire vibrer, cette douche qui aujourd'hui encore, dans la langue populaire, symbolise la thérapeutique physique de la folie (celle des autres; pour soi-même, on pose l'indication d'une cure de sommeil). Mais la bienfaisante ondée tiède dont nous sommes coutumiers dans nos salles de bain ne peut donner aucune idée du Niagara glacé qui suffoquait le patient sous haute pression: «La hauteur moyenne (du réservoir) est de 10 à 15 mètres, correspondant à une pression de une atmosphère à une atmosphère et demie. La pomme (. . .) doit avoir 3 centimètres et demi à 4 centimètres de diamètre, pour donner issue à une colonne liquide de même volume (. . .) La température la plus convenable est celle comprise entre 8 et 12 degrés centigrades.»

Dans quel climat polémique Leuret appliquait-il la douche? En voici une illustration, sous la plume d'Esprit Blanche: «(Il est des hommes qui) se complaisent dans la haute opinion qu'ils ont d'eux-mêmes, et s'obstinent à donner le fruit de leurs pénibles élucubrations pour les limites de l'art. M. Leuret est de ce nombre.»

Si animées que fussent alors les controverses scientifiques, pareil ton n'était pas coutumier. Leuret s'était contenté de traiter de fous ses détracteurs: «Qu'un médecin, avouant qu'il ne sait rien sur la nature et le siège de la maladie à traiter, au lieu d'agir physiquement, ait pour but de combattre des idées par des idées, des passions par des passions; que, pour faire renoncer à des conceptions folles, à des hallucinations, il administre la douche, ou seulement qu'il menace de l'administrer, dès lors il cesse d'agir suivant la méthode reçue, il exerce des cruautés. Ce n'est assurément pas là conclure avec justesse. Je m'étonne que des hommes, dont la profession est de guérir ceux qui déraisonnent, tombent eux-mêmes dans une contradiction aussi palpable.»

Le médecin donc «ne sait rien sur le siège de la maladie» et «combat des idées par des idées». Voilà la doctrine de Leuret. C'est plus qu'il n'en fallait pour déchaîner un ouragan de protestations.

«En s'obstinant, sans aucune bonne raison, à nier que le cerveau, oui, le cerveau seul soit l'instrument positif de la pensée. . . . M. Leuret s'est tout simplement dévoué à un mysticisme que ne comporte plus l'instruction de notre époque. . . .

«Soutenir qu'on ne rencontre ni inflammation des méninges, ni hyperémie du cerveau dans la folie simple, c'est vouloir donner absolument pour caractère à cette maladie de manquer de lésions physiques.

Si l'état actuel de nos connaissances ne permet pas toujours de saisir le rapport intime qui unit les fonctions intellectuelles et les actes matériels de tout l'appareil encéphalique, cela tient d'abord à . . . l'insuffisance de nos moyens d'investigation.»

Protestations haineuses, disions-nous: c'est encore Esprit Blanche, qui rejette ainsi Leuret dans les ténèbres de l'obscurantisme idéaliste. La confusion scientiste, dont il se fait le héraut, entre le matérialisme et un organicisme naïf avait un bel avenir devant elle.

C'est le *Traitement moral de la Folie* qui est ainsi réfuté. Ouvrons-le à notre tour.

«Première proposition. – S'il est vrai que la folie dépende d'une altération de l'encéphale, on ignore complètement en quoi consiste cette altération.

«Deuxième proposition. – Le traitement moral, généralement mis en usage, n'est considéré que comme un auxiliaire du traitement physique (C'est-à-dire clysterium donare, postea seignare, ensuitta purgare. Ce n'est pas une boutade, c'est littéralement vrai: «des évacuations sanguines, des exutoires et des purgatifs») (M.G.).

«Troisième proposition. – Chez les aliénés, l'intelligence et les passions ne peuvent être ramenées à leur type régulier sans le secours du traitement moral; et ce mode de traitement est le seul qui ait une influence directe sur les symptômes de la folie. . . .

«Quant à l'altération qui serait la cause immediate de la folie, je nie que personne l'ait indiquée. S'il en existe une, *elle doit être semblable à celle qui produit les rêves*, qui amène les fausses convictions des individus raisonnables, *qui excite les instincts et les passions* (souligné par nous), elle ne se manifeste jamais par des caractères physiques, et la nature nous en est complètement inconnue. . . .

«. . . La croyance généralement reçue qu'une lésion matérielle et visible du cerveau est la cause de la folie a détourné la plupart des médecins d'aliénés de l'emploi d'un traitement moral énergique. C'est là une faute grave: le cerveau des aliénés n'est visiblement malade que chez les aliénés dont la folie est compliquée d'altération dans les fonctions appelées organiques. . . .

«. . . La médecine morale est donc entrée dans une mauvaise voie; on l'a, sans aucun motif valable, subordonnée à l'anatomie pathologique; il faut l'en dégager et lui donner tout le développement dont elle est susceptible, car c'est à ces conditions seulement qu'elle se montrera efficace dans le traitement des maladies mentales.»

Ce texte fournit à la psychiatrie moderne son titre de propriété sur le domaine qu'elle occupe. Elle peut l'invoquer victorieusement dans les deux procès de mitoyenneté que lui intentent, à sa droite et à sa gauche, «les moralistes» et «l'anatomie pathologique», les psychologues et les somaticiens. Anatomopathologiste éminent, Leuret connaît le cerveau beaucoup mieux que la plupart de ses contradicteurs, et met beaucoup moins d'ambition à prétendre le modifier. Mais il pressent, à propos des «passions», l'existence d'un inconscient normal. Ou du moins, il s'avise qu'un même appareil psychique détermine la dynamique normale, *«celle qui produit les rêves»*, et les productions pathologiques. Peu importent les naïvetés de vocabulaire.

La géniale intuition qui s'exprime ainsi, loin d'être un éclair dans la nuit, animera une conduite thérapeutique toute nouvelle où le médecin répudie la psychiatrie botaniste, refuse de décrire la folie comme un corps étranger, et accepte, nous le verrons, d'établir consciemment une relation avec son malade.

«On comprend sous la dénomination de folie ou aliénation mentale plusieurs états fort différents les uns des autres, et qu'il importe de bien distinguer pour les traiter convenablement. . . .

«On a pourtant essayé, dans ces derniers temps, de n'en faire qu'une seule et même maladie; c'était une nouveauté malheureuse et qui nous aurait reportés bien au-delà des temps hippocratiques. *Mais ceux qui ont eu cette prétention savaient, j'en suis sûr, mieux qu'ils ne disaient, et, dans la pratique, ils se gardaient bien d'appliquer leur doctrine.*»

Voilà, semble-t-il, dans le jardin de l'antipsychiatrie, une pierre bien ajustée.

L'exercice de la psychiatrie met en cause non pas une personnalité mais deux. C'est Leuret qui l'a découvert, et il l'a dit avec quelle force! Et c'est pour cette raison même qu'il renonce aux satisfactions verticales de la philanthropie.

«Tel autre, plus irritable, vous en voudra, croyant que vous vous opposez à ses desseins? Eh bien! qu'il vous en veuille! Est-ce donc pour votre satisfaction personnelle que vous soignez des aliénés? est-ce pour être toujours accueilli par un sourire de reconnaissance ou d'amitié? Alors laissez là la médecine mentale, car vous y trouverez de continuels mécomptes.»

«Si le souvenir du service que vous lui auriez rendu ne parvenait pas à dissiper son ressentiment: eh bien! qu'il vous haïsse, mais qu'il soit guéri!»

N'étant pas philanthrope, il n'espère pas de reconnaissance, et s'il accepte le risque de l'ingratitude, ce n'est pas pour sculpter sa propre statue, c'est pour demeurer jusqu'au bout thérapeute en contrôlant ses propres réactions: «J'eus soin que, dans ma réponse, il ne vît aucun ressentiment, ni même aucun souvenir de nos querelles passées.»

Quant aux sentiments et aux désirs inconscients du malade envers le médecin, Leuret les utilise avec une lucidité qui n'apparaît jamais mieux que lorsqu'il les frustre. Il manifeste alors les formes d'un sadisme qui a pu donner le change aux philanthropes, mais dont en réalité il ne perd jamais conscience. Et il s'en explique d'une façon qui non seulement le justifie, mais fait de lui un précurseur auquel notre temps seul pouvait rendre justice.

«Rappelez-vous que, près d'un malade, vous n'êtes pas homme, mais que vous êtes médecin; et que l'on attend de vous, non pas des égards, de la politesse, de bons procédés, mais la guérison.»

On a tort de ne pas lire Leuret. Il a donné à la littérature psychiatrique quelques-unes de ces «bonnes pages», de ces textes robustes, dignes d'une anthologie et dont le moins qu'on puisse dire est que les temps ultérieurs n'en ont pas été très prodigues. Et la vigueur de son français est soutenue par celle de sa pensée.

Mais c'est une pensée solitaire. Elle ne trahit ni n'exerce d'influence. Si elle peut trouver un écho, ce n'est pas en son temps, c'est, au style près, dans le nôtre. Mais Leuret est mort en 1851, sans avoir jamais été médecin de la Salpêtrière, poste qui consacrait un psychiatre.

Cinq ans devaient encore s'écouler avant la naissance, hors de France hélas, d'un autre anatomiste du système nerveux. Lui aussi quitterait la salle d'autopsie pour s'attacher à «l'altération qui produit les rêves, qui excite les instincts et les passions» et «ne se manifeste jamais par des caractères physiques». Celui-là allait établir, irréversiblement cette fois, qu'on ne fait pas de bonne psychiatrie avec de bons sentiments.

IV SYMPOSIUM

The History of Provision for Health and Welfare

A. Cherubini
Siena (Italy)

Nascita delle assicurazioni sociali in Italia (1860–1920)

Le assicurazioni sociali nascono all'incontro di una triplice esperienza: la benefica od elemosiniera, la mutualista e l'assicurativo-contrattuale. In Italia il primo momento, quello assistenziale, acquista minor valore. Il suo impianto rimane infatti, a preferenza, d'ordine privatistico ed inserito in interessi religiosi, o meglio clericali, chiesastici. Durante l'occupazione francese seguente alle campagne napoleoniche, prende un certo vigore il processo di secolarizzazione dell'assistenza pubblica, ed il principio 'legale' comincia a farsi una qualche strada (seppure scompagnato ormai da quei fini 'sociali', che la Rivoluzione gli voleva attribuire), ma tuttora incerta e restia.

Il Codice napoleonico sancisce infatti la piena autonomia della proprietà privata e una libertà politica a vantaggio della classe dirigente, borghese. Il soccorso continua perciò a vedersi sotto specie filantropica. Anche se il puro ritorno al passato (nelle dottrine e nei metodi) invocato dagli spiriti 'restaurazionali' si rivela impossibile, e certe conquiste rimangono, tuttavia l'arresto è senz'altro notevole lungo il cammino. Il potere municipale amministrativo serba funzioni ispettive e di controllo, non tutti i patrimoni (già confiscati) vengono restituiti alle Opere pie, l'obbligo del ricovero ospedaliero rimane sancito per i poveri affetti da malattia acuta ecc. Ma il liberismo giudica pericoloso il soccorso legale. Poichè il 'quantum' dei salari – egli ragiona – viene determinato dal minimo che occorre per vivere (la cosidetta 'legge di bronzo'), ogni forma di assistenza legale, riducendo un tale minimo, ottiene solo di ridurre proporzionalmente il salario. Nessun beneficio verrà quindi ai lavoratori, mentre lo Stato dovrà moltiplicare le proprie vessazioni per fronteggiare la caduta dei salari con l'aumento dei sussidi. Unico resultato, quello di falsare la concorrenza, dacchè le industrie meno produttive riusciranno avvantaggiate da questa sorta di integrazione salariale.

E' pur vero altresì come dalla stessa 'rivoluzione industriale' nascano vari stimoli tesi al superamento delle trame assistenziali. La protezione già offerta dalle 'corporazioni' si annulla con la scomparsa di queste, proprio mentre la mano d'opera subisce un violento processo di salarizzazione, e nelle fabbriche le condizioni del lavoro si fanno ancor più disastrose. Le città 'industriali' divengono superaffollate, pur restando prive di ogni misura igienica. La facilità del contagio facilita le grandi epidemie, le cui ragioni vengono sempre più e meglio evidenziate dalle inchieste sanitarie. La percentuale dei lavoratori dell'industria scartati alle chiamate di leva è altissima e preoccupante. La medicina del lavoro identifica le malattie professionali, il danno di una fatica eccessiva (per l'individuo e la stessa economia aziendale); di un'alimentazione scadente, nonchè il peso finanziario della morbosità e della moralità nelle classi lavoratrici. Nè la beneficenza può certo valere da unico rimedio. La libera iniziativa – sia dettata dalla filantropia laica che religiosa – più non basta ai nuovi problemi. La propaganda socialista invita alla coscienza e alla solidarietà di classe, mentre denuncia le origini sociali cella miseria. Le correnti politiche liberali puntano allora le proprie carte sulla mutualità, o meglio sopra un'interpretazione liberale appunto dell'associazionismo operaio.

La 'rivoluzione' industriale, abbiam visto, ha rotto l'ordinamento corporativo, lasciando la mano d'opera priva di ogni tutela in fatto di lavoro. Addirittura anzi la legge vieta agli operai di associarsi per la difesa dei 'pretesi interessi comuni'. Maggiori possibilità di resistere hanno le associazioni volte ad altri fini, di aiuto scambievole, già presenti – seppure in forma embrionale – dalla seconda metà del Settecento. La classe operaia allora volge al movimento mutualistico sia per fini politici (che oggi meglio diremmo: sindacali) che assistenziali. In effetti, forme associative operaie basate sul principio solidaristico possiamo trovarle anche prima di questo periodo, eredi della struttura corporativa (mai del tutto tramontata, malgrado gli editti di scioglimento), ed anzi un vero momento di passaggio fra momento corporativo e mutualistico non è ben distinguibile nel tempo. Ma talune differenze di propositi e di meccanismi valgono a colmare sul piano concettuale ogni lacuna. Una vera trama mutualistica mai è presente nel tessuto corporativo, o mai presente nella sua interezza: non obbligo contributivo fisso in rapporto alle prestazioni obbligatorie; non diritto positivo quindi, azionabile entro i termini di statuto e regolamento; soccorso non fisso, predeterminato (caso mai vario in rapporto al danno, fisico od economico), ma relato alle capacità del fondo ed attribuito in seguito ad apprezzamento discrezionale; assenza in genere di una 'riserva' dacchè i fondi raccolti vengono spesi o distribuiti nel corso dell'anno.

Il mutualismo assume invece queste caratteristiche: compito di prevenire il danno, invece di aspettare che arrivi l'indigenza; diritto che insorge all'accertamento obbiettivo del fatto (evento), prestazione fissa e non subordinata a un apprezzamento discrezionale sulla gravità del danno, costituzione di un fondo permanente per via di contributi regolari in lieve accedenza al fine di costituire la riserva, struttura del fondo diversa e secondo gli scopi (ripartizione per il settore malattia, capitalizzazione in varie forme per la pensionistica d'invalidà e vecchiaia, ecc.). Le procedure vengono tratte dall'esperienza dell'assicurazione 'contrattuale' o privata, i cui primi (antichi) esempi si hanno nel commercio marittimo, e che nel XVIII secolo, contemporanea allo svilupparsi degli studi statistici (tavole di mortalità), principia ad occuparsi anche del settore 'vita'. Per quanto riguarda l'Italia la prima compagnia nasce a Milano nel 1825, subito anch'essa manifestando gli inconvenienti altrove riscontrati, e che tengono lontana la classe operaia dalla tutela privatistica: frequenza dell'inganno, scarsa protezione accordata all'assicurato nei confronti dei famigliari, norme troppo minute, premi eccessivi.

Nel XIX secolo l'assicurazione contrattuale cerca di coprire anche il settore degli infortuni sul lavoro e della malattia comune, oltre che la pensionistica per invalidità e vecchiaia. Nell'industria, l'imprenditore qualche volta partecipa al premio assicurativo, sia per spirito filantropico che per tentare forme più strette di vincolo operaio a vantaggio dell'azienda. Il settore 'malattia' è quello più difficile da tutelare, perchè mancano tavole statistiche sufficientemente elaborate. Fra gli antesignani della ricerca possiamo ricordare il nostro Prospero Balbo che nel 1791 pubblica il suo 'Saggio di aritmetica politica', e possiamo ricordare come, già a questa data, Torino è fra le poche città in cui si compila un registro nosologico della morbilità, seppure molto incompleto (nome e mese soltanto, escludendo età, sesso, genere di malattia, esito in guarigione o morte). È solo intorno al 1820 comunque che vengono compilate le prime tavole di morbilità, desumendole da rilevazioni dirette, invece che da rapporti proporzionali istituiti con le tavole di mortalità. Ma si tratta di tabelle ancora inadeguate, destinate a provocare il fallimento di non poche società mutue, ragion per cui le assicurazioni private o preferiscono non avvalersene (escludendo la copertura del rischio) o se ne avvalgono nelle parti a loro favorevoli.

In questo modo, le assicurazioni contrattuali più evidenziano i loro difetti e limiti: intenti di lucro e premi troppo elevati, frodi e abusi, scarsa partecipazione operaia (data anche la scarsezza del reddito), ecc. Come tali, esse quindi si mostrano inefficaci per il problema operaio, e proprio mentre questo si va facendo più acuto e grave. Dopo questa premessa di carattere generale, sarà più facile seguire lo sviluppo dei sistemi mutualistico e previdenziale in Italia.

Il mutualismo qui nasce nella seconda metà del XVIII secolo. Dopo il 1770 le corporazioni vengono abolite in Lombardia, in Toscana, nel Veneto, o di fatto sovvertono compiti e strutture. Seppure con notevole ritardo, la rivoluzione industriale produce d'altronde gli effetti conosciuti: salari scarsi e precari con facile disoccupazione, peggioramento almeno sul piano psicologico delle condizioni di vita e di lavoro, e così via. Gli operai tentano allora nuove forme associative per proteggersi da certi rischi, che limitano od escludono la capacità di lavoro e quindi la possibilità di guadagno. I lavoranti calzettai di Torino già nel 1737 hanno una Cassa di soccorso malattie, cui versano contributi regolari. Sempre a Torino nel 1738 viene costituita una Unione Pio-Tipografica, e nello stesso anno nasce a Venezia la Società di mutuo soccorso fra i compositori. Esempio forse più concreto è quello fornito dal Pio Istituto Filarmonico, fondato nel 1783 tra i professori di musica nazionali dell'orchestra del Teatro della Scala. A Firenze, la Compagnia dei Pennatori o Scardassieri dell'arte della lana, soppressa nel 1785, viene ricostituita nel 1794 sotto forma mutualistica. Con il nuovo secolo, il numero delle Società aumenta. Nel 1822 nasce una società mutua tra i falegnami, nel 1827 fra i lavoranti addetti alle fabbriche di porcellana in Doccia (Toscana). Altre seguono. Persiste ancora un certo spirito di categoria, corporativo, che ne impedisce lo sviluppo in senso orizzontale. I compiti rimangono incerti fra la beneficenza e la mutualità, e largo è il ricorso ai soci protettori, che ovviamente chiedono, in contropartita, il disinteresse politico e cioè l'acquiescienza alla politica dei governi. Lo sviluppo è quanto mai limitato ad alcune regioni, e zone, e mestieri.

Verso il quinto decennio del secolo, la fisionomia accenna a cambiare. Nel 1848 – nascendo da una società mutua di calzolai – viene fondata a Pinerolo, in Piemonte, una Società Generale degli operai, cui aderiscono le Casse particolari. L'iniziativa è sostenuta dalla borghesia d'avanguardia, liberale, e ostacolata dai conservatori, che accusano di propositi rivoluzionari, antimonarchici e di 'principi antisociali'. Anche il clero l'ostacola, sia per l'appoggio fornito dai liberali più accesi (democratici) che dalle mancate esclusioni di iscritti in base a criteri religiosi e simili.

In questi termini, o analoghi, si configura anche l'atteggiamento dei governi italiani. Il mutuo soccorso viene considerato utile come valvola di scarico ad una beneficenza sempre più impegnata e meno bastevole, e viene considerato come stimolo al risparmio ed all'ordine. Si pensa inoltre che possa servire da remora alla costituzione di società d'altra natura (politiche e sindacali) più pericolose e peggio controllabili, specie dove costituite di soli operai. Lungo una tale prospettiva, esso viene quindi sollecitato ed aiutato, ma sempre nel timore che i sodalizi tendano all'autonomia di classe, all'attività 'sovversiva' delle istituzioni. Così l'aiuto viene interrotto a metà, sostituito dalla diffidenza (con i relativi controlli, intralci burocratici, ecc.) ed il mutualismo perde in efficacia. La politica borghese va contro le leggi statistico-attuariali (che altrove sostiene), insistendo per un numero ottimale d'iscritti sui 200, col resultato d'impedire una ripartizione adeguata del rischio. E nega qualsiasi forma obbligatoria d'iscrizione (di cui già si parla) nel timore che – disponendo la continuità dei premi – si rafforzi la richiesta di un 'diritto al lavoro' non più sostanziato di sole parole. Per il mutualismo derivano difetti d'impianto anche assicurativi: procedimenti errati nel rapporto contributi/prestazioni, chiusure di bilancio alla taverna, difettoso ricambio delle generazioni. . . . Lo stimolo esercitato verso una maggiore solidarietà di categoria è comunque indubbio, al pari del ruolo assunto nell'educazione civile e patriottica, specie dopo che nel 1841 Mazzini fonda la 'Unione degli operai italiani', quale sezione della giovane Italia, onde studiare le questioni congiunte alla 'organizzazione e alla retribuzione del lavoro'.

Il mutualismo trae vigore dal clima risorgimentale e si avvia a perdere il suo carattere negativo di frammentarietà, dapprima nel 'libero' Piemonte, dove Carlo Alberto ha nel 1848 abrogato gli articoli del Codice penale contro 'qualunque associazione di più persone organizzate in corpo', e dove nel 1835 le Società di mutuo soccorso raggiungono il numero di 85 (la metà circa di quante ne esistano in tutta Italia).

Sempre in Piemonte, le Società operaie di Pinerolo, Tortona, Casale, Novi Ligure riunite a convegno sotto la volte dell'Associazione generale di mutuo soccorso e d'istruzione degli operai torinesi, approvano sei articoli di aggregazione e l'anno seguente organizzano un convegno cui partecipano 36 sodalizi piemontesi. Nel 1853 si svolge ad Asti il I° Congresso delle Società operaie del Piemonte, per discutere l'educazione popolare, la reciprocità di trattamento, la pensionistica d'invalidità e vecchiaia. L'intervento delle società liguri (mazziniane) introduce temi politici, originando così un contrasto, destinato a produzze feroci lotte intestine. Nel 1860 in Italia si contano 181 società mutue, nel 1867 se ne contano 573 e circa 900 nel 1870, sempre divise in due tronchi: l'uno che accetta (numericamento più modesto) di 'far politica', e l'altro che vi si rifiuta, il primo dominato dai mazziniani, il secondo dai moderati. Nella sfera mazziniana rimane però un limite da superare. Gli elementi che, nel suo principio, partecipano alla mutualità, in genere appartengono all'artigianato od ai settori più colti e progrediti della mano d'opera. Il basso proletariato gli sfugge o ne è sfuggito. Così la propaganda mazziniana, ispirata al solidarismo, perde vigore e avanza quella socialista.

Nel 1878 si calcolano 351.000 iscritti, nel 1885 le società sono circa 4.500 con 780.000 soci circa. Scopo comune, l'assistenza di malattia (sussidio economico, in molti casi assistenza sanitaria gratuita o semigratuita, in un minor numero medicinali gratuiti o con parziale rimborso), cui si aggiungono altri fini diversamente rappresentati: pensioni o sussidi continuativi agli inabili al lavoro (per malattia, per cronicità) e agli infortunati sul lavoro, pensioni (o meglio, promesse di pensione) ai vecchi ed ai superstiti dell'assicurato, attività edilizia popolare, mutuo insegnamento, cooperative di consumo ed anche di produzione, ecc. Le dimensioni sempre maggiori del fenomeno suggeriscono alla classe di dirigente di occuparsene più da vicino, sul piano legislativo. Il progetto è quello di attribuire la personalità giuridica alle società operaie di mutuo soccorso e la relativa legge viene emanata in data 15 aprile 1886, in realtà incontrando scarso favore per gli scarsi vantaggi (certe esenzioni fiscali, gratuito patrocinio, facoltà di possedere beni mobili e immobili) di fronte ai limiti statutari (esclusione della pensionistica d'invalidità e vecchiaia) ed ai pericoli d'ordine politico (interventi delle autorità governative).

Così, al 31 dicembre 1894 le società 'riconosciute' sono pari a 1.156 (17,2 per cento) e pari a 1500 circa (23,7 per cento) al 31 dicembre 1904 con 269.377 iscritti sopra un complesso di circa 6500 Casse con 950.000 soci (di cui 77.000 donne). Poichè lo stesso numero di soci lo troviamo ancora al 31 dicembre 1894, la conclusione appare scontata: il mutualismo, dopo un periodo di rapida espansione, principia a ristagnare, sia perchè non riesce a coinvolgere il proletariato a più basso reddito, sia perchè non riesce a tener fede alle sue promesse (valgano le pensioni d'invalidità e vecchiaia), sia per altri motivi. Non a caso, già coi primi anni del secolo XIX il movimento operaio – convintosi ormai che il puro volontariasmo non serve a proteggere la classe – si avvia a chiedere misure 'obbligatorie' di previdenza sociale.

In questo settore, ben poco l'Italia aveva fatto durante il secolo precedente e fino ai suoi ultimi anni. Cavour prende qualche iniziativa in proposito. Con legge 28 luglio 1861 riordina le Casse per gli invalidi della marina mercantile e con legge 15 luglio 1859 istituisce una Cassa di rendite vitalizie per la vecchiaia, aperta a ogni cittadino e del tutto volontaria, con l'esclusione di qualsiasi concorso statale. La pensione, al compimento di una determinata età, non poteva superare le lire 1200 annue, e ciò al fine di evitare ogni 'speculazione' dei ricchi, bensì non vengono accettati versamenti inferiori alle 5 litre, e quindi nemmeno i poveri possono avvalersene. Le società di mutuo soccorso le si schierano contro e d'altronde la legge mai viene attuata, al punto da ricordarla oggi soprattutto per due clausole singolari, cioè non comuni: l'accettazione degli stranieri (con riferimento ai numerosi italiani immigrati od esuli in Piemonte) e il diritto per la moglie di accedervi fuori del consenso maritale.

Durante il governo della 'Destra storica', iniziative del genere ancor più ristagnano. Nel 1869 viene costituita la 'Commissione consultativa sulle istituzioni di previdenza e sul lavoro', con lo scopo di raccogliere elementi e preparare progetti di legge sulle Casse di risparmio, le società di mutuo soccorso, le cooperative di vario genere, nonchè di studiare le questioni relative alla pensionistica operaia, all'igiene industriale, all'apprendistato, ecc. Ma i principi puramente liberali (e liberistici), cui il governo s'ispira, non consentono grandi voli. Il ministro Minghetti tiene bene a precisarlo, nel presentare il suo progetto dell'anzidetta Commissione. Criteri validi in materia sociale sono 'prestare incoraggiamento e aiuto ... (ma non) inframmettersi direttamente in un campo dove soltanto la libera spontanea iniziativa dei cittadini deve spiegare la sua efficace operosità. Il Governo non può entrarvi se non per rimuovere alcuni ostacoli ... principalmente quelli i quali dipendono dalla mancanza di una provvida ed opportuna legislazione.'

Il clima parrebbe mutare con l'avvento al potere della 'Sinistra', dopo il voto del

18 marzo 1876. Il Ministro dell'interno Nicotera nomina subito una Commissione per la riforma delle opere pie, la cui situazione si va rivelando sempre più disastrosa. Nel gennaio 1877 il deputato Mancardi propone di ricostituire, con qualche modifica, la Cassa per le pensioni vitalizie di cui alla legge del 1859. Nel marzo 1878, il deputato Pericoli illustra alla Camera un suo progetto di legge per la tutela degli infortuni sul lavoro.

Nulla però segue di concreto. Depretis cerca di guadagnar tempo sulle promesse elettorali, rimanda allo studio delle Commissioni. L'egual cosa accade per i seguenti progetti in materia infortunistica: quello del giugno 1880 presentato dai deputati Minghetti-Luzzatti-Villari, e quello del giugno 1881 presentato dal Berti di concerto con lo Zanardelli. Si affiancano, destinati alla medesima fine, altri progetti sull'assicurazione di vecchiaia (novembre 1881), sulla regolamentazione degli scioperi, sul riconoscimento giuridico delle società di mutuo soccorso, sul lavoro delle donne e dei fanciulli.

L'ultimo quarto del secolo è caratterizzato da un maggior vigore del processo d'industrializzazione, specie nel settore dell'industria pesante, che vale però ad accrescere la sperequazione economica regionale; ed è caratterizzato da un aumento cospicuo e generale dei prezzi, mal compensato dalla curva pur ascensionale dei salari. Nuovi 'rischi' poi – abbiamo veduto – si accendono, inerenti alla salute (infortunio, malattia professionale, patologia da usura, abbandono igienico) ed al lavoro (disoccupazione). Il primitivo assenteismo liberale è quindi costretto a cedere, ma la via scelta è dapprima ben lontana da quella di un progresso franco e illuminato.

I progetti di cui abbiamo fatto cenno guardano a certi aspetti della questione sociale, ma in pura funzione conservatrice: distogliere gli operai dalle teorie sovversive o controllare l'attività dei loro sodalizi, ben più e prima che adoperarsi per un proficuo regime previdenziale. La tesi di fondo rimane quella di un associazionismo libero, con l'esclusione di qualsiasi forma di 'obbligo'. Un eventuale concorso (finanziario) dello Stato è visto solo in modo occasionale e breve, dovendo il finanziamento resultare a carico esclusivo delle categorie interessate, o più esattamente a carico dei soli beneficiari, gli operai, poichè l'industria, in fase di espansione non potrebbe – si afferma – sopportarne l'onere senza grave discapito per il processo produttivo.

Nei confronti degli infortuni i progetti di legge si basano – più o meno – sull'inversione della prova, quando non si limitino semplicemente ad accrescere quantitativamente la responsabilità degli imprenditori e dei proprietari, senza però derogare dal diritto comune. Nei confronti della pensionistica, il ricorso è a un tipo di 'assicurazione popolare', però affidata a un Istituto pubblico. Il capitale d'impianto di tale assicurazione potrebbe avvalersi di accorgimenti particolari; gli utili derivanti dall'impiego dei depositi giudiziari, i biglietti di banca non presentati al cambio, l'avanzo della rendita del Fondo per il culto.

Malgrado la mitezza dei propositi, tutti i progetti vengono del pari respinti, e infine il Berti è costretto a dimettersi. Il programma viene ripreso in modo più fiacco ancora dal ministro che gli succede, il Grimaldi. A parte il riconoscimento giuridico delle società di mutuo soccorso, è solo varata una legge sul lavoro dei fanciulli (febbraio 1886), comprensiva anche di norme regolanti il lavoro femminile. Interessante è ricordare come, durante quest'ultimo dibattito, diverse voci si levarono, inascoltate, per proporre l'astensione dal lavoro delle puerpere lungo un certo periodo di tempo. Maggior cura viene invece posta alla previdenza di alcuni pubblici dipendenti. Nel dicembre 1878 si crea un 'Monte delle pensioni per gli insegnanti elementari', nel 1881 viene istituita una 'Cassa delle pensioni civili e militari a carico dello Stato'. Nel 1883, su base volontaristica, nasce la 'Cassa nazionale di assicurazione per gli infortuni degli operai sul lavoro'.

Respinto dal Senato il secondo disegno di legge Berti sulla responsabilità vicile, del pari basato sull'inversione della prova (1882), la Cassa di cui sopra viene istituita, mediante convenzione fra il Ministero dell'agricoltura e alcuni istituti di risparmio, come Ente morale autonomo, amministrato dalla Cassa di risparmio di Milano, con il compito di stipulare, in via facoltativa, contratti individuali o collettivi, per la copertura degli infortuni sul lavoro, in cui l'incapacità lavorativa superi i 30 giorni. Le spese di amministrazione sostenute dagli istituti fondatori, la rinuncia alle imposte governative ed altri servizi gratuitamente concessi fanno sperare che – resultanto i premi più bassi – più facili siano le iscrizioni. L'indennità per gli operai è pari a 300 giornate in caso di morte o d'invalidità permanente, e fino alla metà in caso d'invalidità temporanea.

Le iscrizioni però scarseggiano. Al 31 gennaio 1886 sono state stipulate appena 483 polizze per 18.091 operai con L. 60.519,38 di premi. La clausola dei 30 giorni minimi (d'incapacità al lavoro) è tolta e il Ministero dispone che in tutti gli appalti per conto dello Stato sia fatto obbligo agli appaltatori di assicurare direttamente i propri operai o di subire una ritenuta dell'1 per cento sul prezzo, in prò dell'assicurazione effettuata direttamente dallo Stato.

Malgrado ciò l'iniziativa continua a stentare. Nel 1893 sono assicurati 125.119 operai, che salgono a 160.772 nel 1898, mentre gli infortuni resultano invece notevolmente accresciuti dal 16,68 al 78,08 per mille. La convinzione che necessita mutare cammino ed instituir l'obbligo assicurativo, si è fatta pressochè generale. L'esperienza tedesca in proposito viene attentamente seguita. Non si è avverata alcuna di quelle previsioni catastrofiche che il liberismo ortodosso aveva avanzato, e una qualche teorica del socialismo della cattedra si fa strada anche in Italia. Il movimento operaio si è del pari convinto che occorre passare dalla volontarietà all'obbligo.

In un primo momento, le organizzazioni di classe – strette dalla contraddizione di fondo tra riforme e rivoluzione – avevano espresso un aperto rifiuto verso qualsiasi legislazione borghese, anche favorevole, solo chiedendo una completa autonomia d'azione. Le stesse correnti politiche moderata e repubblicana rifiutano all'inizio leggi previdenziali, solo invocando aiuti per la libera mutualità. Quindi repubblicani e democratico-radicali principiano ad avvicinarsi con minor disagio (o con maggiore interesse) a certi temi classici di un sistema previdenziale 'organizzato', quali apposite leggi, istituti nazionali, partecipazioni contributive dei datori di lavoro e dello Stato. All'opposizione intransigente – in questo periodo che ancora manca di un vero 'partito' socialista – rimangono solo gli anarchici e gli operaisti i quali, al III Congresso della Confederazione operaia lombarda (1883) e in altri Congressi continuano a sostenere come il problema operaio debba seguire strade diverse dal Codice borghese, e quindi respingono i progetti di legge Berti come ogni altra legislazione sociale, in quanto destinata inevitabilmente a favorire il capitalismo e a retardare e contenere la lotta di classe.

I 'socialisti', che stanno nascendo proprio attraverso una differenziazione progressiva (e quindi definitiva) con gli anarchici puri e gli operaisti intransigenti combattono anch'essi i programmi governativi, ma non perchè lesivi in sè della lotta di classe, bensì nella misura in cui si presentano parziali, inadeguati, o addirittura consapevolmente nemici delle più vive esigenze operaie. In luogo di un rifiuto aprioristico, chiedono interventi dello Stato per soluzioni reali, ed anche realistiche (occorrendo). Tipico il giudizio del Costa, discutendosi nel 1884 il programma del ministro Berti: 'esso non è il nostro, ma ci spiana la strada'. La nascita ufficiale del partito socialista (1893) è a questo riguardo fondamentale, con la dichiarazione di un 'diritto . . . alla sicurezza sociale dell'esistenza'. Dalle colonne della rivista del partito, la 'Critica sociale', Bissolati spiega come la pressione del movimento operaio organizzato deve esercitarsi per costringere la borghesia a varare leggi indispensabili di materia sociale, nel campo del lavoro e della previdenza. L'azione dello Stato ormai viene richiesta ed anzi pretesa perchè siano dichiarati taluni diritti (al lavoro, al soccorso in mancanza di lavoro) e taluni doveri (obbligo assicurativo, esclusivo carico dell'impresa negli infortuni sul lavoro, onere esclusivo o prevalente della medesima e partecipazione statale nella pensionistica, ecc.). Il Congresso socialista del settembre 1900 già introduce un sistema protettivo a maglie serrate. Sulla base di questi impulsi (senz'altro prioritari e decisivi) anche le correnti liberale-progressista e perfino quella cattolica si avvicinano a tesi analoghe, seppure – ovviamente – meno impegnate. La 'Rerum novarum' (1891), pur con tutti i suoi limiti, contiene pur sempre un invito per lo Stato ad operare contro le tendenze assenteistiche del liberismo integrale, anche se preferisce tuttavia insistere sulla persuasione morale in luogo della legge. Di conseguenza, nella pratica, il problema divien quello di sollecitare i padroni perchè volontariamente iscrivano i loro operai alle società assicurative private contro l'infortunio, per ora escludendo l'obbligo assicurativo; ma un passo notevole verso una dimensione diversa della previdenza è ad ogni modo compiuto.

I difetti del sistema benefico-assistenziale pubblico e privato essendosi ormai fatti palesi e intollerabili, viene approvata la legge 'organica' di riforma delle Opere pie nel 1890. La legge, pur senza accogliere il 'diritto al soccorso', stabilisce però una serie di trasformazioni, che rendono (ma soprattutto dovrebbero rendere) il settore più vigile e operante. Ormai però la beneficenza, in ogni sua forma (ivi compresa la 'legale') si rivela incapace di affrontare gli aspetti sempre più gravi della questione sociale, ed anche il mutualismo si mostra sempre meno adatto a rispondere positivo ai bisogni crescenti delle masse popolari, specie nei settori dell'invalidità e della vecchiaia.

In Germania il Bismarck ha frattanto creato una vasta rete di assicurazioni sociali obbligatorie, con il concorso padronale e dello Stato, convincendo che l'economia nazionale – lungi dal trarne un danno – ne ha ricevuto un grosso vantaggio, ed altresì convincendo, dati alla mano, che il movimento operaio, pur avendo accresciuto i propri consensi al partito socialdemocratico, in realtà lo ha spinto verso le vie del gradualismo riformista. Per altro verso, anche in Italia (come altrove), in casi d'infortunio sul lavoro, i tribunali condannano con sempre maggiore frequenza e pesantezza i datori di lavoro ad indennizzi onerosi, tanto più da quando le testimonianze operaie in tribunale divengono più esperte e sicure e decise. La tesi dell'obbligo assicurativo conquista quindi uno spazio sempre più largo, per trasferirsi nella legge istitutiva del 1898.

In Italia, per il settore ovviamente infortunistico, di obbligo assicurativo e di premi a carico esclusivo dell'impresa, si parla per la prima volta nel 1890 (progetto Miceli), ma l'altalena parlamentare segue senza nessun costrutto. Il 13 aprile 1897 il ministro Guicciardini presenta infine il suo progetto che, approvato dopo accanita discussione dai rami delle due Camere con varie modifiche (non però sostanziali), diviene la legge 17 marzo 1898 n. 80, la quale sancisce:
(1) l'obbligo assicurativo nei confronti del rischio professionale per talune categorie di lavoratori (dell'industria), il premio ad esclusivo carico delle imprese, le sanzioni penali per la violazione della norma;
(2) l'indennizzo comunque attribuito, anche dove non venga dimostrata la responsabilità civile dell'imprenditore, fuori dalle condizioni che prima la escludevano (colpa operaia, caso fortuito, forza maggiore) o la ponevano in dubbio (indisponibilità economica dell'impresa, litigi interminabili);
(3) l'affiancamento di un servizio pubblico, il quale ha il dovere di accogliere qualsiasi proposta di assicurazione, anche quelle rifiutate dalle compagnie private, seppure dietro certe garanzie di correttezza e di solvibilità.

L'industria trae un vantaggio notevole, conoscendo in anticipo l'onere economico (che può così riflettere sui prezzi) ed evitando le ripercussioni gravi di eventuali disastri. E la base di un nuovo istituto (il 'previdenziale') è sicuramente posta nel diritto alla prestazione che sorge, 'ex lege', seguendo il rapporto di lavoro, indipendentemente dalla volontà stessa dell'operaio e senza che gli venga richiesto alcun adempimento formale. Anche i limiti e i difetti della legge furono subito manifesti: il campo di applicazione eccessivamente ristretto alle industrie di maggiore pericolosità, con l'esclusione del settore agricolo (e delle malattie professionali, soprattutto in Italia ormai da tempo identificate nei loro rapporti con il lavoro esercitato); libera scelta dell'assicuratore mantenuta, con grave danno della Cassa nazionale, che si vede fare una concorrenza spesso illecita e scaricare addosso i rischi più gravi; indennità non solo stabilite in aliquote minori di quelle che avrebbe attibuito il Codice civile, ma stabilite in aliquote troppo misere (specie considerando che vien tolta la facoltà di intentar causa per una qualsiasi colpa padronale); copertura del rischio affidata alla stipula del contratto, per cui – verificandosi l'omissione o verificandosi il mancato pagamento dei premi – all'operaio non rimane che intentar causa per ottenere quanto la legge (e cioè, ormai, il disposto assicurativo) gli avrebbe assegnato.

Nello stesso anno 1898, dopo vari inutili precedenti tentativi, viene altresì approvata l'istituzione di una Cassa nazionale di previdenza per la vecchiaia e l'invalidità degli operai, concepita come una sorta d'istituto di Stato per le assicurazioni popolari. Il fondo iniziale è costituito con vari cespiti (cinque milioni sulla somma dei biglietti consorziali definitivi prescritti per conseguenza della legge sull'abolizione del corso forzoso, cinque milioni sulla somma degli utili netti e disponibili delle Casse di risparmio), quindi accresciuto con altri cespiti di eguale natura. Le entrate ordinarie della Cassa sono rappresentate da una terza parte degli utili netti annuali delle Casse postali di risparmio, dall'importo delle eredità vacanti devolute allo Stato e analoghi. L'iscrizione è del tutto libera e volontaria, aperta ai cittadini italiani d'ambo i sessi che attendano a lavori manuali, ovvero prestino servizio ad opera o a giornata. Il contributo minimo è di lire sei annue, versabile anche a rate non minori di 50 centesimi; il contributo massimo è di lire 100. Per ciascun iscritto, la Cassa concorre con un'aliquota, che non potrà comunque superare le lire 12 annue. La pensione di vecchiaia è attribuita a 60 od a 65 anni di età, quella per invalidità purchè siano trascorsi almeno cinque anni dall'iscrizione.

La Cassa è aperta ai lavoratori agricoli. La donna maritata ed il minore possono iscriversi anche senza l'altrui consenso, e notevoli facilitazioni vengono concessi nell'ordine fiscale. Le sue capacità di espansione si rivelano tuttavia modestissime: nel 1903 appena 126.640 iscritti, che salgono ad appena 241.329 nel 1907. A questa data siamo già ben entro quello che vien detto 'periodo giolittiano'.

Con il febbraio 1901 si forma il ministero Zanardelli, in cui Giovanni Giolitti assume la carica di ministro dell'interno. Nel novembre 1903 Giolitti diviene presidente del Consiglio per rimanere tale, salvo brevi parentesi, fino al marzo 1914. Il giudizio sull'uomo è controverso: per taluni riformista d'accatto (il minimo necessario a conservare il potere e tener calmo il popolo), impegnatissimo nel ridurre ogni questione politica a faccenda amministrativa, corruttore di uomini e di sistemi; per altri, forse lo spirito più intelligente e illuminato che l'Italia abbia visto nella propria recente storia. E' un fatto innegabile comunque che il periodo 'giolittiano' è segnato da un notevole sviluppo economico, e per certi aspetti sociali: aumento dei salari (della produzione, del commercio, del benessere) nel clima di una libertà sindacale prima sconosciuta, diminuzione notevole della mortalità, bilanci statali chiusi in attivo per vari anni.

La questione sociale viene in primo piano, insieme con lo studio dei mezzi per risolverla. Senza dubbio certe riforme (o modificazioni) sono intese quale strumento per battere il socialismo prorompente e rafforzare le istituzioni borghesi, riconquistando le masse lavoratrici allo Stato, ma sarebbe ingiusto negare anche un'esigenza di giustizia nell'uomo e nella sua politica. Il 'filosocialismo' giolittiano delle origini è senz'altro un mito, ma non gli rimangono indifferenti talune esigenze – per cui il socialismo combatte – di una più valida democrazia. I socialisti, dopo la grande battaglia di fine secolo, pensano in maggioranza ad una conquista graduale dello Stato, ad un inserimento progressivo nelle sue maglie tramite l'allargamento del suffragio (a suffragio in ultimo universale) e una legislazione sociale adeguata. Le riforme legislative come criterio dell'azione socialista è il proposito evidente di Turati, nella convinzione (tuttora positivistica) di una ineluttabile vittoria finale. Da una parte i bisogni concreti della classe operaia, dall'altro lo sviluppo dello Stato democratico, e quasi per una spontanea dialettica, a termine, la costruzione socialista. A livello di principi, la teorica può risultar discutibile, ma negli effetti pratici i risultati giungono innegabili, seppure dopo un certo periodo di tempo, quando il 'periodo' giolittiano è ormai chiuso e la guerra ha portato nuovi stimoli. Bensì questo va senz'altro detto e ripetuto: l'elaborazione concettuale di una previdenza sociale a largo raggio, allo scadere del 1914, può dirsi ormai in Italia un fatto compiuto.

I socialisti dapprima puntano soprattutto sull'estensione all'agricoltura della tutela infortunistica e del probivirato, sull'assicurazione obbligatoria per l'invalidità e vecchiaia, sull'istituzione di una Cassa di maternità. Qualche incertezza e remora rimane per il settore malattia e disoccupazione, che si vedrebbe volentieri il primo affidato ancora alla mutualità (opportunamente sovvenzionata) ed il secondo agli organismi professionali, pur nel quadro dell'obbligo (ambedue i settori) e del concorso padronale e statale. Si tratta però di incertezze sempre meno decise (e decisive). Solo gli 'integralisti' continuano a negare qualunque forma di legislazione sociale, universalmente priva di qualsiasi merito. Bensì per quanto è debole il loro diniego, suona abbastanza forte la voce dei 'socialriformisti' i quali, dopo la scissione (Bissolati) dal Partito socialista insistono sulla materia, chiedendo al loro Congresso romano del dicembre 1912: statizzazione dell'assicurazione infortuni, estesa all'agricoltura; assicurazione obbligatoria per l'invalidità e la vecchiaia, con il triplice contributo (operaio, padrone, Stato) e speciali disposizioni per la piccola proprietà e l'artigianato; coordinamento degli istituti relativi all'invalidità e vecchiaia con quelli benefici del settore specifico; avviamento dell'assicurazione obbligatoria contro tutte le malattie professionali e quelle, comunque causate, che colpiscono in modo più frequente e grave certe lavorazioni; integrazione della previdenza libera contro le malattie attraverso le società di mutuo soccorso ed i sindacati di mestiere; estensione dell'assicurazione di maternità (e di malattia) a tutte le lavoratrici; sussidi integrativi per la disoccupazione involontaria, in attesa di un giudizio sull'esperimento inglese di assicurazione obbligatoria.

La Confederazione generale del lavoro si colloca sulla stessa linea delle richieste socialriformiste, però con punte che più tendono all'obbligo generalizzato (e la pari opposizione dei sindacalisti rivoluzionari). Radicali e repubblicani condividono anch'esse le istanze dei socialriformisti, con minor vigore. I cattolici, dopo la parentesi della 'democrazia cristiana' di Murri, tornano a risentire maggiormente delle spinte interne conservatrici. Il loro programma sociale si presenta vago e generico, seppure sollecitato dalla spinta popolare. Bensì questa riman sempre tale da sospingerli, quasi loro malgrado, da criteri previdenziali di 'persuasione' verso un rispetto più denso dell' 'obbligo'. Ciò soprattutto quando Giolitti, venutogli a mancare l'appoggio socialista, si avvicina ai cattolici, con proposito di usarli quali freno (alle richieste socialiste) e di recuperarli allo Stato borghese. Il processo è così certo e deciso, che perfino l'opposizione costituzionale ('di Sua Maestà') deve concedergli. Conservatore in politica e progressista in economia, Sonnino presenta nel 1906 un disegno di legge sull'ispettorato del lavoro, approvato nei singoli articoli (e poi respinto a scrutinio segreto), e nel 1913 un progetto di pensioni obbligatorie per la vecchiaia.

Le società medesime di mutuo soccorso si accorgono di non poter più reggere ai bisogni crescenti della classe operaia, senza profondi mutamenti della struttura 'assistenziale'. Il Congresso nazionale della previdenza già nel 1904 fa voti perchè la Cassa nazionale infortuni e quella di previdenza si uniscano in un forte Istituto, destinato a provvedere agli infortuni, alla vecchiaia, alla maternità, alla disoccupazione, ecc., gestito in maniera democratica (rappresentanze delle Società mutue e previdenziali nella direzione ed amministrazione). Anche i medici chiedono urgenti riforme, e un vasto programma d'interventi non solo per le malattie sociali ma tutti gli aspetti sanitari della questione sociale (igiene delle fabbriche, alimentazione, abitazione, vestiario . . .). Di contro a questo sviluppo del pensiero previdenziale, è tuttavia doveroso ammettere come scarseggiano le realizzazioni, salvo forse nel settore del pubblico impiego (dove speciale interesse vien serbato alla pensionistica).

Con legge 29 giugno 1903 (e quindi con T.U. 31 gennaio 1904, praticamente in vigore fino al 1935) vengono portate alcune modifiche alla legge sugli infortuni nel lavoro. I principi informatori restano identici: obbligo di assicurare per l'azienda e la Cassa nazionale, all'infuori di quello che sia il comportamento dell'operaio o dell'imprenditore; onere ad esclusivo carico dell'impresa in varia misura secondo la classe del rischio; nullità dei patti in contrario; libertà di scelta fra i soli istituti autorizzati e con preciso riferimento ai patti di polizza, ecc. Il campo i applicazione diviene assai più vasto, fino ad includere talune categorie di lavoratori agricoli, e vengono cresciute le indennità (che, su richiesta dell'Istituto, l'impresa è in obbligo di anticipare). I medici condotti e ospedalieri a loro volta sono obbligati a certificare sulla natura e sulle conseguenze dell'infortunio, e gli ospedali sono tenuti al ricovero (salvo il rimborso delle spese). Protetti gli eventi che inducono inabilità superiore a cinque giorni, purchè la medesima non risulti inferiore al 5 per cento. Viene costituito un Sindacato obbligatorio siciliano di mutua assicurazione per gli infortuni sul lavoro nelle miniere da zolfo (1904) e un Sindacato obbligatorio marittimo meridionale per l'assicurazione contro gli infortuni sul lavoro della gente di mare (1905). La Cassa nazionale infortuni continua a trovarsi notevolmente svantaggiata nei confronti delle libere compagnie assicuratrici, costretta com'è ad accettare ogni sorta di rischio ed a subire una concorrenza spesso sleale. Nel 1903, essa comunque già può annoverare 421.363 assicurati. Purtroppo facili e frequenti le frodi.

Scarso il progresso nel settore invalidità e vecchiaia. L'obbligo d'iscrizione viene sancito per talune categorie: operai dipendenti dall'industria privata, come quelli delle tramvie intercomunali (4 per cento del salario a carico dell'operaio e 4 per cento dell'impresa), delle costruzioni navali (contributo di lire 6 a carico del proprietario); operai dipendenti da enti locali; operai dipendenti da amministrazioni statali (manifatture tabacchi, silurificio, zecca, uscieri addetti agli uffici giudiziari, ecc.), per cui la contribuzione – paritetica o meno – chiama sempre ad ogni modo in causa il concorso statale. Anche altre categorie principiano ad avvantaggiarsi di contributi analoghi, e così, per fare un esempio, lo Stato interviene con un concorso annuo di lire 130.000 (180.000 dal 1914) per l'iscrizione alla Cassa nazionale di previdenza di certo personale ausiliario (ruolo commessi degli uffici di registro e delle ipoteche). Ma, per la gran parte dei beneficiari, l'iscrizione alla Cassa riman libera e volontaria, e quindi il suo intervento scarsamente efficace.

Nel 1910 viene istituita la 'Cassa di maternità', per sussidiare le operaie di cui alla legge sul lavoro delle donne e dei fanciulli del 1907 in occasione di parto o aborto. L'onere è diviso in parti eguali fra padroni ed operaie, lo Stato concorre, e l'iscrizione si decide obbligatoria. Nel 1912 si crea l'Istituto Nazionale Assicurazioni, col proposito (poi deluso) di affidargli il monopolio delle assicurazioni sulla vita. Nel 1913 i vari istituti di previdenza marinara vengono riuniti, e la gestione della loro Cassa è affidata alla Cassa nazionale di previdenza.

Con il regolamento generale di sanità del febbraio 1901 poteva dirsi nata la medicina scolastica. Anche la prevenzione degli infortuni viene potenziata con le leggi che riguardano l'esercizio delle strade ferrate, delle tramvie, delle miniere, ecc. Nel 1902 la Direzione generale di sanità presso il Ministero degli interni viene completamente riorganizzata. Nel 1904, la legge sugli alienati disciplina per la prima volta in modo organico la materia. Un nuovo testo unico delle leggi sanitarie è approvato nel 1909. Dal 1901 al 1909 si succedono varie leggi sulla risicultura e sulla distribuzione gratuita del chinino: lo Stato avoca a sè la fabbricazione, la vendita e la distribuzione del chinino per i lavoratori delle zone malariche e per i loro famigliari che partecipano ai lavori aziendali. Nel 1904 sono create le Commissioni di assistenza e beneficenza, al fine di rendere più agile (ed agevole) il settore, anche per quanto ne riguarda gli aspetti sanitari. Nel 1905 la profilassi delle malattie veneree è completamente separata dal regime di polizia (d'ora in poi solo riferito alla prostituzione). Regolamenti speciali vengono dettati sui lavori insalubri, e del 1913 è la legge che regola l'esercizio delle farmacie. Si affiancano norme sul riposo settimanale (1907), sul lavoro delle donne e dei fanciulli (1902 e 1907), sull'Ufficio del lavoro (1902) e sull'Ispettorato del lavoro (1912), sull'abolizione del lavoro notturno nella panificazione e pasticceria (1908), ecc. E si affiancano il diritto di sciopero nonchè l'allargamento del suffragio.

Malgrado tutte queste realizzazioni, è oggi doveroso concludere come il settore previdenziale rimanga nel 'periodo' quello relativamente più trascurato. L'elaborazione concettuale verso un sistema di previdenza organico e largo è fuori discussione, ma – forse per l'intervento bellico – i fatti non seguono ancora. Le malattie professionali restano escluse, malgrado fin dal 1901 sia stata nominata, dal Ministro della Pubblica Istruzione Baccelli, una Commissione per lo studio degli specifici argomenti assicurativi. Così l'agricoltura resta fuori dalla protezione infortuni, malgrado i continui inviti che da ogni parte giungono ad operare in questo senso, e malgrado i progetti di legge che dal 1907 si susseguono. La Cassa nazionale infortuni continua a dibattersi in notevoli difficoltà e ad invocare inutilmente un regime di monopolio (nel 1914 i suoi iscritti sono 662.845). La Cassa nazionale di previdenza nello stesso 1914 annovera appena 532.046 iscritti, sicchè la tutela contro l'invalidità e vecchiaia è quasi per intero delusa. Nulla o quasi viene fatto o prospettato sul piano assicurativo per la salvaguardia delle malattie comuni, le sole iniziative concrete resultando prese, come abbiam visto, sul piano assistenziale. La disoccupazione involontaria è parimente trascurata.

Specialmente grave la mancata protezione infortunistica in agricoltura. A giustificarla s'invocavano molteplici difficoltà. Come inquadrare le migrazioni interne (ad esempio delle mondariso)? L'agricoltura, in crisi permamente, non avrebbe potuto – si affermava – sopportarne i costi, e prima quindi sarebbe stato necessario accrescere la produzione. Dato il profitto minimo della rendita fondiaria, ormai incompressibile, i costi (premi) sarebbero altrimenti destinati a scaricarsi sul magro o magrissimo salario bracciantile. Data l'alternanza delle mansioni, difficile inquadrare il rischio professionale, e più facili invece le frodi e disagevole il controllo. D'altronde – si concludeva – nell'agricoltura, i rischi si presentano forse del pari numerosi, ma certamente meno gravi. Di contro, si dichiarava l'aumento degli infortuni e della loro gravità anche nel settore agricolo, solo mascherati dalle minori denuncie, per l'ignoranza delle plebi rurali. La necessità di arrestare l'esodo dalle campagne imponeva provvedimenti risolutivi, il lavoro ne avrebbe tratto un aumento di produttività. Nè poteva ancora sostenersi la vergogna di una sperequazione tanto vistosa nei confronti dell'industria, essendo ancora nell'agricoltura fermi alla dimostrazione della 'colpa' padronale.

Una certa responsabilità deve attribuirsi anche all'inerzia delle masse contadine, e una responsabilità notevole ai partiti democratici, maggiormente sensibili alle istanze deli operai industriali. Malgrado queste considerazioni ed altre ancora, il giudizio di fondo sul 'periodo giolittiano' non cambia. Frammentarietà e disordine permangono in molte iniziative. Giolitti resta fedele alla tattica di concedere episodicamente e solo quando si riveli indispensabile, senza mai, per nessun motivo 'anticipare'. Bensì la grande 'maturazione' sociale vi si compie, sul piano della persuasione dottrinale e della sensibilità politica. Lo schema del volontarismo si rompe, per dare spazio alle richieste pressanti di un sistema protettivo obbligatorio, organicamente ed armonicamente concepito. In effetti, un vero studio sulla previdenza sociale nell'età giolittiana mai finora è stato pubblicato in Italia (e l'A. del presente saggio si ripromette di farlo quanto prima). Tutti gli storici che hanno scritto sulla 'socialità' di quegli anni, si sono limitati o quasi ad esaminare la legislazione del lavoro, trascurando il capitolo delle assicurazioni sociali. Affermando la contemporaneità di un pensiero che rapido e concreto si evolve, ma frattanto non si realizza, l'A. deve quindi quasi chiedere di essere creduto – almeno per ora – un poco sulla parola. La guerra dapprima sospende e quindi accelera il processo realizzatore.

Fino al 1917, salvo talune urgenti disposizioni a favore dei pescatori dell'Adriatico, impediti di scendere a mare e così indennizzati con un fondo speciali sul bilancio dello Stato, o salvo altre sporadiche disposizioni a favore dei militari invalidi, abbiamo solo provvedimenti d'occasione: nel 1916, ad esempio, una somma di lire 160.000 sul bilancio statale in prò delle Casse mutue che danno sussidi per disoccupazione; nel 1915 un nuovo regolamento sui premi e le indennità della Cassa nazionale infortuni, che sostanzialmente ripete il vecchio; ancorà nel 1915 l'obbligo assicurativo per l'infortunio lavorativo viene esteso alla gente di mare appartenente agli equipaggi delle navi mercantili (il servizio viene eseguito direttamente dallo Stato). Quindi la situazione contadina precipita. Nei campi sono rimasti a lavorare donne e vecchi e fanciulli, e gli infortuni crescono. I salariati agricoli poi non riescono a sostenere l'ascesa dei prezzi. E già si teme che una smobilitazione – più o meno vicina – delle forze armate aumenti in modo vertiginoso il numero dei disoccupati.

La legge 23 agosto 1917 n. 1450 (quindi modificata con legge 20 marzo 1920, n. 297) istituisce quindi l'assicurazioni contro gli infortuni sul lavodo in agricoltura. Assicurati di pieno diritto, dai 15 ai 65 anni compiuti, sono tutti i lavoratori, fissi ed avventizi, maschi e femmine, addetti ad aziende agricole e forestali, nonchè i proprietari, mezzadri, affittuari, loro mogli e figli (anche naturali) che prestino abitualmente opera manuale nelle rispettive aziende. Anche i sorveglianti sono inclusi, entro certi limiti di retribuzione. La capacità lavorativa deve resultare ridotta di oltre il 10 per cento e l'astensione dal lavoro protrarsi per più di dieci giorni. Le indennità, salvo quella giornaliera, seguono l'età e il sesso, attribuite in capitale o versate alla Cassa nazionale di previdenza che le converte in rendita vitalizia (ove questa resulti almeno di 500 lire annue). Organi gestori, le Casse mutue fra le aziende agricole e forestali, ed altre, e la Cassa nazionale infortuni (con gestione separata dall'industria) e le Società private autorizzate. Qualsiasi medico il quale per primo visiti l'infortunato, ha l'obbligo della denuncia e della certificazione, e l'infortunato ha l'obbligo di sottoporsi al controllo medico richiesto.

Le malattie professionali sono ancora escluse e le indennità giungono minori di quelle attribuite agli operai dell'industria. Bensì più meritevoli – nei confronti dell'industria – risultano alcuni criteri informatori. Il settore agricolo è coperto quasi per intero, in parte includendo anche il lavoro autonomo. La tulela è realizzata in modo pienamente automatico, non cioè legata alla stipula di un contratto, ad una denuncia preventiva, alla registrazione di presenze o salari. I lavoratori sono rappresentati nei 'Comitati di liquidazione' (organi autonomi indipendenti dall'Istituto assicuratore). Il sistema contributivo si svincola dal salario per agganciarsi alla (pur ipotetica) produttività aziendale.

L'assicurazione obbligatoria per l'invalidità e la vecchiaia viene instaurata con D.L. Lgt. 21 aprile 1919 n. 603, bensì già fin dal 1917 era stato sancito l'obbligo nei confronti di tutti i lavoratori (circa 800.000) addetti agli stabilimenti ausiliari, requisiti dal governo per la produzione di materiale bellico. Ora soggetti all'obbligo divengono la maggior parte dei prestatori d'opera (alle altrui dipendenze), per un totale di circa 10 milioni, pari al 40 per cento della popolazione superiore ai 15 anni: operai ed impiegati, senza distinzione di sesso o nazionalità; ivi compresi i coloni e mezzadri con le loro famiglie (gli impiegati fino a 350 lire e quindi fino ad 800 lire il mese). I contributi sono paritetici, riscossi a mezzo marche relative a sei classi di salario. Requisito minimo per la vecchiaia: 65 anni e 240 marche. Requisito minimo per l'invalidità: perdita della capacità di guadagno di almeno 2/3 e 120 marche. La gestione è affidata alla Cassa nazionale di previdenza, che prende il nome di 'Cassa nazionale per le assicurazioni sociali'. La raccolta dei fondi è basata sul premio 'medio' e non, come prima, individuale. Carattere 'solidaristico' che, insieme al superamento del lavoro 'manuale' in senso stretto, segna la via nuova che dovrebbe percorrere la previdenza. Per ogni pensione lo Stato contribuisce con 100 lire annue, prendendo a proprio carico il periodo militare 1915–20. Al 31 dicembre 1921 i fondi assommano ad un miliardo, per 217 milioni di contributi riscossi nell'anno. Il sistema finanziario è quello a 'capitalizzazione'.

Con gli stessi decreti del 1917, che prescrivevano l'obbligo assicurativo contro l'invalidità e vecchiaia per i lavoratori addetti agli stabilimenti ausiliari, un sesto dei contributi veniva destinato ad un Fondo per la disoccupazione involontaria, amministrato dalla Cassa depositi e prestiti. Di lì a poco ulteriori disposizioni furono emanate per aiutare gli operai rimasti privi di lavoro, causa la deficienza di energia elettrica. Ad armistizio concluso, con D.L. Lgt. del dicembre 1918 (e seguenti) si imponeva in certi casi ai datori di lavoro di corrispondere un'indennità di licenziamento. Quindi vennero emanati il D.L. Lgt. 17 novembre 1918 n. 1911 sul collocamento della mano d'opera e il D.L. Lgt. 5 gennaio 1919 n. 6 sopra i sussidi per la disoccupazione involontaria.

I sussidi traevano dal reddito nazionale, iscritti nel bilancio dello Stato che in proposito stanziava un centinaio di milioni, affidati in periferia ad Uffici particolari. Bensì, mostratosi il congegno troppo oneroso, fu scelta la via dell'assicurazione obbligatoria con D.L. 19 ottobre 1919 n. 2214, in vigore dal l gennaio 1920. La norma iniziale si riferiva a tutti i lavoratori subordinati di cui alla legge per l'invalidità e vecchiaia. La gestione era affidata ad un Ufficio nazionale per il collocamento e la disoccupazione, creato presso il Ministero del lavoro. Come organi periferici funzionavano le Giunte provinciali e le Casse professionali. Queste ultime si presentavano di due specie, facoltative e obbligatorie, ambedue provviste di amministrazione autonoma, in cui i lavoratori avevano rappresentanze eguali a quella dei datori di lavoro e dello Stato.

Nel novembre 1921 l'assicurazione obbligatoria contro la disoccupazione viene estesa ai dipendenti non operai delle aziende private, e l'esperienza del sistema, così parzialmente affidato all'autocontrollo – dopo un primo periodo d'incertezza e confusione – sembrava avviarsi verso resultati concreti. Nel 1920 e 1922 è istituito rispettivamente il fondo delle pensioni invalidità e vecchiaia per il personale dipendente dai pubblici esercizi di telefonia e per quello dipendente dalle esattorie e ricevitorie delle imposte. La Cassa di maternità viene irrobustita nella sua funzione.

I sussidi salgono da 631.790 lire nel 1918 (aliquota a carico dello Stato di lire 152.868) a lire 4.518.600 nel 1921 (aliquota a carico dello Stato lire 422.256). Il risultato contabile purtroppo è un disavanzo, perchè non si sono parimenti graduate le entrate, ma i profitti industriali presentano margini così alti che lo sbilancio non poteva (e doveva) impensierire.

Con D.L. Lgt. 23 agosto 1917 è nominata una Commissione di studio per la tutela della malattia, che redige due schemi di legge: il primo limitato a qualche riforma nel settore infortunistico ed assistenziale (dei quali però rispetta le trame esistenti), il secondo deciso a proporre l'adozione di un sistema integrale di assicurazioni sociali. Scelta quest'ultima linea, il 16 dicembre 1919 viene così definito un progetto realmente innovatore, composto di 134 articoli, che si propone di assorbire nel medesimo criterio (e in strutture armoniche) i rischi conseguenti 'alla interruzione e cessazione della capacità di lavorare' (malattia, invalidità, morte), da qualsiasi causa originati, escludendo ogni trattamento di privilegio. L'obbligo assicurativo è previsto per tutti i lavoratori subordinati, ed anche per quelli autonomi entro certi limiti di reddito. La gestione del servizio malattia è affidata alla mutualità. Principi e strutture del ricovero ospedaliero vengono adeguate al servizio assistenziale (sanitario). Il finanziamento è plurimo (datore di lavoro, lavoratore, Stato ed anche Enti locali). Le funzioni di soccorso sanitario ai poveri passano agli Istituti di previdenza sociale, i quali all'uopo si avvalgono di medici generici e specialisti, nonchè di tutte le farmacie della circoscrizione, assumendo in certe condizioni un chiaro diritto ad aprire o gestire farmacie proprie. L'istituto previdenziale del pari provvede all'assistenza ospedaliera, nonchè 'all'assistenza per la maternità e pei bambini'. L'obbligo di astensione dal lavoro è proposto nelle ultime sei settimane di gravidanza e nelle prime sei settimane dopo il parto.

Il fascismo tronca questo processo, subito allineandosi alle posizioni più conservatrici del padronato industriale ed agrario. Il 27 marzo 1923 la Confederazione generale italiana dell'industria tiene un Congresso sulle assicurazioni sociali e la istruzione professionale. Le conclusioni alle quali giunge si rispecchiano integralmente nel primo tempo della della politica fascista, fino al 1927. Nel secondo tempo, dopo la promulgazione della 'Carta del lavoro' sotto il segno della 'collaborazione di classe' nello 'Stato corporativo' viene sancito il passaggio dalla impostazione liberistica ad un regime autoritario borghese. Sotto la specie della classe dominante, il cambiamento è più formale di sostanziale. Per quanto considera i resultati, esso deve giudicarsi invece ulteriormente negativo, togliendo anche gli ultimi fermenti di uno sviluppo organico e affidato ad un controllo interno (democratico) delle prestazioni.

Bibliografia

Per qualsiasi riferimento bibliografico, valga rinviare ai miei studi di storia della previdenza sociale: *Fondamenti storici del sistema previdenziale. Teorie politiche ed economiche fino al 1848*, Milano, Giuffrè, 1957; *Dottrine e metodi assistenziali dal 1789 al 1848. Italia-Francia-Inghilterra*, Milano, Giuffrè, 1958; 'Realtà della medicina sociale dalla sua storia', in *Enpas*, 1958, **6**, 27; *Profilo del mutuo soccorso in Italia, dalle origini al 1924*, 1961, **1**, 15; 'Preludi di medicina sociale in Germania (secolo XVIII–XIX)', in *Difesa sociale*, 1961, **4**, 19; L'assistenza pubblica quale momento storico delle assicurazioni sociali in Germania', in *Enpas*, 1962, **2**, 189; 'Note sulle origini delle assicurazioni sociali in Germania', in *Rivista degli Infortuni e delle Malattie Professionali*, 1963, 1–2, 3, 4–5, 6 *passim*; 'Per una storia dell'assistenza pubblica in Italia', in *Previdenza sociale*, 1963, 3, 4 *passim* e 1964, 3, 5 *passim*; *Dialettica assicurazioni sociali in Italia, nel secolo XIX*; 'Due lezioni sulla storia della previdenza in Italia (dal mutualismo operaio alla corporazione fascista', in *Enpas*, 1966, **2**, 199; 'Introduzione storica alle assicurazioni sociali in Italia. Le premesse. Da Crispi a Giolitti', in *Rivista degli Infortuni e delle Malattie Professionali*, 1967, **3–4**, 609; 'Idem. Il 1898. Assicurazione obbligatoria contro gli infortuni e Cassa nazionale di previdenza', in ibid., 1968, **3–4**, 657; 'Idem. Il ventennio fascista 1923–1943' in ibid., 1969, 731; 'Idem. L'assistenza di malattia dal 1900 al 1915', in ibid., 1972, **1**, 70; 'Politica ed economia nella prima esperienza mutualistica italiana', in *Rivista Italiana di Sicurezza Sociale*, 1963, **1**, 474; *Il problema sociale e il mutuo soccorso nella stampa senese (1860–1893)*, Siena, Accademia degli Intronati, 1967; 'Il significato dell'esperienza tedesca nelle origini della previdenza sociale', in *Sociologia internationalis*, 1969, **1**, 103; 'Beneficenza diritto e politica nella prima storia previdenziale', in *Previdenza Sociale*, 1969, **2**, 257; 'Note intorno alla previdenza sociale nell'epoca giolittiana', in ibid., 1970, **3**, 719. 'Note sulle assicurazioni sociali gestite dall'INAIL e dall'INPS nel periodo 1923–1943' in ibid., 1972, I, 3. Nella 'Rivista degli infortuni e delle malattie professionali' sono in corso di pubblicazione due studi su 'La tutela della maternità 1900–1922' e 'L'assistenza di malattia' dal 1915 al 1921.

Ruth G. Hodgkinson
London (Great Britain)

Provision for health and welfare in England in the nineteenth century

British provisions for health and welfare in their present connotation and complexity, and their quality and quantity, date back to our industrial and social revolution which began in the latter half of the eighteenth century. They arose to meet the exigencies of industrialization and urbanization, scientific and technological advances, wars, inflation, economic crises and social upheaval. They stemmed from the problems of unhealthy environmental conditions, disease, poverty, squalor, malnutrition, alcoholism, prostitution, infanticide, the disruption of former family life and relationships. These and all the attending psychological disturbances were the price of economic expansion, the rapid increase in population and the imbalance in the population dispersion.

As social dislocation, public ill health, occupational hazards exploded in the nineteenth century so both the necessity for, and the provision of health and welfare measures increased. Economic prosperity raised the standard of living after mid-nineteenth century and this in itself heightened awareness to problems and needs, augmented desiderata and subsequently the question of 'rights'. So reform gathered momentum, ever widening in range and inclusiveness by the beginning of the twentieth century.

Being the pioneer of the modern age, Britain could not learn from precedents or benefit from others' mistakes. Politically and administratively she was ill-equipped. She had no recent experience of State paternalism or Enlightened Despotism. Therefore neither government nor the people felt strongly that the State was under any obligation to provide for the amelioration of health or living conditions. State intervention was unpopular for generations. To the majority of people it remained a necessity and did not become a principle. At the beginning new ideas, new philosophies emerged through several reasons; later many evolved as an answer to a few hard facts and situations.

Early economist-philosophers must be mentioned briefly insofar as that with their theories for economic expansion they included the suggestion that self-interest of the labouring classes would encourage them to better their own conditions. Sam Smiles, the apostle of working-class self-help, used this idea when he preached to the workers over half a century later. But two philosophers particularly influenced social policy, or more correctly thought and activity, for only in the Poor Law was there any real policy based on theoretical principle. Bentham, with his ideas for legal and administrative reforms which were to produce the greatest happiness of the greatest number by making operational the simple choice mechanism of self-interest, and Malthus, with his population theory, were to provide a long-lasting undercurrent of influence on nineteenth-century developments. What was read into, or attributed to their philosophies affected State and individuals, and had more far-reaching effects and consequences than is generally realized. On the other hand, we must beware of attributing too much to the philosophers. There was in the early nineteenth-century transitional stage of our history much groping for ideas and theories, but it was in the dark or half-light of disorganization and upheaval.

Practical thinkers and doers had more immediate impact. A pragmatic nation fairly quickly recognized the economic cost of ill-health. A high percentage of destitution was attributable to sickness and the Poor Rate was a heavy burden on the ratepayer. Charity was costly. An unhealthy and maimed labour force retarded productivity. Economic expansion also depended on the high mobility of labour and this was impeded by the settlement clauses and supplements in aid of wages of the old Poor Laws. The new middle-class industrialist and the new parliamentarian were converted to the necessity for certain reforms. More slowly they and others in society were, for example, made aware of the consequences of an uneducated people on national health and prosperity. There was interaction and involvement on practical planes throughout. And always there was the strong immediate motivating force that triggered off activity: parliamentary reform, municipal reform, an epidemic, a public movement or a working-class agitation.

Parallel, there began in the eighteenth century and gathering great momentum in the nineteenth, the strong element of humanitarianism. It manifested itself first in an awareness of social malaise and a reappraisal of its causes, and then found more positive expression. Evidence of this humanitarianism was demonstrated by collective and individual thought and activity. Even men like Chadwick and Farr, producing hard facts and impersonal statistics, elaborated or interspersed their writings with an appeal to human emotions and sentiments, and rights. Such is not acceptable practice today. Religious principles were evoked by some reforming groups and these added weight to cold calculated reasoning. And there was also a large group of men and women who were pure humanitarians or practical philanthropists. Late in the nineteenth century, dependent to a great extent on the rise of a powerful working-class movement and middle-class political and social reformers, as well as on a more liberal Parliament, there was a change in attitude to the functions of government.

But it must be emphasized that in Britain there was always a strong dual system of voluntary and State activity. It is important to recognize the significant role charity has played in our provision for health and welfare. And to appreciate achievements as a whole, it is essential to bear in mind the interdependence of thought, of activity; the interaction between abuses, between reforms, and the involvement of many men or movements in several spheres. A recognition of connecting links, of broad contexts and of perspective is very necessary to a deeper understanding of ideas, people and events.

There never existed an all-embracing theory or policy for health and welfare, but there were many large areas where problems became so acute that members of Parliament felt moved, or the government was driven to intervene. The key to activity lay first, in information, that is, a realization of the problem; and second, in the practical possibility for provision or reform. Lack of activity on the part of the State was not always due to callousness or conservatism. Before there can be any new provision or redress of an abuse, attention must be created, both on local and national levels. And there must be an awareness on the part of the community, society as a whole, as well as by the authorities. The dissemination of information on a wide scale is therefore absolutely essential.

The means for fulfilling these desiderata became available simultaneously with their need, and partially indirectly, because of them. Some social and health problems grew to such dimensions that they became blatantly obvious, such as the state of the industrial conurbations. But for the overall picture the climate for investigation and revelation was being created. There was a seeking for knowledge and enlightenment. Politics, religion, philosophy, science were all caught up in the drive for intellectual curiosity. There resulted a cross-fertilization of ideas and interests and then a move toward rationalization. This spirit of general and particular questioning linked to the new humanitarianism and the beginning of specialization, the development of the new sciences, industrial technologies and new philosophies all required accurate information. Enlightened men and practical reformers needed the weapon of statistical and hard facts. A vague humanism or sentimentality would not suffice for the new age. Quantitative analyses, their publication and circulation were imperative. Our modern mathematical techniques and survey tools were only in embryo; nevertheless it is noteworthy how much was accomplished by crude methods and untrained investigators. They were adequate to set in motion reforms which had a cumulative effect and steadily progressed towards comprehensive health and welfare services.

To describe and discuss ameliorative legislation, or the work of individuals, whilst overlooking the background which made both possible would preclude a true understanding and honest evaluation of developments. During the late eighteenth and early nineteenth centuries an awareness of social disruption due to the effects of the long Napoleonic Wars and industrialization was created by unrest among the poor and labouring classes. In addition some medical men and industrialists reacted. But obscurantist governments were frightened for decades by fear of revolution and remained obtuse to the necessity for, and inevitability of reform despite the realization that the changes which were taking place were irrevocable. The philanthropically-minded and the benevolently-interested amateur became the dedicated, informed reformer. Individual strength was augmented by societies. As governments moved slowly, individuals or societies acted first. Workers united but generally for political ends or shorter working hours; they remained unaware of their ill-health, or felt political reform would bring redress in all spheres. Of far greater consequence for immediate health and welfare measures were the societies and associations organized all over the country by educated men. These took the form of learned societies interested in many aspects of society and living, or were established for a special purpose. In the former category were the Statistical Societies founded from the mid-thirties, and the Literary and Philosophical Societies, some dating back to the eighteenth century. By far the most influential organization was the National Association for the Promotion of Social Science established in 1856 with the help of the London Statistical Society. To this belonged everyone interested in any field of health and social welfare. From the middle of the century many more specialist societies arose:

the Epidemiological Society, the many public health organizations such as the Health of Towns Association, societies for organizing the housing of the poor and London workhouses. Their number is enormous and their importance cannot be overestimated. Many men and some women belonged to several groups, they both learned and taught in different spheres so there was great cross-fertilization of ideas.

The transactions or reports published provided a mine of information. Suggestions and practical schemes for reform were compelling. They acted not only as pressure groups on the government but also as consultants for public investigations. Members frequently sat on government inquiries, for the numbers of knowledgeable, albeit still self-trained men on whom the government could draw, were few until late in the century. All the influential societies contained a large number of doctors. The London Statistical Society had a medical committee to investigate health problems and also gave grants for research. The growth of professionalism furthered the need and the means for investigation and dissemination of information. Medical men in addition, had their own societies such as the Medical Officers of Health and the Poor Law Medical Officers, fighting not only for recognition and higher pay but providing a new force for positive health programmes. The British Medical Association had several committees dealing with State doctors and public health problems. Indeed, by the 1870s the Public Health Committee of the B.M.A. had become so influential, that together with the Social Science Association, it was predominantly responsible for the Royal Sanitary Commission of 1869–71 and subsequent public health legislation.

Not only were there large national societies, but local organizations were widespread, aiding national movements or providing information for a special sphere or on problems particular to one area. The establishing and growth of such a large number of societies to provide information and ideas was a new departure in our history and equally important for reform as the other innovation, the large-scale government inquiry.

In addition to all the information collected by the pressure groups there were the facts and pictures presented by the novelists; Charles Dickens probably did more than any other single person to enlighten the general public and force attention of the country as a whole on every social problem. And there were individual investigators: Kay-Shuttleworth who with his survey of the Manchester working population in 1833, provided the first modern 'scientific' analysis, and there were Henry Wyldbore Rumsey, Florence Nightingale and many others during the mid-century. Henry Mayhew in the 1850s produced four large volumes on London life and labour. In the nineties he was followed by Charles Booth with his equally massive survey.

Closely connected with first desiderata for reform, those of providing information, drawing attention to needs and creating a general awareness of conditions, is the supply of adequate, swift and cheap means of communication. Here railway construction helped to solve many problems, although it also created others. Another contribution was made by the vast quantity of reading material that became available through technological advances. With growing need and desire for articulation, furthered by progress in education, there arose the possibility and demand for newspapers, broadsheets and journals. Mayhew claimed to have published the first Blue Book in twopenny numbers, and Dickens published on the cheap and popular instalment system. Every sector of the community made use of the press, and winning the battle for a cheap and free press was a significant factor in nineteenth-century progress on many fronts. Most pertinent to our subject, the *Lancet* may be singled out as an example of the power of the press, and it also illustrates so many factors which contributed to health and welfare. The journal aided improvement in medical education, knowledge and reform. It was typical of the rise of professionalism. It provided a voice for medical men great or humble, it encouraged doctors to play their part in many spheres of social and health improvement and it tried to inform and influence the government. The detailed and lengthy reports of its own team of investigators compelled the government to undertake inquiries which were followed by legislation. Such was the case with the *Lancet* inquiries in the sixties into workhouse sickwards, followed later by investigations into occupational disease and the sweated trades, into hospitals and medical education.

So all the voluntary investigations, publications and demands of societies, individuals and press were of incalculable value in putting pressure on the government. Societies frequently strengthened their cause by sending informative petitions to Parliament, ministers, government boards or departments. They prodded the cumbersome and slow-moving officialdom into activity and provided the knowledge or skills not yet required or possible, in government departments. Collaboration of the government with the expert was imperative and here doctors were essential for public health or industrial health investigations. With the growth of other occupational specialists such as civil engineers, and new technologists, these too became indispensible to inquiries and then to the positive programme of health and welfare provision.

As always in Britain, State and private initiative marched together, each necessary and often complementary to the other. Because the connected problems of insanitary towns, conditions of labour, poverty, disease and ignorance grew in complexity, government interference became imperative, and it was based on government investigation. The State established and firmly secured the system of inquiry by Select Committee or Royal Commission. These alone had finance and scope of sufficient dimensions. They were imbued with seemingly authoritative power. Their findings were less liable to bias or dramatization and they had to be accepted by Parliament as comprehensive, accurate and authentic. So was achieved a vast accumulation of facts and figures covering aspects of health, poverty, housing, education, institutional medical care, working conditions in factories, mines and sweatshops, and medical education and practice. Frequently one inquiry helped another, some investigators were used in different fields, just as many reformers participated in several movements. Occasionally revelations of an inquiry had dramatic consequences. Legislation generally resulted, often belatedly or inadequate, but the initial step set in motion further activity, and amending or more comprehensive Acts followed. When these established a special authority or department, reports were required from the staff. The Assistant Poor Law Commissioners provided a wealth of facts and the Commission undertook its own investigations when an urgent or special problem arose. The Annual Reports of John Simon when he was the Medical Officer of the Privy Council covered every aspect of health and welfare. These were compiled from the reports of his own special investigators who were often chosen because of the research papers they had presented to societies and because they had begun to specialize in different fields.

The greatest source of authoritative information and the greatest single and sustained influence on reform emerged from the Registrar General's Office which came into operation in 1837. The statistics and the reports formed a continuous mine of information on births, marriages and the causes of death. For forty years, from 1840–80 Dr. William Farr appended long explanatory essays sometimes including original research material of his own. He not only interpreted figures but popularized public health and industrial health questions. There was no field in social medicine which he did not enlighten, and frequently he advocated reform measures. His statistics bore out Engel's more lurid and dramatic descriptions of England in the 1840s. Progress in medical nosology was influenced by his insistence on more exact definition of diseases and he demonstrated the urgency for improving medical institutions, education and the status of the medical profession. And Farr associated closely with Chadwick and Simon, the heroes of the nineteenth-century public health and State medical services.

Although government and people were gradually and thoroughly made aware of problems, solution was hampered by the absence of agreement on the form which activity should take. Not only was there no clear overall social and health policy, but prevailing ideas differed regarding any single field. Philosophers and economists preached the virtues of self-help and enlightened self-interest. *Laissez-faire* in industry and commerce was to apply to non-State intervention in social and health matters. Even the working class believed in the virtues of self-help. It has therefore been maintained that the State only stepped in when problems became acute as with poverty or in times of epidemic, and that Britain only found answers to demands, and remedied evils, when compelled by sheer urgent necessity.

I hope that I have already demolished these views in showing that there was sustained interest and inquiry. Had we probed further we would have seen that there were men, not theoretical philosophers, but practical thinkers, who had far-reaching ideas well ahead of their time and beyond the immediate bounds of possibility. Rumsey long campaigned not only for reforms in public health and the Poor Law medical service, but also for the unity of all health services, the use of the expert and strong centralization under a Ministry of Health. The giants, Chadwick, Simon and Shaftesbury wrote and worked all their lives for a far greater, and at the time, unacceptable State intervention and the provision of social services.

Whatever the theories for or against government interference, adequate provision for health and welfare was impeded by many factors. First, was the financial restraint imposed by the Treasury, partly through obscurantism and partly on account of the heavy outlay for military and colonial purposes. Second, the poor could not afford a better quality of food, clothing or housing. The abolition of food adulteration for example, depended not only on science or conscience but on the labourers' pay. Third, tools, equipment, materials or men were not available. Safety of machinery, sanitary environment of factories, employment of women and children in mills, and working hours, could and did come under government scrutiny, as did occupational hazards of the sweated trades. But so much depended on invention and technological improvement; and when advances came, many legislative measures became superfluous. The abolition of sweated labour owed more to technological innovation than to legislation, as did an increase in wages. It also indirectly furthered environmental improvement, for with the growth of large-scale industry and better pay, the necessity for carrying out unhealthy work in the home or a family sharing a single damp, foul room was slowly eliminated. And education played a part on two fronts.

Institutional medical care was investigated and condemned, but could only improve with advances in medical science and practice, and the training of a competent nursing service. Architectural design and standards had to advance, materials such as washable cotton and metals to replace wood, had to be introduced. Iron bedsteads were known in the eighteenth century, just as steam pumps and iron pipes for water supply, but immediate and universal use was delayed to a great extent by cost. The gigantic area of public health improvement depended not only on government interference but on science and technology, training in many new skills and supporting services. Many specialists or special bodies had to be found. The amateur had to become a professional. Medical science and technology had to progress: bacteriology and epidemiology followed, they did not precede nineteenth-century public health measures. Whatever the legislation, the adoption of a discovery or application of a skill, or even compliance with an Act of Parliament, was hampered by cost, and closely allied, by the conservatism of local authorities or employers.

So many factors have to be taken into account in analysing the provisions for health and welfare. Legislation gathered momentum after mid-century simultaneously with the scientific revolution and the increase in national wealth. Developments were cumulative and complementary; reforms aroused attention to the need for more. And so much depended on education. It was necessary not only for training experts and workers, but also for creating an awareness of the public of health hazards, of the need for personal hygiene, of general cleanliness. Education forms a trilogy with public health and industrial health. Another factor to be borne in mind was that at the beginning of the nineteenth century the composition of both central and local government was an anachronism. A landed aristocracy at the top, with a chaos of local authorities jealous of their rights below, were matched in inefficiency by the countless ad hoc bodies established for dealing with such problems as water supply, sewage disposal, street lighting and paving.

Therefore the first parliamentary Reform Act of 1832 was the prerequisite of all future State activity. This began the long continuous process towards liberalizing the constitution and the gradual inclusion of all sections of the community in central government. The reform of local government followed with the Municipal Corporations Act of 1835, and again throughout the nineteenth century there was continuous progress. After mid-century and particularly after 1870, an incorruptible and efficient civil service was established. This depended greatly on a wider provision of education as did the staffing of the many new government departments. As the sphere of government interference and responsibility increased, as the departments swelled in numbers by the twentieth century, the recruitment of administrative staff and experts would have been impossible without first primary education and then special training of men from many sectors of the population.

From mid-century there was a change in attitude to the functions of government both by parliament and people. The stage was set for the large volume of statutory measures for health and welfare which was to follow. Public and private investigators were set in an irreversible trend to maintain constant awareness. The fear of violent revolution which had for over fifty years lurked in the background and frightened rulers away from liberalism was subsiding. The wealthier members of society realized that many social problems urgently needed remedying for they affected them from an economic point of view and healthwise. The growing number of humanitarians recognized that neither philanthropy nor self-help were adequate. So the ruling classes tolerated and sometimes furthered improvements in public health, occupational health and working conditions, medical care and institutional improvements, although frequently, even among reformers, no measure was to infringe on economic expansion.

Five main groups of legislation will be discussed. First, the Registration Acts, beginning in 1836, at first imperfect and inadequate, were essential to progress in public health, the medical profession and medical research, child welfare, the safety of work and occupational disease. Later amending Acts required more and more information, so there developed a significant use of vital statistics. And, as already mentioned, Farr's monumental studies analysing census returns which were appended to the Registrar General's Reports, provided a real breakthrough for all medical and public health fields.

The second group of government measures formed the nucleus of our modern Welfare State. Through the Poor Law the 'politics of poverty' were learned. It is from the Poor Laws that our State medical and so many welfare services evolved. The Poor Law Amendment Act of 1834 was forced on the Government through growing social dislocation, the pressure of the high cost of maintaining the poor, the ever-increasing number of destitutes, and the philosophers demanding that old chaotic measures be rationalized. And economists wished to increase the mobility of labour so necessary to rapid industrialization. Attributing poverty to inherent moral vice, legislation was based on deterrence. By prohibiting outdoor relief for the able-bodied, fear of the workhouse was to encourage people to work. Although the New Poor Law was so condemned for its harshness and the hardship inflicted by its principle of less-eligibility, the administration of the Act provided the model for future government activity: strong centralization, salaried public servants responsible to a small partly autonomous government Board, and rationalization of local authorities, i.e. the grouping of parishes into Unions under Boards of Guardians. Local and central efficiency was imperative for any successful State activity in the nineteenth century because problems increased in complexity and ideas on their solution were only in a formative stage. The inefficient, corrupt former system gave way to over-rigid centralization, although there was full measure of local responsibility. Throughout the century much suffering was caused because relief policy was so narrowly conceived, and unbending local authorities kept their eyes on the Poor Rates. The principle of strong centralization remained anathema to the upper classes.

Although change in circumstances and thought made many statutory amendments necessary, the Act of 1834 predominated throughout the nineteenth century. Its inelasticity and many shortcomings were in part attributable to the faulty diagnosis of poverty. Strictly limiting its provisions to the absolute pauper, no help was permissible for the prevention of destitution. Sickness was a significant factor contributing to poverty, and sick paupers formed a high percentage of the total. No Medical Service was written into the Act; it was developed by the Poor Law Commission and its successors. Therefore without any initially prescribed rigidity, a service could evolve and improve as need dictated. National uniformity was never quite achieved; yet the provision for the destitute sick, the innumerable rules and regulations of the central board, provided the nucleus of our National Health Service. The sick were exempt from the workhouse order, and allowances were made for varying characteristics. Availability of care and treatment depended on this and on medical science and practice, and not only on Poor Law orders. Part-time District Medical Officers and Workhouse Medical Officers were appointed. Salaries were pitifully low. Records had to be kept and reports made. The Poor Law Medical Officers became the public vaccinators and generally were the overworked medical men who took charge in time of epidemic. Growing in number to over 4,000 by the end of the century, they formed associations to fight not only for better pay, conditions and status, but also to improve the care available to their patients. They were largely responsible for the change in attitude to poverty, drawing attention to the correlation between disease and destitution, so that the sick were gradually regarded differently from the able-bodied paupers.

The horrors of the workhouse became notorious. The 'Bastilles' were grossly overcrowded with no amentities. Inmates were subjected to rigid discipline, complete isolation from the outside world, poor diets and the most menial of jobs. Although the buildings grew in size and number to accommodate the vast population requiring indoor relief, supply never kept pace with demand. At first the sick were mixed in the general wards but by mid-century special sick wards or separate wings were added. Nursing was still atrocious as this was left to old women inmates generally paid in drink. Few institutions had resident doctors. So large had the workhouse hospital service become in the sixties that it provided 80 per cent of all hospital beds in the country. The *Lancet* wrote that here lay 'the real hospitals of the land'.

The greatest proportion of the mentally ill also came under Poor Law provision, and one in ten paupers was a lunatic. The Government Commissioners in Lunacy with the Inspectorate and Visitors did much to obtain better classification, separation and improvement in the workhouses where the majority of the insane were housed, and to encourage their removal to a County Asylum and later to special institutions.

The last three decades of the century witnessed great improvement in State hospital provision and for this much credit is due to the detailed inquiries of the *Lancet* and the Poor Law Board in the 1860s. Better qualified doctors and a more competent nursing service were introduced, and improved infirmary buildings and amenities. The Great Metropolitan Poor Act of 1867 is the only one of the eighteen Poor Law Statutes passed between 1834 to 1870 which was devoted to medical aspects, and from it stemmed the large specialist hospitals for infectious diseases and the mentally ill. Developing from the Metropolitan Asylums Board which was established, and whose functions were also applied to the country the year following, there gradually emerged specialized care for the aged and the children and all those inadequately covered by private endeavour or rejected by the voluntary hospitals. Most important: before the turn of the century the non-destitute began to be catered for by the State, and for many categories of sickness this was the only institutional care available. A complete hospital service emerged, including sanatoria and institutions for the handicapped. Voluntary provision could not keep pace with need and the State medical services grew to gigantic proportions. Unfortunately they still retained the stigma of coming under the Poor Law authorities until 1929, despite the creation of the Ministry of Health in 1919.

Closely connected with poverty and the Poor Law medical service was the third area of State intervention, public health. Both fields are linked in their formative years by one of the leading reformers of all time, Edwin Chadwick. The ideas, work and influence of this giant cannot be over-estimated. From 1834 to 1848 his was the inspiration and guiding hand in all Poor Law activity. His transference from Poor Law to Public Health is significant. Beginning as a leader in rationalizing poor relief and reducing the claims of poverty through principles of centralized control, he progressed to becoming the initiator in the provision of effective minima for environmental health. Once again doggedly and unflinchingly he fought for efficient administrative machinery. From his desiderata for poor relief and public health the whole conception of public obligations altered, and in his career can be traced the change in ideas from misdiagnosis and repression to prevention of poverty and disease. He was so effective because he based his ideas and demands on his own vast amount of research and first-hand experience. To him scientific investigation, statistics, strong centralization, the use of the expert, was the new method necessary to meet new circumstances. He applied this first serving the Poor Law Commission and then later the General Board of Health. He provided the long despised prototypes of future government departments. He had been Bentham's pupil, and Bentham had in the 1820s thought of a Ministry of Health and a Ministry of Preventive Services. Even before he entered Poor Law service, Chadwick had recognized that poverty was closely linked with sickness, and then he learned that poverty and sickness were closely allied to the problem of environmental health.

So he was responsible for the pioneer inquiry into living conditions of the poor, undertaken in the late thirties by three Assistant Poor Law Commissioners. The 1838–39 reports pointed out the economic cost of poverty and disease: sickness entailed loss of earnings of employment to the individual, the employer lost his labour force, the expense of medical care and funerals, and the burden to the parish of bereaved families. Therefore ill health had to be prevented for economic, as well as humanitarian reasons. Chadwick followed this inquiry with his monumental Sanitary Report of 1842, the first national investigation in modern concept, and which has had repercussions all over the world, probably to this day. He also presented a lengthy separate report on burial problems. From Chadwick's surveys stemmed further government inquiries, private societies, and in 1848, the Public Health Act. This instituted the General Board of Health consisting of three non-medical, but dedicated men. Chadwick had had able lieutenants particularly Dr. Southwood Smith, Dr. Kay-Suttleworth and Lord Shaftesbury. He had made good use of Poor Law Medical Officers' reports and informative complaints. The cholera epidemic of 1831–32 had seen the setting up of inefficient temporary central and local boards of health. Under the Act of 1848 permanent local boards were established which could appoint Medical Officers of Health. It took a generation before many of the largest cities complied, and the first Medical Officer of Health had a department of one. By the end of the century there were 1,450 Medical Officers of Health with ever-growing numbers of assistants and specialized departments. The early local health officers were pioneers for public health improvement, for they, like the Poor Law Medical Officers, knew the needs of the poor and lived with their problems.

Chadwick had envisaged District Medical Officers who, independent of private practice and with special qualifications and responsibilities, should initiate sanitary measures. The first General Board of Health survived only until 1854. It fell dramatically because of Chadwick's unpopularity and the opposition to strong centralization. Leadership in the public health movement now passed to John Simon. The foundations for reform had been solidly laid and under Simon developed to great dimensions. Both men were inflexible, indefatigable, courageous and great public administrators. But whilst Chadwick believed that sanitary engineering was a panacea for many ills, partly because curative medicine seemed inadequate, Simon, as a doctor, turned more to medical knowledge and activity. And it must be remembered that medical science and practice in his era were just beginning their revolutionary development.

Among Simon's outstanding contributions to public health were his Annual Reports to the Privy Council. These covered every aspect of social medicine such as cholera, diarrhoea, dysentery, diphtheria, tuberculosis, occupational disease, diets of the working class, hospital hygiene, housing and nutrition. Simon was aided by inspectors who provided reports on their special investigations. Ancillary inspectorates attached to other government departments helped to provide a comprehensive picture of environmental conditions and needs, and the consequences were cumulative. There were the Factory Inspectorate (1833) the Prisons' Inspectorate (1835) the Anatomy Inspectorate (1839) and in the fifties Inspectors of London Water Sources, London Lodging Houses, Noxious Trades and Burial. Lunacy Commissioners had been appointed in 1828 and Charity Commissioners in 1854. In the seventies Port Sanitary Authorities were established, a Metropolitan Board of Works and public food analysts. All these made great inroads on the principle of self-reliance and aroused animosity to increasing bureaucracy and State paternalism.

From 1858 the central health authority came under the Privy Council, and after 1871, the Local Government Board. The pressure and agitation of societies and individuals were continuous. Parliament demonstrated that it had been converted to interference, by public health becoming a political issue and by the many official investigations undertaken. The 1850s and 1860s saw many Nuisances Removal Acts and sanitary regulations which culminated in the Public Health Act of 1875. Renewed vigorous activity was triggered off by the cholera epidemic of 1866. The Sanitary Act of that year, the Public Health legislation of 1871–72 and particularly the Royal Sanitary Commission of 1869–71 paved the way for this outstanding consolidating Act. The compelling and informative massive reports illustrated the chaos of authorities, the overlapping of functions and cogently pointed out the great need for rationalization and for uniformity in administration. A Ministry of Health was suggested and ignored. But one of the new departures was that local authorities might establish hospitals, and although the start was slow, several hundred were built by the end of the century. The Public Health Act was one of Simon's outstanding achievements, but he retired from public office in 1876 frustrated and disgusted by the parsimony and Poor Law mentality of the Local Government Board. During his last years he had devoted himself assiduously to sponsoring State-aided medical research.

After 1875 government measures in the public health field were involved more with individual abuses: river pollution, canals, the sale of horsemeat, milk supply, the drink trade and the provision of parks. Whilst earlier dedication was to ensure adequate and pure water supplies, sewage disposal and environmental improvement, housing now became a primary concern. Common lodging houses, insanitary housing and the institution of baths and washhouses had received attention from the forties, but in the last decades of the century there was an increasing insistence on the removal of domestic nuisances, the repair and upkeep of houses and some attempt to get rebuilding. The legislation of 1885 and 1890 introduced inspection and compulsory land purchase. But local authorities were vacillating and weak, and inspection was resisted. The problem of the slum was too great. It became a powerful issue in local politics at the turn of the century. So did community provision of social services. Here, Joseph Chamberlain, when he was Mayor of Birmingham, gave a lead in the eighties with his 'gas and water socialism'.

A conclusion that can be drawn from a review of British public health activity is that there was continuous thought, inquiry and progressive development. Reform did not come merely at a time of crisis or as an answer to an emergency; although dilatory, it was sustained.

We have seen that by the middle of the nineteenth century the irreversible trend of State commitment to health and welfare policy had been launched, and that objection to interference or dogmatic insistence on *laissez-faire* in these areas was receding. The fourth sphere of government involvement, that in working conditions, was again via central regulation and the employment of an efficient inspectorate and public servants. Through Poor Law, public health and factory reform the paternalistic State became accepted, and in time unquestioned, as the vehicle for curbing abuses and the promotion of welfare on an ever-widening scale. With intervention in industry the government was treading on the most controversial ground, for the absolute freedom of employer and trader was regarded as imperative for economic expansion, and therefore national prosperity. Early reformers like Cobbett might fulminate against the nation's wealth being based on the labour of 300,000 little girls, but the nation's wealth was put above the nation's health, and the dependence of one on the other was accepted only by a relative few and not even contemplated widely.

The original factory legislation was instigated by humanitarians and especially enlightened industrialists, many of the latter entering the reformed Parliament after 1832. Some established their own model factories and villages. From the humble and ineffectual first Act of 1802 which was aimed at saving pauper apprentices from their cruel fate in northern textile mills, the factory movement progressed through sustained agitation and minor statutes to that of 1833. This really marks the beginning of effective factory legislation. The employment of children under nine was prohibited and the hours of work of young persons under eighteen was limited to twelve hours per day. Four Factory Inspectors were appointed, and Certifying Factory Surgeons were to provide certificates proving the age of children between nine and thirteen. Through the trojan work of Lord Shaftesbury and his ceaseless campaigning, the Mines Act of 1842 forbade the employment of women and boys under ten from working underground. The way was prepared for State control of adults by boys of fifteen not being allowed to be in charge of machinery. During the next decades Mines Inspectors were appointed and regulations extended so that they paralleled factory reforms. In the mid-forties women in textile mills were for the first time included in the same category as young persons, machinery was to be safeguarded and not to be cleaned while in motion. The Ten Hours Act of 1847 was a landmark, but men were excluded, so that the statute only became effective when the working day was limited to 6 a.m. to 6 p.m., or 7 a.m. to 7 p.m. with a two hours' break. These hours remained legal until 1937. Factory regulations were extended in the late sixties to include small workshops, and covered unregulated industries such as metal, tobacco, printing, paper, glass, copper. Restrictions were placed on dangerous trades. By 1870 over 100,000 workers came under the survey of the factory inspectors.

In 1878 a grand consolidating measure was passed (following closely behind the 1875 Public Health Act) and forty-five Acts were compressed within one statute. The Factory Inspectorate was also greatly augmented. Subsequent legislation concentrated on dangerous and sweated trades, and an increasing number of industrial diseases became notifiable to the Chief Inspector. Workmen's Compensation was introduced in 1897 and was widely increased in the following twenty years. The new century also ensured the eight-hour day in coal mines, the establishing of Labour Exchanges, as well as Shop Hours and Minimum Wage Acts. In 1911 came the National Insurance Act. Lloyd George's measure, augmented by Churchill's the year following, was a great culmination and also the twentieth-century starting point of the Welfare State. It was the first step in meeting the accumulated needs of unemployment, poverty and disease which were so forcefully pointed out in the monumental reports of the Poor Law Commission of Inquiry of 1906–9. More government directives and provision were imperative.

Meanwhile industrial medicine was becoming occupational health. The father of English industrial medicine was Charles Turner Thackrah, who in 1832 published a comprehensive study of working conditions and their effect on health. John Simon was greatly influenced and in the 1860s instigated investigations into lung disease among industrial workers. From then on the Factory Inspectorate interested itself in the problems of specific industrial diseases of which lead poisoning was the most common. Legislation for protection against lead, arsenic and mercury poisoning followed. Lead poisoning was made notifiable in 1899 and intensive studies were undertaken hereafter into conditions in the lead trades. Corresponding activity was shown in other dangerous trades. In 1896 a doctor, Arthur Whitelegge, was for the first time made Chief Factory Inspector and two years later a Medical Inspector of Factories was appointed. The work of Dr., later Sir Thomas Legge, achieved world renown in the twentieth century. By the first decade, the Factory Inspectorate consisted of 200 persons and there were 2,000 factory surgeons. The State cognisant of its duty was involved in preventing conditions in industry which were conducive to the high rate of sickness and mortality as well as impaired health. But again so much awaited progress in industrial technology and medical science.

Allied and essential to all aspects of health and welfare are medical science and practice. And it was to this sphere that another field of State activity was devoted or had indirect influence. As with all scientific and technological advances there was pre-eminently indigenous development, but frequently the rate and the direction was determined from outside. There can be no doubt that government and independent inquiries into environmental and industrial health hastened scientific medical investigation and stimulated special spheres of work. The statistics of the

Registrar General on the incidence of, and deaths from, tuberculosis, all the fevers and epidemic diseases, were a spur to research. But whilst medical science moved from miasmatic to germ theory, whilst the bitter controversy raged between contagionists and non-contagionists, sanitarians and public activity forged ahead in combating the diseases most common to the nineteenth century. And the rise in the standard of living played its part in the fall of the death rate from 22 per 1,000 in 1850 to 16 per 1,000 in 1900. Bacteriology did not emerge significantly until 1880. The last epidemic of cholera was in 1866; Koch isolated the vibrio in 1882. Tuberculosis began to decline from the 1830s; Koch discovered the bacillus in 1883. Medical exploration in the preventive field in the eighteenth and nineteenth centuries must not be belittled, but save for smallpox vaccination, the impact of discovering preventive or remedial agents, was not great until very late. It must not be overlooked that the State doctors, the Poor Law Medical Officers, were the public vaccinators (vaccination was the first universally free medical service) and that the Medical Department of the Privy Council sponsored medical research in areas beyond immediate preventive medicine and epidemiology. In 1913 the government established a Medical Research Committee and the Medical Research Council was founded in 1919.

Although the medical profession was itself responsible for the very necessary advances in education, practice and organization, the State played a significant, though often dilatory part. To a great extent this was due to dissension within the profession and, save for the Anatomy Act of 1832, because only a few laymen were interested in controversies over legislation. This began with the Apothecaries Act of 1815 with its regulations for medical education and qualification, and rules for practice. The general practitioner evolved from the apothecary, but quackery continued for many decades. The Medical Act of 1858 introduced medical registration, and only doctors holding a double qualification in medicine and surgery could be registered. Also the General Medical Council was founded to investigate practice and education and propose improvement in both. The statute with its subsequent amendments assured a higher and more uniform standard of medical care. The State doctors had to possess the double qualification and be registered. But it was not until 1888 that special public health training and the Diploma in Public Health were required of city Medical Officers of Health. Another generation passed before these were made a universal rule.

The government was also very procrastinating compared with those of other countries in prescribing for the training and regulation of women midwives. There was no supervision until 1872 and it was not until 1902 that the Midwives' Act demanded proof of adequate training, registration and regulation of practice. But improvement in personal and public hygiene helped to reduce maternal suffering and mortality, particularly as progress in obstetrics and hospital antisepsis were not really significant until the very end of the nineteenth century. In the care of the mentally ill or insane, government intervention came early and continuously. During the eighteenth century much publicity was given to the problems of lunacy. Throughout the nineteenth century classification was improved, County Asylums were provided and special institutions were built. The Lunacy Commissioners were excellent public servants, dedicated to alleviating miserable and often reprehensible conditions. They were particularly anxious to get the insane removed from workhouses and check the abuses of the private licensed houses where such a large proportion were lodged. Their Annual Reports and recommendations did much to implement medical innovations, particularly in more humane treatment. Indeed, humane treatment of the insane was one of the major advances made by Britain in the nineteenth century. Although the care of the mentally ill never kept pace with the need, the late nineteenth century witnessed the transition from custodial to an attempt at remedial care, and during the last years special schools for retarded or handicapped children, and training for the young and adults, was made available in State institutions.

I round off this survey of State activity as I began, by alluding to one field which was implicit, in, and imperative for all progress in the people's health and welfare. Without education no advance in any direction would have been possible. Limiting the hours of work and prohibiting the abuse of child labour meant children had time to attend school. Enlightening the parents led to a change in their attitude, and raising their wages obviated the dependence on the child's pittance to augment the family income. The French Jacobins had demanded 'universal, compulsory, gratuitous and secular education'. The English ruling classes were frightened for decades by the ideals of revolutionaries. Only in 1833 was the first grant given for voluntary schooling by the Board of Trade. But in 1838 Dr. Kay-Shuttleworth reported on the inefficiency of schools and the depressing facts of the monitorial system. In 1846 the parliamentary grant was raised to £100,000 and a five years' apprenticeship of 'pupil teachers' was initiated. Public opinion began to accept State aid and supervision, but still opposed the idea of a State educational service. In the fifties another central committee, the Department of Education under the Privy Council, was established, and towns were empowered to levy rates for education. A commission of inquiry revealed that State-aided and inspected schools were superior to private schools but the report did not recommend compulsory education; public antagonism was still too strong. During the sixties it became glaringly patent that English education lagged behind that of the Continent and the U.S.A. So the demand for a national system grew, and the parliamentary Reform Act of 1867 made urgent the problem of educating the masses. Two million children were not attending school at all. In 1870 national primary education was instituted and from this developed the gradual provision of compulsory and then free education, culminating in 1902 with one of the greatest constructive measures of the nineteenth century. Sir Robert Morant was primarily responsible. County and city councils were made the local authorities in charge of all primary, secondary and technical education, and had to form local education committees. For the first time public money was available to ensure properly paid teachers and a standardized level of efficiency for all children alike.

As some measure of the nineteenth-century achievement the dramatic fall in the death rate could be quoted, but even at the end, one-third of the population were still living below subsistence level and one-third of the male population was unfit for service in the Boer War. The Booth and Rowntree surveys and particularly the famous Poor Law Commission inquiry of 1906–9 drew attention to the incredible amount still to be done to secure adequate provision for the health and welfare of the people. But, partly owing to all the investigations, partly as cumulative effect and interaction of previous measures, and partly due to the growing political liberalism of the ruling classes and the rise of effective working-class politics and pressure, the twentieth century was ushered in with a spate of government activity. Some of this has already been mentioned. Children were provided with school meals, a school medical service and free clinics. Over 4,300 medical officers served the education authorities. The 'Children's Charter' set up juvenile courts, the probation system, and forebade the imprisonment of children. In 1908 Old Age Pensions were introduced, in 1909 Labour Exchanges and a Housing and Town Planning Act. The 'People's Budget' of 1909 had as its object a more equal distribution of wealth, heavily taxing the rich to pay for the reforms for the poor. In 1911 the working class could insure for the emergencies of sickness and unemployment. But by then, however inadequate, a complete pattern of health and welfare services had emerged on which the Welfare State could be built. The trend, as the need, was irreversible.

In England the dual system of State and voluntary activity is very strong. And as a nation there has existed a very laudable strain of philanthropy. Also in the past the State looked to private or self-help to supplement its own provision, and to a significant degree it still does. Taking the Poor Law as only one example: this restricted assistance in order to foster frugality and self-help by encouraging the poor to join clubs, benefit societies and savings banks. In some areas of the country, particularly in the North, people were so fiercely independent that they preferred quacks and other forms of medical care to State or charitable aid.

The central Poor Law administration did its utmost to promote the idea of medical self-help but failed miserably. Through this it was first realized that it was difficult to maintain a strict demarcation between poor and pauper, and that for meeting the contingency of sickness, it was impossible. From the mid-thirties Guardians and Poor Law Medical Officers were admonished to introduce sick clubs to increase self-reliance. Rules and regulations for guidance were circularized. But subscriptions, however low, were beyond the means of the poor, especially in hard times. The collection of money was difficult and spasmodic. Medical Officers were extremely poorly paid and most were hostile. In the forties the early State-sponsored form of medical club was abandoned.

Meanwhile, particularly in Wales and Cornwall, members of the labouring class banded together to establish their own self-supporting sick clubs or Field Clubs, giving non-members medical care on loan. In the iron-mining centres clubs had existed for accident or occupational disease for a long time, and included some relief for unemployment caused by sickness. Some mine-owners formed unique contributory schemes. Another type of club was established in rural areas by the clergy or landed gentry. Patronage and financial aid of honorary members was vital because the contributions required of the poor were so low. Sickness benefit, less than wages, was given, and the sick were attended by a doctor whom they could choose from a panel. Few of these clubs lasted long, and where they survived were changed into friendly societies, dropping medical care but maintaining sickness benefits.

The strictly medical club disappeared after the forties. Many of the combined benefit-medical clubs continued until the sixties and some longer. But attending protracted illnesses could ruin a doctor and the poor complained frequently of inadequate treatment and insufficient medicines. The inability of members to maintain subscriptions and the misuse of the clubs by those who could afford to pay higher contributions hastened the decline of this type of self-help. The

British Medical Association had a Friendly Society and Sick Club Committee which began a campaign for higher pay: a five-shilling capitation fee. Because of the battle between doctors and clubs, wholesale medical resignations followed, and an uneasy relationship continued until the problem was partially resolved by the National Insurance Act.

Abortive health insurance Bills had been introduced in Parliament in the late eighteenth century, and in 1786 a National Friendly Society had been proposed. This had been abandoned for its 'compulsory' principle. In the nineteenth century Dr. William Farr urged a government system of health insurance, because he regarded friendly societies as unsatisfactory financially, and a government system would reduce expenditure on poor relief.

But throughout the Victorian era workers who could, and wished to provide for sickness, joined benefit societies or savings banks. Both grew in importance with the increase in prosperity and confidence of the lower classes. From the thirties deposits in savings banks increased enormously. None of the ordinary benefit and friendly societies provided for medical attendance for families, but these organizations were far the most successful, and it was to them that the majority of labourers looked for provision not only for sickness but for old age and unemployment, so that they would not fall on Poor Law relief. Although some friendly societies were old the great stimulus began in the 1840s. Doctors also seemed willing to assist. They were successful because accounts were strictly kept and a health certificate was required of prospective members. Men in unhealthy occupations were excluded. The Friendly Societies Act of 1875 ensured greater protection to savings. Up to the seventies the largest item in the expenditure of Friendly Societies was for sickness benefit. Burial was also provided for. But there were still far too many small societies whose deficits were high. For rationalization of insurance and complete development, this great movement in working-class self-help again had to await the National Insurance Act. By that time there were over four million insured wage earners in Friendly Societies and millions more in insurance societies for death benefit, thrift clubs and burial clubs, besides those who were members of building societies or enjoyed help from Trade Union benefit funds. By the 1920s Friendly Societies alone had 7 million members with funds amounting to £91 million.

Self-supporting dispensaries were occasionally connected with a friendly society and over a hundred existed by the end of the eighteenth century. Much was heard of them in the 1830s when an Association for the Encouragement of Dispensaries existed. Some had as many as 2,500 members and afforded treatment to over 1,500 of them per year. A period of quiescence followed, but provident dispensaries revived in the sixties and many new ones were started, particularly in London, in the next decade. This was through the efforts of the Charity Organization Society to re-organize Metropolitan poor relief and charitable medical relief. The British Medical Association and the *Lancet* came out in favour, maintaining that there was a general failure of the medical system. The hospitals they demonstrated were for acute cases, the outpatients dealt only with trivial cases. Charity could not pay for the rest, and State relief was inadequate. Mutual assurance was the only answer. The self-supporting dispensaries consisted of honorary members and the working class, but chiefly the latter. The honorary fund covered building and maintenance costs, and the members' funds provided for medical costs. Because the workers contributed such a large proportion of the money, they were provided with better medical care than was offered by a pure medical charity, and there was also choice of doctor.

The provident dispensary system was popular because income was assured in time of sickness, and treatment and medicines could be obtained without delay. Further, retaining their independence meant much to the poor. Doctors also received a salary which they did not from the public dispensaries. Benefit societies paid a subscription proportionate to their members, and sometimes the Poor Law authorities purchased tickets of admission, for this helped to reduce the pressure on the Poor Rates. Although the dispensaries were run by respectable committees and gave efficient service, their growth was retarded by the unwillingness or inability of the poor to contribute regularly, and generally it was the class just above them who subscribed.

But the weakest members of society were never successful in providing for themselves. Yet these suffered most from sub-normal health and malnutrition, and infectious diseases and debilitating complaints attacked them first. They joined the submerged class when sickness overwhelmed them. A distinct demarcation between poor and indigent could not be achieved by State, charitable organizations or self-help. None of these systems was adequate individually and their functions frequently overlapped. 'Integration in a State medical system for the poor with comprehensive Public Health provision would alone make medical relief efficient' (cf. Ruth G. Hodgkinson, *The Origins of the National Health Service*, London, 1967, p. 619).

Last we turn to charitable help for those who could not help themselves. Here, pre-eminent, stands the voluntary hospital service. Again, as with State Poor Law medical care an attempt was made to differentiate between the deserving poor and the outcast pauper. The general voluntary hospital system was founded in the eighteenth century for the treatment of the sick poor. It depended entirely on charity and the gratuitous services of doctors, and provides the finest single illustration of British philanthropy. By the end of the eighteenth century there were about 4,000 beds in the country (2,000 of them in London) for a population of nine million. Both figures had doubled by mid-nineteenth century and medical education relied greatly on the teaching in voluntary hospitals. With the tremendous increase in population and sickness there came an ever-growing demand for the extension of buildings and the erection of new ones. Financial insecurity was a permanent burden and reached its height by the end of the nineteenth century, by which time all kinds of money-raising stratagems had to be resorted to. From the middle of the century small cottage hospitals staffed by general practitioners were founded by local charities. These, however, expected a small contribution from patients.

The voluntary hospitals mitigated the hardship caused by the restrictive State provision. They also became an auxiliary in providing for the indigent when workhouse infirmaries were overcrowded. Many Boards of Guardians subscribed to a hospital for a certain number of pauper patients, and this was particularly common in large cities and in London. In the late thirties Guy's Hospital, for example, took thirty at 10s. 6d. per head. However, an accusation was levelled against the hospitals that they prevented the development of the self-supporting clubs and dispensaries. On the other hand, as the large general hospitals restricted themselves to acute and accident cases, barring the old, the very young, maternity cases and those suffering from infectious and venereal diseases, the State hospitals had to cater increasingly for these categories. It must not be forgotten that very few sick from the middle or upper classes sought treatment in a hospital until the very end of the nineteenth century.

The exclusion of so many from the general hospital, as well as the growing needs of medical education and specialization encouraged the founding of specialist hospitals. They had begun in the eighteenth century but after the mid-nineteenth century grew in great numbers. These were, however, established by doctors and were therefore under their control, but they relied on charitable contributions, or donations from grateful patients. At the turn of the century the voluntary hospital system was providing 80,000 beds and the public-controlled, 150,000. By this time the financial difficulties of the voluntary hospitals, their obsolete geographical location, the frequent overlapping of functions between them and the State hospitals, called for a serious review of the whole field of institutional care. Reform and rationalization were imperative.

Closely connected with the voluntary hospital and sometimes almost an out-patients' department, the public dispensary originated at the end of the eighteenth century. Frequently a doctor, including the most distinguished, served in both hospital and dispensary. The medical profession often founded these stations for the ambulant sick poor, particularly those for special diseases. Dispensaries were popular because patients were also visited in their homes, and because treatment and medicines could be obtained quickly without the formality or stigma of going through the parish. They were dependent on voluntary subscriptions and grew in size in the nineteenth century. A large number of new dispensaries were established in the sixties. After mid-century Poor Law Guardians sometimes founded dispensaries, or more often they contributed annually from the poor rate to those already in existence. Because of this the public dispensaries complained that they were being abused and doctors complained that they saw twice as many patients as a District Medical Officer. Wealthier people also began to make use of the dispensary and helped to drain medical and financial resources. Many of the Metropolitan dispensaries had a few thousand patients a year and also provided them with free medicines. Like the voluntary hospitals they fell into straitened circumstances and had to resort to all kinds of expedients for raising money. However, by the end of the century 100,000 sick poor were benefiting from their help.

But in the nineteenth century not only sickness, but many other aspects of living were creating problems which ever kept in advance or relief. So out of the new humanitarianism, great philanthropy, uneasy consciences and increasing general awareness of the social malaise, innumerable charities arose for combating adverse circumstances and every human misfortune. There was a vast increase in charities after the 1860s and this synchronized with advance in political liberalism, change in philosophy, and paralleled the growth in prosperity and State activity. It was not maudlin sentimentalists but practical philanthropists whose work and wealth created a significant movement, which has been described as assuming the 'dignity of a great work and a noble science'. Many societies were directly responsible for investigations and reports, and many were founded because of these, in answer to an urgent need. By far the most influential was the Charity Organization Society, established in 1869. This speedily organized twenty-eight district committees in London and then spread to the provinces, where it had eighty-five branches by the nineties. Today it is the Family Welfare Association. A pioneer in its aims, it was founded to co-ordinate charitable activities and provide some semblance of policy and co-operation. It was maintained that there existed a great deal of harmful indiscriminate relief, and that to rectify abuses means must be found for seeking out only the deserving poor. As philanthropy had to be disciplined the Charity Organisation Society investigated over a thousand other societies. It became famous for its inquiries and for the information that was passed on, and especially for the training of social workers in casework. A lecture system was inaugurated to augment practical training, and by the end of the century payment for teachers and advisers had been instituted. Through the C.O.S. social work became a profession. For the deserving individual the organization found employment, offered loans and provided letters of admission to a hospital. On a national scale, it tried to further social reforms such as housing, public health and education. Aiding the poor without almsgiving was scientific philanthropy in its modern concept.

Allying closely with the C.O.S. were the Visiting Societies. Many were founded and organized by women, such as those for visiting workhouses, slum dwellings, the poor and prostitutes. These were the case-work and group-work societies, always originating in one area to meet a local need or specializing in a particular field of welfare. From them and the C.O.S. developed a branch of social work regarded as so vital in the twentieth century. There were innumerable organizations founded for different purposes by every religious group. Bible and missionary societies were a very necessary complement to the meagre State provision for education, particularly in the earlier nineteenth century. To aid the forgotten poor and distressed, were charities for the blind, deaf and dumb, for cripples, orphans and the aged. There were nurseries for helping working mothers, women's training schools for cookery and domestic work, and homes for unemployed needlewomen and servants. Philanthropic societies assisted the clergy, foreigners, naval and military personnel and ex-prisoners. Refuges and night shelters were provided for the homeless. And to conclude the list in a typical Victorian strain, there were societies for the Preservation of Life, Health and Morals. Two of the best-known survivors of philanthropic endeavour are the Christian Mission founded in 1865 which became the Salvation Army in 1878 and Dr. Barnardo's Homes, established in 1870.

Throughout the nineteenth century emigration was regarded as a powerful means of getting rid of what the Colonial Office called the 'redundant mass'. And a great many organizations, religious and secular, were devoted to providing for passages and settlement in the colonies and the United States. The detailed ledgers of these societies reveal the vast sums expended each year, and the reports show the tremendous amount of work undertaken. But the labouring class did much itself to escape from the sordid life to which many felt themselves condemned. The men and women who left England were often the young and most enterprising, but of those who remained, thousands joined temperance societies, education groups, and other self-help organizations. The whole working-class movement is too vast to be included here. The co-operative movement, trade unionism and political activity grew in strength, organization and power with the rise in the standard of living, the growing self-consciousness of the worker and the emergence of the paternalistic State.

So we have seen how the State, self-help and philanthropy together contributed to provide for the health and welfare of the people. Complementing, augmenting and overlapping each other, all had strong motives and filled a need. How much of the past still lingers with us both in problems and their solutions, and how much of the uniquely British tri-partite system? Yet great progress was achieved in the nineteenth century through the ever-increasing awareness of problems new or old, the growing possibility for their amelioration, the rise of professionalism, the expert, the revolution in invention and technological innovation and the full measure of reforming heroes. As desiderata were constantly rising, and philosophy and principles changed, the rise in the standard of living never seemed to be adequate. Demand and supply in health and welfare can never be equated. Would the State have done more had there been less independent and voluntary effort? Was public provision, rationalization, efficiency and the equitable distribution of help delayed by these? Considering the prevailing philosophy, social and economic theory, a restrictive Treasury and practical administrative shortcomings, probably not. We were well into the twentieth century before it was widely recognized that the real wealth of a nation is the *total* health of the nation.

J. C. Sournia
Paris (France)

Le développement des institutions de sécurité sociale en France

Les médecins remarquent avec étonnement que dans l'histoire de nos sociétés occidentales la protection de l'individu contre la maladie, contre ses épreuves physiques et les débours financiers qu'elle impose est une réalisation relativement récente; elle n'a même pu se développer à l'échelle des nations que depuis quelques décennies, c'est-à-dire depuis que la science médicale dispose de thérapeutiques efficaces.

Auparavant, la protection que la société proposait en France aux déshérités du sort visait autre chose que la maladie: elle cherchait d'abord à assurer le vivre et le logement, et nos hôpitaux du moyen âge n'avaient pas d'autre ambition. Puis au XVIIe siècle devant l'augmentation du nombre de pauvres, Louis XIV créa l'Hôpital Général qui devait assurer le renfermement des mendiants, certes pour les protéger contre l'infortune, mais aussi pour protéger la société contre eux, comme possibles fauteurs de troubles. Aux XVIIIe et XIXe siècles, avec la naissance des manufactures et des fabriques la protection des classes inférieures visa d'autres buts: le maintien de l'ordre dans une population qui assurait sa main d'oeuvre à l'industrie, et si possible la stabiliser. Enfin à notre époque la Constitution française reconnaît à tout citoyen le droit au travail et le droit à la santé.

Cette évolution des mentalités se lit très bien lorsque l'on passe des travaux du Comité de Mendicité de l'Assemblée Constituante de 1789, à ceux de la Commission de l'Assistance et de la Prévoyance Publique de la IIème République en 1850, et à ceux de la Commission des Affaires Sociales, Familiales et Culturelles de l'Assemblée Nationale de 1972.

Une longue maturation législative a été nécessaire avant que la santé du citoyen soit garantie par l'Etat. La protection contre la maladie s'est inscrite la dernière dans un contexte plus large de protection sociale, dont l'élaboration s'est faite au milieu d'événements politiques, économiques et sociaux si intriqués, que l'histoire de l'assurance-maladie ne peut pas être dissociée des autres formes d'assurances sociales. C'est ce cheminement des esprits et de la réglementation que nous essaierons de tracer, dans une opposition ininterrompue d'idéaux et d'intérêts, et dans des conflits qui durent encore entre réformistes et immobilistes.

I. JUSQU'EN 1945: TRAVAIL ET SÉCURITÉ ÉCONOMIQUE

1°. On trouvera en épreuve non jointe un exposé chronologique des principales étapes de l'évolution de la législation en matière de sécurité, mais les *circonstances sociales* de la période envisagée doivent surtout être rappelées.

A la veille de la révolution de 1848 qui devait profondément bouleverser la France, le pays n'avait pas encore subi la transformation industrielle qui déjà avait changé la Grande-Bretagne et l'Allemagne Occidentale. Néanmoins les hauts fourneaux se multipliaient, les mines se groupaient en grandes compagnies, les tissages se développaient dans le Nord, et les sociétés de grands travaux, qui se consacraient d'abord aux canaux sous la Restauration et Louis Philippe, allaient bientôt stimuler l'activité bancaire grâce aux chemins de fer.

L'évolution industrielle de la France au XIXe siècle et jusqu'à la deuxième guerre mondiale fut caractérisée par sa lente croissance qui n'altéra profondément ni l'activité relative de l'industrie et de l'agriculture (la France resta sur les plans économique, politique et démographique un pays à prédominance rurale), ni les rôles respectifs de la grande et de la petite industrie (même si les grandes firmes augmentaient, les petites prédominaient en nombre), ni les relations respectives des classes sociales: malgré le développement des classes moyennes (commerçants, professions libérales, fonctionnaires) l'inégalité de statut dans la communauté entre le patron et l'ouvrier restait radicale. L'obsession du citoyen était la propriété, grande ou petite: c'était à la propriété que se jugeait l'indépendance et la liberté de l'homme, l'obsession du manoeuvre était l'achat d'un petit atelier, le tâcheron agricole visait l'acquisition d'un lopin, le contremaître voulait devenir petit patron.

Dans cet univers mental, le travail salarié était ressenti comme l'avilissement de l'individu, et il n'est pas rare de voir sous la plume des écrivains de l'époque, Proudhon, Fourier, Saint-Simon, Marx, des comparaisons entre le statut d'ouvrier et celui des serfs de l'Ancien Régime. Au moins l'esclave était logé et nourri par son maître, ses vieux jours étaient assurés, le maître avait intérêt à le maintenir en bonne santé, alors que l'ouvrier était laissé à lui-même avec un salaire permettant la survie de justesse, l'ouvrier était renvoyé sans façon à l'occasion d'un écart de conduite, d'une maladie, ou de l'âge. Aucun lien de solidarité n'unissait patron et salarié, l'un disposait sur l'autre d'un pouvoir discrétionnaire. Il fallait attendre 1901 pour que Millerand, député socialiste, pût tenir à la Chambre des Députés des propos qui eussent été séditieux quelques décennies plus tôt: «Rien semble-t-il n'est plus équitable, et l'on ne paraît guère le contester sérieusement, que de demander au patron d'inscrire à ses frais généraux l'assurance et l'amortissement de son personnel humain, comme il y inscrit l'assurance et l'amortissement de son matériel et de ses machines.»

En 1848 cette «équité» n'avait pas cours, et à cette époque arriva en France le mot «paupérisme» né en Grande-Bretagne. La misère n'était cependant pas un phénomène nouveau en France, elle existait déjà sous l'Ancien Régime, mais elle prit à cette époque un aspect nouveau qui la rendit plus spectaculaire. Le paupérisme apparut dans les esprits comme un phénomène dû à la fois à la ville et à la machine.

De cette interprétation découlèrent plusieurs phénomènes historiques, dans le domaine qui nous intéresse.

D'abord l'idée se développa peu à peu dans la société que la paupérisation et l'insécurité des travailleurs étant liées au progrès de l'industrie, la misère n'était sans doute pas toujours le résultat de la paresse et du vice, contrairement à une opinion qui fut toujours très répandue: dès lors l'industriel avait le devoir d'y remédier, au moins en partie.

Ensuite, deuxième idée généralement admise, c'était l'ouvrier de l'atelier et de l'usine lié à la machine qui avait besoin des secours prioritaires pour ses vieux jours, alors que le travailleur aux champs était beaucoup moins exposé aux risques d'accident et aux aléas de l'emploi, et nécessitait moins de secours. Une attention beaucoup plus grande fut portée à la misère urbaine qu'à la rurale, d'autant que les ouvriers s'organisèrent plus vite et s'agitèrent davantage que les paysans: les remèdes sociaux furent plus vite élaborés pour les travailleurs des usines que pour ceux des champs.

Pour illustrer ces tournures d'esprit, rappelons qu'il fallut attendre 1899 pour que fût votée une loi portant sur les accidents du travail dans l'agriculture, et encore ne visait-elle que «les exploitations dotées d'une machine mue par une force autre que celle des hommes et des animaux»: en clair, les accidents du travail survenant dans les fermes employant des chevaux ne justifiaient pas de réparation!

Enfin il n'est pas possible, pour retracer le climat social dans lequel se déroula ce siècle, de ne pas évoquer ce qui se passait au delà des frontières de la France. Les législations sociales progressèrent en Belgique, en Grande-Bretagne, en Allemagne, en Italie à des rythmes presque semblables, mais avec certains décalages dans le temps, et chaque pays influença son voisin. En France, ce fut nettement la politique de Bismarck, inaugurée en 1883 pour des motifs plus politiques que sociaux, qui marqua le plus les esprits, et il est piquant de suivre dans les Débats de la Chambre les périphrases employées pour désigner les réalisations prussiennes: en effet, on était alors en pleine obsession «revancharde», et toute référence directe à la législation allemande eût été aussitôt marquée d'opprobre.

2°. Sur cet arrière-fonds économique, social et mental, une législation sociale fut peu à peu mise sur pied avec prudence, au milieu d'innombrables hésitations, et je voudrais maintenant détailler les *oppositions qui freinèrent cette construction.*

L'attitude des patrons doit d'abord être étudiée car dans la Société et à la Chambre ils avaient plus de poids. Leurs idées étaient loin d'être claires et uniformes, et nous verrons que les ouvriers n'étaient pas plus unanimes.

Dès les années 1830 certains patrons avaient formé, d'abord dans le Nord de la France, des «caisses de secours» destinées à venir en aide aux ouvriers malades ou à leur famille en cas de décès, et à assurer une modique retraite à certains d'entre eux. Ces caisses de secours avaient des caractéristiques qu'il faut énumérer: elles étaient nées de l'initiative du patron, mais si certains d'entre eux avaient cru bon d'en créer, ils n'entendaient pas y être forcés, la caisse était le témoin de la liberté de l'entreprise, et le milieu du siècle fut marqué par l'opposition du patronat à toute forme d'obligation légale dans ce domaine. Le refus de l'obligation était la marque du libéralisme économique qui inspirait la France, alors que toute obligation eût été la voie ouverte au socialisme et au communisme. Ce problème de l'obligation souleva des tempêtes que nous imaginerions mal actuellement.

La caisse répondait à des buts très mitigés. Il faut y voir l'une des manifestations du christianisme social qui naquit à cette époque sous sa forme moderne, mais le patronat entendait aussi en faire un instrument de fixation pour un personnel qui changeait trop volontiers de patron. Le bon fonctionnement de la caisse de secours était un facteur attractif pour le personnel, il évitait les départs de fantaisie, et il était aussi un élément de chantage pour inciter le travailleur à une «bonne conduite» et aussi à un bon rendement: en effet les cotisations versées par l'ouvrier ne lui étaient pas restituées s'il était renvoyé.

Les caisses de retraite étaient alimentées essentiellement par les cotisations des ouvriers fixées par les patrons, c'est-à-dire en fait par un prélèvement sur les salaires, et la gestion des fonds était assurée par la direction de l'entreprise. Le problème de l'emploi et du placement des fonds ainsi recueillis agita les esprits pendant tout le XIXe, on opposa constamment le système de retraite par capitalisation au système par répartition, les ouvriers n'entendant pas que leurs cotisations fussent placées en actions de sociétés anonymes dont ils condamnaient l'existence!

Finalement le principe de ces caisses découlait d'un paternalisme, ou plutôt d'un système de «patronage» qui poussait le patron pour retenir son personnel, à construire dans le même matériau des locaux d'habitation de type «coron» pour maintenir la morale familiale, et des églises pour maintenir la religion.

Cependant ces libéralités intéressées n'étaient à la portée que des grosses entreprises, et les petites ne pouvaient pas se les permettre, même si elles en voyaient la justification et l'utilité. Aussi certains esprits envisagaient comme possible l'intervention de l'Etat dans un domaine intéressant la collectivité, comme ils trouvaient légitime que l'Etat vienne au secours des salariés que la mauvaise gestion d'une caisse de secours laissait sans ressources (les sommes versées restant propriété de l'entreprise), ce qui ne fut pas rare. Mais appeler l'Etat au secours n'était pas sans danger, et l'on vit pendant un siècle le patronat partagé, en matière de sécurité sociale, entre des désirs difficilement conciliables: se rendant compte qu'il ne pouvait pas tout faire tout seul, il envisageait la participation de l'Etat, à laquelle il se refusait cependant au nom de la doctrine sacrée du libéralisme.

En face, la tactique du monde ouvrier ne fut ni cohérente, ni continue, ni toujours logique. La Révolution ayant fait disparaître les ghildes d'entraide qui existaient dans certains compagnonnages, on les vit ressurgir dans le courant du siècle sous la forme de mutuelles; mais le système mutualiste se chercha longtemps, les premières expériences en furent malheureuses et restèrent rares en France. Ce n'est qu'en 1898 que, les esprits ayant évolué et les ouvriers ayant mûri, la promulgation de la loi qui devint le code de la Mutualité lui assura dans le pays une très grande popularité.

Lorsque les patrons créèrent leurs premières caisses de secours, ils essayèrent d'y associer leurs ouvriers, mais ceux-ci ne se prêtèrent jamais de gaieté de coeur à ce qu'ils appelaient une complicité. Eux aussi étaient partagés sur le caractère obligatoire de toute cotisation, qu'elle fût ou non accompagnée d'une cotisation patronale, eux aussi hésitaient sur le rôle à donner à l'Etat qui pouvait ou bien se substituer au patron et donc le devenir, ou au contraire protéger l'ouvrier contre le patron. Ceci explique que des réalisations législatives comme les lois créant la Caisse Nationale de Retraite pour la Vieillesse (1850) et la Caisse Nationale d'Assurances contre les Accidents du Travail (1868) ne suscitèrent aucun enthousiasme dans les milieux ouvriers, et finalement furent peu suivies d'effet.

Tout au long du siècle les discussions eurent lieu sur les retraites dans les réunions syndicales. L'analphabétisme ne conférait pas une claire vision sur les problèmes de gestion, ou sur la différence entre capitalisation et répartition, l'ouvrier voyait seulement que sous le prétexte d'alimenter une caisse qu'il connaissait mal en vue d'une retraite hypothétique, on diminuait son salaire. Toute participation à un système réglé par la loi devenait à ses yeux la participation contrainte à un système social qu'il récusait. On vit au nom des principes les plus sacrés s'opposer d'une part les révolutionnaires radicaux qui voulaient d'abord détruire le capitalisme pour instaurer un monde sans accidents de travail, où la communauté prendrait soin des vieux travailleurs sans qu'ils aient cotisé à une retraite, et d'autre part les réformistes qui préféraient des lois assurant une sécurité imparfaite, à l'absence de loi. Jules Guesde s'opposait à la Chambre et dans les réunions ouvrières à Jean Jaurès, la C.G.T. contredisait la C.G.T.U., les partis socialistes étaient divisés. Jusqu'au milieu du XXème siècle l'unité du monde ouvrier ne se réalisera jamais sur ces questions.

Si les classes extrêmes étaient éloignées l'une de l'autre sur bien des principes, leurs oppositions n'avaient rien de farouche puisqu'en elles-mêmes les dogmes n'étaient pas unanimement reconnus. Par contre on peut dire que les classes moyennes, les petits propriétaires, les commerçants et artisans, les professions libérales, les médecins présentaient une belle unanimité contre tout système de protection sociale, qu'il s'agisse des assurances contre le chômage et les accidents du travail, ou des retraites ouvrières et paysannes votées en 1910. Certes elles rechignaient à ces lois qui leur imposaient des charges alors qu'elles n'en attendaient aucun avantage, mais leur opposition venait aussi de leur attachement indéfectible au libéralisme. La protection assurée par la collectivité devenait une atteinte à la responsabilité et à l'initiative individuelle, elle menaçait les conceptions de l'homme et de la société qui avaient toujours été à la base de notre civilisation.

De la morale on passe volontiers au moralisme, et un médecin était l'interprète d'une grande partie de son milieu lorsqu'il écrivait en 1929: «l'Allemagne a perdu la guerre pour avoir endommagé son système nerveux avec les Assurances Sociales.» Cette même tournure d'esprit qui durait encore entre 1940 et 1945 attribuait aux allocations familiales et aux congés payés la mollesse du peuple français et ses malheurs de 1940.

3°. *Si la législation se développa cependant*, en dépit d'une opposition composite mais incoordonnée, ce fut grâce à l'action opiniâtre de personnalités diverses qui se succédèrent pendant cent ans. Les uns, dès le Second Empire étaient des hommes inspirés par le plus pur christianisme social. Les autres étaient de ces personnalités politiques libérales qui se rencontrèrent en France sous tous les régimes et sous les gouvernements de toutes teintes, issus de partis les plus variés, ceux qui s'appelaient eux-mêmes les «républicains de progrès». D'autres encore, plus discrets, étaient de hauts fonctionnaires; on peut d'ailleurs constater que, inspirateurs discrets des orateurs publics, ils furent les constructeurs des institutions actuelles, témoignant d'une persévérance dont les personnages politiques étaient incapables.

Avec prudence et avec une remarquable continuité de vue, ils poursuivirent une oeuvre législative, génération après génération, qui couvrait de nombreux domaines. Et surtout ils surent placer sous la garantie morale et financière de l'Etat des institutions où on le voyait intervenir avec crainte. Finalement, par l'intermédiaire de la loi, c'est bien l'Etat qui assure à tout citoyen, patron ou ouvrier, la garantie d'une égale répartition des charges et des avantages de toute assurance sociale.

A la veille de la deuxième guerre mondiale, la protection sociale du travailleur français était acquise sur de nombreux points. Ses horaires de travail étaient réglementés. Des indemnités lui étaient versées en cas de chômage. Une retraite lui était assurée au-delà de 65 ans. Une assurance le couvrait et garantissait sa famille en cas d'accident de travail ou de maladie professionnelle. Une politique nataliste avait inspiré une loi sur les allocations familiales.

Certes beaucoup de progrès restaient à faire: les sommes versées étaient généralement insuffisantes même si elles diminuaient l'insécurité du travailleur, et certaines catégories de citoyens n'en bénéficiaient pas encore. En tout cas certaines idées étaient définitivement admises sur lesquelles on ne reviendra plus, telles que la solidarité entre employeurs et salariés dans le versement et la gestion des cotisations, la garantie donnée par l'Etat au fonctionnement du système, et l'obligation faite à tous par la loi d'y participer: il avait fallu un siècle pour y parvenir.

II. APRÈS 1945: SANTÉ ET SÉCURITÉ

1°. Ce n'est pas le lieu ici de décrire comment, année après année, furent complétées après 1945 les lacunes que la sécurité du salarié présentait encore en 1939. Je rappellerai simplement *l'effort législatif et règlementaire considérable* qui fut entrepris par les gouvernements de la Libération, en 1945 et 1946.

Les mentalités politiques et sociales n'étaient plus celles de l'avant-guerre, les structures syndicales avaient changé, les partis conservateurs avaient provisoirement disparu de la scène politique au profit d'organisations libérales, en particulier la démocratie chrétienne joua un rôle considérable dans les premiers gouvernements de la IVe République. Enfin on peut rappeler que le Général De Gaulle était lié aux milieux patronaux du Nord de la France, dont nous avons vu le dynamisme dans ce domaine dès le milieu du siècle précédent.

Même si la loi sur l'Assistance Médicale Gratuite date de 1893, même si certaines mesures d'assurances médicales avaient été instaurées après 1930, on peut dire que les aspects médicaux des assurances sociales ne prédominaient pas dans la législation en dehors des accidents du travail et des maladies professionnelles. A partir de 1945 la branche «assurance maladie» va prendre une place grandissante.

2°. Pas plus que dans les périodes précédentes, on n'assistera à une unanimité populaire, rassemblant toutes les classes et toutes les professions dans le souci commun de la *protection de l'individu contre les charges financières imposées par la maladie*. Au contraire tous les particularismes se manifestèrent.

Les ordonnances de 1945 avaient cependant émis le principe d'un régime unique d'assurance maladie, en réalité les choses se passèrent différemment. Les travailleurs salariés avaient déjà leur institution, mais de nombreuses professions ne voulurent pas s'y rallier, les unes pour sauvegarder les systèmes dont elles étaient dotées depuis longtemps (par exemple dans les chemins de fer et les mines), souvent de type mutualiste, les autres pour échapper aux taux des cotisations qu'elles jugeaient trop élevées bien qu'acceptées par les employeurs et les salariés.

Ainsi vit-on naître, à côté du régime général, des régimes qui s'y rattachèrent sur certains points (régimes dits «particuliers»), et d'autres pleinement autonomes (régimes dits «spéciaux»). Le particularisme français ne simplifia pas les choses, et la multiplicité des régimes crée bien des difficultés de gestion.

Alors que les travailleurs salariés agricoles étaient couverts pour le risque maladie depuis 1935, il fallut attendre 1960 pour que les exploitants acceptent une garantie dans ce domaine. Enfin le régime instauré par la loi du 12 juillet 1966 pour les commerçants, artisans et professions libérales ne s'imposera pas sans de vives résistances des bénéficiaires, et il est encore soumis de leur part à d'incessantes retouches. En 1972, la presque totalité de la population vivant sur le territoire français est protégée par un régime d'assurance maladie: la maladie n'est plus la hantise qu'elle a été si longtemps pour le travailleur.

3°. Suivant la tradition née dans le pays depuis plus de 120 ans, la *gestion du risque maladie* est assurée par des caisses très décentralisées, dont le ressort correspond généralement à un département: l'Etat exerce sur elles une tutelle qui, minutieuse sur certains chapitres, est plus libérale sur d'autres, mais il veille scrupuleusement au respect de tous les droits des assurés et à une stricte observation des lois et règlements.

Mais la composition du conseil d'administration des caisses a subi de nombreuses variations. On a vu que les ouvriers, un siècle plus tôt, hésitaient à leur assurer leur participation, puis qu'ils y entrèrent avec des réticences atténuées par le temps. En 1945 leur représentation fut fixée dans le régime général, d'après des arguments valables, aux deux tiers des conseils, les employeurs disposant de l'autre tiers; le système ne fonctionna pas sans de nombreuses difficultés, aussi en 1967 grâce à une argumentation non moins valable, fut mis en oeuvre le paritarisme qui donna une représentation égale d'une part aux organisations d'employeurs, d'autre part aux grandes centrales syndicales des salariés. Le patronat qui redouta si longtemps l'intervention de l'Etat dans la gestion des caisses car il y voyait sa propre dépossession, s'est donc vu restitué en partie en 1967 le rôle dont il avait été dépouillé en 1945.

On ne saurait évoquer la gestion des Caisses d'Assurance Maladie sans évoquer la place qu'y tiennent leurs médecins. En effet la plupart des régimes se sont dotés d'un corps de médecins-conseils qui contrôlent la justification des prestations en nature et en espèces versées par les caisses, jouent le rôle d'experts en matière d'incapacité et d'invalidité, sont les conseillers des assurés pour qu'ils jouissent de la totalité de leurs droits, et aussi les conseillers des caisses en matière d'action sanitaire et sociale (oeuvres sociales de toutes natures, octroi de prestations supplémentaires à certains malades, participation à l'équipement hospitalier et sanitaire du pays, etc. . . .). La situation administrative de ces médecins, pharmaciens, chirurgiens-dentistes au sein des caisses est différente selon les régimes, et a varié avec le temps.

4°. On ne saurait imaginer d'assurance-maladie qui n'implique pas la participation, ou du moins la *collaboration du corps médical*. Qu'en est-il en France, et comment les événements se sont-ils déroulés?

Dans la première partie a été évoquée l'attitude des classes moyennes et des professions libérales en France à l'égard de tout système de protection sociale, elle a été celle des médecins et dans une certaine mesure elle l'est encore: position de défense du libéralisme qui fut longtemps d'hostilité et de refus de participation. La profession de médecin a toujours été considérée comme individualiste au plus haut point: le médecin est seul devant ses responsabilités de diagnostic et de traitement, ses techniques professionnelles sont celles d'un artisan travaillant seul, sa formation universitaire, ses revenus et le prestige qui l'entoure, l'intègrent à la bourgeoisie. N'employant pas de personnel, il n'est ni patron ni ouvrier. Au siècle dernier il était le maître de ses honoraires, il fixait à sa guise ceux qu'il demandait aux riches, et trouvait normal de soigner gratuitement les indigents, mais il n'entendait subir dans ce domaine aucune contrainte extérieure: ce mode de pensée fut celui de la profession jusqu'à une date récente.

Une première atteinte à ce principe fut portée par la loi de 1893 sur l'Assistance Médicale Gratuite, une deuxième par une loi suivant la première guerre mondiale sur les soins aux pensionnés militaires: dans les deux cas une administration se chargeait de régler aux médecins les honoraires justifiés par les soins donnés à certaines catégories de malades. Ce fut le début du système du «tiers payant» qui inspire toujours aux médecins la même appréhension.

En effet l'entente directe, coutume selon laquelle les honoraires seraient fixés par accord entre le médecin et le malade est l'un des éléments de cette «charte de la médecine libérale» dont on commença à parler lors des premières discussions sur l'assurance maladie dans les années 1930 entre les médecins, les caisses et l'administration. Cette charte comportait également le libre choix de son médecin par le malade, le respect du secret médical, la liberté de la thérapeutique par le médecin, toutes notions qu'aucun projet d'assurance-maladie en France n'a jamais menacées.

En fait au nom de la prétendue entente directe, le corps médical a toujours défendu le droit de fixer ses honoraires à son gré, possibilité que toute intrusion d'un organisme tiers entre le médecin et son client interdit définitivement.

Nous ne pouvons relater ici toutes les péripéties qui illustrèrent les discussions entre les syndicats médicaux, les organismes sociaux et les représentants des pouvoirs publics, discussions qui durent encore après quarante ans, et qui furent illustrées d'innombrables assemblées professionnelles, de scissions bruyantes et de réconciliations clandestines, de l'intrusion épisodique de l'Ordre des Médecins, organisation de type corporatif créée en 1940 par le gouvernement de Vichy.

Peu à peu se mit en place, à partir de 1960, un système de conventions où les honoraires étaient réglés par des accords entre les Caisses d'assurance maladie et les syndicats de médecins soit par convention départementale, soit par convention individuelle. Enfin le 29 octobre 1971 a été signée une convention nationale entre les principaux régimes de sécurité sociale et les confédérations médicales: le maintien des caractéristiques essentielles de la médecine libérale est garanti à la profession, mais les honoraires sont fixés après discussion à l'échelon national contrôlé par l'Etat, et non plus par l'initiative de chaque médecin. Sur ces bases, la presque totalité des médecins de France est désormais conventionnée, et assure ses soins à des tarifs négociés à la presque totalité de la population.

Cette convention n'a évidemment marqué qu'une étape dans une évolution dont nul ne peut prévoir le cours.

III. REMARQUES

Au terme de cette histoire résumée des législations sociales en France quelques remarques sur le passé s'imposent, et aussi quelques interrogations sur l'avenir.

La lenteur de cette élaboration doit d'abord être soulignée. Depuis les caisses de secours du premier tiers du XIXe siècle jusqu'à une couverture contre les principaux risques assurée à toute la population française, un siècle et demi s'est écoulé. Bien des projets de loi ne furent acceptés que par la génération suivante, car les initiateurs généreux ne trouvèrent que tardivement le public qui les comprit. Bien des institutions décidées ne fonctionnèrent pas, bien des textes restèrent lettre morte, bien des règlements subirent des modifications et aboutirent à des résultats différents de ceux escomptés, tantôt heureux, tantôt malheureux. Bien des oppositions dues à la méfiance ou au conservatisme social trouvent de nouvelles manières de se perpétuer.

Et pourtant le système a progressé; de la charité on est passé lentement à l'assistance, puis à l'assurance; le citoyen dispose dans le pays d'une protection presque suffisante contre le chômage, la misère, l'accident, la vieillesse, la maladie. La sécurité n'est plus comme autrefois un luxe lié à la propriété, elle est un droit du citoyen.

Cette sécurité a grandi en même temps que le pays se développait, mais elle a été aussi un facteur de développement. L'industrialisation que l'on accusait de provoquer le paupérisme a fait naître de nouvelles conditions de travail, leur évolution et celle du droit du travail est indissociable de la vie de la sécurité sociale; accroissant le bien-être et améliorant la santé, elle améliore le travail et la production, elle prolonge la vie de l'individu, et contribue à l'enrichissement de la communauté dans tous les domaines. Capital et travail ne sont plus séparés par l'asservissement de naguère, mais solidarisés par des soucis communs, leurs rapports ne sont plus ceux que décrivaient Marx ou Proudhon; selon l'école à laquelle on appartient, on conclura que la sécurité sociale assure la survie du capitalisme, ou qu'elle suscite un capitalisme humain.

Enfin dans le domaine médical, le système français actuel assure une distribution de soins de type libéral, avec une gestion de type communautaire. Il assure au citoyen la possibilité de se faire soigner avec des frais supportables pour n'importe quelle affection et par le médecin de son choix, et il donne au médecin une rémunération suffisante: la médecine française ne pourrait plus se passer de la sécurité sociale.

On pourrait dire que les institutions actuelles donnent satisfaction à la population française, médecins et malades, si elles étaient stables, ce qui ne semble pas le cas. Bien des inquiétudes subsistent, qui tiennent surtout au coût croissant de la santé auquel se heurtent la plupart des pays industrialisés. Aucun système de sécurité sociale ne saurait prétendre à la longévité, tant nos sociétés et nos conceptions évoluent vite, et tant sont rapides les progrès de nos techniques médicales.

Huw W. S. Francis
Leeds (Great Britain)

Discussion

May I say how great a pleasure it is for me also to participate in this session of the Congress. Not only is it the first session of the International Congress to be devoted to the social history of medicine, but Professor George Rosen is President of the Society for the Social History of Medicine, and our opening speaker, Dr. Ruth Hodgkinson, was a member of the small group of people, of whom I was one, who came together in 1970 to launch the Society in this country. My English Chairman has also made distinguished contributions to the development of my own speciality, community medicine.

By coincidence today is also an historical occasion in the development of the National Health Service, since it is the day of publication of the proposals on the Management Structure for the Reorganization of the Service, which is planned for 1 April 1974.[1] In the machinery which produced these suggestions I happen to have been a small cog. One must say that historical knowledge is more than useful in such a situation, but historical sensitivity does not ease, but adds to the stress of such participation.

Dr. Hodgkinson, in her excellent opening remarks, rightly referred to *trends* in the nineteenth-century social history of medicine, and of the growth of science as being one of those important trends. This is quite true; but nineteenth-century science requires rather careful scrutiny. The great English sanitarian, Sir John Simon, published his book on pathology in 1850[2] – the first systematic textbook in English, and the first to introduce the ideas of Virchow to the United Kingdom – lest his notoriety as a public health reformer should sully his scientific reputation.[3] If the trend alone is observed, the extent to which 'science' was a kind of ideology in Victorian times might be missed. There is also a danger of which Dr. Hodgkinson, from her scholarly knowledge of Edwin Chadwick and Thomas Hodgkin, will be well aware. The emphasis on *trends* obscures the complex patterns of inter-personal relationships which underlie them. The distinguished, if controversial, English historian, Sir Lewis Namier (who was not English by birth) revolutionized our ideas of the course of English politics in the eighteenth century, in two works based on a meticulous, painstaking analysis of biographical data about the then Members of the House of Commons.[4,5] Such studies would be rewarding in the social history of medicine; two examples will suffice:

First, let us look at William Pulteney Alison, who between 1820 and 1856 successively held the Chairs of Medical Jurisprudence, the Institutes of Medicine (or physiology), and the Practice of Medicine at the University of Edinburgh. He was noted, not only for direct personal philanthropy, but also in the advocacy of social reforms. Amongst the earliest of his pupils was James Philips Kay (later Sir James Kay-Shuttleworth), who was both a colleague of Chadwick in the preparation of his great Report of 1842, and later became the first Secretary of the Commission of the Privy Council on Education – effectively the first English senior civil servant directly concerned with education.[6] But in addition three of Alison's later pupils were members of the Royal Sanitary Commission of 1869–71 (which led to the great Public Health Act, 1875). These were: William Stokes (senior) of Dublin; Sir Henry Acland, Regius Professor of Medicine at Oxford; and, Sir Thomas Watson, a Professor of Medicine in London.[7]

Now what I find of even greater interest is that Alison was, as a young man, a keen student under the Scottish philosopher Dugald Stewart who wished Alison to succeed him in the Chair of Philosophy (not a unique occurrence in Scottish medicine).[8] But Lord Palmerston, who as Home Secretary in 1854 tried to prevent the fall of the first General Board of Health, was also a student of Dugald Stewart, before completing his university work at Cambridge.[9] How much in English social development do we owe directly or indirectly to Dugald Stewart?

Second, Octavia Hill, who did much social good in the foundation of The National Trust, in housing and social work reform was the grand-daughter of Thomas Southwood Smith, and was deeply influenced by him.[10]

Let us turn, however, to two other trends.

Sir Edwin Chadwick, when a young man was the friend and secretary of Jeremy Bentham, 'the most typical of the English Utilitarians'.[11] Now English Utilitarianism was both a programme of social action, and an ethical philosophy. Its basic ethical proposition was that the greatest good was that action which produced the greatest happiness of the greatest number. Much policy-making is explicitly, and a great deal of management thinking is implicitly, utilitarian. This is now the subject of much critical comment; as Professor Stuart Hampshire, the Warden of Wadham College, Oxford, put it significantly in this year's Leslie Stephen Lecture at Cambridge: '. . . To others, and particularly to many of the young in America and in Europe . . . it seems now obvious that the large-scale computations in modern politics and social planning bring with them a coarseness and grossness of moral feeling, a blunting of sensibility, and a suppression of individual discrimination and gentleness, which are a price that they will not pay for the benefits of clear calculation. Their point is worth considering: perhaps it can be given a philosophical basis . . .'.[12]

Hampshire is not alone in his rejection of utilitarianism. John Rawls of Harvard has recently published his massive – and long expected – argument for the re-examination of 'distributive justice',[13] and in a tempestuous, occasionally injudicious, series of essays and lectures the literary don, F. R. Leavis, has fired many broadsides into the hull of what he calls 'technologico-Benthamism'.[14] Clearly the course of this trend may – perhaps must – change if medical practice is ready to progress.

I must mention a trend which seems to me to be underestimated in studies of Victorian and Edwardian social medicine, namely religious belief. One of the first bits of legislation in this century which led to the welfare state was the establishment of a school medical service, by a sub-section only of an Act of 1907. The catalyst which led to this service was the publication in 1903 and 1904 of two articles by Major-General Sir John Frederick Maurice, who had been Director of Recruiting at the War Office during the Boer War. He drew attention to the very low state of health and fitness of a high proportion of those who volunteered for military service. The story is usually told as a soldier's natural concern for national defence. This is certainly part of the truth. What has not been appreciated is that J. F. Maurice stood in a line of social and religious commitment. His father, of whom he wrote an outstanding biography, was Frederick Dennison Maurice, a well-known Victorian divine, and the founder with Charles Kingsley and J. M. Ludlow of the Christian Socialist Movement. His grandfather Maurice Maurice had been assistant to Joseph Priestley at the Hackney Unitarian Chapel. Priestley was so radical in his political views, that suspected of Jacobinism, he spent his last years in voluntary exile in Philadelphia.

As a footnote to this story, one should add that the 1907 Act was passed by that Liberal House of Commons, which was the high-water mark of the political influence of the 'Non-conformist Conscience'. However, the son of J. F. Maurice took action similar to his father. He was Major-General John Barton Maurice, and when Director of Operations at the War Office, accused Lloyd-George in an article in the *Daily Telegraph* of misleading the Commons about the strength of the Army, a concern shared by father and son. In the 'Maurice Debate' which followed early in 1918, the 'official Opposition' divided the House against the Government for the only time during the 1914–18 war, irrevocably splitting the Liberal Party, and leading to its decline.[15]

My second and last example of a religious influence in nineteenth-century social history is the important book by William Booth of the Salvation Army, *In Darkest England and the Way Out* published in 1890. It was based on the experience of social work of the Salvation Army itself, and in part on the researches of his unrelated namesake Charles Booth. It was written with the help of W. T. Stead, and Catherine Booth, his wife. In fact the greater part of it was composed in her sick-room, as she lay dying of carcinoma of the breast, for which she had rejected the surgery advised by Sir James Paget, and even any anodyne, until the last few weeks of her illness, so that her mind should remain clear.[16,17] The book raised the concern of many ordinary middle-class and citizen readers about 'the submerged tenth' and also was partly responsible for stimulating others, like Seebohm Rowntree,[18] to action and to further social enquiries.

The four discussion points I have tried to expound – the use of 'science' as an idealogy, the need for a biographical analysis, the promptings to revise our view of the utilitarian ethic, and the religious influences in Victorian and Edwardian social thought – lead in one direction. Social policies of all kinds must be strongly imbued both in conception and in action, as Professor Titmuss has recently reminded us,[19] by altruism. This is true of medicine, if it is to continue truly humane. Perhaps today, of all days, this should be said.

References

1 *Management Arrangements for the Reorganised National Health Service*, London, H.M.S.O., 1972.
2 SIMON, J., *General Pathology*, London, 1850.
3 LAMBERT, R., *Sir John Simon*, London, MacGibbon & Kay, 1963.
4 NAMIER, L., *The Structure of Politics at the Accession of George III*, London, Macmillan, 1929.
5 NAMIER, L., *England in the Age of the American Revolution*, London, Macmillan, 1930.
6 BLOOMFIELD, B. C. (ed.), *The Autobiography of Sir James Kay-Shuttleworth*, University of London, Education Libraries Bulletin Supplement 7, 1964.
7 MACKINTOSH, J. M., *Topics in Public Health*, Edinburgh, Livingstone, 1965.
8 *Dictionary of National Biography.*
9 RIDLEY, J., *Lord Palmerston*, London, Constable, 1970.
10 POYNTER, F. N. L., *Proc. R. Soc. Med.*, 1961, **55**, 381.

11 FINER, S. E., *The Life and Times of Sir Edwin Chadwick*, London, Methuen, 1952.
12 HAMPSHIRE, S., *Morality and Pessimism*, London, Cambridge University Press, 1972.
13 RAWLS, J., *A Theory of Justice*, London, Oxford University Press, 1972.
14 LEAVIS, F. R., *Nor Shall my Sword*, London, Chatto & Windus, 1972.
15 FRANCIS, H. W. S., in preparation, 1972.
16 COLLIER, R., *The General Next to God.*, London, Collins (Fontana), 1968.
17 BRAMWELL-BOOTH, C., *Catherine Booth*, London, Hodder & Stoughton, 1970.
18 BRIGGS, A., *Seebohm Rowntree*, London, Longmans, 1961.
19 TITMUSS, R. M., *The Gift Relationship*, London, Allen & Unwin, 1970.

I. Galdston
Brooklyn, N.Y. (U.S.A.)

Evolving of medical care in the U.S.A.

It was Ortega y Gasset who made the astute observation that any issue which at any given time is uppermost in the minds of the populace is already forty years past its prime significance. Karl Marx in his writings on the revolution of 1848 appears to have been of the same opinion.

Odd as this judgment may appear to be, it is actually easy to comprehend and to accept. For it stands to reason, and is confirmed in history, that by the time prime ideas percolate down from the level of their origin to those of the masses, new issues have arisen and new ideas have emerged and these tend to override the antecedent ones. One might, without being cynical, say that mankind never really solves its problems; they are rather displaced by new ones.

How to provide medical care and service to the sick has been a problem since the beginnings of human existence. History shows that the ways in which the sick were treated and dealt with, by whom, how, and under what economic arrangements, have differed from region to region and changed from age to age.[1] However, the provision of medical care and service became a highly significant and increasingly pressing problem mainly during the last 200 years, and mostly during the last half century. Its emergence can be traced to the development of modern industrial civilization.

Three factors contributed to the intensification of the medical care problem: the crowding of many persons into industrial centres; the development of what has been so aptly termed the Crowd Diseases; and the late developed competence of medicine to deal effectively with a host of diseases, mainly those that are infectious in aetiology.

The need for medical care increased as larger and larger masses of human beings were, so to say, distanced from the earth and subjected to multiphased inimical ecological disorganization.

With the masses' increasing need for medical services there emerged an agitation for what has been variously termed either 'state' or 'socialized medicine'. The essence of this agitation is for the provision of every form of medical service, initially for the poor but later for all persons; this, under the aegis of, and financial administration by, government.

The long history and ultimate (almost universal) success of this agitation is competently recounted in the New York Academy of Medicine publication entitled *Social Medicine, Its Derivations and Objectives*. The socialization of medicine has not yet entirely prevailed in the United States, the last bastion of individual enterprise. But all signs point to its ultimate victory.

Whether the socialization of medical services can, does or will benefit either those who render the services or those who receive them is irrelevant to my thesis. Henry Sigerist, who once was an enthusiastic proponent of socialized medicine, on the basis of study and experience later changed his mind somewhat. But, wise or otherwise, the universal socialization of medical services appears to be inevitable. This movement is energized by the vis-a-tergo of compelling social necessity. Though not every 'social necessity' necessarily and inevitably yields a social benefit, its actualization is by definition inescapable. *If not eventuated* it was not a compelling social necessity.

Accepting the inevitableness of the socialization of medicine, the question to be asked is: why is the medical profession so largely 'in opposition'? Why are they so agitated about it? The only plausible explanation for this seemingly irrational and futile behaviour appears to me to lie in Ortega's observation that whatever issues are uppermost in the mind of the populace (the medical included) are already forty years past their prime significance.

Yet the inevitable, though inevitable, is modifiable. The form and pattern of its realization can be affected by pressures from many directions. Those who concern themselves with the administrative issues involved in rendering medical services within a socialized scheme are in a sense conditioning the inevitable. Their efforts are valuable and in a measure effective. But for the medical profession, as well as for the recipients of its services, the administrative issues – i.e. who pays, how much, under what conditions, to whom, and for what – are not really now of uppermost importance. Important are such problems as how one is to *practise* medicine within the socialized pattern, and what are the medical problems which the profession and the public are even now facing, and will be facing in much greater measure in the near future – problems deriving from the phenomenal technological revolution which we are undergoing.

I will have relatively little to say about problems in rendering medical services within the socialized scheme, save only to observe that what appears to have changed most are the sources of payment and the ways in which payment is obtained. Otherwise, medicine in the socialized scheme is practised much in the ways previously followed in private practice – but not as successfully, and that chiefly for two reasons: the load of patients is too heavy, and, even more important, the character of the new patient is of a new and different order.

'Character' is not a very informing term. But what terms are more descriptive? I have elsewhere called the new patients 'Proletbourgs', and justified this term in the following argument. Modern medicine is historically a derivative of the social and economic developments initiated and fostered by the entrepreneur class. Specifically, modern medicine was engendered by the growth of cities, by the development of modern commerce and industry, by the rise and proliferation of the middle class, of the professional and functionary groups, and of the proletariat.

It was in the larger cities, the principal commercial and government centres, that the great universities were first founded. In certain of these, namely, Salerno, Bologna, Padua, Montpellier, and Salamanca, there developed great schools of medicine. Here too there were established notable hospitals. Here gathered the new class of *entrepreneurs*, the *bourgeoisie*, the town and city dwellers, the merchants, crafts masters, apprentices, and common workers. And with them emerged the growing masses of civil and clerical functionaries, forerunners of the modern bureaucrats. It is in these centres, proximate to the universities and hospitals, inspired and animated by the new learning emanating therefrom, and responsive to the needs and demands of the more numerous and wealthy new class of citizens (the *bourgeoisie*), that the modern patterns of medical practice had their origins. Here, the cardinal elements of free choice, fee for service, and the confidential relations of patient and doctor, were crystallized, and thereafter acquired the sanction of established principles.

Today medicine, as society itself, is confronting a new class, *entrepreneurs* of another order, and far more numerous than was even the middle class. I call them *proletbourgs*, for they are in effect derivative from the proletariat of past times, now grown akin to the *bourgeoisie*. They are a product of our mounting and spreading affluence. Also, they are better informed, more articulate, and financially more competent than were their proletarian ancestors. They know what medicine has to offer and they rightly believe that they are entitled to its benefits.

It is this new order of medical consumers who today crowd our hospitals and tax our medical personnel and resources, wanting to be treated for and relieved of those illnesses and physical disabilities the like of which their elders years past would have carried and suffered their whole life through.

These patients constitute a new class of medical consumer different from those we have known before. They are unlike the traditional poor and the familiar prosperous. They are not the historical middle class. Not infrequently these patients are boxed in by constricting material, social and cultural circumstances, within which they can manoeuvre but little. With such patients, one is in most instances restricted to the practice of that order of medicine which is descriptively to be termed restitutional.

This order of practice requires its practitioners to know a great deal more than they do now about the family, about sociology, economics, group dynamics and culture in general. More important, with the afore-described patients, solo practice is not likely to prove adequate, by which I do not intend to argue *for* group practice, that is, the clustering of a variety of specialists in one centre, desirable though that may be. What I intend to affirm is that the physician will need to be one among several co-operating professionals, all of whom are concerned with and participate in the treatment of the patient. Among these 'other professionals' I would count social workers, visiting nurses, nutritionists, and psychologists. Such would be the basic team, interacting as a team, in the treatment of the patient, and I can perceive that while the physicians' services in diagnosing disorders and prescribing treatment will remain very important, the services of the other professionals will, in the long run, count for most. It will be they who in effect will actualize recovery, and foster prevention – providing of course the patient is willing and co-operative.

Traditional, historic, private-solo-practice, never developed team practice, save only with other medical specialists. But then, how long ago was it that social workers, and the other members of the envisaged basic team appeared on the medical scene? Not further back than the early decades of the present century. In this connexion, it is worth noting that what is described above is in effect the *schema* for Russian medical service. I limit myself to the term *schema* because it remains as such, not having as yet been actualized.

How one is to practise, i.e. to render medical service within the socialized pattern, is so patently clear and challenging a problem that one is impelled to wonder why so little study and experimentation has been applied toward its resolution. I am, of course, aware of the medical prepayment programmes, the so-called Union Clinics and other forms of contract-medical group practices. These help spread the financial costs of service, frequently however, at the expense of quality. But these are not the forerunners of the service patterns suited to the requirements of socialized practice. The latter are yet to be worked out.

I would like to believe that medical educators are fully cognizant of this challenge, but the recent comment of a newly appointed Dean of one of our country's leading medical schools chills my hopes. His high priority, he affirmed, is for 'a lot more basic research and biologic science'. He said nothing on how the findings in basic research are to be made applicable and useful to the communal man within the ambient of socialized medicine.

Here I want to turn to the medical problems which are likely to confront us in the near future (some of which indeed are already present now), deriving from the phenomenal technological revolution we are experiencing.

In my paper, entitled 'The Pathogenicity of Progress', I set forth the proposition that, *every innovational technological change which man has experienced since time immemorial has brought with it grievous consequences*. It now appears that the greater and the more rapid the technological changes, the more grievous are the possible consequences. These persuasions are shared by a host of distinguished historians and sociologists (see *Daedalus*, winter 1965). I want to cite two passages from this issue of *Daedalus*. Professor Eric Weil wrote: 'Science and its offspring, technology, have come to stay, and we shall have to live with them. The question is, first, how we are to do so without producing more and more split personalities, particularly among the best educated and most serious people, and, second, how we are to prevent those drunk with this new power from exercising in our name the acquired mastery over nature and history in order to dominate us for domination's sake.'

Oscar Handlin wrote: 'The people who are simultaneously delighted with additional years of life expectancy and terrified by the bomb, are in no position to strike the balance of their gains and losses in happiness. In their confusion, they wonder whether the price of the gadgets which delight may not be servitude to the remote and alien few who control the mystery.'

I am, at the present, less concerned with the *global* menace of the new technologies. I want rather to reflect on what *new order of medical disabilities* is likely to be incidental to the new technologies, *disabilities* likely to result from the ecological upset which the new technologies will unquestionably further effect in our immediate world and in our everyday living. In these respects the challenge to medicine is not only to adapt its practices to the age of computers, electronic diagnostic tools, synthetic chemotherapeutic agents, the marvels of tissue and organ transplantation, the webs of bureaucracy and government medicine, et al., but also to study, to anticipate and to become prepared to meet the miseries and sicknesses that will perforce come in the wake of the new technological innovations.

Zbigniew Brzezinski of Columbia University published in the July 1966 *Foreign Affairs Quarterly Review* a most luminous article titled 'Tomorrow's Agenda'. His thesis is so proximate to my own that I am prompted to cite him freely. His premise is that in the second half of the twentieth century the developed nations, given new scientific and social developments, will face a real threat to the continued existence of man as a spontaneous, instinctive, rather autonomous and even somewhat mysterious being. A social revolution already in progress is likely to be shaped by the widespread adoption of automation and cybernetion for social and economic reasons. Man's environment, and man himself, will more and more be subject to purposive control and manipulation. Our society will be fundamentally transformed. Our concepts of work and leisure will most likely undergo a basic reversal, leisure becoming a burden and creative work a privilege of the gifted few. The relationship between employment and way of life will be revised. Retirement and unemployment, the basic social functions of trade unions, and of government welfare operations, will most likely undergo radical revision. The relationship between earning and consumption will be blurred, with the prospects of arbitrary standards to assure a minimum [but relatively high] level of consumption. Within such changes, how is the integrity and freedom of man as an individual to be preserved? Given the trends and medical sciences, as a physical being man will become more malleable, and as a personality, subject increasingly to external manipulations. The more man is thus manipulated and programmed, the increasingly more denatured he is likely to become. The extended result is likely to be personal and political alienation and a pervasive sense of seemingly purposeless lives.

All of these are likely eventuations. They are concomitants of the new technologies and carry with them the prospects of a host of new medical problems. Medicine therefore must seek to anticipate them, ultimately to meet them, and to deal with them effectively. On these scores too medicine must be prepared to intelligently counsel government and other social groups and organizations. All this calls for, among other things, a critical look at present-day medical education, in order to assess whether, and how, we can in time educate and train physicians competent to meet the emergent medical needs of the new society and whether, in the larger sense, we can effect and, in the world of our professional concerns, see to it that 'the penalties and compensations which things owe to one another [in a changed ecology] are paid out in time and in good coin' (Anaximander).

References

1 I have sketched this in my paper 'Doctor and Patient in History'. Much information on these scores is to be found, though scattered, in Puschmann's *History of Medical Education*, translated and edited by Evan H. Hare, London, 1891; also in Julius Petersen's *Hauptomomente in der Geschichtlichen Entwikelung der Medicinischen Therapie*, Copenhagen, 1877.

2 GALDSTON, IAGO (ed.), New York, The Commonwealth Fund, 1949.

W. Kock
Stockholm (Sweden)

The social history of medicine in Sweden

Nowadays Sweden is said to be regarded in many quarters – and rightly so – as a sort of social laboratory, in which solutions to various social problems are tested. This has been especially true in the field of medicine. But the road to this state of affairs has been very long in Sweden, a country with a harsh climate, remote from the great centres of culture, where the people have had to struggle hard to profit from the country's natural resources and were long satisfied with such subsistence as the soil, the forest and the iron-ore mines could provide. It was not until relatively late in the nineteenth century that the rate of industrialization increased and an economic boom took place which transformed Sweden from a poor country to one of the ten richest countries in the world.

The earliest records of the art of healing in Sweden may be studied – partly by analogy with observations from the other Scandinavian countries – in runic inscriptions, sagas, legends, the poetic Edda, chronicles, archaeological finds and observations of popular medicine. The primitive beliefs in all manner of magical beings only slowly relinquished their hold on the Scandinavian peoples. In olden times, life was short, and infectious ailments and deficiency diseases wreaked great havoc, but, of course, ordinary internal ailments also occurred then as now, together with a number of nervous and mental diseases. The short expectation of life set its mark on the panorama of disease. Witchcraft (with the aid of runes), mysterious chants and *sejd* (from the Icelandic word *seidr*, denoting a form of witchcraft found among the Nordic peoples, by which the future could be read, sickness could be cured, etc.) played important parts in the battle against disease, even after people had learned to make use of the healing powers in the three realms of nature.

In the earliest Swedish provincial laws, we encounter at a surprisingly early date the qualifications expected of the practitioners of the healing art who were to be regarded as professional men in their capacity as *läkare*. The word *laeknir* or *lackir* (= *läkare*, healer, doctor) is common to all the Nordic languages; it is of Celtic origin and means 'he who blesses'. In the Södermanland and Uppland laws, a knowledge of surgery was stipulated. Thus, in the Uppland law of 1296, it is stated that a *läkare* in the legal sense of the word must 'have demonstrated his ability to heal knife wounds, fractures in wounds, severed limbs or double wounds from stabs straight through the belly'. The laws also made mention of the fees. According to the Västgöta and Hälsingland law, the fee 'for the healing of a thrall [was] 3–4 öre [at that time 4 öre was the ordinary price of an ox], for minor wounds 4 öre and for more serious wounds, such as castration, a severed hand or foot, an eye poked out, a tongue, nose or ears cut off 8 öre'.

The Nordic peoples took a tolerant attitude to the question of the doctor's legal responsibility. Thus, an Icelandic law dating from the Viking period says: 'If a man cauterizes or bleeds anyone in order to heal him or performs any act in order to heal another, for the purpose of giving him a cure and not ill-health, he shall risk no punishment, even if the other man dies of it or suffers injury'.

THE MIDDLE AGES AND THE VASA PERIOD

During the Middle Ages and far into the Vasa period (1523–1654), the art of healing was practised in Sweden by bath attendants and barber-surgeons, who came from abroad – mainly from Germany – and by the representatives of 'monastery medicine'. From the finds made at the monasteries of Alvastra, Varnhem and Vreta, we know that the medicine practised in the monasteries was by no means restricted to 'decoctions of herbs and ointments' but also included surgical operations, though, of course, besides bleeding and cupping, only such procedures as could be classified as simple 'external' surgery, such as the treatment of fractures. The quality of the barber-surgeons who came to Sweden was very variable. They generally worked in cottage hospitals and regulations for them were issued in 1571 by Johan III. Stockholm had already had a guild of barber-surgeons since 1496.

It proved to be extremely difficult even for King Gustav Vasa (1496–1560), who is usually called 'the founder of the nation', to attract foreign doctors to Sweden and even more difficult to induce young Swedes to study medicine abroad on scholarships and afterwards to settle down to practise as doctors in their native country. For financial reasons, such young doctors could only count on getting employment at court and in the service of noblemen. It is true that the first university in Sweden (Uppsala) was opened in 1477, but it was closed from 1517 to 1595 and it was not until 1595 that a chair of medicine was established there. However, this chair was not occupied until 1613 (by Johannes Chesnecopherus).

A few foreign doctors appeared fleetingly at the courts of Gustav Vasa and his sons, but they did not usually stay long. There was also a barber-surgeon and an apothecary, who had to supplement his meagre income by making sweets on ceremonial occasions. A royal herb garden was laid out at Stockholm Castle and a special gardener, brought from Holland, was given the task of distilling aromatic waters from the herbs and spices grown in this garden. It is typical of the contemporary situation that in his last illness the king had to be attended – right down to the last few days – for lack of a doctor, by the Rector of St. Nicholas (Storkyrkan), who had studied medicine at Wittenberg, alongside his theological studies, a barber-surgeon and an apothecary. In spite of – or perhaps because of – the drastic multiplicity of drugs administered to him, in accordance with the custom of the time, combined, as we know, with spiritual ministrations, the great king died – tired, worn out with hard work, tormented by toothache, impaired hearing, marked arteriosclerosis, etc., in addition to the acute illness of which he died – an intestinal ailment of uncertain nature.

If this was the situation of the head of the state, it was naturally even worse for his subjects. Apart from the treatments recommended in popular medicine, the information to be garnered in the 'medical books' was of great importance at this period. The first major work of this kind to be written by a Swede was Benedictus Olai's *Een Nyttigh Läkere-Book* (A Useful Book of Medicine), which was published in 1578 by Sweden's first doctor of medicine (trained abroad).

The history of the Swedish hospitals goes back to the *sälohus* of olden times (hospices along the roads for weary and sick travellers), the *helgeandshus* (hospices for the poor and sick established in the Middle Ages, usually in the towns, and mainly to be regarded as poorhouses and charitable institutions), and the asylums, which were originally intended for lepers. However, there seems to have been no great difference between these categories and towards the end of the Middle Ages they were all called asylums.

It is interesting to note that, despite the importance of the monastic system in this sphere in Sweden (which was still a Roman Catholic country at this time), these establishments were run by superintendents appointed by the secular authorities (in the towns the municipal authorities). Although they were always regarded as having to some extent an ecclesiastical character, the Church generally had no control over their administration. Their finances were based on the tithes, donations, alms and contributions from certain societies and guilds, which provided assistance for the sick and the infirm.

Of course, the Reformation proved to be a serious blow to the medical services in Sweden. However, its effects were mitigated by Gustav Vasa's wise ruling in 1528 that the hospitals were not to be deprived of the property and revenues which had hitherto facilitated their existence. In 1533 the administration of the hospitals was regulated by an 'Ordinance for *Helgeandshus* and Asylums'.

During the Middle Ages, there were in Stockholm, in addition to a *helgeandshus*, what was called 'Örian House' (a leper hospital), a hospice for travellers, a cottage hospital and a madhouse – but not all of them at the same time. In 1531 the king ordered that they should be amalgamated to form a hospital, and located in an old Franciscan friary on Riddarholmen. When the plague broke out in 1549, the king's personal fear lest the infection should spread to the nearby royal palace would seem to have been conducive to his ordering that the sick should be transferred to the Danvik asylum, which dated back to medieval times (in later years it was best known as a madhouse). However, the transfer did not take place until 1557–58. The conditions in the Stockholm hospitals were extremely unsatisfactory for a long time and this problem was not solved until the middle of the eighteenth century.

The first proposal to set up a teaching hospital was made as early as 1561 by Vilhelmus Lemnius, a Dutch doctor who had immigrated to Sweden. It is regrettable that this far-sighted proposal – which also included suggestions for the organization of the medical system, the collection of indigenous medicinal plants, the setting up of pharmacies, the fixing of drug prices and measures against charlatans – was not to be realized for 200 years and then only in parts, including the question of the hospitals.

Among the milestones on the way to the present organization of Sweden's social welfare, public health and medical care, I may mention the efforts which were made in the reigns of the next few rulers. Thus Johan III (Gustav Vasa's second son) emphasized the importance of the municipalities taking over control of certain parts of the medical service and the social-welfare work, but again the increased influence for the Church and the clergy.

THE SEVENTEENTH CENTURY

Swedish medicine had its first period of greatness in the seventeenth century. This period was by no means dominated by the many royal physicians-in-ordinary and court doctors who were to be found in Sweden in the reigns of Gustaf Adolf II and Queen Christina, nor exclusively by the members of the medical faculties at the universities (now two in number, as the University of Lund came into existence in 1668). It was native Swedes, who were thoroughly trained and had gained experience in long periods of study abroad, who created this period in the history of medicine in Sweden. Four names are particularly prominent in this connexion: Olaus Rudbeck the elder (1630–1702), who demonstrated his discovery of the lymphatic system in 1652; Petrus Hoffvenius (1630–82), who was also a professor at the University of Uppsala and who introduced clinical instruction at the bedside on a modest scale; Urban Hiärne (1641–1724), chemist, mining expert, physician-in-ordinary and founder of Swedish hydrotherapy; and Johan von Hoorn (1662–1724), the medical officer of health in Stockholm and the founder of Swedish midwifery.

This century also saw the establishment of the first emergency hospital in Sweden – not in Stockholm but in Falun. This hospital was intended for the clerks and the miners at Stora Kopparberg, the mining company which is the oldest limited liability company in the world.

One of the most important events in Swedish medicine in this century occurred in 1663. In that year, four Stockholm doctors addressed a petition to the King-in-Council – it was granted on 16 May – asking for permission to form a 'Collegium medicorum' for mutual support and to counteract the disorder and the abuses which had hitherto characterized the practice of medicine in Sweden. This Collegium was to develop into the authority which supervised the medical system in Sweden and until 1809 in Finland also. Its first President was one of the founders – Grégoire François Du Rietz, physician-in-ordinary to Queen Christina. We may say that in its way the Collegium had the functions which are now carried out by the National Board of Health and Social Welfare, the Swedish Society of Medical Sciences and the Swedish Medical Association, i.e. it was simultaneously a civil service department, a scientific forum and a professional organization.

Thus, the Collegium medicorum (later the Collegium medicum) was to exercise control over all the practitioners of the healing art, including doctors, surgeons, apothecaries, and midwives, to conduct examinations in certain cases and in any case to grant *licentia practicandi* to both Swedish and foreign citizens. 'With the exception of those who, like *doctores medicinae*, have previously practised medicine for some years under the Swedish crown, all those concerned are to pass an *examen practicum*, conducted by the Collegium in the presence of a learned magistrate.' The other duties of the Collegium included the control of fees, the preparation of a Swedish pharmacopoeia, assisting in fixing the prices of drugs and the combating of infectious and dangerous diseases.

The ordinance on medical care issued in 1663 was superseded by the 'Medical ordinances or privileges which the King-in-Council has granted to the Collegium medicum' (30 October 1688). But as the apothecaries and the surgeons considered themselves unfairly treated, the printing of the ordinance was stopped and the ordinance was revised, with the result that the new medical ordinances were not sanctioned until 1698. They were published in 1699 but were dated ten to eleven years earlier. These 'medical ordinances of 1688' were to form the basis of the medical systems of Sweden and Finland for very many years to come.

In addition to the supervision of the medical practitioners and, to some extent, of the practice of medicine itself, the ordinances also mentioned that a college of anatomy was to be established for the furtherance of the study of medicine. The study of botany was to be encouraged, as well as the cultivation of indigenous herbs. The apothecaries were to undergo examinations and their shops were to be inspected. Surgeons were forbidden to treat internal ailments in places where doctors were available.

The position of the Collegium was made difficult by the vagueness of the regulations, the weakness of its authority and the lack of support from the medical faculties. However, new instructions led to some improvement and also to new tasks.

No real faculty of medicine existed at Uppsala University until some time in the 1620s. There were then three professorships – nearly 150 years after the founding of the university. The professors had widely different and very extensive subject fields and the students were more attracted by theology, philosophy, languages and the natural sciences than by medicine. Scholastic medicine, based on Hippocrates, Galen and the Arabian writers, still predominated in the first half of the seventeenth century. Humoral pathology flourished. However, medicine of a more scientific nature gradually reached even remote Sweden; it was represented, *inter alia*, by the anatomy of Vesalius and the teachings of Paracelsus.

Gustav Vasa's third son, Charles IX, who succeeded Johan III, carried on the traditions of his father's reign in the field of social welfare and decided in 1605 that the sick should be cared for in the asylums and the poor in the 'parish workhouses'. This seems to have been the first attempt in Sweden to separate the care of the sick from the maintenance of the poor. In 1624, Gustaf Adolf II, the great warrior king, directed that an asylum should be set up in every province, instead of the badly run asylums in the towns. Of great importance were the 'Rules and regulations on the treatment of beggars and poor persons who are really in need of alms and likewise that of tramps and idlers', which were issued in 1642 during the reign of Queen Christina and which set the standard for the next 100 years. Both the asylums and the cottage hospitals in the countryside were to be supervised by both the secular and the ecclesiastical authorities.

The obligation of the parish to take care of its poor had already been emphasized at an early date, and this system was maintained even after the Reformation. The provision for the poor consisted in the sick and the infirm being admitted to asylums or workhouses. Other persons incapable of working had to beg, but begging was not permitted until a certificate or pass – the 'beggar's pass' – had been issued, generally by the ecclesiastical authorities. It was valid for begging within a certain district. Regulations on the provision for the poor were issued in the Church Regulations of 1571, the above-mentioned Begging Ordinance of 1642, the Canon Law of 1686 and an ordinance of 1698.

THE EIGHTEENTH CENTURY

In Swedish history, the eighteenth century was a period marked by military complications, economic difficulties, political antagonisms, difficult social conditions and – during the later half of the century – a considerable cultural advance. We may speak of a second period of greatness in the field of medicine. Its leading figures were men like Nils Rosén von Rosenstein (1706–73), who breathed new life into the subject of paediatrics, for which he became internationally famous, Carl von Linné (Linnaeus) (1707–78), who gained world-wide fame as a botanist but was also, like Rosenstein, Professor of Medicine at Uppsala. Abraham Bäck (1713–95), who in his capacity as President of the Collegium medicum was for forty-three years a leading medical administrator and also physician-in-ordinary to several Swedish kings, and Olof af Acrel (1717–1806), the father of Swedish surgery. All these men had travelled widely to study medicine and had transplanted their observations in foreign countries into their poverty-stricken native country.

The position of the Collegium medicum was strengthened during this century. This strengthening was assisted, to begin with, by the efforts made by the members of the organizations which came into existence to combat epidemics – first the 'Health Collegium' which was founded in 1721 and later dissolved and then, in particular, the 'Health Commission', which was appointed in 1737 and which existed until 1766. In 1763, the Collegium medicum was given new instructions, which enlarged its sphere of activity in many ways – to cover the supervision of the doctors, the superintendence of the national state of health, public health measures (including the conservation of the environment, in that they were to 'investigate the unhealthiness of certain districts, trades and professions'), the conditions in the hospitals and even the promotion of veterinary science. In 1774 these duties were further increased, although funds sufficient for these purposes were not placed at the disposal of the Collegium, nor was sufficient support provided by the Government. Amongst other things, the Collegium was now to propose candidates for all posts as district medical officers and to see that the poor received medical treatment and free medicine in both town and country.

The end of the eighteenth century saw the introduction of a very important amendment into the Collegium's instructions. It was to mark – at least officially – the end of the long-standing conflict between the surgeons' society and the doctors' society, which had at times been very bitter. The surgeons' society (the 'Barbers' Office'), which is referred to for the first time in 1685 as the 'Surgical Society', was headed by a national director-general of surgery and had had a hard fight for its existence. The struggle became increasingly uneven and came to an end when the King-in-Council issued new instructions to the Collegium medicum in 1797, by which the 'Surgical Society' was dissolved and its functions were taken over by the Collegium, in which, however, the surgeons were also to have seats and vote. The Collegium was to consist of a President, a Vice-President and eight assessors, four of whom were to be doctors and four surgeons. In addition, there were to be some administrative staff. The Collegium was also to supervise the practice of surgery and consequently also the manufacture of surgical instruments in Sweden. Its position was also strengthened, as regarded the prosecution of doctors for negligence in the practice of their profession.

It was the internationally famous Olaus Rudbeck the elder who took the initiative in the establishment of Sweden's first teaching hospital. But the little 'nosocomium academicum' in Uppsala was not brought into being until 1717 by Professor Lars Roberg, after Charles XII had sanctioned the enterprise. It fell into decay relatively soon but flourished once more to some extent under the direction of von Rosenstein. At the beginning of the century similar plans had been afoot in Lund, which had become a university town in 1668. However, the problem there was solved by the eventual establishment of a small county hospital in 1768. By that time, however, the hospital problem had naturally begun to come to the fore in Stockholm.

It was symptomatic of the difficult economic situation in Sweden, which was then impoverished by many military campaigns, that neither the State nor the City had any funds available for so important a purpose as the establishment of a hospital in Stockholm. However, in this connexion I may point out that even internationally the establishment of the great hospitals went along with the increasing urbanization which was especially characteristic of the eighteenth century. The philanthropic ideals of the time were also of great significance in this connexion (cf. the Charité Hospital in Berlin, Guy's, St. George's, and the London Hospitals in London and King Frederik's Hospital in Copenhagen).

The struggle for the hospital in Stockholm passed through many stages. Petitions were submitted to both the 1731 and the 1734 Parliaments by Nils Boy, the then Medical Officer of Health in Stockholm, and to the Parliament of 1738–39 by Samuel Gustaf Stierneld, who was then a lieutenant but later became a field-marshal. Thus these men had in mind both the poor people of the city and the sick soldiers of the garrison. Parliament discussed the matter extensively, but the essential thing was the collection of money, for which purpose the future hospital was granted certain privileges. The methods adopted certainly seem particularly strange by modern standards. The most important source of income was a private lottery. In addition, contributions were collected privately in many ways, such as fees for every Swedish comedy acted and voluntary collections at weddings and christenings, when people could be expected to be in a happy mood and therefore inclined to be generous. Both Bäck and Acrel also published pamphlets to stimulate interest in the establishment of the hospital.

In 1748, King Fredrik I instituted the first Swedish orders of knighthood – the Order of the Seraphim (still the most distinguished), the Order of the Sword and the Order of the North Star. In this connexion it is noteworthy that the statutes of the Order of the Seraphim included a rule – which naturally derived from the medieval orders of chivalry – that the Knights of the Seraphim should supervise hospitals and poorhouses. In the same year the Chapter of the Order also drew attention to the necessity of establishing a hospital in the capital and announced that it had at its disposal 50,000 copper riksdalers for this purpose. Eight Knights of the Seraphim were appointed to deal with the problems which were thought to be associated with the building of the hospital. This gave the hospital its name, *Serafimerordens-lazarettet* (the Hospital of the Order of the Seraphim), which was later shortened to *Serafimerlazarettet* (The Serafimer Hospital). It was opened on 30 October 1752 in a nobleman's manor-house which had been bought for the purpose and rebuilt as a hospital. This was a red-letter day in the history of Swedish medicine. Unfortunately, this national hospital, serving both Sweden and Finland, had only eight beds, four for men and four for women. It was considerably enlarged in several stages and at its peak, in the 1940s, it had 500 beds. It is still in operation, although on a reduced scale. It has for long, with good reason, been known as the stronghold of Swedish medicine, on account of both its high standard of treatment and its teaching.

Although the Serafimer Hospital was fairly soon improved (it received its first grant from the national budget in 1783 – from the 'tobacco duty'), it must have been quite inadequate to serve both Sweden and Finland. It was therefore only natural that the people in the provinces should regard their obligation (laid down in 1754) to make financial contributions to the hospital in Stockholm as unduly burdensome. In 1765 they succeeded in getting permission to use the funds instead to set up and maintain hospitals in the provinces. Among the oldest Swedish hospitals after the Serafimer Hospital are those at Kalmar (1754), Mariestad (1762), Gävle (1767) and Lund (1768).

In 1756 – when a medical fund of 15,000 silver riksdalers annually was also set up – the Swedish Parliament (Riksdag) attempted to take the initiative in providing care and protection for the unfortunates in society – the patients admitted to the 'crown asylums'. The discussions in the Estates resulted in orphanages and asylums being placed under the control of the 'Estates Deputation on Asylums and Orphanages' (1757). A royal ordinance in 1763 laid down the criteria for admission to the asylums. Apart from persons merely in need of maintenance, the persons to be admitted included 'lunatics, imbeciles and such wretches as are suffering from contagious or incurable diseases, such as cancer, falling sickness, leprosy, etc.'

The Riksdag of 1765–66 dissolved the Deputation on Asylums and Orphanages and set up a 'Directorate-General', whose functions were taken over in 1773 by letters patent by two Knights of the Order of the Seraphim, who were thus to constitute the national board supervising the asylums and orphanages, and after 1776 the general hospitals as well. These two Knights had a Director-General to advise them. The first Director-General was Olof af Acrel. In a royal rescript of 1774, it was further emphasized that the asylums were primarily intended for lunatics and patients with serious physical ailments.

In 1787 King Gustaf III instituted a subdivision of the Order of the Seraphim – 'a guild which, on behalf of the Order, will superintend and carry on the management of Orphanages, Asylums and General Hospitals in the Kingdom'. In the instructions given to this important guild in 1791, it was provided that there should be an asylum and a general hospital in each county, all of which were placed under the control of the guild. This laid the foundation of an organized hospital system in Sweden, but it should be remembered that for a long time the connexions with the central medical authorities were very loose.

Many of the institutions which dated back to the Middle Ages and which numbered the mentally ill among their protégés were eventually closed. In 1756 there were forty-two such institutions in the kingdom (four of them in Finland). In 1774 it was decreed that the smaller asylums should be closed and instead larger ones should be set up in every province. There were a number of changes in their organization. Curiously enough, as regarded the care of the mentally ill, the system of administration by the Guild of the Order of the Seraphim lasted until 1877, when the National Board of Health became the responsible authority.

In this connexion, it should also be remembered that, according to the instructions given in 1797 to the Collegium medicum, hospitals and institutions 'intended for lunatics, inoculation against the smallpox, midwifery, etc.' were to be superintended by the Collegium, as regarded the practice of medicine. The doctors were to send in annual reports to the Collegium.

If we consider the hospital situation almost at the end of the eighteenth century (1798), we shall find that the position was as follows. There were twenty-one county hospitals in Sweden proper and five in Finland. The number of patients was 2,240, half of whom were suffering from venereal diseases. The mortality in that year was eighty-two. The costs amounted to only 2,212 riksdalers. In addition to these hospitals, there were certain medical establishments in Stockholm, including the Royal Hospital (i.e. the Serafimer Hospital), which at that time had eighty beds, the 'Public Inoculation House', which was founded in 1766 and where variolations against smallpox were performed, the 'Public Lying-in Hospital', which was founded in 1775 and where 400–500 babies were delivered annually, the 'Pro Patria Lying-in Hospital', which was founded in 1774 and which could accommodate 111 women in childbed, and a number of small military hospitals and special establishments (belonging to certain occupational categories). One could, of course, also include the Danvik Hospital, which had a clientele of chronically ill patients, paupers and lunatics. In 1798, 287 paupers were being maintained there, while the number of 'lunatics' in the whole country was 1,004.

In 1716, Stockholm acquired its first professorship of anatomy, which was, however, only held for a short time. In 1749, Abraham Bäck became Professor of Anatomy and lectured at the Royal Academy of Science. From 1756 to 1779 the chair of anatomy and surgery was held by Roland Martin (1726–88). In 1761, a professorship of obstetrics was instituted and its first holder was David Schulz von Schulzenheim (1732–1823). In the same year a professorship of natural history and pharmacy came into existence and was held by Peter Jonas Bergius (1730–90). All these professorships were dependent on the Collegium medicum and were instituted for the training of medical students, journeymen barber-surgeons, student apothecaries and student midwives.

THE NINETEENTH CENTURY

In David Schulz von Schulzenheim, who took no part in public life for some years during Gustaf III's period of absolute rule in protest against the prevailing political conditions, the Collegium medicum found in 1809 a dynamic and far-sighted President, although he was seventy-seven years old when he was elected. He proposed the appointment of the 'Medical Committee', which was commissioned by the Estates in 1810 to prepare a draft bill for general and improved medical care in Sweden. He also enforced a change in the organization of the Collegium which placed it on a par with the other state departments. One of the reasons for this change was the placing of the Army medical service under the superintendence of the Collegium. The name was changed too, and in 1813 the 150-year-old Collegium medicum was re-named the 'Health Collegium'. According to the instructions issued in 1815, the duties of the Collegium were to be divided between the civilian branch and the military branch. The Collegium's tasks included being responsible for 'the supervision and control of the state of health, the medical care and the nursing' of both the civilians and the military in peace and war. But there were important exceptions from the Collegium's supervision; the lecturers at the universities and the Guild of the Order of the Seraphim, which still had supreme control over the national hospitals, clinics for venereal diseases and lunatic asylums – an authority which, as far as the hospitals and clinics were concerned, was not transferred to the Health

Collegium until 1859. The Collegium was also to take an active part in the prevention and cure of epidemics and venereal diseases, to supervise inoculations against small-pox, to exercise a measure of control over matters of environmental and occupational hygiene and to superintend the practice of 'cattle medicine', i.e. veterinary science. The Collegium was also responsible for supervising the activities of baths attendants, barber-surgeons, dentists and midwives and for superintending the pharmacies, the supply of drugs, the pharmacopoeia and the prices of drugs. It also had to deal with questions concerning the Army medical services and forensic medicine, which constituted an important part of its duties. It was also to be the supervisory authority for the Karolinska Institute (founded in 1810), the Pharmaceutical Institute and several other institutions.

On the initiative especially of Professor Erik Carl Trafvenfelt (1774–1835), there came into existence in 1810 the 'Institute for the training of army doctors' (later called the Karolinska Institute), chiefly on account of the unfortunate experiences of medical care in the field during the war in Finland in 1809. The professorships mentioned above were the forerunners of this Institute, which was originally intended for the training of army doctors and barber-surgeons. An intense dispute was carried on for a large part of the nineteenth century between the representatives of the Uppsala Faculty of Medicine in particular (especially Israel Hwasser) and those of the Institute (especially Jöns Jacob Berzelius). In spite of the many famous men on its teaching staff, it was a long time before the Institute acquired the right to grant the degree of licentiate of medicine and (from 1874) to hold disputations for the doctorate. It did not receive the right to grant the degree of Doctor of Medicine until 1906. By that time, it had already been entrusted, as a famous medical school, with the task of awarding the Nobel Prize for medicine, in accordance with the terms of Alfred Nobel's will.

Among the great names in Swedish medicine in the nineteenth century were four men who worked at Karolinska Institute: Anders Retzius the anatomist (1796–1860), Jöns Jacob Berzelius the chemist (1779–1848), Carl Johan Ekströmer the surgeon (1793–1860) and Magnus Huss (1807–90), who was the first doctor in Sweden to give clinical instruction in internal medicine. The last two, who gave practical instruction at the Serafimer Hospital, which became the Institute's medical school, were also Presidents of the Health Collegium.

What was the situation in the hospital sphere in 1813, when the Health Collegium came into existence? Sweden then had thirty-three general hospitals (and a clinic for venereal diseases at Danvik in Stockholm) with a good 700 beds. There was one hospital bed for every 3,437 inhabitants and about 4,000 patients were admitted each year. Thus, in spite of the considerable developments, the numbers involved were still very small.

In 1817, the county hospitals came under local administration in the form of management committees, one for each county, with the provincial governor as permanent chairman. However, the Guild of the Order of the Seraphim appointed the doctors and managers proposed by the management committees and continued to act as the national board of control, especially as regarded finance. But the administration was passing more and more into the hands of the Health Collegium, which finally assumed control, as I mentioned above, in 1859. In 1877 the Health Collegium became the National Board of Health under a board consisting of the Director-General and four members, all doctors appointed by the King-in-Council.

The setting up of the county councils in 1862 was of very great importance for Sweden. These councils were empowered to make decisions, *inter alia*, about public health matters in the counties and soon they began to show great interest and to be involved in medical care. Thus, a further 1,158 hospital beds were added in the period 1865–76.

It may be asked what a Swedish county hospital looked like 100 years ago. Some information on this point may be derived from the inspection reports submitted by the divisional heads who carried out inspections on behalf of the Health Collegium. We may select the county hospital in Falun in 1867 as being representative of the provincial hospitals of the time in densely populated districts. In 1867, Kopparberg county had 177,195 inhabitants and the only public hospital was that in Falun. It was situated in the town centre and consisted of a two-storey stone building with an attic storey, which had formerly been used as an asylum. The offices were on the ground floor, where there were also bathrooms and five wards. The central part of the building was occupied by accommodation for a nurse – one room and a kitchen – and three wards. The corridors were dark and narrow. Two of the wards held six beds, three held four beds, one held three or four beds and the remaining one three beds. The cubic space per bed varied between 825 and 1,043 cubic feet. The upper floor contained accommodation for another nurse, the doctor's consulting room, the operating theatre and ten wards with altogether forty-two beds. All the wards communicated with each other. There were two wards for private patients in the attic, which was otherwise mostly used for storage.

On the lower floor, the hospital also had a ward for the treatment of patients with venereal diseases, with fifteen beds divided among three or four rooms. Patients with internal and external diseases were not separated in the wards. The wards were fairly lofty and light, but the ventilation was inadequate and unfortunately the hospital was plagued with vermin. The rooms were heated with tiled or iron stoves and lit by candles or paraffin lamps. The water was brought in from outside, as was the bath water sometimes, when the hospital's well did not yield a sufficient supply. The buildings in the courtyard included storage space, a morgue and a stable. The hospital had seventy-eight beds altogether, i.e. one for every 2,218 inhabitants. The hospital did its own catering, which was in the hands of the housekeeper (unlike many other hospitals, where the catering was done by contractors). The beds were made of iron or wood, the bedlinen was plentiful, the drinking vessels were of pewter or copper and the dinner service was of chinaware. The surgical instruments were good for the period.

The staff consisted of a doctor, a manager, a chaplain, two nurses, a housekeeper, four maids and a female janitor and their annual salaries varied between the doctor's 1,600 riksdalers and the janitor's 96 riksdalers. The manager received 800 and the nurses 300 riksdalers *per annum*. The cost of each patient was calculated to be, on the average, 88.9 öre. The average number of days each patient stayed was 42.1 in the hospital wards and 61.4 in the venereal-diseases ward – somewhat high figures in comparison with the national averages (cf. Table 1).

As regarded the treatment of the mentally ill, I may mention that in the 1820s the Estates proposed the establishment of central asylums, a proposal which was supported by the Guild of the Order of the Seraphim. Accordingly, the crown asylums began to be closed down and in 1840 there were only eight of them left. The treatment of the mentally ill in Sweden was regulated in its entirety by a statute in 1858.

TABLE 1 Falun Hospital in 1867

Number of beds: 78 (1 bed per 2,218 inhabitants of the county)
Space per bed: 825–1,043 cubic feet

Staff	*Number*	*Annual salary, riksdalers*	
Doctors	1	1,600	
Managers	1	800	
Chaplains	1		
Nurses	2	300	
Housekeepers	1		
Maids	4		
Female janitor	1	96	
Cost per patient: 88.9 öre			
		General ward	*Ward for venereal diseases*
Average length of stay per patient, days		42.1	61.4

As I have already mentioned, the maintenance of the poor in Sweden had been regulated by several statutes since the Church Regulations of 1571. Yet it was not until the 1847 Poor Relief Act that there were regulations in this field which applied to the whole country. However, it still proved to be difficult to secure similar standards of poor relief in different municipalities. It was only in the present century that a better system was established in this field.

Poor relief was, of course, originally the only public assistance there was and it included the care of the aged, medical treatment, child welfare and unemployment assistance. However, certain forms of social insurance also have a long history. In this field the medieval craft guilds began to provide a certain amount of financial support for their sick members by arrangements which resembled the modern health insurance. However, it was not until the nineteenth century that real health insurance schemes outside these guilds began to be formed and they were closely connected with popular movements, such as the Free Churches, the temperance movement and the labour movement. In 1891 the Swedish state began to subsidize these schemes.

THE TWENTIETH CENTURY

The twentieth-century developments in the field of public health and medical care have, of course, been many-sided and very intensive and therefore I can only give you a few glimpses of them here. In 1901 the King-in-Council issued a regulation to the effect that the National Board of Health should continue to supervise the medical services and the establishment of the general hospitals and to act as a forum for complaints concerning medical treatment. The county councils – in the towns the municipal councils – were otherwise responsible for the general hospitals, but the National Board of Health was to carry out inspections, when necessary. The hospital doctors, whose positions had long been somewhat insecure and who had not even had the right to decide on admissions to hospital, were now to be appointed by the Crown. The assistant doctors who were now beginning to appear in hospitals were to be appointed for three years. The increasing degree of specialization was also beginning to make it necessary to establish several medical posts at the same hospital. The first provincial hospital to have separate doctors for medicine and surgery was Falun Hospital (in 1897).

It would be going too far to discuss here the many other regulations and ordinances which governed the work of the hospitals and the medical services in the years that followed. A typical feature of the development has been the co-ordination of social welfare, public health and medical care, which has been manifested in the merging of the National Board of Health in 1967 into the National Board of Health and Social Welfare (which at present has a doctor as its Director-General). In this connexion, I may also mention that the regulations for giving social assistance were tightened up in the Public Assistance Act of 1918 and that the amalgamations of municipalities which took place in 1952 and in the 1960s increased the possibilities of standardizing, as between the municipalities, the methods used in social-welfare work.

Rather than follow up all the laws and ordinances in this field, it would seem to be more interesting to consider the actual problems, as regards the expansion of Sweden's public health and medical services, and some of the reforms which have been made. When the National Board of Health, which is probably the oldest body of its kind in the world, celebrated its 300th anniversary in 1963, Dr. Arthur Engel, who was then Director-General, set down some interesting views on current problems. One of the aims in the development of the medical services is that the specialization now in progress and the centralization resulting from it should not be driven so far as to make specialist treatment no longer available for every patient in the country. The continually rising costs of medical care naturally increase the demand for the rational organization of the institutional care in particular. In this connexion, I may also mention that 'the philosophy of medical care' entails the integration of the somatic and mental health and medical services and the provision of an unbroken chain of treatment from prophylactic measures to rehabilitation and the resumption of the patient's contributions to society. This has led to the public health and medical services being transferred almost entirely from the state to the county councils, who are, of course, intimately acquainted with the problems of medical care and have a suitable population basis.

Dr. Engel took the initiative, single-handed, in drawing up the plan for regional hospital services, a plan which has attracted international attention and has now come into operation following a Riksdag decision in 1960. The plan was put forward in 1958. Dr. Engel himself has written as follows: 'This plan deals with the expansion of hospital care within the county-council areas and analyses the degree of specialization which should best be brought about in the main hospital of the region [the central hospital] and then the specialized care which calls for a greater population basis than a county council has to offer.' The plan is based on the division of the country into medical regions, each with about one million inhabitants and with a regional hospital equipped with departments for certain specialities, such as neuro-surgery, neurology, thoracic surgery, cardiology, plastic surgery, paediatric surgery, urology, radiotherapy (cancer clinics) and dermatology.

The principal data for the existing hospitals, according to the latest available statistics (for the period 1959–68) are shown in Table 2. In addition, there are cottage hospitals and nursing homes for somatic and psychiatric treatment, hospitals and homes for epileptics, institutions for mentally retarded children, special hospitals and nursing homes. In 1968, the period of treatment for all somatic illness was 19.1 days and in the general hospitals 14.1 days.

TABLE 2 Institutions for medical care in 1968

Type of hospital	*Number*	*Number of beds*	*Admissions during the year*
General hospital, type 1 (at least 1,000 beds for the somatic treatment of the acutely ill)	8	14,054	264,508
General hospital, type 2 (500–999 beds)	24	20,613	434,378
General hospital, type 3 (hospitals, sanatoria and isolation hospitals with less than 500 beds). The no. of beds for the somatic treatment of the acutely ill refers to the total no. of beds at the hospital, minus the no. of beds for psychiatric and chronically ill patients.	102	25,737	466,696
Other hospitals of the general hospital type (homes for the disabled, seaside sanatoria, the National Social Insurance Board's independent institutions, hospitals for rheumatic diseases and large private hospitals)	17	1,989	17,406
General hospitals for psychiatric treatment	28	23,955	48,893

In addition, there are cottage hospitals and nursing homes for somatic and psychiatric treatment, hospitals and homes for epileptics, institutions for mentally retarded children, special hospitals and nursing homes.

Period of treatment: For all somatic treatment 19.1 days.
For the general hospitals 14.1 days.

The mental health services have, of course, been regulated by a number of ordinances since 1858 and control of them has now passed from the state to the municipalities. The Swedish word *hospital* (lunatic asylum), with its traditional associations, was used until 1929, when it was changed to *sinnessjukhus* (mental hospital). From 1960 onwards, these hospitals were called *mentalsjukhus* (mental hospitals) and since 1967 they have been called *lasarett för psykiatrisk vård* (hospitals for psychiatric treatment). The formal intention was to emphasize the integration of the psychiatric treatment with the somatic treatment – the endeavour to regard the mentally ill as 'ordinary' patients and to give the patients admitted to the psychiatric wards access to the technical resources of the general hospitals.

The expansion of the medical services has, of course, resulted in a need for more teaching hospitals. At this point it is perhaps appropriate to say something about the origins of the Swedish teaching hospitals.

The Serafimer Hospital was for long the most important teaching hospital. The Uppsala hospital, which began as a *nosocomium academicum*, was merged in 1867 with the present University Hospital (*Akademiska sjukhuset*). The small county hospital in Lund developed into the now very large teaching hospital there. The Sahlgrenska Hospital in Gothenburg, which originally came into existence in consequence of a donation by Anton Niclas Sahlgren, the managing director of the Swedish East India Company, was opened in 1782. It was planned from the beginning as a teaching hospital but did not become a university hospital until 1954; it is now one of the largest in Sweden. The General Hospital in Malmö was founded in 1857 but became a teaching hospital in the 1940s as a result of the shortage of clinical places for the medical students at Lund. The plans to supplement the Serafimer Hospital in Stockholm with another teaching hospital were put forward as early as 1905 but were not realized until after the Riksdag decision of 1927, when the Karolinska Hospital was founded (it was opened in 1940). In addition, in recent years prospective doctors and other medical personnel have also been given instruction at several other hospitals (in Stockholm at the Söder and Danderyd Hospitals and during 1972 at the newly built Huddinge Hospital). The increased demands for clinical places for students which medical training has entailed in recent years have meant that even the general hospital in Umeå, which was founded in 1785, has also been given the status of a teaching hospital (in 1959). The 'medical school' at Linköping, where the general hospital was originally founded in 1778, now also provides clinical instruction.

Here I should perhaps say something about the training given to those who were and are responsible for the treatment provided at our hospitals. The long-standing division of the Swedish medical profession into university-trained doctors and surgeons trained on handicraft lines did not come to an end in 1797. However, the 'master barber-surgeons' were given the designation of *chirurgie magister* and became members of the Collegium medicum, i.e. they became, in a sense, registered 'doctors'. Candidates for the degree of *chirurgie magister* had to be apprenticed to a master barber-surgeon for three years and then undergo an examination set by the Collegium medicum. They then became *chirurgie studiosus*, which entitled them to hold certain minor posts. If they wished to proceed further, they had to study for another four years (including six months at the Serafimer Hospital and periods of service at the School of Anatomy and the Lying-in Hospital in Stockholm).

Medical training in Sweden made only slow advances. For example, it was regulated in the statutes of Uppsala University in 1625 and 1626 and the rules included in the new statutes in 1655 continued to apply until 1852. Students who wished to devote themselves to medicine had first to secure a broad education in the humanities; they were compelled to take a degree in the Faculty of Theology and afterwards another in the Faculty of Arts and Sciences. Only then did their real medical studies begin.

In the middle of the eighteenth century, the purely medical examinations included a *disputatio exercitii gratia*, an *examen theoreticum* (for the first degree), an *examen practicum* (for the degree of licentiate of medicine) and a *disputatio pro gradu* (for the doctorate).

According to the statutes which replaced the old university 'constitutions' in 1852, a prospective doctor must first pass an examination in medicine and philosophy (including the natural sciences); however, this requirement was abolished in 1907. In 1861, the *chirurgie magister* degree was abolished and it was decided that the faculties alone should take charge of the examinations for the first degree, while the candidates for the licentiate of medicine should sit for their examinations either at the faculties or at the Karolinska Institute. In 1874 the Institute was given the right to hold examinations for the first degree. Women have had the right to pursue medical studies since 1870.

The oath which was formerly sworn by all doctors was abolished in 1887. The oath usually sworn by doctors abroad was introduced into Sweden at an early date, both as a doctor's oath on receipt of an academic degree and as an affirmation with the character of a professional oath. It is uncertain when these oaths were introduced; presumably it was during the seventeenth century. There was also the 'written witness's oath sworn by doctors employed in the public service', which had a practical purpose, in that, in virtue of this oath, certain medical officers did not need to confirm their certificates by oath in court in medico-legal cases. This practice dated from 1758.

The present century has seen the introduction of a number of reforms in the training of doctors in Sweden. The latest measure – in 1969 – replaced the licentiate of medicine with what is called the 'medical degree'. The basic medical training was reduced from six and a half to five and a half years. The subjects included in the degree are those internationally accepted. The degree is followed by 'further training', which for those who have gained their medical degrees under the new system comprises general service for twenty-one months (six months each in medicine, surgery and non-institutional care and three months in psychiatry), after which comes specialist training or training for general practice. The new list of specialities includes thirteen specialities with sub-sections.

The training of nurses in Sweden is not of long standing. The old 'minders of the sick' were not replaced by trained nurses until the nineteenth century. Training for nursing was first given by the Deaconess Institute in Stockholm, which was founded in 1857. The first two pupils in a secular school of nursing were admitted in 1867 to a little school at 'the new hospital in Uppsala' organized by the 'Association for the Voluntary Care of Wounded and Sick Soldiers in the Field'.

The present nurses' training (decreed by the Riksdag in 1965), leading to state registration, does not follow the 'apprenticeship system' which exists in many places and was also formerly in use in Sweden. The Swedish training lasts two and a half years, alternating between theoretical and practical courses, and provides opportunities for further training in various specialist fields and in administration.

The shifts in the population basis and especially the working population's need of easily accessible medical treatment have played important parts in the planning of the medical services. The population pyramid, with its increasing number of old people, has necessitated investment in wards for long-term care, as well as the renovation of our old people's homes. The newest of these homes have the character of hotels for retired people, in which, however, medical care can only be provided for short periods. Considerable sums have been invested in the district-medical-officer system, including the group practices, which have received extensive technical equipment and increased staffs. The company and industrial medical services – together with other medical services connected with the workplaces – have proved to be very important. In this field, Sweden has the oldest traditions in Europe, on account of the medical services provided for employees as early as the beginning of the seventeenth century by Stora Kopparberg AB, the oldest limited liability company in the world (it dates from the thirteenth century). In this field, we were aware at an early stage of the importance of prophylactic measures, including health checks, together with inspections of workplaces and attention to environmental questions. Considerable effort is now being devoted to work in the latter field.

Though the health insurance offices are of long standing in Sweden, it was only realized in the present century that more efforts should be made to promote health insurance. In 1910 a bill was presented to bring in compulsory health insurance. However, it did not go through and state-controlled, voluntary insurance came into being. The ordinance on recognized health insurance offices, both central and local, was not promulgated until 1931. However, the allowances made by these offices were far too low and the 1946 Riksdag decided to introduce compulsory health insurance as from 1950. Following the English pattern, the government decided to make the compulsory sickness benefit the same for all, although voluntary supplements were to be available. The General Health Insurance Act was passed in 1947 but did not come into force until 1 January 1955. On that date the recognized health insurance offices became public health insurance offices. As from 1963, they were called public social insurance offices and they now have other functions, including dealing with pensions. The sickness benefit paid to employees is graded according to income, in the same way as in industrial injury insurance, most of which has been taken over by the social insurance offices. These offices, which are to be regarded as government organizations, are supervised by the National Social Insurance Board (*Riksförsäkringsverket*), and their decisions may be appealed against to the National Social Insurance Court. Although modifications were introduced in 1970, the social insurance office pays part of the cost of medical treatment, the entire cost of treatment in a public ward at a local hospital and of journeys undertaken in connexion with medical treatment, and part of the cost of medicines (at present the patient pays a maximum of 15 crowns per prescription made out at the same time as the examination). In some cases, the social insurance office pays the cost of dental treatment (special insurance for dental treatment does not yet exist in Sweden), physiotherapy and convalescent care. In addition to health insurance, the system includes sickness-benefit insurance, with basic sickness benefit, supplementary benefit and an allowance for children.

Among the social reforms which have been widely discussed is the 'seven-crown reform', introduced in 1970, which means that a patient who consults a medical officer or attends an outpatient department is guaranteed the right to have carried out all the examinations necessary for establishing the diagnosis (including X-ray examinations and laboratory tests) and the treatment resulting therefrom (although not medicine) for this amount, which cannot, however, be reclaimed from the social insurance office. A committee is now investigating whether this scheme can be extended to cover the patients attending private practitioners, whose importance for the health services has lately been officially attested after long discussions. However, such an extension would presuppose that these doctors, like the hospital doctors, would in some way be paid a full salary.

TABLE 3 Some data on the Swedish medical system

	1870	*1960*	*1968*	*1970*
Doctors	560		9,840 (124 per 100,000 inhabitants)	
Nurses (entitled to pensions from the Government Pensions Institute)	—		27,770	
Midwives	1,864		1,860	
Hospitals	83		890 (all categories)	
Beds in hospitals (including mental hospitals)	6,055		128,324 (somatic and psychiatric treatment)	
Admissions to hospitals (including mental hospitals)	28,672		1,291,444 (all hospitals)	
Total cost of medical treatment		2.3 milliard crowns		9.7 milliard crowns
Per cent of gross national product		2.4		6.6
Average cost per patient		972 crowns		3,500 crowns (1971)
Cost per inhabitant		319.60 crowns		1,208.70 crowns (1969)
Government expenditure on public health, medical care and social welfare, in accordance with the 1972 budget proposals				2,730 milliard crowns (an increase of 350 million over 1971)

The 'seven-crown reform' has naturally increased the burden on non-institutional care, which is nevertheless cheaper than institutional care, which has almost led to a financial crisis. The reason for this critical situation is not clear-cut. One may point out that instruments and technical equipment have become more expensive, that the shortage of doctors and certain other medical staff in Sweden has resulted in the inefficient use of hospital wards and that there has been a considerable increase in the cost of administration. In addition, the working hours of the staff have been reduced. It must therefore be in everybody's interests that as much medical treatment as possible should be transferred to the non-institutional sector.

Some statistics illustrating the conditions 100 years ago and today in the Swedish medical system are given in Table 3. The overwhelming increase in the cost of medical treatment in Sweden may be indicated by mentioning that in 1960 it amounted to 2.3 milliard crowns or 2.4 per cent of the gross national product (GNP). By 1970 the cost had increased to 9.7 milliard crowns or 6.6 per cent of the GNP. The estimate for 1975 is 12 milliard crowns or 6.6 per cent of the GNP. Nevertheless the number of beds and the number of days in hospital have not appreciably increased. While the average cost per patient admitted was 972 crowns in 1960, it had risen to 3,500 crowns by 1971. If we consider the cost per inhabitant, this was 319:60 crowns in 1960 and 1,208:70 crowns in 1969. The cost of running a large Stockholm hospital (Söder Hospital) increased from 38.2 million crowns in 1960 to 107.8 million crowns in 1970, despite the fact that its medical services were fairly unchanged. It hardly seems to be possible to say that the quality of the treatment has increased in proportion, from the patient's point of view.

As I mentioned by way of introduction, Sweden is today in many respects a social laboratory. It is to be hoped that in this laboratory – with the help of many keen intellects – we shall find the formula which will allow us to retain, within the limits imposed by the available resources of finance and staff, the high standard which, despite all the difficulties, has long been regarded as characteristic of Swedish medical care.

Bibliography

BJÖRCK, P., 'Mentalsjukvården', *Medicinalväsendet i Sverige 1813–1962* (ed. W. Kock), Stockholm, 1963, pp. 243–80.

BJÖRKQVIST, E. and FLYGARE, I., 'Den centrala medicinalförvaltningen', *Medicinalväsendet i Sverige 1813–1962*, Stockholm, 1963, pp. 7–102.

ELMÉR, Å., *Svensk socialpolitik*, Lund, 1969 and 1970 suppl.

ENGEL, A., 'Medicinalväsendets aktuella problem', *Medicinalväsendet i Sverige 1813–1962*, Stockholm, 1963, pp. 667–91.

HJELT, O. E. A., *Svenska och finska medicinalväsendets historia 1663–1812*, Helsingfors, 1891–93.

HOLMSTRÖM, L.-G., 'Sjukvården fyra gånger dyrare på tio år', *Expressen*, 15 December 1971.

KOCK, W., *Kungl. Serafimerlasarettet 1752–1952*, Jönköping, 1952 (with references).

KOCK, W., 'Lasaretten och den slutna kroppssjukvården', *Medicinalväsendet i Sverige 1813–1962*, Stockholm, 1963, pp. 158–242.

KOCK, W., 'Läkare- och kirurgyrkets förening i Sverige', *Sv. läk. tidn*, 1942, **39**, 2466–75.

KOCK, W., *Medicinhistoriens grunddrag*, Halmstad, 1955.

KOCK, W., 'Svenska läkareeder', *Med. fören. tidskr.*, 1939, 276–83.

RABO, MÄJT, personal communication (on the modern Swedish training of nurses).

SCHULZ VON SCHULZENHEIM, D., *Tal om den offenteliga vården . . .*, Stockholm, 1801.

Socialstyrelsen & Universitetskanslersämbetet: Information om den nya utbildningen av läkare, *Statistisk Årsbok für Sverige* (Statistical Abstract of Sweden), Stockholm, 1971.

TOTTIE, M. and JANZON, B. (eds.), *Regional Hospital Planning* (in honour of Arthur Engel), Stockholm, 1967.

H. Schadewaldt
Düsseldorf (West Germany)

Die Entwicklung der staatlichen Gesundheitsfürsorge in Deutschland

Die hippokratischen Ärzte, denen man durchaus zugestehen darf, dass sie zum ersten Mal in der Geschichte dem wissenschaftlichen Prinzip in der Heilkunde zum Durchbruch verhalfen, haben die Medizin folgendermassen deklariert: ,,Die ärztliche Kunst umfasst drei Faktoren: die Krankheit, den Kranken und den Arzt.“ Eigentlich erst in der Aufklärungszeit hatte man dann erkannt, dass dieser Definition als quartum comparationis auch noch die *Gesellschaft* zugeordnet werden muss, und das berühmte Werk des in Rodalben bei Pirmasens geborenen Johann Peter Frank (1745–1821) ,,System einer vollständigen medicinischen Polizey“, geschrieben in der letzten Dekade des 18. Jahrhunderts, bildete sozusagen den Ausgangspunkt einer neuen Bewegung, die neben der Individualmedizin die sogenannte *Sozialmedizin* ins Leben rief, die später als öffentliche Gesundheitspflege oder im angloamerikanischen Sprachraum als ,,public health movement“ Aufgaben einer Staatsmedizin übernahm, bis sie in der zweiten Hälfte des 19. Jahrhunderts besonders als Folge der Industrialisierung der europäischen Völker eine eigenständige Bedeutung im Rahmen der Gesamtmedizin erhielt.

Nur in Deutschland – und das ist vielleicht bezeichnend – hat es Diskussionen darüber gegeben, ob man diese neue Disziplin als Grenzgebiet der Medizin und der Soziologie als *Sozialmedizin* oder, wie dies insbesondere einer ihrer grossen deutschen Vorkämpfer Alfred Grotjahn (1869–1931) propagierte, besser und zutreffender als *Sozialhygiene* zu bezeichnen habe. Obwohl darunter zweifelsohne genau das Gebiet verstanden wurde, was im ausserdeutschen Sprachraum als Sozialmedizin verstanden wurde, hat diese besondere deutsche Wortschöpfung zu manchen Missverständnissen Anlass gegeben, zumal Grotjahn die Sozialhygiene noch unter dem Generalnenner der Hygiene unterzubringen versuchte, obwohl er schon deutlich sah, dass neben die *soziale Hygiene* als Lehre von der Erhaltung und Förderung der physischen Wohlfahrt des Volkes – so die Definition von Alfred Nossig (geb. 1894) – die *soziale Pathologie* zu treten habe, als die Betrachtung der Beziehungen jeder Krankheit zur sozialen Umwelt, wie dies Grotjahn selbst in dem von ihm herausgegebenen ,,Handwörterbuch der sozialen Hygiene“ im Jahre 1912 betonte.

Die soziale Hygiene war danach eine ,,deskriptive Wissenschaft von der Lehre von den Bedingungen, denen die Verallgemeinerungen hygienischer Kultur unter der Gesamtheit von örtlich, zeitlich und gesellschaftlich zusammengehörigen Individuen und deren Nachkommen unterliegen“.

Im Gegensatz zu dem deutschen Grotjahn hat der Österreicher Ludwig Teleky

(1872–1957) bereits 1909 in seiner Wiener Antrittsvorlesung das von ihm richtig als *soziale Medizin* bezeichnete Gebiet klarer und umfassender umrissen, und seine Definition, wie er sie auch den 1914 erschienenen ,,Vorlesungen über soziale Medizin“ in der Einleitung voranstellte, sei daher an dieser Stelle angeführt:

Die soziale Medizin ist das Grenzgebiet zwischen den medizinischen Wissenschaften und den sozialen Wissenschaften. Sie hat die Einwirkung gegebener sozialer und beruflicher Verhältnisse auf die Gesundheitsverhältnisse festzustellen und anzugeben, wie durch Massnahmen sanitärer oder sozialer Natur derartige schädigende Einwirkungen verhindert oder ihre Folgen nach Möglichkeit behoben oder gemildert werden können. Ihre Aufgabe ist es auch, anzugeben, wie die Errungenschaften der individuellen Hygiene und der klinischen Medizin jenen zugänglich gemacht werden können, die einzeln und aus eigenen Mitteln nicht im Stande sind, sich diese Errungenschaften zunutze zu machen. Sie hat den Ärzten das wissenschaftliche Rüstzeug zu liefern, dessen sie bei ihrer Tätigkeit auf dem Gebiete der sozialen Versicherung und der sozialen Fürsorge bedürfen. Auch die Wandlung in der Stellung des Ärztestandes sowie die hier sich geltend machenden Entwicklungstendenzen hat sie zu studieren.

Grotjahn sah offensichtlich die soziale Medizin sehr viel enger, weil er darunter in erster Linie den Fragenkomplex der Versicherungsmedizin verstand und ihr die soziale Pathologie als Versuch einer Lehre von den sozialen Beziehungen der menschlichen Krankheiten zur Seite stellte, während er die soziale Hygiene als Oberbegriff verstand. Während Teleky aber unter sozialer Medizin nicht nur die gesamte Medizinalstatistik mit Morbiditäts-, Mortalitäts- und Letalitätszahlen, Geburtenhäufigkeit und Militärtauglichkeit verstand, sondern auch sogenannte Wohlstandsstufen, Verschiedenheiten der körperlichen Beschaffenheit von Säuglingen, Kindern und Erwachsenen, Beurteilungen der Krankenkassenleistungen, den Einfluss der Arbeitslosigkeit auf den Krankenstand und schliesslich auch die gesamten Gewerbe- und Berufskrankheiten darunter subsumierte, wollte Grotjahn gerade die letzteren, die häufig nur je einen einzelnen Arbeitnehmer oder bestimmte Gruppen betrafen, aus seinem Gebiet der sozialen Hygiene herausgenommen und als eigene Disziplin behandelt wissen.

Grotjahn konnte damals in der Tat mit Recht betonen, dass sich die soziale Medizin nicht so sehr den akuten, auffälligen und die Behandlung nachdrücklich fordernden Erscheinungen zuzuwenden habe, sondern sich vor allem mit den ansteckenden chronischen Krankheiten, wie Tuberkulose und Geschlechtskrankheiten, befassen müsse. Er warnte die Hygiene davor, nur eine reine ,,Komforthygiene“ zu werden, ihr Ziel müsse vielmehr nicht die ,,Gesundheit einiger Bevorzugter, sondern die Verallgemeinerung der hygienischen Kultur sein, unter einer Gesamtheit von örtlich, zeitlich und gesellschaftlich zusammengehöriger Individuen und deren Nachkommen“. Es liegen eine Reihe von scharfsinnigen Arbeiten vor, deren Autoren diese deutsche Sozialhygiene von der französischen und angloamerikanischen sozialen Medizin abzugrenzen versuchen um auch die Unterschiede zur Medizinsoziologie auf der einen Seite und zur Umwelthygiene auf der anderen Seite deutlich zu machen und sie auch gegenüber der public health, der öffentlichen Gesundheitspflege, abzugrenzen und auszuweiten.

Im deutschen Sprachraum dürfte Salomon Neumann (1819–1908) 1847 der Erste gewesen sein, der in seinem Buch ,,Die öffentliche Gesundheitspflege und das Eigenthum“ gefordert hat:

Dass der grösste Teil der Krankheiten nicht auf natürlichen, sondern auf gesellschaftlichen Verhältnissen beruht, bedarf keines Beweises. Die medizinische Wissenschaft ist in ihrem innersten Kern und Wesen eine soziale Wissenschaft, und solange ihr diese Bedeutung in der Wirklichkeit nicht verifiziert sein wird, wird man auch ihre Früchte nicht geniessen, sondern sich mit der Schale und dem Schein begnügen müssen. Die soziale Natur der Heilkunst steht über allem Zweifel.

Erste Auswirkungen dieser Vorstellungen, dass die Medizin nicht nur für den einzelnen Patienten, sondern auch für ein Kollektiv von Arbeitern oder Bürgern genutzt werden müsse, sind die frühen Krankenkassen, wie sie in den Knappschaftsvereinigungen und den Zunftkassen des Mittelalters existierten und wie sie auch bei den Seefahrern bekannt waren. Aber dies waren mehr genossenschaftliche Hilfsvereine, und sehr viel später als in England und Frankreich, nämlich zu Beginn der Revolution von 1848 in Deutschland, ist man sich darüber klar geworden, dass die Heilkunde auch über das Individuum hinausgehende Aufgaben der allgemeinen Wohlfahrtspflege haben müsse, die nicht mehr von Armenärzten und Armenkassen geleistet werden konnten, sondern die auf einem Anspruch des Bürgers auf Erhaltung oder Wiederherstellung seiner Gesundheit als einem der kostbarsten Güter beruhte. Die Aussage des deutschen Philosophen Arthur Schopenhauer (1788–1860) „neun Zehntel unseres Glücks beruhen auf Gesundheit“ zeigt diese besondere Bedeutung der Gesundheitspflege, die auch ein dem Pessimismus huldigender Denker voll anerkannte.

Es besteht kein Zweifel, dass wesentliche Impulse von der vom 26 jährigen Rudolf Virchow (1821–1902) und seinem Freunde Rudolph L. Leubuscher (1821–61) während der Revolutionsmonate 1848–49 ins Leben gerufenen Zeitschrift „Die medicinische Reform“ ausgingen. Darin hatte Virchow, ein liberaler, in seiner Jugendzeit sogar wohl als revolutionär zu bezeichnender Demokrat direkte Verbindungen zwischen der Medizin und der Politik postuliert und letztere sogar als eine „Medizin im Grossen“ bezeichnet. Von der Überzeugung ausgehend, dass viele, ja sogar die meisten Krankheiten aus sozialem Elend entstünden – seine Beobachtungen während der Fleckfieberepidemie in Oberschlesien 1847 mögen dafür Pate gestanden haben –, forderte er von der Medizin, dass sie sich auch als eine soziale Wissenschaft verstehe und folgte damit den Argumenten von Neumann, der die medizinische Wissenschaft als eine im besonderen Masse und notwendigerweise soziale Wissenschaft bezeichnete ua ue, und den Vorstellungen von Jules Guerin (1801–86), der 1848 wohl zum ersten Mal in einem Artikel in der „Gazette médicale de Paris“ von „médecine sociale au corps médical de France“ gesprochen hatte und vorschlug, die bisher voneinander ungenügend abgegrenzten Gebiete der Medizinalpolizei, öffentliche Hygiene und Staatsmedizin unter dem neuen Namen „Sozialmedizin“ zusammenzufassen.

Aber Virchow blieb sozusagen ein Rufer in der Wüste, denn nach der Niederschlagung der 48er Revolution und der Institutionalisierung der Restauration traten andere Probleme in den Vordergrund, die in der Medizin insbesondere von der Bakteriologie aufgeworfen wurden, während in der Politik ein gesamtdeutscher Nationalismus sich ausbreitete.

Die Virchowsche Vorstellung, dass ein Grossteil der Krankheiten durch soziale Misstände ausgelöst oder verschlimmert werden könnte, wurde durch die Entdeckung der verschiedensten Krankheitserreger auch für die bisher als Armenkrankheiten bekannten Seuchen, wie Tuberkulose und Typhus, in den schatten gestellt, und die 1876 erfolgte Gründung des Kaiserlichen Gesundheitsamtes in Berlin zeigt deutlich, dass der Akzent der offiziellen Gesundheitspolitik nunmehr nicht mehr so sehr im sozialen Bereich als in der Aufklärung der Ursache epidemischer Erkrankungen, deren Prophylaxe und möglicher Bekämpfung lag.

Ich selbst bin in einem historischen Kapitel zusammen mit Paul Diepgen (1878–1966) und George Benno Gruber (geb. 1884) über „Der Krankheitsbegriff, seine Geschichte und Problematik“ im „Handbuch der allgemeinen Pathologie“ auf diese Frage eingegangen, besonders aber sei auf die hervorragende Arbeit von George Rosen (geb. 1920) „What is Social Medicine“ im *Bulletin of the History of Medicine*, von 1947 verwiesen, wo dieser ganze Komplex ausführlich diskutiert wurde. Nach wie vor wird man auch das Werk von Alfons Fischer (geb. 1873) „Geschichte des deutschen Gesundheitswesens“ von 1933 konsultieren müssen.

Die divergierenden Auffassungen des liberalen Demokraten Virchow, der von einer Verbesserung der sozialen Lage der unterprivilegierten Schichten wesentliche Erfolge für die Bekämpfung der verschiedensten Krankheiten erwartete, und dem mehr konservativen Emil von Behring (1854–1917), der noch 1893 diese Präponderanz sozialmedizinischer Vorstellungen zu Gunsten von epidemiologischbakteriologischen Verhütungsmassnahmen verwarf, zeigen, wie stark bei der Beurteilung der Bedeutung der Sozialmedizin auch die jeweilige politische Einstellung mitwirkte. Tatsächlich darf man feststellen, dass im Gefolge der unerhörten Fortschritte der Bakteriologie in den letzten Dezennien des 19. Jahrhunderts die soziale Komponente weitgehend in den Hintergrund trat und erst mit dem Wirken dreier bedeutender Sozialhygieniker, dem schon erwähnten Grotjahn als dem ersten Professor für Sozialhygiene an einer deutschen Hochschule und hauptsächlichsten theoretischen Vorkämpfer, Adolf Gottstein (1857–1941) als einem mehr in der Praxis beschlagenen Gesundheitspolitiker und dem zuerst in Wien und dann in Düsseldorf wirkenden und durch das Dritte Reich zur Emigration gezwungenen Teleky seine Protagonisten fand.

Aber kehren wir, bevor wir das Wirken dieser drei bedeutenden deutschen Sozialmediziner betrachten, noch einmal zu den Fakten in der Zeit des 19. Jahrhunderts zurück. Erste Bemühungen um eine soziale Besserstellung der unteren Klassen dürften in den Reformen des Freiherrn Heinrich Friedrich Karl vom Stein (1757–1831) 1808 zu sehen sein, dessen Gesetze die Bauernbefreiung mit sich brachten, zugleich aber auch die absolute Verfügungsgewalt über den Privatbesitz.

Aber wie und wann stellte sich überhaupt in Deutschland die soziale Frage? Noch bis zum Ende des Ersten Weltkrieges galt in Preussen das sogenannte *Dreiklassenwahlrecht*, das auf der Grundlage von Eigentum und Grundbesitz aufgebaut war, das aber bereits 1817 in Württemberg durch das allgemeine gleiche Wahlrecht ersetzt worden war, das auch Otto von Bismarck (1815–98) dann für die Wahlen zum Deutschen Reichstag nach 1871 durchgesetzt hat. Die an sich durchaus sozial gemeinten Steinschen und Hardenbergschen Reformen hatten dazu geführt, dass gerade der Grundbesitz als absolutes persönliches Eigentum angesehen und damit der Grundstücksspekulation Tor und Tür geöffnet werden konnte. Damit war ein erstes Problem der späteren sozialen Frage aufgeworfen. Ein zweites entstand aus der zweifelsohne später als in England und Frankreich in Deutschland eintretenden Industrialisierung, die eine Zeitland von nationalen Vorstellungen der Errichtung eines geeinten deutschen Reiches, ebenso wie in Italien, in den Hintergrund gedrängt wurde.

Aber wie Tutzke in einer eindrucksvollen Studie zeigen konnte, sind auch schon im 19. Jahrhundert auf diesen Versammlungen immer wieder sozialhygienische Themen ausführlich erörtert worden, so in Vorträgen über die sogenannten Volkskrankheiten, über die Gesundheitsförderung, über die Entwicklung der Humanitätsanstalten oder die Kulturaufgaben der Volksbäder. Auch die Alkoholfrage ist von den verschiedensten Seiten aus beleuchtet worden.

Aber die deutsche Medizin ist interessanterweise an in anderen Ländern brennenden Fragen wie der Kinder-, Frauen- und Nachtarbeit zunächst einmal vorbeigegangen. Erst die Schrift des Elberfelder Industriellen Friedrich Harkort (1793–1880) 1844 ,,Bemerkungen über die Hindernisse der Civilisation und Emancipation der unteren Klassen" machte auf die inzwischen drängender gewordene soziale Frage aufmerksam, und als ein Paukenschlag darf das 1847 von Karl Marx (1818–83) und Friedrich Engels (1820–95) verfasste ,,Kommunistische Manifest" angesehen werden, dem dann als erster wesentlicher Beitrag aus der Feder eines Arztes die schon erwähnte, 1847 veröffentlichte Monographie von Neumann ,,Die öffentliche Gesundheitspflege und das Eigentum" folgte. Seine These, dass Krankheit nicht auf natürlichen, sondern auf künstlich erzeugten gesellschaftlichen Verhältnissen beruhe, spielt heute in der Bundesrepublik in der neomarxistischen Diskussion wieder eine grosse Rolle und war zweifelsohne ein Ausfluss der Beobachtungen der verschiedenen Aufstände sozial benachteiligter Gruppen, wie sie Gerhart Hauptmann (1862–1946) in seinem Drama ,,Die Weber" in dichterischer Weise geschildert hatte. Ihr folgte der berühmte Bericht von Virchow über die Hungertyphusepidemie in Oberschlesien vom Jahre 1848, der zum ersten Mal als Prophylaxe gegen derartige Katastrophen für alle Volksschichten *Bildung mit ihren Töchtern Freiheit und Wohlstand* forderte und behauptete, dass eine vernünftige Staatsverfassung das Recht des Einzelnen auf eine gesundheitsgemässe Existenz unzweifelhaft feststellen müsse. Dies war wohl der erste klar ausgesprochene Versuch, von der bisherigen karitativen Armenpflege zu einer staatlich gelenkten allgemeinen Wohlfahrtspflege zu gelangen, und die gleiche Forderung hatte auch Neumann gestellt, als er verlangte, dass man statt der *Barmherzigkeit,* die man als Grundlage der Armenkrankenpflege propagiert hatte, für diesen wichtigsten Teil der öffentlichen Gesundheitspflege das *Recht* als oberstes Prinzip aufstellen müsse und dass ein Rechtszustand erzeugt werden müsse, der die Gnade entbehrlich machen, ein Rechtszustand, der den Besitzlosen ihr einziges Eigentum, ihre Gesundheit, sichere. Damit ist zum ersten Mal von Neumann, Virchow und dessen Freund und Mitstreiter im Rahmen der ,,Medicinischen Reform" Rudolph Leubuscher das *Recht auf Gesundheit* postuliert worden, das eigentlich erst nach dem Zweiten Weltkrieg und vor allem im Rahmen der Verlautbarungen der Weltgesundheitsorganisation allgemeine Anerkennung fand. Hatte schon die Weltgesundheitsorganisation den Gesundheitsbegriff als körperliches, seelisches und soziales Wohlbefinden deklariert, so ist neuerdings in Deutschland von seiten der regierenden Sozialdemokratischen Partei das erweiterte Schlagwort von der *Lebensqualität* in die Diskussion geworfen worden, die es für jeden Bürger dieses Staates wesentlich zu verbessern gelte.

In der Revolutionszeit von 1848 hat man sich in erster Linie mit der damals unwahrscheinlich langen Arbeitszeit beschäftigt und ihre Beschränkung auf 8

Stunden pro Tag gefordert, während sie tatsächlich in der Regel 10, in vielen Fällen 14, ja sogar bis zu 16 Stunden betragen haben dürfte. Bereits in der niemals in Kraft getretenen Verfassung des Deutschen Bundes vom 28. März 1849 wurde die Reichsgewalt ermächtigt, im Interesse des Gesamtwohls allgemeine Massregeln für die Gesundheitspflege zu treffen, und es wurde eine Zentralorganisation des gesamten Medizinalwesens des Reiches verlangt, wie es 1876 mit der Schaffung des sogenannten Kaiserlichen Gesundheitsamtes in die Tat umgesetzt wurde, wenn es auch schon ab 1808 in Preussen ein spezielles Ministerium der Geistlichen, Unterrichts- und Medizinalangelegenheiten gab, in dem kein Geringerer als Wilhelm von Humboldt (1767–1835) mit grossem Erfolg tätig geworden war. Ein eigentliches Gesundheitsministerium gibt es dagegen in Deutschland erst nach dem 2. Weltkrieg sowohl in Ost wie in West. Kurze Zeit, von 1919–23, gab es in der ersten deutschen Demokratie ein Ministerium für Volkswohlfahrt, wo der bedeutende deutsche Sozialmediziner Gottstein als Ministerialdirektor die Leitung des preussischen Medizinalwesens übernommen und wesentliche fortschrittliche Entwicklungen angebahnt hatte.

Neben diesen parlamentarischen Bemühungen, die allerdings durch die Insuffizienz des Frankfurter Parlaments bald zum Erliegen kamen, gab es zwei weitere Gruppen, die sich für die Institutionalisierung der sozialen Medizin einsetzten. Das waren einmal die in jener Zeit zahlreichen, aus dem Boden schiessenden sogenannten Gesundheitspolitischen Vereine, zum andern Mitglieder der 1822 gegründeten Gesellschaft Deutscher Naturforscher und Ärzte, die 1865 zum ersten Mal eine neue Sektion für Medizinalreformen gebildet und 1867 eine weitere Sektion für öffentliche Gesundheitspflege etabliert hatte. Kurze Zeit später, 1869, begann die erste eigentliche Zeitschrift, die „Deutsche Vierteljahresschrift für öffentliche Gesundheitspflege" zu erscheinen, und damit wurden auch starke Impulse von seiten der Ärzte selbst und nicht nur der Politiker offenkundig. Inzwischen hatte sich Preussen unter Bismarcks Führung – er war 1862 Ministerpräsident geworden – für die kleindeutsche Lösung unter Ausschluss Oesterreichs entschieden, und 1867 wurde der Norddeutsche Bund begründet, der 1869 die erste, auch für Fragen der öffentlichen Gesundheitspflege wesentliche Gewerbeordnung verabschiedete. Sie war nun keineswegs die erste deutsche Manifestation der Fürsorge für die ärmeren Bevölkerungsschichten. Schon 1845 war ihr eine preussische Ordnung vorausgegangen, in der der Gesundheit der Arbeiter besondere Bedeutung zugemessen wurde. Aber natürlich war dies nur ein Tropfen auf den heissen Stein, und erst die 1862 von Ferdinand von Lassalle (1825–64) gegründeten Arbeitervereine machten die Offentlichkeit unermüdlich und unablässig auf die besonderen Probleme der mit der Industrialisierung einhergehenden sozialen, psychologischen und gesundheitlichen situation einer neuen Klasse, eben der Proletarier, aufmerksam.

Es mutet uns im übrigen heute etwas merkwürdig an, dass noch nach dem Ersten Weltkrieg 1919 Edmund Fischer ein „sozialhygienisches Friedensprogramm" für die ganze Welt vorschlug, das er in 12 Punkte gliederte:

1. Obligatorische Durchführung der Schulpflicht in allen Ländern.
2. Einführung der allgemeinen Fachschule.
3. Verbot der Erwerbstätigkeit für Kinder unter 15 Jahren.
4. Beschränkung der Arbeitszeit für Arbeiterinnen an Sonnabenden auf 4 Stunden.
5. Verbot der Beschäftigung von Frauen in besonders gesundheitsschädigenden Betrieben.

6. Schutzbestimmungen für Frauen vor und nach der Niederkunft.
7. Einführung der Mutterschaftsversicherung.
8. Festsetzung der Arbeitszeit für alle Arbeiter auf 8 Stunden täglich oder 48 Stunden wöchentlich.
9. Grundsätzliches Verbot der Nachtarbeit.
10. Grundsätzliche Gewährung einer zusammenhängenden Ruhepause von mindestens 36 Stunden wöchentlich.
11. Herabsetzung der Arbeitsdauer in gesundheitsgefährlichen Betrieben auf weniger als 8 Stunden.
12. Verbot der Heimarbeit für gesundheitsgefährliche Arbeiten ebenso wie für die Herstellung von Lebens- und Genussmitteln.

Ferner sollte überall eine Versicherung gegen Arbeitslosigkeit, Krankheit, Betriebsunfälle und eine Invaliden- und Hinterbliebenenversicherung eingeführt werden.

Diese Forderungen waren jedoch zum Teil schon recht alt. Sie erschienen bereits in der „Medicinischen Reform" von Virchow und Leubuscher, wo auch ein nationales Gesundheitsministerium gefordert worden war. Die Gewerbeordnung des Norddeutschen Bundes brachte auch mancherlei Rückschritte, so z.B. die sogenannte Kurierfreiheit, für die vor allem Virchow energisch eingetreten war und die nunmehr auch Laien den Zugang zur Krankenbehandlung ermöglichte und die damit schweren Schaden gestiftet hat. Auch die Subsumierung der ärztlichen Berufe unter die Gruppe der Gewerbetreibenden muss als eine gewisse Fehlbeurteilung der ärztlichen Tätigkeit angesehen werden und hat viele Jahrzehnte lang die Gemüter bewegt. Positiv darf man die Bestimmung einer besonderen staatlichen Approbation für Ärzte und Apotheker, die bereits seit 1845 in Preussen bestand, ansehen, die aber schon in zahlreichen deutschen Ländern durch Bestimmungen wesentlich älterer Medizinaledikte eingeführt worden war. Weiter waren die Forderungen nach einer fortlaufenden Gesundheitsstatistik, einer modernen Gesundheitsgesetzgebung, insbesondere was die Impfpflicht betraf, und nach einer Reorganisation des öffentlichen Gesundheitswesens positive Impulse, und der Ruf nach einer Institution, die eine einwandfreie Medizinalstatistik zu erstellen in der Lage wäre und sich sachkundig zu Medizinalgesetzen äussern könne, führte schliesslich zur Errichtung des Kaiserlichen Gesundheitsamtes am 16. Juli 1876. Dass ihr zweiter Präsident der ehemalige praktische Arzt Robert Koch (1843–1910) werden sollte, hat diesem Amt besondere Bedeutung verliehen, und bis heute spielt das nunmehr Bundesgesundheitsamt genannte Institut für die öffentliche Gesundheitspflege und die Medizinalgesetzgebung eine bedeutende Rolle.

Inzwischen hatte sich im übrigen auch eine erhebliche Verschiebung in der Bevölkerungsstruktur ergeben. Lebten noch 1812 76,8 pro Cent der Bevölkerung in Baden auf dem Lande und nur 23,2 pro Cent in der Stadt, so hatte sich das Verhältnis 1900 zu 58,6 pro Cent auf dem Land und 41,4 pro Cent in der Stadt verändert. Der Steinkohlenbergbau, das Hüttenwesen und in aller Welt bekannte Unternehmen wie Krupp, 1861, und Borsig, 1868 begründet, mit ihren hunderten und tausenden von Arbeitern führten zu neuen Problemen und warfen die sogenannte soziale Frage erneut auf.

Hatten bereits die idealistischen Philosophen in den ersten Dezennien des 19. Jahrhunderts für allgemeine Volksrechte plädiert, so Johann Gottlieb Fichte (1762–1814) das Recht eines jeden Bürgers auf Existenz und Friedrich Wilhelm Joseph von

Schelling (1775–1854), die These vertreten, dass das Leben Freude und nicht Schmerz mit sich bringen müsse, so fanden die unteren Volksklassen in den sogenannten Materialisten, in Marx, Ludwig Feuerbach (1804–72), Jacob Moleschott (1822–93) und Ludwig Büchner (1824–99) beredte Anwälte, die die zuerst in Frankreich als solche erkannte soziale Frage nun auch in Deutschland diskutierten. Wenn Lorenz von Stein (1815–90) 1888 die Auffassung vertrat, dass die Sorge für die Bedingungen der Erhaltung der Gesundheit sowie für die Heilung der Krankheiten nicht mehr von dem Besitz eines Kapitals abhängig sein dürfe, so waren damit die Gedanken einer *Volksversicherung* vorweggenommen.

Aber diese Postulate hatte bereits der deutsche Reichskanzler Bismarck wenige Jahre vorher unterlaufen. Er hatte, die konservative Richtung behauptete, aus echtem sozialem Verantwortungsgefühl, die Sozialdemokraten glaubten eher, um damit ihrer Partei und ihrem wachsenden Einfluss den Wind aus den Segeln zu nehmen, und die Katholiken behaupteten, als Ausfluss des Kulturkampfes, 1883 die ersten bis heute beispielhaften Sozialgesetze durchgesetzt, die Krankenversicherung der Arbeiter, die freilich nur für einen beschränkten Kreis von sozial Schwachen in Frage kam, und die 1888 erlassenen Gesetze zur Arbeitslosen- und Invalidenversicherung. Da in der Tat Bismarck der Kolonialpolitik der anderen europäischen Mächte nur zögernd folgte, hatte vielleicht ein liberaler Politiker wie der Hallensische Medizinprofessor Ernst Kohl Schütter (1837–1905), wie Dietrich Tutzke (geb. 1920) betonte, nicht Unrecht, wenn er behauptete, dass zu seiner Zeit in Deutschland nicht in erster Linie *Kolonial- sondern Sozialpolitik* betrieben würde.

Um dem Verlangen nach einer eindeutigen Statistik zu entsprechen, freilich auch als Ouverture für den bald einsetzenden Kulturkampf mit der katholischen Kirche–der Begriff stammte übrigens von dem demokratischen Abgeordneten Rudolf Virchow –, hatte Bismarck bereits 1874 das Standesamt eingeführt und im gleichen Jahr die für das gesamte Deutsche Reich geltenden Impfgesetze verabschieden lassen. Zwar war in Preussen bereits auf Veranlassung des Freiherrn vom Stein schon 1805 ein Königliches Statistisches Bureau begründet worden, doch waren die Angaben, auf die es sich stützen konnte, alles andere als zuverlässig. Erstmals 1839 erschien eine amtliche Schrift über die Zusammensetzung der preussischen Bevölkerung, und erst im Jahre 1843 konnte eine erste Veröffentlichung über die Zahl der Geburten, Eheschliessungen und Todesfälle in Berlin veröffentlicht werden, während dann im Jahre 1845 die statistischen Tabellen des preussischen Staates mit der Angabe der Zahl der Ärzte, Apotheker, Hebammen, Tierärzte und Krankenanstalten von W. Dieterici erschien.

Inzwischen aber hatten die von der sozialen Not besonders Betroffenen, die Arbeiter, zur Eigeninitiative gegriffen. Denn wenn bis zum Jahre 1850 z.B. der Eigenheimbau für die Arbeiter noch durchaus üblich war, nahm die nun zunehmende Bodenspekulation und die hektische sogenannte Gründerzeit nach dem Kriege 1870/71 gegen Frankreich den Arbeitern selbst jede Möglichkeit, ihr bescheidenes Kapital zu investieren und führte etwa von 1860 an zur Etablierung der sogenannten Mietskasernen, deren muffige Enge der Berliner Lokaldichter Heinrich Zille (1858–1929) und die grosse deutsche Künstlerin Käthe Kollwitz (1867–1945) drastisch dargestellt haben. Der Versuch, ,,eigentumslose Arbeiter in arbeitende Eigentümer" zu verwandeln, schien also gescheitert. Er ist im Zweiten Weltkrieg mit grösserem Erfolg wieder aufgenommen worden, aber unter anderen Vorzeichen erheben sich jetzt in Deutschland neue Diskussionen über Sinn und Wert der individuellen Eigenheime gegenüber grösseren Wohngemeinschaften, die nicht zuletzt auch aus psychologischen und sozialen Gründen ihren Propagandisten Vorteile zu versprechen scheinen. Auch in diesem Zusammenhang spielen Fragen der Grundstückspreise bei uns wieder eine ganz erhebliche Rolle, und zahlreiche aus dem Ausland importierte Modelle werden zur Zeit lebhaft diskutiert.

In diesem Zusammenhang sei auf das Wirken des deutschen Arztes Daniel Gottlob Moritz Schreber (1808–61) hingewiesen, der Ende der 40er Jahre die Kleingartenbewegung, die inzwischen in Deutschland den Namen Schrebergarten erhalten hatte, inaugurierte, die so auch den ärmeren Bevölkerungsschichten ein Wochenendleben in gesundheitlich vertretbarer Umgebung ermöglichen sollten. Ihr standen die sogenannten ,,Arbeiterkolonien", erstmals im Jahre 1862 zur Diskussion gestellt, zur Seite, und dieser ,,Schrebergarten" ist sicherlich eine spezifisch deutsche soziale Einrichtung geworden, während es weder in Frankreich noch in England oder Italien entsprechende Einrichtungen gibt.

Schon 1819 ist im übrigen in Württemberg ein weiteres interessantes Sozialmodell erprobt worden. Damals wurde eine Gemeinde Korntal gegründet, die vollständige Eigentümerin des Grundbesitzes blieb und jedes Mitglied der Gemeinde verpflichtete, den Grund und Boden nur an die Gemeinde wieder zu verkaufen. Dieser Ort ist rasch zu einer besonderen Blüte gediehen und ist heute ein Mittelpunkt industriellen und kulturellen Lebens, wobei allerdings bestimmte pietistisch-protestantische Richtungen bei der Entwicklung dieses Modells eine wesentliche Rolle spielten.

Mit der Einrichtung des Kaiserlichen Gesundheitsamtes 1876 und der Verabschiedung der ersten Sozialgesetze, wie der Krankenversicherung für Arbeiter und der Arbeitslosen- und Invalidenversicherung von 1883–88, hatte das Deutsche Reich zweifelsohne in gewisser Weise die Initiative auch für eine sozialmedizinische Gesetzgebung übernommen. Aber schon vorher, 1865, war der Apotheker Max von Pettenkofer (1818–1901) zum ersten Ordinarius für Hygiene in Deutschland an der Universität München ernannt worden, und er hatte sich bereits mit dem wichtigsten Problem der sozialen Medizin, mit den Umweltbedingungen der arbeitenden Bevölkerung intensiv auseinandergesetzt. Er ist den Fragen der Wasserversorgung, der Kanalisation, der Wohnraum- und Städtehygiene ebenso nachgegangen wie dem Fäkalien- und Müllabfuhrproblem. Aber Pettenkofer hat mehr die natürliche Umwelt und nicht so sehr die sozialen Verhältnisse in Erwägung gezogen. In diesem Punkte war in Fortsetzung der Virchowschen Gedankengänge Eduard Reich (1836–1919) 1862 mit einem Werk ,,Betrachtungen über die Erkrankungen der Gesellschaft" hervorgetreten, und er hatte in Fortsetzung der aufklärerischen Gedanken, wie sie Johann Peter Frank in seinem ,,System der allgemeinen medicinischen Polizey" vertreten hatte, die Notwendigkeit des Lehrens der Gesundheitspflege betont und in seinem 1870 erschienenen ,,System der Hygieine" besonders hervorgehoben, dass er unter Hygiene die Gesamtheit jener Lehren verstehe, deren Anwendung die Erhaltung der individuellen und sozialen Gesundheit, der Sittlichkeit, der Zerstörung der Krankheitsursachen und die Veredlung des Menschen in physischer und moralischer Beziehung bezwecke: ,,Will man eine Bevölkerung glücklich und gesund erhalten, muss man zunächst Teuerung und Hungersnot verhüten". Er pries die amerikanischen Gartenstädte, in denen die Arbeiter die Freiheit des Landlebens und zugleich alle Vorteile einer Weltstadt geniessen würden, als der Weisheit letzter Schluss. Wir kennen inzwischen die Problematik derartiger Satellitenstädte, wo sich die zurückgelassenen Ehefrauen einsam fühlen und wo sich kein eigentliches städtisches Leben entwickeln kann.

Wir wiesen schon darauf hin, dass das Interesse an den sozialen Fragen und an dem sogenannten öffentlichen Gesundheitswesen mit der aufkommenden Bakteriologie in andere Richtung gelenkt wurde und die Umweltverhältnisse weniger Interesse erregten, als die ätiologischen Faktoren der Infektionskrankheiten, deren Bekämpfung nunmehr unter Robert Kochs Leitung auch zum Hauptanliegen des Kaiserlichen Gesundheitsamtes wurde. Erst nach der deutschen Revolution 1918 traten wieder mehr die sozialhygienischen Aspekte in den Vordergrund, und für ihre Verbreitung in der sogenannten Weimarer Republik waren vor allem drei Persönlichkeiten von ausschlaggebender Bedeutung: Alfred Grotjahn, Adolf Gottstein und Ludwig Teleky, die als die eigentlichen Begründer der modernen Sozialhygiene im deutschen Sprachraum angesehen werden können. Alfred Grotjahn hatte bereits in der Kaiserzeit den Mut gehabt, nach seinem Medizinstudium noch soziologische Studien, vor allem bei dem Berliner Nationalökonom und sogenannten Kathedersozialisten Gustav von Schmoller (1838–1917), zu absolvieren, und er hat sich frühzeitig der Sozialdemokratischen Partei zugehörig gefühlt. 1896 liess er sich in Berlin als praktischer Arzt nieder. Ein erster Versuch, sich 1902 für das neue Fach der Sozialhygiene – zu habilitieren, scheiterte am Einspruch des damaligen Hygienikers Max Rubner (1854–1932) und es gelang Grotjahn erst 1912, die akademische Laufbahn einzuschlagen. Es war das Jahr, in dem er sein Hauptwerk „Die soziale Pathologie" veröffentlichte, in der er noch einmal nachdrücklich das neue, dann erstmals nach dem Ersten Weltkrieg von ihm als Ordinarius vertretene Fach propagierte:

Die Sozialhygiene als deskriptive Wissenschaft ist die Lehre von den Bedingungen, denen die Verallgemeinerungen hygienischer Kultur unter der Gesamtheit von örtlich, zeitlich und gesellschaftlich zusammengehörigen Individuen und deren Nachkommen unterliegt. Die Sozialhygiene als normative Wissenschaft ist die Lehre von den Massnahmen, die die Verallgemeinerung hygienischer Kultur unter der Gesamtheit von örtlich, zeitlich und gesellschaftlich zusammengehörigen Individuen und deren Nachkommen bezweckt.

Zeit seines Lebens blieb er der Überzeugung, dass soziale Hygiene und Sozialismus Geschwister seien, und auf dieser Basis sind seine Vorstellungen von der Sozialisierung der Medizin zu verstehen, die ihm viele Gegner verschafft haben und die ihm auch heute noch in der westdeutschen Ärzteschaft zweifelsohne kaum Freunde eintragen würden. So hatte er 1921, inzwischen Abgeordneter des Deutschen Reichstages der SPD geworden und zum Ordinarius für Sozialhygiene gegen den Willen der Fakultät an der Berliner Universität ernannt, Forderungen erhoben, wie sie heute in den sozialistischen Ländern, in Schweden und in England zum Teil in die Tat umgesetzt wurden, wie sie aber in der Bundesrepublik Deutschland noch äusserst heftig umkämpft sind: „Übernahme des gesamten Heil- und Gesundheitswesens in den Gemeinbetrieb unter Beseitigung jeglicher privatkapitalistischer Wirtschaftsform, Vereinheitlichung des sozialistischen Versicherungswesens und seine Ausdehnung auf alle Volksangehörige, Übernahme und Ausbau der Krankenanstalten, Ambulatorien, Polikliniken und gesundheitlichen Fürsorgeeinrichtungen sowie aller sonstigen, der öffentlichen Gesundheitspflege dienenden Einrichtungen in Stadt und

Land, Eingliederung der Ärzte, Hebammen und des übrigen Heil- und Krankenpflegepersonals in die Gesamtorganisation des Heil- und Gesundheitswesens unter planmässiger Verteilung auf Stadt und Land bei sorgfältigster Berücksichtigung der Arbeitsteilung und Arbeitsersparnis sowie Zuhilfenahme aller technischer Hilfsmittel, Sozialisierung der Apotheken und aller Stätten der Herstellung, des Handels und des Vertriebs von Heilmitteln und Sanitätswaren, unentgeltliche, würdige und gleichartige Totenbestattung in der Form der Beerdigung oder Einäscherung nach erfolgter ärztlicher Totenschau, Erlass eines Irrengesetzes, das Unterbringungszwang und Freiheit der geistig Gestörten und Minderwertigen regeln sollte, Organisation eines umfassenden, von wählbaren Amtsärzten durchzuführendes Gesundheitsdienstes in den Gemeinden unter Führung eines Reichsministeriums für Volksgesundheit".

Grotjahn war also der Auffassung, dass das deutsche Gesundheitswesen vereinheitlicht werden müsse: „Ein einheitliches, in sich geschlossenes Medizinalwesen ist also die erste Forderung, die gestellt werden muss", so betonte er in einem spektakulären Vortrag im Verein der Sozialistischen Ärzte in Berlin im Dezember 1919. Darin kam wiederum seine Überzeugung zum Ausdruck, dass in dem Augenblick, wo die Familienversicherung der Krankenkassen gesetzlich verankert würde, die Sozialisierung des Heilwesens aktuell und mit ihr auch die der Apotheken gleichzeitig erfolgen müsse. Aber er räumte auch ein, und diese Probleme haben sich auch in unseren Tagen dann bei derartigen Sozialisierungsmassnahmen ergeben: „Eine solche Sozialisierung wird allerdings nicht ohne heftige Erschütterung hergebrachter Zustände vor sich gehen können."

Weiter sprach er sich für „soziale Versicherung und Bevölkerungspolitik, Bekämpfung der dem Volksganzen und dem Bestand der Gesellschaft gefährlichen Ausdehnung des Geburtenrückganges durch eine gesteigerte soziale Hygiene zwecks Menschenersparnis durch Beseitigung aller Hemmungen der Elternschaft und der Frühehe durch eine Begünstigung der kinderreichen Eltern auf Kosten der ledigen, kinderlosen und kinderarmen Personen vermittels Steuer-, Erbschafts-, Lohn-, Siedlungs- und Versicherungsgesetzgebung" aus. Schon die letzten Punkte zeigen, dass er keineswegs ein überzeugter orthodoxer Sozialdemokrat war, der auf marxistischer Basis stand, sondern durchaus eigene, originelle Beiträge zur Frage der modernen Gesundheitspolitik beizutragen sich erlaubte. So war er im Gegensatz zur damaligen SPD, die eine Aufhebung des sogenannten Abtreibungsparagraphen 218 forderte, der den nicht medizinisch indizierten Abort unter Strafe stellte, der Auffassung, dass zum Schutze der Volkssubstanz, wie er sich ausdrückte, dieses Gesetz erhalten bleiben müsse. Er war ein Propagator einer fast sektiererhaft anmutenden vegetarischen Ernährungsform, weil er die wirtschaftliche Autarkie Deutschlands glaubte befürworten zu sollen. Aber trotz dieser verschiedenen, von rechts und links gleichermassen angegriffenen Theorien blieb er der grosse theoretische Anreger, dem sozusagen als mehr praktisch orientierter Kollege Adolf Gottstein zur Seite zu stellen ist.

Ebenso wie Grotjahn war auch Gottstein viele Jahre lang Praktiker in Berlin, bis er zu seiner eigenen Überraschung auf Grund seiner verschiedenen Arbeiten 1905 zum Leiter des Medizinalwesens der damals noch selbständigen Stadt Charlottenburg vor Berlin ernannt wurde und im März 1919 mit der Leitung des preussischen Medizinalwesens im Volkswohlfahrtsministerium beauftragt wurde. Unter seiner

Ägide wurde das deutsche Hebammengesetz 1922, das Gesetz zur Bekämpfung der Tuberkulose 1923, das Reichsgesetz für Jugendwohlfahrt 1924 und das besonders wichtige Krüppelfürsorgegesetz im gleichen Jahr ins Leben gerufen. In diesem Jahr musste er aus Altersgründen sein Amt aufgeben und wirkte noch bis ins Dritte Reich, das ihm allerdings eine weitere publizistische Tätigkeit ab 1937 unmöglich machte. Seine Monographie über die „Epidemiologie", 1937 abgeschlossen, hat besondere Bedeutung für die Sozialmedizin erhalten, und er war neben Grotjahn sozusagen der mehr praktisch und auf die politische Durchführbarkeit bedachte Vorkämpfer der deutschen Sozialhygiene.

Im ersten Heft der im Juli 1919 begründeten „Zeitschrift für soziale Hygiene, Fürsorge und Krankenhauswesen" hatte Gottstein den Leitartikel übernommen und dabei darauf aufmerksam gemacht, dass Pettenkofer und seine Schüler den Einfluss der unbelebten Welt auf die Gesundheit der experimentellen Erforschung zugänglich gemacht hätten, damit aber die individuelle Hygiene und damit die der Vermögenden stärker gefördert habe als die der weniger bemittelten Kreise. Der Bakteriologie machte Gottstein im übrigen den Vorwurf, dass über der parasitären Exposition der krankheitsfördernde Einfluss von Disposition und Konstitution und damit von sozialen Misständen zu gering erachtet worden sei, und als wichtiger Satz aus seiner Arbeit sei hier zitiert:

Der Ausgangspunkt jeder sozialhygienischen Betrachtung ist aber der Satz, dass Krankheitsbedrohung, Krankheitsentstehung, Krankheitsverlauf und Krankheitsausgang, jedes für sich oder gemeinsam, je nach der sozialen Lage einer Bevölkerungsschicht recht erhebliche Abweichungen zeigen, und aus diesem Satz folgt, dass auch die Massnahmen zur Verhütung der drohenden und zur Bekämpfung der entstandenen Krankheiten als Massenerscheinung mit diesem Zusammenhang zu rechnen haben.

Er machte ferner darauf aufmerksam, dass man die soziale Bedeutung einer Krankheit nicht nur an der Mortalitätsstatistik ablesen könne, denn

soziale Einflüsse verändern im einen Fall nur die Zahl der Erkrankungen, ohne dass das Verhältnis der der Erkrankung Erliegenden beeinflusst wird. Ein zweites Mal ist die Neigung zur Erkrankung zwar für alle Schichten die gleiche, dafür aber sind Verlauf und Ausgang verschieden.

Und ausserordentlich modern mutet seine Forderung an, die sämtlichen Mitglieder der Krankenkasse einer planmässigen periodischen Untersuchung, also den erst jetzt nach dem Zweiten Weltkrieg in vielen Ländern eingeführten Vorsorgeuntersuchungen zu unterziehen.

Eine besondere Leistung Adolf Gottsteins war die 1920 erfolgte Errichtung dreier Akademien für Staatsmedizin in Breslau, Charlottenburg, und Düsseldorf. Gottstein hatte nämlich während der Jahre seiner Charlottenburger Tätigkeit feststellen müssen, dass auch die Amtsärzte auf dem Gebiet der Sozialhygiene und Gesundheitsfürsorge nicht ausreichend unterrichtet waren, weil sie in erster Linie mit gerichtsmedizinischen und von der Bakteriologie beeinflussten hygienischen Problemen vertraut gemacht wurden. Dabei war für den Sitz der Berlin–Charlottenburger Akademie natürlich die Aktivität Gottsteins selbst von grösster Bedeutung. In Düsseldorf hatte sich sein Freund, der Direktor der damaligen Kinderklinik der Medizinischen Akademie Arthur Schlossmann (1867–1932) energisch dafür eingesetzt, während die Vorgeschichte der Breslauer Akademie leider ganz bis heute nicht geklärt werden konnte. Für alle drei Akademien war ein gleichartiger Lehrplan festgelegt worden, der Grundzüge der sozialen Hygiene mit Bevölkerungspolitik, Vererbung und Eugenik, Anthropometrie sowie praktische Übungen auf dem Gebiete der Stadthygiene, der Gewerbehygiene und Berufskunde verlangte und weiter soziale Pathologie mit Demonstrationskursen, Mutter-, Säuglings- und Kinderberatungswesen, Schulhygiene und Kinderorthopädie ebenso umfasste, wie die Beratung auf dem Gebiete der Tuberkulose und Geschlechtskrankenfürsorge sowie der Prostitution. Auch die Fürsorge für Geisteskranke, Schwererziehbare, Schwachsinnige und Gefangene war vorgesehen und eine Einführung in die Grundzüge der Staats- und Kommunalverwaltung mit praktischen Übungen in Fürsorgestellen und Besichtigungen einschlägiger Institutionen.

Gemeinsam mit seinen Freunden Teleky und Schlossmann gab Gottstein nach seiner Pensionierung das grosse *Handbuch der sozialen Hygiene* heraus, das noch bis in den Zweiten Weltkrieg hinein als vorzügliches Quellenwerk galt. Mit Vorliebe beschäftigte er sich mit statistisch-mathematischen Fragen, und auf der Grundlage dieser Arbeiten ist er seinerzeit zu einem erbitterten Gegner der enthusiastischen Lobpreisungen des Behringschen Diphtherieheilserums geworden, weil er glaubte, dass die damals vorgelegten statistischen Beweise ungenügend seien. Er hat sich damit sehr viele Feinde gemacht und auch im eigenen sozialhygienischen Lager manchen Widerspruch gefunden. Seine These jedoch, dass vielleicht für das spektakuläre Absinken der Diphtherietodesfälle nicht das Heilserum allein, sondern eine entsprechende Virulenzabschwächung des Diphtheriebazillus verantwortlich sein könne, wird heute allgemein akzeptiert, wenn auch seine scharfe Gegnerschaft gegen die Serumtherapie inzwischen nur noch historisch gesehen werden kann.

Als dritten im Bunde darf man den Österreicher Teleky betrachten, der nicht müde wurde, für die Eigenständigkeit der von ihm, dem internationalen Sprachgebrauch entsprechend, ,,soziale Medizin" bezeichneten Disziplin zu plädieren. Es war Gottsteins Verdienst, ihn 1920 als Leiter für die soeben errichtete Akademie für Sozialmedizin in Düsseldorf zu gewinnen, und hier hat er ganze Generationen von Amtsärzten ausgebildet und einen detaillierten Lehrplan für soziale Hygiene, soziale Pathologie, Gesundheitsfürsorge, Organisations- und Gesetzkunde und praktische Arbeit in den Fürsorgestellen aufgestellt. Er war allerdings wohl mehr Gelehrter als Lehrer und hatte nicht die leichte Hand, die Führung einer so inhomogenen Akademie, die sich noch dazu einer gewissen Gegnerschaft von seiten der deutschen Universitäten erwehren musste, verlangte. Im Dritten Reich wurden die Akademien sofort aufgelöst und sind erst nach dem Kriege in der Bundesrepublik wieder entstanden, allerdings inzwischen auf Düsseldorf als einzige Zentraleinrichtung konzentriert.

Seine Tätigkeit wurde von Schlossmann unterstützt, der als Abgeordneter im preussischen Landtag ebenfalls ständig die Bedeutung der sozialen Medizin in prophylaktischer und wohl auch kurativer Hinsicht betonte und der sich besonders zu Fragen der Mütter- und Säuglingsfürsorge sowie der Krüppelgesetzgebung äusserte, und man darf in der Tat die Fürsorge für Säuglinge und mit angeborenen Leiden behaftete Kinder in der Deutschen Republik von 1919–33 als vorbildlich für Europa betrachten.

Mit der Machtergreifung durch Adolf Hitler (1889–1945) wurde das Wort ,,sozial" allgemein suspekt und alle entsprechenden Institutionen sofort aufgehoben und die

Sozialmedizin zu Gunsten einer völlig andersartigen Ideologie, der Rassenlehre, vernachlässigt. Im Sinne eines modernen Sozialdarwinismus wurde nicht mehr die Hilfe für die sozial Schwächeren oder gar für an, wie man früher glaubte, vererbbaren Krankheiten Leidenden forciert, sondern eine besondere Art Eugenik bis zur sogenannten Euthanasie, der Vernichtung lebensunwerten Lebens, verfolgt.

So war es ein mühseliger und langsamer Neubeginn nach 1945, der erst allmählich dazu führte, dass an den deutschen Universitäten wieder Lehrstühle für Sozialmedizin eingerichtet wurden, und erst in jüngster Zeit hat die neue Approbationsordnung das Fach „Sozialmedizin" obligatorisch gemacht und in seinen Prüfungskatalog entsprechende Fragen aufgenommen.

Freilich besteht zur Zeit in unserem Land die Gefahr, dass im Zuge einer etwas einseitigen Betrachtung diese Probleme ideologisiert werden und die solide wissenschaftliche Basis, die wie in allen Disziplinen der Medizin auch für die öffentliche Gesundheitspflege die conditio sine qua non ihrer Existenz darstellt, da und dort verlassen zu werden scheint.

Vor allem ist die Diskussion über die Vor- und Nachteile einer sozialisierten Medizin, die optimale Behandlung in den Krankenhäusern, die Vorsorgeuntersuchungen und die Rehabilitation sowie die Massnahmen für Säuglinge, Kinder und alte Menschen in heftigster Weise entbrannt, doch scheint die Mehrzahl der deutschen Ärzte zur Zeit an der freien Arztwahl für den Patienten und am freien Beruf des Arztes festzuhalten, wobei interessanterweise die alten Postulate des Freundes von William Harvey (1578–1657) und des englischen Lordkanzlers Francis Bacon (1561–1626) meist ohne Bezugnahme auf ihre historischen Hintergründe wieder aufgenommen werden, dass die Heilkunde nämlich drei Aufgaben habe: Die Gesundheitserhaltung, die Krankenheilung und die Lebensverlängerung.

J. L. Brand
Bethesda, Md. (U.S.A.)

Discussion

It has been a considerable pleasure to attend the two symposia on the history of provision for health and social welfare presented at this international congress. The very knowledgeable and capable speakers, both in Wednesday's session and that of this morning, have in a remarkably brief span of time sketched some of the major steps in the development of public responsibility for medical care in their respective national traditions. Dr. Galdston's paper, in discussing the evaluation of medical care in the United States, has also moved directly into some of the major current issues concerning Americans and the American medical profession, as our own country deliberates the changing role of the Federal Government in the provision of health services.

The systems we have heard described have constituted alternative traditions and solutions – varying organizational patterns of health services – which have emerged from the particular social, economic and political conditions of the countries concerned. As one of the other panel discussants in the first session mentioned, I too regret that it has not been feasible to include in these sessions an historical paper on the development of health services in Eastern Europe. There is, of course, available in English, Henry Sigerist's *Medicine and Health in the Soviet Union*, although it is over twenty-five years old. We also have the more recent sociological studies of Mark Field of Harvard University, and the 1969 descriptive study by the Weinermans, *Social Medicine in Eastern Europe*, which gives a synopsis of the current systems of social medicine in Czechoslovakia, Hungary and Poland. It is to be hoped that additional historical studies of the development of health service programmes of countries which have moved through different patterns of social and political organization will become available, both to historians as well as to those who administer national health service systems. Among the comparative data on which we need more historical background, for example, are: (1) The points of first entry into existing medical care systems, as influenced by national tradition. (2) The interrelationship of stated national health goals, at different periods in a country's history, with various regional and local traditions. (3) Historical approaches to the evaluation of medical care. (4) The provision, at various historical periods, of health services for minority groups and how such services were affected by regional sub-culture patterns. (5) The influence of the medical profession in different countries in extending and/or opposing the development of local or federal responsibility for the personal health services.

You will have observed by now that it has been difficult for some of the symposia speakers and discussants to view their subjects as medical historians, rather than as medical administrators or medical sociologists actually concerned with present-day developments in social medicine. In writing his preface to the symposium on *Medical History and Medical Care*, held two years ago in London, Lord Cohen of Birkenhead pointed to a goal of that 1970 meeting as the need to find out 'how far such historical studies help to provide a future perspective, capable of contributing to the solution of contemporary problems'. And in noting this, Lord Cohen cited Sir Winston Churchill's observation, 'The farther you look back, the farther forward you can see'.

Even as a historian, I sometimes think that too much can be expected of the practical uses of history or of the historical examination of contemporary social problems. It is, perhaps, easier to justify historical research personally in terms of the intrinsic satisfactions which come from reconstituting the past – from making patterns out of fragments – rather than with a certainty that it will lead to forecasting steps to an optimum future. For, as you are all well aware, historians bring to their reconstructions of the past their own assumptions of causality – basic assumptions such as whether or not the passage of years is co-ordinate with human progress; whether or not history is primarily determined by great men. Some historians have based their examination of the past on assumptions of natural selection, many others on economic determinism, and also on the primary importance of geographic and natural resources.

Still another body of those who write history are afflicted by the disease of 'presentism', who either consciously or unconsciously believe that their age has arrived at the final truth, and who toss brickbats at their predecessors in trying to evaluate their actions, without attempting to discern the contemporary values of those they write about.

I make this very brief excursion into historiography, because the historical study of provision for health and social welfare is a subject particularly vulnerable to moral judgment. One of the major questions which arises when one examines historically the nature and degree of commitment of a society to public health sanitary programmes, personal health services, or national health insurance programmes, is the allocation of resources. The historian of national health and welfare programmes must range deeply into economic, social and political history and must deal directly with the question of allocations of resources and alternative decisions. It is difficult, for example, to evaluate national decisions which may lead to the provision of better standards of nutrition or housing, as alternatives to the provision of medical care, for the aged or for the whole population. Even more crucial choices confront many developing countries, whose limited resources are sought for capital equipment and industrial development. In the industrialized Western nations an increased demand for medical services is confounded by the elaboration of biomedical technology, increased manpower needs and spiralling costs of medical care.

The subject we discuss historically today is clearly one implicit with moral and philosophical issues, through which the historian must proceed carefully, and, at minimum, in awareness that his own value system will inevitably enter into the selection and analysis of source materials.

The two symposia this week on the history of provision of health and social welfare constitute an auspicious beginning. It is to be hoped that future meetings of the Society for the Social History of Medicine will continue with selective historical examination of this important subject, and will develop new perspectives for cross-national interchange.

V CONGRESS THEME

Medicine and Society

A. Pazzini
Rome (Italy)

La professione medica nella Grecia d'Ippocrate

Da quanto risulta da notizie che, isolate, sembrano avere una importanza relativa e contingente, ma che riunite costituiscono un complesso notevole documentario, l'esercizio della professione medica in Grecia all'epoca di Ippocrate risulta suddivisa in tre sezioni.

E cioè: la medicina sacrale; un esercizio empirico; uno veramente medico secondo regole ben disciplinate, di scuola.

E cominciamo dall'esercizio della medicina nei templi.

L'esistenza di una medicina basata sulla interpretazione divina della malattia, sulla possibilità di guarigione solo per 'grazia ricevuta' attraverso l'intercessione del sacerdote, è certa anche in Grecia, come a l'inizio di tutte le grandi civiltà.

Notizie anteriori al culto ufficiale di Asclepio, esistono, sia pure frammentarie.

Il culto medico dei primi greci era un culto solare. Apollo manda la peste, dardeggiando i suoi raggi come saette, e diviene guaritore quando cessa di essere pestifero.

Altre notizie ci mostrano una Igiea identificabile con Atena-Hygieia, documentata da Pausania e da Plinio a proposito di una statua che lo scultore Pyrros scolpì per incarico di Pericle.

Una Panacea, prima di essere ritenuta figlia di Asclepio, sarebbe anch'essa preesistita, quale attribuzione di Atena Paionia con un culto proprio.

Da queste poche notizie si può prospettare una specie di Olimpo medico greco, esistente prima della assunzione di Asclepio, l'originario principe della Tessaglia abile, secondo Omero, a guarire le ferite, divinizzato come figlio di Apollo, rappresentando la parte guaritrice della pestifera divinità.

Fu verso la fine del VI secolo che il culto famigliare di questo principe, entrando nella ufficialità, uscì dalla nativa Tessaglia, e, attraverso il Peloponneso, giunto in Epidauro fu unito a quello preesistente di Apollo, e di lì passò in Attica, in Eleusi, a Paro, a Coo, a Creta, a Rodi e in Asia minore, dove ebbe il celebre tempio di Pergamo.

E fu nei templi che ebbe rigoglio la medicina sacrale, il che per altro non significa che prima della loro costruzione (che fu tarda) non esistesse il culto.

Negli asclepiei che Luciano chiama 'la bottega del nume', era una medicina miracolistica ad essere esercitata, ed in essi, come Aristofane riferisce, non ci si faceva scrupolo di ricorrere al trucco dal sacerdote camuffato da Asclepio che, di notte, distribuiva i suoi consigli, svegliando i postulanti addormentati intorno alla sua cella.

Ed Elio Aristide, nelle sue epistole, ci mostra gli asclepiei come una consorteria om merciale tramandantesi i 'clienti' dall'uno all'altro fino a che, malati come prima, non fossero stati a dovere spennati.

Ben differente era la medicina esercitata e tramandata nella famiglia degli Asclepiadi, discendenti di Esculapio, Podalirio e Macaone, suoi figli. Ben differente anche se talvolta con lo stesso nome si indicavano tanto i sacerdoti dei templi quanto ifamigliari. Anche Platone, nominando Ippocrate, aggiunge 'quello degli Asclepiadi'.

Dalla famiglia naturale di Asclepio, infatti, attraverso i figli e i figli dei figli, si tramandava l'insegnamento della medicina come retaggio strettamente famigliare, segreto di casta, inviolabile. Da questa famiglia uscì Ippocrate, al quale la storia riconosce la istituzione della medicina 'clinica' come la definisce Plinio o 'Fixa' come è definita dagli ippocratici stessi, col significato di una scienza razionale, basata su di un dottrinario, frutto di studi, di ragionamento e di esperienza.

A questa famiglia di medici si dovette il retto esercizio ufficiale della medicina che i contemporanei lodarono ed ammirarono.

Stretti nell'unità del ceppo famigliare, questi Asclepiadi costituirono la vera scuola, legati dal vincolo di una sacralità di culto famigliare che ne costituiva una specie di religione, di segrete conoscenze dottrinarie e di attuazioni pratiche, inibita agli estranei fino a che Ippocrate, con l'espediente dell'istituto dell'adozione non ne permise l'ammissione con la stipulazione di un atto legale e il vincolo sacro di un giuramento.

Ebbe così origine una vera medicina di scuola, con il suo 'corpus' dottrinario, con le sue leggi morali e scientifiche, con un unico criterio di interpretazione definito 'razionale' basato su le leggi di natura che regolavano la costituzione e il funzionamento dell'umano organismo in sè, in quanto connesso con l'ambiente ed in relazione stretta tra psiche e materia.

Fu, questa mirabile concezione, assai ammirata dalle menti superiori dell'epoca, tanto da divenire parametro di ragionamento da un Socrate, un Platone, un Aristotele i quali lo trasportarono in campo di politica, sociologia, di giurisprudenza, di filosofia.

Ora, la stessa denominazione di Asclepiadi ha generato confusione (come ho accennato) tra i sacerdoti degli asclepiei e gli appartenenti alla famiglia di Asclepio e quasi si son volute vedere scuole mediche, in questo senso così nobile dove, come vedemmo, si esercitava una medicina miracolistica.

Ben differente l'esercizio dell' una e dell'altra. Probabilmente, tuttavia, unico può essere stato il ceppo, dal quale, a un certo punto, un ramo si potè essere staccato, seguendo la parte culturale che fu inizio della scuola, e l'altra, la parte rituale, forse anche più redditizia, allorchè il culto del proavo Asclepio, ufficialmente divinizzato, ebbe l'onore della erezione di templi frequentati da folle di postulanti.

Accanto a queste due forme di esercizio professionale che abbiamo ora considerato, esisteva una classe di medici empirici.

L'esistenza di una medicina empirica, professata da personale addestrato soltanto da una elementare pratica, è documentata da numerose attestazioni rinvenibili sia da molteplici passi di opere del 'Corpus' sia nell'intero libro della 'Legge' del Corpus stesso, sia in chiari riferimenti di autori non medici quali Platone, Aristotele e altri.

E' Platone specialmente che nel dialogo 'Le leggi' ci presenta al vivo questa classe che distingue dai medici veri con la designazione di 'servi dei medici' dai quali hanno imparato con la consuetudine di vita, alcuni rudimenti di semplice pratica. E ce li dipinge come persone arroganti, indaffarate a correre a curare l'uno e l'altro, assolutisti nelle cure, schivi nel trattare con i pazienti perchè ignoranti della vera medicina.

Peggio ancora ce li dipinge la 'Legge' del 'Corpus': istrioni, ignoranti legati tra loro dalla loro stessa insipienza. Ed è singolare il fatto di ritrovare in questo scritto ippocratico, le stesse invettive scagliate da Plinio contro la 'turba crassantium' dei medici del suo tempo, e il rammarico stesso che non esistano leggi che puniscano i loro misfatti.

Ora è superfluo dedurre da questa indignazione, che l'Autore non se la può prendere contro i medici usciti dalla propria scuola e cioè dagli Asclepiadi, anche perchè nello stesso tempo sono accennati i principi educativi per formare un vero medico conformemente al giuramento cui la 'Legge' appare intimamente legata.

Altra testimonianza dell'esistenza di una medicina empirica è data dalla frase del primo aforisma dove è detto 'experientia fallax' dove a questa parola erroneamente si è attribuita la traduzione di 'esperimento' nel significato moderno e non quella di Aristotele, quando distingueva la 'scientia' dalla 'experientia' col significato di empirismo.

Sorge ora il problema di poter stabilire quando queste tre maniere di esercitare l'arte medica ebbero inizio.

Per quanto riguarda la medicina sacrale essa corrisponde, come dissi, ad un culto solare identificato in Apollo generatore della peste.

I culti solari sono, nella storia dell'umanità, i più antichi e quindi non databili. Più netti riferimenti con la mitologia egiziana (nella identità della formazione della favola di Asclepio e di Imotep) accertano che come collegamenti di cognizioni mediche, dovettero esistere, tra la medicina egiziana e quella greca dell'epoca della Odissea, come indubbi influssi di arte si riscontrano tra i primi templi greci e quelli egiziani, così collegamenti dovettero esistere anche nel culto medico.

Inoltre, l'introduzione nel mondo mitico greco di personaggi 'eroici' appartenenti al mondo minoico, cicladico, egeo con attributi medici, guaritori del tipo di Epimenide di Cnosso, Talete di Cortina, Melampo, Eracle ed altri, fa supporre un confluire di tradizioni preelleniche.

Parimenti difficile è poter definire quando abbia potuto aver origine la medicina empirica, essendo l'empirismo uno degli aspetti essenziali della conoscenza umana solo in seguito organizzata in una classe di esercenti allorchè si affiancò alla medicina ufficiale delle scuole dalla quale trasse quelle cognizioni cui prima ho accennato.

Per quanto concerne il sorgere di quest'ultima, per consenso unanime, sia delle fonti coeve e della storia stessa la quale è l'unico giudice umanamente imparziale ed infallibile nei suoi giudizi, è ad Ippocrate che si riconosce questo merito.

Così attestano Platone, Socrate (per tramite di Platone) Aristotele, Sorano di Coo, Plinio che attinse alle fonti greche-alessandrine e latine, Galeno, Eroziano, Dioscoride, Celso il quale, come Plinio, attinse alle più antiche testimonianze ed infine tutto il mondo culturale del classicismo e di conseguenza tutti gli studiosi delle epoche posteriori.

Senza minimamente dubitare di quanto l'intera storia ha decretato, è sempre lecito di rendersi ragione di come i fatti si siano svolti.

E' più che noto, ed unanime la critica moderna è d'accordo, che la provenienza delle opere del 'Corpus' è alessandrina, i cui bibliotecari raccolsero per ogni dove scritti, appunti, brani, saggi filosofici, relazioni, lezioni, e persino opere appartenenti ad altre scuole anche di contrari indirizzi.

Non sfuggì a quei raccoglitori il fatto di trovarsi in possesso di materiale così eterogeneo e spesso dubbio, onde non esitarono, in una prima cernita inizio di una futura critica, di collocare gli scritti più dubbi, in instanze speciali cui posero l'indicazione di 'ta ex ploion'.

Su questo materiale in seguito lavorarono gli studiosi chiosatori.

Non sta a noi ora, nè sarebbe la sede opportuna, ripercorrere le vie compiute da gli studiosi ippocratici antichi e moderni per giungere a conclusioni (che del resto possono essere sempre opinabili) su la attendibilità o meno degli scritti del 'Corpus' in quanto a genuina provenienza del maestro.

Uno spiraglio, tuttavia, sembra potersi dire aperto, dalla scoperta fatta del papiro greco detto 'L'anonimo londinese' il quale riporta le opinioni dei più antichi medici circa la natura delle malattie, Ippocrate compreso.

Orbene, è con non poca meraviglia che si può notare come unanime fosse il consenso di medici anche anteriori ad Ippocrate, di scorgere nel fattore alimentare e nel conseguente digestivo, la causa patologica.

Così si esprimono Eurifone, Erodico di Cnido, Alcamone di Abido, Timoteo di Metaponto, Erodico di Selimbria ed altri.

Ippocrate si inserisce in questa schiera aggiungendo che dai 'residui' dei cibi, oltre i 'mali succi' indiziati da gli altri, si generano anche i 'venti' e che sono questi i veri responsabili delle malattie.

E' chiaro che da qui sorge il concetto della medicina 'pneumatica' onde Ippocrate fu definito in antico, non il medico umoralista, ma il fondatore della medicina pneumatica.

Nella collezione delle opere contenute nel 'Corpus' una ve ne è che rispecchia in pieno queste idee ed è il 'De prisca medicina', opera dedicata alla dieta e poi ripresa con ampliamenti e completamenti e dottrinari dell'autore dei tre libri della dieta.

La perplessità consiste nel constatare la esiguità dei concetti che furono a base di tutta la dottrina ippocratica ed una specie di piatto inserimento col solo aggiungersi della produzione dei 'flati' ad una comune accezione dell'idea patogenetica vigente a quel tempo.

Della autenticità delle idee riportate dall'Anonimo, ci è garante Platone il quale, facendo dissertare di medicina il suo Timeo, ripete gli stessi concetti, mentre della autenticità del 'De prisca medicina' ci è garante il ritrovare in essa gli stessi concetti dell'Anonimo.

Tale fu l'inizio della dottrina ippocratica, e già Polibio, come lo stesso Anonimo riporta, ne perfeziona e ne completa le idee.

Ma Ippocrate fu l'anima della medicina stessa, fu il creatore di una scuola cui infuse la sua forza di pensiero, sì che la scuola fu lui e lui la scuola, cui egli dette lo spirito vitale sufficiente per valicare vittoriosamente, venticinque secoli di storia.

G. Sacino
Barletta (Italy)

La professione medica in epoca romana

'Salus publica suprema lex' 'Il passato si trova e non s'inventa'

S. DE RENZI

Plinio afferma che per tutto il tempo che decorse dalla fondazione di Roma (754 av.C.), fino all'arrivo del primo medico straniero, Arcagato (219 av.C.), i Romani stettero senza medici, se non senza medicina.

Di contro, Dionigi di Alicarnasso, lo storico e retore greco vissuto nel I sec. av.C., asserisce che anche prima della venuta del suddetto medico peloponnesiaco altri medici erano esistiti nella città. In una pagina della sua 'Storia antica di Roma' (IX–70) egli, infatti, scrive che nell'anno 453 av.C., in occasione di una pestilenza, furono tanti i morti che 'non bastavano ai malati i medici'; e, poco più oltre, aggiunge che 'molte famiglie, per scarsezza di curanti, furono distrutte'.

Ad un accurato vaglio di queste due opinioni, sicure entrambe, ma così differenti tra di loro, quella del grande Naturalista romano, che pure merita di essere tenuta nel debito conto, appare intessuta d'incongruenze e di contradizioni, in conseguenza del fatto che se è vero – com'è vero – che nell'elenco dei Collegi istituiti da Numa Pompilio non figura alcun collegio di medici, e che la medicina al tempo della Roma dei Re e della Repubblica non aveva al suo servizio medici pubblici, provenienti da scuole d'insegnamento ed ufficialmente riconosciuti dallo Stato, è altrettanto vero che in quelle remote epoche vi erano persone che s'intendevano di praticare le cure (quali che esse fossero!) a chiunque ne avesse bisogno: è norma inderogabile che dovunque vi sono malati, là vi debbono essere, per necessità, persone capaci di prestare la loro opera per tentare di debellare il male.

Non meno ambigua della precedente, si è appalesata, alla luce della critica moderna, l'affermazione di Dionigi, scritta in un'epoca in cui i medici erano già venuti a Roma. Infatti, non v'è da credere che quelli che egli chiama col nome generale di medici e poco dopo indica col semplice appellativo di 'curanti', fossero medici nel senso ufficiale dell'espressione.

In massima parte, essi erano medicastri, mestieranti volgari, impostori, che applicavano rimedi di oscuri e bizzarri effetti, e medicamenti, in parte magici, in parte derivati dalla loro fantasia.

Persone, cioè, che s'intendevano sopratutto di medicare e che, occasionalmente si erano dedicate all'esercizio della medicina, profittando della caotica situazione che s'ingenera durante una pestilenza.

Per lo più, era gente di bassa condizione, simile all'artigiano, praticona di cure in generale per una specie di tradizione terapeutica, che fra le altre cose, non apparteneva al numero dei cittadini romani di nascita e che proveniva dalla Siria, dall'Egitto, e specialmente, dalla Grecia. Gente, per la verità, abbagliata dalla luce del nascente splendore della città dei Quiriti, che emigrava dalla propria terra in cerca di migliore fortuna.

Veri e propri periodeuti, come si nota, che in nulla si differenziavano dagli stregoni, dai fattucchieri, dagli empirici tutto fare e dai ciarlatani di piazza, i quali forniti di abbondante coraggio e di altrettanta avidità di lauti guadagni, giravano per le vie di Roma anteponendo alla teoria l'esperienza pratica e vendendo, con profitto, filtri amorosi, medicamenti abortivi, belletti per le donne da postribolo, unguenti lenitivi per atleti e gladiatori.

Gli epigrammi di Marziale contro il medico Simmaco che andò a visitarlo ed i pungenti strali di Plauto e di Giovenale contro questi briganti, sono chiara testimonianza della loro crassa ignoranza, della loro boria, e del loro difettoso comportamento morale nella società romana.

Tipico rappresentante di questa ciurma, fu Arcagato, figlio di Lisania, famoso, invero non sappiamo ancora bene se più per la sua non comune destrezza nello squarciare il corpo dei cittadini romani o per la sua glaciale insensibilità verso di essi. All'inizio, com'è noto, questo carnefice venne esaltato, poi, ben presto, fu ignominiosamente cacciato, e, forse, linciato addirittura.

Quanto sin qui detto, non deve meravigliare, in quanto, in quell'arco di tempo, la medicina altro non era che una semplice raccolta, disordinata e stereotipata di nozioni empiriche che provenivano dal vicino popolo etrusco e che si tramandavano oralmente senza che venissero insegnate in qualche scuola.

D'altro canto, chiunque, in quel tempo, era mosso dall'ardente sete di guadagno (piaga di ogni tempo e di ogni luogo!), poteva esercitare liberamente la nobile arte d'Ippocrate. Per professarla non occorreva alcun permesso superiore, nè si teneva in alcun conto l'intervento dello Stato, che allora, ignorava qualsiasi forma di controllo sull'attività professionale mediante esami. Bastava che qualsiasi persona si spacciasse come medico e già poteva darsi all'esercizio sanitario. Occorrerà attendere l'epoca di Silla, per vedere promulgata nel IV secolo la legge Aquilia, che puniva l'ignoranza e le sue disastrose conseguenze. A ciò, s'aggiunge il fatto che il cittadino romano, nato per gl'immediati bisogni della guerra e per il rispetto delle patrie tradizioni, non intendeva affatto occuparsi di un'arte esercitata in modo così avvilente da una simile accolita di avventurieri, sedicenti medici.

Conseguenza inevitabile di tale andazzo, fu che la medicina non era molto quotata in quei remoti tempi.

Ma, dopo quanto sin qui detto, non v'è a credere che l'esercizio della medicina nell'antica repubblica poggiasse solamente sulla pratica empirica.

Particolare appoggio esso trovò anche nel suggestivo fascino della religione che, a quanto sembra, bene si adattava all'ingenua mentalità di quella rozza ed altera schiatta, la quale, credente nel superstizioso lasciato in eredità dai primitivi popoli italici, riteneva che tutti i mali fossero castighi e flagelli delle divinità, onde rimedi più efficaci non potevano essere che soltanto le preghiere, i sacrifici, gli scongiuri.

Fu questa loro cieca credenza nel soprannaturale e nel mistico, che, all'inizio, dette ampio sviluppo alla medicina teurgica o jeratica.

Praticata nell' 'aedes sacra' o 'fanum' degli Asclepiadi di Asclepio, essa rappresentava qualcosa di più del concetto di casta, qualcosa che andava al di là del concetto aristocrate nel senso della leggenda.

Nell'esercitarla, i sacerdoti di Esculapio la poggiavano oltre che sull'elemento soprannaturale e su di un vasto senso di meraviglioso anche sull'interpretazione mistica di qualsiasi profilassi e terapia, sul miracolo da invocare nel momento dell'insorgenza di ogni male, specialmente, sull' 'incubatio', atto religioso, che, forse, nessun beneficio recava al malato se non quello di procurargli l'illusione di una immediata guarigione o di una risoluzione del male di là da venire.

Una numerosa serie di formule speciali, di pratiche curative bizzarre, di strani gesti e di procedimenti tratti dall'astrologia e dalla magia, completavano il loro compito.

Ma, la medicina sacrale non ebbe lunga vita. Pure essendosi rivelata di qualche utilità reale, come provano la grande quantità di ex voto d'iscrizioni, e di donaria rinvenuti fra i suoi ruderi, col passare dei secoli, tramontava in Roma lo splendore degli aedes Aesculapi, che, per lungo tempo erano valsi, forse, ad illudere la buona fede degl'ingenui romani. Templi e case andarono man mano scomparendo, e si ridussero ad un lurido luogo di raccolta di schiavi, di malati buttati in quegli squallidi carnai dai padroni di casa, che si volevano liberare del peso si qualche servo malato.

Maggiore credito, a quanto ci è dato supporre, riscosse, per la componente affettiva egoistica che aveva alla sua base, la medicina 'patriarcale'. Era praticata comunemente dai 'paterfamilias', i quali secondo quel che può desumersi dagli scritti di M. P. Catone, il 'De medicina domestica', disgraziatamente perduto, ed il 'De re rustica', dovevano comportarsi non soltanto da sacerdoti, censori, amministratori edili, rappresentanti politici della gens, ma anche da medici, qualora la necessità lo richiedesse.

Da quei suddetti opuscoli del tipo dei moderni vade mecum, si rileva che quella da loro esercitata, era 'una medicina alla buona, quasi in pantofole, che si riduceva per lo più, alla medicina del vino, del cavolo, dell'aceto' (Puma), delle lesioni traumatiche, delle fratture, delle coliche in generale, dell'occlusione dei vasi del fegato, della milza, ed anche del cancro (?) 'Una medicina paciaccona da racconti biblici, edulcorata ed adattata al gusto di certe pubblicazioni tendenti a ridurre tutto lo scibile medico terapeutico ad un solo arsenale di soli digestivi, analgesici, ansiolitici' (Puma).

Se la medicina patriarcale, vera medicina sui generis, bene si adattava alla mentalità del ceto medio e del popolino di rango inferiore, non poteva soddisfare, invece, quella dei nobili romani.

Ad essi, superbi com'erano per natura, ripugnava l'idea che tutti quei medicastri, e con loro, i paterfamilias, i sacerdoti di Esculapio dovessero all'occorrenza interessarsi alla salute pubblica o a quella dei propri congiunti.

In caso di malattia, essi ricorrevano all'opera degli schiavi o 'medici domestici seu familiares seu captivi seu servi a valetudinario egizi, siriaci, elleni, che come si rileva dalla letteratura, dall'epigrafia e da alcune leggi romane, abbondavano nell'antica Roma, per il fatto che l'esercizio sanitario era considerato indegno per il cittadino romano. Questi, infatti, non ammetteva mai che un uomo azzimato e togato, qual'era il civis romanus, dovesse trascorrere intere giornate in una botteguccia a preparare unguenti per i gladiatori, beveraggi amorosi per le donne di postribolo, o a praticare salassi.

'All'epoca della Roma repubblicana, l'ars sanandi, era per lo più, nelle mani di costoro o meglio alla mercè delle famiglie patrizie, che secondo il costume di quei tempi, avevano cura d'istruirli, di accrescerne le loro cognizioni di medicina iscrivendoli ad una scuola d'insegnamento privato di medicina, per poi rivenderli, come c'informa Platone, a prezzi molto elevati per la vasta conoscenza dimostrata da essi nell'arte di sanare'.

Così affrancati, divenivano liberti o 'medici manumissi'.

Con questo nuovo titolo, essi potevano esercitare liberamente la professione senza temere alcun controllo del governo. Ciò malgrado, nel praticarla, essi facevano a gara fra di loro per portare ad un più alto livello la medicina, considerata, allora, degna di un operaio. Ne è prova sicura, la singolare abilità professionale dimostrata da A. Musa, che, da schiavo, divenuto, poi, liberto, seppe conquistarsi onori e fama per avere ridato la vita ad Augusto, colpito da una severa malattia di fegato dopo il ritorno, nel 23 av.C., da una spedizione militare. Oltre che di questa libertà, essi godevano anche dell'ambita cittadinanza dello 'jus quiritum', venivano esonerati dalle pesanti tasse: dovevano, però, rispettare talune norme.

A quanto sembra, i modesti effetti della loro opera svolta sia in privato sia nell'ambito della vita romana, non tardarono a farsi sentire in un momento molto difficile per l'esercizio della medicina. Col volgere dei secoli, infatti, la professione medica assunse, sia pure molto lentamente, un nuovo aspetto e venne tenuta in maggiore considerazione dagli stessi cittadini romani, i quali, come ben dice il Pazzini, non esitarono più a vedere in essa 'un vile mestiere ma l'espressione di un'arte vera e propria'.

Chiara testimonianza di questa sua riabilitazione, ci offrono non solamente le numerose citazioni di medici generici, di medici schiavi, liberti, che si trovano nella letteratura, nell'epigrafia, nelle leggi di Roma ma anche l'opinione del divino oratore arpinate, che, in vari punti delle sue maggiori opere 'De Divinatione', 'Tusculanae I', 'De Officiis I, 42', include la medicina fra le 'artes honestae'. Non poca è la meraviglia che in lui si suscita, allorquando egli constata che già, a quel tempo, andavano istituendosi scuole d'insegnamento della medicina e comparendo medici che precorsero la specializzazione in maniera tanto perfetta. Vi erano, infatti, chirurghi che praticavano la paracentesi, l'estrazione della pietra, la plastica delle palpebre affette da ectropion, e con loro, quelli che si dedicavano alle malattie della testa, quelli che operavano la cataratta, le fistone in generale, gl'internisti, ed infine, gli odontojatri, la cui tecnica, in questo campo, raggiunse, talvolta, tanta perfezione e precisione, da vederne preparate non poche a perfetta regola d'arte.

E non basta. Ulteriore prova della sua maggiore reputazione, ci viene data, sopratutto, da un più vivo interessamento dell'autorità governativa nella disciplina dell'esercizio sanitario. Infatti, in breve spazio di tempo, i medici vengono ad emanciparsi prima dallo stato di schiavi, e, poi di liberti; diventano 'cives pleno jure'. Negli ultimi tempi del basso impero, anche se insorgono invidie, rivalità, inimicizie fra i medici per sopraffarsi, per brillare a qualunque costo, anche a prezzo di veleno o di sangue, la loro dignità acquista maggiore rispetto, e si completa fino al punto da raggiungere lo stato di 'primus inter pares' ed il titolo di 'praesulis spectabilis, perfectissimus vir, clarissimus vir'.

Oltre a tali privilegi, viene loro concesso il diritto di fare parte della nobiliare 'comitiva primi ordinis', la loro personalità trova posto nel 'Corpus Juris Justinianaei', e, quel che più conta, è il fatto che viene loro conferito il titolo di 'Archiatra'.

Com'è noto, il titolo di 'archiatra' era assai comune all'epoca di Costantino

(II–III sec.d.C.). Sin da quel tempo, costituiva e rappresentava una categoria di Medici bene definita, anche se non sappiamo con certezza quale significato e quale validità avesse tale titolo prima d'allora. Pare, che quello riferito da Galeno per Andromaco corrispondesse al 'superpositus medicorum' dell'epigrafia del tempo dei Flavi.

Gli Archiatri si dividevano in 'Palatini' ed in 'Popolari'.

Quelli 'Palatini' erano Medici con la lettera Maiuscola, e, generalmente venivano nominati dal governo, il quale provvedeva a fornire loro le ricompense e gli onori derivati dalla loro carica. La loro scelta, il loro numero, l'avanzamento nel grado, spettavano unicamente all'arbitrio del sovrano, nelle cui grazie dovevano subito entrare dopo avere ricevuto il suo beneplacito. Dovevano provvedere non soltanto alla sua salute, ma anche a quella dell'intera famiglia imperiale e di tutte le persone addette al disbrigo dei vari uffici nella corte.

Nel 'concistorium principis', corrispondente al Consiglio di Stato dei nostri tempi, essi occupavano il primo posto, ed al pari di tutti gli altri ufficiali superiori conviventi nella regia, godevano della 'comitiva primi ordinis', che era il massimo grado della nobiltà e della carriera professionale.

Godevano di molti privilegi, tra cui l'auxilium restitutionis con il quale avevano diritto al risarcimento danni subìti dai loro beni durante la loro assenza per servizio militare o per accompagnare l'imperatore nelle spedizioni di guerra. Venivano anche esonerati dal pagamento delle tasse (piaga di tutti i tempi!). Non potevano, però, assumere incarichi civili al di fuori della regia (Codex l. x, tit. LXIV) e nè offrire ospitalità ai militari di transito per la città. Fatto di rilevante importanza, è che nessun tribunale poteva citarli, o spiccare loro mandato di cattura per arrestarli. Nessuno, poi, poteva offenderli: se ciò, qualche rarissima volta, accadeva, il trasgressore veniva punito con grave pena e con ammenda pecuniaria elevata dal giudice competente, che elaborava un'istruttoria del tutto particolare, atta ad assicurargli la piena libertà.

Raggiunti i limiti d'età, venivano collocati a riposo dallo Stato, pur conservando sempre il titolo di 'ex archiatra'. Un apposito 'Collegio degli Archiatri', provvedeva alla loro sostituzione, dopo un profondo sondaggio delle capacità professionali del nuovo candidato.

Rispetto agli Archiatri palatini, maggiore interesse storico presentano quelli Popolari, per l'obbligo che avevano d'insegnare anche la medicina, per questo chiamati 'Archiatri Scolastici' secondo la dizione del Brian, inclusa, successivamente, con pari termine da S. Reinach nel *Dictionnaire des Antiquités* di Daremberg e Saglio s.v. 'Archiater'.

Che questo compito spettasse loro, lo prova una legge di Costantino inserita nel Codice di Giustiniano (l. x, t. LII, lex VI) in cui gli Archiatri popolari sono messi alla pari con i grammatici, con i professori di lettere (esercenti letterari), e con i dottori anche nei riguardi di vari provvedimenti, privilegi, esenzioni da oneri fiscali, retribuizione.

Anch'essi, come quelli palatini, godevano di speciali privilegi, come si legge in talune leggi riportate nel Codice di Giustiniano ed in quello di Massimiano, dov'è testualmente scritto che 'Exceptis qui liberolium studiorum antistites sunt et qui medendi cura funguntur, decuriorum decreta, immunitas tribuni potest'. Fra questi benefici, era incluso anche quello che concedeva loro la facoltà di accettare o di rifiutare gli onori concessi dallo Stato per i medici che insegnavano. Tale beneficio, si legge nel Corpus Juris di Teodosio.

Espressioni queste, l'una diversa dall'altra, riportate nel Codice di Giustiniano, molto significative per dimostrare la loro attività didattica ed il loro diritto di essere retribuiti dallo Stato. La prima dice: 'quo facilius liberalibus studiis et memoratis artibus multos instituant'; la seconda: '. . . mercedes etiam et salaria reddi iubemus.'

Com'è noto, essi vennero istituiti nel 370 all'epoca di Valente e di Valentiniano. Corrispondevano ai Medici condotti moden. Per questo, avevano l'obbligo di visitare gratuitamente tutti i cittadini romani poveri, gli artigiani, i piccoli commercianti riuniti in 'collegia corpora comunis', la classe dei coloni 'plebs rustica', che era superiore agli schiavi ma inferiore ai liberti.

Essi non dipendevano dallo Stato, ma dal Municipio, esattamente, come ai nostri giorni. Il Municipio, infatti, proponeva il medico aspirante archiatra; successivamente, il Collegio o 'Ordo Archiatrorum' (da non confondersi con l'Ordine dei Medici, come erroneamente interpreta il Pinto a pagina 90 della sua opera) prendeva in esame il curriculum professionale del candidato, ammettendolo, dopo accurato vaglio, nel suo 'Ordine' vero seminario di tecnica, in cui si cercava di mantenere viva la fiaccola dell'arte medica con la cultura, con la preparazione ferrata, e, sopratutto con la dedizione.

La loro opera professionale, svolta nell'ambito dell'archiatria con notevoli disagi per la pesantezza del lavoro intrapreso, veniva retribuita in parte con denaro versato dall'autorità governativa, in parte con franchigie varie, come ad esempio, l'esenzione da obblighi di cariche pubbliche, dalla legge degli alloggi, dalle ordinarie vie del tribunale in caso di giudizio, dall'arruolamento dei figli nelle file dell'esercito, e dalle tasse. In caso di giudizio o di arresto, evenienza ancora più rara della prima, venivano giudicati con speciali formalità e con talune cautele.

Il loro numero era uguale a quello dei rioni dell'antica Roma: 17. Di questi, 14 per i rioni della città, 1 per la città di Porto, 1 per il Sisto, portico di convegno o scuola addirittura, dove si riunivano filosofi, letterati, uomini di cultura, ed 1 per la Casa delle Vestali. Antonino Pio (66–161 av.C.) portò a 10 il numero di questi esercenti nelle grandi città, a 7 nelle medie, a 5 nelle altre. Anche nelle 'civitates', ampie circoscrizioni dello Stato romano, essi svolgevano la loro attività professionale.

Concludendo, da quanto abbiamo sin qui riferito, emerge chiaramente che l'esercizio della medicina, praticato da quei nostri Colleghi antenati nella città dei Quiriti, pur sorto da umili origini ed in stato di schiavitù, di scarsezza di serietà professionale, di coerenza morale cristiana, e, sopratutto, di preparazione, di onestà, di dignità e di umanità, con il trascorrere dei secoli, si nobilitò, come provano la concessione della cittadinanza romana ad essi fatta all'epoca di Giulio Cesare ed i vari clamorosi onori, di cui resta tipico quello di una statua eretta sul Campidoglio ad Antonio Musa. Poi, un po' per volta, la dignità della classe sanitaria aumenta, vengono le alte cariche a corte, fattiva si fa l'ingerenza del Medico palatino negli affari di politica, sino a quando la professione medica assurge a così alto prestigio da penetrare in tutti gli strati della società romana con una varia gamma di Medici dei nobili, dei ricchi, dei poveri, dei ginnasi, dei gladiatori, e, finanche, dell'esercito e delle navi.

Ma, fatto ancor più interessante, è che sin da quei remoti tempi, la 'Città dei barbari' mirò, con i mezzi allora a sua disposizione, a tutelare la persona e la professione sanitaria; sin da quell'epoca, infatti, i Medici rappresentarono una classe salvaguardata dalla legge, circondata, non raramente, dalla stima e dalla fiducia dei cittadini romani, sino a rivestire, nell'età imperiale, le più alte cariche dello Stato.

Ultima privilegiata posizione sociale da essi raggiunta, fu quella di vedersi inseriti nella società con l'alto onore di avere una più giusta legislazione, ufficialmente riconosciuta: condizione più favorevole di questa, non poteva essere loro concessa.

H. M. Koelbing
Zurich (Switzerland)

Professional ethics in the writings of some early modern surgeons (sixteenth to eighteenth centuries)

SUMMARY

In the early modern period, the bulk of practical medical work in European countries lay in the hands of surgeons. These were primarily craftsmen, held in low esteem by the learned physicians and at the same time exposed to the reckless competition of quacks. Therefore, responsible surgeons – e.g. Pierre Franco (*c.* 1504–78), Fabricius Hildanus (1560–1634), Lorenz Heister (1683–1758), William Cheselden (1688–1752), Thomas Kirkland (1722–98) – endeavoured fervently to raise professional standards and to establish lines of conduct that were in keeping with the importance of the surgeon's task and would, at the same time, enhance and maintain his social status.

From the end of the Middle Ages until 1800, even in advanced countries the bulk of medical practice lay in the hands of surgeons, not of physicians. The surgeons were primarily craftsmen; they were held in low esteem by the learned doctors and had to struggle hard for professional recognition – hence the famous statement of an English surgeon at John Hunter's death (1793): 'He alone made us gentlemen.'[1] On the other side, they were exposed to the reckless competition of all kinds of empirics, bloodletters, itinerant stonecutters, oculists, etc. Responsible surgeons, therefore, endeavoured to raise professional standards – in terms of knowledge, of technical skill and of conduct – in order to make their art and the men who practised it respectable and reliable. If such a surgeon wrote a textbook or published his medical observations, his aim was not just to give technical instruction or scientific information; his purpose was as much to state what good surgery was like and how a good surgeon should behave in order to be recognized as such by profession and laity. Therefore, in many surgical writings of the sixteenth, seventeenth and eighteenth centuries, ethical considerations play an important part. The most notable example of this I know is Lorenz Heister's *Chirurgie* of 1719,[2] but I shall try and give you some additional instances, too.

Let us begin with a Frenchman: Pierre Franco, born around 1504 in Turriers-en-Provence. He came to Switzerland as a Calvinist refugee and died in Lausanne in 1578.[3] Franco was certainly the most experienced cataract surgeon of his time, and an extremely skilled operating surgeon in general. For instance, he did the first suprapubic cystotomy in operating for vesical calculus (sectio alta) in the case of a ten-year-old boy when he could not seize the stone by the ordinary, perineal approach. But although he was, of course, very happy with the success of his bold intervention in what seemed to be a hopeless situation, he was far from recommending the procedure he had invented: the risk of general complications (in our terms: of peritonitis) would be too great; the traditional perineal technique was safer.[4] Safety, not brilliance or novelty, is, for Franco, the hallmark of good surgery.

For the sake of his patients' safety and also, but clearly to a lesser degree, in the interest of the operating surgeon's reputation, Franco deplores the fact that doctors, and even many surgeons leave the most difficult form of medical treatment, namely the major surgical interventions such as lithotomy, herniotomy or cataract couching, to ignorant mountebanks, even impostors. He admits that the reluctance of physicians and respectable surgeons to undertake interventions which may turn out fatally is to some extent understandable: '. . . s'il advient que un patient meure entre les mains du *médecin*, il est toujours excusé en partie. Aussi est l'*appothicaire*. Le *chirurgien* qui ne exerce ceste partie, est aussi excusé aucunement. Mais nous, si ce qu'aurons entrepris ne succède toujours si heureusement qu'on voudroit . . . *on nous appellera meurtriers et bourreaux*, avec contrainte bien souvent de gaigner les champs: ne considérant point que Dieu l'a ainsi préveu. . . .'[5]

But in spite of these risks, well-trained and responsible surgeons have the duty to operate, and learned physicians must have, at least, such knowledge of surgical conditions and techniques as to be able to judge for themselves whether an operation is indicated at all and whether, if it is indicated and done, it is done properly. We might put it like this: It is Pierre Franco's conviction that *every member of the medical profession is to some extent responsible for the state of the whole of medical practice in the community at large*. In the second place only, he appeals to the political authorities that they protect their people from incapable and dishonest empirics.

Half a century later than Franco and for quite different, purely professional reasons, a German surgeon came to Switzerland and settled here: Fabricius Hildanus (Wilhelm Fabry von Hilden, 1560–1634), who became eventually City Surgeon (Stadt-Wundarzt) of Berne.[6] (At all times, Swiss prosperity, intellectual as well as economical, depended considerably upon immigrants!) For Fabricius, very much as for Franco, the basis of professional ethics is the Christian belief that you are responsible before God for all your dealings with your fellow-men. In practical terms, the worst flaws of a practitioner, the very signs of irresponsibility, are ignorance and avarice. Much more than Franco, however, Fabricius Hildanus stresses the *obligation of political authorities* to promote the training of good practitioners and to prevent malpractice by incompetent empirics including the more vulgar variety of Paracelsians '[die] falschen, verlogenen und unerfahrenen Chymisten'.[7] In a letter of 1618 to Philibert Sarrazin (Philibertus Sarazenus), a Genevan physician practising in Lyons, he complains of the medical activity of the hangman of Berne, who had treated in one instance a respectable woman with a potion that did her no good at all but caused her violent headache and blindness. (This may well have been an attack of acute glaucoma precipitated by a mydriatic.) The case was made still worse by the patient's refusal to accept what Fabricius himself believed to be the supreme remedy for eye disorders: the truly sight-saving seton in the neck (Haarseil). 'What do you say, please', he asks his learned friend, 'of these men that sink to such – shall I call it imprudence or negligence? – that even here and in the neighbouring most splendid States they authorize not only the most inexperienced and incompetent people but also the filthiest hangmen to practise medicine and surgery and apply internal and external remedies without any restriction?' – 'You see, my dear Sir, how mighty the Prince of Darkness is, so that he even may strike with blindness the mental eyes of those who should give light to all . . .'.[8]

During the next hundred years, the picture of surgical practice as a playground for irresponsible and avaricious ignorants did not, at least in Germany, change very much. This is testified by the complaints of Lorenz Heister (1683–1758) in the preface to his textbook *Chirurgie*. (Although the 'Vorrede' to the first edition is dated – in the second edition of 1724 – 1 October 1718, the book, according to the title-page, came off the press only in 1719!) Heister himself, M.D. and professor of anatomy and surgery at the universities of Altdorf near Nürnberg and later of Helmstedt (Braunschweig), united in his person medical learning and surgical craftsmanship. Surgery was to him a science (Wissenschaft) as well as a craft (Kunst). The ideal surgeon, as he emerges from his book, is an educated man, who reads Latin and French, and already his appearance, his manners as well as his clothing, show him trustworthy: 'Es soll sich auch ein Chirurgus allezeit manierlich und suber, so wohl in seinen Geberden als Kleidung verhalten.'[9]

The difficult question of *the surgeon's truthfulness* is repeatedly discussed in Heister's book. On the whole, Heister states, the surgeon should keep to the truth as much as possible; he should neither exaggerate the gravity of a case in order to enhance his own importance, nor conceal the real dangers of a disease, an injury or an operation from the patient's friends. On the other hand, he must by no means deprive the patient himself of his hope – 'dieweilen durch die allzu grosse Kümmernuss und Furcht die Sache nur schlimmer wird, durch die Hoffnung aber kein Schaden noch Uebel verursachet werden kann.'[10] Thus, the surgeon has to care for the *emotional well-being* of his patients as well as for their physical safety.

If we turn now to the remarks on surgical practice that Heister's contemporary William Cheselden (1688–1752) has included in his *Anatomy of the Human Body*, we find a different tone prevailing: the activity of incompetent surgeons is mentioned casually, when Cheselden relates brief examples of mischief done by 'a bold unthinking surgeon' or 'an injudicious blood-letter',[11] but no longer can their existence prejudice the rank and reputation of a first-rate surgeon such as Cheselden himself. So it seems at least, but we must be careful in comparing Cheselden with Heister and take into account the brevity of the former's style and, perhaps, the general English tendency to understatement. Nevertheless, we may take it for granted that not only in France, but also in England, surgery enjoyed, already in the first half of the eighteenth century, a higher status than in Germany.[12]

In the second half of the eighteenth century, operative techniques were so much improved that, according to Thomas Kirkland (1722–98) of Ashby-de-la-Zouch (Leics.), 'almost every one who undertakes the cure of external disorders becomes an expert operator',[13] and this within a year or so. Operative surgery appears now, in 1783, as that field of medical practice where fame and reputation are most easily gained, and Kirkland deems it necessary to warn of the neglect of conservative surgical treatment: 'Every blockhead can amputate a leg; but how much more praise-worthy is he whose skill enables him to effect a cure and preserve the limb?'[14] Really good knowledge of this less spectacular 'medical surgery', however, cannot be acquired without many years' study and experience.

Hardly more than two centuries earlier, Pierre Franco had to tell surgeons that, for the patients' sake, they must operate; now Thomas Kirkland must remind them *not to specialize in operating* – a remarkable change indeed. There is, of course, a common denominator: the insight that the responsible way is not the easiest one.

Responsible conduct includes a particular kind of truthfulness: *the honest self-critical evaluation of success and failure.* In his matter-of-fact way, Cheselden makes this perfectly clear. For instance: 'I have, in three different subjects, taken stones out of the loins, which had made their way from the kidneys through the muscles to the common integuments, where, upon opening the skin only, the stones appeared with a quantity of matter and urine. We have heard of operators who have cut for the stone in the kindeys; but I will venture to affirm that those cases were no other than these, *tho' unfairly related.*'[15] Cheselden himself gives a short, but careful statistical survey of the successes and losses in 213 lithotomies carried out by himself at St. Thomas's Hospital, London, following his own method, the so-called 'lateral operation for stone'.[16] This account may be regarded as an early example of valuable medical statistics, which set an example for the future. But what is more: it is evidence of Cheselden's honesty. And this – I mean *the personal example* – was, and still is the best way to promote professional ethics.

References

1 GARRISON, FIELDING H., *An Introduction to the History of Medicine*, 4th ed. (1929), reprinted 1960, p. 347.

2 See the forthcoming M.D. thesis of Rüdiger Korff (University of Zurich), 'Das Berufsethos des Chirurgen Lorenz Heister'.

3 For the life of Pierre Franco, see Eugène Olivier, *Médecine et Santé dans le Pays de Vaud des origines à la fin du 17e siècle*, 2 vols, Lausanne, 1962; KOELBING, HULDRYCH M., *Renaissance der Augenheilkunde 1540–1630*, Berne and Stuttgart, 1967.

4 FRANCO, PIERRE, *Petit Traité contenant une des Parties principalles de Chirurgie laquelle les Chirurgiens hernières exercent*, Lyon, 1556, reprinted separately by *Revue de Chirurgie*, Paris, 1884.

5 FRANCO, PIERRE, *Traité des Hernies*, Lyons, 1561, new edition with introduction by Edouard Nicaise, Paris, 1895, p. 165 (italics according to original).

6 The most exact account of Fabricius Hildanus' life is given by Erich Hintzsche in *Wilhelm Fabry von Hilden*, Gründlicher Bericht vom heissen und kalten Brand (Hubers Klassiker der Medizin und der Naturwissenschaften, **4**) Bern and Stuttgart, 1965.

7 FABRY VON HILDEN, WILHELM, *Von der Fürtrefflichkeit und Nutz der Anatomy*, new edition by F[riedrich] de Quervain and Hans Bloesch (Veröffentlichungen der Schweizerischen Gesellschaft für Geschichte der Medizin und der Naturwissenschaften, **10**) Aarau und Leipzig, 1936, p. 53, and *passim*.

8 FABRY VON HILDEN, WILHELM, *Opera quae extant omnia*, Frankfurt a.M., 1646, p. 1026, epistola 92, 15 April 1618.

9 HEISTER, LAURENTIUS, *Chirurgie*, Nürnberg, 1719, p. 14.

10 Ibid., p. 17.

11 CHESELDEN, WILLIAM, *The Anatomy of the Human Body* (1st ed., London, 1713), 9th ed., London, 1768, pp. 89, 158. For the life of Cheselden, see Zachary Cope, *William Cheselden*, 1688–1752, Edinburgh and London, 1953.

12 HAESER, H[EINRICH], *Lehrbuch der Geschichte der Medicin*, 2nd ed., Jena, 1853, p. 767: 'Am traurigsten war es um die Chirurgie noch bis zur Mitte des achtzehnten Jahrhunderts in Deutschland bestellt, indem sie sich fast ausschliesslich in den Händen ungebildeter Empiriker befand.' See also Garrison, op. cit., p. 341.

13 KIRKLAND, THOMAS, *An Inquiry into the Present State of Medical Surgery*, 2 vols, London, 1783/86, vol. I, p. 4.

14 Ibid., p. 12 f.

15 CHESELDEN, op. cit. (note 11), p. 260.

16 Ibid., pp. 332–33.

E. Fischer-Homberger
Zurich (Switzerland)

The First World War and the crisis of medical ethics

It is well known that doctors during the First World War did sometimes treat the so-called war-neurotics in an astonishingly inhuman way. War-neuroses included not only hysteroid suffering but more severe shock ('shell-shock') as well. But war-neurotics were all called hysterics (whereby an affinity of hysteria with malingering was admitted) and treated rather brutally with cold water,[1] punishment-drill,[2] denying of leave,[3] provoking of fear,[4] or application of painful electric currents[5] which occasionally led to death.[6] When the patients then preferred returning to the front instead of undergoing further medical care this was considered proof of the treatment's success.[7] Sending the patients back to the front was in itself considered a good treatment of war-neurosis.[8] It is therefore not surprising that when in November 1918 revolution broke out among the German soldiers many doctors had to flee from their former patients.[9] In Austria the electric treatment of war neurotics caused the so-called Wagner-Jauregg Prozess after the war (1920). Complaints were received from former military patients against half a dozen neuropsychiatrists, including Wagner-Jauregg. In the expert report which Sigmund Freud had to write on this occasion he accused Wagner-Jauregg and his colleagues for not having defended their patients but having done them wrong during the war.[10]

These events grew out of a fundamental uncertainty about medical ethics. The doctors who mistreated their patients in the First World War did not consider themselves unethical. They just adhered to a new form of medical ethics whose aim it was not to care primarily for the sick individual but for their endangered country. The uncertainty about medical ethics had existed long before the outbreak of the First World War. But it was during that war that for the first time its practical effects became visible on a large scale.

Medical interest for human society had powerfully arisen in the eighteenth century, the age of enlightenment. A systematically hygienic way of thinking was the most important result of this development. Medicine then no longer was concerned merely with isolated individuals in need of medical help, but with whole groups of patients. Even individual problems – as those of children, cripples, soldiers, mothers, and poor people – began then to be viewed as group problems. Consequently, medical care was applied not only to the sick individuals, but to that whole group. Preventive medicine was a logical extension of this concept. Instead of treating innumerable individuals ill of the smallpox, society could be freed from that calamity by prevention. Variolation and Jenner's vaccination are thus true consequences of the enlightenment.

Ethical problems did not arise then. The hygienic care for society was entirely in the interest of all the individuals constituting this society. Sometimes, of course, hygienic measures brought about some restriction of individual liberty. But objections raised on these grounds against hygiene did not appear reasonable. Thus the great enlightenment hygienist Johann Peter Frank said that hygienic measures interfered with individual liberty no more than taking away dangerous toys from children.[11]

During the first half of the nineteenth century the situation remained more or less the same. The sanitary movement in England and the medical reform in Germany brought no grave ethical problems.[12] It still seemed evident that hygiene was not contrary to anybody's individual interest. It must be kept in mind how wretched and precarious the hygienic situation was at that time. Hygienic measures were able to provoke enormous effects. Even if there occurred unfavourable secondary effects of such measures to the well-being of single individuals – such as a few deaths from vaccination – these were by far outweighed by the tremendous benefits they brought to the majority of others. The success of hygienic thinking gradually convinced doctors that care for society was their ethical duty as well as care for individuals.

This situation changed with the advent of Charles Darwin's theory of evolution. The survival of the fittest was then recognized as being favourable to the species. The succumbing of the feeble in the struggle for life, was recognized as an advantage to a community. In this framework medicine at once seemed but to add to the ruin of the human species. Medicine helped the sick. But were not the most feeble human beings the most prone to sickness? Should not just these be abandoned to their fate for the sake of the human species? Had not hygiene, which was primarily concerned with the well-being of society, to warn against an unreasonable keeping-alive of the feeble?

Alfred Russel Wallace (1823–1913) who had worked out the theory of evolution at about the same time as Darwin, was the first to apply it to human society. And he soon found that human ideals seemed to oppose the aim of evolution: by helping the helpless and curing the sick they opposed the power of natural selection.[13] Francis Galton (1822–1911) who was Darwin's cousin, also applied Darwin's theory to the human species. His practical conclusions made him later on the founder of eugenics. Darwin, in his *Descent of Man* (1871) discussed Wallace's and Galton's views. Human beings used to take care of 'the imbecile, the cripples, and the sick', he wrote. Vaccination 'had preserved thousands who from a weak constitution would formerly have succumbed to smallpox. Thus the weak members of civilized societies propagate their kind. No one . . . will doubt that this must be highly injurious to the race of man.'[14] But, interestingly enough, neither Wallace nor Darwin nor Galton thought that care for the sick and weak should be suppressed on these grounds. Wallace tried to interpret mercy and pity as evolutionary high-level behaviour raising the level of human ethics above the level of nature red in tooth and claw. He therefore saw no need of suppressing it.[15] And Darwin wrote: we could 'not check our sympathy, if so urged by hard reason, without deterioration in the noblest part of our nature. . . . Hence we must bear without complaining the undoubtedly bad effects of the weak surviving and propagating their kind. . . .'[16]

Galton's practical conclusions applied only to promotion of a first-rate offspring. This he called eugenics. He did not consider suppressing feeble contemporaries by eugenic measures.[17] There were, however, 'Darwinians' who did not agree with Darwin as to the social consequences of his system. Thomas H. Huxley (1825–95) for instance blamed his contemporaries for trying to oppose nature and nature's laws in the name of outmoded right and morals. They were not open-eyed enough to see that Darwin's theory was a scientific discovery which necessarily resulted in a revolution of ethics and practical life.[18] Other followers of Darwin took the same view. Thus Darwin's theory became 'Darwinism'. Eugenics became more aggressive towards the sick. This can be said of the German form of eugenics, for instance of German 'Rassenhygiene'.

'Rassenhygiene', racial hygiene, arose towards the end of the nineteenth century with Alfred Ploetz (1860–1940) and Wilhelm Schallmayer (1857–1919). Its way was prepared by the works of the German Darwinian Ernst Haeckel (1834–1919), the poet–philosopher Friedrich Nietzsche (1844–1900) and the economist and politician Alexander Tille (1866–1912). Haeckel helped to encourage Schallmayer by getting him the first prize in a competition on 'Natur und Staat', state and nature, which he had established himself. Tille had translated Nietzsche's 'Thus spoke Zarathustra' into English. This book is, of course, the cradle of the German superman (Uebermensch). He adored Nietzsche and largely based his book on Nietzsche's writings.[19] He severely criticized the English for being too humanitarian to draw the ultimate conclusions from their own knowledge. Galton, Wallace and other English scientists, Tille wrote, were too much biased in favour of the Christian commandment of charity to perceive that the theory of evolution had its impact on ethics too.[20] Darwin's theory called for a new code of ethics ('Das neue Ideal') which Tille called 'Entwicklungsethik' after the English expression 'evolutional ethics'.[21] Evolutional ethics necessarily contradicted traditional humanitarian ethics which concentrate on the individual.[22] Tille was no medical man. But Alfred Ploetz was. Ploetz applied the new thought to medicine, especially hygiene. The word 'Rassenhygiene' was most probably coined by him.[23] Ploetz criticized doctors for doing the contrary of what the theory of evolution required. Clinging to their antiquated humanitarian beliefs originating in Christianity they neglected their duties towards the human species.[24] Treating individuals was not good in itself. Traditional individualistic hygiene did things which resulted in a negative selection and thus acted contrary to the aims of racial hygiene.[25] Discussing war, Ploetz deplored the fact that traditional warfare brought a greater risk for the brave and tough than for the weak.[26] Ploetz was clearly aware of the ethical conflict which this concept would produce for doctors. He saw the solution of this conflict in placing the evolutionary aim above individual well-being.[27]

Willhelm Schallmayer, extensively quoting Nietzsche and Tille, stressed this point.[28] Like Ploetz, Schallmayer paid particular attention to the negative selective effects of modern warfare and of medicine adhering to its traditional ethics.[29] An ethical revolution was to come. Like Huxley, Schallmayer stated that one had not yet drawn practical conclusions from the theory of evolution. The twentieth century, he hoped, would be destined to do so.[30]

But a sound practical reason why the individual patients' welfare should be disregarded by their doctors was still missing. The great project of the race-hygienists could not yet be realized. The majority of doctors were not yet sufficiently motivated to join the new religion. The anger provoked by the traumatic neurotics taking social insurance money instead of working for the country was not sufficient to mobilize enough people to carry out Schallmayer's ethical revolution.[31]

This situation changed rapidly with the onset of the First World War. The epidemic of war-neurosis, shell-shock, etc., which rendered thousands of German soldiers unfit for battle was to be the cause of the change. The classic symptom was trembling, but many other sufferings were diagnosed as 'war-neuroses'. War-neurosis, a descendant of traumatic neurosis was considered a serious threat to the nation, obviously for military but also for economic reasons. For, if all those diagnosed as war neurotics had to receive public indemnity, this would have meant the economic breakdown of the country as well. This aspect of war-neurosis was all the more stressed because a tremendous increase of the collective values of community existence with priority over the value of individual existence was a characteristic of that war. Of course, such a rising of 'social' ethics above 'individual' ethics is a characteristic of wars in general. If it has not been instrumental in starting a war it usually gets instituted during the war. In the 1914–18 war other reasons reinforced the arrangement. Social Darwinism in its popularized aggressive forms played a considerable rôle in starting and conducting that war. As individuals had to prove themselves worthy to live in the struggle for life, nations had to prove their right to existence in war. For many Germans the First World War was even destined to prove the superiority of the German nation and, correspondingly, its right to expansion.[32] And, since one of the signs of such superiority was the development of social ethics[33] and another was winning the war, there was scarcely an escape from the thought that every German had to sacrifice himself for the nation.

Under the pressure of these political, military and conceptual circumstances, doctors tended to give up traditional individual ethics and to adopt social ethics. They felt themselves cowards and traitors if they gave way to pity for their neurotic patients. They feared to add to the negative selection of war by taking those with nervous breakdowns away from the front. Like Adolf Struempell (1853–1925)[34] and Ernst Kretschmer (1888–1964)[35] they felt they had to become 'educators' of their patients, that their treatment had to be pedagogical. So there was nothing wrong with treatments resembling or being punishment. Besides, 'Darwinian' ethics had resembled ethics of warfare from the beginning. The Swiss psychiatrist Auguste Forel (1848–1931) compared the good doctor to the good officer long before the World War.[36]

Thus the inhuman way in which doctors sometimes treated their patients is less to be viewed as sadistic behaviour or a consequence of ethical decay. Would it have been but this, we would probably lack the extensive discussions leaving the many written documents on which this paper rests. One need not discuss sadism or decay. What one does discuss is a new ethics. And the inhumanity so far described was based on medical ethics becoming dominant at that time. The crisis which medical ethics had started to experience in the nineteenth century had now become manifest. The word 'crisis' can be understood in different ways. It can mean upset or turning-point. In which sense did medical ethics undergo a crisis in the First World War?

People took different views after the war. The discussions about ethics were lively then. Some upheld evolutionary or social ethics. Their efforts, unfairly but somehow inevitably[37] politicized, eventually led to the medical murders which took place during the Second World War in Germany[38] for instance. In Soviet Russia which became an independent social system during the First World War the new kind of ethics now called 'socialistic ethics', are accepted to this day. Hippocratic ethics are considered an antiquated form of medical ethics. There too the ethical concept has been invaded by politics. Being a political activist is a foremost duty of a doctor in a communist country.[39]

Other people, such as Oskar Hertwig (1849–1922),[40] Robert Gaupp (1870–1953)[41] and Ernst Mayer[42] of Berlin, took the First World War crisis for a perturbation and pleaded for a return to traditional ethics after the war.[43] Traumatic neurosis played an important rôle in the ethical discussions between the two wars, as war neurosis had been important in the ethical developments during the war.[44]

Today we too usually adopt traditional individualistic ethics, especially when looking at the German and Soviet experiments. But we should be aware that the old unhappy alternative of individualistic ethics *versus* social ethics might emerge again in a new situation. An empirical answer based on two cases will perhaps not be sufficient then. We should by that time know also theoretically why we have decided for the dominance of individualistic ethics. This will help us to give our answer before politicians have given it for us.

ACKNOWLEDGEMENTS

I should like to thank Professor E. H. Ackerknecht, my parents and Mr. James M. Walsh, C.M.G., O.B.E., former British Consul General, for their help in translating this paper.

References

1 FORSTER, E., 'Hysterische Reaktion und Simulation', *Mschr. Psychiat. Neurol.*, 1917, **42**, 317.

2 WAGNER, 'Die Dienstbeschädigung bei nerven- und geisteskranken Soldaten', *Z. Ges. Neurol. Psychiat.*, 1917, **37**, 235.

3 FOERSTER, O. (Discussion at the 'Kriegstagung', Munich, 1916), *Verh. Ges. dt. Nervenärzte*, **8**, 167; KRETSCHMER, E., 'Die Gesetze der willkürlichen Reflexverstärkung in ihrer Bedeutung für das Hysterie-und Simulationsproblem', *Z. Ges. Neurol. Psychiat.*, 1918, **39**, 372.

4 MUCK, O., 'Heilungen von schwerer funktioneller Aphonie. (Methode: Erzeugung eines Angstschreis durch vorübergehend endolaryngeal herbeigeführte Kehlkopfstenose.)', Feldärztliche Beilage zur *Münch. med. Wschr.*, **63**, 1916, 441 (193).

5 KAUFMANN, FRITZ, 'Die planmässige Heilung komplizierter psychogener Bewegungsstörungen bei Soldaten in einer Sitzung. Feldärztliche Beilage zur', *Münch. med. Wschr.*, 1916, **63**, 802(354)–804(356); FORSTER, op. cit., 1917, p. 317; WAGNER, op. cit., 1917, pp. 234–35; CIMBAL, WALTER, 'Die Zweck- und Abwehrneurosen als sozialpsychologische Entwicklungsformen der Nervosität', *Z. Ges. Neurol. Psychiat.*, 1917, **37**, 417–18.

6 WAGNER, op. cit., pp. 234–36. Cf. also, FISCHER-HOMBERGER, ESTHER, 'Der Begriff des freien Willens in der Geschichte der traumatischen Neurose', *Clio Medica*, 1971, **6**, 130–31.

7 FORSTER, op. cit., pp. 322–23.

8 NAEGELI, OTTO, *Unfalls- und Begehrungsneurosen* (Neue Deutsche Chirurgie, Bd. 22), Stuttgart, 1917, pp. 154–55; LILIENSTEIN (Discussion at the 'Kriegstagung'), *Verh. Ges. dt. Nervenärzte*, 1916, pp. 178, 182; POENITZ, KARL, *Die klinische Neuorientierung zum Hysterieproblem unter dem Einflusse der Kriegserfahrungen*, Berlin, 1921, p. 24.

9 KRETSCHMER, ERNST, *Gestalten und Gedanken*, Stuttgart, 1963, p. 94.

10 ELLENBERGER, HENRI F., *The Discovery of the Unconscious*, New York, 1970, pp. 470, 837–38.

11 FRANK, JOHANN PETER, *System einer vollständigen medicinischen Polizey*, 3rd ed., Vienna, 1786, vol. 1, pp. xx–xxiii.

12 ROSEN, GEORGE, *A History of Public Health*, New York, 1958, pp. 192 ff.; ACKERKNECHT, ERWIN H., 'Beiträge zur Geschichte der Medizinalreform von 1848', *Arch. Ges. Med.*, 1932, **25**, 61–183 and 'Zur Geschichte der medizinischen Ethik', *Praxis*, 1964, **53**, 578–81.

13 WALLACE, ALFRED RUSSEL, 'Die Entwickelung der menschlichen Racen unter dem Gesetze der natürlichen Zuchtwahl', (first published 1864) in *Beitraege zur Theorie der natürlichen Zuchtwahl*, essays, trans. by A. B. Meyer, Erlangen, 1870, pp. 346–79, esp. pp. 356–57, 375–76.

14 DARWIN, CHARLES, *The Descent of Man and Selection in Relation to Sex*, London, 1871, vol. 1, p. 168.
15 WALLACE, op. cit.
16 DARWIN, op. cit., pp. 168–69.
17 Cf. for instance GALTON, FRANCIS, *Inquiries into Human Faculty and its Development*, London, 1883, pp. 331–37.
18 HUXLEY, THOMAS, *Ethik und Entwickelung. Die Zukunft*, 1893, **4**, 103–10, 167–77.
19 TILLE, ALEXANDER, *Von Darwin bis Nietzsche. Ein Buch der Entwicklungsethik.*, Leipzig, 1895, pp. 210 ff., 231: 'Nicht nur fort sollst du dich pflanzen, sondern hinauf!'; p. 234: 'Und wen ihr nicht fliegen lehrt, den lehrt mir – schneller fallen' (Nietzsche).
20 Ibid., pp. viii–x, 29, 50–52, 74–75, 110–13, 151–52.
21 Ibid., pp. x, 17, 22, 206–41. Cf. also TILLE, ALEXANDER, 'Charles Darwin und die Ethik', *Die Zukunft*, 1894, **8**, 302–14.
22 Ibid., pp. 10, 21, 40, 112–13, 142, 180–205.
23 PLOETZ, ALFRED, *Die Tüchtigkeit unserer Rasse und der Schutz der Schwachen. Ein Versuch über Rassenhygiene und ihr Verhältnis zu den humanen Idealen, besonders zum Socialismus*, Berlin, 1895, p. 5.
24 Ibid., pp. 147, 187–88.
25 Ibid., pp. 2–3, 13, 207–8.
26 Ibid., pp. 61–63, 147.
27 Ibid., p. 13.
28 SCHALLMAYER, WILHELM, *Vererbung und Auslese im Lebenslauf der Völker* (Natur und Staat, 3), Jena, 1903, pp. 152–53, 227, 243.
29 Ibid., pp. 111–21, 146–52, 302–3.
30 Ibid., pp. ix–x.
31 FISCHER-HOMBERGER, ESTHER, 'Ursachen der traumatischen Neurose von der "Railway Spine" bis nach dem Ersten Weltkrieg', *in press*.
32 STRUEMPELL, ADOLF, *Die Schädigungen der Nerven und des geistiges Lebens durch den Krieg*, Leipzig, 1917, p. 3; 'Feldmarschall Hindenburg hat einmal den Ausspruch getan, dass dasjenige Volk den Endsieg erringen werde, welches die besten Nerven habe.' Cf. also, VON SALIS, J. R., *Weltgeschichte der Neuesten Zeit*, 2nd ed., Zürich, 1962, vol. 2, p. 45; ELLENBERGER, op. cit., p. 235.
33 SCHALLMAYER, op. cit., p. 250.
34 STRUEMPELL, op. cit., pp. 4, 15–16, 28.
35 KRETSCHMER, op. cit., 1918, p. 384. Cf. also FORSTER, op. cit., pp. 312–13, 372, 381.
36 FOREL, AUGUSTE, 'Ueber Ethik', *Die Zukunft*, 1899, **28**, 574–87.
37 The socialist Ploetz and the more nationalistic authors Tille and Schallmayer already used their theories to support their political views. Cf. their works mentioned above, also: TILLE, ALEXANDER, 'Deutsche Darwinisten als Sozialethiker', *Die Zukunft*, 1894, **8**, 510–21; AMMON, OTTO, *Der Darwinismus gegen die Sozialdemokratie. Anthropologische Plaudereien*, Hamburg, 1891.
38 Cf. DOERNER, KLAUS, 'Nationalsozialismus und Lebensvernichtung', *Vischr. Zeitges.*, 1967, pp. 121–52.
39 SCHUERER, ELISABETH, *Die Intelligenz in der Sowjetunion*, Berne, 1970, pp. 101–2; ACKERKNECHT, ERWIN H., review of *Das hippokratische Ethos. Untersuchungen zu Ethos und Praxis in der deutschen Aerzteschaft*, Halle, 1967. *Schweiz. Arzteztg.*, 1970, **51**, 834–35.
40 HERTWIG, OSCAR, *Zur Abwehr des ethischen, des sozialen, des politischen Darwinismus*, 2nd ed., Jena, 1921 (first edition 1918).
41 GAUPP, ROBERT, *Die künftige Stellung des Arztes im Volke*, Ansprache an die Studierenden der Medizin der Universität Tübingen, 23 October 1919, Tübingen, 1919, p. 9.
42 MEYER, ERNST, *Die Krisis des deutschen Aerztestandes. Eine soziologische Untersuchung*, Berlin, 1924.
43 There have been, of course, authors of German language who took similar views during and before the war already. Cf. MOLL, ALBERT, *Die ärztliche Ethik*, Stuttgart, 1902, p. 425; GRUBER, MAX, 'Vererbung, Auslese und Hygiene', *Dt. med. Wschr.*, 1909, **35**, 2052; BUMKE, OSWALD, *Ueber nervöse Entartung*, Berlin, 1912, pp. 64–66; ASCHAFFENBURG, GUSTAV (Discussion at the 'Kriegstagung'), *Verh. Ges. dt. Nervenärzte*, 1916, pp. 180–81; STRASSER, CHARLOT, 'Ueber Unfall- und Militärneurosen', *Corr.-Blatt Schweizer Arzte*, **47**, 1917, 273–74.
44 Especially the so-called 'Herrschende Lehre' of Bonhoeffer and His stimulated such discussions. Cf. BONHOEFFER, KARL and HIS, WILHELM, 'Beurteilung, Begutachtung und Rechtsprechung bei den sogenannten Unfallneurosen', *Dt. med. Wschr.*, 1926, **52**, 179–86; RIESE, WALTER (ed.), *Die Unfallneurose*, Stuttgart-Leipzig, 1929; CIMBAL, WALTER, *Die Neurosen des Lebenskampfes*. Berlin-Wien, 1931, p. vii.

R. de Rosa
Karlsruhe (West Germany)

The discipline of the medical profession in the eighteenth-century practice of penance

INTRODUCTION

According to Gilbert Murray a great part of the history of modern medicine is a story of emancipation from the dead hand of Hippocrates and Galen. In our age we may be able to say that this emancipation has been accomplished and that the new methods of research, based on observation and experiment, prevailed definitively. But one little treatise attributed to Hippocrates still expresses the aim of the medical profession in the modern world – the Oath. The Declaration of Geneva, which was adopted after the war by the third General Assembly of the World Medical Association in a mood of purification and regeneration, following one of the most terrible crises of human civilization, accepted the principles of the Hippocratic Oath completely.

Emancipation from tradition in the scientific field and acceptance of it in the moral sector seems also to characterize the medical profession. This sets its members in a very special position of giving a valuable contribution to the solution of the big political problems of modern mass society, where new forms of social control have to replace a vanishing community culture.

The history of medicine considered in a broad sense and not separated from the framework of its social connexions provides the best way of becoming conscious of such a task.

THE EIGHTEENTH CENTURY

The new methods of modern scientific medicine were developed together with the principles of liberalism during the age of enlightenment by the aristocratic society of the eighteenth century. The basic philosophical renewal of the age was produced by a medical scholar, John Locke, who, with his *Essay Concerning Human Understanding* (1690) set the foundation of the empirical epistemology and opened the way to the rational elaboration of experience.

The rationalizing thought of the empiricism passed into France where it was further developed by the Encyclopaedists and spread abroad through the medium of the French language which has superseded Latin as the *lingua franca* of intellectual Europe.

Quesnay, also a physician, stimulated the ideas of Adam Smith on free trade and on the laissez-faire system which, as long as small self-adjusted units governed the field, proved to be efficient and favourable to general progress. The liberal trade-bourgoisie arose. Meanwhile the expropriated lands of the monasteries were granted to a new class of landowners who treated their holdings as a source of revenue rather than as a mark of responsibility.

In this way the social conditions for the development of empirical sciences, free from the influence of scholastics, were established: Thomas Sydenham, a friend of John Locke, published his *Observations on Acute Diseases* (1676) and G. B. Morgagni, eighty-five years later, his splendid work *De Sedibus et Causis Morborum*.

The diminishing authority of the Church was gradually replaced by the authority of science. But science had an aristocratic character and was not in a condition, like religion, to perform an integration of society on deep levels. It had also, because of its theoretical nature, no possibility of becoming a source of any kind of practical process, 'since it has not for its end the good to be attained by action', as Aristotle pointed out. And so, while the laissez-faire system, with its lack of insight into the social background induced increasingly a fatal disintegration, the duty of preserving a certain harmony of valuations, institutions and education, without which society cannot function, was left still to the Church.

As concerning the Catholic Church, which had in many respects maintained a pre-capitalistic and pre-individualistic interpretation of Christianity and was, for this tradition, in a better condition to understand the needs of a social order beyond individualism, an almost universal control was exercised through the practice of penance.

THE DOCTRINE OF CONFESSION

The relief of a burdened conscience by the open acknowledgement of its guilt is an instinct of natural piety and has been often expressed with the help of medical metaphors: Isaiah compares the sinner to a woman with child near the time of her delivery and Origen speaks of the confession as a kind of necessary vomiting after indigestion. The principle of confession became established as a law of nature and was introduced in the ecclesiastical discipline together with the practice of penance.

Penance (poenitentia) has a history of its own and underwent different meanings during the centuries. In the eighteenth century the affirmation of the Council of Trent was valid, penance being 'truly and properly a sacrament instituted by Christ our Lord for the benefit of the faithful to reconcile them to God as often as they shall fall into sin after their baptism.'

In the primitive Church the penance was public and was applied mostly for public offences. According to Gratian a penitent presented himself before the Bishop clothed in sack-cloth with naked feet and eyes cast down on the ground. After the Council of Châlons held in 813 by order of Charlemagne, the private penance was extended to more and more cases until it had become universal with Innocent III, who, at the fourth Lateran Council (1215) with the celebrated Canon known (from the words with which it commences) as the Canon 'Omnis utriusque sexus', ordered general sacramental confession at least once a year. From this date on, secret sins were followed by secret penance, and the purging, rather than the punishing effect of the sacrament was stressed. According to the Catechism of the Council of Trent, to receive the sacrament of penance three things were necessary: (1) sorrow (contritio) for sins committed, along with a purpose to commit them no more; (2) an entire confession (confessio) of all sins committed; (3) the performance of the penance (satisfactio) enjoined by the confession.

Possible satisfactions were, besides fasting, alms, abstinence, the repeating of a certain number of Ave Maria's, Pater Nosters, Credos, the wearing of hair shirts, self-flagellation, etc. The alms referred to whatever might be expended for the benefit of our neighbour: to give money, clothes and food, to furnish personal assistance, to wait on the sick, to pray for the confession of sinners.

The absolution was mostly conceded instantly with tacit understanding that the penance would be forthwith performed.

It was surely not easy for the priests to ensure by confession the immediate guidance and governance of conscience. There were two basic problems: (1) the theoretical study of the moral theology; (2) the practical application of the law in every particular case.

THEORETICAL SOURCES

The theoretical instruction of the confessor required the reading of the Holy Scriptures, the knowledge of all canons, decrees, edicts of the Church and the constant study of the many exegetical and critical works of the Fathers. A systematic arrangement of the immense material was to be found in the special treatises of moral theologists.

One of the most profound and diffused treatises of the eighteenth century was compiled by St. Alfonso de Liguori who also made observations of some psychiatric importance on scrupulosity. St. Alfonso maintained, like the Jesuits, that in doubtful cases a man might follow an opinion, of the soundness of which he was not convinced, provided always that the said opinion were defended by some author of repute (conscientia probabilis).

Such an attitude might give to the Confessor a free area of interpretation. But probability, which had been accepted in the methods of science and medicine, could not be accepted without fail in the moral code of conduct. On the contrary, probability had been increasingly reduced by the Popes, who, like Alexander VII in 1665 and Innocent XI in 1679, had rejected many probable opinions of the Fathers as false, and had narrowed severely the freedom of interpretation. In this way it was possible for authors, following the tradition of Roman law, to give the confessor a very clear code of ethics.

In the treatise of Gury we find a very plain formulation of condemned acts for the medical profession which partially recalls the simplicity of the decalogue.

The doctor sins gravely in the following cases: (1) If he should attempt to treat a serious sickness without adequate competence. (2) If in the case of grave and unusual sickness he does not take extra special care. (3) If he makes use of insufficiently tested medicaments merely to try them out. (4) If, without having adequately diagnosed the case, he dares to use dangerous remedies which could endanger life or limb. (5) If, having recognized the danger in which a sick person is, he does not make himself available to the patient, day or night, and use all means necessary to cope with the sickness. (6) If he does not allow the consultation of other physicians when he should, or if he does call in others more because of his friendship with them than for their medical expertise. (7) Or equally if he calls in other consultants unnecessarily and at great expense to the patient or if he acts on the advice of such consultants when it is contrary to his own opinion. (8) If he continues treatment of a patient merely for the financial gain; making unnecessary visits for which he makes a charge; or if he overcharges for his visits. (9) If to favour friendly chemists he prescribes unnecessary medicines. (10) If he performs or provides the means for an abortion. (11) Finally a doctor is guilty of grave sin if he fails to warn a patient of the seriousness of his illness, so that he may receive the last sacraments.

But for all the clearness of the moral treatises it appeared necessary to give the priests more practical instruction which, being based upon the theoretical conclusions, might better reflect the casuistical situation, the *hic et nunc* of the confession. For this reason and also because the practitioners could have had neither the money to buy nor time to read the voluminous works of moral theology, they were supported in their office by practical manuals which as abridgements of the moral treatises were often compiled in the form of a dialogue between confessor and penitent.

THE PRACTICAL SOURCES

St. Alfonso edited two such abridgements, one in Latin for confessors in general, and one in Italian, more concise, for confessors in rural areas. A famous collection of aphorisms for the practice of confession had been edited after the Council of Trent by Emanuel Sa, a learned Portuguese Jesuit, who taught philosophy at Coimbra. A very popular manual of the eighteenth century was the 'Praxix Confessionalis' of the Capucine Corella, originally in Spanish but soon diffused in Latin.

Corella, following the systematics of the 'Codex Justinani' added to the first part of his manual concerning the usual sins against the precepts, a second part 'About the Obligations Concerning the Sins of Priests, Judges, Advocates and Physicians in their Office', with the aim of instructing the confessor about the special sins of the various professions.

Usually the Penitents preferred to minimize the importance of such professional sins and accused themselves with a very general formula: 'Me accuso de defectibus commissis in meo officio' – 'I accuse myself of the faults committed in my professional state'.

The well-instructed confessor was able to put particular questions and to oblige the penitent to speak the whole truth about his professional transgressions. As an example I quote from Corella's dialogue between confessor and physician:

Physician I confess to having neglected the further study of my art since I qualified as a doctor.

Confessor Even if a doctor had a very good training he is obliged to follow the further development of his art in order to cure adequately difficult diseases for which his early training does not provide. He is also obliged to avoid taking care of too many patients, which would impede his ability to give adequate attention to the patients in his care, and to improve his art by study. Further it is not possible for his conscience to allow him to prolong treatment either for financial gain or because of carelessness.

Physician I confess to having neglected the care of the poor.

Confessor Did you run your surgery in a place where you received a special salary with the obligation to assist the poor? Because in this case you sin more gravely if you do not assist them.
Physician No, my surgery is a private one.
Confessor Was there at the place another physician with said obligation? In this case you were not obliged to take care of the poor, although it would be a duty of piety to assist them in any case.
Physician No, there was no other physician at the place.
Confessor Were the poor then in grave necessity?
Physician Oh yes, indeed.
Confessor Charity obliges the doctor to assist the poor gratis, if they are in great need.

Such a particular social control of the medical profession which was carried out in the time of high religious authority is not possible in a society which is mainly defending individual interests and leaving a final integration to the natural harmony of interests.

The inhibitions determined by the Civil law are insufficient not only because they are based on the mere probability of a proceeding action but also because of the very grave obstacles which the court meets in handling actions against members of the medical profession. In this respect it is regrettable that some '*ethical*' articles regulating the inter-relationship of the members of medical associations have a strong corporative character and represent an undemocratic impediment to a better integration of the medical profession into the community.

Bibliography

ARISTOTLE, *The Nicomachean Ethics* (D. P. Chase), Oxford, 1847.
BINGHAM, J., *Origines Ecclesiasticae*, London, 1840.
BUCKLEY, TH. A., *A History of the Council of Trent*, London, 1852.
BUCKLEY, TH. A., *The Catechism according to the Decree of the Council of Trent*, London, 1852.
GURY, J. P., *Compendium Theologiae Moralis*, Paris, 1851.
LANDON, E., *A Manual of Councils of the Holy Catholick Church*, London, 1846.
LEHMKUHL, A., *Casus Conscientiae*, Freiburg, 1913.
LIGUORI, ST. A. DE, *Theologia Moralis*, Rome, 1767.
LIGUORI, ST. A. DE, *Homo Apostolicus*, Regensburg, 1862.
MORINUS, J., *De Sacramento Poenitentiae*, Paris, 1651.
MURRAY, G., 'The Value of Greece to the Future of the World', in *The Legacy of Greece*, Oxford, Livingstone, 1922.
RUSSEL, B., *History of Western Philosophy*, London, 1946.
ST. THOMAS AQUINAS, *Summa Theologica* (Faucher), Paris, 1887.

I. Veith
San Francisco, California (U.S.A.)

On privileged communication: a comparative study of two medical cases

'and whatsoever I shall see or hear in the course of my profession, as well as outside my profession in my intercourse with men, if it be what should not be published abroad I will never divulge, holding such things to be holy secrets.'[1]

Everyone here will know that this exhortation is a quotation from the Hippocratic Oath. It is one of the few statements that has not been hotly debated as to authenticity or justification. It means in the words of the translator W. H. S. Jones: 'The physician must not gossip, no matter how or where the subject matter for gossip may have been acquired; whether it be in practice or private life makes no difference.'[2]

With this comment, Professor Jones, goes beyond the original injunction. He excludes all manner of gossip from the physician's repertoire of conversation, whereas the Oath itself restricts as secret only 'What should not be published abroad'.

In this fashion, Jones interprets the injunction somewhat like the Chinese code of medical ethics – which is of uncertain date and authorship and probably stems from an aphoristic compilation of Sung dynasty (tenth century) writings. Here we read: 'Examine the patient carefully and never speak of what you experience in his house not even to your wife.'

No one can tell with any assurance what was the actual relationship of the Hippocratic Oath to the totality of the *corpus hippocraticum*. In fact, as Professor Jones states, this relationship is 'unknown and, indeed unknowable', although Edelstein, on the other hand, offered specific theories.[3] We also do not know how representative the Oath was of Greek thought; whether it was taken by all the practitioners of medicine, or perhaps only by the members of a select medical guild. Besides, it is unknown whether the Oath had a binding force beyond its moral sanctions: Was it taken literally as an oath, or simply interpreted as – again in Jones' words – a 'counsel of perfection?'

In China the injunction of the ethical precepts was obviated by the peculiar way in which in former times physicians were selected: in our way of speaking they were given a chance to 'make a bid'. Several physicians were invited to examine the patient, make a diagnosis, suggest a specific therapy, and the one was retained whose diagnosis and therapeutic suggestions were most pleasing to the patient, to his family or to his friends. In such a procedure many more than 'the doctor's own wife' became familiar with the patient's illness and the goings-on in his house.

Taken literally, the Hippocratic Oath, as well as the Chinese code, deprive the physician of a most tempting subject of conversation. But somehow, although few among the public know of the Oath or the traditional injunction to medical silence, it is taken for granted that whatever goes on between the patient and his doctor assumes a state of privileged communication, similar to that with a lawyer or a priest and they react with dismay at the breach of silence.

If we wonder whether the details of the Oath have any noticeable influence upon doctors of today, we are interested to see if the physician in earlier times actually abided by the injunction of privileged communication.

Transgressions of the rule of privacy can rarely be found in the writings of Hippocrates, since case histories had not yet come into general use. In those few histories in the *Epidemics* in which names were mentioned, a tendency towards anonymity is perceptible. The few individual patients listed are devoid of identification as to their age, local origin, and family so that scarcely any conclusion as to their identity could have been drawn.

Later in the Graeco-Roman antiquity we find that Galen of Pergamon, although a devout admirer of Hippocrates, could not resist the temptation inherent in being physician to the intellectual and imperial elite. His case histories on the illness and recovery of Emperor Marcus Aurelius and the famous peripatetic philosopher Eudemus appeared in full detail. That in both cases Galen's own opinion and regimen had differed sharply from those of his colleagues added considerable spice to the pleasure in his disclosures. However, it needs to be stressed that Galen's revelations concerning the illnesses of these prominent patients, were directed not to the general public but to other physicians who were presumably bound by the code of professional confidence.

There have, of course, been other medical men in history who could not resist the temptation of writing detailed descriptions of the illness and final days of illustrious patients. Such physicians incurred severe criticism for what the world of their contemporaries considered blatant indiscretion. This criticism sharpened, because some publications expanded beyond the purely medical aspects and included descriptions of the patient's political life, as it was influenced by the course of his illness. Specific examples at hand are the two histories that were written about the last illness of King Frederick II of Prussia and the publication of excerpts from the Diary of Lord Moran, as they refer to his observations of his eminent patient Winston Churchill.

The personality and illness of the Prussian king were so striking that they gave rise to two monographs from the pens of the last two physicians who attended him. One appeared in 1786, the year of Frederick's death, in several instalments in a Prussian medical journal, entitled *Beiträge zur Natur-und Arznei-Wissenschaft*,[4] a publication designed for medical scientists, to which the lay readers and the court gossips did not normally have access. The author of this monograph was Dr. C. C. Selle, Professor of Medicine, physician to the Charité Hospital, and member of the Royal Academy of Science at Berlin. Dr. Selle had been one of Frederick's several personal physicians who had been replaced by the more flamboyant and famous Dr. Johann Georg Zimmermann, a compatriot and student of Albrecht von Haller. After an honourable and successful career in his native Switzerland, Zimmermann had been called to the Royal Court at Hanover to become personal physician to the King of England, George III. It was from Hanover that Frederick the Great called Zimmermann to his sickbed in Potsdam, as he expected that the famous Swiss physician might be able to restore his sadly deteriorated health.

In this expectation he was mistaken. The art of medicine of the eighteenth century was powerless to cope with the king's complex ailment. As has happened so often in the history of medicine, all of the king's physicians – including the knowledgeable monarch himself – had viewed each of his many symptoms as a separate entity, an opinion which contributed neither to the cure, nor even to the alleviation of the king's lifelong suffering.

Dr. Selle had modestly entitled his publication about his royal patient a 'Case History of the last blessed King of Prussia, Frederick the Second, Majesty', and confined himself to medical observations. So far as the title and most of the contents are concerned, Selle had presented an impersonal case history. Throughout this description of the king's illness we find evidence of Selle's profound admiration for the personality of his illustrious patient. To quote one of the initial paragraphs:

The constitution of the King was so powerful and his medical conduct so simple that one could observe the very movements of nature as it resisted a severe illness for a considerable period of time under the most unpropitious circumstances. It was therefore possible to distinguish the changes actually brought about by the use of medication. In this respect is it possible for the physician to derive instruction from the natural and unimpeded course of an illness.

Selle's subsequent summary of Frederick the Great's symptoms reveal in their totality the actual nature of a disease, which during his lifetime was as yet unknown and therefore not treatable as a whole. In Selle's matter-of-fact description we read that even in his early years the king had suffered from a significant weakness and sensitivity of his stomach, so that he frequently vomited all he had eaten. In his later life, although he ate voraciously and digested well, he continued to suffer from so irritable a digestive tract that he had to be purged repeatedly, although he was also subject to attacks of spontaneous diarrhoea.

In addition to that the king was beset at an early age by recurrent attacks of gout and haemorrhoids; and as the former – gout – became regular, the physicians attempted to cure it by treating the haemorrhoids with venesection and mild purges. At the age of thirty-six the king suffered a transitory attack of hemiplegia which underwent a spontaneous remission and never recurred. So much, Dr. Selle found out from interviews of court personnel; and only at the age of seventy-five, did the king feel inclined to inform him of the details of his medical history. It was at a time when he was feeling relatively well and when he suffered only from occasional and transitory weakness and colics, which he attributed to his haemorrhoids but which were mostly caused by the wear and tear of old age and his greatly weakened power of digestion. So much we gather from Dr. Selle's tactful and professional 'Case History'.

How different was the story published by his successor, the famous Dr. Zimmermann, which makes the doctor part of the title and obtrudes his personality upon the attention of the reader. In short, this book is entitled: *Dr. Zimmermann's Conversations with the late King of Prussia.*[5]

It is an old cliché that no man is a hero to his valet. Similarly few men are heroes to their personal physician, especially when the physician concentrates all his skill and attention upon his one patient as is the case with the court doctor, who gets to know his patient in his somatic configuration and intimate habits as well as in his social and psychological make-up. In ordinary life and among ordinary men, the doctor will tell his patient to maintain a certain diet, to stop smoking, to control his alcohol intake, and to take his medication according to schedule. All the doctor can do is to hope that the patient will follow his orders. A personal physician and a court physician is present if the patient follows or transgresses his orders. He is present in those many moments when his charge ceases to be a patient and conducts himself as any man, with ideas that bear no relation to his illness; and frequently they may be of so private a nature that the doctor should not even – as the Chinese suggested – 'share them with his wife'. But the temptation to acquire vicarious status by knowing so much about the private thoughts and oddities of behaviour of as illustrious a patient as Frederick the Great, so irresistibly dazzled Zimmermann as to tell it all in his letters to various friends. These friends saw no reason not to enhance their own status by withholding these invaluable bits of intimate information about the great king and published them without Zimmermann's permission as 'Fragments about Frederick the Great'. This placed Zimmermann in the embarrassing position of denying the correspondence altogether or of making the best of his indiscretion by publishing the contents of his letters in his book about his conversations with the dying king. Obviously the subsequent publication that was much criticized was based on a diary that Zimmermann kept during his stay at the Prussian Court.

By way of contrast to the publication of Dr. Selle I wish to cite a few passages from Dr. Zimmermann's *Conversations with the late King of Prussia*, which he had admittedly spiced with 'several curious particulars and anecdotes of that extraordinary prince'.

Naturally the information of Dr. Selle's notes and a multitude of court personnel was available to Zimmermann who did not refrain in his book from expressing his mild amusement at the foibles of his illustrious patient. Where Selle had simply stated that King Frederick had always eaten large quantities of food, Zimmermann felt it incumbent upon himself to detail the somewhat ludicrous eating spree upon which the king had embarked during his physician's temporary absence.

At three in the afternoon I found the king in the most painful situation: every thing was changed and become worse. When in good humour, he had taken his medicine of dandelion and drank coffee: after this, he had applied from half after three in the morning till seven, to public business. Great part of the morning he had spent in eating, for as soon as I left him, a plate of sweetmeats, composed of sugar, whites of eggs, and cream, had been brought him, one of which I ate, and found the cream very sour. His majesty ate the whole plateful for his breakfast; and afterwards strawberries, cherries, and cold meat. At eleven his servants found great difficulty in getting him on horseback. He remained there three hours, in the great garden of Sans Souci, galloped almost the whole time, and returned very much weakened and exhausted. When he sat down to table he had no appetite; and immediately after dinner he was seized with a vomiting.

At three o'clock of the next day the king was again attacked by a colic, the consequence of indigestion; and he was in very bad humour. At dinner he had eaten plentifully of fresh eels. . . .

Zimmermann's book contains many convincing references to the king's own medical acumen which often made him a partner in treatment rather than a mere patient. Initially the king denied that he was suffering from dropsy although he actually was sufficiently conversant with that affliction to recognize it when it could no longer be denied. Thus later he observed: 'I have reflected a good deal upon what you said yesterday, respecting the dropsy, which from your hints I have reason to apprehend. I am now convinced you are right; for I pressed my legs with my finger, and the part remained hollow. This is an evident symptom of the dropsy.'

Although the king's observation was absolutely correct in describing pitting oedema, Zimmermann tried to comfort him by assuaging the fear caused by that symptom. Frederick, however, was convinced of the sad state of his health and replied: 'O! do not speak to me of hopes!'

Dropsy and ascites were actually symptoms of one devastating disease from which the king had suffered since he was a youth: the symptoms included generalized and ever-worsening ascites, gastric colics, violent sweating, severe headaches and accelerated pulse; he furthermore suffered from painful limbs, and dark red urine. It is this last-named symptom which confirms the clue that was suggested by Hunter and Macalpine's brilliant study on *George III and the Mad-Business.*[6] In their totality, the symptoms obviously prove that Frederick the Great, like his blood relative George III, was a sufferer of porphyria.

Unlike Dr. Selle who confined his 'Case History' to medical observations, Zimmermann also published his non-medical conversations with the king and included his patient's political views. It is here where he leaves the strict confines of medical reporting, and exposes himself to sharp criticism. In fact, leading personalities even a century later have called him vain and self-serving, and the well-known Berlin physician Ernst Ludwig Heim spoke of him as a fool and an egotist.[7]

The keeping of a diary must be an enormous temptation for physicians to highly placed personalities. This becomes evident from the hotly debated book on Churchill[8] which was derived from the diary notes of his personal physician Lord Moran.

Needless to say, both publications, that by Zimmermann and by Lord Moran would seem to be in contradiction to the earliest Greek and Chinese injunctions about privileged communication. But, beyond this, both publications have much in common: both described patients who were of extraordinary stature, highly placed in public and political life, subject to hostility as well as to fanatic devotion. Both Frederick the Great and Churchill had considerable medical knowledge, at least so far as their own persons were concerned, both wanted to be consulted about their treatment and followed it only if they were convinced of its rationale. Both men, furthermore, had outstanding personal foibles, even in their bedroom attire, which their physicians did not forget to detail. Frederick the Great, even in bed wore his large tri-cornered hat which he politely doffed upon his physician's entrance; his other garments were shabby and spotted by snuff. In contrast to the formal behaviour but shabby and unkempt appearance of the king, Churchill is pictured by his physician as having been extremely uninhibited in the presence of his doctor. He made elaborate preparations for bed, wearing a silken vest, and using various creams for his face and head, and dosing himself with sleeping tablets at night and pep pills in the morning. Unlike Dr. Zimmermann, Lord Moran served as a general friend, confidant and sounding-board to the Prime Minister, and we learn from his book that for several years England's fate was guided by an ailing man who had to persuade himself with the utmost energy that he was fit to do his job and that his continued service would be for the good of his country.

Zimmermann attended the king for less than a year, not long enough to develop even a trace of the personal affection and devotion that are so evident in Lord Moran's diary notes about his patient. But, in spite of this admiration and devotion in Lord Moran's twenty-five years of service to the great man, there is, as the anonymous, but apparently English reviewer in the *New York Times* book review[9] stated 'something morbid about publishing so clinical a record of a great man; possibly something "unethical" as Americans put it'. Now, in both these cases, the books about Frederick the Great and Churchill, we all may have our thoughts about ethics and the inviolability of privileged communication but, as medical historians we must welcome as treasures these publications as the purest source material that may ever become available to us.

References

1 HIPPOCRATES, vol. I, The Loeb Classical Library, with an English translation by W. H. S. Jones, London and Cambridge, Mass. Harvard University Press, 1948. *The Oath*, p. 301.

2 Comment by W. H. S. Jones, translator of the Oath, loc. cit.

3 EDELSTEIN, LUDWIG, 'The Hippocratic Oath: text, translation and interpretation', *Bull. Hist. Med.*, Baltimore, Johns Hopkins Press, 1943, supplement no. 1.

4 'Krankheitsgeschichte des Höchstseeligen Königs von Preussen Friedrichs des Zweyten, Majestät', *Neue Beiträge zur Natur-und Arznei-Wissenschaft*, teil III Medizinische Beobachtungen, nr. 12, S. 152, ed. by C. G. Selle, Berlin, 1786, pp. 152 ff.

5 ZIMMERMANN, J. G., *Doctor Zimmermann's Conservations with the late King of Prussia, when he attended him in his last illness and a little before his death. To which are added several curious particulars and anecdotes of that extraordinary Prince*, trans. . . . London, 1791.

6 HUNTER, R. and MACALPINE, I., *George III and the Mad-Business*, London, Allen Lane, Penguin Press, 1969.

7 KESSLER, *Der alte Heim*, Leipzig, 1879, vol. 2, p. 32.

8 MORAN, LORD, *Churchill, Taken from the Diaries of Lord Moran: The Struggle for Survival 1940–1965*, Boston, Houghton Mifflin Company, 1966.

9 *New York Times*, 13 May 1966.

Y. Nakagawa
Osaka (Japan)

Medical thought and society: a historical interpretation

Health care problems have in many countries become critical year by year. Medical historians should and could analyse the structure of this critical situation and contribute to give some solutions. In my view the present critical situation of health care problems could be understood as a discrepancy in principle between demand and supply. In 1946 the World Health Organization declared in the Constitution of Health: 'the enjoyment of the highest attainable standard of health is one of the fundamental rights of every human being without distinction of race, religion, political belief, economic or social condition.' Since that time, health care has come to be dealt with as a problem of human rights, and the government has come to be responsible for providing health care for the entire population. However, medicine has never had the experience of providing health care for the entire population. What medicine can do is to meet such demand only by expanding and rationalizing the hitherto employed principles. However, amazingly the rising health care demand is always overwhelming such endeavours to meet increasing demands. Furthermore, the skyrocketing rise of health care costs will soon make it a heavy burden on public finance. Considering these consequences, the principles of modern medicine are seemingly approaching the terminus in their applicability, and a fundamental change in medical thought is now needed.

Many distinguished medical historians and medical sociologists state that medicine is a social institution. Based on this assumption, and considering the quantity and quality of health care of the past, we can make a new interpretation of medical history. The aim of this paper is to present a possible frame of reference, that is, a new way of enquiring into periods of the history of medical thought or medical methodology.

The period division which I propose is: the period of court medicine, the period of private practice medicine, the period of hospital medicine, and the period of social medicine. In this division, instinctive medicine, magic medicine, and religiously delivered medicine are put out of consideration.

Firstly, what I termed court medicine is the medicine applied to the situation whose major concern was the health care of the court, and which at the same time was available to other groups in limited amounts. The clients of this medicine were small definite numbers of privileged persons, and the duty of health care personnel was to preserve the health of their clients. Practically, the recognition and the treatment of minor ailments and feeblenesses were main objectives, because health itself was not considered to be a medical problem. Methodologically speaking, such objectives could be realized by means of natural historical approach, because the health care personnel would spend the major part of their time with their clients observing successively the ways of daily life, identifying causative conditions of the ailment and offering means to correct it. All experience and knowledge were gathered and formed from the viewpoint of natural history. In this context, for instance, the nature of Hippocratic medicine and why Hippocratic medicine had been so highly esteemed in ancient times and the Middle Ages could be clearly understood. For example, the concept of natural healing power corresponds implicitly to the assisting attitude of healing personnel in court. They considered disease as a manifestation of the healing process, not as an offensive entity for the body. Here we recall a phrase in the Hippocratice Corpus: 'I will follow that system of *regimen* which, according to my ability and judgement'. The word regimen was written in Littré's text díaíta (life or mode of life) which was a synonym for medicine at that time.

Secondly, what I termed private practice medicine is the medicine which had arisen in the process of urbanization. There have been many kinds of private practitioners in the history of medicine, but what I call private practitioners here are health care personnel developed as liberal independent professionals in the latter Middle Ages. The philosophy of this medicine places emphasis on the relationship between one physician and one client, accordingly, on a closed relationship excluding the third party. In this context, stress was placed rather on moral treatment, and knowledge of the physician as a scholar was sought outside of the physician–client relationship. To be a physician or to be a doctor was considered to be an advantage for securing the client's confidence. This is the reason why so many physicians were pioneers in natural science from the sixteenth to eighteenth centuries.

Thirdly, what I called hospital medicine is designed to offer health care for large indefinite numbers of sick indigents in the hospitals. In this situation, because history taking was limited more than in the case of court medicine or private practice medicine, healing personnel had come to treat disease and the patient separately. Contrasting to an old medical aphorism; 'Socrates and an idiot should not be treated with the same treatment even if both had the same symptoms', it became to be said that Socrates and an idiot should be treated with the same treatment when both had the same symptoms. That is, the hospital medicine rather ignores individual difference of the patients, but is concerned with the difference of diseases. Moreover, because hospital medicine treated mainly severe cases, diseases were well ripe for easier identification. With such a way of recognition, hospital medicine developed as a science and offered many techniques to conquer diseases. We really have conquered many diseases, but we are hearing louder and louder voices demanding health care in every place. Of course, fortified endeavours have been taken in every country, but they have always been surmounted. For instance, specialization or super specialization which is an evidence of development in hospital medicine, rather lowers efficiency and raises the cost, that is, specialization differs from the divisions of labour which have been introduced in industry. Thus, the more inclination to specialize, that is, to attain higher standards of medicine, the more serious the shortage of health manpower and health care finance. Adding to these, the attitude of being mainly concerned with the recognition of disease and putting the patient aside, has given rise to detached objectivism in medical care. All these tendencies show that hospital medicine has been originally and fundamentally designed for offering medical care to a large indefinite number of sick indigents. This number does not include the entire population, but only enlarges it to some extent. Sooner or later, the latter manoeuvre will fall into a dilemma.

To overcome a dilemma or the present difficulties in health care, we should expect the fourth medicine, named social medicine, which will be designed and constructed to offer health care to the entire population of definite number. In this medicine the key concept will be ill health. Contrasting to the concept of disease as actual abnormality within the body, the concept of ill health refers to actual and possible abnormality in relation to the patient's external life conditions. Methodologically, ill health can be elucidated namely by means of ecological approach, as once Dr. I. Galdston mentioned in his book entitled *Meaning of Social Medicine* (1954). When the shift (Aufheben) to social medicine shall be completed, medicine will become a social institution in the full sense of the word. We are now in this transition.

A. Terzioğlu
Munich (West Germany)

Die Ilkhanischen Krankenhäuser und die Einflüsse der islamischen Medizin auf Byzanz zu dieser Zeit

Während der mongolischen Expansion im 13. Jh. wurden in Asien und Europa viele Städte zerstört und die zivilisatorischen Werte völlig mißachtet. Die Schrecken der mongolischen Verwüstung sollten aber dennoch nicht dazu verleiten, den positiven Beitrag zu übersehen, den das Mongolenreich zur Berührung der islamischen Kultur mit den europäischen und fernöstlichen Kulturen beigetragen hat. Obwohl die Einflüsse der islamischen Medizin in China schon von der T'ang-Zeit (618–906) an besonders zur Zeit der Sung-Zeit (960–1126) vorhanden waren, wurden die islamischen Einflüsse in der Mongolenzeit noch wirkungsvoller.[1]

In der als Yüan-Zeit genannten mongolischen Epoche wurden medizinische Abhandlungen der islamischen Ärzte ins Chinesische übersetzt. Eine dieser Übersetzungen war das „Hui-hui yao-fang" genannte Werk.[2] Zu dieser Zeit fanden auch die islamischen Arzneizubereitungen und Rezepturen in die Hofbibliothek Eingang. In der Staatsbibliothek von Peking existieren heute noch 36 Bände mit islamischen Rezepten.[3] Die Einflüsse der islamischen Medizin kamen meistens über das islamisch-türkische Kulturzentrum Samarkand nach China. Schon Tschingiz Khan (1155–1227) ließ sich in Samarkand von einem islamischen Augenarzt behandeln.[4]

Die Arzneimittelanwendung durch das Sirup genannte Getränk wurde im Jahre 1268 aus Samarkand nach China gebracht.[5]

Zur Zeit der Mongolen wurden in China mindestens drei Krankenhäuser nach islamischem Muster errichtet.[6] Diese Krankenhäuser wurden von islamischen Ärzten geleitet. Eines dieser islamischen Krankenhäuser stand in der Sommerresidenz des Kubilai Khan Shang-tu (= Ciandu) in K'ai-p'ing fu.[7]

An diesem Krankenhaus sowie an das andere islamische Krankenhaus in Ta-tu (Peking) waren je ein Medikamentenamt angeschlossen. Diese beiden islamischen Krankenhäuser existierten seit 1292.[8] Das größte islamische Krankenhaus war das Kuang-hui-sze genannte Krankenhaus in Peking.[9] Dieses Kuang-hui-sze war ein Hofkrankenhaus. Dort wurden kaiserliche Leibwächter sowie in Peking ansässige Mongolen durch die dort angestellten islamischen Ärzte behandelt.[10] Nach Ming-Wong[11] wurde diese Anstalt in Peking im Jahre 1270 errichtet. Es muß eine Gründung des Kubilai gewesen sein. Es ist durchaus möglich, daß diese islamischen Krankenhäuser in Peking, in Shang-tu, in Ta-tu von islamischen Architekten nach seldschukischem Muster gebaut worden sind, wie es bei den ilkhanischen Krankenhäusern in Kleinasien und Persien der Fall war.[12] Nach Angaben von Yang-Yü[13] gehörten die mohammedanischen Ärzte zum Kaiserlichen Medizinalamt.

Im Jahre 1339 waren unter den neun Hofärzten im Kaiserlichen Palast vier islamische Ärzte tätig.[14] Die islamischen Ärzte hatten aber auch den Wert der chinesischen Medizin erkannt. Zur Zeit der Ilkhane fand die chinesische Pharmakologie, Pulslehre und Alchemie ihren Weg über die islamische Medizin in den Westen. Das von dem chinesischen Arzt Kao Yang im 13. Jh. verfaßte Werk über die Geheimnisse des Pulses, Mochüeh, wurde zur Zeit der Ilkhane (14. Jh.) ins Persische übersetzt, sowie mit Kommentaren versehen. Diese persische Übersetzung hat den Titel „Tanksuq nameh il khan dar fanun ulum khata-i", Das Buch der Merkwürdigkeiten des Ilkhan über die Art und Weise der chinesischen Wissenschaft.[15]

Die Ilkhane, die nach der Teilung des Tschingis-Khan's Weltreiches die mongolische Herrschaft in Persien, Irak, Afghanistan und einen Teil von Kleinasien fortsetzten, haben Zuder Berührung der seldschukisch-islamischen und fernöstlichen Kulturen mit den europäischen Kulturen wegen ihrer geopolitischen Lage am meisten beigetragen. In Aserbaidjan, nahe der Stadt Maraga, wurde schon zur Zeit der Hulâgu Ilkhan im Jahre 1259 ein großes Observatorium errichtet. Unter Leitung des türkisch-islamischen Astronomen und Arztes Nasired-Din Tusi haben in diesem Observatorium in Maraga zahlreiche Wissenschaftler aus verschiedenen Ländern gearbeitet. Auch der Chinese Fao-Mun-Tschi, genannt Sing-Sing (= Arif = Gelehrte), war hier tätig.[16] Obwohl zur Zeit Hulâgu Ilkhans auch chinesische Ärzte am ilkhanischen Hofe tätig waren,[17] wurden die islamischen Ärzte bevorzugt. Die bedeutenden ilkhanischen Veziere wie Sa'd-ed-Din und Raschid-ed-Din waren islamische Ärzte, die zuerst als Hofärzte den ilkhanischen Herrschern dienten.[18]

Der bekannte islamische Arzt und Astronom Qutb ad-Din Mahmud ibn Mas-ud aš-Širazi, der ein Schüler von Nasir ed-Din Tusi war, hatte im Auftrage von Argun Ilkhan eine Landkarte von Vorderasien angefertigt. Qutb ad-Din hatte für die Vorbereitung dieser Arbeit mit dem Genuesen Buscarello di Ghizalfi die anatolischen Küsten untersucht.[19]

Zur Zeit Ghazan Khan's waren die Ilkhanen zum Islam übergetreten. Mit ihm begann auch eine große Bautätigkeit. Besonders Täbriz wurde zu einer glanzvollen Stadt unter der Herrschaft Ghazan Khan's. Er hielt im Jahre 1295 seinen Einzug in Täbriz und stieg in dem Palast ab, der von Argun Khan (1281–92) im Dorfe Sham westlich von der Stadt auf dem linken Ufer des Adjitschai erbaut worden war.[20] Vier Jahre später begann der Bau des von ihm gegründeten Krankenhauses.

DAS KRANKENHAUS VON GHAZAN IN SHAM (Nahe von Täbriz)

Nach seiner Rückkehr vom Feldzug in Syrien hatte Ghazan Khan vom Jahre 1299 n. Chr. an mit der Errichtung vieler Bauwerke begonnen.

„Zu seiner Begräbnisstätte bestimmte er das schon erwähnte Sham. Hier wurde ein Gebäude errichtet, höher als Gunbad (Grabmal) des Sultans Sandjar in Marw (Merw), das bis dahin als das höchste Bauwerk der islamischen Welt galt. Neben diesem Mausoleum, das von einer Kuppel überwölbt wurde, lagen eine Moschee, zwei Medresen (eine schafi'itische und eine hanefitische), eine Herberge für die Saiyiden (Dar al-Siyadat), ein Krankenhaus, ein Observatorium, ähnlich wie das in Maragha, eine Bibliothek, ein Archivgebäude, ein Haus für die Verwaltung dieser Anstalten, eine Zisterne für Trinkwasser und ein Badehaus für heiße Bäder. Wakfgüter, deren Einkünfte sich auf 100 Tuman Gold beliefen, wurden zur Unterhaltung dieser Gründungen bestimmt. An jedem Tor der neuen Stadt wurde eine

Karawanserai, ein Markt und ein Badehaus erbaut. Obstbäume wurden aus fernen Ländern herbeigebracht."[21]

Im Jahre 703 (1304 n. Chr.) wurde Ghazan Khan mit großem Pomp in dem Mausoleum zu Sham beigesetzt.

Die prächtigen Bauten Ghazan Khans im Dorfe Sham (der heutigen Vorstadt Kara-malik) sind vollkommen verschwunden. Schon im Jahre 1611 hatte Schah-Abbas die Materialien der Ruinen von „Sham-Ghazan"[22] für den Bau einer Festung verwandt.

Zur Zeit des Ghazan Khan (1295–1303) wurden in der anatolischen Stadt Sivas das Dārû's -Siyyâdat-i Ghāzaní genannte Armenhaus sowie von seinem Vezier Raschid ed-Din ein Krankenhaus (Dar al-Schifa) mit einer Apotheke (Darû Khâna) in Hamadan errichtet.[23]

DAS KRANKENHAUS VON SULTANIYA (in der Nähe von Täbriz) gegr. 1305

Der Bruder und Nachfolger des Ghazan Khan, Oldjaytu, hatte weitere Krankenhäuser errichtet. Eines dieser Krankenanstalten war das im Jahre 1305 in Sultaniya gegründete Krankenhaus. Es gehörte einem aus Moschee, Medrese, Mausoleum von Oldjaytu, Apotheke, Palast u.a. Bauten bestehenden Baukomplex an.[24]

Das für den Schah Schudja von Ali bin Husein Alâ ül-Kazvini in Persisch geschriebene allgemeine Geschichtsbuch behandelt im Kapitel Oldjaytu Khan auch das Krankenhaus von Sultaniya und die neben dieser Anstalt vom Vezier Raschid ed-Din (oder Raschid üd-din) gegründete Armenküche (Imâret).[25]

DAS KRANKENHAUS VOM VEZIER RASCHID ED-DIN IN TÄBRIZ

Der islamische Arzt Raschid ed-Din Fazlullah, der seit 1298 den Ghazan Khan und seinen Nachfolgern Oldjaytu und Abu S'aid bis 1318 als Vezier diente, hatte mit Hilfe islamischer, indischer, chinesischer und abendländischer Gelehrter ein „Cami'ül-Tevarih" genanntes monumentales Geschichtswerk geschaffen.[26]

Angeregt vielleicht durch seinen Landesherren, schuf Raschid ed-Din im Jahre 1310 eine Universitätsstadt in Täbriz, die sogar den alten Komplex übertraf. Sie enthielt 24 Karawanserails, 1500 Geschäfte, 3000 Häuser, spezielle Viertel für die Studenten, die sich aus allen Ländern dort trafen, Krankenhäuser, Apotheken und Gärten. An Gediegenheit und Größe übertraf diese Universitätsstadt alle vergleichbaren Einrichtungen.[27]

Diese Rab'-i Raschidi genannte Universitätsstadt lag östlich von Täbriz am Hang von Kuh-i Veylan. Obwohl diese prächtigen Bauten heute nicht mehr existieren, gibt die Stiftungsurkunde[28] dieser Anlage wertvolle Hinweise. Dort wurden für die Studenten aus verschiedenen Ländern getrennte Wohnquartiere untergebracht. Die türkischen Studenten und Akademiker, die in dieser Rab-i Raschidi untergebracht waren, sind vorwiegend Architekten, Wasserbauingenieure, Gartenarchitekten, Maler, Goldschmiede und Kalligraphen gewesen. Ihre Namen wie Kuttun Boka, Olcay, Tok Timur, Ayatur Timur lassen erkennen, daß sie vorwiegend uigurische Türken waren.[29] Die Uiguren waren im chinesischen Teil des mongolischen Reiches auch Hofbeamte und Gelehrte. Der Präsident der Han-lin-Akademie in China war ein Alin Tämür genannter Uigure.[30]

In dem großen Krankenhaus dieser Universitätsstadt Rab-i Raschidi waren 50

Ärzte aus Ägypten, Syrien, Indien und China tätig.[31] Der Direktor dieses Krankenhauses war Muhammed ibn ul-Nilî. Die bis heute erhaltenen Briefe von Raschid ed-Din beweisen, daß in dieser Universitätsstadt in Täbriz auch ein Studentendorf für griechische Studenten vorhanden war.

Vezier Raschid ed-Din schrieb an seinen Sohn Djelal ed-Din, der in Anatolien als Gouverneur tätig war, daß er in der von ihm gegründeten Universitätsstadt (Rab-i Raschidi) in Täbriz viele Dörfer für Ausländer, darunter auch für Byzantiner, gegründet habe. Er möchte, daß sein Sohn 40 byzantinische Familien nach Täbriz schicken solle, damit er sie dort ansiedeln könne.[32]

Die jährlichen Steuern, welche Byzanz an die Ilkhane zahlen mußte, wurden für die 6.000 Studenten dieser Universität ausgegeben.[33] Die byzantinischen Studenten haben in der Universität Täbriz nicht nur Medizin sondern auch Astronomie studiert. Sie haben mehrere islamische Werke ins Griechische übersetzt.[34] Der byzantinische Priester Isaak Argyros hatte auch einige astronomische Werke aus dem Arabischen ins Griechische übersetzt.[35] Zur Zeit der Ilkhane waren die islamischen Einflüsse auf Byzanz besonders in der Medizin sehr stark. Der aus Trapezunt stammnede byzantinische Arzt Gregorios Chioniades war zu dieser Zeit in Persien. Später hatte er einige persische Werke in die griechische Sprache übersetzt. Als Beispiel könnte man unter anderem das „Antidotoi ek persias" genannte Werk angeben, welches von ihm aus dem Persischen übersetzt wurde.[36]

In dem „Asile-u Acvibe-i Raschidi" genannten Werk von Raschid ed-Din wurden viele Fragen von ausländischen, darunter auch von byzantinischen Ärzten gestellt und von ihm beantwortet. In diesem Werk wird der Arzt Raschid ed-Din von dem byzantinischen Gelehrten als ein noch größerer Gelehrter als Aristoteles und Platon beschrieben. Dieses bis jetzt nicht beachtete Werk befindet sich in mehreren Handschriftexemplaren in der Hagia Sophia-Bibliothek in Istanbul (Nr. 2180), in der Bibliothek der Selimiye Moschee in Edirne (Nr. 1930), in der National-Bibliothek Teheran (Mecelle-i Mihr. VIII, N 4–5) und in der Topkapi-Schloß-Bibliothek in Istanbul (Ahmed Salis Nr. 1930).

Dieses Werk enthält die Antworten auf die Fragen der ausländischen Gelehrten aus Arabien, Chowaresmien, dem östlichen Turkestan (Khotan), Sind (Multan) und Byzanz. Diese Fragen wurden von diesen ausländischen Gelehrten brieflich mitgeteilt. Diese Briefe und die Antworten zu diesen Fragen hat der ilkhanische Herrscher Oldjaytu mit seinem Vezier und Arzt Raschid ed-Din diskutiert. Diese Teile des Werkes stammen aus dem Jahre 1311 (710 H.). Die Fragen der byzantinischen Gelehrten und die Antworten des Raschid ed-Din umfassen in dem Handschriftexemplar der Hagia Sophia-Bibliothek in Istanbul etwa 43 Seiten.[37]

Raschid ed-Din hatte einige der Fragen der byzantinischen Ärzte ausführlich beantwortet. Zu den für ihn einfach erschienenen Fragen 2, 3, 4 und 5 hat er ganz kurze Erklärungen gegeben. Zu Frage 1 hat er dagegen eine 15 Seiten umfassende Antwort dargelegt. Die Fragen der byzantinischen Ärzte und die Antworten zu diesen Fragen sollen hier ganz kurz erwähnt werden.

Frage 1: Was für eine Beziehung gibt es zwischen der menschlichen Seele und dem Blut? Warum hat menschliches Blut rote Farbe?
Antwort: Blut ist nicht mit dem Leben identisch, aber wenn die Seele den menschlichen Körper verläßt, wird auch das Blut nicht zirkulieren. Das eigentliche Grundprinzip ist die Bewegung. Wo es Bewegung gibt, existiert auch Wärme. Damit kann man das Geheimnis der Existenz des Blutes erklären. Wenn das Leben den menschlichen Körper verläßt, sind Bewegung und Wärme nicht mehr vorhanden und

deswegen zirkuliert auch das Blut nicht mehr. Die rote Farbe des Blutes dient als Maßstab, um den normalen oder anormalen Zustand festzustellen. Das Blut kann seine Farbe verändern.

Frage 2: Die menschlichen Sinne sind in der Zahl fünf. Warum gibt es aber anstatt fünf nur vier Elemente?

Antwort: Diese Frage habe ich in meinem Latâi 'if al haqaiq" genannten Werk im Abschnitt Risâlat al-fayd wa'l fayyad behandelt.[38] Fahr ed-Din Razi hatte darüber in seiner Abhandlung al-Mabâhhith al-Mašriqiya seine Gedanken mit den Zitaten aus Avicenna (Ibn Sina) dargelegt. In diesen Quellen kann man die Antwort zu dieser Frage finden.

Frage 3: Jedes Wesen braucht einen Raum, wo es existiert. Wenn die menschliche Seele ein einfaches Wesen wäre, hätte sie auch einen Raum gebraucht. Aber die Seele befindet sich im menschlichen Körper. Wenn die Seele den menschlichen Körper verläßt, existiert der menschliche Körper ohne sie trotzdem. Wenn die Seele sich im menschlichen Körper befindet, ist sie ein Wesen. Wenn die Seele den menschlichen Körper verläßt, existiert die Seele weiter, aber sie hat mit dem Wesen nichts mehr zu tun. Wie kann man die Frage erklären?

Antwort: Die Seele braucht keinen Raum (Hayyiz). Die Seele sowie der menschliche Körper existieren unabhängig voneinander. Seele und Geist existieren vor der Vereinigung im menschlichen Körper. Sie werden aber auch, wenn sie den menschlichen Körper verlassen existieren.

Frage 4: Die menschlichen Nägel haben mit den Haaren viele Ähnlichkeiten. Sie können wieder wachsen, wenn sie abgeschnitten sind. Die Haare sowie Nägel riechen genauso, wenn man sie im Feuer verbrennen würde. Also sind sie ähnliche Produkte der Natur. Warum haben die menschlichen Haare in verschiedenen Rassen unterschiedliche Farbe, obwohl die Nägel bei jedem Menschen einheitliche weiße Farbe haben?

Antwort: Die Dinge, die einige Ähnlichkeiten haben, müssen nicht alle in jeder Hinsicht gleiche Eigenschaften besitzen. Es gibt Dinge, die gleiche Farbe haben, aber sonst völlig verschieden sind.

Frage 5: Die Tiere unterscheiden sich von den Pflanzen dadurch, daß sie sich bewegen können. Die Menschen haben mehr zusätzliche Bewegungen als die Tiere. Obwohl die Tiere ihre Ohren bewegen können, warum sind die menschlichen Ohren nicht beweglich? Einige Tiere können sogar ihre Schwänze bewegen. Wie können Sie diese Frage erklären?

Antwort: Der Schöpfer muß einen Grund gehabt haben, warum er die Geschöpfe so geschaffen hat. Die Menschen können mit ihren Händen die Fliegen wegjagen, während die Tiere dies mit ihren Schwänzen tun. In der Natur wird kein Organ untätig bleiben. Wenn Sie dieses Prinzip begreifen, werden Sie selbst Antwort auf derartige Fragen finden.

Frage 6: Gott (Allah) ist König der Könige. Ein König wird erst als König anerkannt, wenn er ein Land mit Bevölkerung besitzen würde. Wo hatte Gott der Herr als König der Könige sein Reich und seine Untertanen, bevor er den Himmel und die Erde geschaffen hatte?

Antwort: Alles fängt mit Gott an. Er ist Schöpfer. Er ist ewig. Bevor unser Raum und unsere Zeit geschaffen wurde, gab es ohne Zweifel ein anderes Universum und Geschöpfe, die wiederum von Gott geschaffen wurden. Darüber haben wir keine Kenntnisse. Dies bedeutet aber nicht, daß Gott früher kein anderes Universum geschaffen hat. Wir können nicht über unsere Raum- und Zeitvorstellung hinaus die früheren oder späteren Schöpfungen Gottes begreifen. In dieser Beziehung sind unsere geistigen Vorstellungen und unser Verstand nicht absolut, sondern relativ, das heißt, daß sie von gegebenen Umständen abhängig sind.

Frage 7: Gott hat unsere Welt nach seinem Willen geschaffen. Warum vernichtet er wieder seine eigenen Schöpfungen nach seinem Willen? Wenn Gott diese Vernichtung gegen seinen Willen tut, dann hat er keine Allmacht. Da man ihn nicht als unfähig und unvollkommen bezeichnen kann, wie kann man diese Frage erklären?

Als Antwort zu dieser letzten Frage der byzantinischen Ärzte weist Raschid ed-Din darauf hin, daß er diese Frage in seinen Abhandlungen Risâla fi hašr al-adjsâd va ibtal al-tanâsukh und Risâla fi'l djabr va'l-l'qadar, die in sein Werk Miftah al-tafásir gehören, eingehend behandelt hat.[39]

Zu diesem VIII. Abschnitt des ,,Asile-u Acvibe-i Raschidi" hat ein namentlich nicht genannter byzantinischer Arzt eine Einleitung geschrieben. Nach dieser Einleitung kann man folgende Rückschlüsse ziehen:

1. Dieser byzantinische Arzt war zu dieser Zeit in Täbriz im Dienste von Raschid-ed-Din tätig. Er hatte die Fragen der byzantinischen Ärzte zusammengestellt, die Antworten des Raschid ed-Din zu diesen Fragen auf griechisch übersetzt und nach Konstantinopel geschickt. Es ist durchaus möglich, daß dieser byzantinische Arzt Gregorios Chioniades war.
2. Nach Ansicht dieses ,,Frenk tabibi" genannten byzantinischen Arztes war Griechenland früher Geburtsort der Medizin, Naturwissenschaft und Philosophie. Aber zu dieser Zeit konnten nur Raschid ed-Din und die Gelehrten in Täbriz diese schwierigen Fragen beantworten. Nach seiner Ansicht würden sogar Aristoteles und Platon gerne zu dem Studentenkreis des Raschid ed-Din gehört haben, wenn sie zu dieser Zeit gelebt hätten.

Diese Einleitung beweist, daß zur Zeit des ilkhanischen Veziers Raschid ed-Din Täbriz das medizinische und kulturelle Zentrum der damaligen Welt war, welches islamische Einflüsse nach Byzanz und anderen Ländern ausstrahlte. Es ist schade, daß diese Universität, sowie die anderen ilkhanischen Krankenhäuser verschwunden sind. Aus der ilkhanischen Zeit ist nur ein Krankenhaus in Amasya (Türkei) bis heute gut erhalten geblieben.

DAS KRANKENHAUS VON AMASYA, gegr. 1308 n. Chr.

Dieses Krankenhaus in Amasya wurde im Jahre 1308 n. Chr. von Anber bin Abdullah gegründet. Der Gründer war ein Sklave der Gemahlin des Oldjaytu Ilkhan Mehmed (1304–16) gewesen. Diese Angaben und das Gründungsdatum sind der dreizeiligen arabischen Gründungsinschrift des Krankenhauses zu entnehmen.[40]

Baulich hat dieses Krankenhaus die Merkmale der typisch seldschukischen Architektur, wie es bei dem Nured-Din-Krankenhaus (1154) in Damaskus und bei anderen türkischen Krankenhäusern aus der seldschukischen Epoche in Kayseri (1204), in Sivas (1217) und in Divrigi (1229) der Fall ist. Das aus sieben großen Sälen und zwei Zimmern bestehende Krankenhaus hat eine Größe von 24,5 m × 35 m. In den Sälen sind keine Kaminstellen zu finden. Nach der Restaurierung nach dem Erdbebenschaden im Jahre 1912 wurde man aber auf Rohrleitungen aus Ton aufmerksam. Weil neben diesem Spital auch ein Bad besteht, ist man zu dem Ergebnis gekommen, daß dieses Spital von der aus dem Bad durch die Rohrleitungen kommende Warmluft erhitzt würde.[41]

Nachdem die Stadt Amasya im Jahre 1393 den osmanischen Türken gehörte, haben die in diesem Krankenhaus berühmten osmanischen Ärzte wie Schükrullah (gest. 1488), Halimi (1516), Merzifonlu Atufi (*ca.* 1516), Mehmed bin Lütfullah (15. Jh.), gearbeitet. Der türkische Arzt Sabuncuoğlu Scheref ed-Din bin Ali, der 77 Jahre nach der Gründung dieses Krankenhauses geboren wurde, war der berühmteste Mediziner dort gewesen, welcher 14 Jahre lang in diesem Spital gearbeitet hatte. Wie er in seinem Werk ,,Mücerrebname" angibt, wurden in dieser Krankenanstalt neben anderen Kranken auch Irre medizinisch behandelt.[42] Sabuncuoğlu

Scheref ed-Din hat außerdem ein berühmtes chirurgisches Buch „Kitab-elCerrahiyye-i Khaniye" im Jahre 1465 für den türkischen Sultan Mehmed Fatih verfaßt. Wie seine anderen Werke hat er auch diese Abhandlung in türkischer Sprache geschrieben. Laignel-Lavastine[43] und E. Blochet behaupteten, daß diese chirurgische Abhandlung von Sabuncuoğlu aus dem Persischen übersetzt wurde.[44] Aber diese Behauptung stimmt nicht. Zwar hat Sabuncuoğlu von Ebul Kasim Zehravis „at-Tasrif" vieles übernommen, aber er hat auch an 40 Stellen eigene wissenschaftliche Überlegungen dargelegt.[45] Über das in der Pariser Bibliotheque Nationale existierende Handschriftexemplar dieses Werkes wurde von P. Huard und M. D. Grmek eine Veröffentlichung herausgegeben.[46]

Dieses heute noch existierende ilkhanische Krankenhaus in Amasya ist nicht nur medizingeschichtlich, sondern auch baugeschichtlich von besonderer Bedeutung. Die baulichen Eigenschaften dieses Krankenhauses beweisen, daß die ilkhanischen Krankenhäuser nach seldschukischem Muster von seldschukischen Architekten erbaut wurden. Viele seldschukische Krankenhäuser waren auch in der ilkhanischen Epoche in Betrieb. Raschid ed-Din hatte nicht nur in Täbriz, Sultaniya, Hamadan und Erdebil[47] neue Krankenhäuser errichtet, sondern hat auch das seldschukische Krankenhaus in Schiraz „Dar al-Schifa-i Muzafferi" reorganisiert und dort Mahmud Ilyas als Arzt angestellt.[48]

In Schiraz wurde von dem ilkhanischen Herrscher Abud Said (1316–36) ein weiteres Krankenhaus errichtet.[49] In zwei Inschriften am Khan Ortmah, welcher vom Statthalter des Sultans Uwais (aus der Dynastie von Djalairiden) Amir Amin al-din Mirdjan in Bagdad 760 Hg. (1359 n. Chr.) gegründet wurde, ist der Dar al-Schifa (Krankenhaus) am Bâb al-Gharabah erwähnt worden. Aus dieser Inschrift geht hervor, daß der Angehörige des ilkhanischen Herrschers Oldjaytu Amin al-Din Mirdjan für dieses Krankenhaus und Madrasa viele Immobilien als Waqf stiftete.[50] Dieses Krankenhaus in Bagdad war höchstwahrscheinlich eines der letzten ilkhanischen Krankenhäuser.

Die Glanzzeit der Ilkhanen hat nicht lange gedauert. Nach dem großen Arzt, Historiker und Staatsmann Raschid ed-Din, der am 18. Juli 1318 ermordet wurde, endete diese Glanzzeit.[51]

Anmerkungen

1 RALL, JUTTA, *Die vier großen Medizinschulen der Mongolenzeit, Stand und Entwicklung der chinesischen Medizin in der Chin- und Yüan-Zeit*, Wiesbaden, 1970, S. 28, 32; CH'EN YUAN, *Western and Central Asians in China under the Mongols*, Los Angeles, 1966, S. 103; vgl. LIN T'IEN-WEI, *Sungtai hsiang-yao mou-i shih-kao*, Hongkong, 1960.

2 LEE, T'AO, 'Chinese medicine during the Chin (1127–1234) and Yuan (1234–1368) eras', *Chinese Medical Journal*, 1955, **73**, S. 241–58.

3 RALL, JUTTA, a.a.O., S. 30.

4 NESEVI, M., *Sîretu Celâleddin Mengübirti*. Hrg. O. Houdas, Paris, 1891, S. 41; vgl. SPULER, B., *Die Mongolen in Iran*, Leipzig, 1939, S. 441.

5 Dieses Wort Sirup kommt von dem arabischen Scharab oder Scharbat. Auf Chinesisch wurde dieses Wort Scharbat zu Scheli-pieh; vgl. SABURÔ, MIYASHITA, *Sôgen no i-ryô*, Kyôtô, 1966, S. 159.

6 MIYASHITA SABURÔ, a.a.O., S. 160.

7 CH'EN YUAN, a.a.O., S. 60; MIYASHITA SABURÔ, a.a.O., S. 160.

8 RALL, JUTTA, a.a.O., S. 30.

9 MIYASHITA SABURÔ, a.a.O., S. 160; RALL, JUTTA, a.a.O., S. 30.

10 RALL, JUTTA, a.a.O., S. 30.

11 MING WONG, 'Les Doctrines Médicales Chinoises et leur Evolution sous les Mongols', *Clio Medica*, 1971, **6**, 4, S. 287.

12 Uber die Tätigkeit der ausländischen Architekten im Dienste der Mongolen sind die Quellen sehr dürftig. Nach Angaben Wilhelm von Rubruks errichtete Meister Wilhelm aus Paris am Eingang des mongolischen Schlosses in Quara-Quorum einen Baum aus Silber, zu dessen Wurzeln vier Löwen aus Silber lagen; vgl. SPULER, B., *Geschichte der Mongolen*, Zürich-Stuttgart, 1958, S. 135.

13 FRANKE, HERBERT, *Beiträge aus der Kulturgeschichte Chinas unter der Mongolenherrschaft*, Wiesbaden, 1956, S. 34, 72.

14 MIYASHITA SABURÔ, a.a.O., S. 160.

15 RALL, S. J., 'Zur persischen Übersetzung eines Mo-chüeh, eines chinesischen medizinischen Textes', in *Oriens Extremus*, 1960, 7/2, S. 152.

16 D'OHSSON, M., *Histoire des Mongols*, Amsterdam, 1852, Bd. 3, S. 265; KÖPRÜLÜ, M. FUAD, 'Maraga Rasathanesi', in *Belleten*, 1942, Bd. 6, 23–24, S. 221; DILGAN, HAMIT, *Büyük Türk Âlimi Nasireddin Tusi*, Istanbul, 1956, S. 9.

17 SPULER, B., *Die Mongolen in Iran*, Leipzig, 1939, S. 441.

18 SPULER B. a.a.O. S. 440–41.

19 TOGAN ZEKI VELIDI 'Argun Hanin kullandiği "Garb Denizi" haritasina dair', *Türk Yurdu*, 1952, Bd. 26, 2, S. 45–48; FASÂ'Î, *Fars-nâme-i Nâsiri*, Teheran, 1313, Bd. 2, S. 140–41; KÖPRÜLÜ, M. FUAD, a.a.O., S. 221.

20 MINORSKY, V., 'Täbriz', in *Enzyklopädie des Islam*, Leiden–Leipzig, Hrsg. Houtsma, 1934, bd. IV, S. 634.

21 MINORSKY, V., a.a.O., S. 634; vgl. POPE, A. U., *Persian Architecture*, London, 1965, S. 171; WILBER, D. N., *The Architecture of Islamic Iran*, New-Jersey–Princeton, 1955, S. 17 und S. 190; SARRE, F., *Denkmäler persischer Baukunst*, Berlin, 1910, Textband S. 27.

22 Eine eingehende Beschreibung dieses stolzen Baues findet sich im 'Ikd al-Djman von Badr al-Din al-Aini (+1431), der den Bericht der Gesandtschaft des Mamluken-sultans el-Nasir zur Zeit des Ilkhan Abu Sa'id benutzt hat.

23 WILBER, D. W., a.a.O., S. 190.

24 ÜNVER, SÜHEYL, *Seldschuk Tababeti*, Ankara, 1940, S. 41.

25 ALI b. HUSEIN ALA ÜL-KAZVINI, TARIHI ALI SELDSCHUK, *Hagia Sophia Bibliothek in Istanbul*, Nr. 3019, 2. Abschnitt, Blatt (Varak) 89; vgl. ÜNVER, SÜHEYL, a.a.O., S. 41.

26 JAHN, KARL, *Histoire Universelle de Rashid al-din*, I. Histoire des Franks, Leiden, 1951 (Introduction).

27 POPE, A. U., *Persian Architecture*, London, 1965, S. 172; ELGOOD, CYRIL, *A Medical History of Persia and the Eastern Caliphate*, Cambridge, 1951, S. 311–12.

28 Diese Stiftungsurkunde (Vakfiya-i Hvaca Raschid ed-Din) befindet sich im Kitah-hana-i Milli Malik-Bibliothek in Teheran Nr. 1233.

29 ESIN, EMEL, 'Quelques aspects des influences de l'art des anciens nomades Eurasiens et de l'art du Turkestan prè-islamique sur les arts plastiques et picturaux turcs', in *First International Congress of Turkish Art. Communications presented to the Congress*, Ankara, 1961, S. 104–5.

30 FRANKE, HERBERT, a.a.O., S. 6.

31 RASCHID ED-DIN FAZLULLAH, *Mukatebat-i Raschidi* (*Letters of Rashid al-din*) Hrg. Muhammed Shafi, Lahor, 1948, S. 183.

32 *Mukatebat-i Raschidi*, S. 63.

33 *Mukatebat-i Raschidi*, S. 183.

34 Vgl. GUILLAND, R., *Essai sur Nicéphore Grégoras*, Paris, 1926, S. 72; KÖPRÜLÜ, FUAD, a.a.O., S. 225.

35 SUTER, H., *Geschichte der Mathematiker und Astronomen der Araber*, Leipzig, 1900, S. 29, 161; KRUMBACHER, K., *Geschichte der byzantinischen Literatur*, München, 1897, S. 622, u. 623

36 TERZIOĞLU, ARSLAN, 'Einflüsse der islamischen Krankenhäuser auf die abendländischen Hospitäler', in *Belleten*, 1970, Bd. 34, 133, S. 151, 160.

37 Hagia Sophia Bibliothek in Istanbul, Nr. 2180, S. 264b–86b.

38 Eine Abschrift dieser Abhandlung des Raschid ed-Din existiert in der Hagia Sophia Bibliothek in Istanbul unter der Nr. 3833.

39 Die Abschriften dieser Werke von Raschid ed-Din sind in den Suleymaniye (Istanbul) und Manisa Bibliotheken vorhanden.

40 GABRIEL, A., *Monuments Turcs d'Anatolie*, Bd. 2, Paris, 1934, S. 49–50.

41 ÜNVER, SÜHEYL, *Tip Tarihi Yilliğimiz I*, Istanbul, 1966, S. 13–14.

42 SABUNCUOĞLU, SCHEREF ED-DIN, Mücerrebname. Fatih Kütüphanesi in Istanbul, Nr. 3546, Blatt 130a.

43 LAIGNEL-LAVASTINE, *Histoire Générale de la Médecine*, Paris, 1936, S. 509.

44 KILICOĞLU, VECIHE, *Cerrahiye-i Ilkhaniye*, Ankara, 1956, S. 4.

45 ÜNVER, SÜHEYL, *Cerrahiye-i Ilkhaniye*, Istanbul, 1939, S. 8, 9; KILICOĞLU, V., a.a.O., S. 4.

46 HUARD, P. und GRMEK, M. D., *Le Prémier Manuscript Chirurgical Turc, redigé par Charaf ed-din* (1465), Paris, 1960.

47 TOGAN, Z. V., 'Raschid ed-Din', in *Islam Ansiklopedisi*, Bd. 9, Istanbul, 1963, S. 708.

48 *Mukatebat-i Raschidi*, S. 352–56; Dieses seldschukische Krankenhaus in Schiraz wurde im Jahre 1210 (607 H.) vom türkischen Fürsten Atabeg Ebu Bekr b. Sa'd-i Zengi gegründet. (Devletşah: Tezkire-i Devletşah, Ankara, 1963, Bd. I, S. 324).

49 WILBER, D. N., a.a.O., S. 191.

50 Vgl. SARRE, F. und HERZFELD, E., *Archäologische Reise im Euphrat und Tigrisgebiet*, Bd. 2, Berlin, 1920, S. 188, 189, 191.

51 JAHN, KARL, 'Dogu ile bati arasinda bir Ortacağ kültür Merkezi: Tebriz', in *Review of the Institute of Islamic Studies of Istanbul University*, vol. IV, parts 3–4, 1971, S. 32–33.

H. E. Müller-Dietz
Berlin-West (Germany)

Zur Geschichte des Marine- und Landtruppen-Hospitals in St. Petersburg

Mit einer breiten Klinikfront reicht die Leningrader Militärärztliche Akademie „S. M. Kirov" im Vyborger Bezirk bis an das rechte Ufer der Neva, zwischen der Abzweigung der Grossen Nevka und der Litejnyj-Brücke. Vor über 170 Jahren (1798) entstand an dieser Stelle, nach den Vorbildern der Berliner Pépiniere und des Wiener Josephinums, die St. Petersburger Mediko-chirurgische Akademie. Einer ihrer ersten Rektoren war Johann Peter Frank, der auch hier seine Pläne zur Reform des medizinischen Unterrichts verwirklichen wollte.[1] Er musste dem einflussreichen, aus Schottland stammenden Sir James Wylie (in Russland Jakov Vasil'evič Villie genannt) weichen, der das russische Militärmedizinalwesen organisierte und lange Zeit hindurch leitete.[2]

Die neue Akademie fasste die Aufgaben der kleineren medizinischen Lehranstalten in Moskau, Petersburg und Kronstadt sowie des deutschen „Chirurgischen Instituts am Kalinkin-Krankenhaus"[3] zusammen und wurde zur grössten Ausbildungsstätte des Russischen Reiches, vorwiegend für Truppen- und Marineärzte. Ihren guten Ruf hat diese Hochschule, 1881 in „Militärärztliche Akademie" (Voenno-medicinskaja Akademija) umbenannt, bis heute behalten. Leider sind ihre reiche Bibliothek, ihre Archive und Sammlungen dem historisch interessierten Ausländer verschlossen.

Für das ganze 19. Jahrhundert ist die Geschichte der Anstalt durch ein Werk gut belegt, das anlässlich des Centenariums der Gründung von N. P. Ivanovskij[4] herausgegeben wurde. Beschreibungen von G. G. Skoričenko,[5] G. Prozorov,[6] M. Heine[7] und anderen ergänzen diese Übersicht. Doch die Mediko-chirurgische Akademie war seinerzeit keine völlige Neuschöpfung. Sie baute auf den Schulen an den grossen Petersburger Hospitälern und am Kalinkin-Krankenhaus auf. Auch von diesen Anstalten kann man aus verstreuten Angaben in der zeitgenössischen Literatur ein recht anschauliches Bild gewinnen. Fast nichts aber ist aus dem zugänglichen Schrifttum über die Baugeschichte der Vorläufer der Akademie zu erfahren – des Marine- und des Landtruppen-Hospitals, von ihrer Gründung durch Peter den Grossen bis zur Eingliederung in die neue Mediko-chirurgische Akademie. Die spärlichen Angaben darüber wurden hier für die erste Hälfte des 18. Jahrhunderts zusammengestellt und mit einigen Abbildungen illustriert.

Reimers[8] nennt die Lage der Akademie „zweckmässig gewählt, da dieser Stadttheil einer der ruhigsten und geräuschlosesten Gegenden der Residenz ist". Realistischer formuliert es Georgi,[9] wenn er meint, der Vyborger Bezirk sei „der unansehnlichste Theil der Stadt, und die meisten seiner Einwohner beschäftigen sich auch ländlich mit Gärten, Vieh u.s.f." Noch um die Mitte des 19. Jahrhunderts gab es in diesem Bezirk nur 55 steinerne Häuser, ein Fünfzigstel aller Steingebäude Petersburgs.[10] Bis 1717 waren hier erst 350 Höfe gebaut worden, fast ausschliesslich klein und aus Holz, während die ganze Stadt bereits 4.250 Anwesen umfasste. Zu 90 Prozent bestand die Bevölkerung der „Vyborger Seite" aus Soldaten und Unteroffizieren, Handwerkern, kleinen Angestellten und Krämern.[11] Die Hospitäler waren von einer Zuckersiederei und Brauerei und einer Werft eingefasst. In unmittelbarer Nähe befand sich die „Kosaken-Vorstadt" mit ihren schmutzigen, baufälligen Hütten, deren Einwohner die Petersburger Baukommission 1739 summarisch als Diebe bezeichnete.[12] Für eine grosse Krankenanstalt war also die Umgebung recht triste. Noch 1784 gab es in dem Bezirk nur eine Strasse, die parallel zum Ufer verlief und stellenweise gepflastert war. Sie musste den 2.000 ständigen Bewohnern genügen.

Diese ungünstige Lage ist kein Zufall. Bei allen Plänen, die Peter, seine Baumeister und seine Nachfolger für die Struktur der Stadt entwarfen, blieb der Vyborger Teil ausserhalb der eigentlichen Stadtgrenzen. Hier, vor den „Mauern", sollten Friedhöfe, Schlachthäuser, Gewerbebetriebe, Speicher, Krankenhäuser und Asyle angesiedelt werden. Ausserdem wollte Peter das Marinehospital so weit an das Wasser bauen, dass die Verwundeten von den Schiffen direkt in die Krankenzimmer getragen werden konnten. Daher wählte der Zar diesen abgelegenen Platz, trotz der Entfernung zu den Verwaltungs- und Versorgungszentren, trotz sumpfigen Bodens und ständiger Bedrohung durch Überschwemmungen.

Die Literaturangaben über das Datum der eigentlichen Gründung beider Hospitäler sind widersprüchlich und schwanken, je nach der Definition, zwischen 1710 und 1720. In Moskau hatte Zar Peter 1706 ein grosses Militärhospital eingerichtet und ihm eine chirurgische Schule mit anatomischem Theater für die Versorgung der Armee und der jungen Marine angeschlossen. Es steht fest, dass der Zar ähnliche Pläne schon sehr früh auch für die 1703 gegründete Festung und Stadt Petersburg hatte. Zunächst jedoch benötigte er alle Mittel und Arbeitskräfte für den Ausbau der Befestigungsanlagen, für den Bau der Admiralität (der Werft), des Stückhofes (der Geschützgiesserei) und fester Gebäude für die Unterbringung des Hofes, der Truppen und der Beamten. Die medizinische Versorgung der ersten Einwohner und der vielen Bauarbeiter war äusserst mangelhaft. Sie wurde durch einige Wundärzte und durch 18 Hütten, die als Revierstuben für Kranke hergerichtet waren, improvisiert. Eine Improvisation war offensichtlich auch die Benutzung zweier leerstehender Kasernen-Baracken am sumpfigen Ufer der Nevka (dort, wo heute das Hotel „Leningrad" steht).

Die ersten, das Lazarett betreffenden Anordnungen des Zaren an seinen Generalzeugmeister P. B. Sumarokov übermittelt uns Čistovič.[13] Am 2. August 1710 erhielt Sumarokov den Befehl, alle kranken Soldaten unter seine Aufsicht zu nehmen und in diesen Kasernen zu sammeln. „Die Kasernen, in denen jene Soldaten liegen sollen, sind zu inspizieren und zu reinigen, damit es immer sauber ist, und die schwarzen Hemden der Soldaten sollen gewechselt und gewaschen werden, damit sie weiss sind." Das war der Anfang der einen der beiden Anstalten, des Hospitals für die Landtruppen. Im nächsten Jahr (November 1711) ergingen, da die Baracken wohl nur bedingt brauchbar waren, detaillierte Anordnungen, in denen es heisst: „. . . auch sollen die Kasernen inspiziert und gereinigt und, wo sie schadhaft sind, repariert werden. Vor den Fenstern sind Verkleidungen aus Leinwand anzubringen, die man mit Öl, oder was sonst geeignet ist, bestreichen soll. In diesen Kasernen sind unverzüglich Öfen und Kamine zu setzen, und jedem Soldaten ist ein Lager mit einem Strohsack zu bereiten. . . .“ Der Befehl, kranke und verwundete Soldaten in diesem Lazarett aufzunehmen, wurde im Juni 1716 nachdrücklich und unter Aufzählung aller Einheiten, für die die Anstalt zuständig war, wiederholt.

Im Mai des gleichen Jahres (1716) findet sich in einem Befehl an Sumarokov die interessante Anweisung, für die kranken Soldaten der Petersburger Garnison die eine Hälfte des Hospitals zu reservieren, die an der Kleinen Neva liegt, und die andere Hälfte dem Kriegskommissariat zur Disposition zu überlassen. Hier erst deutet sich die Teilung des Hospitals an, denn diese zweite, östliche Hälfte wurde dann zum Admiralitäts- oder Marinehospital.

Für die folgenden Jahre überschneiden sich die Angaben. Im Frühjahr 1715 liess der Monarch, wie Staehlin[14] und Golikov[15] berichten, dort den Platz für den Bau des neuen Land- und Seehospitals säubern und legte feierlich, in Gegenwart aller Militär- und Zivilbeamten und der Geistlichkeit, den Grundstein für die neuen Gebäude. Geplant war ein langgestrecktes, dem Ufer parallellaufendes Gebäude, das durch eine zentrale Kirche getrennt und an beiden Giebelseiten von je einem anatomischen Theater abgeschlossen werden sollte. Der Bauplatz muss neben den Hospital-Kasernen oder zwischen ihnen und dem Flussufer gelegen haben. Wahrscheinlich sollte zuerst der östliche Teil für das Marinehospital fertiggestellt werden, denn die Marinehistoriker beanspruchen 1715 als Gründungsjahr ihrer Anstalt für sich. An dem Admiralitätshospital wurde später auch eine Tafel mit den Worten angebracht, die Peter bei der Grundsteinlegung ausgesprochen hatte und die Richter[16] in etwas holprigem Deutsch wiedergibt: „Hier finde jeder kranke Krieger Beruhigung und Hülfe, die ihm bisjetzt fehlte: Gott gebe nur, dass niemals viele derselben nöthig haben mögen, hieher gebracht zu werden!“ Während der Bauarbeiten wurden, zumindest in den ersten Monaten, die Kasernen auch für die Versorgung von Matrosen und Werftarbeitern genutzt, denn Michajlov[17] fand im Marinearchiv einige Krankeneinweisungen in das Admiralitätshospital aus der Zeit von Oktober 1715 bis 1717.

Es ist nicht ganz korrekt, von einem „Grundstein“ zu sprechen. Wegen des flachen sumpfigen Ufers, und damit die Schiffe mit den Verwundeten direkt an den Gebäuden anlegen konnten, liess der Zar Pfähle in das seichte Wasser rammen und darauf oder dahinter ein steinernes Fundament aufschütten. Auf diesem sollte ein solider Bau aus Stein errichtet werden. Das verzögerte sich jedoch. Entweder hatte eine der vielen Überschwemmungen die Tragfähigkeit des Fundamentes beeinträchtigt oder man brauchte umgehend Ersatz für die baufälligen Kasernen – jedenfalls wurde in den Jahren 1717 bis 1719 zunächst ein langer Fachwerkbau errichtet und als Hospital benutzt. Vielleicht war dem Zaren auch das Geld ausgegangen, denn 1716 erliess er eine Verfügung, dass jedem Offizier, vom Fähnrich bis zum General, bei einer Beförderung ein voller Monatssold zugunsten des Krankenhausbaus abzuziehen sei. Luppov[18] gibt an Hand einiger Dokumente aus dem Leningrader Historischen Archiv an, dass die Fachwerkgebäude im Jahre 1719 fertiggestellt waren, dass im gleichen Jahre befohlen wurde, sie wieder einzureissen und durch Gebäude aus Stein zu ersetzen und dass diese Arbeiten ziemlich rasch vorangingen, denn schon 1721 begann man, die Dächer mit Schindeln zu decken.

Mit dem Bau des Hospitals wurde der aus Lugano im Tessin stammende Architekt

Domenico Trezzini (*ca.* 1670–1734) beauftragt,[19] der 1703 in die Dienste des Zaren getreten war und von dem bis 1726 alle wesentlichen Gebäude der Stadt geschaffen wurden – die Festung mit der Peter-Pauls-Kathedrale und dem Petertor, das Alexander-Nevskij-Kloster, die „Zwölf Kollegien", in denen jetzt die Leningrader Universität untergebracht ist, und viele andere. Mit dem Bau des Hospitals beeilte sich Trezzini so sehr, dass bereits 1723 der eine Flügel, wohl der des Marinehospitals, und 1726 der zweite Flügel fertiggestellt waren. Nur die Kirche in der Mitte dauerte lange und wurde zu Lebzeiten Trezzinis nicht abgeschlossen. Sein Sohn und Nachfolger, Pietro Trezzini, erhielt 1741 den Auftrag, für die Kirche einen neuen Plan auszuarbeiten. Doch auch dieser wurde nicht realisiert, und später baute man den Mitteltrakt zu einem zentralen anatomischen Theater mit Bibliothek um. Offenbar bestand der Zar auf dem raschen Fortgang der Arbeiten, denn aus dem Jahre 1722 ist von Trezzini ein Verzeichnis der Bauarbeiten überliefert, die der Zar befohlen hatte, und in dem es heisst: „Das steinerne Hospital auf der Vyborger Seite, dessen erste Hälfte gedeckt ist, wird heuer fertiggestellt."[20]

Sicherlich bergen die Archive der Akademie auch Bauzeichnungen aus jener Zeit. Sie sind uns nicht zugänglich, und wir halten uns an eine Beschreibung von Petrov[21] für das Jahr 1719. Hier wird noch einmal betont, dass das langgestreckte Steingebäude auf Pfählen mit zwei Flügeln zu beiden Seiten einer Plattform für die Kirche errichtet wurde. Jeder Flügel war zweistöckig und 138,5 m (65 saž.; 1 sažeń = 2,13 m) lang und 17 m (8 saž.) tief. Das Erdgeschoss hatte eine „Galerie". Darunter ist ein durchgehender Korridor an der flusszugewandten Seite zu verstehen, von dem aus alle Krankenzimmer zu erreichen waren. Jeder Flügel hatte in jedem der beiden Stockwerke 15 Räume von 9,20 m (4,3 saž.) Länge. Sie waren im unteren Geschoss 3,30 m (11 Fuss) und im Obergeschoss 3,60 m (12 Fuss) hoch. Die Höhe des Gebäudes betrug 8,50 m (4 saž.) über dem Boden. Jedes Zimmer hatte also eine Grundfläche von ungefähr 140 qm und konnte etwa 25 Patienten aufnehmen. Im Generalreglement für die Hospitäler von 1735[22] heisst es im 12. Abschnitt über den Bau der Krankenräume: „Die Zimmer für die Kranken sind so gross anzulegen, dass in ihnen zwanzig oder dreissig Kranke liegen können." Michajlov[23] gibt an, dass das Marinehospital im November 1723, als es sicherlich noch nicht voll belegt werden konnte, 219 Kranke aufgenommen hatte. An dem Bau waren übrigens 150 Lohnarbeiter beschäftigt; er kostete 6.000 Rubel.

Für einige Jahre fehlen dann weitere Nachrichten zur Baugeschichte der Hospitäler. Wahrscheinlich bestanden Pläne, das ganze Gelände um die Gebäude zu drainieren und trockenzulegen, denn es muss sich bald als hinderlich erwiesen haben, dass beide Teile der Anstalt vom Lande her nur über Dämme zu erreichen waren. Irgendwann war der östliche Teil, das Marinehospital, durch einen rechtwinklig landeinwärts angebauten Flügel erweitert worden. Aus dem Jahre 1732 berichtet Čistovič[24] über einen regen Briefwechsel zwischen dem Kriegskollegium und der Baukommission. Er betraf den Bau eines steinernen Gebäudes für das „Petersburger Hospital", der nur schleppend voranging und trotz zahlreicher Mahnungen und Kontrollen erst 1733 fertiggestellt wurde. Čistovič nahm an, dass es sich hierbei um das Steingebäude für das Landtruppen-Hospital gehandelt habe, und zitiert: „. . . für die Fertigstellung des Fundamentes bis zum 1. Mai und andere Arbeiten sind ausreichend Soldaten von den Feld- und Garnisonsregimentern abzustellen." Das Kriegskollegium beschleunigte die Arbeiten so sehr, dass sie nicht sorgfältig genug ausgeführt wurden. Die Folge war, dass das kaum fertiggestellte Hospital im Frühjahr 1733 abbrannte.

In den Akten erscheinen dann die Hospitäler erst 1739 wieder, als die Petersburger Baukommission, die dem regellosen Wachsen der Stadt durch eine verbindliche Bauklanung Einhalt gebieten sollte, ihre Pläne für die Vyborger Seite bekanntgab.[25] Die Kommission hielt es vor allem für erforderlich, wegen der Brandgefahr die hölzernen und unregelmässigen Häuser der Hospital-Bediensteten zu entfernen. Diese Hütten sollten abgerissen und auf freien Plätzen in grösserer Entfernung von den Steingebäuden wieder aufgebaut werden. Zu beiden Seiten der Hospitäler sollte der Platz jedoch freibleiben.

An das steinerne Landtruppen-Hospital sollte für weitere Krankenzimmer und zur besseren Symmetrie ein neuer steinerner Flügel angebaut werden, ebenso wie beim Marinehospital. Auch ein Garten war für diese Seite vorgesehen. ,,An den beiden Ecken des an der Neva liegenden Hauptgebäudes, die jetzt hölzerne, mit Eisen verkleidete Kuppeln tragen, soll später, wenn die Kuppeln baufällig werden, zur besseren Symmetrie statt der Kuppeln noch ein Stockwerk (appartament) aufgesetzt und darüber eine angemessene Verzierung angebracht werden. Im Hof hinter den Hospitälern soll ein Kanal gezogen und der niedrige Boden auf diesem Hof allmählich mit Erde aufgeschüttet werden. Hinter besagten Hospitalgärten aber soll Platz gelassen und eine Strasse angelegt werden." Bezüglich der Kuppeln und des zusätzlichen Stockwerks meinte Petrov an anderer Stelle.[26] ,,. . . niemand dachte später an die Ausführung dieser Pläne." Weitere Anordnungen der Kommission betrafen den Ausbau der Umgebung der Hospitäler, den Standort neuer Kasernen und den Bau einiger grosser Strassen. Überall, auch unmittelbar neben den Hospitalgebäuden, war der Boden mit Hilfe von Gräben trockenzulegen.

Zehn Jahre später (1749) musste das Marinehospital gründlich überholt werden. Die Fussböden wurden ausgewechselt, die Öfen umgesetzt, Wände und Decken repariert. Neue Gebäude entstanden für Schuppen und Speicher, für die Wohnungen der Angestellten, für den Kommissar, die Wache und die Arrestanten, für eine Brauerei und ein Bad.[27] Doch die Freude an der verbesserten und verschönten Anstalt war nur kurz, denn ebenfalls bei Petrov[28] finden wir den lakonischen Vermerk: ,,In der Nacht vom 4. zum 5. Dezember 1753 brannte das Admiralitätshospital ab."

Weiter soll der Zeitraum dieses Berichts nicht ausgedehnt werden. Wir wenden uns zum Abschluss der Frage zu, ob unsere Vorstellungen von diesen Gebäuden durch zeitgenössische oder wirklichkeitsnahe Bilder zu belegen sind. Die älteste bekannte Abbildung findet sich in dem axonometrischen Plan, den Weber 1720 seinem Journal ,,Das Veränderte Russland"[29] beigegeben hat. Sie zeigt, zwischen Lagerhäusern und einer Brauerei, ein langgestrecktes, eingeschossiges, im Wasser stehendes Bauwerk mit hohem Dach. In der Mitte treten zwei runde Türmchen etwas aus der Baufluchtlinie hervor. Der Datierung nach muss dies wohl die einzige überlieferte Abbildung des Fachwerk-Hospitals sein. Die nachprüfbare Naturtreue anderer Gebäude auf dem Plan lässt darauf schliessen, dass der Zeichner auch das Hospital realistisch abgeschildert hat. Auf einem anderen Bild, einem Panorama der Neva mit Blick nach Osten von Marselius[30] aus dem Jahre 1725, lässt sich in der Ferne ebenfalls das Hospital ahnen, nun aber schon das Gebäude aus Stein. Details sind jedoch nicht zu erkennen.

Frühe Abbildungen der steinernen Bauwerke schienen nicht erhalten geblieben zu sein. Ein Stadtplan von Unvertzagt[31] aus dem Jahre 1737 zeigt schon ungefähr den für die spätere Anlage charakteristischen U-förmigen Grundriss. Analogien zu anderen Schöpfungen des gleichen Baumeisters, den „Zwölf Kollegien“ etwa, sind unsicher, da Trezzini keineswegs einförmig gebaut hat. Eine Bleistiftzeichnung in den Fonds der Leningrader Ermitage zeigt ein langes, zweigeschossiges Gebäude, das auf einem von Pfählen umkleideten Sockel im Wasser steht. Zu beiden Seiten einer unfertigen Kirche erstrecken sich zwei durch Rondelle mit Türmchen abgeschlossene Flügel mit je 31 Fensterachsen – ebenso vielen, wie das an seiner Stelle stehende Klinikgebäude heute noch aufweist. Der linke Flügel (das Landtruppen-Hospital) hat zum Wasser hin zwei und der rechte Flügel (das Marinehospital) fünf Türen. Das Blatt ist nicht signiert, trägt aber eine handschriftliche Legende:

Daß große Steinerne Hospitahl, worin / die in der Mitte komende Kirche noch nicht / aufgebauet, und unter Dach gebracht worden, / als welches, des schlechten Terrains wegen, / auch niehmahel aufgebauet werden / wird.

Die Zeichnung gehört zu einer Serie gleichartig beschrifteter Blätter,[32] die dem schwedischen Kammerjunker F. W. von Bergholtz zugeschrieben werden, der durch sein Tagebuch[33] bekannt geworden ist und der sich im Gefolge des späteren Zaren Peter III. von 1742 bis 1746 in Russland aufgehalten hat. Das Sockelgeschoss der Kirche, das Trezzini jun. 1741 oder 1742 begonnen hatte, verweist die Entstehung des Bildes in die gleichen Jahre. Wie schon erwähnt, geriet der Bau der Kirche immer wieder ins Stocken, bis er endlich ganz aufgegeben wurde. 1746 hat Trezzini noch weitere Varianten für die Gestaltung der Hospitalkirche vorgelegt, von denen Korolkov[34] zwei veröffentlicht hat.

Aus der Leningrader Ermitage stammt ein Hinweis auf eine ganz ähnliche Kollektion im Schwedischen Nationalmuseum. Nachforschungen ergaben, dass Bergholtz 1746 offenbar eine umfangreiche Sammlung von Stichen und Architektur-Zeichnungen, von denen 400 noch erhalten sind, von Russland nach Stockholm gebracht hat. B. H. Hallström[35] hat die Geschichte der Sammlung und die einzelnen Stücke anschaulich beschrieben. Auf den Bauzeichnungen sind zum grossen Teil die gleichen Sujets dargestellt wie in der Leningrader Kollektion. Die Stockholmer Blätter sind aber zumeist grösser und koloriert. Das Petersburger Land- und Marinehospital wirkt stilisiert, weist aber die gleichen Elemente und Abmessungen auf. Die Legende darauf – von derselben Hand geschrieben wie auf dem Leningrader Blatt – lautet:

Facade / Des, von dem Höchst Seeligen Keyser, Peter, dem Grossen, Erbaueten, Grossen Hospithals, von Stein / in St:Petersburg, auf der anderen seite, des Newa Strohms, gegen, dem Gies Hause über.
A. Die angelegte, aber außer Dach gebliebene, und nicht ausgebauete Kirche.
B. Daß Hospithal von der Land Milice.
C. Daß Hospithal, von denen See Bedienten.

Als jüngste Abbildung sei die subtile Darstellung auf dem mit grösster Feinheit ausgeführten axonometrischen, Machaev[36] zugeschriebenem Plan aus dem Jahre 1753 erwähnt. Der Künstler hat sich jedoch in manchen Details nicht an die Wirklichkeit, sondern an den Plan gehalten und den Realitäten der Bauentwicklung vorgegriffen. In seiner Zeichnung ist die Kirche schon fertiggestellt. Prächtige Gärten erstrecken sich hinter den U-förmigen Gebäuden. Noch stehen sie im Wasser und noch sind die Pfähle des Fundaments zu erkennen. Aber die Struktur zeigt schon die Form der späteren Klinikgebäude, wie sie aus den Abbildungen des späten 18. und des 19. Jahrhunderts geläufig ist und sich bedingt bis heute gehalten hat.

Wer ohne Zugang zu den Archivalien einen Blick in die Baugeschichte der Petersburger Hospitäler zu werfen versucht, muß Lücken in Kauf nehmen. ,,Möge die That dem guten Willen entsprechen und die unmögliche absolute Vollständigkeit der Darstellung, in der Schwierigkeit des Auffindens aller Urkunden, eine gerechte Entschuldigung finden" (W. M. Richter[37]).

Literatur

1 MÜLLER-DIETZ, H., 'Johann Peter Frank und die Reform des Medizinstudiums in Petersburg', in *Verhandl. d. XX. Intern. Kongr. Gesch. Med.*, Hildesheim, 1969, S. 98–102.
2 MÜLLER-DIETZ, H., 'J. Wylie und die Mediko-chirurgische Akademie in St. Petersburg. Zum 200. Geburtstag von Sir James Wylie', *Clio Medica*, Oxford, 1969, **4**, 99–107.
3 MÜLLER-DIETZ, H., 'Das Kalinkin-Institut, eine, deutsche medizinische Hochschule in St. Petersburg', *Med. hist. J.*, Hildesheim, 1968, **3**, 310–27.
4 *Istorija Voenno-medicinskoj Akademii za sto let (1798–1898)* (Geschichte der Militärärztlichen Akademie in hundert Jahren 1798–1898), Hrsg. N.P. Ivanovskij, S. Peterburg, 1898.
5 SKORIČENKO, G. G., *Stoletie Voennogo Ministerstva, 1802–1902.* Bd. IX: *Imperatorskaja Voenno-medicinskaja (mediko-chirurgičeskaja) Akademija. Istoričeskij očerk* (100 Jahre Kriegsministerium, 1802–1902. Bd. IX: Die Kaiserliche Militärärztliche (mediko-chirurgische) Akademie. Historischer Abriss), 2 Teile, S. Peterburg, 1902 und 1910.
6 PROZOROV, G., *Materialy dlja istorii Imperatorskoj Sanktpeterburgskoj Mediko-chirurgičeskoj Akademii* (Material zur Geschichte der Kaiserlichen St. Petersburger Mediko-chirurgischen Akademie), Sanktpetersburg, 1850.
7 HEINE, M., 'Zur Geschichte der Kaiserlichen Medicinisch-Chirurgischen Akademie zu St. Petersburg', *Med. Ztg. Russlands*, 1850, **7**, 349–52, 357–60 und 364–68.
8 REIMERS, H. V., *St. Petersburg am Ende seines ersten Jahrhunderts*, 2 Theile, St. Petersburg, 1805, S. 128.
9 GEORGI, J. G., *Versuch einer Beschreibung der Rußischen Kaiserlichen Residenzstadt St. Petersburg und der Merkwürdigkeiten der Gegend*, St. Petersburg, 1790, S. 127.
10 POSSART, P. A. F., *Wegweiser für Fremde in St. Petersburg*, Heidelberg, 1842, S. 55.
11 LUPPOV, S. P., *Istorija stroitel'stva Peterburga v pervoj četverti XVIII veka* (Geschichte des Aufbaus Petersburgs im ersten Viertel des 18. Jahrhunderts), Moskva-Leningrad, 1957, S. 28 und 35.
12 *Polnoe Sobranie Zakonov Rossijskoj Imperii* (Vollständige Gesetzsammlung des Russischen Reiches), 1. Sammlg., Sanktpeterburg, 1830, Bd. X, Nr. 7874.
13 ČISTOVIČ, JA., *Očerki iz istorii russkich medicinskich učreždenij XVIII stoletija* (Skizzen aus der Geschichte der russischen medizinischen Institutionen im 18. Jahrhundert), Sanktpetersburg, 1870, S. 225.
14 STÄHLIN, J. V., *Originalanekdoten von Peter dem Großen*, Leipzig, 1785, S. 225.
15 (GOLIKOV, IV.), *Dejanija Petra Velikogo, mudrogo preobrazitelja Rossii* (Die Taten Peters des Grossen, des weisen Reformers Russlands), Bd. 5, Moskva, 1788, S. 34 f.
16 RICHTER, W. M., *Geschichte der Medicin in Russland*, Bd. 3, Moskwa, 1817, S. 17.
17 MICHAJLOV, S. S., *Medicinskaja služba russkogo flota v XVIII veke* (Der medizinische Dienst in der russischen Flotte im 18. Jahrhundert), Leningrad, 1957, S. 56 f.
18 LUPPOV, S. P., loc. cit. (Nr. 11), S. 34.
19 LISAEVIČ, I., *Pervyj architektor Peterburga* (Der erste Architekt Petersburgs), Leningrad, 1971.
20 KOROLKOV, M., 'Die Architekten Trezzini', in *Starye gody*, Sanktpetersburg, April, 1911, S. 34.
21 PETROV, P. N., *Istorija Sankt-Peterburga s osnovanija goroda, . . .* 1703–1782 (Geschichte St. Petersburgs seit der Gründung der Stadt . . . 1703–1782), S. Peterburg, 1884, S. 172.
22 *Polnoe Sobranie . . .*, loc. cit. (Nr. 12), bd. IX, nr. 6852.
23 MICHAJLOV, S. S., loc. cit. (Nr. 17), S. 62.
24 ČISTOVIČ, JA., loc. cit. (Nr. 13), S. 228 f.
25 *Polnoe Sobranie . . .*, loc. cit. (Nr. 12), bd. X, nr. 7874.
26 PETROV, P. N., loc. cit. (Nr. 21), S. 387.
27 PETROV, P. N., loc. cit. (Nr. 21), S. 520.
28 PETROV, P. N., loc. cit. (Nr. 21), S. 541.
29 (Weber, F. Ch.), *Das veränderte Rußland*, Frankfurth, 1721.

30 MARSELIUS, CH., *Prospet de la Citadelle Saint Petersbourg.* 1725 (Bibliothek der Akad. Wiss. UdSSR, Handschriften-Abteilung, Leningrad).
31 UNVERTZAGT, G., Plan der Kayserl. Residentz Stadt St. Petersburg. 1737 (Bibliothek der Akad. Wiss. UdSSR, Handschriften-Abteilung, Leningrad).
32 *Pamjatniki russkoj kul'tury pervoj četverti XVIII veka v sobranii gosudarstvennogo ordena Lenina Ermitaža* (Denkmäler der russischen Kultur des ersten Viertels des 18. Jahrhunderts in den Sammlungen der Staatlichen Ermitage 'Leninorden'), Katalog. Hrsgg. von V. N. Vasil'ev und V. M. Glinkin, Leningrad–Moskva, 1966.
33 BERGHOLTZ, F. W. V., 'Tagebuch (1721–1725)', in *Magazin für die neue Historie und Geographie,* hrsg. von Anton Friedrich Büsching, 19. Theil, Halle, 1785, S. 3–202; 21. Theil, Halle, 1787, S. 178–360.
34 KOROLKOV, M., loc. cit. (Nr. 20).
35 HALLSTRÖM, B. H., Russian architectural drawings in the National Museum, Stockholm, 1963.
36 *Plan stoličnogo goroda S. Peterburg* (Plan der Hauptstadt St. Petersburg), 1753 (Bibliothek der Akad. Wiss. UdSSR, Handschriften-Abteilung, Leningrad).
37 RICHTER, W. M., loc. cit. (Nr. 16), Bd. 3, S. iii.

P. Gelmetti
Bologna (Italy)

Un nosocomio dallo strano nome: 'L'Ospedale della Morte' di Bologna

Il vero spirito della speoalità, inteso come fraterno e disinteressato soccorso al prossimo che soffre, è di natura prettamente cristiana e la locanda, nella quale il Samaritano condusse il mercante ferito dicendo all'oste 'ricoveralo, abbi cura di lui e metti tutto sul mio conto', si può considerare il primo vero ospedale.

La Parabola del Buon Samaritano sta alla base di una nuova concezione medica: da essa prende origine quella che in seguito sarà definita assistenza medica sociale.

Molti anni, però, dovranno trascorrere prima di poter vedere la costruzione di un grande nosocomio e ciò avvenne proprio in Italia.

'Prima fra tutte istituì un xenodochio; in esso raccolse malati che giacevano nelle piazze e ristorava le membra dei poveri, consunti dai languori e dall'inedia.'

Così, in una lettera inviata ad Oceanio, si esprimeva S. Girolamo ammiratore entusiasta di Fabiola la quale, com'è noto, aveva fatto costruire in Trastevere il primo ospedale sorto in Occidente.

Ad esso ne fecero seguito molti altri ed anche Bologna non fu seconda ad altre città sia italiane sia estere.

Essa, infatti, nel 1200 possedeva circa novanta 'hospitali' che all'inizio, però, avevano la funzione di luogo di ristoro per pellegrini affaticati, stanchi, con il fisico logorato ed a volte ammalato causa il lungo viaggio.

Solo in seguito assunsero una vera e propria funzione ospedaliera, pur rimanendo, spesso, edifici piccoli ed angusti perchè ricavati da vecchie costruzioni.

I primi due edifici costruiti espressamente per tale uso furono quelli che presero il nome di Ospedale della Vita e di Opedale della Morte.

L'Ospedale della Vita, antecedente al suo confratello, fu fondato, quasi certamente, nel 1260 dalla Compagnia dei Battuti istituita dal beato Riniero (o Rainiero) Fasano (o Fagiani) de'Barcobini da Perugia del Terzo Ordine di S. Francesco.

L'Ospedale della Morte, invece, fu fondato il 20 Luglio 1336 dalla Compagnia dei Divoti dello Spedale di S. Maria della Morte, chiamata in seguito Arciconfraternita di S. Maria della Morte.

Questa compagnia di laici si era assunto come primo impegno la cura degli infermi, ma, in seguito, ebbe altri compiti fra cui l'incarico di confortare ed assistere i condannati a morte e di seppellire i giustiziati.

I condannati a morte erano condotti sul luogo dell'esecuzione della pena capitale da Divoti che dal 1292 avevano avuto il titolo di Confraternita e poi, fino al 1351, si chiamarono Confrati Divoti di Maria.

In tale anno, dal milanese Giovanni Naso Vescovo di Bologna e da Giovanni Visconti, per l'incarico assunto di seppellire i giustiziati, ottennero anche l'autorizzazione di confortarli e di assisterli prima della morte.

Per tale ufficio, assunsero il nome di Confratelli della Morte e tale denominazione la ereditò anche il loro ospedale.

Nel 1586, con Breve di Papa Sisto V, la Compagnia di S. Maria della Morte venne dichiarata Confraternita, privilegio che la Compagnia di S. Maria della Vita aveva già ottenuto nel 1582.

Il Bosi, nel suo libro 'Archivio patrio di antiche e moderne Rimembranze felsinee', ci fornisce utili notizie della suddetta Confraternita:

Questa spirituale Congregazione eretta in Bologna aveva per istituto di visitare i prigioni, e di confortare i condannati alla pena di morte, il che nel 1351 venne ad essa concesso da Giovanni Naso Vescovo nostro. In tale anno i Confratelli di detta Compagnia recarono a compimento la chiesa di S. Gio. Battista decollato presso la Montagnola, in quello spazio di terreno che ora è occupato dal giuoco del pallone, dando ivi cristiana sepoltura a chi lasciava la vita sul patibolo. La qual Confraternita della Morte recavasi processionalmente alla detta chiesa in ogni ultima settimana dei mesi onde recitarvi i sette Salmi Penitenziali, e v'ascoltava Messa per l'anima de' defunti giustiziati. – In seguito essa Compagnia con Breve del Pontefice bolognese Gregorio XIII, ottenne di poter liberare dal carcere un condannato a morte nell' anniversario della decollazione di san Giovanni (29 Agosto), purchè il condannato non fosse reo d'eresia, nè di lesa Maestà, nè sacrilego, nè incendiario di chiese, e di Luoghi Pii, nè falsatore di monete. E se in tale anniversario non eravi nelle carceri alcun dannato alla morte, se ne dimandava uno fino a quel giorno, nel quale facevasi libero.

Nel 1433 (31 agosto) dal Senato, e da Marco Vescovo d'Avignone Governatore di Bologna fu dato a questa Arciconfraternita il privilegio e la sopraintendenza di condurre, ordinare e disporre i viaggi delle Processioni per Bologna colla B. V. di san Luca nelle Rogazioni Minori (questo privilegio fu confermato da Clemente VII nel 1524; da Pio IV nel 1562; e da Pio V nel 1567) e questo fu il primo anno in cui la detta santa Immagine venne recata a Bologna, e quivi trattenuta con solenne triduo.

Nel 1592 nel seno di detta venerabile Confraternita, per Breve di Clemente VIII, venne eretta una Congregazione detta 'di Carità', destinata a visitare settimanalmente le carceri, a provvedere di vitto i carcerati, e sollecitare le loro cause criminali, e a dare tutte le disposizioni necessarie alla nettezza e sanità. I Statuti di tale Congregazione furono fatti ed approvati da Monsignor Alfonso Paleotti, mentre era Coadiutore dell'Arcivescovato di Bologna al Cardinal Gabriele.

L'Arciconfraternita di S. Maria della Morte era composta da laici che avevano funzioni diverse: alcuni reggevano ed amministravano l'Ospedale, altri l'Oratorio per cui i primi facevano parte della 'Compagnia larga dell'Ospedale', i secondi della 'Compagnia stretta dell'Oratorio'.

Il 9 Luglio 1798 l'Arciconfraternita di S. Maria della Morte si sciolse; il 31 Gennaio 1799 fu chiusa la Chiesa; il 2 Giugno 1801 fu soppresso l'Ospedale.

Questo Nosocomio dallo strano nome, la cui costruzione ebbe inizio il 20 Luglio 1336, aveva sede nel Vicolo della Morte[1] ove, in seguito ebbe sede anche la 'Speziaria della Morte',[2] che, all'inizio, corrispondeva all'antico ingresso dell'Ospedale della Morte.[3]

Il suo costruttore, l'architetto Antonio Bernardino Trebigli, detto il Terribilia, curò, poi, anche l'erezione dell'attiguo e famoso Archiginnasio.

L'unico a porre un dubbio circa l'esattezza della data riguardante la costruzione dell'Ospedale della Morte, è il Guidicini il quale scrive:

. . . Che l'approvazione della Compagnia sia del 1336 è probabile, ma non si crede che la sua prima instituzione fosse diretta ad aprire un Ospitale per infermi, ma bensì che il suo primo, e vero Instituto fosse di confortare li condannati a morte, ed eccone le ragioni. Nel libro dei memoriali, sotto l'anno 1338 si trova registrato il testamento di Samolino Pavanesi il quale fa un legato alla Compagnia della Morte, servendosi di questa espressione: – 'Item Societati, qui vadunt ad Iustitiam'. – La medesima espressione si vede in altri atti susseguenti, sicchè pare che questo fosse il suo vero, e primo istituto. Così in un'atto del 1339 si legge: – 'Hospitali devotorum qui associant homines ad Iustitiam', – pare quindi che solo nel 1339 avessero formato l'Ospitale. Così in altro atto del 1340 si legge: – 'Bartholomeus de Argile Prior Societatis Battutorum de Morte, et misericordia, qui vadunt ad justitiam.'

Fatta questa precisazione, il Guidicini, nel suo libro 'Cose notabili della città di Bologna', prosegue con dettagliati particolari nella storia di questa Compagnia e del suo Ospedale:

Nel 1350 il 26 novembre si trova che la Compagnia comprò per ampliare e aggrandire l'ospitale da Domenico detto Mengo, e da Giacomo del fu Venturino fornaro, una casa sotto 'S. Michele' dei Lambertazzi, che confinava da due lati coll'Ospedale, e dagli altri con gli eredi di Giovanni Ospitatore di Desio Bualelli, con una casa dei frati degli Apostoli e colla via pubblica.

Fu data una nuova ampliazione all'Ospitale pochi anni dopo, essendochè per questo fine compra la Compagnia li 26 luglio 1364 da Graziano, e Francesco del fu Artinisio di Franceschino Artenisi una casa piana sotto S. Xfro dei Geremei, che confina coll'Ospitale da due lati, e la via pubblica dagli altri lati, pagata lire 100 rogito Francesco del fu Lorenzo Costa.

Nel 1377 1 Marzo l'Ospitale comprò da Lucchino del fu Bartolino della Cura una casa piana sotto S. Vito dei Lambertazzi, presso l'Ospitale, e in via pubblica da tre lati, per lire 200. Rogito Stefano di Giacomo Ghisilardi.

Li 13 Ottobre 1394. Gli Anziani decretarono a favore dell'Ospitale che si chiudesse con muro certa viazzola turpissima e disonesta tra l'Ospitale, e 'S. Michele dei Lambertazzi', e quella tener chiusa, e incorporata a detto Ospitale. Rogito Giacomo Toschi, Giacomo da Castel de Britti e Pietro Urselli.

Antonia di Giovanni Bambaglioli moglie di Matteo Gessi vendette li 11 gennaio 1430 una casa per lire 120 all'Ospitale posta sotto S. Xfro del Ballatoio in confine dell'Ospedale, degli eredi di Enrico Felicini, e della via pubblica, la qual casa fu demolita a comodo dell'Ospitale, rogito Frigerino S. Venanzi. Confinava colla detta casa della Gessi quella degli eredi Felicini, la quale anche essa sarà stata comprata per ampliare l'Ospitale, ma di questo acquisto non se ne trova memoria.

Nel 1433 li 4 aprile, per ampliare l'Ospitale fu demolita la Chiesa di san Remigio di proprietà della Chiesa di S. Appolinare di Seravalle, che era stata venduta ai Battuti per lire 200, rogito d'assoluzione del prezzo fatto dal notaio Frigerino di Savenanzi.

Il Giovedì 19 agosto 1434 a ore 20 fu ultimato conduzione dell'acqua della fonte Remonda all'Ospitale della Morte, che fu usata da molti per la sua bontà, a modo che i Dazieri del vino se ne ingelosirono, e vi si opposero perchè ne soffrivano, e tanto si adoperarono che fu rovinato il condotto. Vedi Ghirardacci.

Nel 1435 era già fatto il portico dalla parte di S. Xfro del Ballatoio.

Susseguentemente li 4 aprile 1433, il Priore di S. Apolinare di Seravalle assolse l'Ospitale della Morte di lire 200 per saldo della Chiesa di S. Remigio già demolita dall'Ospitale, ed incorporata nella nuova fabbrica di detto Ospitale, rogito Frigerino Savenanzi.

1544. Dimissione fatta da Ippolita figlia, ed erede del fu Cesare dalla Nave con il consenso di Francesco del fu Giovanni Aspettati suo marito a favore dell'Ospitale di una casa sotto S. M. dei Cartari, che confinava i beni della morte essendo successori del dottor Filippo da Milano, gli eredi di Francesco Salimbeni successori degli eredi di Giovanni Arrigoni, altri beni dell'Ospitale, la via pubblica, per lire 600. Rogito Melchiore Beroaldi. La detta casa servì per la nuova fabbrica dell'Ospitale.

1550 3 Giugno. Cessione alla Morte di Alessandro del fu Pietro Bianchi di testare le ragioni ad esso spettanti sopra una casa, che li 30 marzo passato Bianchi aveva acquistata da Ippolita del fu Cesare dalla Nave, vedova di Francesco Aspettati, è posta sotto S. M. dei Carrari, confina gli eredi di Nascentore Nascentori, l'Ospitale, certa viazzola verso detto Ospitale, e Scipioni Vasselli mediante l'Androna, per lire 650. Rogito Giovanni Beroaldi.

1566 30 Marzo. Convenzione fra la Compagnia della Morte, e Antonio di Bernardino Trebigli per la fabbrica da farsi sopra le volte del portico della Chiesa della Morte, dove eran già le scuole di medicina. Rogito Francesco Barbadori. Li 22 dicembre la fabbrica del portico della Morte era finita.

Nel 1436 fu deciso dai devoti di fare l'Oratorio il quale dopo esser stato ampliato fu riaperto li 15 agosto 1585. Questo vecchio Oratorio fu destinato ad infermeria per le donne, e gliene fu sostituito un nuovo che si aprì nel 1719.

Lo Statuto della Compagnia della Morte e dell'Ospitale della Morte fu concentrato in quello della Vita dietro Reno, dove furono trasportati gli ammalati, restando qui un ambiente con alcuni letti, e cocchietti per accorrere ai bisogni di feriti, e pericolati.

1124. Chiesa dedicata alla B. V. detta della Compagnia della Morte. Li 21 o 22 gennaio 1427 questa Chiesa fu benedetta e dopo fu posta la prima pietra fondamentale del portico dal pillastro d'angolo verso la piazza mentre nevicava essendo rettore della Compagnia Bernardino Muletti notaro, priore Ciro Alfrapadore, e massaro Giovanni di Nicolò Carlini speziale.

Li 10 settembre 1524, l'Ornato accordò all'Ospitale suolo pubblico per fare un portico, che dalle case dei PP. di S. Michele in Bosco condotte da Nascentore Nascentori, e cioè per pertiche 12, arrivasse ad attaccarsi a quello che restava avanti la porta principale della Chiesa della Morte. Questa concessione farebbe credere che il portico fatto nel 1427, cominciasse dall'angolo della via del Pavaglione, e terminasse d'avanti la porta della Chiesa.

Nel 1565 li 30 marzo, passarono convenzioni con Antonio del fu Bernardino Trebigli architetto per la fabbrica nuova da farsi sopra le volte del portico della Chiesa dell'Ospitale dov'erano già le scuole di medicina. Rogito di Francesco Barbadori.

Nel 1569 Pio V ordinò regolamenti per le lettere di cambio, e fissò il portico davanti all'Ospitale della Morte per loggia del cambio, ordinando che detto portico dovesse dirsi Loggia del Cambio. Nel 1735 la Chiesa fu rimodernata.

Nell' 1600 circa sotto il portico vecchio della morte vi si tenne per poco tempo il Pavaglioncino ossia lo smercio dei Bozzoli coltivati in Città.

Li 30 agosto 1433. Marco Vescovo Avignonese, e Governatore di Bologna destinò il Rettore, Priore, Massaro e Uomini della Compagnia della Morte, al governo dell'Immagine della B. V. di S. Luca e in conferma della concessione fattagli dagli Anziani e Collegi di poter portare la detta S. immagine alla Città di Bologna processionalmente, e collocarla nella Chiesa dell'Ospitale per qualunque bisogno della Città, concedendo alla Compagnia di far fare un armadio, entro il quale debba conservarsi detta immagine dalla Chiesa del Monte della Guardia e munirlo di tre chiavi, una da stare presso il Gonfaloniere o Priore degli Anziani pro tempore, l'altra presso la Priora di S. Mattia e la terza presso il Rettore della Morte. Ordinava ancora che ogni anno in perpetuo nella prima domenica di luglio detta immagine per gli uomini di detta Compagnia fosse portata a Bologna, ed incontrata alla porta dagli Anziani e Reggimento, da tutte le compagnie, clero e popolo di Bologna assieme a tutte le reliquie dei Santi della Città ecc. poi fare processioni portandola in qualche Chiesa destinata a ciò, ivi cantandovi la messa solenne, e poscia per detti uomini riportata al suo luogo solito accompagnata come sopra dal clero e popolo sino alla porta di Saragozza. Di quì ebbero principio le processioni che poi si fecero per le rogazioni minori, li quattro giorni precedenti alla solennità dell'Ascensione, funzione che per l'ultima volta fu regolata da questa Compagnia secondo l'antica consuetudine sotto il Priorato del conte Domenico Levera. L'ultimo Priore della Compagnia della Morte fu il marchese Francesco di Guido Pepoli essendosi sciolta, e preso possesso dei beni della medesima, non che della Congregazione dell'Ospitale li 9 luglio 1798 dal Governo.

Le Rogazioni minori furon continuate trasportando la B. V. dal Monte della Guardia, alla Chiesa di S. Pietro, di dove si conduceva processionalmente il lunedì, martedì e mercoledì alle Chiese destinate per cantarvi messa solenne; uso che fu levato e d'allora in poi la S. immagine stette per tutti i giorni delle Rogazioni esposta alla venerazione dei fedeli sull'altar maggiore della Cattedrale, di dove è tolta soltanto il mercoledì dopo pranzo per dare la benedizione sulle scale di S. Petronio.

La Chiesa fu chiusa li 31 gennaio 1799 e affittata ad uso di magazzeno di mobili, e di libraria. L'Ospitale fu soppresso, e decretata la sua unione a quello della Vita dietro Reno li 2 giugno 1801, e li 8 susseguente si cominciò il trasporto degli ammalati, e feriti al nuovo Ospitale. L'Oratorio della Compagnia, e parte delle infermerie furono occupate da una fabbrica di seterie, e da falegnami.

La conforteria, o assistenza ai condannati cessò col cessare della Compagnia. L'ultimo assistito secondo l'antico ordine fu Domenico Benedetti da Palazolo stato Fiorentino decapitato li 10 settembre 1796 sotto il Priorato del conte Pietro Aldrovandi.

Clemente VIII con bolla delli 11 aprile 1592 soppresse la Prefettura Generale della custodia dei Guardiani delle Carceri, e ordinò che in ogni Città dello stato Ecclesiastico, l'uffizio del Custode delle prigioni fosse applicato a quella Compagnia Spirituale, che fosse stata solita di esercitare uffizi di carità verso i poveri detenuti. Alfonso Paleotti coadiutore della Chiesa Vescovile di Bologna dichiarò per la più degna secondo la mente Pontificia la Compagnia della morte rivestendola della Prefettura dell'ufficio di custodia, e del diritto di deputare i Guardiani delle Carceri.

Resta a dirsi che questa Compagnia ebbe li 11 aprile 1592 la Prefettura ed ufficio della custodia e deputazione dei guardiani delle carceri. Il primo custode detto poi Capitano delle Carceri nominato dalla Confraternita della Morte fu Meo Nanni eletto li 9 giugno 1592, l'ultimo fu Giovanni Battista Presciuti confinato li 18 luglio 1796.

1123. Porta con scala immediata, che ascende alli trapiani, e sopra le volte del portico della Morte, dalla parte del fianco di S. Petronio.

Li 15 settembre 1620 l'Ospitale della Morte locò al Collegio degli Artisti sette stanze, ossia scuole per anni tre, e per annue L. 100 rogito Giovanni Pini.

Li 24 settembre 1623 fu fatta locazione di alcune case, botteghe, e stanze ai Presidenti del sacro Monte di Pietà per ergervi il così detto Monte, o della scala, dietro l'annuo affitto di L. 1050, rogito Vittorio Barbadori. Nel 1681 continuava ad esservi il detto Monte, che occupava il fabbricato sopra il portico inclusivo quello dalla parte della Compagnia degli Orbi nella via Foscarari.

L'Ospedale della Morte, 'per i poveri febricitanti', era diviso in tre classi: per gli uomini, per le donne e per i feriti.

Il termine 'poveri-febricitanti', si riferiva agli ammalati acuti poichè gli statuti escludevano categoricamente dal ricovero i malati cronici e quelli contagiosi.

Il 15 Settembre 1620 il suddetto Ospedale affittò al Collegio degli Artisti sette stanze ad uso di scuola per tre anni.[4]

Il 23 Agosto 1742, Papa Benedetto XIV, 'motu proprio', istituì nell'Università di Bologna una Scuola di Chirurgia Pratica denominata 'dell'ostensione delle Operazioni Chirurgiche dei Cadaveri' prescegliendo a professore di essa 'vita sua natural durante' Pier Paolo Molinelli (1702–64).

Si trattava di un doppio corso di venti lezioni ciascuno che si teneva d'inverno, prima nell'Ospedale di S. Maria della Vita[5] e poi nell'Ospedale di S. Maria della Morte.

Dette lezioni erano facilitate specialmente perchè presso l'Ospedale della Morte, oltre ai cadaveri dei detenuti, era possibile avere anche quelli dei giustiziati che, come si usava dire, venivano 'dati all'anatomia' o 'dati all'anatomia secreta' o 'dati all'anatomia pubblica'.

Certi cadaveri, inoltre, venivano concessi per ricerche anatomiche o per preparazioni particolari che non venivano eseguite pubblicamente e ne venne dato anche uno ad un assistente per preparare uno scheletro.

Comunque è accertato che dal 13 Ottobre 1541 al 24 Gennaio 1725, per studi anatomici, vennero consegnati 38 cadaveri fra cui tre di donne.

Come si può notare, questo ospedale, oltre che per la cura degli ammalati, fu importante anche per le lezioni che si tennero[6] e per i primi studi anatomici che vennero eseguiti.

Esso, infine, ebbe notorietà perchè frequentato da diversi illustri medici fra cui: l'iniziatore della chirurgia plastica scientifica Gaspare Tagliacozzi (1546–99) studente praticante fino al III anno di medicina; Giovanni Battista Cortesi (1553–1634) garzone barbiere a 16 anni, ottenne un posto di assistente e si laureò; il celebre studioso dell'orecchio Antonio Maria Valsalva (1666–1723); l'anatomico Giovanni Antonio Stancari (1668–1748); il grande anatomo-patologo Giovanni Battista Morgagni (1682–1771) vi intraprese gli studi anatomici; l'anatomico Gaetano Fattorini (1716–97) ed altri.

Dopo tante gloriose esperienze, il 2 Giugno 1801 l'Ospedale di S. Maria della Morte venne fuso con quello di S. Maria della Vita per costituire il Grande Ospedale che il 24 Giugno 1801 assorbì altri piccoli Spedali e precisamente quelli di S. Francesco; di S. Maria dei Servi, detto di S. Biagio; della Trinità; di S. Antonio Abate, detto 'degli Sportini'.[7]

Nel 1814 il Grande Ospedale, eretto in Via Ripa di Reno, prese il nome di Ospedale Maggiore e ciò si trova scritto nella prima pagina dei 'Regolamenti disciplinari per l'Ospedale Maggiore stabiliti dalla Congregazione di Carità in Bologna': 'Titolo Primo. Determinazioni preliminari. Lo Spedale, che ora chiamasi Grande Spedale della Vita, e della Morte si chiamerà per l'avvenire Spedal Maggiore della Città di Bologna. Questa denominazione sarà posta sopra la porta dello Spedale.'

Verso le ore 10 del 24 Luglio 1943, durante il primo bombardamento aereo americano di Bologna, l'Ospedale Maggiore venne semidistrutto e reso perciò impraticabile.

Dopo molti anni di sistemazioni provvisorie e frammentarie dei vari reparti, nel 1963 l'Ospedale Maggiore, confortato dalla più moderne attrezzature sanitarie, rivide finalmente la luce fuori Porta S. Felice, in Via Emilia Ponente N^{0} 31, costruito nell'area un tempo denominata 'Prati di Caprara'.

Oggi, così, a Bologna nel modernissimo Ospedale Maggiore prosegue ininterrottamente l'opera di assistenza e cura degli ammalati iniziata oltre sette secoli or sono in quel nosocomio che portava lo strano nome di Ospedale della Morte.

Notes

1 Attuale Via de' Musei.

2 In seguito fu chiamata prima Farmacia della Morte, poi Farmacia del Pavaglione (nome attuale) e fu situata in principio del portico anzichè in fondo, come in origine.

3 La Speziaria confinava con l'infermeria degli uomini a cui si accedeva attraverso la farmacia stessa. Solo in seguito, quando il Trebigli costruì il nuovo edificio, l'ingresso dell'Ospedale fu spostato nella adiacente Via de'Foscherari.

4 L'affito fu stabilito in L. 100 l'anno.

5 Nell'Ospedale di S. Maria della Vita erano conservati i 250 ferri chirurgici, di cui 70 in argento, fatti costruire a Parigi sotto la direzione del celebre Lapeyronie e donati a Papa Lambertini dal Re di Francia Luigi XV.

6 L'insegnamento universitario era praticato in ambedue gli ospedali fino dalla seconda metà del 1500.

7 Lo Spedale di S. Francesco e di S. Biagio erano antichi ospizi per pellegrini; lo Spedale della Trinità era un convalescenziario per i malati dimessi dagli Ospedali della Vita e della Morte; lo Spedale di S. Antonio era una istituzione nosocomiale fondata e gestita dai Fatebenefratelli (detto anche Spedale degli Sportini dal soprannome che avevano i Fatebenefratelli per il fatto che andavano alla questua con una sporta.).

Bibliografia

BOSI, G., *Archivio patrio di antiche e moderne Rimembranze felsinee*, Bologna, Tipografia di Antonio Chierici da S. Domenico, 1853, vol. I.

BOSI, G., *Archivio patrio di antiche e moderne Rimembranze felsinee*, Bologna, Tipografia di Antonio Chierici da S. Domenico, 1855, vol. II.

BRONZINO, G., *Notitia doctorum*, Giuffrè Editore, Milano, 1962.

BUSACCHI, V., 'L'Ospedale della Morte', in *Sette secoli di vita ospitaliera in Bologna*, Cappelli Editore, Rocca S. Casciano, 1960.

DALL'OSSO, E., *Appunti sulla storia degli ospedali e cliniche di Bologna*, Luigi Pozzi Editore, Roma, 1956.

FANTI, M., *L'Archiginnasio*, Bologna, Coop. Tipografia Azzoguidi, 1907, vol. II.

FANTI, M., *L'Archiginnasio*, Bologna, Azzoguidi Soc. Tip. Editoriale, 1963, vol. LVIII.

FANTUZZI, G., *Notizie degli scrittori bolognesi*, Bologna, Nella stamperia di S. Tomaso d'Aquino, 1790, tomo VIII.

FRATI, L., *Opere della Bibliografia Bolognese*, Bologna, Zanichelli Editore, 1888, vol. I.

GALLASSI, A., 'Richerche e studi su Riniero Fagiani De' Barcobini fondatore dell'Ospedale della Vita', in *Sette secoli di vita ospitaliera in Bologna*, Cappelli Editore, Rocca S. Casciano, 1960.

GELMETTI, P., 'La prima cattedra di medicina operatoria in Bologna: Manoscritti inediti di Pier Paolo Molinelli', in *Giornale di Batteriologia, Virologia ed Immunologia ed Annali dell'Ospedale Maria Vittoria di Torino*, Ciriè, Tipografia Cav. Giovanni Capella e Figli, 1968, vol LXI, no. 11–12.

GENTILI, G., 'Ospedali non più esistenti a Bologna', in *Sette secoli di vita ospitaliera in Bologna*, Cappelli Editore, Rocca S. Casciano, 1960.

GIACOMELLI, R., *Il cuore di Bologna*, Tamari Editore, Bologna, 1968.

GUIDICINI, G. B., *Cose notabili della città di Bologna*, Bologna, Società Tipografica dei Compositori, 1870, vol. III.

HIRSCH, A., *Bibliographisches Lexikon der Hervorragenden Aerzte*, Wien und Leipzig, Urban e Schwarzenberg, 1885.

MAZZETTI, S., *Repertorio di tutti professori antichi e moderni della famosa Università e del celebre istituto delle scienze di Bologna*, Bologna, Tipografia S. Tommaso d'Aquino, 1847.

MEDICI, M., *Della vita e degli scritti degli anatomici e medici fioriti in Bologna*, Bologna, Tipografia S. Tomaso d'Aquino, 1889.

PAZZINI, A., *Bibliografia di Storia della medicina italiana*, Milano, Istituto Editoriale Italiano Bernardo Carlo Tosi, 1939.

PIETRA, G. C., *Origine dei nomi delle strade piazze porte in Bologna*, Bologna, Tipografia delle scienze di Giuseppe Vitali, 1868, vol. I.

PIETRA, G. C., *Origine dei nomi delle strade piazze porte in Bologna*, Bologna, Stabilimenti Poligrafici Riuniti, 1933.

SABENA, V. e MARAGI, M., 'Dall'Ospedale della Vita all'Ospedale Maggiore', in *Sette secoli di vita ospitaliera in Bologna*, Cappelli Editore, Rocca S. Casciano, 1960.

SARTI (de'), L., *Thesoro delle Indulgenze di Bologna*, Editore G. Rossi, Bologna, 1589.

SIMILI, A., 'Ospedali della vita e della morte a Bologna', in *Rivista Ospedaliera*, Roma, Tipografia Consorzio Nazionale, 1957, no. 1–2.

SORBELLI, A. e SIMEONI, L., *Storia della Università di Bologna*, Bologna, Nicola Zanichelli Editore, 1944, vol. I.

SORBELLI, A. e SIMEONI, L., *Storia della Università di Bologna*, Bologna, Nicola Zanichelli Editore, 1947, vol. II.

A. M. Luyendijk-Elshout
Leiden (The Netherlands)

The Caecilia Hospital in Leiden (1600–1972)

A tourist arriving in Leiden can leave his car in a dilapidated square situated behind a busy street lined with shops. As the traveller inches the nose of his car toward a crumbling wall still showing the blackened outlines of a chimney, the old car-watcher shuffles alongside. He raises a hand and points aloft to the high pointed roof of the ruin before which they are standing. 'This', he says, 'is Boerhaave's famous hospital.' Siste viator!

If the tourist's curiosity is aroused, he strolls to the low entry in the Vrouwensteeg, the name given to the alley when the long-since demolished Vrouwenkerk (Church of Our Lady) still graced it. The green door carries a small sign. The text reads: 'St. Caecilia Gasthuis. Originally Augustinian Convent 1465. After the Reformation, Madhouse and Pest-house with quarters for pensioners. In 1636 Collegium Medico-Practicum, best known for the teaching of Professor Boerhaave (18th century) at the sickbed. Royal Dutch Tourist Association ANWB.'

If he rings the bell and anyone comes, he finds himself in a narrow alley. On his right there are a number of small buildings, each with a green door provided with a peephole, the old madhouse cells. To his left is the municipal storehouse, where the peat and wood supplied to the poor were kept. At the end of the alley there is an entrance on the right, admitting him to the large square garden surrounded on three sides by high-roofed buildings and closed off on the east by the pensioners' houses.

On the south side, if he takes the trouble to search, he will find the entrance to the *Boerhaavezalen*, the wards where Boerhaave taught. The handsome Burgundian outer staircase has disappeared, but the doorway is still intact. The wards themselves have high ceilings, and the light falling through the arched windows placed high in the walls throws shadows on the old tiles of the floor. The oaken ceiling is carried by heavy beams resting on double corbels. Art historians consider these two wards to be the best surviving examples of seventeenth-century hospital construction in The Netherlands.

On the north side of the garden is the impressive building in which the regents' room was situated. Their peeling coats-of-arms still hang above the door.

Like Hofmeier[1] in 1966, the traveller will leave the Caecilia complex with a feeling of melancholy. The historian will feel belligerent. Is it permissible for a building of such great historical value to be allowed to fall into this state? The municipal storehouse has completely lost its roof. The artists and young bohemians who live in the complex, many of them clandestinely, complain of falling rubble. The city of Leiden is poor. The university prefers to maintain its institutional neutrality. The structure is on the list of the National Department of Monuments, but this department is behind schedule and hampered by a lack of funds.

Even a brief consideration of these facts brings the historian to a point at which he passes beyond history and enters a very difficult field, one involving new questions. It seems more than likely that historians in all fields and in all countries are about to be, or have already been, confronted with these questions.

The Caecilia Gasthuis is not a unique case. All over The Netherlands, and apparently in other places as well, historical monuments are succumbing to neglect. This holds less for ornate palaces than for the more modest buildings with an unusual structure and great historical value. One of the results of this neglect of remarkable buildings, most of which are located in the old centres of cities, is that whole districts are being demolished and depopulated. The process affects not only churches, schools, patrician residences, and courthouses, but also the small houses of simple people built in the distant past. The loss of so many buildings makes a district unlivable. The small local shops disappear with their customers; supermarkets, banks, and warehouses take the place of homes, cafés, and nursery schools. Small neighbourhood parks become parking areas. Before long, the district is no longer fit to live in or to work in. It looks lifeless and mutilated.

This is the fundamental problem underlying the restoration of the Caecilia Gasthuis. If this building is to serve a useful function, the livability of the district around it must be guaranteed. In other words, the entire area will have to be examined as a whole to determine whether the intended function is consistent with the overall developmental pattern.

The historian starting to work from this angle comes into contact with the sociologist, the city planner, and also with the people living in the district, in this case *de Kamp*, the central point of which is formed by the Caecilia Gasthuis. It has slowly become evident that the present plan to reconstitute the complex as a new museum for the history of science would be quite satisfactory if the factor of the livability of the district is taken into consideration. This would mean, for instance, opening the garden to the public – so that children could play in the convent garden as they once did long ago – and converting part of the municipal storehouse into a café with a terrace for outdoor tables.

But at the same time the building will have to be restored in a way that satisfies the criteria for a museum, including proper conservation and protection of the contents. And it must also satisfy modern standards concerning the display of material having permanent value for the general public. To avoid having a slumbering museum, there should be space for special exhibitions dealing in particular with current problems in terms of their historical background. The exhibition *From Witchdoctor to Medical Doctor* held in Haarlem in the spring of 1972 has shown that such exhibitions can draw a large attendance.

A museum set up on this basis can do much to increase the living quality of the district, and the visitor strolling through the restored wards could also, for instance, follow the history of Leiden astronomy and physics illustrated by objects of which the present Museum for Science has an abundance but no space to exhibit.

A university with as rich and varied a history as the University of Leiden should unquestionably lend its full weight to the execution of a plan that will preserve for posterity the work of the very men who were responsible for its fame.

The importance of finding a suitable function for a historical monument in relation to the livability of a district is also shown by the successful way in which the St. Elizabeth Gasthuishof, also situated in *de Kamp*, has been restored and given a constructive function. As I shall show in discussing the history of the Caecilia Gasthuis in more detail, from the historical point of view these two hospitals were built according to two entirely different principles. The St. Elizabeth Gasthuis was originally a house with grounds around it, which was bought by a private group in 1428 and converted into a women's hospital on a plan conceived entirely in the medieval tradition. For one thing, a chapel was added, the altar of which was consecrated in 1433 by the Bishop of Utrecht. The priest was entrusted with the spiritual care of the patients, and mass was said daily. There was also an open communication between the chapel and a ward, so that the sick paupers could follow the service.[2]

In the course of time, as for the Caecilia Gasthuis, quarters were built for pensioners. The pensioners bought a place in the Gasthuis for a sum which was partially determined by the individual's age, thus providing the hospitals with a certain source of income.

The entire arrangement – wards with altar, pensioners' quarters, and facilities for the care of the aged – is reminiscent of the Hôtel Dieu of the French city of Beaune. The St. Elizabeth Gasthuis was a Dutch example of this form of medieval care. In carrying out the restoration, which is now almost completed, the architects have managed to preserve the ancient character of the *gasthuis* and still adapt the function to the character of the district and present-day needs. The St. Elizabeth Gasthuis has become the Sint Elizabeth Gasthuis Hof:[3] a complex consisting of quarters for old people with a charming garden and provisions for the nursing and rehabilitation of elderly patients. The nursing staff is quartered in the pensioners' houses. The chapel and wards have been returned to their original form.[4] Tourists can visit the complex without disturbing the patients.

We must now ask just what the importance of the Caecilia Gasthuis is from the historical point of view, and why it is so imperative that its historical cachet be preserved when the complex is restored. To answer these questions we must examine the factors that led to the conversion of the St. Caecilia Convent, which until 1586 had been inhabited by the Augustian nuns, into a pest-house and madhouse.

In the middle of the sixteenth century the Low Countries were at war with Spain. Toward the end of this period, when the domains under the Spanish hegemony had developed into an independent nation, trade flourished in the liberated regions. In 1575 the Spanish siege of Leiden was lifted by the troops of William of Orange. The city began to grow rapidly, and soon felt the need of adequate accommodation for the sick and insane. The latter were still to be seen roaming the streets, as in the Middle Ages, clothed in red tabards with the municipal coat-of-arms embroidered on the sleeve,[5] the charges of the city. But at this time Calvinism had replaced Catholicism as the state religion, and this meant a change in the philosophy underlying the care of the sick and the poor. In the Middle Ages both fell under the same category of charitable work, but Calvin drew a distinction between the care of the poor and the care of the sick, and he also made a separation between those suffering from pest (infectious diseases) and those with other sicknesses.[6] This concept is reflected in the seventeenth-century hospitals of The Netherlands.

In the northern Netherlands, the altar and the beds were separated in the now secularized hospitals. The House of Charity became a hospital, usually with individual rooms which could be heated separately and would prevent 'poisoning' of one patient by another.[7]

With the coming of the Reformation the cloisters were emptied in Leiden, as in other places. The municipal authorities then made ground available for a hospital behind the Vrouwenkerk in *de Kamp*. When objections were raised to this terrain, it was exchanged for the St. Caecilia Convent just to the north, which covered a large rectangular area[8] and could be converted into a hospital.

To insure an adequate reconstruction of the convent complex, the authorities consulted the Medical Faculty of the University of Leiden. At that time, the Faculty consisted of three professors, Joannes Heurnius (1543–1601), Gerard de Bont (1537–99), and Pieter Pauw (1564–1617). Their report, which dates from 1598, has survived, and in it we find indications for the reconstruction which were adopted by the architect.[9] The report itself reflects a distinct tendency to hold to Calvinistic ideas where it came to hospital construction. The city authorities themselves had already intended to separate the infectious diseases from the other diseases. According to the recommendations, the rooms for the 'pest patients' (in other words, cases of infectious disease) should have high ceilings and be well ventilated, and provide for the isolation of the patients. In this they based themselves on the experience of the Italian physicians, among them Joannes Philippus Ingrassia, and also on the Nürenberg physician Joachim Camerarius. They therefore specifically proposed that in the 'pest wards' the windows should be situated high in the walls and opposite each other, so that there would be a draught guaranteeing a supply of fresh air. There were to be no more than six to eight beds in each ward, placed in such a way that the patients could not see each other. Above the beds a gallery was to be constructed on which the blankets and sheets could be aired.

The insane, on the contrary, were to be placed as far away as possible from the other patients in small rooms – 'the darker the better' – each provided with a small toilet facility and a hatch through which food could be passed. The idea that the mentally diseased should be kept in the dark derived from Classical Greek medicine and was referred to by Celsus, who became popular during the Renaissance. This advice was consistently applied in later years, as the designs for the reconstruction of the Caecilia Gasthuis show. When it was completed, men like Franciscus de le Boë Sylvius and Herman Boerhaave stood on the galleries of the pest wards and visited the sick in their isolated beds.

It is from the Caecilia Gasthuis that we know the oldest publications north of the Alps of case histories with autopsy reports. The first publication of thirty autopsy reports, some of them prefaced by a description of the clinical picture, was prepared by Ottho Heurnius (1577–1652),[10] the oldest cases dating from before 1636, the year in which clinical teaching was introduced. The earliest report is from 1617, and describes the clinical course of what was probably a case of pneumonia in a child. A whole series of autopsy reports was later incorporated into the work of Th. Bonet.[11] A second and longer series was published by Franciscus de le Boë Sylvius (1614–72); these reports had been collected by his student Joachim Merian in 1659, 1660 and

1661, and appeared in Sylvius' *Opera Medica.*[12] In the supplement to this work, which comprises 160 cases, the use of medicaments is discussed in detail, and in a second supplement, entitled *Collegium Nosocomicum*, thirty-three autopsy reports are given. Justus Schrader,[13] who also studied under Sylvius, published a number of autopsy reports dating from the same period. The importance of the clinical teaching in the Caecilia Gasthuis has been amply demonstrated by G. A. Lindeboom in his contribution to *The History of Medical Education*[14] 1972, particularly in relation to the teaching of Herman Boerhaave.

But we are more concerned here with the hospital's fate when, after Boerhaave, clinical teaching deteriorated and the *gasthuis* was visited only by the municipal doctors. It was not until 1787 that the Collegium Clinicum[15] was re-established, and it soon became evident that the Caecilia's accommodation fell far short of the standards set by the rapidly developing field of medicine. Only two rooms in the whole complex were suitable for the admission of patients!

On 22 September 1797, Meinard Simon du Pui (1754–1834), who had been appointed ordinary professor of practical medicine and obstetrics in 1795, made a request to be allowed to set up a small ward with six beds in the Caecilia Gasthuis for the treatment of poor maternity or surgical patients.[16]

But despite many efforts and much improvisation, and even with the use of space in the nearby St. Elizabeth Gasthuis, it proved to be no longer feasible to treat surgical patients and perform deliveries in the Caecilia Gasthuis. All it could be used for was a *collegium casuale*, an out-patient department for minor surgery.[17] In 1799 the Caecilia Gasthuis was abandoned as Collegium Clinicum, and the now more highly differentiated clinical teaching was distributed over buildings in other parts of the city. The Caecilia Gasthuis remained open only for mental cases until 1810, when it again came into use as a municipal hospital. In 1884 the care of the insane was transferred to the St. Joris Gasthuis at Delft. In 1868, part of the Caecilia hospital was converted into municipal workshops, and five years later it was officially abolished as a municipal hospital, the institution being combined with the school of clinical medicine in the new University Hospital on the Steenstraat.[18] Part of this building now houses the National Museum for the History of Science.

The former gasthuis remained in use as a workshop, but a long, sombre period of decay had set in. Today, in 1972, The Caecilia Gasthuis complex is a collection of slum buildings in *de Kamp*, a disintegrating monument, a disgrace to both the city and the University of Leiden. But it must not be forgotten that it was collaboration between the city and the university that brought the Caecilia Gasthuis into being. And it was collaboration between professors and the municipal physicians that brought the clinical school it housed to widespread fame in the world of medicine. Herman Boerhaave in particular, by his custom of teaching at the sickbed, 'made a celebrated institution of the simple, twelve-bed Caecilia Gasthuis in the heart of the old city of Leiden'.[19] As long ago as 1936, Barge drew attention to the need for restoring this valuable monument.[20] Since then, many voices have been added to his plea that the building be saved.

The road leading to the present plan to save the Caecilia complex and to use it as a Museum for the History of Science has been long and difficult, and even now the moment for the commencement of the restoration has not yet arrived. In this time of depersonalization and commercialization of our cities, when they are becoming less and less livable, the historian must commit himself to the support of every effort for the preservation of fundamental values. These essential values of course do not solely concern tourist attractions; they mean the preservation and maintenance of historically developed parts of cities and individual buildings whose intrinsic value contributes to the wellbeing of the inhabitants. Seen in this light, a plea for the preservation of the Caecilia Gasthuis in Leiden cannot be considered a mere giving way to historical sentiment. The entire project should be seen as part of the duty of city and university to put all of their resources into the realization of the plan to preserve an internationally important monument of the history of medicine, to the benefit of the people belonging to that same city and university.

References

1 HOFMEIER, H., 'Ein Besuch in Boerhaave's Krankenhaus zu Leiden', *Med. Monatschr.*, 1966, 5, 218–20.

2 LEVERLAND, B. N., 'Het Sint Elisabeth Gasthuis in de Kamp', *Jaarboekje voor Geschiedenis en Oudheidkunde van Leiden en Omstreken*, Leiden, 1970, pp. 51–68.

3 VAN DONGEN, M. A., 'Van Sinte Elisabetten Gasthuis tot Sint Elisabeth Gasthuishof', ibid., pp. 79–88.

4 VAN OERLE, H. A., 'Het plan voor de restauratie van het St. Elisabeth Gasthuis en het hof van zessen in de Kamp', ibid., pp. 69–78.

5 LIGTENBERG, CHR., *De armenzorg te Leiden tot het einde van de 16e eeuw*, [thesis], Utrecht, 1908, p. 100.

6 DOUMERGUE, E., 'Jean Calvin', *Les hommes et les choses de son temps*, Lausanne, 1917, vol. 5, p. 257.

7 UHLHORN, G., *Die Christliche Liebesthätigkeit seit der Reformation*, Stuttgart, 1890, bd. III, p. 100.

8 VAN OERLE, H., 'De bouw van het St. Caecilia Gasthuis in de Camp te Leiden', *Jaarboekje voor Geschiedenis en Oudheidkunde van Leiden en Omstreken*, Leiden, 1941, pp. 63–81.

9 VAN HOUT, JAN, *'Armboecken' 1574–1852*, Municipal Archives, Leiden, MS. 2296, fols. 13, 14.

10 HEURNIUS, OTTHO, *Historiae et Observationes quaedam rariores ex praxi et diario*, Supplement to Heurnius' edition of Joh. Fernelii *Universa Medicina*, Trajecti ad Rhenum, 1656.

11 BONETI, TH., *Sepulchretum sive Anatomia Practica ex cadaveribus morbo denatis, proponens historias et observationes omnium corporis humanum affectuum ipsorum causas reconditas revelans etc.*, Geneva, 1700.

12 DE LE BOË SYLVIUS, FRANCISCUS, *Opera Medica, hoc est Disputationum Medicarum Duas, Methodo Medendi Libri duo, Ideae Novae Proxeos Medicae Libri Tres, ad eosque Appendix variaque alia Opuscula*, with two supplements: *Casus Medicinales Annorum 1659 60, 61, quos ex ore CL. Sylvii calamo excepit Joachimus Merian, Ph. et M.D. ac Phys. Moeno. Francof. una cum Remedics Sylvianis; itemque Collegium Nosocomicum ab Authore habitum; cum Appendice de Formulis quibusdam Remediorum ad varios affectus ab eodem praescriptis*, Venice, 1736.

13 SCHRADER, J., *Observationum Anatomico-Med. Decades quatuor; denique Cadavera Balsamo condiendo modus studio.* Supplement to W. Langly, *Observationes et Historiae omnes et singulae e'Guilelmi Harvei libello De Generatione Animalium excerptae etc.* Amstelodami 1674. Typei Abrahami Wolfgang.

14 O'MALLEY, C. D. (ed.), *The History of Medical Education*, UCLA Forum Med. Sci. no. 12, Los Angeles, University of California Press, 1972.

15 MOLHUYSEN, P. C., *Bronnen tot de Geschiedenis der Leidsche Universiteit*, Res. Cur. Den Haag 1923, vol. 6, p. 326.

16 WOUDSTRA, D., 'Meinard Simon Du Pui (1754–1834), stadsmedicus te Kampen (1780–1788), en te Alkmaar (1788–1791). Eerste Leidse hoogleraar in de praktische chirurgie en verloskunde (1791–1826)', *Kamper Almanak*, 1969–70, pp. 1–55.

17 The out-patient book in manuscript form is kept in the Department of Anatomy of the Leiden University Medical Centre.

18 JONGSMA, M. W., *325 jaar Academisch Ziekenhuis Leiden*, Lochem, 1963.

19 DANKMEIJER, J., 'Is Boerhaave's Fame deserved?', *Analecta Boerhaaviana, Vol. VI: Boerhaave and his Time*, ed. by G. A. Lindeboom, Leiden, 1970.

20 BARGE, J. A. J., *De stichting van het Academisch Klinisch Onderwijs te Leiden voor 300 jaren*, Leiden, 1937.

P. Reznikoff and D. Reznikoff
New York (U.S.A.)

Changes in therapy in a two hundred year old hospital (New York Hospital 1771–1971)

New York Hospital was granted a charter by King George III in 1771. It is the oldest hospital in New York City and the second oldest in the northern hemisphere. We thought it would be of interest to review the records of this institution to see what treatments were used during various periods of the Hospital's existence and to note the relation of changes of therapy to advances in general medical knowledge.

The first fairly complete records of the medical cases, with which this report will deal, began in 1809. Previous to this time detailed descriptions of the patients admitted to the hospital and their treatment were not kept or are not available.

A study of the therapy employed in the hospital during the first hundred years may be discouraging to a modern physician. However, one must remember Lester King's admonition that when we study the history of medicine we must avoid the fallacy of presentism – judging the past by present standards. We should ask ourselves how we would have treated a patient in the first part of the nineteenth century without thermometers, sphygmomanometers, X-ray machines, chemical, haematological and bacteriological laboratories, electrocardiography, antibiotics, steroids and all the armamentarium we have inherited and are constantly acquiring.

It is generally believed that for a good part of the nineteenth century, certainly during the first fifty years, therapy for most medical disorders consisted of bleeding, purging, blistering and the constant use of calomel and emetics. It is true that these agents were consistently used but a considerable number of other drugs and procedures were employed perhaps for better or probably for worse. As far as calomel administration is concerned, even in the present century we are told by one of our professors of medicine who contributed a chapter on malaria in the third edition of Cecil's *Text Book of Medicine* published in 1933; 'Calomel is the best purgative.'

Before we present some of the therapeutic measures used in a few illustrative diseases we should mention that for most conditions the same remedies were prescribed regardless of the illness.

Incidently it is of interest to note that New York Hospital had a Pharmacopoeia in 1816, four years before the first United States Pharmacopoeia was published.

CARDIAC DISEASE

In the first third of the nineteenth century the diagnosis of cardiac disease was not very specific. In most cases calomel and squill, morphine and many forms of blisters to the precordium were prescribed. Among the latter was a liniment of tincture of capsicum and camphorated oil, and emplastrum vesicans which apparently contained a potent blistering agent. In some cases a seton, consisting of a thread inserted under the skin of the cardiac region and pulled through was employed as a counterirritant to alleviate pain.

Cupping appeared in the medical records about the beginning of the 1830s. The first mention of the use of the stethoscope in a cardiac case is found in an 1829 record but was not in common use for several years.

In the 1830s more precise diagnoses of cardiac conditions were made such as pericarditis, hypertrophy and dilatation, hypertrophy and anasarca, congenital heart disease, pericardial effusion. Not until 1880 does the diagnosis of aortic cardiac disease appear and in 1890 endocarditis is recorded. In 1901 valvular disease is noted.

However, the treatment for many years was not varied appreciably from the calomel, squill, morphine routine until digitalis was added early in the 1830s. Bleeding was rarely ordered after the middle of the last century but as late as the 1940s occasional phlebotomies were performed for plethora.

Some other medications were tried such as Dover's powders (ipecac and opium), tartar emetic (antimony potassium tartrate), Hoffmann's anodyne (compound spirit of ether). In 1880 a patient received a tincture of aconite plaster 'to reduce the size of the heart'. In 1890 some patients were given strophanthus instead of tincture of digitalis and in 1901 oxygen began to be utilized. While calomel, given with sodium bicarbonate and digitalis was still the basic therapy of the 1910 period, a salt-free diet and mercurial diuretics were now fairly routinely prescribed.

It is with a feeling that one is living in modern times that in the Cornell Conferences of Therapy (1946) we learn that sulfonamides and finally penicillin were the treatments for bacterial endocarditis. In 1947 acute coronary accidents were treated as cases of shock. In 1953 anticoagulants, especially for thrombo-embolic conditions were employed. In 1951 disorders of rhythm were receiving much attention and there were many discussions about the relative merits of digitalis, quinidine, procaine and other drugs for arrhythmias. It is of interest to note that in 1955 an angiocardiogram was considered important before a pericardium was tapped. The implantation of pacemakers and cardiac surgery brings us to modern times.

The concern which the physicians of the old New York Hospital had for their patients can be illustrated by the attention which was paid to the toxic effects of their medicaments. Digitalis was discontinued if the patient vomited. Mercurials were stopped if ptyalism occurred and for this complication gargles, mouth-washes and occasionally applications of caustics to the gums and strong solutions of alum were used.

In addition to medications and dietary restrictions it is of interest that orders were recorded to raise the head of the bed to help the patient breathe, and for shock, warm baths, sinapism (mustard) and hot bricks to the feet, mustard paste to the epigastrium. As supportive measures alcoholic drinks were given quite freely not only in cardiac disorders but in almost all medical conditions. In most cases wine, gin, brandy and towards the end of the 1800s whisky was prescribed.

DROPSY, OEDEMA, ASCITES

Before specific diagnoses were made to establish the cause of fluid retention, certainly in the first part of the nineteenth century, conditions such as 'dropsy', 'anasarca', 'ascites' were all treated in much the same way. Diuretic concoctions such as apocynum cannabinum (Indian hemp), decoction armorac (horseradish root), in addition to calomel, squill, jalap, ipecac, tartar of antimony and potassium, digitalis, sweet spirits of nitre, tincture of iodine (orally) and a host of other drugs were employed to rid the body of fluid. Strong cathartics such as castor oil were given.

Even in those early days tapping was employed for ascites and various medicaments were rubbed into the extremities and on the abdomen such as ointment of mercury and camphor, pulvis jalap compositus, and liniments (for example a mixture of colchicine, squill and oil of camphor).

After 1834 the urine was examined for albumen indicating to the physician that fluid retention might be due to nephritis. In 1850 the specific gravity of the urine was determined. Other diuretics were employed such as cream of tartar, linseed tea, and the patient's legs were bandaged in many cases. Bleeding was occasionally used as late as 1850. With more modern diagnostic measures available the cause of water retention began to be treated (1870) then as now with salt restriction, diuretics and digitalis.

It is interesting to note the diets employed in the early days of the hospital. The charts list barley water, generous diet, milk, farinacious diet, arrowroot, chicken soup. Alcoholic beverages were almost routinely dispensed – ale, cider, brandy, wine, gin, porter.

DYSENTERY, DIARRHOEA, ENTERITIS

One of the most frequent reasons for hospitalization in the first half of the 1800s was 'dysentery'. About 1850 'colitis' began to be the diagnostic term for many diarrheal conditions. The drugs usually ordered for this complaint were calomel, opium, jalap, tartar emetic, castor oil, laudanum, Dover's powders, morphine and spirits of Mindererus (ammonium acetate solution). Ammonium carbonate, and lead acetate combined with opium were also frequently prescribed. Some patients were requested to drink freely of mucilage of gum acacia. Abdominal poultices and rubrifacients were used routinely. Enemata, called injections, were commonly employed – ipecac, starch and tincture of opium, tincture of opium and arrowroot, anodyne enemata, the composition of which is not given, and solution of alum. In some cases silver nitrate and chalk mixtures were added to the starch enemas. In 1850 opium suppositories and leeches were used for anal pain as well as cupping of the lower abdomen.

Although the relations between alcoholic excesses and the diarrheal condition was noted, still orders for brandy, port and wine were prescribed in most cases, in addition to a diet of arrowroot and occasionally milk. In 1869 beef tea and whisky were given to a patient.

In 1890 a patient with tubercular dysentery had the following therapy: astringent diarrheal mixture, creosote mixture, mustard paste to the abdomen, lead and opium pills, laudanum, and a diet of milk, lime and beef juice.

As will be noted subsequently under the diagnosis of Phthisis, all tuberculosis patients were given cod liver oil beginning in 1850 and cod liver oil and malt later in addition to other medicaments.

FEVER

Not until about 1835 were fevers classified as remittent or intermittent or just plain fever. However, the therapy was the same regardless of the cause. By 1870 the diagnosis of 'fever' was no longer used. Patients were grouped under the probable cause of the fever.

The most common medication prescribed for all fevers, certainly after 1825, was quinine sulphate. Before this cinchona bark was ordered from which quinine was isolated in 1820. Other drugs frequently employed were Fowler's solution (potassium arsenite), ammonium carbonate, aloes, calomel, Dover's powders, ipecac, antimony tartrate, ammonium acetate, morphine sulphate, jalap, infusion of amara (a bitter) and an infusion of serpentaria (snakeroot). In the 1870s potassium iodide and salicylic acid were added. In 1880 a patient with fever and a large spleen had tincture of iodine painted over the left upper quadrant of the abdomen.

By 1910 the customary treatment of malaria was quinine and calomel and magnesium sulphate were the cathartics of choice.

In addition to drugs patients were given warm baths, tepid vinegar baths, the head was cupped and also treated with cold applications, and extremities with hot fomentations and brandy. Mustard was applied to the feet, belladonna plasters to the chest and also leeches.

Diets for fever differed during various periods. In the early days of the hospital a regular house diet was usual but later, one finds diets of milk and bread, snakeroot tea, soups, gruel, wine whey, beef tea, chicken soup, tea, chicken, lime water. Meat was definitely prohibited especially in the latter half of the nineteenth century. In most cases ale, porter, brandy, wine and whisky were ordered.

HEPATITIS AND CIRRHOSIS

Hepatitis was a frequent diagnosis in the early days of the hospital. Cirrhosis and icterus were occasionally mentioned.

In addition to the medications generally employed in all conditions one notes the following drugs – squill, spirits of nitre, juniper, strychnine sulphate, potassium sulphate and for sedation potassium bromide and chloral. When necessary paracentesis was ordered and as might be expected, for pain over the liver, blistering, cupping and leeches were the treatments prescribed.

In 1880 patients received cod liver oil and malt, Blaud's pills and calomel, and the diagnosis for most cases was catarrhal jaundice.

In more recent times (1948) hepatic insufficiency was the term used, and bed rest, a high caloric diet usually low in fat and vitamin K were prescribed. Later multivitamins were usually ordered. In severe precomatose states steroids were given to some patients. Of course alcoholic beverages were strictly forbidden.

However, in the nineteenth century alcoholic beverages were ordered and diets recorded were barley water slightly acidulated, lime water, milk, farinacious foods and arrowroot.

NEPHRITIS

The first diagnosis of nephritis in the records of the hospital was noted in 1837. In 1850 a urine determination was reported which indicated that a microscopic examination was made. The urine contained triple phosphates, ammonium urates and an abundance of blood corpuscles. The reaction was alkaline and the specific gravity was 1.025. However, such urine examinations were not performed routinely for many years to come.

In addition to the usual medications such as aloes and calomel, a pill called triplex, containing potassium citrate, bicarbonate, and tartrate was ordered as a diuretic. Also recorded during the ensuing years were oil tiglii (croton oil), potassium iodide, nitroglycerine, citrate of caffeine, urethane for convulsions, potassium acetate, bicarbonate of soda, chloral for suspected high arterial tension (1890), strophanthus and digitalis for dyspnoea, ascites and oedema. In 1901 heroin and paraldehyde were prescribed and in 1910 veronal and chloroform for convulsions.

Catheterization of the bladder is recorded in 1841. Cupping over the kidney as well as blistering and in some cases phlebotomy as late as 1910 was ordered. Considerable effort was made to produce diaphoresis by such agents as vapour baths (1855), hot air baths (1869), hot packs (1890) and diaphoretic medications such as Dover's powders, whisky in hot water and spirits of aromatic ammonia.

Diets increased in importance with time, for example: arrowroot (1841), farinaceous diet (1869), milk diet, restriction of fluid, oyster broth, beef tea, eggs (1890), chicken, no red meat (1901), Karrell diet (milk), a salt-free diet, restriction of fluids (1910).

In 1869 a patient was advised to reside in lower altitudes.

CENTRAL AND PERIPHERAL NERVOUS SYSTEM DISORDERS

In reviewing the records of the old New York Hospital, disorders of the central nervous system were apparently frequent and results of the treatment seem to be as frustrating as they are sometimes now. In the first part of the nineteenth century, and even later, the terms apoplexy, paralysis, arachnoiditis or irritatio spinalis were often noted.

While the medications used in most medical cases were also prescribed in central nervous system disorders such as calomel, Dover's powders, strychnine, jalap, aloes, morphine, potassium iodide, quinine, mercurial inunctions inside of the thighs and axillae, extract of ergot (1869) extract of belladonna (1869), chloral hydrate (1901), other measures were also employed such as cupping to the temples, venesection, mustard sinapism, blistering of various regions of the body, stimulating enemas, shaving of the head and application of ice, liniments to the spine, friction of the paralysed limbs and of the back, seton to the back of the head, and leeches. In the 1840s and 1850s electricity of various types was used.

In the latter part of the nineteenth century more accurate diagnoses were made such as paraplegia due to syphilis, thrombosis of the middle cerebral arteries, pachymeningitis, meningitis, cerebral haemorrhage. For these disorders milk diet was the rule and alcoholic beverages were liberally dispensed.

In 1855 neuralgia of the face was treated by various procedures such as surgical severance of the infraorbital nerve, cautery of the infraorbital foramen, stramonium leaves applied to the face and treatment of decayed teeth. In 1879 electricity was tried for neuralgia of the face and also of the feet. For the latter condition the feet were wrapped in a saturated solution of sodium bicarbonate. Tincture of iodine was applied, cautery was used and salicylic acid was prescribed.

In 1890 thoracic neuralgia was treated with flaxseed poultices, potassium iodide, cautery, and in 1900 a patient with alcoholic neuritis received galvanic battery stimulation, massage, splints to the back of his knees, and exercise of his feet and hands.

The treatment of meningitis in modern times is of course dependent upon the advent of antibiotics, sulfonamides, penicillin and for tuberculous meningitis streptomycin, isoniazide and para-aminosalicylic acid.

PHTHISIS (TUBERCULOSIS)

Tuberculosis was one of the most frequent diagnoses of the old New York Hospital. This condition was listed as phthisis. As one reviews the charts of these patients it seems clear that therapy did little to help these patients and probably made them worse.

Expectorants, cathartics and attempts to alleviate the symptoms were the usual therapeutic procedures. Peruvian bark, potassium bitartrate, opium, squill, antimony, morphine, quinine, inhalation of iodine, creosote, Stoke's expectorant, cod liver oil (1850), stramonium, ammonium carbonate, fluid extract of ergot for haemorrhage, potassium iodide, creosote mixture, 4 per cent cocaine, codeine, inhalation of creosote were the main remedies as late as 1890. Even in 1910 calomel and sodium bicarbonate were frequently employed. For chest pain blisters, flaxseed poultices were ordered.

Before 1835 the main diet was milk and soups. From 1835 to 1850 orders for a nourishing diet, arrowroot, chicken soup were common. To the diet wine and porter were added. In 1890 egg noggs were in vogue and in 1910 the customary diet ordered was a salt free, light diet without meat but with fruit.

Throughout the records we note such items as 'good nursing', 'make patient as comfortable as possible', 'rest'.

In 1910 the sputum was examined for tubercle bacilli, fluid from a paracentesis was injected into a guinea pig, lumbar puncture was practised and the spinal fluid was examined for tubercle bacilli.

Today with anti-tuberculosis chemotherapy, the entire picture of disability and prognosis in this disease has changed.

PNEUMONIA

Pneumonia was one of the frequent diseases which brought patients to the hospital from its earliest days.

It is beyond the scope of this paper to enumerate the great number of drugs used for this condition. Those most frequently noted were: antimony tartrate, Dover's powders, a great variety of expectorant mixtures, potassium carbonate for fever, calomel, opium, morphine, squill, syrup of Tolu, ipecac, ammonium carbonate, codeine cough mixture, digitalis, cod liver oil, malt, heroin, inhalation of creosote, various gargles and mouth washes, caffeine sodium salicylate.

For the frequent occurrence of herpes, benzoinated oil was applied to the lips.

The chest was blistered and leeches were used frequently. In 1856 an oiled skin jacket sometimes with spirits of turpentine was placed on the thorax or a vaseline-based liniment. Tincture of iodine was frequently applied to the affected side (1879) and also turpentine stupes.

After 1856 bleeding in pneumonia was a rarity.

Oxygen began to be used in 1890.

The first mention of the use of the stethoscope in pneumonia appears in a record dated 1836. By 1839 chest examinations were more complete and flatness on percussion and 'crepitus' rales are noted in the charts.

Diets were the same as in other conditions – milk, light diet and the exclusion of meat. Some physicians continued to prescribe brandy until 1930 and digitalis was employed almost routinely up to that time.

In 1920 sputum began to be typed by the mouse method and blood cultures were taken in dextrose broth as well as on agar. Anti-pneumococcus serum given intravenously often resulted in severe chills and temperatures of 107 degrees. In 1929 a more refined serum (Felton's serum) was available. A concentrated horse serum was produced by Lederle and required sensitivity tests before administration.

In the 1920s following World War I, Dakin's solution (sodium hypochlorite) was employed after thoracotomy for empyema, a frequent complication of pneumonia.

A few patients were subjected to bronchoscopy in 1930 in an attempt to remove plugs from the air passages and promote adequate drainage.

These then were the treatments for pneumonia before antibiotic therapy was introduced.

POISONING

Patients were admitted to the hospital not infrequently because of 'poisoning' either accidental or suicidal. Some of the more common ones and their treatment might be noted, as follows:

Laudanum and opium, zinc sulphate as an emetic, the use of a stomach pump, cold applications to the head and mustard to the feet, mucilagenous fluids, arrowroot diet and enemas (1840–50). In addition, in 1869–79 potassium bromide and potassium bromide and chloral were ordered if sedation was necessary. An interesting note in 1841 reads 'keep patient awake by the free use of a cane'. In 1879 a physician adds 'try to break habit'.

For arsenic poisoning, flaxseed tea and gruel diet (1840) was ordered. In 1890 lavage of the stomach with or without an oxidizing agent was tried. After World War II BAL (British Anti-Lewisite) was the remedy for arsenic as well as for mercury poisoning. Before that mercury poisoning cases received symptomatic therapy. A patient in 1890 had a milk diet, atropine and a poultice over the lower abdomen for 'difficult' urination. The records of New York Hospital do not indicate that sodium thiosulphate, a frequent therapeutic agent for arsenic or mercury poisoning, was used to any extent. In 1946 lavage with 10 per cent sulphoxolate and 5 per cent sodium bicarbonate was ordered.

Carbon monoxide poisoning or 'coal gas poisoning' (1880) was treated with digitaline, croton oil, cupping, and inhalation of oxygen. Catheterization was usual. In 1910 a patient was phlebotomized and in 1946 caffeine and artificial respiration (7 per cent CO_2 and 93 per cent oxygen) were most commonly used.

Barbiturate poisoning became rather frequent by 1946. The orders in the charts read as follows: keep air passage open, intramuscular neo-synephrine, oxygen inhalation, intravenous dextrose, lavage with 1:5000 potassium permanganate being careful of aspiration. In 1953 this therapy was still used but definite directions for suction from upper air passages, caffeine for stimulation, penicillin as a prophylactic and pulmonary ventilation were employed in the treatment.

Carbolic acid poisoning in 1890 was treated by washing the stomach, and giving the patient saccharated lime and flaxseed tea. In 1946 the orders were olive oil, cod liver oil, cotton seed oil, castor oil, vegetable oil, white of egg, gastric lavage with 10 per cent glycerine.

RHEUMATISM

A review of the admissions during the nineteenth century indicates that the diagnosis of rheumatism was one of the most frequent made and the remedies used were many.

Some of the drugs ordered in the first part of the last century were antimony and potassium tartrate, salicylic acid, tincture of colchicum, wine of colchicum, tartaric acid, potassium iodide and, of course, calomel, Dover's powders, opium and many of the usual medications commonly used at that time for most conditions which have been listed previously. Phlebotomies were ordered until 1837.

However, considerable attention was paid to the treatment of the local conditions and what we call physical measures – blisters, steam baths (1809–34), cupping, scarification over the seat of pain, vesicants, warm baths, tincture of capsicum, liniments of various types, direct friction, strapping, leeches, poultices, electro-magnetism (1845), arnica, passive motion (1845).

After 1850 joints were painted with iodine, lead acetate lotion was applied to a painful joint and chloroform and from that time on until well into the twentieth century – methyl salicylate.

In the 1850s a solution of Rochelle salt as an alkaline wash was frequently ordered, and in the 1860s a lotion called Fuller's was wrapped around the joints and by 1870 patients were using crutches on discharge from the hospital.

In 1890 mustard baths and sodium salicylate were noted and some other items applied to the joints were – oil of wintergreen (methyl salicylate), belladonna and glycerine, ice poultices, flaxseed poultices, chloral and camphor liniment and cautery. Salicylates were discontinued if a patient complained of a ringing in the ears.

Patients with gonorrheal rheumatism were treated with an ice poultice, oil of sandalwood, wrapping the joint in a rubber bandage, belladonna liniments, sodium salicylate, lead and opium wash, mercurous chloride applied to the joint with an ice poultice and joints painted with iodine.

By 1900 a distinction was made between joint involvement and synovitis although the term synovitis was noted as early as 1850; but the treatment of the two conditions was not materially different.

In 1910 it was customary to bake involved joints, meat was prohibited in the diet, sodium bicarbonate was given with sodium salicylates presumably so that the patient could tolerate the salicylates. An alkaline mixture called Lambert's was frequently employed. Also in 1910 plaster casts were ordered as well as crutches. It is interesting to note that in 1930 methyl salicylate was applied with red flannel.

In 1947 in the Cornell Conferences on Therapy it was pointed out that salicylates act as a suppressive not as a curative agent and the prophylactic value of sulphonamides was discussed in rheumatic fever.

SYPHILIS

Syphilis was a common diagnosis from the earliest days of the hospital. In the first part of the eighteenth century, muriate of gold, mercurials and iodides were the treatments in use. Ulcerations were touched with silver nitrate solution.

By 1910 'blood for Wassermann' appears on the charts. Mercury inunctions and mercury salicylate orally seemed to be the common remedy and in 1920 salvarsan was given intravenously and intraspinally.

In 1947 bismuth and neoarsphenamine were the usual medications and penicillin according to the Cornell Conferences on Therapy was considered experimental. Potassium iodide was thought to have a possible value in cardiovascular syphilis and fever therapy was still used in syphilis of the central nervous system. By 1950 penicillin was accepted as the therapeutic agent for syphilis.

TYPHOID

Typhoid fever was one of the diseases responsible for the admissions of many patients to the hospital from its earliest days until the first decade of the twentieth century.

While therapy was obviously of a palliative nature until our recent acquisition of chloramphenicol some of the therapeutic measures recorded in the records may be of interest. The most commonly mentioned drugs and treatments were: ammonium carbonate, mixture cretae (calcium carbonate), Dover's powders, starch and opium enemas, olium ricini, spirits of Mindererus (ammonium acetate solution), quinine sulphate, calomel, antimony tartrate, phlebotomies, ipecac and in 1880 digitalis.

However, the most significant part of the treatment of typhoid fever was attention paid to the diet and to alcoholic beverages. From 1809 to 1840 arrowroot, wine whey, infusion of serpentaria (snakeroot) for a beverage and wine were ordered. In 1841 brandy and wine were used as stimulants. Beef tea, eggs, milk, farina, rice and whisky are noted in the charts in 1870; sherry (1880), extract of malt, no potatoes in diet (1890), fluid diet (1901).

In 1910 Dr. Conner's Typhoid Diet was the routine order. This consisted of cream soups, bread and butter sandwiches, chicken gravy and rice.

In 1920 high calorie diets were ordered, as much as 3,575 calories including two eggs, nine slices of bread and butter, oatmeal gruel, milk, cream, custard with cream, and scraped beef.

The danger of cross infection was apparent for in 1879, 'every stool should be disinfected' was an order and netting was placed over the beds at the beginning of the present century as a protection against fly contamination of other patients.

Cold baths were used for hyperpyrexia and one of the important concerns was the avoidance of bed sores.

TYPHUS FEVER

Typhus fever was one of the most prevalent diseases afflicting New York City in the first half of the nineteenth century.

The horrible conditions which prevailed on the ships carrying the immigrants who arrived in the City of New York and the filthy tenements in which they lived were mainly responsible for this malady which resulted in virtual epidemics. Many of the

New York Hospital patients came from prisons where sanitary conditions were indescribably bad.

Patients were first given 'purification treatment' which consisted of thorough sponging of the body usually with dilute vinegar. The treatment was the same as for most febrile diseases.

As an example the following are the orders for a case in 1836: (1) antiphlogistic treatment consisting of venesection, 12 ounces of calomel, antimony powders, cups to temple, cold effusions to head, blister to neck, effervescing droughts, diet of gruel and arrowroot; (2) pulv. gum camphor and pulv. opii; (3) snakeroot infusion, Dover's powders at bedtime. In the 1840s ammonium carbonate seemed to be the drug of choice. After 1856 very few cases were reported.

SOME GENERAL OBSERVATIONS

Many notations appear in the records for conditions which were not seen as often as those enumerated.

In 1890 for cases of abortion, fluid extract of ergot and douches of hot bichloride of mercury, tannic acid or carbolic acid were ordered.

By 1840 anaemic patients received iron. Certainly some patients were rendered anaemic by phlebotomies. By 1890 the term pernicious anaemia is seen among the diagnoses and Fowler's solution (potassium arsenite) was the medication of choice.

Patients with peritonitis were transferred to the Surgical Service probably about the 1900s. Dr. Fitz of Boston first recognized acute appendicitis in 1886.

In 1880 urine was examined for sugar in a patient with pruritis vulvae.

As early as 1809 lime juice, fresh vegetables and fresh meat were given for scurvy.

In 1920 hot saline irrigations were used for acute tonsillitis because gargles were considered of little value. Fifty years later gargles are still ordered.

A review of the treatments of medical diseases for a century and a half of the 200 years of New York Hospital's existence would justify the conclusion that most of the therapy was based on clinical experience or more likely upon authority rather than on science.

It is interesting to note that the quarrel between the scientific and the clinical in the practice of medicine still goes on unabated. For example Crichton states that the expression 'in my clinical experience' is a phrase that usually introduces a statement of rank prejudice or bias. Ring responds that 'clinical experience is the foundation of research'.

Certainly much of our present practice will be considered unscientific by future physicians as more knowledge accumulates.

It might be well to heed Lester S. King's definition of scientific medicine. He says 'scientific medicine does not depend on gadgets or tests or on sharply precise results; neither does it imply the capacity to cure the patients. It does require the ability to examine the data, to seek connexions between them, to find an explanation, and in all these processes to apply critical acumen.'

Whether the practice of modern medicine is influenced by clinical experience or by scientific advances, there is not much difference between our present New York Hospital physician and his nineteenth-century predecessor in his main purpose – to help his patients. It is heartwarming to read the lament of a house officer in the

1850s when his patient showed no improvement with his best efforts. He wrote 'the patient is becoming discouraged and so am I'.

Bibliography

KING, LESTER S., 'The Development of Scientific Medicine', in *Mainstreams of Medicine*, University of Texas Press, 1971, pp. 133–51.
CRICHTON, *New Engl. J. Med.*, 1971, 285, 1491.
RING, *New Engl. J. Med.*, 1972, 286, 324.

A. E. Brade
Copenhagen (Denmark)

Everyday life at the Royal Frederic's Hospital in Copenhagen

The reason for having taken your attention to a subject, which in the history of international medicine may seem peripheral, is that this hospital became of importance at the beginning of the Listerera. As is well known, Joseph L. Lister (1827–1912)[1] used for the first time his antiseptic method of carbolic-acid-bandage on 12 August 1865 in the Royal Infirmary of Glasgow, but very soon he got into difficulties, as his colleagues did not recognize the importance of this discovery introducing a new era. In July 1869 the Danish professor Mathias Hieronymus Saxtorph (1822–1900)[2] came to Glasgow in order to study medicine under Lister. He found out that it was possible to create a surgical department free from hospital infection, and the method proved to be successful. After his homecoming he introduced the antiseptic method at the Frederic's Hospital and on 18 July 1870 he wrote his world-famous letter to Lister, making a brief statement of the great and practical importance of the Lister-method. In extract the letter runs as follows:

My dear Sir,

It is now nearly a year since I left Glasgow where I had the opportunity of seeing how the antiseptic treatment of wounds is to be carried out. Every surgeon who has seen the remarkable results of this treatment must feel it his duty to imitate you, and dress the wounds after your principles. I therefore, as soon as I came home, adopted your method, and have used it continually since that time. . . . All the compound fractures which I had to deal with last year . . . have healed without the least suppuration in the fracture itself. . . . I feel so much indebted to you for what I have learnt in seeing you employing the antiseptic dressing, that I thought it my duty to let you know how things went on in my hospital practice; and I am happy to say that I never tried any innovation which answered so admirably as this treatment of wounds. Believe me, my dear Sir, ever yours

Saxtorph

This letter, which also contained a description of the most difficult cases treated successfully by Saxtorph using Lister's method, was published by Lister on 27 August of that year in the *Lancet*. It is obvious that this initial approval of the value of the method from the leader of a great surgical department on the continent, helped the Lister's method to break through.

Five years later Lister visited Saxtorph in Copenhagen and here he was present both at a ward round in the Frederic's Hospital and at a clinical lecture by Saxtorph.

The hospital, which Lister visited in 1875, was built in 1757 as a four-winged building with two double-storey mainbuildings, two single-storey wings, and two double-storey pavilions facing the streets. The closed yard was laid out as a garden.

The oldest known engraving of the hospital witnesses with its inscription: 'Solatur et instruit' about its twofold duty: to relieve and to educate.

When a patient arrived, he was taken to the inspection-room, where the physician on duty decided whether the patient should have a bath or not, and had him dressed in the hospital clothes, marked: K.Fr.H., which according to a standing joke at the hospital meant: 'Come fresh home', 'King's fresh help troops' [auxiliary troops] etc. Then the patient was taken to his ward, where he was examined, a case record was written, and the physician on duty indicated the provisional treatment. If a patient's temperature-card blew down just as he was put into bed, it was thought to mean that he would come home again.

As is the case with many buildings, which were constructed by clever architects, the wards were pretty rooms in good proportions, with sufficient space between the beds and between the two rows of beds. By night they were not well illuminated, only a few gas-lights being available, but small oil-lamps provided with green shades, placed on the tables beside the beds, gave a very comfortable impression. If a patient was being treated by compresses of arnica, which were boiled in a bag in a special apparatus, a mild, aromatic and old-fashioned smell spread through the ward.

The beds (eight to fourteen in each ward) were situated on one side with the bed-head towards the windows, and the patients there, lying in an incessant draught from the windows, had but the view of those towards the opposite wall. Those lying there got the light from the windows right in their eyes. Their view, however, was pleasant. Some of the patients had to be put close to the big stove, and the fire-screens did not always protect efficiently against the heat. The patients therefore nearest the stove were almost roasted, whereas it was difficult for the most distant ones to keep warm. The air in the wards could be stuffy for several reasons, and it was obvious that airings had to take place. The most effective method was to open all windows, resulting in a furious draught. However, it was also possible to lower half outward the upper part of the windows so that the stale air slipped out without cold air being admitted to the patients in the beds beside the windows. For the sake of ventilation there was also a shutter in the ceiling, which could be opened by a long pole. This usually resulted in a lot of dust being blown into the face, as it was used very seldom.

It was not very quiet in the wards. At 6 a.m. the ward-mistress started to make the patients ready, and see that everything should be in order before the ward round. At 7.30 a.m. the chief surgeon and the assistant surgeon, graduates and students, entered ward P and from there proceeded to the other wards. At each bed the patient was examined and the case-book was dictated to one of the graduates. There was not much time, but the patients never had the impression of being neglected – on the contrary they often had the feeling, that 'my case is especially interesting, as the professor dictates so much about me'. From 9 to 10 a.m. there were clinical lectures or questions and answers for the teams of students preparing for the next examination, and much of this instruction took place in the wards. Even the examination often took place in a ward.

When all this was over dinner was served. It was prepared in the central kitchen of the hospital and from here taken to the wards in baskets, pots and pans, whereafter it was heated in the small kitchen attached to each ward. After dinner harmony spread and one made oneself comfortable – especially at Christmas.

The wards were separated from each other by cross-passages from the garden to the backyard, so that there might be a whistling draught, when both doors were open. It was a very good form of ventilation, the necessity of which you will understand when you hear to what extent these passages were used. I hereby quote a description of 1895:

For each person using his eyes, those kitchens forming the only domestic offices are the greatest horror. Such a kitchen is common to 4 wards, each provided with 8 to 10 patients, and it consists of a corridor of about 1½ metres broad and 20½ metres long, being used first of all as a passage from both sides and then giving shelter to the most curious collection of objects for everyday use and activities. On a small kitchen-range is boiled water, milk, gruel; is made tea, coffee, chocolate etc., for all the patients from the four wards; just opposite the kitchen-range is a still smaller sink in which all the patients' plates, cups, spoons, forks etc. are washed, but also their spitting-mugs and urinals. The sink is leaning towards the wall on one of the two toilets, which are placed in the kitchen with special caution. A safe vis a vis one of the toilets is used as a pantry, in another smaller cupboard the milk is kept in open jugs; on the nails and pegs of the wall uncovered are placed dish-towels, jugs, brooms, scoops, coffeepots and cups. Above the kitchen-range a kiln to air sheets and body-clothes is found; besides the kitchen has a cupboard to the patients' dirty linen, another to the girls' coats and on the remaining surface of the wall stretchers are hanging, being used to carry the patients out into the open air, and racks on which from time to time about 30 students hang their coats. If one imagines all these things gathered on about 40 square metres you will have a picture of one of the hospital's tea-kitchens. . . .

Worst of all was the fact that the bed-pans from the wards necessarily had to be carried through the kitchen in order to be emptied in a little sidewing in the backyard. Here was too a barrel for food-leavings and there was keen competition between the farmers from the neighbourhood in order to be the one who got permission to get these food-leavings, which formed an excellent pig-food.

Now one might think that such a kitchen was anything but comfortable. Nevertheless there was a particular kind of a cheerful atmosphere in the small room. The ward-mistresses, the charwomen and the night-mistresses had their coffee there, and also the cat appreciated a rest on the kitchen-range. The cockroaches fled in big quantities, when their activities in the dark were suddenly disturbed by a ray of light. In the kitchen there was always an odd, mixed smell, the strength of which was in inverse proportion to the charwoman's cleanliness.

After the clinical teaching had finished at 10 a.m., the surgeons could start to operate. The operating-room was practically always called 'The Church' because it was used on Sundays and on festivals for divine services. The patients were taken up there by the hospital-officials or by the graduates. For their transport baskets or a stretcher were employed, and the patient was closely wrapped in woollen blankets. The basket was covered in some cases by a cover, which was necessary as the patient often had to be carried to the operating-room through the garden. The staircases, up which the patients had to be carried were so narrow and steep, besides having several landings, that it was quite a study beforehand to decide whether the patient should be transported with the head lying in one direction or the other, as he could easily slide out of the basket.

If there were more operations the patients on their stretchers were placed in a long row upon the landing outside the operating-room, each accompanied by his ward-mistress, who tried to encourage him. From the operation one could hear the rattling of instruments and the professor's monotonous dictation for the case-record, now and then interrupted by plaintive sounds or horrifying cries, which were terrifying for the waiting patients. When the operation had finished the professor came out dressed in his operating-clothes, drying his hands on a towel, looked at the row outside and said with a low voice: 'The next one'. Then the patient nearest the door was carried inside, and the other ones moved one place forward. This was a patient's experience in the year 1900.

The operating-room was very small, but it was beautiful, supplied with an amphitheatre for the audience and with overhead lighting. During an operation it might happen that one of the listeners was requested to 'pull the rope' in order to clean the air. Then he opened a long and small groove into the wall and pulled in a thick rope with the result that the big window giving overhead-light on the operating-table pulled up, kept in balance by a lead – and the fresh air from above together with old dust from the loft poured down. When there were many students there was not much space. But one often succeeded in sitting between the legs of those who had got seats in advance.

A barrier kept the listeners at a distance and for this there was good reason, as that part of the room reserved for the professor and his assistants was very small. Besides the operating-table and several chairs for the professor and people especially invited, there were three tables for books, dressing materials, bottles, dishes, etc., and for instruments. Later on the space was further reduced by arrangement of a sink with water from taps and outflows from three china-dishes – a very big improvement, but not even with hot water. Hot water was supplied by a small instrument of twisted pipes, which were put into connexion with the cold-water-wire and heated by small gas-lights under the pipes. This hot water was used when a patient needed wine, mixed with hot water to stimulate after an operation. If otherwise one needed hot water it had to be carried from the washhouse or from the bathhouse, brought through the garden and emptied into a barrel in a room opposite the operating-room.

Water was a great problem for the hospital. It was taken in buckets from the pump in the yard, but it was not clean as the hospital had been built on filled-up-earth. It was well supplied with organic components, such as mosquito-caterpillars, tadpoles, leeches and small fishes, to say nothing of eels, which it was impossible to keep out of the pumps. This water could only be used for house cleaning. The drinking water, however, was little better although it was taken from some lakes outside Copenhagen, led into the town by underground pipes, made by outbored Pomeranian pinewoods. It is not strange that people unwillingly drank water and preferred beer.

The patients were cared for by the ward-mistresses. For decency's sake only widows were employed in this job and their age had to be between thirty and fifty, and it was required that they were Lutherans and able to read so that in the evenings they could read edifying works to the patients. They wore their own clothes and lived in the wards in a small compartment the breadth of two beds. In this apartment there was just room for a bed, a chair and a chest of drawers. In the wall into the wards were little windows enabling them to look into the wards. Working hours were from 6 a.m. to 10 p.m. and they must not leave the wards except for extraordinary necessity, and they must not have their children with them. For cleaning work they were helped by the so-called charwomen, and by night they were replaced by night-mistresses. The old ward-mistress had no more important or independent tasks. Therefore they were not fitted to follow the antiseptic development, and in 1885 they were replaced by real nurses. There were, however, many splendid personalities among these ward-mistresses, marked by the sense of discipline and moderation of that time, but in a high degree keeping their character and dignity.

In the loft, slightly illuminated through a little window between the tiles, there were two wards each provided with three beds. These were to be used by surgical patients, who also had an infectious illness, or for patients who disturbed the others in the big ward. Here the 'miss' nursed her patients with never-failing care and with good-humoured kindness and in the evenings after the round, she baked apple-cakes for them on a little kitchen-range out on the loft. It was placed close to her wardrobe, and her chest of drawers and close to the little toilet. After the end of a day's work she could retire to her room, which had the slanting roof as a ceiling and of which the walls were boards. It got light from a window, cut out towards the backyard in order to make room for the bed, in front of which was a small table. But she was satisfied with life. Indeed she was still able to have guests in there – on her twenty-five years' jubilee she had three guests for coffee, but then one was unable to move in there and one of them had to remain standing.

The thought of the horror in case of fire on the staircase leading to this loft, seemed not to have occupied anybody till Inspector Teisen in 1891 placed a fire escape leading from a window down the roof to the garden. The garden was planted with trees, bushes and flowers, and far from the noise of the town it lay silently and harmoniously, surrounded by beautiful buildings. It was most attractive in the different seasons, but used most often by the patients in summer and in autumn. In good weather the patients were moved on stretchers out into the garden as soon as they were well enough. Especially in visiting hours there was a colourful life in this garden. The chief surgeon of that time, Oscar Bloch (1847–1926), was very happy seeing the patients feed the birds, and for further amusement he requested the hospital's joiner to make a pigeon-house, which because of its size did not transform the garden to another Place of St. Marcus, a great disappointment for the chief surgeon. Neither was a little playground lacking for the youngest patients. When the patients had been put to bed and everything was quiet in the wards it was peaceful for the staff to sit in the garden on a beautiful summer evening to have tea, talk and sew.

Numerous and dearest memories are attached to Frederic's Hospital as the old, charming hospital with its delightful garden and its beautiful buildings. Both physicians, ward-mistresses and inspectors, artisans and hospital officials remembered this hospital with great veneration, built at a time when medicine groped blindly, but still functioning in the beginning of this century, when radical changes had to be made by the installation of X-ray apparatus, establishment of laboratories for bacteriological research, etc. Much romance is attached to this hospital in spite of its evident defects. About 1900, however, it had to be admitted that it was hopelessly antiquated. In 1910 the last patients were removed from the old Frederic's Hospital to a new building, the present State Hospital. A chapter in Danish hospital service had finished.

Bibliography

BLOCH, OSCAR, 'Erindringer fra Det gamle Frederiks Hospital', *Gads Danske Magasin*, Copenhagen, 1925.

GOTFREDSEN, EDV, *Det kongelige Frederiks Hospital*, Copenhagen, 1957.

GOTFREDSEN, EDV., 'Det kongelige Frederiks Hospital. Tohundredåret for dets Oprettelse', *Tidsskrift for Sygeplejersker*, 1957.

GREDSTED, FR., *Det kongelige Frederiks Hospital 1757–1907. Et Jubilaeumsskrift*, Copenhagen, 1907.

THERKILDSEN, J. M., 'Minder fra Frederiks Hospital', *Medicinsk Forum*, 1950.

J. A. Ross
Liverpool (Great Britain)

Medicine in the years of reform

Britain was dominated by the European War and its aftermath until about 1820, so that the years of reform can be said to extend from 1820 until 1880, when Victorian society became relatively static. The great year of reform was in 1832 when the reformers won their first victory; on the continent the reformers had to do battle in 1848 during that year of revolutions, which met with less success than the bloodless reform in England. These years were a constant anxiety to the governing class in all European countries; the bogy of workers' revolts was always present and in England the Chartist movement was held to be a menace to peace and to security of property.

It is a great watershed between the old society and the new, dividing the old world from modern technology.[1] Reform cannot take place without ideas; but it was not a desire for change that brought the changes but the Industrial Revolution had been, and was bringing about a slow metamorphosis, slow, because a change from past conditions and thought is, as always, far from easy. If the ideas of the past are to be denied, men must substitute others to take their place, itself a slow, and sometimes painful process. Most of the changes were derived from discoveries made outside the universities, which for a large part were still set firmly in the old world. In the early part of the nineteenth century, the Fellows of Cambridge and Oxford colleges were simply biding their time until they received a Church preferment and the contribution of such men to real learning was mediocre in comparison with their numbers. Much of the real technical knowledge was produced outside the universities. It was not surprising that the Royal Society was called the Royal Society of London, i.e. the city of London.

In some respects the Dissenting Academies did for the nineteenth century what Gresham College did for the seventeenth. The universities gave more attention to science after the Moderns had defeated the Ancients and Richard Bentley[2] had made science theologically respectable in the eighteenth century as Bacon had done in the seventeenth.[3] Science had always been suspect and you will recall that Harvey's practice declined after *De Motu Cordis* was published; similarly in the nineteenth century, Thomas Young,[4] the last of the Polymaths, and William Prout[5] avoided the label scientist in case their medical practices suffered. For science and technology to advance, proper professional guidance, leadership and research were necessary. Wise men were worried at the lack of professional organization and even later in the century the Prince Consort was concerned. The nineteenth century, however, believed in Progress with a capital P and it was thought that this could be achieved by education. The reformers sought to bring about a golden world in an Iron Age, but reforms often misfired and were even unworkable, such as the 1834 Poor Law Act.

Medicine with a long professional tradition had certain advantages but traditions themselves could sometimes be stultifying and delay reform. One encouraging factor was that medical works could, with propriety, be written in the vernacular instead of Latin because most medical terms had been anglicized in the eighteenth century.[6] It is significant that the great Newton published his *Principia* in Latin in the seventeenth century and his *Optics* in English in the eighteenth.

An important event in medical education was the passing of the Apothecaries Act of 1815 which gave the Apothecaries a large control of licensing men who became general practitioners. Many hospitals insisted on a houseman having the licence of the Society of Apothecaries even when otherwise suitably qualified. The improvement was necessary because many of the lower members of the profession had been illiterate and incompetent men, persisting well into the nineteenth century; some could hardly read and write. Parry-Jones describes some of these men who kept private mad-houses,[7] men so ignorant that they punished the inmates and so evil that they signed false certificates.

A much better technical education was now being given to the young doctor. The dispensaries had opened their doors to students[8] and lectures were given by members of the medical staff; from some of these, hospitals were founded which took students. Such an institution was the Liverpool Dispensary from which the Liverpool Medical School originated.[9] Another great advance was the foundation of medical schools associated with the great London teaching hospitals in the early years of the nineteenth century. Early in the nineteenth century an attempt was made at Cambridge to alter the medical curriculum.[10] At that time the works of Galen were still required reading.

These changes produced a different and a better type of doctor, as exemplified by Dr. Thorne of Trollope's Barset novels and Dr. Lydgate of George Eliot's *Middlemarch*.[11] Trollope vividly describes the different types of medical men. Conservative patients did not always like the change from the best type of 'talented, observing and educated men' to men like Dr. Thorne, despised by some of his colleagues for charging less than they did and for keeping a dispensary; nevertheless he was a better doctor being a product of the new system, but then even Dr. Thorne probably did not use a stethoscope.

To paint a picture of medical education, I propose to refer to the lives and work of two men, who spanned this period. They were both distinguished physicians in their day but neither made an original discovery; both were representative of soundly trained physicians of their day.

The first of the two is James Richard White Vose, born in 1811 the son of James Vose, M.D., a well-known Liverpool medical man, one of the first teachers of medicine at the Liverpool Dispensary, the real origin of the Liverpool Medical School. I wish to describe his training. First he was admitted to Downing College, Cambridge, in 1827 but took his degree in Edinburgh where he was elected President of the Students' Society, known as the Royal Medical Society.

Young Vose went to Paris early in 1832 which was at that time a Mecca for medical graduates. He also visited German clinics but we know a good deal about his sojourn in Paris[12] because we have his manuscript notes of lectures, cases, etc. It is carefully written with a meticulous index at the beginning. This book has never been published.

Vose particularly records his gratitude for the kindness of M. Mayer without whose influence he might, as a stranger without a diploma, have been excluded. Vose attended the cases under Mayer's charge in the wards of La Charité and attended lectures at the École de Médecine. Cruveilhier and Andral were his teachers and he reports the lectures given by both and also the demonstrations of cases and post-mortem material.

Cruveilhier's life covered our period. He carried Bichat's ideas into Pathology and his *Atlas of Pathology* was splendid. He made several original descriptions such as that of disseminated sclerosis, progressive muscular atrophy and also Duchenne palsy (Cruveilhier's palsy).

Gabriel Andral also spanned the period and he was the successor of the Professor of Medicine – François Broussais. It is odd that Vose only attended one of Broussais' lectures. Broussais wrote the work *Physiological Medicine* showing a completely didactic, authoritative point of view, a sort of modified Brunonian theory stating that life depended on irritation.[13] Treatment therefore must consist of depletion – by blood-letting, purges, emetics or leeches. It is a well-known fact that during Broussais' tenure the import of leeches to France went up by leaps and bounds. Perhaps Vose did not approve of Broussais' theories? Few did in his later years and Andral himself could not stomach such an exclusive system, because Andral was an eclectic and was too intelligent to accept any hard and fast rules. Andral made considerable contributions to haematology, and was one of the first, too, to consider that gangrene might be due to a nutritional defect. Vose made notes of his lectures and those on physical signs are very full, no doubt because Andral was an authority as editor of Laënnec's work. Andral was one of the first to discourage blood-letting. Vose also describes one of Dupuytren's cases.

I cannot give a description, as I would wish, of Vose's account of the cholera epidemic of 1832 in Paris – part of the terrible pandemic. Vose was an eye-witness and a medical participant.

There are a few rather pleasing little drawings in the book made by Vose in March 1832, including one showing the brain and spinal cord of a pigeon.

He was also interested in the electricity generated in a torpedo fish, an interest presumably derived from Cruveilhier's well-known interest in Comparative Anatomy. Incidentally, at the top of one of the pages there is one of the only personal notes in the manuscript and that is Vose's laundry list. Vose's final notes concerned cases seen in London hospitals and also notes about the purchase of instruments in London and a number of prescriptions.

On returning home to Liverpool, Vose was physician at the Northern Dispensary and later the Infirmary. He also showed an interest in mental disorders because he attended Haydock Lodge, outside St. Helens, a private mental asylum drawing its patients from Lancashire, but also from much farther afield, for example, the county of Anglesey. Incidentally, Haydock Lodge was only closed down in 1969.

In 1859, Vose had reached the summit of his career and was elected F.R.C.P. and also President of the British Medical Association when the association met in Liverpool. The success of the meeting was largely due to Vose.

I wish to refer now to a man who spans the latter part of the period – Frederick Thomas Roberts who was born in Cardigan in 1840. He had a period of apprenticeship in Carmarthen in 1852 and went to the Medical School in Liverpool transferring to University College in 1858, graduating M.B. in 1863 and proceeding to the M.D. degree and the M.R.C.P. diploma later. He was a pupil of Sir William Jenner, most of whose pupils were profoundly influenced by his teaching and personality.

Roberts was appointed assistant physician to the Northern Hospital, Liverpool, and it was during this period that his ability as a teacher was shown because the number of students registering at that hospital considerably increased during his tenure of office.[14] He was particular to tabulate disease – history, etiology, pathology, diagnosis and treatment. Sometimes students laughed at this but more often found it useful particularly at examinations. It was his pen that was of most importance in establishing his position as a teacher. His *Handbook of the Theory and Practice of Medicine* was published in 1873, and reached its tenth edition in 1909. It was an epoch-making book – one of the first really modern textbooks for students and practitioners. It 'reduced to order and sequence the chaotic masses of information acquired by various reading and practical observation'. Roberts returned to London to become Assistant Physician to University College Hospital and also the Brompton Hospital. He was elected F.R.C.P. in 1877 and was also a Censor of the Royal College of Physicians.

His book was of special value to students but in early days he did not accept the germ theory – diseases such as diphtheria were ascribed as due to 'specific poisons', although in other respects he was in advance of his time. It was one of the books which set the firm of H. K. Lewis Ltd. on its feet.[15] In the preface of his first edition Roberts thanks Mr. Lewis for his help and guidance. It was an achievement also because as he says in the preface he had been stricken by a sudden illness when he was producing the book and he received help from two or three colleagues, one of whom was William Gowers.[16] It was written with 'accuracy and precision' which a reviewer in the *Practitioner* stated was 'a faithful representation of modern medical beliefs and practices which would earn him the gratitude of very many students and practitioners by the apparent limitless expansion of the field of medical knowledge'.[17] This was written ninety-nine years ago.

Frederick Roberts was a really gifted teacher and I am sure that it was he who was one of the magnets that attracted so many Welsh students to University College Hospital, a tradition that persists to this very day. Roberts says that he would have been better rewarded as an operatic singer and this may indeed have been true because he had a beautiful voice, like many Welshmen, and he was much in demand as a singer on social occasions. It is true to say that Roberts by his teaching and his writing made an impact on medical education which has scarcely been duly recorded because, as often happens, the changes in Medicine were so rapid in his later life that his work became outmoded. I quote from Roberts' address to the Liverpool medical students[18] – 'But even if you do not possess the requisite talent for discovery, there is still quite sufficient in the mere honourable practice of your profession to enable you to create names for yourselves, that shall remain long after you have passed away.'

In conclusion – I believe that the Reform Years form a great division between the old world and the new, that is our own age of Modern Technology. To bring the world into the new age, changes in education were a necessity. I have tried to illustrate these educational changes by describing the work of two representative doctors, one in the early part of the period and one at the end.

ACKNOWLEDGEMENTS

I am indebted to Mr. L. M. Payne, Librarian of the Royal College of Physicians, and also to W. R. Merrington Esq., F.R.C.S.

References

1 PERKIN, H., *The Origins of Modern English Society*, London, Routledge & Kegan Paul, 1969.
2 WHITE, R. J., *Dr. Bentley – A Study*, London, Eyre & Spottiswood, 1965.
3 HILL, CHRISTOPHER, *The Intellectual Origin of the English Revolution*, Oxford University Press, 1965.
4 WOOD, ALEX, *Thomas Young*, Cambridge University Press, 1954.
5 BROCK, W. H., 'The life and work of William Prout', 1965, *Med. Hist.*, **9**, 101–26.
6 ROBERTS, Ff., *Medical Terms, their Origin and Construction*, 5th ed., London, 1971.
7 PARRY-JONES, W. L., *The Trade in Lunacy*, London, Toronto University Press, 1972.
8 COPE, SIR Z., 'The influence of the free dispensaries upon medical education', *Med. Hist.*, 1969, **13**, 29–36.
9 ORMEROD, H. A., *The Early History of the Liverpool Medical School*, Liverpool University Press, 1953.
10 ROOK, ARTHUR (ed.), *Cambridge and its Contribution to Medicine*, London, Wellcome Institute of the History of Medicine, 1971.
11 ROSS, J. A., 'Medicine in Barset', *Med. Bull.*, October 1961.
12 VOSE, J. R. W., Paris Notebook in manuscript, 1832.
13 GARRISON, F. H., *History of Medicine*, Philadelphia, 1914.
14 Minutes of the Northern Hospital, Liverpool.
15 EDWARDS, G. W. (Messrs. H. K. Lewis Ltd.) Personal communication.
16 ROBERTS, F. T., *A Handbook of the Theory and Practice of Medicine*, London, 1873.
17 Review in the *Practitioner*, quoted in the Centenary Volume of Messrs. H. K. Lewis Ltd.
18 ROBERTS, F. T., Introductory Address, School of Medicine, Liverpool, 1868.

J. D. Holmes
Mwadui (Tanzania)

Medical students, societies and teaching in eighteenth-century Edinburgh

The first medical professorship at the University of Edinburgh was founded in 1685 but it was not until 1726 that the Professors of Botany, Anatomy, Chemistry and the Practice of Physic were constituted as the Faculty of Medicine. At the same time pressure was exerted to establish a hospital 'for maintaining and curing sick poor . . . which would coincidently mean that students in Physick and Surgery might hereby have rather a better and easier opportunity for experience'.[1] The first six beds of the Infirmary were opened in 1729 and from that time students did have 'opportunity for experience' as the following extracts from letters, journals and printed works show.

Alexander Monro *primus* received his early education in Edinburgh where his father was a member of the Incorporation of Surgeons. He became an apprentice of his father, John Monro, who helped 'by assisting dissections, furnishing books and chemical vessels; putting the sick pensioners of the town under his care and obtaining of the Physicians and his Brethren to let him attend their patients in uncommon cases – he attended the Demonstrations of Pharmaceutical Plants exhibited every Summer by Mr. George Preston; a course of Chemistry which Dr. James Crawford sometimes gave and the dissection of the human body which was showed once in every two or three years by Mr. Robert Elliot'.[2] Afterwards in 1717 he went to London, Paris and Leyden for further experience before returning to Edinburgh in 1719 to set up in practice. Monro was fortunate to come from a family who lived in Edinburgh and so was spared the problem of finding lodgings and wondering what were the best courses to attend. His father was very much aware of the value of a medical school to the city and he went out of his way to ensure that his son received a good education. Most students, however, came from outside Edinburgh and had to find lodgings. John Moultrie came to Edinburgh in 1746 from South Carolina and managed to find a house 'where there is seven sober young students'[3] which cost him £5 10s. per quarter. Twenty-five years later, Thomas Parke from Pennsylvania wrote 'the afternoon I spent looking for lodgings, which I found very dear . . . I took a room on the first floor for which I am to pay £12 per quarter'.[4] It was in a large house and comfortable but 'they take in a large number of lodgers . . . there being no less than 10 of us when we are all at home'.

At the same time Thomas Ismay from Yorkshire boarded 'with an old gentlewoman opposite the Colledge. Her husband had been dead some years; he was a professor in the Colledge . . . there are two gentlemen in the house who board also' and he paid £10 per quarter 'which is the lowest one can get boarded in a genteel manner'.[5] In 1771 Sylas Neville from East Anglia 'went to several lodging and boarding houses, many of them very dirty . . .' before finding suitable accommodation.[6]

On his arrival in Edinburgh in 1764 from Philadelphia, young Benjamin Rush spent his first days 'waiting upon the Professors in the College, and as the classes had set down, I procured Tickets from each of them to attend their lectures. Having procured lodgings I began my studies immediately with all the diligence and vigour I was capable of.'[7] 'Waiting on the Professors' usually entailed presenting letters of introduction from a previous student. Rush took one for Dr. William Cullen from John Morgan who had graduated at Edinburgh in 1763. Cullen 'having read the letter, took each of us by the hand welcomed us to the College . . .'.[8] Benjamin Franklin also gave a letter to Rush but he took care to warn him that 'letters of recommendation may serve a stranger for a day or two, but where he is to reside for years, he must depend on his own conduct which will either increase or totally destroy the effect of such letters'.[9]

The professors would often suggest which courses to attend and when John Moultrie went to see Dr. Andrew StClair, who had then retired from the professorship of the Institutes of Medicine, he was advised to attend Anatomy and Materia Medica only during his first year. Dr. Black and Dr. Monro advised Sylas Neville 'that attending a Surgeon's shop or the Clinical lectures would be of no service the first year'. Thomas Parke first met all the professors socially and attended their introductory lectures, which were open to all students as an advertisement. Since the income of the Professors was derived from the three-guinea fee from each student it was obviously advantageous to attract as many students as possible to their classes. Parke recalls 'At 8 AM Dr. Home accosted the medical tribe in his appartment in the most important and engaging manner he was capable of, which to be sure was not much. At 9 AM Dr. Cullen, the inimitable Cullen I say, addressed his Class in the warmest manner words could express. . . . Dr. Black delivered his Introduction to his Chemistry at 10 AM – good language and very instructive but I blush for his delivery – at 11 AM the sensible Gregory gave a pathetic discourse on the advantages of the Institutes of Medicine. . . . 1 PM went to *Dr. Monro*'s Anatomical Theatre where I beheld the greatest collection of med: students (upwards of 200) and the most elegant theatre there is in any one place in Europe I suppose, the Dr. is certainly the best orator . . . then at home till 4 PM when I went to Dr. Young's Introductory lecture to his course of midwifery – a tolerable discourse but I blush for his delivery . . . .'

After two weeks of term Parke decided to attend only Cullen's lectures and Gregory's clinical lectures. Rush on the other hand attended the courses of 'Anatomy, Chemistry, the Institutes of Medicine, Natural Philosophy and the Clinical Lectures at the Royal Infirmary'. He confided to John Morgan 'I find it a painful piece of labour to attend these lectures as I should and I am now more fully convinced than ever how much sleep you must have sacrificed in transcribing those volumes of learning you carried with you to America.'[10] His energy was limitless, as his later life was to show and during his first summer in Edinburgh he was 'reviving my knowledge of the Latin language and in the study of the Mathematicks, under a private tutor. . . . I likewise made myself master of the French language & acquired so much knowledge of the Italian and Spanish languages as to be able to read them.'[11]

Most of the lectures lasted for about one hour but Monro seems to have been an exception because Parke records 'attended Monro on the Brain, began at 10 AM and lecturing until ¼ after 2 PM – the longest and most minute lecture I have ever heard'. Sylas Neville mentioned that Monro had 'finished his course, which is a very long and full one and would not have been over these 2 months if he had lectured only an hour at a time'.

Samuel Bard from New York decided not to attend Midwifery because 'it is a class which intrudes so much upon the others, by being obliged to set up whole nights, and thus rendered unfit for Business the next day'.[12] He records that during his second year at university in 1764 'Dr. Cullen has lately entertained me much by some private Lectures he gives to those who attend him for a second year . . . we are convened at his own house once or twice a week, when after lecturing for an hour, we spend another in an easy conversation upon the subject of the last evening's lecture and everyone is encouraged to make his remarks and objections with the greatest freedom and ease . . .'. Sylas Neville and some friends arranged for a private course of anatomical demonstrations for Mr. Innes, who was Monro's official Dissector. Innes was eager to help students because when Neville first approached him with a problem 'he seemed pleased at my going to him, saying that many students, when they do not understand anything at first, are apt to pass it by and think no more about it'.

Students had to listen to the content of the lectures and try to make some sensible notes for later use, although the Professor of Rhetoric prohibited the taking of notes. Sylas Neville apparently was able to take copious lecture notes and a fellow-student wondered how a new student 'not yet acquainted with the profession can take the lecture so full'. The secret was that he took 'a great deal of the principal observations but not near the whole lecture, for tho' I write very fast and contract much, I cannot write shorthand'. Thomas Parke cultivated the friendship of a Dr. Watson from London who 'had facility and ease with which he writes shorthand' and hoped thereby to get a good copy of Cullen's lectures. Samuel Bard stated in 1763 that his rough notes of Cullen's account of the vitriolic acid 'which are taken from his mouth' amounted to twenty quarto pages 'which if I was to attempt to copy and correct would be considerably increased; this exercise of copying my notes is a task I reserve for the Summer'. Others copied and expanded their notes whilst the lectures were still fresh in their minds; Parke for example spent most evenings writing out lectures and borrowing other students' notes 'I intend to copy some cases from them'. Thomas Ismay in 1771 requested his father to send him a 'Hundred or two of Quills . . .' because he used so many 'as I write five or six sheets of paper every day'. He spent at least four hours writing out lectures every evening. Samuel Bard used his evenings to do some practical anatomy 'In order that I might be enabled to go over his [Monro's] lectures with advantage, I bought some old bones which I met with by accident . . . I frequently to improve myself in this fundemental part of my profession, study comparative anatomy, by dissecting in my own room the parts of Quadrupeds and yesterday dissected the Brain of a sheep and today an ox's eye.' One of the drawbacks of studying anatomy at Edinburgh was the perpetual shortage of bodies for dissection. 'The people of this place, are so superstitious and bigotted, that a student would shun the risk of being banished, if not of his life, if it was known he had a bodie in his possession . . . for this reason I am obliged to content myself with the dissection of Quadrupeds which is but a poor substitute. Some days ago I injected a dog in order to trace the blood vessels.'[13] Some students went to London to gain experience in practical anatomy. The bodies that were obtained in Edinburgh came in the most part from executed criminals; Neville saw two men hanged on 15 September 1773 and then went along to the college to see the dissection.

One advantage of several students living together in one lodging house was that topics of mutual interest could be discussed at mealtimes and in the evenings. In January 1772 Thomas Parke reports 'our lodgers, 10 in number, have agreed never to speak any English in the Dining room – but always Latin and French . . . this agreement bids fair to make us understand the Latin and I think will be useful to us all'. At the same time he also records that 'from supper 'till 12 spent in attendance at our Weekly Society for improvement in Medicine – which seems as if it might be of considerable use'. In all he records five meetings of 'our Society' but gives no idea of the form of the meetings other than that they 'met and disputed'. He had, however, been taken as a visitor to two of the student medical societies, the Chirurgico-Medical Society 'where I heard them dispute upon medical subjects' and the Physico-Medical Society 'some sensible members among them tho' I cannot say I heard anything very instructing'. He was afterwards introduced to the Medical Society 'where I was much entertained, I think it much the best society of any here, more sensible members in it.'

The Medical Society of Edinburgh, or the Royal Medical Society as it has been familiarly known following its Royal Charter of Incorporation in 1778, was founded in 1734 when six students 'having employed themselves in the dissection of a body . . . agreed to spend a social evening together at a tavern – After supper it was proposed by one of the company, that his little society should meet once a fortnight . . . that a dissertation, in English or Latin on some medical subject at the choice of the Society, should be composed and read'.[14] Samuel Bard became a member of this Society on 30 April 1763 and he said 'It now consists of between 20 & 30 members who meet every Saturday evening in a room in the Infirmary, where they dispute upon medical subjects in the following manner – each member has about six months beforehand a set of papers given him to write a comment on consisting of a practical case, a question on some medical point and an Aphorism of Hippocrates. Every Saturday a set of these papers are produced and read before the Society by the Author, having circulated for a week before amongst the members who come prepared with objections and the Authors with arguments to defend their papers. In this exercise of disputing we spend about 4 hours and I really think to very good purpose, for we are obliged to muster our whole stock of knowledge to defend our opinions, which are never allowed to pass without being thoroughly examined, and as there are always a number of members who are near graduating, and men of real knowledge, we young members are not allowed to be carried away by false reasoning, or led into errors instead of truths.'

The Society continued to prosper and in 1775 it was asking for funds to build a Hall of its own 'it is acknowledged by all who are acquainted with the University of Edinburgh that the assiduity and ardour in study which is so remarkable in the greatest part of the students of medicine, has been especially excited and supported by the Medical Society' as the *Scots Magazine* put it.[15] The Hall, which was opened in April 1776, was '30 feet long and twenty feet broad, and there are two rooms besides in the building, one for a library, the other for Chymical and Philosophical experiments'.[16]

George Logan writing home to his brother in America in 1778 mentioned that he was a member of three medical societies 'from which I assure you I have received as much improvement as from any one professor. In one of these societies the Latin language is spoke with great fluency and ease.'[17] It would be interesting to know to which Society he was referring because six years previously Sylas Neville had been taken to the Medical Society and was not impressed 'the undigested matter they throw out tends more to perplex than to increase medical Knowledge and as much time which might be better employed is lost in attendance, writing papers, preparing questions, etc. I do not think I shall ever petition for admission. A little while before they break up, they dispute in Latin upon an Aphorism of Hippocrates, but very little is generally said and such latin!' A year later he had changed his mind and petitioned for admission because of 'the advantage and probability of increasing my knowledge in Medicine by being present at the debates'.

Students were aware that too much study was a bad thing; after four weeks of hard study, Thomas Parke wrote 'my way of passing my time does not agree quite so well with me as I could wish – as I do not use sufficient exercise'. He started to take long walks about the town and down to the Port of Leith. George Logan managed to have several trips around the countryside – including one to the Highlands. Sylas Neville records many visits to the theatre and at the end of his first year in Edinburgh '. . . went (with friends) to no less than 3 brothels, not with any bad intention but merely from curiosity. In an Edinburgh brothel dirtiness and vice are combined'.

For a student to be allowed to take the M.D. degree at Edinburgh he had to have attended courses in Anatomy, Chemistry, Botany, Materia Medica and Institutes of Medicine over a period of three years and to have spent at least one year at Edinburgh. However, many students did not intend to graduate, only coming to attend the lectures of one man. Between 1790 and 1800 there were 5,594 matriculations in Medicine at the university but only 394 medical graduates. In order to graduate the student had first to have a 'certificate of the lectures' which he had attended and this had to be presented before he was allotted his examinations. The student had also to write a thesis in Latin; when John Ravenscroft from Viriginia presented his first draft to Dr. Gregory in March 1770 he was told to rewrite it 'I will be obliged in a manner to do it all over afresh and writing two or three times over 15 folio pages is na sma' drink.'[18] Many students found it difficult to write in Latin and Ravenscroft reports a 'disputing pedant who reads Latin with me and has the knack ere I'm aware of drawing me into a dispute; we commonly begin in Latin, but it is not very long before plain English becomes the vehicle of sentiment between us'. Dr. John Brown, who was later to achieve some notoriety on account of his Brunonian Theory of Medicine, 'maintained himself and a young family while a student by teaching the Latin Language and translating English theses into Latin for those graduates who were unable to do it for themselves'.[19] The thesis had to be presented as a printed book and Sylas Neville records in September 1776 'was at the Printing Office correcting the press until 10 o'clock'.

As for the examination itself Bard recalls 'on the first day I had not the distant hint what was to be the subject of my tryal, I went in trembling and Dr. Cullen after desiring me to set down, began my examination by asking me some general definitions as "Quid est medicina?" My next tryal was writing commentaries upon two of Hippocrates' Aphorisms and defending them against old Dr. Monro and Dr. Cullen. My last private tryal was writing commentaries upon two practical cases . . . during all these tryals, my exercises were written in Latin, and I was obliged to defend them in the same language.' Sylas Neville reports Dr. Cullen as saying that 'they had rejected two gentlemen this year (1775) on account of language'.

After the lectures, studying and examinations were over the young doctor returned home and remembered his time at Edinburgh. John Morgan in his thesis of 1763 hoped '. . . in the distant reaches of America, there will come to my mind, and relive for me, from time to time, the beloved memory of my studies at Edinburgh, where all that delights and improves the mind is available'.[20] Benjamin Rush stated before leaving Edinburgh '. . . the public lectures and private conversations of the professors not only gave me many new ideas, but opened my mind to enable me to profit by reading and observation'.

Surely this is the ultimate aim of any education system and it would appear to be fairly satisfactorily fulfilled at Edinburgh during the eighteenth century.

References

1 ANON, *An Account of the rise and Establishment of the Infirmary or Hospital for the sick-poor, erected at Edinburgh*, Edinburgh, 1730.

2 ERLAM, H. D., 'Alexander Monro *primus*', *Univ. Edinb. J.*, 1954, pp. 77–105.

3 *Univ. Edinb. J.*, 1931, **4**, 271–74.

4 PARKE, THOMAS, 'Journal' M.S. in Historical Society of Pennsylvania Library.

5 'Letter from Thomas Ismay', *Univ. Edinb. J.*, 1936, **8**, 57–61.

6 *The Diary of Sylas Neville*, ed. Basil Cozens Hardy, London, 1950.

7 RUSH, BENJAMIN, 'Scottish Journal', M.S. in University of Indiana Library.

8 RUSH, BENJAMIN, Letter to John Morgan, 16 November 1766.

9 *Lancet*, 1967, **ii**, 423.

10 RUSH, BENJAMIN, Letter to John Morgan, 16 November 1766.

11 RUSH, BENJAMIN, *Autobiography*, ed. G. W. Corner, Princeton University, 1948.

12 BARD, SAMUEL, Letters to his father, John Bard, 1762–64, M.S. in New York Academy of Medicine.

13 Ibid.

14 LETTSOM, J. C., 'Some Account of the late John Fothergill M.D.', in *Collected Works of Dr. John Fothergill*, London, 1783.

15 *Scots Magazine*, 1775, **37**, 416.

16 *Scots Magazine*, 1776, **38**, 339.

17 George Logan Letters, MS. in Historical Society of Pennsylvania.

18 LYON, D. M., 'A student of 1765–70', *Univ. Edinb. J.*, 1951, **48**, 186.

19 RUSH, *Autobiography*, op. cit.

20 'John Morgan's Medical Thesis, "Pus Production" Edinburgh 1763', trans. M. W. Smith, *Trans. Stud. Coll. Phys. Philadelphia*, 1965, **32**, 123.

L. A. Falk and N. A. Quaynor-Malm
Nashville, Tennessee (U.S.A.)

Early Afro-American medical education in the United States: the origins of Meharry Medical College in the nineteenth century*

The origins of Meharry Medical College, Nashville, Tennessee, are examined here in the context of black social-medical history. Meharry is one of two predominantly black medical schools in the United States. The name comes from its original donorship family. It has produced nearly half of all the black physicians ever to graduate in the United States. Its 100th anniversary now approaches in another period of great social change such as the one which attended its birth.

These origins can be traced along two streams. One is that of Methodist Church history, in its relation to slavery and to slaves. The other is the stream of black medical history within the context of general black history, especially in the roles of the healers, patients, and the community.

MEDICAL HISTORY OF THE BLACK HEALER

The history of the black doctors of the U.S.A. and the Caribbean is dealt with only modestly in English language medical history journals.[2-10] We have been struck by how much of the material revolves around white viewpoints. Few medical cultural inheritances from Africa to the U.S.A. have been traced in them.

Black people called doctor have been identified in the U.S.A. as early as the seventeenth century,[11-16] but slaves, especially males, were forbidden the healer role by law in at least several states.[14,16] This was stated in the laws as necessitated by the fears they would poison their masters or other persons. In addition, the healers' mobility was too useful for a potential insurrectionist. Finally, learning in general was feared, especially in Negroes. In 1844, a Tennessee Court ruled that slaves should not practise medicine for fear that 'such doctors might foment insurrection', in the following case:

> Macon was the owner of . . . Jack, and permitted Jack to go about the country practicing medicine. . . . He was indicted . . . the defendant [Jack] was an obedient, exemplary slave, and a most extraordinary character, and all his time was occupied in attending the calls of diseased persons. . . . The court . . . charged the jury that a

* This is the second paper in our Black Medical History series. The first[1] used the word 'Negro'. Since that time the word 'black' has become generally preferred usage.

This work is from the Department of Family and Community Health, Meharry Medical College, and was presented to the 23rd International Congress of the History of Medicine, London, England, 5 September, 1972. The studies are supported, in part, by grants from the Carnegie Corporation and from the Public Health Service.

slave had no right to practice medicine under any circumstance – verdict of guilty . . . the defendant having been fined one dollar, appealed. (Macon v. State of Tennessee). . . . Later, the judgement was affirmed: the legislature was guarding against . . . insurrectionary movements on the part of the slaves. . . . A slave under pretense of practicing medicine, might convey intelligence from one plantation to another, of a contemplated insurrectionary movement; and thus enable the slaves to act in concert to a considerable extent, and perpetrate the most shocking massacres . . . it was thought most safe to prohibit slaves from practicing medicine altogether.[17]

The slave owners in Tennessee had cause to be nervous. Slaves had tried to revolt over the years and they became increasingly restive in the nineteenth century.[18]

Free blacks were not permitted to vote or hold office in Tennessee after 1834, and life was made increasingly difficult for them,[19] their mobility being especially feared. A key measure of that period was the attempted colonization of Negroes back to Africa or to Haiti by the American Colonization society and its state affiliates.[20] In Western Tennessee there was more concern with the elimination of the free Negro than elsewhere in that state. Enforced colonization of free blacks was combined with laws that limited their movement in an effort to keep them away from slaves.

East Tennessee had considerable anti-slavery sentiment in the early part of the nineteenth century. One expression of this was a strong abolitionist movement. The first periodical in America devoted entirely to the abolition of slavery was founded in 1819 at Jonesboro, Tennessee, entitled the *Manumission Intelligencer*; edited by Elihu Embree, it was part of the activities of an abolitionist group.[21] It was succeeded by the *Emancipator*, and then by *The Genius of Universal Emancipation*, edited by Benjamin Lundy, the mentor of the better-known abolitionist William Lloyd Garrison.

Slave-holding had been forbidden by the popular and powerful Methodist Church in Tennessee, meeting near Nashville in 1808, and Methodist slaveholders were not allowed to preach or lead prayers. It must be realized that there were about twenty times as many *non*-slave-owners as there were slave-owners among the whites. Some tens of thousands of slaves were allowed to become Methodists and attend the same churches as did whites. Another expression of abolitionism was the widespread petitioning by many counties of the Tennessee State legislature to ask it to abolish slavery. While slaveholding power increasingly prevailed as the nineteenth century wore on, slaves were escaping, alone or in the 'Underground Railroad'. By 1844, slave-owners had become the dominant power in the South. The Methodist Church South broke off as a segregated branch of Methodism, justifying and practising slaveholding.

The restrictions on the free blacks grew.[22] Indeed, we do not yet have the names of any free black doctors in antebellum Tennessee. There were, however, a number of free black physicians elsewhere in the U.S. Some were so significant medically and socially, we intend to report on them in a subsequent paper, especially on a remarkable group of them who were abolitionists and leading intellectuals, social and political leaders in the U.S.A. These include Doctors James Still, William Wells Brown, David Ruggles, James McCune Smith, John Rock and Martin Delaney.

CIVIL WAR

Slaveowner power grew. In 1861, the South seceded. Nashville, Tennessee was occupied by Federal (Union) troops in 1862 and remained so until the Civil War ended in 1865. Slaves escaped. So did some free blacks and unionist southern whites. Epidemics occurred. All looked to the union army for help in increasing numbers. Many were sick, hungry, aged and disabled. Provision of hospital care, food programmes and education became necessary. In 1863, the slaves were freed by President Abraham Lincoln's Emancipation Proclamation, but the Proclamation excluded Tennessee until the matter was voted upon by that state. The formal freeing of the 275,000 slaves in Tennessee came in 1865 upon vote within the state legislature. It was Jubilee!

RECONSTRUCTION

The Freedman's Bureau became the southern Negro's *de facto* government.[23,24,25] The Union Army and church groups worked together in Negro education and health care. We have this story in the words of J. M. Walden, Bishop of Cincinnati, Ohio diocese of the Methodist Episcopal Church:

> In 1866, as corresponding secretary of the Freedmen's Aid Society of the Methodist Episcopal Church, I called at General Fisk's head-quarters in Nashville to consult about housing our opening school-work in that city; and he turned over to us a large building known as 'the Gun Factory'. Early in the war the Confederate authorities had seized it for the purpose of establishing a manufactory of arms, but they were not given time to consummate the purpose. That this building should be first used as a school house for the freedmen instead of a Confederate gun-factory, as had been proposed, is still an interesting fact. This was not Government property as in the case of the hospital buildings devoted to the Fisk School; hence its use was temporary. But here was the early and rude seat of the school which, during the nearly twenty-four years, has grown into the Central Tennessee College. The use of the Gun Factory, through General Fisk's agency, not only gave an impulse to the school, but determined its location in the southern section of the city, which has been a great advantage.[26]

CENTRAL TENNESSEE COLLEGE AND ITS MEDICAL DEPARTMENT

Along with the Quakers and Congregationalists the Methodists rallied to the aid of the freed blacks.[27] A Nashville school for black people was opened in 1865 by Rev. G. H. Hartupee in the basement of a church, Clark Chapel, named in honour of Bishop David M. Clark. Since almost all the freed slaves were illiterate, having been prohibited by law from receiving schooling, education was an urgent function of the church and of the public schools. Soon thereafter, Meharry Medical College's parent institution, Central Tennessee College, was founded. It took over many of the health and education functions of the Freedmen's Bureau.

TENNESSEE ANNUAL CONFERENCE OF THE METHODIST EPISCOPAL CHURCH

Rev. R. S. Rust, Secretary of the Freedmen's Aid Society of the Methodist Episcopal Church, along with several of his colleagues conceived Central Tennessee College for higher education of freed blacks, at the first Annual Conference of the Methodist Episcopal Church in Tennessee in 1866.

A Conference Aid Society, to supplement the National Freedmen's Aid Society of the Methodist Episcopal Church was formed. The resolutions adopted will give the flavour of the meeting:

1. That we acknowledge it to be the duty of the Church to provide for the education of the Freedmen's children and will do all in our power to aid in this good work.
2. That we approve of the organization of the Freedmen's Aid Commission of the Methodist Episcopal Church, that we will cooperate with it in our several fields of labor and pray that the Divine blessing may attend it.
3. That we rejoice in the establishment of the Central Tennessee College for the general and theological Education of Coloured People and will give it all the aid in our power.
4. That when day schools are not established by the Freedman's Bureau, or the aid Societies operating in the fields to which we are assigned, we deem it the duty of the Pastor, if practicable to see that such schools be opened.
5. In view of the urgent demands made upon us for the establishment of schools for the Freedmen in our bounds, as well as throughout the South, we earnestly appeal to our friends at the North to contribute liberally to the funds of the Freedmen's Aid Society of the Methodist Episcopal Church, that it may be able to respond to the calls so imperatively made upon it.
6. We also recommend the organization of a Conference Aid Society, auxiliary to the Freedmen's Aid Society of the Methodist Episcopal Church. . . .[28]

In 1866 then, Central Tennessee College was founded. After a year, Rev. John Braden replaced G. H. Hartupee as its President.[29]

The period following the end of hostilities was one of epidemics and malnutrition. White and the few black doctors were extremely pressed to meet the emergency needs of the sick and war-injured. Yellow fever, cholera, smallpox and other epidemics came in waves, and endemic diseases such as malaria, typhoid and dysentery abounded. It was not long before the need for medical training of blacks came to be perceived. A 'Medical Department' of the new Central Tennessee College was discussed. A family of Illinois abolitionists of Irish ancestry named Meharry (brothers Hugh, Jesse, David, Samuel and Alexander) gave $500 to help such a medical department start, and provided more in their wills.[30]

THE MEDICAL EDUCATORS

In the final months of the Civil War, a friendship had developed between a white northern Army Medical Corpsman, G. W. Hubbard, and a Confederate Army Surgeon, Dr. W. G. Snead (sometimes spelled Sneed). Dr. Snead was originally from Nashville, while John Hubbard had been born in New Hampshire and came to Nashville in 1864 under Methodist auspices. He joined Sherman's Army, marched through Georgia, taught the 110th U.S. Colored Troops and then was mustered out of the service. A third member of the group, name unknown, joined Dr. Snead and Mr. Hubbard on the trip back to Nashville. This unnamed third member of the trip became seriously ill. Dr. Snead and John Hubbard took it upon themselves to help get him well again. After a hard search they found a black woman to nurse him, under Dr. Snead's direction. To replenish the trio's funds, which were running very low, Hubbard secured employment. He had been trained as a teacher at the New Hampshire Methodist Conference Seminary and found a teaching position at the Belle View Public School in Nashville.[31] Thus, Dr. Snead and Mr. Hubbard were able to meet expenses and to take care of their friend, seeing him completely recovered. He, in turn, then took over George Hubbard's income-earning role in order to enable Hubbard to enter medical school, Hubbard's expenses being advanced by the two friends. This plan worked out well, and in 1876 young Hubbard graduated from Nashville Medical School (now Vanderbilt University School of Medicine).

The doctors had been planning to open a medical school for black students. These ideas were in line with what Reverends Rust, Walden and Braden of the Methodist Church had been working on. Hubbard accepted the initiative to build the college.

MEDICAL DEPARTMENT OF CENTRAL TENNESSEE COLLEGE

In 1875, classes in Anatomy and Physiology were organized under Dr. Snead for some undergraduates of Central Tennessee College. The graduation of Dr. Hubbard from medical school gave the plan the needed impetus. The school was designated the Medical Department of Central Tennessee College and was formally chartered in October 1876. Hubbard and Snead were joined by seven other white teachers on a part-time basis that first year.

The course consisted of two terms of five months each. Admission requirements were that students be of good moral character and able to pass a satisfactory examination in 'the common English branches'. To graduate, the student must have attained the age of twenty-one, studied medicine two full terms and attended two full lecture courses, the last of which was to be done at Meharry Medical College. The students were all males at first. They were required to pass a satisfactory examination on all of the branches laid down in the course, and present 'an acceptable original thesis on some medical subject'.

Tuition was ten dollars a term in advance; board and other expenses were about eight dollars a month; the graduation fee was ten dollars.[32] The first entering class consisted of eleven students, all ex-slaves. The only medical graduate in the class of 1877 was J. W. Jamison, a native of Nashville, whose picture we have, but little else. He is known to have practised, and prospered, in Topeka, Kansas. All his original classmates had to drop out because of poverty, illness or other reasons at some time or other during the two years.

However, three more graduated in 1878. They were John S. Bass, John C. Halfacre and Lorenzo Dow Key. It was at this time that the first commencement exercises for the medical department were held. The President's remarks included the following: '. . . I congratulate you tonight, first because you are recognized as men. You were born slaves, the recognized property of others; your bodies, intellects, moral natures were under the absolute control or guidance of your master.'[33]

The curriculum was a thoroughly Anglo-Saxon white medical one, with textbooks like Gray's *Anatomy*, Dunglison's *Medical Dictionary* and Meig's *Diseases of Children.* (We have found no reference to the medical writings of the Methodist Church's founder, John Wesley. Wesley's book *Primitive physick* is not mentioned in the school's catalogues.) If any voodoo or conjuring was practised by the ex-slave medical students, it has not been reported. However, religion and the role of preacher were clearly part of these healers' roles. Active Christianity was assumed by all concerned. Several of the early Meharry graduates were part-time ministers and religious leaders in their communities.

The diseases of the times are discussed in the students' graduating theses. One of the graduates, Lorenzo Dow Key, presenting a discussion on malaria, stating: 'Malaria was derived from two Latin words which mean bad air. It is supposed that air in certain portions of this and other countries, is filled with germs that are formed by the decomposition of animal and vegetable matter and it is thought by a large number of writers on the subject that persons who inhabit these districts, take into their systems during respiration, these germs which enter the circulation. . . .'[33] This account is from a small 'Proceedings'. It speaks of the large audience which had assembled to witness Meharry's first commencement.[34]

Dr. Bass practised later in Murfreesboro, Tennessee (near Nashville), Dr. Halfacre in Nashville itself, while Dr. Key migrated to Greeneville, Texas. Henry Alonzo Napier had been in this class also, but had to drop behind due to illness. He did graduate in 1880, but died young. Napier was the name of a white plantation owner and is identifiable as that of an English family. There is a story we have been unable to confirm, or disprove, that Henry Alonzo Napier had been told by his white father to attend medical classes at the University of Nashville Medical School (later Vanderbilt), but that the white students protested his presence.[35] John Hubbard was alleged to be in the class and to have been outraged by the injustice, vowing to start a medical school for blacks as a result. (The University of Nashville Medical School had started in 1851, founded the same year as the *Nashville Journal of Medicine and Surgery*. That school divided ultimately, one part becoming the current Vanderbilt University Medical School, the other joining with the University of Tennessee in Memphis, leaving Nashville entirely.)[36]

By 1879, Meharry produced eight medical graduates. One of them, Henry T. Noel, had previously earned a D.D.S. and became the first black faculty member of Meharry. Others of this class spread out geographically for their practices as follows:

TABLE 1 Name and Place of Practice of Meharry Medical Graduates – 1879

Name	*Place of Practice*
George M. Anderson	Memphis, Tennessee
James P. Andrews	Chattanooga, Tennessee
Joseph H. Ballard	Indianapolis, Indiana
William P. T. Jones	St. Louis, Missouri
John F. McKinley	Austin, Texas
Burgess E. Scruggs	Huntsville, Alabama
James E. White	Not determined

This southeast regional spread then became a national and an international one, including the Caribbean and Africa. Class sizes increased and the duration of training lengthened to three, and then four years.[37] A Dental Department started in 1886 and several early graduates held both degrees.

The 1882 graduating class numbered eight, and it included Robert F. Boyd, perhaps the greatest Meharry graduate of the century. He already had a master's degree and in 1887 also received a Meharry dental degree. He is treated at some length in a forthcoming history of Meharry by Dr. Harold West, President Emeritus, but we must mention here that he became a leading faculty member, practitioner and fund raiser for Meharry. Dr. Boyd was the first black doctor to open an office in Nashville* and he was the first black doctor in Tennessee to perform an abdominal operation. He was appointed at different times Professor of Hygiene (presumably the predecessor of the Department of Family and Community Health), Professor of

* His advertisement in the *Fisk Herald* in1884 says 'Office Open All Night'.

Physiology, Anatomy, Chemical Medicine, Diseases of Women, Clinical Medicine and then of Surgery at Meharry. He was president from 1895 to 1897 of the National Medical Association, the organization of black physicians in the U.S., founded after the American Medical Association and almost all state and county societies persistently banned black physicians from membership. Dr. Boyd became an honorary member of the Royal Society of Anthropology, London, England. He died in 1912 at the age of fifty-four.[38]

Two somewhat younger Meharry graduates became pioneer black medical editors. Dr. Miles Vandahurst Lynk, Meharry class of 1891, practised west of Nashville in Jackson, Tennessee, and founded the first Negro medical journal in America in December, 1892. Called the *Medical and Surgical Observer*, it appeared as a thirty-two page monthly and developed a national circulation, at some financial sacrifice by Dr. Lynk. Dr. Lynk also founded the Medical College of Western Tennessee, which survived until 1909.[39]

The second distinguished editor was Dr. C. V. Roman, Meharry class of 1890. He practised in Dallas, Texas, became president of the National Medical Association in 1904, Professor of Ophthalmology at Meharry, founded the *Journal of the National Medical Association* in 1912, and wrote one of the few books about Meharry.[40] Medical history interests are evident in his writings.

Dr. Boyd's class of 1882 included three women who reached junior class status (Henrietta Davis, Florence Holmes and Julia Thomas), but they did not graduate. The first woman to graduate was Georgia E. L. Patton, whose picture we also have. She practised promptly after graduation in Liberia. She became ill, returned to Memphis in 1895, practised there, became Mrs. Georgia E. L. Patton Washington and died in 1900.[41] The proportion of women in Meharry has increased greatly since this time.

A Dental School opened in 1886, a Pharmaceutical College in 1889.

RECONSTRUCTION AND REACTION

The period immediately after the Civil War was marked by a flowering of black and poor white power in southern political affairs. Public education was introduced, mental hospitals and other humane measures were developed. However, the former slaveowners counter-attacked. Ideologically, they whipped up the poor whites to racism, including fear that Negroes would rape their wives and daughters, and fear of Northerners. Economically, they reclaimed their lands and introduced the sharecropping system, thereby binding both blacks and poor whites again to them. Politically, they worked successfully so that in 1876 the Tilden-Hayes agreement prematurely withdrew Federal troops from the South. This left force and power in the hands of the large landowners, who used terrorist groups such as the Ku Klux Klan, and then increasingly regained state and county government power. The Northern capitalists allied themselves with the plantation-owner 'gentlemen', and a mercantile class arose dependent on Northern capital.

Thus, the very year that Meharry was founded, the alliance against the Negro asserted itself. As the century wore on, white racism became shriller ideologically, more repressive legislatively and more violent, so that lynching, mutilation and systematic segregation and repression of the Negro increased. The Negro was disenfranchised through thinly veiled measures such as 'poll tax' and 'literacy' laws.

'Jim Crow' legislature was enacted, forbidding blacks and whites from doing almost anything public together, such as riding together in public transport. Schools were strictly segregated and black schools' budgets were slim. Black patients would not be seen by doctors in their offices, except perhaps during segregated hours and in a separate undersized waiting room. Hospitals would either not admit Negro patients or would have a special ward in the basement for blacks, almost always inferior to that for whites.

In these circumstances, the black doctor first had to be willing to suppress many normal attitudes of self-respect and independence. To get through training required financial and other kinds of approval by 'Mister Charlie' (the white men with power in the community). Then, the role expected was that of the educated 'pacifier', so that lynchings, beatings, robbings, and various other misdeeds done to the black community did not result in reprisal. The churches taught the blacks to be all-suffering – and segregated them in all-black churches.

Negro doctors patched the wounded and tried to keep the society stable and avoid conflict. Technological knowledge and skills were stressed. Hard, uncomplaining work became the lot of the Meharry graduates. In the cities, they developed Negro hospitals to counter the segregated wards of the white hospitals, plus their own inability to obtain hospital privileges. Separate Negro medical societies held their own professional and social meetings and published their own state and local journals.

Booker T. Washington, who obtained money for Tuskegee Institute in return for opposing the vote for Negroes, was dominant in this period. We have been unable to locate any great black physicians whose general social and intellectual role is equivalent to that of the abolitionist physicians of the early part of the century. Some doctors, such as R. F. Boyd, responded in a way which helped make the new winds of self-respect blow harder and cleaner. It was W. E. B. Dubois, historian and sociologist, who called out clearly for equality to be asserted by black people. Dubois founded the Niagara (New York) movement which later became the National Association for the Advancement of Colored People. He wrote and talked profusely on topics including health and social affairs.

MEHARRY'S LATER ROLE

We will not follow Meharry into the twentieth century in this paper except for a few final comments. In 1900, Central Tennessee College changed its name to Walden University. The Flexner report in 1910[42] found seven medical schools for Negroes including: Howard University, Washington, D.C.; Meharry; Flint in New Orleans; University of Western Tennessee, in Memphis; and the National Medical College, in Louisville, Ky. Flexner said, 'Meharry at Nashville and Howard at Washington are worth developing . . .'. This is what happened, and they are the only two still surviving.

Meharry graduates went predominantly into black practices, in urban and rural black communities, but some conducted research and became medical teachers. By 1956, there were forty-eight black physicians in Nashville. Of them, ten were certified Board specialists.[43] Meharry graduates were to be found in almost every major community of the United States by then, and in many communities in the Caribbean and Africa.

It was not until 1954 that the Supreme Court of the United States struck down legally segregated education – in the case of Brown vs. the Board of Education. Only then could the first white student be legally admitted to Meharry. Fairly soon, the student body included 20–30 per cent whites, and its faculty about 33 per cent. A period of doubt followed. Would predominantly black schools continue? Would they close down and would their students gain admission to white schools? Would Vanderbilt University School of Medicine take over Meharry?

The limitations of our white society promptly demonstrated themselves. The black community then surprised not only whites, but many of themselves by entering a phase of 'black power' and 'black consciousness'. This meant developing their own goals, their own identity and their own leadership, whether or not these suited the white majority. Many Meharry medical students and faculty members joined in the 'sit-ins', 'freedom rides', desegregation of health services and other civil rights demands in the 1950s and 1960s.

In 1966–67, a faculty renaissance occurred with the projection of an exciting statement of mission. The school's mission was set as the achievement of excellence in education, research and service to the black, brown, red, yellow and poor white communities. Problem-solving learning in health care delivery models designed for the future (e.g. as family health teams in health centres) were projected to be part of all students' experiences. A major health services research programme was begun.

With new energy and confidence, growth spurted ahead in 1968. By 1972, the College's budget had been quadrupled, employing 2,100 people. Consumer-involvement, rural and international community health, primary and comprehensive care educational models have been developed.

Perhaps the next hundred years will be equally or more significant for Meharry and its communities of health protection throughout the world.

ACKNOWLEDGEMENTS

Appreciation is expressed to: the Director of the Wellcome Institute of the History of Medicine, the librarians and other staff; Drs. George Rosen and Francisco Guerra for references; Dr. Harold West, President-emeritus of Meharry Medical College; Mr. William Fort, Assistant to the President; Mr. Sylvester Walker, history graduate student at Fisk, and an assistant in our Department; Ms. Gloria Leath, Librarian of the Department of Family and Community Health; Librarians at the Fisk University, Methodist Higher Education Board, Methodist Publishing House and the Tennessee State Archives; Ms. Mayche White and Ms. Kala Ladenheim, Teaching Assistants; Ms. Joyce Foley, Ms. Gloria Drake, Ms. Carolynn McGowan, MS. Lornetta Taylor, and others of our staff; other colleagues and to my wife, Joy. Professor Henry E. Sigerist has been my life-long model in medical history.

References

1 The first paper in this series was Leslie A. Falk, 'The Negro American's health', *Medical Care*, 1966, **4**, 171–77. The bibliography in U.S. Negro history and of Negro health status may be useful.

2 FARMER, H. E., 'An account of the earliest colored gentlemen in medical science in the United States', *Bull. Hist. Med.*, 1940, **8**, 599–618.

3 SWADOS, FELICE, 'Negro health on the ante bellum plantations', *Bull. Hist. Med.*, 1941, **10**, 460–72.

4 DOW, THOMAS W., 'Primitive medicine in Haiti', *Bull. Hist. Med.*, 1965, **39**, 34–52, esp. pp. 35–36.

5 BOUSFIELD, M. O., 'An account of physicians of color in the United States', *Bull. Hist. Med.*, 1945 **1**, 61–84.

6 GUERRA, FRANCISCO, *American Medical Bibliography, 1639–1783*, New York, Lathrop-Harper, 1962, 885 pp.

7 MORAIS, HERBERT, *The History of the Negro in Medicine*, 3rd ed., Washington, Association for the Study of Negro Life and History. *International Library of Negro Life and History:* World distribution by International Corporation, Miami, Florida, U.S.A. The bibliography is rather curiously organized, but is extensive. The illustrations in the book are profuse.

8 MORAIS, ibid., pp. 142–44, 285–86.

9 MILLER, KELLY, 'Historic background of the Negro physician', *J. Negro Hist.*, 1916, **1**, 101.

10 WOODSON, C. G., *The Negro Professional Man and the Community*, Washington, Association for the Study of Negro Life and History, 1934, p. 5.

11 WARING, JOSEPH I., *A History of Medicine in South Carolina, 1670–1825*, So. Carolina Medical Association, 1964, p. 69. Caesar 'achieved the popular name of Doctor'. He was a slave freed for disclosing his cures.

12 RUSSELL, J. H., *The Free Negro in Virginia*, Baltimore, 1913, p. 53, quoted in Ulrich Phillips, *American Negro Slavery*, Appleton and Co., 1918, pp. 263–64, 322.

13 DUFFY, JOHN, *The Rudolph Matas History of Medicine in Louisiana*, vol. 1, 1958, pp. 324–25.

14 BLANTON, WYNDAM E., *Medicine in Virginia in the Seventeenth Century*, 1930, vol. 1, p. 172. Vol. 2 on the eighteenth century, pp. 173–77, 193, gives a summary, based especially on Phillips.

15 GUERRA, op. cit., pp. 113, 121, 661.

16 NEWBELL, PUCKETT N., *Folk Beliefs of the Southern Negro*, Chapel Hill 1926, reprinted by Dover Book Co., 1969. See esp. pp. 177 ff.

17 CATTERALL, HELEN T., *Judicial Cases Concerning American Slavery and the Negro*, New York, Octagon Books, 1926–37, vol. 2, pp. 520–21. Vol. 4 Humphreys, pp. 421–23.

18 BENNETT, JR., LERONE, *Before the Mayflower: A History of the Negro in America 1619–1964*, Chicago, Johnson Publishing Co., 1961, pp. 111–13. We are grateful to Sylvester Walker, history assistant in our Department for further information concerning these episodes. Aphtheker's work on slave revolts is basic and classic.

19 WOODSON, CARTER GODWIN, and WESLEY, CHARLES H., *The Negro in Our History*, Washington, Associated Publishers, 1922, p. 106.

20 PATTERSON, CALEB PERRY, *The Negro in Tennessee 1790–1865*, Austin, University of Texas, 1922, p. 186.

21 Ibid., pp. 108 ff.

22 Ibid., pp. 103 ff.

23 There is a great deal known about the Freedman's Bureau, including its Kentucky-Tennessean branch. A classic account is in W. E. B. Du Bois' *The Souls of Black Folks*, 1903, ch. II, pp. 23–41, available as a paperback reprint from Fawcett World Library, New York. See also *Educational Efforts of the Freedman's Bureau of Tennessee* by Joy H. Falk, Vanderbilt University Department of History Library, Nashville, Tennessee, 1969, 52 pp., footnotes and bibliography.

24 REYBURN, ROBERT, *Type of Disease Among The Freed People of the United States; Consolidated Reports of Sick and Wounded Free People and White Refugees Under Treatment from 1865 to June 30, 1872, by Medical Officers on Duty in Bureau of Refugees, Freedmen and Abandoned Lands*, Washington, D.C., 1891. (Available in Fisk University Negro Collection.) Data are given on deaths by cause, common infectious diseases, and by type of services provided.

25 CARR, ELLEN LILLARD, *The Struggle of the Freedmans' Bureau to Effect Social Rehabilitation in Nashville and Davidson County*, M.A. Thesis Dept. of History, Fisk University, 1967, 178 pp. This is a study based on thorough primary source searches.

26 *The Christian Educator*, 1890, p. 30.

27 JOHNSON, HENRY MORRISON, *The Methodist Episcopal Church and the Education of Southern Negroes, 1862–1900*, Ph.D. Thesis, Yale University, 1939. Available in the Methodist Board of Higher Education Library, Nashville, Tennessee.

28 Methodist Episcopal Church, *Northern Annual Conference Records, 1866–1888*, Tennessee State Library Archives. Copy provided by Rev. A. M. Anderson of Clark Memorial Methodist Church, Smyrna, Tennessee.

29 BRADEN, MARY E., *John Braden – A Pioneer in Negro Education*, Morristown, Tennessee, Triangle Press, 1935, 31 pp.

30 MEHARRY, FRANCES, *The Meharry Family*, Lafayette, Indiana, Indiana Printing Co., 1925.

31 MORAIS, op. cit., p. 44.

32 *Central Tennessee College Bulletin*, 1876, available in Methodist Episcopal Higher Education Board Library, Nashville.

33 *Bulletin of Meharry Medical College*, 1950, 80th Anniversary Issue, **42**, 14, Nashville, Tennessee, Commencement address of Rev. John Braden, 1878, the first such statement. The entire address is a moving statement, well worth reading.
34 *Central Tennessee College Bulletin*, 1878.
35 Dr. O. Davis of Oklahoma, a graduate of Meharry in 1901, was the source. (Told to L.A.F. at Oklahoma MeDePhar Annual Meeting, 1971.)
36 *Central Tennessee College Bulletin*, 1879.
37 MORAIS, op. cit., p. 67.
38 *Bulletin, Meharry Medical College*, op. cit.
39 LYNK, MILES V., *Sixty Years of Medicine: An Autobiography*, Memphis, Tenn. Twentieth Century Press, 1951.
40 ROMAN, CHARLES V., *Meharry Medical College, A History*, Nashville, Tennessee, Nashville Baptist Publishing House, 1934.
41 HUBBARD, JOHN, 'Dr. Georgia E. L. Patton Washington', *The Christian Educator*, 1901, pp. 5–6.
42 FLEXNER, ABRAHAM, *Medical Education in the United States and Canada*, New York, Carnegie Foundation for the Advancement of Learning, 1960, pp. 180–86, reprint of the original edition.
43 REITZES, DIETRICH C., *The Negro and Medicine*, Cambridge, Mass., Harvard University Press, 1958, pp. 316–28.

E. Lutzker
New York (U.S.A.)

The London School of Medicine for Women: origin: important contributions to medicine by a few graduates

Contemporary society, with its own active issues and concerns, forgets the bitter moral, legal, and social battles waged by earlier generations to secure rights that today are taken for granted. But betterment does not just happen. It has to be fought for. And often it is fought against odds that require not only intensity of purpose, but also firm belief in the ability of people to change once they are persuaded and become convinced of the justice and logic of a particular cause. One striking instance of this is the account of women's struggle to acquire medical education in Britain in the nineteenth century.

Just a little over one hundred years ago one lone woman, Sophia Jex-Blake, applied for admission to the University of Edinburgh for a medical education which would entitle her to practise medicine legally in Britain. Men and women from all walks of life and from all levels of society became involved in this social and professional issue – should women be trained to practise medicine in England? Her simple application to the medical faculty of the University of Edinburgh set off a battery of conflicts that raged for years.

When it became known that the university had refused permission for one woman to attend classes in botany and in natural history, four other women joined Sophia Jex-Blake and the application was renewed. The group was then allowed to make arrangements for classes separate from men. In October 1869, the five women were admitted to the required preliminary examinations, which all of them passed. With the consent of every governing body in the university, the women were then accepted for formal matriculation and subsequent 'instruction for the profession of medicine'.

On 12 November 1869, the following regulations were issued officially and inserted in the Calendar of the University where they re-appeared annually for the next several years.

(1) Women shall be admitted to the study of medicine in the University.
(2) The instruction of women for the profession of medicine shall be conducted in separate classes, confined entirely to women.
(3) The Professors of the Faculty of Medicine shall, for this purpose, be permitted to have separate classes for women.
(4) Women not intending to study medicine professionally may be admitted to such of these classes, or to such part of the courses of instruction given in such classes as the University Court may from time to time think fit and approve.
(5) All women attending such classes shall be subject to all the regulations, now or at any future time in force in the University, as to the matriculation of students, their attendance on classes, examinations or otherwise.

(6) The above Regulations shall take effect as from the commencement of session 1869–70.[1]

After matriculation, they were duly inscribed as *Cives Academiae Edinensis*, which committed them to promise obedience to college discipline.

During the first session the women did so well that the latent opposition to them began to come out into the open. Some professors refused to teach them; male students mobbed them; university authorities withdrew their commitment to them on the tenuous grounds that they had exceeded their powers in admitting them in the first place. More than five years of continuous anxiety, frustration, and doubt about whether they would be permitted to complete their medical education at the University of Edinburgh came to an end. During those years they had to pay four times more in fees to the professors than the male students paid. Their admission had opened a Pandora's box of every possible kind of resistance at every level of the university's complex administrative structure and particularly from the Medical Faculty and its male medical students, as well as from the medical profession and the general public.

The medical profession argued that women doctors were not needed and were not wanted. Their objections appeared widely in newspapers and medical journals. In response there were some enlightened doctors and some sections of the population who maintained that the profession's objection to women doctors was motivated by their fear of the competition they would face if women practised medicine; and that their lofty rhetoric only obscured their need to prevent any encroachment on the 'male preserve' they were determined to retain.

The superior academic performance of this handful of women, whose names appeared on honour lists in every subject during every semester of those five years, served only to exacerbate the general hostility. Newspapers (with the rare exception of one or two), medical journals, editorials, news items, letters to the editors from some segments of the public, vociferously condemned the five women who had sought to become doctors and to serve their sex at a period in medical history when the practice of obstetrics and gynaecology was left to untrained midwives and when male doctors were often disinterested, inexperienced, and uninformed in these branches of medicine. High maternal and infant mortality figures did little or nothing to change the attitude of male doctors toward the practice of obstetrics and gynaecology, and this despite the fact that their own wives, families and friends fell victim to the prevailing practice of the time. Infant mortality was often as high as, and sometimes even exceeded maternal mortality, but these calamities brought little improvement in the broadest sections of the medical profession.

Although imperfectly understood, the feeling prevailed among doctors and laymen, supported by current religious institutions, that since childbirth was a physiological process, it should proceed without medical interference which was called 'meddlesome midwifery'. In fact Sir Anthony Carlisle, an eminent surgeon, told a Select Committee that 'it is an imposture to pretend that a medical man is required at a labour'.[2] Even the President of the Royal College of Physicians stated in a letter that the practice of midwifery was 'an act foreign to the habits of a gentleman of enlarged academic education.'[3] Consequently, is it any wonder that the feeling prevailed, if mother and child survived, God be praised! If not, God's Will be done! When an attending, usually untrained, midwife saw that her patient was not delivering normally, and that things were taking a difficult turn, she would call for a doctor, but most often too late to save the life of the mother, the child, or both.

For young girls of the family who were in the house during their mother's labour pains, the experience must have been traumatic when things went wrong. Was this what they must expect when they grew up and married and had children of their own? In the days when most women gave birth to their children at home, they were often made to assist the midwife and so they were eye-witnesses of the long hours of labour and the uncontrollable cries of their mother's agony. Is it any wonder that the thought crossed the minds of some of these girls that some day they would train as nurses, midwives, and even doctors so that they might alleviate the suffering they had seen when their own mothers brought children into the world? And when mother and child died, the anguish these children experienced at first hand must have left indelible scars on their memories!

Whether the five women who began the fight for medical education had been witnesses, unwilling or frightened participants in such heartrending events is not known. Nevertheless they showed total dedication in the face of the barriers hurriedly contrived against them, and the determination and fortitude to break through and to achieve the complete education available to men students at the University of Edinburgh.

At that time a medical degree could be obtained either from a recognized British university or from one of the nineteen British Examining Boards named in the Medical Reform Act of 1858, which had set up a General Council of Medical Education and Registration of the United Kingdom. Under this Act, every legally qualified practitioner's name must be recorded in a Register. Those already in practice in 1858 who had received their medical education in foreign countries or in colonial universities were entitled to be registered. The General Medical Council was not required to conduct qualifying examinations.

The Act of 1858 had been passed before the admission of women into medical schools or medical societies. The framers of the Act had aimed at controlling medical qualifications to save the public from the quackery that was rampant at that time. There is no evidence that the exclusion of women was calculated or intended. The Act consistently used the word 'persons'. But it was not easy in 1869, when this group of five pioneers began their campaign, to persuade the public that women were indeed 'persons'!

Under the Act's provision permitting the names of those already in practice to be entered in the Medical Register, Elizabeth Blackwell (1821–1910) provided the first wedge for the five other women. She had been graduated from a medical college in Geneva, New York, in 1849, the first woman in America to do so. She had already practised medicine in New York City for about seven years when she came to England in 1858. She was the first woman to be registered on 1 January 1859 under that Medical Act. And so a precedent came into being.

But the apple-cart was upset when Elizabeth Garrett (1836–1917) began her study of medicine in 1860. She was required to attend one of the teaching bodies controlled by the nineteen agencies listed in the Medical Act of 1858. After several rejections she was finally accepted at Apothecaries Hall whose rules explicitly stated that no one who met the conditions of study could be refused admission to its examinations. She met difficulties that male students did not face. For example, she was barred from attendance at some classes and had to engage private teachers for those subjects. She had to leave the Middlesex Hospital where she was getting clinical training. The male students at that hospital objected – reportedly, because of her superior work. But, nevertheless she completed her studies in 1865, her name was entered in the Medical Register and she was licensed to practise.

Some medical authorities resented this second wedge. They considered the rules of the Apothecaries Society too loose, and contrived with its Master and Wardens to change those rules so as to prohibit the substitution of private instruction for class instruction. This feeling was expressed by the *Medical Times and Gazette*, a leading medical journal:[4]

For ourselves, we hold that the admission of women in the ranks of medicine is an egregious blunder, derogatory to the status and character of the female sex, and likely to be injurious to the highest degree to the interests and public estimation of the profession which they seek to invade. By insisting on the attendance of all students at the public-class delivery of anatomical lectures, and in the public-class dissecting room, the only possible guarantee of uniformity of teaching will be obtained, and, at the same time, a difficulty will be placed in the way of female intrusion which it will not be easy for women of character, and clearly none else are eligible, to surmount. We hope, however, that the Court of Examiners will not stop with the erection of the barrier we suggest, but that they will distinctly *refuse to admit any female candidate to examination* unless compelled by a legal decision from the bench; and we also hope that they will be supported in such refusal by the Master and Wardens of the Society, as well as by the profession out-of-doors. [Italics added.]

I shall not relate here the details of the indignities suffered by these women in the streets, in the classrooms, and from the University of Edinburgh itself, which finally ousted them despite their excellent academic performance, or perhaps because of it. By 1871 five more women had joined the original pioneers. The reconstituted group of ten, upon legal advice, brought suit against the Senate of the University in March 1872, and in July 1872, won the verdict. Their suit, however, failed to name the University Court; and the Senate alone was not empowered to allow the women to continue their education to completion. On this technicality the university appealed against the verdict and in July 1873 won a reversal by a seven to five vote. All legal expenses of the women's case, and the university appeal, the amount of £848 6s. 8d., were imposed on the women.

Sophia Jex-Blake and her friends then decided to broaden their appeal, basing it on their inherent right to study medicine, and addressing themselves to Parliament and to public opinion. In April 1874 'A Bill to Remove Doubts as to the Powers of the Universities of Scotland to Admit Women as Students and to Grant Degrees to Women' was introduced. Adroit manoeuvering by hostile members of Parliament extended debate on this and other related bills until August 1876, when royal assent was finally given. But even then, the universities, medical schools, and examining agencies retained the *option* to admit women at their discretion. The final version of the bill was *permissive* and not *mandatory*. The extent to which prejudice permeated the Parliamentary debates is very revelatory. Again, space does not permit concrete instances of this; but I can only suggest that Parliamentary Debates, 3rd series, 1874, vol. 219; 1876, vols. 222; 226; 230; 1877, vol. 233; 1878, vol. 238–240, be read by those who still need to be convinced of the barriers these indefatigable women had to overcome in the nineteenth century to open the medical profession to women.

One cannot but wonder at the courage shown by Sophia Jex-Blake who had initiated the struggle in Edinburgh and who now determined not only to complete her own medical education but also to make it possible for other women to acquire one without going through the soul-searing experiences she had undergone. It was she who conceived the idea of creating a medical school for women in London. During her search for a medical school that would admit women, she became acquainted with Dr. A. T. Norton of St. Mary's Hospital. Why not organize a medical school in London for women, staffed by recognized lecturers from existing schools, she asked him? She was encouraged also by Dr. F. E. Anstie, another supporter of women in medicine.

And so, an organizational meeting was held at Dr. Anstie's house on 22 August 1874, and a provisional committee of registered medical practitioners only was set up. Dr. T. King Chambers of Scotland, Dr. Anstie, Dr. Norton, Sophia Jex-Blake, Edith Pechey, Mrs. Isabelle Thorne were present and it was unanimously resolved that '. . . a school be founded in London with a view to educating women in medicine and enabling them to pass such examinations as would place their names on the Medical Register'. It was decided to open the school on 12 October 1874 – less than two months away, and to call it the London School of Medicine for Women. Sophia had won many friends in Edinburgh during the agitation stirred up by the campaign there and financial help came from them and others in London who had become interested in the school's aims. The venture was supported by Charles Darwin, Thomas Henry Huxley, Henry Fawcett and James Martineau, to mention a few only.

Sophia also undertook to find quarters for the school. On 15 September 1874, she signed a lease on the building at 30 Henrietta Street that was rumoured to have been the residence of King George IV's mistresses. She personally supervised the many alterations that had to be made. On 12 October 1874, fourteen students arrived and began their studies. Their names were:

Mrs. Isabel Thorne	Sophia Jex-Blake
Edith Pechey	Alice Ker
Mrs. Marshall	Annie E. Clark
Mrs. Foggo	Miss Vinson
Miss Rorison	Edith Shove
Elizabeth Walker	Agnes McLaren
Miss Waterston	Fanny Butler

The unfortunate and tragic death of Dr. Anstie three days before Sophia signed the lease on the building probably precluded formal opening ceremonies and an inaugural lecture. Dr. Norton stepped in to accept the post of Dean and to devote himself to the school at a time when 'prejudice against the movement was strong and active, and it required much courage and determination' on his part to do so. Nine additional students enrolled in the first year, bringing the total to twenty-three. A three-year plan of study was worked out on a basis of rotation of subjects, as follows:

1874–75:	Winter session:	Anatomy; practical anatomy; physiology; chemistry
	Summer session:	Botany; materia medica; practical chemistry; comparative anatomy; mental pathology

1875–76:	Winter session:	Anatomy; practical anatomy; physiology; surgery; practice of medicine
	Summer session:	Midwifery; forensic medicine; ophthalmic surgery
1876–77:	Winter session:	Practice of medicine; clinical medicine; clinical surgery; pathology

The fourth year was to be devoted to hospital work or to practice in a dispensary, to include practical pharmacy and midwifery, vaccination, etc. The curriculum also included such subjects as zoology, mental pathology and ophthalmic surgery, not required by most of the existing examining boards. Five new students were admitted during the second year.

Despite stringent economy, the cost of running the school was higher than that of most others, one reason being that fees to lecturers were guaranteed, an unusual procedure for that time.

Lord Shaftsbury, an enthusiastic supporter of the School, on 2 June 1875 distributed prizes earned during the preceding session, noting the difficulties the women had been through and adding that not only they but also the medical profession would gain in stature and character therefrom. He believed 'in the inherent right of choice possessed by all persons as to their occupation'.[5] When he awarded the student prizes the following year, Sophia noted the contrast with Edinburgh, where faculty members had twice refused to appear at prize distribution ceremonies if the women were to be present to receive the prizes they had earned.

By midsummer of 1876, when the Enabling Act passed by Parliament emphasized its permissive rather than mandatory nature, it was realized that the school's future depended on two essential factors: first, official recognition by at least one of the nineteen examining boards. This could be achieved only by permitting the school's students to take its examinations. Such permission was flatly refused by all. The second necessary condition was the admission of the school's students to a hospital with at least one hundred beds, for bedside training. Nearby was the Royal Free Hospital which was not a teaching hospital and hence had no students. Nonetheless, its medical staff objected to admitting women students.

Under a Medical Act Amendment (College of Surgeons' Bill) introduced the previous year, the College of Surgeons had approved the opening of its examinations in midwifery to women. Sophia, Edith Pechey and Isabel Thorne applied for admission to these examinations and were accepted. The acceptances were based on the legal advice given to the College of Surgeons which stated that 'it had the power to admit women under its supplementary charter, and could be compelled by legal process to examine and grant certificates . . . that the Medical Act considered the holder of such certificate a licentiate in midwifery and as such, entitled to register'.[6]

When it became known, however, that the women's applications to take the examinations had been accepted, the entire board of examiners resigned. No further examinations were scheduled and no one would agree to serve on that examining board for the succeeding ten years. It was clear that the physicians were not unanimous in approving the legislation, although it had received royal assent in July 1875. By this means the opposition sought to violate existing law. And so, still another door was shut in the women's faces.

In December 1876, the Women's School appealed to the King and Queen's College of Physicians in Ireland to approve its qualifications as a teaching body and to admit its students to examination. They won their appeal, and the College became the first medical college in Great Britain to grant licences for the practice of medicine to women students of the London School of Medicine for Women.

Meanwhile, Sophia Jex-Blake and Edith Pechey, who had been thwarted in all their personal efforts, left for Switzerland in the autumn of 1876 to take medical courses and M.D. examinations in German at the University of Berne. In January 1877, both received M.D. degrees from that university. By that time M.D. degrees from the University of Berne were accepted by the College of Physicians in Ireland. Both women took examinations there in May 1877, and after passing, became Licentiates of the King and Queen's College of Physicians in Ireland (LKQCPI). Their names were entered in the Medical Register at long last, qualifying them for medical practice. And so one of the two important hurdles was overcome.

The second hurdle was cleared in March 1877, when the Royal Free Hospital agreed to admit the women students for bedside training. The School had to agree to pay £400 annually for five years for the clinical teachers of the students, and £315 annually for five years for the use of the hospital for practical training.

With increasing enrolments and both obstacles cleared away, the October 1877 session opened with a brilliant inaugural address by Dr. Edith Pechey. She took it for granted that 'there are no unwilling daughters driven here much against the grain by the commands of inexorable fathers . . . and who must be warned against the distractions of beer and billiards'. . . . She hoped that students would expand their knowledge of all the sciences . . . and would rather believe that they were animated with the desire of leaving the world 'better and richer and wiser for your presence in it' . . . urging them to dedicate themselves 'to do what in you lies, in however and humble and small a way, to further the prevention and cure of disease!'

By 1887 there were seventy-seven students; by 1889 there were ninety-one; by 1892, there were 133. In other words, the number of students had risen from twenty-three at the School's opening, to 159 in 1896. These statistics effectively refuted those who had insisted that women doctors were not wanted, were not needed, and were not capable of completing medical studies and engaging in medical practice. In 1903 enrolment was 318; in 1917, it was 441![7] By any yardstick the school was a tremendous success.

The professional education of women took a giant step forward when the University of London in mid-1877 agreed to admit women to its medical examinations and as degree candidates.

For twenty-three years the London School of Medicine for Women retained its own name and identity. Public and patients came to realize to a greater or lesser degree that a formidable breakthrough had occurred. In 1897, however, the affiliation between the London School of Medicine for Women and the Royal Free Hospital resulted in a change of name to the 'London (Royal Free Hospital) School of Medicine for Women'. The school's origins were thus not entirely submerged.[8] By May 1947, however, that name was abandoned and replaced by 'The Royal Free Hospital School of Medicine'. The word 'women' was deleted where it appeared.[9] The origin of the London School of Medicine for Women has become obscured with the passage of time and is by this time lost to the present generation.

The following are a few of the accomplishments of the pioneers who began the campaign in Edinburgh and founded the London School of Medicine for Women in 1874, and of others who received their medical education there.

Sophia Jex-Blake opened the first hospital for women and children, staffed and directed by women, in 1886 in Edinburgh, on the earliest battleground of that bitterly fought struggle.

Dr. Edith Pechey (1845–1908) was the first woman to go to India as a fully qualified doctor who had no connexion with religious missions. She arrived in Bombay in 1883 and in 1886 was appointed First Physician in charge of the Cama and Albless Hospital there. She carried on effective campaigns among the Indian people for widespread and higher education for girls and women and for their admission to medical colleges, especially to the University of Bombay. Before the Cama Hospital was completed, she opened a dispensary for women and children in the poor section of Bombay where her services were urgently needed because Indian tradition forbade the examination or treatment of girls and women by male doctors. During the devastating cholera and plague epidemics that raged from 1896 in Bombay, and until her retirement from India in 1905 – after twenty-two years there – she participated in house-to-house visitations with flying squadrons of soldiers and disinfection groups, and was assigned to the Mohammedan areas of the city because among them especially, prohibitions were very strict against the females receiving medical treatment from male doctors. The anti-cholera and anti-plague vaccines created by Waldemar M. Haffkine in 1893 and 1897 respectively, and administered by her, saved thousands of lives. She married Herbert M. Phipson, a naturalist in 1889 in Bombay. Their country home in Nasik Road, about 100 miles north of Bombay, was expanded into the Pechey–Phipson sanatorium where poor families of Bombay could occupy the twenty-odd cottages for a month, free of cost, and so escape the unbearable heat of Bombay during the hot seasons. The women of India wove by hand a beautiful carpet for her when she retired to show their gratitude for her services to them.

Matilda Chaplin (1846–83) received her M.D. in Paris in 1872 and in Britain in 1880. She married her professor, William Edward Ayrton (1847–1908) who was also her cousin; he was a student of Lord Kelvin and a pioneer in electrical engineering. With him she went to Japan when he was appointed to the Imperial College of Engineering in Tokyo. She continued her work in Japan where she made a study of the physical stature of the Japanese people and its effect on the state of their health and their reaction to medical treatment.

Mrs. Isabel Thorne (1836–1917) had lived in China for many years before her return to England. Her only daughter died there due to the inadequate medical attention available to women and children at that time. She was convinced that more women doctors were needed and joined Sophia Jex-Blake's group to study chemistry, anatomy, hygiene and midwifery. She became Honorary Secretary to the London School of Medicine for Women and dedicated herself to its success although she had already earned her own medical degree. She wrote a history of the school up to 1904. Her daughter, May Thorne, also became a doctor and continued the family association with the school. It was she who performed surgery on Edith Pechey-Phipson in her last and fatal illness of diabetes and cancer.

Little is known about Helen DeLacey Evans, one of the original pioneer group of five women. She married Alexander Russel, Editor of the *Scotsman*, whose sympathies were with the medical pioneers and who put his newspaper at their service thereby helping to create public opinion in their favour.

Other students of the School who distinguished themselves were Edith Shove who won prizes there in every session in almost every subject. She engaged in the practice of medicine and was appointed medical officer to women post-office clerks, an acknowledgement of her competence.

Dr. Annie McCall started the first prenatal clinic for pregnant mothers in the 1880s.

Dr. Janet Campbell, D.B.E., contributed to a decline in infant and maternal mortality.

Dr. Alice Mary Corthorn headed the plague hospital in Poona, India, and was awarded the Kaiser-i-Hind medal for outstanding work during the plague epidemic of 1896. It is a mystery that my searches for her obituary in many libraries have remained unsuccessful.

Mary Sharlieb got her M.D. from the University of London in 1888 – the first woman to do so. She had done some medical work in Madras and returned to London for health reasons. Sir James Paget, a supporter of women doctors, referred his gynaecological patients to her. She was also one of the first women magistrates and worked in juvenile courts on the Lunacy Commission at Holloway Prison for women. She organized children's clinics and lectured throughout the kingdom on venereal diseases. King George V bestowed the title of Dame of the British Empire on her. She wrote a book of her reminiscences before she died in 1930.

Jane Walker pioneered in the treatment of tuberculosis. She was one of the first doctors in Britain to believe in open-air treatment for patients and had great faith in rehabilitation through appropriate work therapy. In 1901 she opened the East Anglian Sanatorium.

Dr. Maude Abbot was acclaimed for her work in coronary diseases.

Dr. Elsie Inglis served in Serbia during World War I.

Dr. Jane Walker of Yorkshire got an M.D. in Brussels, and her name was placed in the London Medical Register in 1884. She went to Vienna for more study. The University of Leeds awarded her an Honorary title of LL.D.; in 1931 King George awarded her the Order of Companion of Honour.

Drs. Agnes McLaren, Isabella Mears (died 1937, aged eighty-two), Marian Erskine, Isabel Venters, were members of the first graduating class of medical students at the London School of Medicine for Women.

Dr. Maud M. Chadburn was a gynaecological surgeon and cancer specialist, educated at the London School of Medicine for Women but got her medical licence in 1893 through the Guild of Apothecaries. She was senior consulting surgeon supervising a staff of thirty and was on the surgical or obstetrical staff of several hospitals. In 1924 she was one of the four surgeons who promoted radium treatment for uterine cancer.

Dr. Christine Murrell died in 1933, just as she was to be seated as the first woman elected to the General Medical Council of Great Britain.

Almost all women who sought medical educational opportunities of the same quality as men had been at some time or other associated with the London School of Medicine for Women. The names of a very few only are given above. Much more research – in archives that have been overlooked, will doubtless yield the names of many more.

Notes

1 *The Nineteenth Century Review*, July 1877, Edinburgh and London, 1878; *Medical Women, an Historical Sketch*, by Right Hon. James Stansfeld, M.P. Also, *University Calendar*, p. 260.
2 KERR, JOHN MUNRO *et al.*, *Historical Review of British Obstetrics and Gynaecology: 1800–1950*, Edinburgh, 1954, p. 332.
3 Ibid., p. 332.
4 23 February 1867, p. 199.
5 *The Times*, 3 June 1875.
6 *Br. med. J.*, 1876, pp. 77–78.
7 ANDERSON, LOUISA GARRETT, *Elizabeth Garrett Anderson*, London, 1939, p. 287.
8 Prospectus, University of London, Royal Free Hospital School of Medicine, Session 1962–63, p. 16.
9 Alterations to the Charter of the London (Royal Free Hospital) School of Medicine for Women, referred to in the Foregoing Order in Council, p. 2, at the Court at Buckingham Palace, the 21st Day of May, 1947. The King's Most Excellent Majesty in Council.

D. D. Gibbs
Lichfield (Great Britain)

Recommendations of Sir John Floyer on the education of a physician

Though the seventeenth century was marked by great political and religious events and the scientific achievements of the period have earned it the title of 'the century of genius', by contrast, formal education provided by schools and universities in England changed remarkably little. Stuart education was not much different from Tudor, with its basis in the Latin curriculum which continued into and through the eighteenth century. Despite trenchant criticisms and proposals for reform in school education emanating, among others, from Sir Francis Bacon, Milton and at the end of the century, from John Locke, English grammar schools seemed impervious to change, and formal teaching at the universities retained much of its medieval character (Watson, 1968).

Detailed contemporary comments on the education and training which he considered appropriate for a physician in the early eighteenth century are to be found in the writings of Sir John Floyer (1649–1734). John Floyer was born in 1649 and was the son of a Staffordshire landowner. His two brothers attended the local grammar school at Tamworth, near his home, but illness may have interfered with his own schooling. 'I cannot remember the first occasion of my asthma, but I have been told it was a cold when I first went to school' (Floyer, 1698). Whether he was able to attend school or was taught by a tutor at home, he must have been instructed in subjects conforming to the traditional curriculum, qualifying him at fifteen to matriculate at Oxford University. He entered the Queen's College, graduated B.A., after three years in 1668, and M.D. in 1674.

By 1675, at the age of twenty-six, it is recorded that he lived in Lichfield, the city in which he remained practising as a physician for over fifty years. He retained links with Oxford, taking his doctorate in 1686. He became a member of the Philosophical Society of Oxford. In loyalty to his college he bequeathed it many of his medical books, and more than ten years before his death, he deposited certain of his manuscripts in the newly built College library.

Sir John Floyer was not born into a medical family and neither of his two sons followed him in his profession. He was probably approaching the age of seventy when he wrote *Advice to a Young Student of Physic*, which he dedicated to a grandson named John; however, his hopes for a family succession in the profession of medicine ended, when the boy died in childhood. Although ambitions for his grandson expressed in this essay remained unfulfilled, the writings offer an insight into the views of an experienced clinician on an education suitable for a student of medicine.

Before proceeding to the university at sixteen he recommended the following education: 'Let him continue at school till he can translate any Latin author into English and from the English into proper Latin: and collect French grammar to teach him to speak in commonly. And let him have so much Greek as to construe his Greek testament perfectly; the making themes and verses at school and the criticisms in Latin and Greek are very useless. Let him read Terence, and Erasmus's and Corderius's Colloquies very much, and practice the speaking Latin.' While these recommendations are unlikely to have been comprehensive it is clear that he was satisfied with a curriculum which remains narrowly classical and that the basic training was aimed at producing fluency in Latin. As far as the curriculum was concerned there was no break between school and university. 'To the University he may go at 16 and continue there two or three years and no longer. During that time let him read logic and the Latin poets and the Roman history at first year.'

He justifies the long training in classics partly as a necessity to achieve a broad philosophy and learning as an essential basis for clinical judgment, and partly for more utilitarian reasons. 'We must come to the study well instructed in the learned languages in which Hippocrates and Galen have writ, and the Latin language (in which the modern have writ their books) was as necessary as the Greek.' Rhetoric, music and poetry, ethics, history, grammar and metaphysics he considers 'may be ornaments to physicians and procure them esteem, but not necessary to the art of physic.' He concedes that 'rhetoric may be useful to comfort the melancholic and to encourage the fearful, to appease the angry and furious and persuade the obstinate to the use of medicines', and 'ethics are useful to the physician for governing both his own and his patient's passions'.

By the second year at university he advised the student to study 'natural philosophy and see a course of chymistry and, for his diversion study botany, and get a course of anatomy'. Floyer had a contemporary and essentially Galenic interpretation of the relevance of these preclinical subjects. 'Anatomy shows us the natural and preternatural state of the fluids and solid parts. Botany and chymistry discovers the nature of our medicines by their sensible qualities. Natural philosophy discovers the immediate principles which compose our humours, and the several causes of their alterations and the effects of the external causes on our bodies. Though all these sciences may be in some degree of advantage to the institution in physic, yet many errors have sprung from the introduction of too much of them into the tracts of physic.' Even allowing for some personal vagaries by Floyer in interpreting the place of these subjects in medical training it is apparent that though they could be regarded as equivalents of the basic sciences they were only distantly related.

The books mentioned by Floyer help our understanding of the scope of the subjects he envisaged. Boyle's books are recommended to accompany seeing 'those experiments which are usually taught in a course of natural philosophy' and Lemery should be read while seeing a course of chemistry. In the second year Drake's *Treatise of Anatomy* should accompany a course of anatomy. In the afternoons, visits are to be made to the physic garden and on the subject of botany, 'amongst our new writers, Mr. Ray's History of Plants, and Pomet'. The pre-clinical training for the student who had reached the ages of seventeen and eighteen thus contained a balance between daily practical instruction and learning from contemporary authors.

It was in clinical training that practical teaching was lacking in England and Floyer had no doubt that the student should seek this where it was available. 'At 19 let him go into Holland and there see the practice of physic and chirurgy for two or three years in their hospitals. Any further travelling will be useless.' To remedy the deficient facilities in England he wanted hospitals built for the care of the poor where 'all the young students would see the practice of physic'. ' 'Tis certainly a great defect in the education of physicians in the universities that none of their professors teach the practical part, but only treat their auditors with notions about which all disputes are unnecessary.' In medicine he wanted students to observe all the effects of dispensatory medicines and then to try the prescripts from Bates and Fuller; practical training should also include observations of 'all the curious chirurgical operations and those in midwifery'.

A long reading list is recommended to complement experience in hospital. For instance, he suggested that Riverius's and Etmuller's accounts of the same diseases should be compared. He recommended consulting those 'authors who treat on any single disease they know most of' – the equivalent of monographs – and cites among others Morton's work on fevers, Lower's *Tractactus de Corde*, and his own *Treatise of the Asthma*.

On several occasions Floyer reiterates the absence of any facilities for clinical training in this country. 'Beyond seas the practice of physic will be shown by the professors there, but all time spent by a physician in our universities after two or three years is misspent, there being no college for physicians nor hospitals for practice.' He recommends the student to Holland, and there can be no doubt that he referred to Leyden. In 1714 Boerhaave succeeded Bidloo as professor collegii medico-practici and, from 1720 Herman Schacht helped him, each taking his turn in bedside teaching in rotation for periods of three months. Thus, at the time that Floyer was writing for his grandson in about 1720, clinical teaching was at its peak in Leyden.

Education for the physician was clearly a life-long process in Floyer's estimation. 'He is an ill physician who has no time to study and improve his faculty by . . . finding a more pleasant, shorter and safer method of curing disorders of which he has many experiments; who neglects the writing of the history of such, or any rare experiments, or to record the histories of dissections of diseased bodies, nor keeps an account of some experiments made by others. . . .' The educational value of the post-mortem examination was clearly accepted and he states that 'in chronical diseases we must know the causes by dissection, as is related in Bonet's Sepulchretum'.

In his practice as a provincial physician he was, however, often thwarted in this endeavour, because he was unable to overcome the prejudices of the local population. In advancing understanding of asthma he made two special contributions. He thought that spasmodic asthma was in part due to constriction of the bronchi, and he gave the first detailed description of emphysema from a dissection he performed on a broken-winded mare, relating his findings to human disease. He would dearly have liked to prove that there was the human counterpart of broken-winded horses. He wrote to a colleague in 1710: 'If I could have procured the dissection of such persons as have died of this disease in my neighbourhood, you should have had that evidence too; but my countrymen are averse to such practices, though designed for their good. But I must leave this part of this subject to the young practicers in London, to look for the air-bladders in asthmatics.'

Floyer's membership of the Philosophical Society of Oxford founded by Robert Plot has been mentioned. The minutes of the society contain many accounts of clinical cases, though Floyer does not appear to have been personally involved in the proceedings very much, perhaps because of the distance from Lichfield to Oxford. But, in recognizing the need for the continuing education of a physician it is clear that he put great store on the value of case presentation. When advocating a physician's college he held that those who had received their clinical training should 'be obliged to communicate all the rare cases in practice, or experiments of our own country medicines'.

During the second half of the seventeenth century it has been said that progress in scientific discovery and learning came from the top rather than the foot of the educational ladder (Ashley, 1967). Sir John Floyer was happy to have his grandson moulded by the same narrow schooling as he had received fifty years previously. As a result of his own schooling and university education he developed into one of the 'clinical physicians' who adopted systematic note-taking and case recording and advocated post-mortem examinations. His special contribution concerned pulse timing as a particular aspect of physical examination. The important difference between his own education and that which he advocated fifty years later related to bedside teaching formally arranged on patients in hospital. He was not alone in laying emphasis on this form of clinical education. John Bellers, a Quaker philanthropist, made detailed recommendations in 1714, probably anticipating those of Floyer by a few years, with the object of preventing 'many from travelling to foreign hospitals to learn, when they shall be capable of doing it better at home'. Bellers particularly emphasized that there should be one hospital at each of our two universities: 'they being the great nurseries of our graduated physicians, make hospitals there to be absolutely necessary for their better instruction, by adding practice to their aphorisms and theory'. Floyer is mentioned by Bellers in terms of approbation on the subject of 'exact observations to be made on the pulse'; but it is not known how far their views on clinical teaching in hospitals were reached independently. There were others who held similar views outside the universities. In these institutions apparently little interest was shown in such practical affairs as bedside teaching, which did not become available in Great Britain until 1746 in the wards of the Royal Infirmary in Edinburgh, from Alexander Monro *primus* who had studied in Leyden.

References

ASHLEY, M., *England in the Seventeenth Century*, London, Penguin, 1967.
BELLERS, J., *An Essay toward the Improvement of the Sick*, London, 1714.
FLOYER, SIR J., *A Treatise of the Asthma*, London, 1698.
FLOYER, SIR J., *The Physician's Pulse Watch*, vol. 2, London, 1710.
FLOYER, SIR J., manuscripts [undated].
WATSON, F., *The Old Grammar Schools*, London, Cass, 1968.

P. Romanell
El Paso, Texas (U.S.A.)

John Locke's thoughts concerning medical education

Of all the biographical items about the great English philosopher John Locke (1632–1704), the one that seems to present the biggest difficulty to his many interpreters has to do with the versatility of his interests and writings. Granting that Locke's versatility as an author is not especially peculiar to him when compared with other famous names in his own 'Century of Genius', rather than with ours in the Age of Specialization, the difficulty in his case persists nevertheless. Actually, it has become even more acute of late, simply because the recent acquisition of his copious literary remains in the Lovelace Collection by the Bodleian Library has had the effect of re-opening the whole subject as to the chronology and compass of his interests. What relationship, if any, is there between Locke's thoughts on philosophy in his masterpiece, *An Essay Concerning Human Understanding* (1690), and his thoughts on science and medicine, economics and politics, education and religion?

In 1958, on the basis of some new evidence from Locke's medical manuscripts, I argued in print 'that the secret of Locke the philosopher lies in Locke the physician',[1] in other words, that Locke's medical interest has a greater direct bearing on his general philosophy than his other interests. Subsequently, Peter Laslett had this to say about how best to approach Locke's political thought in his *Two Treatises of Government* (1690): 'Empirical medicine, rather than philosophy, seems to be the model for the man who sets out to comment on political matters. Locke the doctor rather than Locke the epistemologist is the man we should have in mind when we read his work on *Government*.'[2] This is an apt observation as far as it goes, but it does not go far enough. For it is precisely Locke the doctor whom we should have in mind in the first place when we read Locke the epistemologist and his work on the *Understanding*.

Moreover, strangely enough, Laslett contends that '*Two Treatises* is not written on the "plain, historic method" [*sic*] of the *Essay*'.[3] Even were he right, he is inconsistent with his own premise. If 'empirical medicine' is taken as Locke's 'model' as a political theorist, then Laslett does not apparently realize that Locke's 'historical, plain method'[4] in the *Essay* is the very method of 'empirical medicine' *generalized*. In fact, what Locke calls the 'historical, plain method' in the *Essay* is nothing but his own more guarded version of the 'natural history' method of inquiry popular during the English Restoration among the Baconians and the members of the Royal Society. To anticipate the closing part of this paper, it was in its application to medicine that Locke first learned to appreciate the favourite method of observation of his scientific circle, and what he does in the *Essay* is to proceed cautiously to extend in principle its area of applicability to *all* matters of fact (including private matters of prudence and public matters of politics), his reason for the methodological extension being, simply, that all such matters are 'only known by experience'.[5]

Modern European philosophy since Descartes has been so obsessed with the problem of method in epistemology that it is quite understandable culturally why Locke's theory of knowledge is traditionally assumed as the tie of his multiple thoughts. On the other hand, Laslett the political historian is somewhat justified in being suspicious of this Procrustean approach to Locke. Even so, if Locke is all of one piece – and I for one think so – there must be some unity in the variety of his writings. Locke scholars as a rule have been missing the connecting link because they have been looking for it in the wrong place. Partly due to Locke's own fault, they have taken too much for granted that he is an *epistemologist,* when he is at heart a *moralist.*[6] The clearest statement on this score is when Locke concludes in the *Essay* 'that *natural philosophy is not capable of being made a science,*' and 'that *morality* is *the proper science and business of mankind in general*'.[7]

This dual conclusion of his implies that epistemology is handmaiden to morality: *ancilla ethicae.* The conclusion itself in turn reflects that Locke has a *practical* ideal of life. Now, once it is recognized that this practical ideal of life controls the way he thinks in general, then it should be quite evident that it is precisely the very same ideal of life which serves as the connecting link in the chain of his thoughts on sundry subjects. But, from whence his practical ideal of life? This is where Locke's medical background acquires the utmost relevance, because it affords the most direct access to his whole perspective on things. To Locke at least, morality as the proper business of mankind *in general* coincides, in ideal of practicality, with medicine as the proper business of physicians *in particular.* If there is one field of human endeavour which is thoroughly practical, and vitally so at that, literally, medicine is definitely it. Thus, technically speaking, the connecting link in Locke is not so much epistemological as axiological, since his empirical ideal of knowledge itself rests ultimately upon his over-all practical ideal of life.

An excellent way to test and confirm our conclusion regarding the primacy of the practical in Locke is to examine his thoughts concerning medical education, especially since the very subject chosen for the present paper involves the linkage of at least three of his interests: philosophy, medicine, and education. Locke's views on medical education are highly indicative of his pragmatic mentality, and they are important to consider for three main reasons: (*a*) they provide a major source of inspiration for his entire scheme of education; (*b*) they document his negative reaction to the medical curriculum of his times in the late seventeenth century; (*c*) they bear directly on his characteristic way of thinking as a practical empiricist. Let us briefly take up these reasons in order.

To begin with, it is well known that Locke was immensely disappointed with his studies at Westminster School in London and at Christ Church College in Oxford. Reference to this disappointment with his formal education at Oxford is first communicated in an obituary letter by Lady Masham, the earliest informant we have of his life and character. But, her most perceptive remark about him is that he had 'a universal Love of all sorts of usefull Knowledge'.[8] No truer remark could have been made of her beloved friend than this, for it explains succinctly why Locke reacted negatively to his schooling: he found it *useless*, period. The best proof in print of this negative reaction on his part to the standard classical curriculum of his day in England and Europe is, of course, *Some Thoughts Concerning Education* (1693), which is not only the most autobiographical work ever published by our author, but the sole book of his which is marked with the indelible stamp of Locke the physician from cover to cover.

As Locke himself acknowledges at the outset, his treatise on *Education* is 'suited' especially to the sons of the English gentry, whose duty is 'to have the Knowledge of a man of Business' and to be 'Useful in his Country according to his Station'.[9] However, although Locke's programme of education is restricted to a particular class in English society and its method of teaching is restricted to a private tutor, there is no doubt that what he defends educationally fits in perfectly with his own economic interests and sympathies for the business way of life. But, as our specific concern here is how his work on *Education* reflects the medical rather than the economic aspects of his thought, let us rest content for the time being with the bare assertion that both aspects are expressive of his practical ideal of life.

Despite the work's set restrictions as to social class and pedagogical method, Locke succeeds in the *Education* to offer a pragmatic reform of education which, though not altogether original with him, has had great influence on the educational world ever since in one way or another. On the negative side, his reform in education amounts to severe attacks on Learning, Latin, and Logic (the three L's of education in force during his era), on the ground that such subjects of study are of little help to anybody except pedants. On the positive side, his revolt against the alleged 'trash' taught then in school ('trash', incidentally, in the *Education* corresponds to 'rubbish' in the *Essay*) features the all-importance of two things which converge in Locke's ever practical mind – physical education and moral education – the first addressed to the health of the body, the second to the health of the soul. Here we see concretely on the educational plane how Locke the practical physician and Locke the practical moralist join forces in Locke the practical educationist. Time does not permit us to show that his whole 'exercise' theory of education, with its almost Spartan accent on hardiness in the bringing up of children, is based on an analogy with physical education and, consequently, takes its point of departure from his particular medical outlook.

Turning next to the second reason for considering Locke's ideas on medical education, we may say that his negative reaction to the standard medical curriculum of his period is significant, not only because it reinforces his general criticism of the 'book learning' at the time, but because the reinforcement itself comes from the very field of his own professional interest, medicine. Discounting the natural element of bias in Locke, we must assume that as a medical student he knew what he was talking about when he attacked the official curriculum in medicine to which he was exposed at Oxford. What are his objections to it?

Before listing his objections, they all boil down to the same thing he finds wrong with the existing classical programmes of education in general. As should be expected from a man with a practical ideal of life, Locke thinks that what was wrong with contemporary medical training is its lack of practicality, and hence its irrelevance to a physician's calling. To be more specific, Locke accuses it of being (*a*) purely eristic, (*b*) purely speculative, (*c*) purely verbal, (*d*) purely authoritarian, and (*e*) overly anatomical. Practically all of these objections are brought out in his two major medical fragments, *Anatomia* (1668) and *De Arte Medica* (1669). However, as these unfinished manuscripts are the best known of his medical papers, we are going to refer in the sequel to posthumous material of his less generally known. Meanwhile, with respect to the earlier of the two fragments mentioned, let us just comment in passing that his special fear of an overdose of anatomy in medicine has turned out to be unfounded, in view of subsequent clinical advances in the field. Ironically, sometimes a practical man is not practical enough in the long run, but this only proves once more that hindsight is much easier than foresight.

Lest there be misunderstanding of Locke's reform of education – general and medical – it should be made clear immediately that his attack on traditional logic has to do, strictly speaking, with the abuse of logic, that is, with logomachy. At any rate, Locke was apparently tactful enough to be mum about the eristics at his own University at Oxford. But, fortunately, he does record in his journals some priceless instances of the academic practice of 'disputations' at two of the leading medical schools in Europe he visited, Montpellier and Leyden. In his Journal for 1676 there are two entries[10] in shorthand on his reaction to wrangling at the Medical School in Montpellier. The earlier of them says: 'Disputation at the Physick Schoole. *Much* French, *hard* Latin, *little* Logic *and little* Reason.' The later one says more or less the same uncomplimentary thing in different words against 'hogshearing'. The entry in his Journal for 1684 on 'Disputation' at the Medical School in Leyden is telling for another reason, inasmuch as it conveys why he prefers medical education in Holland to its counterpart in France. The reason given is that at Leyden medical studies 'tend most to practise for in disputeing noe one that I heard urged any argument beyond one or 2 syllogisms.'[11] Note the clarion voice of Locke the pragmatist in medicine coming out of the Medical School in Leyden.

Of all the voluminous Locke correspondence, the most important letters from a medico-philosophical standpoint are those he wrote to his friends, the Molyneux brothers – William the lawyer and Thomas the physician. In a letter dated 15 June 1697 to William Molyneux, Locke complains bitterly that the academic systems of medicine dominant in his generation are all built on sheer 'hypothesis', being 'learned, specious, and talkative, but ineffective to its great end, the health of mankind'.[12] And, in an earlier letter dated 20 January 1692/3 to Thomas Molyneux, Locke tells his medical colleague that the speculative systems of medicine battling for supremacy in medical schools at the time – the Galenist, the Paracelsian, and the Helmontian – 'will upon examination be found to be but so many learned empty sounds, with no precise determinate signification',[13] in a word, mere verbiage. Finally, Locke's reaction against authoritarianism in the teaching of medicine comes out perhaps most forcefully in his posthumous work, *Of the Conduct of the Understanding* (1706), where he chides the various medical sects throughout the ages – 'the dogmatists, methodists or chemists' – for making the venerable Hippocrates the Bible of Medicine itself.[14]

The third and last reason why Locke's thoughts on medical education are worth considering takes us to the heart of the matter, namely, the intimate bearing of Locke the physician on Locke the philosopher. As we have seen, Locke has definite ideas as to what was wrong with medical studies in his day, but he also has certain convictions as to how to improve them. All his convictions take their inspiration from Thomas Sydenham (1624–89), the so-called 'English Hippocrates' whom he lauds in a Lovelace manuscript as the 'great Genius of Physick'.[15] In this connexion, one explanation as to why so many scholars have not realized the significance of Sydenham's direct influence on our author is that Locke himself in the *Essay* mentions his close medical friend along with three other 'master-builders' in the 'commonwealth of learning' – Boyle, Huygens, and Newton – great names associated with modern chemistry and physics rather than with modern medicine.[16] But, despite Locke's possibly misleading listing of his Big Four in 'The Epistle to the Reader' of the *Essay*, the biographical fact remains that it is Sydenham the medical practitioner who has more to do with the eventual development of his mind than the other three physical scientists. There are several pieces of evidence which point unmistakably to the direct impact of Sydenham on the medically-inspired mind of Locke, but we will select the one which clinches the case.

In a letter to Dr. Thomas Molyneux, dated 1 November 1692, he pays his memorial respects to Sydenham as an innovator in practical medicine. With an eye to the training of doctors in the future, Locke expresses the hope that many will follow Sydenham's example, 'and by the way of accurate practical observation, as he has so happily begun, enlarge the history of diseases, and improve the art of physick, and not by speculative hypotheses fill the world with useless, tho pleasing visions.'[17]

It is clear from this tribute to his medical mentor that Locke regards Sydenham's 'way of accurate practical observation' as infinitely better than 'that romance way of physick'[18] prevailing in his age. But, what exactly is this method in Sydenham, and how is it restated in Locke's *Essay*? Sydenham's way of *accurate practical observation* in medicine is precisely, word-for-word, Locke's own 'historical, plain method' in the *Essay*.[19] Generalize Sydenham's diagnostic method of 'accurate practical observation' as the proper way to the facts concerning the course and treatment of diseases, and you arrive logically at Locke's 'historical, plain method' as the proper way to *any* facts 'which concern our conduct'[20] and, therefore, are *useful* to know. Can there be any better evidence that Locke's practical ideal of life and knowledge stems directly from his medical interests, especially from his abiding interest in improving the study and art of medicine along Sydenhamian lines?

To sum up, we may conclude from all the foregoing considerations that the special significance of Locke's medical interests for future Locke scholarship lies in their unique value as a new key to Locke.

References

1 ROMANELL, PATRICK, 'Locke and Sydenham: a fragment on smallpox (1670)', *Bull. Hist. Med.*, 1958, **32**, 293.

2 LASLETT, PETER (ed.), John Locke, *Two Treatises of Government*, Cambridge, Cambridge University Press, 1960, p. 85.

3 Ibid., p. 83.

4 FRASER, ALEXANDER C. (ed.), John Locke, *An Essay Concerning Human Understanding*, Oxford, Clarendon Press, 1894, vol. I, p. 27.

5 AARON, R. I. and GIBB, JOCELYN (eds.), *An Early Draft of Locke's Essay*, Oxford, Clarendon Press, 1936, p. 117.

6 The present writer first arrived at this assessment of Locke the philosopher in Patrick Romanell (ed.), John Locke, *A Letter Concerning Toleration*, New York, Liberal Arts Press, 1950, pp. 7–8.

7 Locke, *Essay* (Fraser ed.), vol. 2, pp. 350, 351.

8 MASHAM, DAMARIS, Remonstrant MS., Amsterdam, J. 57a.

9 AXTELL, JAMES L. (ed.), *The Educational Writings of John Locke*, Cambridge, Cambridge University Press, 1968, pp. 112, 197.
10 LOUGH, JOHN (ed.), *Locke's Travels in France: 1675–1679*, Cambridge, Cambridge University Press, 1953, pp. 50, 54.
11 DEWHURST, KENNETH, *John Locke (1632–1704): Physician and Philosopher*, London, Wellcome Historical Medical Library, 1963, p. 261.
12 LOCKE, JOHN, *Some Familiar Letters between Mr. Locke and Several of his Friends*, London, Churchill, 1708, p. 224.
13 Ibid., p. 285.
14 LOCKE, JOHN, *An Essay Concerning Human Understanding*, 2nd American ed., Brattleboro, Thomas *et al.*, 1806, vol. 3, pp. 259–60.
15 Bodleian MS. (Oxford), Locke fol. 21, p. 16.
16 LOCKE, *Essay* (Fraser ed.), vol. 1, p. 14.
17 LOCKE, *Some Familiar Letters*, p. 279.
18 Ibid., p. 284.
19 For this close affinity of methods in Locke and Sydenham, *vide* R. G. Latham (ed.), *The Works of Thomas Sydenham*, London, Sydenham Society, 1848, vol. I, pp. 3–7, 11–24, 27–28.
20 LOCKE, *Essay* (Fraser ed.), vol. I, p. 31.

A. Szallasi
Esztergom (Hungary)

Sociography and hygiene

Ethnic-national literature has always tried to meet its sociographic function in accordance with demands, although this differs greatly with the given people, it is inversely proportional to the population number and the resources. The literature of any people is a literature of human condition at the same time because it contributes to the universal fate of mankind by presenting its own, and the manifestations of the soul are interesting in that they differ in nuances. Certainly, everybody considers the literature of his own nation as characteristic, which it really is. But it follows from the aforesaid inverse proportion that the literature of small peoples is more sociographic than that of the great. This applies at least to the literature of the Hungarians between the two World Wars. It is exciting for every literature to feel and show, to identify itself with and weigh the characteristic and hidden traits, virtues and flaws, opportunities and dangers of its own people.

Why Hungarian social progress fell behind that of West Europe by several phases after the Turkish occupation would require a lengthy historical-sociological explanation. Following World War I, an economically backward small people, detached from the disintegrated Monarchy, petrified almost in a state of feudalism and doped with false illusions, tried to struggle to its feet. The leaders, insensitive to the trends of the times, tried to preserve the obsolete, to save what could not be saved. It was in such anachronistic circumstances that the rural sociologist movement came into being and was feeding on a number of veins; it was intended for exposing poverty as it had existed in the tempests of history, like the natives of a hardly known island of Oceania in the heart of a twentieth-century Europe.

The first steps for making a survey of social backwardness were taken by official circles. The University Seminar of Village Policy was founded in 1920, the Rural Sociological Institute of the Hungarian Society came into being not much later, and the Sociological Institute of the Hungarian Statistical Society was formed in 1926.

The surveys made by these high-sounding bodies were of a statistical nature first of all, and carefully avoided drawing any conclusions in respect to the inequalities of the distribution of landed property. The young group of village-explorer writers, moved by the great author of that time, Zsigmond Móricz, first of all, made their start with a substantially more vehement emotional charge and a greater will to save.

The great days of the movement were in the middle, the second half of the thirties; it was at that time that great works revealing reality were born, and the panorama of a shocking misery was unfolding from interesting folkloristic features. What this populous, talented team of writers starting from many directions needed for harmonizing their intentions was some facility of publication, with clear-cut conceptions of editing. This role was filled with vocational zeal by the periodical *Válasz* (Reply) of György Sárközi. He also launched a sociographical book series in 1936, the *Discovery of Hungary*. The surprises involved in this action stirred up a storm. Luckily for our sociography and literature, it was a masterpiece that appeared on the pages of *Válasz* right at the beginning. Gyula Illyés, who ranks with our greatest personalities since then, gives testimony of this sub-social world more authentically than any official record. His work has become the pregnant yardstick of merciless candour, summing up the social-hygienic conditions like this: '. . . the people of the plains dread diseases not because they might fall out of life in this way, but because they would lose their jobs beyond doubt sooner or later. There is little mercy for the sick. . . . Was disease a shame? Everybody concealed it as long he could. The farm labourers groaned, hissed, complained of pains in their flank, it even happened that they simulated some disease, but they were reluctant to say "I'm sick".'

These farm labourers lived amid dark superstitions and little mercy; they hardly differed from the natives of faraway lands whom it was befitting to pity in the name of humanism even in the Hungary of those days. The tone does not accuse, it only establishes facts; but the facts put down in this work accuse convincingly.

The alarming spread of only-childism incited the village explorers to strike a note that was still more dramatic than their concern for destitution. The only-childism starting from the Ormánság of South Transdanubia was analysed from many angles by a physician living there, with all its depressing consequences. Studying the symptom in the system of co-ordinates of statistical data, it appeared that the alarming drop of the birth rate set in in 1893, and reached the lowest level in 1933. 'Considering all this, it admits of no doubt that the shift to one-childism had proceeded from the stage of consideration to that of resolvedness by the sixties, to be handed down from offspring to offspring merely as a custom later on. . . .'

It was stated officially at the anti-one-childism conference of the Hungarian Sociological Society in 1927 that '. . . until there is improvement in the means of subsistence, and the present pressure of overpopulation decreases, it is untimely to speak of increasing the population and improving the birth rate . . .'. Thus the official circles were afraid of overpopulation even in the shadow of one-childism. The aforesaid physician mentions the correlations between endemic goitre, malaria, and one-childism, as well as the germ-damaging role of inbreeding. '. . . whoever has eyewitnessed what a destruction malaria is able to bring about, has seen that colourless, yellow suddenly collapsing human being who is interested in nothing in his extremely debilitated state. The entire mental niveau of such a person is sinking, and as if his nerves were made of rope, he does not react to any external stimulus. It seems as if he had no other functions than instinctive vegetation, because stimuli of demands no longer get to his brain, and likewise no will whatsoever starts from there. . . .'

Földindulás (Landslide), a dramatic play by János Kodolányi, is an artistic representation of one-childism at Ormánság.

The most restless corner of the country was assigned to Géza Féja in György Sárközi's sociographical map. The revolutionary past and present of this south-eastern spot of discontent spoke to us through him. This is no longer the patient people of the plains, it is the 'liberated' agrarian population whom liberalism '. . . had freed from domestic servitude, but ousted them from domicile by the same gesture, let them earn their bread themselves. But the serfs were not at all prepared and armed for this kind of struggle for life . . .'.

Féja's book is a kind of sociography where even the dreariest figures are inflamed by lyricism. Illustrating the desperate state of social hygiene, he speaks up for the children first of all. '. . . needless to say, the proper feeding of children is out of the question. The children eat the same as the adults, mainly soup, and – if there is any – bread. In summer they eat melons, and there is no variety, no regard to the organism of the child. The school doctors' examinations reveal shocking data. And this applies not only to the proletarian regions. In places where they could afford wholesome food, people are for the most part too ignorant to feed the children properly. . . . And the findings of the medical examinations in schools were like this: Healthy are 25% of the children, normal weight: 40%, underfed 25%. Except in towns, there is hardly any care for mothers and infants. . . .'

A different region is the Matyó district in North Hungary, the most exciting in respect to folklore. The people produce the famous needlework and the seasonal labourers where the contrast of poverty and gaudy clothes is the more striking. The writer of this region, Zoltán Szabó, presents his beloved land without any romanticism. 'The duty was this: to dip the hand into the wounds deeply, so that I get to know from the wounds the tools which cut them. We now feel that fatal negligence, crimes and faults have been committed. One went there with this feeling, and returned with the certainty of all this. . . . But there was no choice after this experience: I had to subordinate the researcher to human feeling sociology to the situation. Diagnosis became the end, research was but the means. . . .'

Tuberculosis decimated the population as a result of insufficient feeding. '31% of the deaths per year occurred at the age of one year, which means that almost one-third of the deaths occurs among infants. Fifteen children under the age of one year die in the village every year on the average, this is about every fourth newborn. Tuberculosis amounts to 20% of all deaths. . . .'

Nor is the picture more cheerful elsewhere. Imre Kovács described the caloric intake of the agricultural labourers like this: 'A constant feeling of want runs through their entire life. Their calorie requirement is not met. In the family the father works hard to earn bread, the mother does hard household work. Their annual work performance is about 385 kilowatt-hours. But this is only the performance of weekdays, and the performance on Sundays and holidays must be added to this, because it is on these days that the farm-hand does the work about the house, such as cutting wood, tilling the contracted land, etc. so we may put the annual muscle-work performance at 400 kilowatt-hours. 6,500 calories are required for covering one kilowatt-hour of muscle-work performance . . . add the calorie requirement of basic metabolism which is daily 1,680 calories for a man of 70 kg. Counted for a family, this is an annual requirement of 6 million calories, while the actual caloric intake is only about 4 – 4 and half million, i.e. less by one-third. . . .'

The work of Géza Féja and Imre Kovács earned imprisonment. 'After the dullness of old monographs which amassed but data, we now bring the substantial, thus the material of our books is a critical attitude in itself, a merciless separation of transient and substantial things, a collecting of values and an autumn fire built up of what is to be burned. We have been walking with open eyes and an open soul: villages, towns, classes, individuals, institutions, superstition and customs passed before our watching eyes, we looked and judged and do not conceal whom and what we found to be wanting . . .', wrote Géza Féja.

The importance of written truths is enhanced by the contrast of given circumstances. Taking this into account when making recollections, we believe that the hygienic situation report of rural sociological literature is of interest also for medical history. In addition to extant statistics the material contributions written with subjective intentions are important documents for judging a bygone era.

L. Stroppiana
Rome (Italy)

The hospital crisis of the sixteenth century and its hygienic and social aspects

Throughout the centuries many complex factors are involved in the evolution of hospital institutes in their most glorious or in their most sad moments. These factors have been examined closely by a number of scholars and they lead me on to a consideration of various occurrences which took place around the year 1500 and which characterized, or rather had influence on the progress of hospital assistance in that period of history.

In examining historic facts I do not intend to set up a trial on history, which often proves to be a sterile practice, or to compile a simple chronology of events, but rather to follow with equanimity the various factors related to the problem. In this way, through a selection of the facts themselves, one can discard the negative factors so as to give weight to those elements which can indicate to us the best road to follow in the future so that one can develop better assistance for the sick.

If, first of all, we consider the various influences on the hospitals in this period we find at least two factors of great importance. One of these is the concept of concentrating the smaller hospitals into one large organism which can develop and better carry out its function of total assistance to the needy; in other words to gather together all those who need assistance, the sick and the poor as well as the vagrant.

The other element which we must consider in relation to the hospital crisis of 1500, which in my view is very important and on which we must concentrate all our attention, is the revision of the concept of assistance in relation to the changing political and social scene. These factors are all tied to the need for relating the running of hospitals to civil organisms, religious orders and local lay administrative bodies.

Seen as a whole these events seem praiseworthy and necessary so as to make assistance more efficient in view of the demands of society, so that it could develop and improve in every direction. But if we look at their results they are open to many criticisms which are related to other elements which have had a negative influence or at least held up the execution of these plans. For example the principle of uniting the small hospitals of the Middle Ages in one building may seem to lead to better assistance, but eventually it is nothing but another way for the prince to display his exterior ambitions. In fact the utility of the building is limited to its exterior; elsewhere sentiments of Christian charity are overcome by the grandiose ideas of the man who has to impose himself on his subjects and who shows off even on this occasion the luxury which surrounds him in his court, in his cities and in his palaces.

But this only shows his complete disinterest in the needs of the ill, something which may be far from his specific field of interest, but which should touch him at least on humanitarian grounds.

Above all princes and lords were preoccupied with handing down their names to future history, but they did not care whether the charity in their hearts was equal to the pomp and glory which surrounded them; on this subject Pazzini says that: their preoccupation was only to '. . . be seen doing good' (Pazzini, 1958, p. 152).

There was a great deal of hypocrisy in the magnificent Renaissance of the dignity of Man who at last was upholding his rights and his thoughts. When it was convenient, dignity and respect for Mankind were forgotten vilely and despicably, and where charity was supposed to reign supreme, dirt and abandonment could be found in its place.

But, as I said, the most important development in this period was the desire to put the hospitals within the sphere of religious and civil administrative organizations. Under this influence the hospitals sought to improve their positions through a battle for reforms in collaboration with lay and religious forces.

In fact in this period one can find the first statutes and regulations concerning hospitals. These are essentially so healthy that some of them were a starting point for those of the modern era. One of the greatest scholars of hospital rights, Emilio Nasalli Rocca, tells us that from the very first they usually seem to be of autonomous inspiration coming from mixed administrative bodies without the participation of the bishops or the civil authorities although, as he says, 'it was still controversial whether these statutes should be approved by the sovereign power'. This is a phenomenon typical of the Renaissance, a period which was full of uncertainties and struggles for supremacy which only served to put a brake on normal evolution and promising premises.

The limits between state and church were not very well defined on the subject of hospital matters. One can find ecclesiastical and lay legislation which is either limited in its specific field, or in contrast with each other, or tacitly allowing the bishop to control such concerns, albeit indirectly. However, generally ecclesiastical rights were in decline compared to what they were in the Middle Ages, but this took different forms from country to country.

In fact between 1400 and 1500 there was a certain contrast, or rivalry between the ecclesiastical authorities and the lay bodies, public or private. This was apparent whenever it was necessary to give directives based on the new principles of law to form a legislation which was in line with and adequate for the new social structures which were in slow evolution.

There were also conflicts of jurisdiction during the transformation of small medieval hospitals into the large centralized hospital of the Renaissance. The government, through its own power and under various pretexts, often ascribed to itself privileges and incomes against the spirit of the ecclesiastical regulations, which, it seems, could be eluded with a certain ease. On other occasions there was a reciprocal agreement, embracing both spiritual and material assistance, which was in harmony with the human and social aspirations of a time which was continually changing.

To understand a more direct civil legislation on the subject of hospitals we can look at the example of France where, with the Reformation, the lay authorities were reigning supreme. In Italy, on the other hand, the supremacy depended on the situation of each individual territory and on the system of government in power.

Examples on this subject are not lacking. If we look at the various Italian states, we can see that the phenomenon was common to all the states where the lay powers and the church were struggling for temporal power, either on the disloyal and hypocrite level of so-called diplomacy, which was really a mirror of ambition and egoism, or on the more open and perhaps more loyal level of open warfare.

To confirm this, I would like to take as an example what was happening in various European countries. In England Henry VIII was decreeing the closure of the monasteries and making hospital assistance a lay concern, in disrespect for Christian concepts, even if Edward VI, in contrast with the policies of his father, founded the first large hospitals of London; St. Bartholomew, St. Thomas of Bridewell and the hospital of Bethlehem. In France hospitals were still being turned over to lay hands by Louis XII with the foundation of the Hôtel Dieu in Paris and Lyon.

By 1500 government representatives were increasing in importance in hospital administration and real regulation was introduced to discipline the internal life of hospitals not only from a political standpoint, but also within the administration.

The Council of Trent in the years 1543, 1562, 1563 (sess. 7, 22, 25) had given bishops the right to visit hospitals, but often rulers prevented them from exercising such a right. That there was dissent between the two authorities was evident if the Council in 1565 and 1576 '. . . besought the princes and the magistrates not only not to impede the episcopal functions, but rather to encourage them'.

The church certainly took on a large task in embarking on a legislative re-organization of the hospitals in spite of being in contrast with the lay state on some principles. Thus the influence of bishops in hospitals was reduced in this period.

In Italy, to take another example, if we examine the situation of the hospitals in Modena, we find that the problem of assistance was resolved in the same way as in other regions and the various institutes were concentrated into one body called the 'Santa Unione'. But this did not happen without contrast between the citizens and the religious authorities on the one hand and the civil authorities on the other. Each of these attributed to itself the prerogative of issuing the degree of constitution of the new body until the whole affair ended with an excommunication issued by the ecclesiastical authorities of the city (Di Pietro, p. 217).

The administrative situation in general reflected on the one hand a real disinterest in the needs of the ill and on the other the impossibility of guarding their interests, so far had bad habits penetrated into the personnel who had the task of assisting the needy. This showed a deformation in the desire for independence which was far from moral, ethic and religious principles and with the administrators frequently abusing their tasks.

When, for example, in 1546 bishop Zerbinato went to the hospitals of the Misericordia, S. Giovanni Decollato and others in Rovigo, he found a situation of evident fraud, so much so that his visits were often not paid for. He found in some hospitals 'beds' made of straw instead of sheets and blankets.

One can say the same thing about innumerable regions and towns where the hospital administrations behaved in the same way, to the harm of the unfortunate inmates.

To eliminate such abuses French and Spanish bishops proposed to the Council of

Trent that the episcopal powers be increased especially as concerned the hospitals which were so far out of their control. In the XXVth sess. de ref. c. 8 the Council enforced the position of bishops giving them the faculty of deposing administrators and selling abandoned hospitals for other pious uses.

In spite of this terrible situation in which administrators had a free hand in making their miserable profits, we have seen that the original inspiration for new hospitals and for new social legislation was conceived for good ends. But good premises do not always lead to good results, especially if good conditions are not available. Programming reforms and their relative institutions is one thing, putting them into practice is another. Thus one can see that if in any historical period an efficient organization is missing, any new legislation is left unenforced with the obvious results.

Often it was left to a few volunteers and even more often to a few individuals to give body and substance to the reform movement. This took place outside the establishment and continued between the two traditional powers, state and church. In fact their rivalry was based on questions of legal right and was far from the need for the creation of a real health service.

Thus we find men who followed the path of a real Christian tradition and whose names have been handed down to history as examples of charity and heroism combined. Even more often we find laymen who dedicated themselves with love and passion to sanitary (or medical) assistance in the real sense of the word and this often led them to the honour of sainthood. They approached and cured people afflicted by all sorts of diseases, even the most unpleasant and repellent kinds, who were usually ignored by good society, as we would call it today, and left to their fate.

Charitable men took it upon themselves to find some kind of help for the needy and to comfort the infirm with loving assistance. They directed most of their attention towards incurables and it is just the work of these future saints that soon inspired organizations in the whole of Italy. It is a second period of charitable concern for the ill which was in contrast with the usual regulations contained in the hospital statutes ordering the institutes to refuse individuals of this type.

I should remember here the impulse given by the interior tranquillity of Bartolomeo Bosco for the hospital which grew up in Genova called Pammatone; Don Juan Ciudad, Portuguese, who became Giovanni di Dio in 1538; Vincenzo de' Paoli (1576); Camillo de Lellis (1590) a nurse in the Roman hospital of S. Giacomo in Augusta who began there his deep changes in the concept of nursing; Fabrizio Pignatelli who founded the hospital of SS. Trinita dei Pellegrini in Rome in 1575; and many others who also founded religious orders and who were raised up to the honour of sainthood later on.

After so many centuries we can calmly present an objective judgement. The sixteenth century marks an important moment in hospital assistance through new schemes of organization and institutional ideas. I would say that it is a moment of transformation of the earlier concepts which considered the character of the ill person who had to be assisted. A new period is certainly beginning in view of the legal position in which the ill find themselves in relation to the special characteristics of hospitals as autonomous institutions with particular privileges.

In this period the desire to improve the organization and the assistance does exist, but unfortunately it is very much conditioned by the contrasts between the two powers, which are continually increasing. This situation and these factors create inevitable struggles and rivalries through the ambition of one side desiring to have supremacy over the other.

This is where widespread application of the reforms met its greatest obstacles which were only overcome by the virtue and constancy of those who, quite outside personal petty interests, were able to impose, even though with limited results, their initiatives of good and charity.

These are, in my view, the most important events which contributed towards the hospital crisis of the sixteenth century. They are negative conditions which must be discarded without second thoughts so as to avoid in future repetitions of the same situation. In this way we can bring a constructive contribution towards the resolution of this ancient problem concerning the hospitals, which is today more than ever the problem of the moment.

I invite you, therefore, to consider seriously how damaging to progress and to evolution generally such situations can be and to concentrate your strength on a real and fruitful collaboration.

Bibliography

CASSIANO CARPENETO DA LANGASCO, O. F. M., 'L'intervento papale nelle concentrazioni ospedaliere del Rinascimento in Italia', in *Atti Primo Congresso Italiano di Storia Ospedaliera*, Reggio Emilia, 14–17 June 1956.

DALL'AGLIO, P. L., L'amministrazione degli Ospedali di Parma dal sec. XIII al XIX', ibid.

DI PIETRO, P., 'Sulla Santa Unione degli Ospedali e delle Opere Pie della Città di Modena nel 1541', ibid.

IMBERT, J., 'Les prescriptions hospitalières du Concile de Trente et leur diffusion en France', ibid.

NASALLI ROCCA, E., *Il diritto ospedaliero nei suoi lineamenti storici*, Milan, 1956.

PAZZINI, A., *L'ospedale nei secoli*, Rome, 1958.

PECCHIAI, P., 'Storia del "privilegium amplum" del 1° luglio 1559 concesso dal Re di Spagna Filippo II', in *Riv. L'Ospedale Maggiore*, no. 6–7, 1913.

PECCHIAI, P., 'La immunità ecclesiastica del 'Ospedale Maggiore di Milano', ibid., no. 5, 1914.

C. Coury and R. Rullière
Paris (France)

Les premiers hôpitaux spéciaux pour tuberculeux

La création d'hôpitaux ou de services spéciaux réservés à certaines maladies n'a pas été initialement motivée par l'idée de regrouper en un même lieu des cas pathologiques comparables afin de pouvoir mieux les étudier ou mieux les soigner. Elle a obéi le plus souvent à des considérations d'hygiène publique et au souci de protéger les sujets sains contre des affections considérées comme communicables. Le cas de la lèpre en a été l'illustration la plus ancienne et la mieux connue. La notion empirique de transmission interhumaine, solidement ancrée dans la croyance populaire, a été déterminante et a précédé de très loin sa démonstration scientifique.

En matière de tuberculose, si l'on fait exception de l'idée qu'a eue Galien de transformer sa propre maison de Stabies en un lieu de cure diétético-climatique pour les cracheurs de sang,[1] à notre connaissance le premier établissement réellement spécialisé a été créé en France. Encore ne concernait-il pas la «phtisie pulmonaire», mais les «scrofules» ou «écrouelles». Dès l'Antiquité, celles-ci avaient acquis la réputation d'être fortement contagieuses, d'autant que leur aspect extérieur était rebutant, leur évolution sévère et qu'elles englobaient certainement des affections ganglionnaires ulcérées ou suppurantes très diverses. A cette période de l'épidémiologie, les manifestations externes de la maladie tuberculeuse primaient sur ses localisations pulmonaires.

Reims, la ville traditionnelle du sacre des rois de France, était depuis le XIe siècle un lieu de ralliement pour de très nombreux porteurs d'adénites cervicales, originaires des différentes provinces et même de l'étranger, qui venaient y chercher la guérison des mains du souverain. On s'explique aisément les problèmes d'hygiène publique qui se trouvaient ainsi posés par la protection contre la promiscuité de malades pérégrinants et dangereux. En 1645, une certaine Marguerite Rousselet et quelques autres rémois charitables consacrèrent une partie de leurs biens personnels – auxquels s'ajoutèrent par la suite des dons, des legs et des aumônes – à entretenir une maison «dite de saint Marcoul» réservée aux scrofuleux. L'exposé des motifs rappelle qu'il s'agissait d'une région «où plusieurs personnes et surtout les enfants en bas âge sont sujets et souvent attaquez du mal d'Ecrouëlles, d'autant plus dangereux qu'il se communique par la fréquentation».

D'après les Lettres Patentes établies sur une proposition de la municipalité de Reims du 18 novembre 1682 et délivrées à Joigny en mai 1683 par Louis XIV, assisté de son ministre Colbert, la mesure avait eu un heureux effet[2]: «. . . Les malades ainsi sequestrez et hors du commun n'ont point communiqué leurs maux

aux personnes saines, plusieurs de ceux qui en estoient atteints ayant recouvré leur santé et trouvé leur guérison dans ladite Maison, par les remèdes qui leur ont été fidèlement administrez. . . .» Ce document confirme la fondation, réglemente l'organisation et prévoit le fonctionnement du nouvel hôpital. Il était prévu de confier l'administration de cet «Hôpital des Incurables de saint Marcoul» à trois personnes, dont un religieux et deux séculiers nommés par le Conseil de la ville de Reims. Les malades devaient être «servis par de bonnes filles qui seront par eux (les Administrateurs) choisies, lesquelles ne pourront être astreintes, reçeuës ny admises en aucune closture et régularité Monastique ny former aucune Communauté régulière». C'était instituer avant l'heure et contrairement à l'usage de l'époque, un corps d'infirmières laïques virtuellement spécialisées dans les soins aux tuberculeux. L'original de ces Lettres Patentes semble avoir disparu; mais ces dispositions royales, dont nous avons eu connaissance grâce à nos collègues lillois les Professeurs Gernez-Rieux et Gervois, ont été enregistrées par le Parlement de Paris le 29 janvier 1684[3] et par la Chambre des Comptes le 29 février de la même année. Elles résument la première mesure de lutte antituberculeuse qui ait jamais été prise par une autorité gouvernementale.[4] Lors de la Première Guerre Mondiale au cours de laquelle il fut détruit, l'Hôpital Saint-Marcoul de Reims, plusieurs fois remanié, était encore le doyen des établissements pour tuberculeux. Or, les «personnes de piété» qui l'ont fondé ignoraient en leur temps l'origine et la nature exacte de la maladie pour laquelle il a été conçu.

En France, l'exemple de Reims fait toutefois figure d'exception. A Paris notamment, au temps de la Révolution, le célèbre rapport du duc de La Rochefoucauld-Liancourt au Comité de Mendicité (1790) établit qu'à l'Hôpital de Bicêtre, à la Salpêtrière et à la Pitié, les scrofuleux porteurs d'écrouelles «et ceux qui ont des humeurs froides . . . sont confondus dans les mêmes salles (que les autres malades) quoi qu'il y en ait plusieurs destinées à ce genre d'infirmités; . . . il se fait une communication continuelle des maux de toute espèce dont ils sont attaqués et chacun a nécessairement bientôt ceux de tous».[5] Le pavillon des enfants scrofuleux fut rétabli le 27 Vendémiaire an IV. Au début du XIXe siècle, le nouvel «Hôpital des Enfans» (1802) était incapable d'accueillir tous les scrofuleux qui durent être évacués à plusieurs reprises sur Forges-les-Bains ou sur Berck. En 1866, le visiteur anglais Simms fait la même remarque à propos de l'hôpital pédiatrique Sainte-Eugénie.[6] Vingt ans plus tard, l'Oeuvre des Enfants Tuberculeux disposait toujours de moyens insignifiants.

Pour ne pas quitter le domaine des tuberculoses externes, rappelons qu'il a fallu attendre un siècle et demi après la fondation de l'hôpital de Reims pour que la vogue de la cure hélio-marine conduise à des situations analogues dans d'autres pays. En 1791, Lettsom et Latham ont créé à Margate la «Royal Seabathing Infirmary for Scrofula»[7]; ouverte à partir de 1796, elle s'en tint rigoureusement à son objectif et n'admit jamais de pulmonaires. D'autres établissements s'établirent par la suite à Torquay, à Bournemouth et en divers points du littoral britannique. En France, en Italie, en Hollande et ailleurs, les hôpitaux de bord de mer se sont multipliés à partir de 1845 (Sète, 1847; Viareggio, 1856; Berck-sur-Mer, 1861; Wykaan See, 1865, etc.).[8]

Les tuberculeux pulmonaires ont bénéficié d'hôpitaux spéciaux à une date beaucoup plus tardive que les scrofuleux. Les premières initiatives prises dans ce sens ont suivi de plus de 200 ans la publication de l'admirable ouvrage de Fracastoro: elles n'en ont pas moins découlé de la notion très répandue dans les pays méditerranéens que la phtisie constituait un grave danger de transmission par voie indirecte ou directe.[9] Il n'y a pas lieu d'évoquer ici l'extrême sévérité des mesures de protection adoptées par les autorités en Italie, en Espagne ou au Portugal dès la fin du XVIIe siècle. Le principe de l'isolement des malades dans une infirmerie spéciale avait été énoncé et parfois matérialisé dans plusieurs villes transalpines, notamment à Lucques en 1737, à Venise en 1772, à Naples en 1776.[10] Dès le milieu du XVIIIe siècle, le grand hôpital romain du Santo Spirito disposait d'un pavillon à part pour les phtisiques et les scrofuleux; ceux-ci bénéficiaient des soins d'un personnel spécialisé informé du caractère contagieux de la maladie; ce véritable service de phtisiologie fut agrandi grâce à l'initiative du Pape Benoit XIV, particulièrement soucieux de l'hygiène publique (Romagnoli). Le fait était suffisamment remarquable pour que Jacques Tenon le souligne dans ses Mémoires sur les Hôpitaux (1788): «On sépare à l'hôpital du Saint-Esprit, à Rome, et en général dans les hôpitaux d'Italie, les pulmoniques des autres malades: on n'a pas toujours la même attention dans nos hôpitaux.... Mon avis, relativement aux pulmoniques, se réduirait à les mettre dans des salles particulières, ne fût-ce que pour empêcher qu'ils n'incommodassent d'autres malades par leur toux, l'infection de leurs crachats purulents, l'idée fréquente qu'ils offrent de la mort....»[11]

Mais l'époque était peu favorable à l'adoption de telles mesures, d'autant que la contagiosité de la phtisie allait être, sinon formellement niée, du moins considérée comme négligeable par rapport au facteur héréditaire; cette réaction néfaste, qui rallia même Laennec, a persisté jusqu'au dernier tiers du siècle, avant d'être ébranlée puis définitivement vaincue par les découvertes de Villemin et de Koch.

A cet égard, les conceptions britanniques ont été en avance sur leur temps et de nombreux établissements pour les maladies de poitrine ont été créés en Angleterre à partir de 1814; mais les premiers hôpitaux strictement réservés aux consomptifs, c'est-à-dire aux tuberculeux, ne sont apparus que vers 1850. L'«Infirmary for Asthma, Consumption and other Pulmonary Diseases» fut fondée à Londres en 1814; appelée par la suite «Royal Hospital for Diseases of the Chest», elle a été rebâtie en 1863 et agrandie en 1885. Bodington dirigea de 1830 à 1840 à Sutton Coldfield une clinique privée qui recevait surtout des pulmonaires. De la même époque datent l'ébauche du célèbre «Brompton Hospital» de Londres (1841),[12] l'«Infirmary for Consumption and Diseases of the Chest», située 26 Margate Street à Londres (1847), le «City of London Hospital for Diseases of the Chest» à Victoria Park (1848), le «Western Hospital for Incipient Consumption and Diseases of the Chest» de Bournemouth (1855).

A une époque où la transmission de la tuberculose, enfin confirmée, était devenue une des principales préoccupations des médecins et des hygiénistes, Lawrence Flick s'est attaché à recenser les institutions qui existaient alors en Grande-Bretagne: en 1890, 18 établissements, capables de recevoir annuellement 6.000 à 7.000 malades, admettaient électivement les affections thoraciques; mais trois d'entre eux seulement, d'une capacité annuelle totale de 275 lits, étaient exclusivement destinés aux tuberculeux.[13]

Aux Etats-Unis, le «Channing Home for Consumptives» (Boston) date de 1857.

Quelques salles spéciales ont été prévues au Bellevue Hospital et au City Hospital de New York, mais le «Chestnut Hill Hospital for Consumption» ne fut créé qu'en 1896.

Vers 1883, s'inspirant des dispositions prises à l'Hôpital Militaire, l'Hôpital Civil de Buenos Aires ouvrit des pavillons spéciaux pour tuberculeux; les médecins argentins se déclarèrent très satisfaits des résultats ainsi obtenus. En Allemagne, l'existence à Berlin d'un service spécialisé et la création des premiers sanatoriums par Brehmer à Görbersdorf (1854), puis par Dettweiler à Falkenstein (1876), était bien loin de satisfaire aux exigences de l'hygiène publique[14]: les malades peu favorisés par la fortune relevaient de soins à domicile ou du régime hospitalier commun. Un hôpital pour enfants tuberculeux a été créé à Moscou en 1887.[15]

En France, la situation était plus fâcheuse encore. Les tuberculeux adultes ne disposaient d'aucun hôpital spécial. Certes, dans la première moitié du XIXe siècle, les phtisiques avaient été dirigés de préférence sur l'Hôpital Necker ou sur la Charité et la Pitié, non par souci de prophylaxie ou d'isolement, mais pour répondre au désir de certains médecins comme Laennec, Louis ou Andral qui désiraient regrouper autour d'eux, dans un but d'étude, les affections pulmonaires qui les intéressaient particulièrement. Mais, dans la règle, les tuberculeux étaient répartis indistinctement entre les divers hôpitaux généraux qui en étaient encombrés et où ils étaient plus ou moins négligés et relégués.[16]

A partir de 1875, de nombreux avis ont pourtant été formulés en faveur de l'affectation d'établissements spéciaux à l'isolement et au traitement des tuberculeux pulmonaires. Parmi les apôtres de cette politique novatrice, il faut retenir les noms de Nicaise, de Trélat fils, de Jaccoud, de Grancher, de Faisans, de Brouardel. L'Hôpital Lariboisière fut le premier de Paris à être doté d'un petit service spécialisé comprenant quatre salles en pavillon: il fut ouvert le 25 décembre 1897. Sur l'initiative de Letulle, des dispositions analogues furent prises l'année suivante à l'Hôpital Boucicaut. Différents rapports présentés en 1903, 1904 et 1905 aboutirent finalement à la création d'un grand service spécialisé de 250 lits à l'Hôpital Laennec; un dispensaire pour malades externes lui fut annexé et Edouard Rist en assuma la direction. Deux autres services furent créés à la même époque à l'Hôpital Tenon et à l'Hôpital Saint-Antoine.[17] L'hôpital sanatorial de Brévannes fut ouvert en 1907,[18] tandis que les enfants atteints de tuberculose pulmonaire étaient dirigés sur l'Hôpital Hérold. En fait, les premières ébauches de sanatoriums avaient été en France, le fait d'une inititative religieuse privée (1878), puis celle de Charles Sabourin (1890).[9] A partir de 1900, la cure hygiéno-climatique s'implantera dans la plupart des pays et fera surgir un nombre sans cesse croissant de sanatoriums de plaine ou de montagne. L'époque archaïque de l'isolement et du traitement de la tuberculose était enfin révolue.

Bibliographie

1 GALIEN *Methoda medendi . . . – De ulceribus, quae in aspera arteria sunt, et in summa ejus parte, ac de lactis, quod apud Tabias habetur, perfectione*, edit. de Froben Bâle, 1561, chapter 12, p. 68.

2 Texte imprimé à Reims en 1684 par P. Lelorain (Bibl. Nat., F. 23614/118).

3 Archives de France, Reg. X 1a 8677, fol. 75.

4 JADART, H., 'L'Hôpital Saint-Marcoul de Reims', *Trav. Acad. Reims*, **111**, 1901–2; LANDOUZY, L., Le toucher des écrouelles – L'Hôpital Saint-Marcoul – Le mal du roi. Assoc. Fr. pour l'Avancement des Sc., Paris, 1907; GERNEZ-RIEUX, CH. et GERVOIS, M., Rapport à la XX° Conférence

Internationale contre la Tuberculose, New York 1969 et manuscrit inédit aimablement communiqué par les Auteurs.
5 Cité par SIGURET, Thèse de Doctorat, Paris, 1907.
6 SIMMS, F., *A winter in Paris . . .*, J. Churchill édit., Londres, 1866.
7 A plan for a charitable institution to be established on the sea-coast, London, 1791.
8 DAREMBERG, G., 'Sur l'établissement dans le Midi d'hôpitaux maritimes pour les phtisiques', *Gaz. Hebd. de Paris*, 1880, p. 584; D'ESPINE, A., 'Sanatoriums maritimes pour enfants', *Congrès International de la Tuberculose de* 1905, Berger–Levrault édit., Paris, 1905.
9 RIANT, A., 'Les hôpitaux spéciaux pour phtisiques', *Ann. d'Hygiène Publique (Paris)*, 1885, **14**, 315–31; COURY, CH., *Grandeur et déclin d'une maladie: la Tuberculose au cours des âges*, vol. 1, Lepetit, S.A., Suresnes, 1972.
10 CASTIGLIONI, A., 'Il concetto della contagiosità della tisi e le legislazione antitubercolare italiana nel settecento', *Rassegna clinico-scientif. (Milan)*, 1927, **11**, 5; FERRARI, A., *Notizie storiche sugli inizi dell'assistenza sanatoriale in Italia*, Minerva Medica édit., Turin, 1949; ROMAGNOLI, G., 'L'evoluzione del concetto della contagiosità et della profilassi della tubercolosi polmonare attraverso i secoli, dall'antichità fino alla scoperta del bacillo di Koch', *Giorn. Batt. Virol.*, 1968, **61**, 233–73.
11 TENON, J., *Quatrième Mémoire sur les Hôpitaux*, 1788, p. 193.
12 BISHOP, P. J., 'The Brompton Hospital and its first medical reports', *Tubercle*, 1967, **48**, 344–55.
13 FLICK, L. F., *Special hospitals for the treatment of tuberculosis*, Philadelphia, Medical Press Company, 1890.
14 KNOPF, S. A., Les sanatoria; traitement et prophylaxie de la tuberculose pulmonaire, Thèse de Doctorat, Paris, 1895.
15 MARKUSON, V. D. et coll., 'Seventy years of the first children's tuberculosis hospital in Moscow (1887–1957)', *Pediatrya*, 1959, **37**, 8, 19–24.
16 HUSSON, A., *Etude sur les hôpitaux . . .*, P. Dupont édit., Paris, 1862, p. 259; GALLET, L., *Un grand hôpital parisien en 1886*, Steinheil édit., Paris, 1887; PETIT, L. H., 'De l'hospitalisation des tuberculeux d'après l'opinion des médecins des hôpitaux de Paris', *Congrès pour l'Etude de la Tuberculose de 1893*, Masson édit., Paris, 1894.
17 'L'oeuvre de l'Assistance Publique à Paris contre la Tuberculose (1896–1905)', *Congrès International de la Tuberculose de 1905*, Berger–Levrault édit., Paris, 1905.
18 THIEL, P. H., L'isolement des tuberculeux des hôpitaux de Paris. La question des tuberculeux adultes de Brévannes, Thèse de Doctorat, Paris, 1909.

H. Dubovsky
Bloemfontein (South Africa)

The early history of the anti-tuberculosis movement

Robert Koch's discovery of the tubercle bacillus in 1882 was followed by scepticism with the diathesis-contagion controversy remaining unsettled. The *British Medical Journal* of that year reports that a speaker at an association meeting 'questioned the connection between these bacilli and the diseases with which they were associated . . . as cause and effect'. The 1886 editions of two standard British textbooks confused the issue. Fagge on medicine cast doubt on the infectivity of the disease.[1] Powell and Hartley's chest diseases stated that 'in the ordinary circumstances of life, phthisis is not an infectious malady'.[2]

THE EDINBURGH SCHEME

The significance of Koch's discovery was recognized by Robert Philip who graduated at Edinburgh the same year. Diverted from studies in gynaecology in Vienna, he returned to Edinburgh in 1883 to commence a career in tuberculosis. A professor of medicine considering the subject exhausted discouraged him. Dissatisfied with existing facilities, Philip with the help of a few professional and lay friends founded the Victoria Dispensary in 1887 as a private venture. Here was the first tuberculosis clinic in the modern concept and here commenced a unique participation by volunteers in disease control.

Tuberculosis caused one-ninth of all deaths in the United Kingdom at that time. Mortality tables for 1907 show it heading the list with 77,850 of a total of 678,851. The extent of the disease in children, a sensitive index of the whole problem, is evident from autopsy and tuberculin studies up to the age of fourteen years done in Vienna. Tuberculosis caused the death in about 40 per cent of 848 post-mortems. The von Pirquet tuberculin test showed that 70 per cent of the eleven to fourteen year group were infected. Thus the tuberculosis movement had a formidable problem.

Next Philip and his group established the Royal Victoria Hospital for early cases in 1894 and a Farm Colony of fifty acres of arable land in 1910. The municipality had added a Pavilion for Advanced Consumptives at the City Hospital in 1906. This tuberculosis complex known as the Edinburgh Scheme with the Dispensary as 'clearing house' attained recognition as the first integrated public health tuberculosis unit.

THE TUBERCULOSIS DISPENSARY[3]

The Dispensary was home orientated. Health Visitors, appointed in 1887, supervised home conditions; arranged home treatment and the clinical examination of contacts known as the 'March Past'. X-rays discovered in 1895 came into general use only years later. The dispensary doctor separated curable and advanced cases for the appropriate institution; a separation which evoked criticism but had the support of Osler; 'to give the best of care to these unhappy victims is a true charity to them, to place them where they seem to be no danger to the general health is a true charity to others'. The collection of statistics and liaison with the municipality were other activities.

Philip campaigned for twenty years before the acceptance by Edinburgh in 1907 of compulsory notification of tuberculosis. A voluntary committee of ladies, the Samaritans, attended to welfare problems.

TREATMENT

Aerotherapy, described as a 'deliberate attempt at increased oxygenation' and regarded as inimical to the bacillus, formed the main treatment. The patient was constantly exposed to fresh air with the bed under the open window. Cold air was regarded as harmless, indeed beneficial, provided the patient was not subjected to temperature changes. Tuberculin discovered by Koch in 1890 was given by injection in high dilution and increasing doses to non-toxic cases. Rest and graduated exercises in the form of work therapy was done. 'While sanatorium life is a life of treatment . . . it should not be an idle existence' (Philip). This principle was continued at the Farm Colony as a conditioner for open employment.

SPREAD OF THE MOVEMENT

Over the first ten years of the century, the example of the Edinburgh Scheme particularly the Dispensary, was followed abroad with local adaptations. Emphasis was, however, placed on the sanatorium rather than the dispensary and the administrative unity of the scheme was lost. Nevertheless, great interest in tuberculosis was aroused in medical circles by Philip's teaching ability. He gave the disease academic status. 'Its teaching is not limited to tuberculosis. It is luminous with principles which give just proportions to the facts of disease. . . .'

The participation by laymen in tuberculosis control was followed abroad by associations. Here are examples of the variety of their activities. The Paddington Dispensary[4] in London was established in 1909 by charitable enterprise led by Miss McGaw, despite some opinion favouring municipal control. A special activity of the Swiss Tuberculosis Association founded in 1902 was holiday colonies for poor children in the mountains, a plan originated by cleric Pasteur Bion. The Swedish Association formed in 1902, promoted health education with a permanent exhibition in Stockholm of pathological specimens, statistics, plans of sanatoria and literature. Germany favoured sanatoria dating from Brehmer's institution at Göbersdorf in 1854 and aided financially by compulsory industrial sickness insurance. Koch[5] made the public health aspects of tuberculosis the theme of his Nobel Prize address in 1905 and paid tribute to the German voluntary movement started in 1895 which largely acted as a pressure group. An annual congress of sanatorium doctors was one of their projects. Norwegian voluntary workers active from 1910 acquired flats for renting to families of cases and arranged domestic help.

Trudeau's pioneer sanatorium at Saranac Lake in 1884 started the movement in America based on state sanatoria. With municipalities taking care of dispensaries, the associations commencing in Pennsylvania in 1892 promoted tuberculosis publicity and education at all levels, which the National Association founded in 1904, continues with publications such as the *American Review of Respiratory Disease*. The Pittsburgh group[6] employed a full-time teacher to lecture school children on tuberculosis. Her advice to 'spit in the gutter . . . where the sun and air may kill the germs' must be viewed against a background of currently acceptable practice. Initial control by adequate provision of spittoons in public places was followed by eradication. Regulations[7] of 1906 for government offices required that 'spittoons shall receive a daily cleansing with very hot water' and that tuberculous employees would 'not be permitted to use the public spittoons but must provide themselves with individual sputum receivers'. 'Tuberculosis Sunday' with talks from the pulpit, launched countrywide on 24 April 1910 with the backing of President Taft stimulated publicity and fund raising.

The man in the street contributed greatly over the thirty years following the bacillus discovery in laying the foundation of modern government tuberculosis control. Carriere,[8] Deputy Director of the Swiss Federal Health Services, commented in 1911 that state tuberculosis control would 'prove too uniform, too rigid, too costly. . . . Private initiative being more adaptable, more capable of varying its methods, more responsive to local conditions, should predominate.' Perhaps you will agree that something of value has been lost in the change to present-day bureaucratic control of tuberculosis.

References

1 FAGGE, C. H., *The Principles and Practice of Medicine*, Churchill, London, 1886, vol. 1, p. 946.
2 POWELL, R. D. and HARTLEY, P. H., *On Diseases of the Lungs and Pleurae including Consumption*, 3rd ed., London, H. K. Lewis, 1886, p. 283.
3 SUTHERLAND, H. G., *The Control and Eradication of Tuberculosis*, Edinburgh, W. Green, 1911, p. 37.
4 Ibid., p. 45.
5 KOCH, ROBERT, 'The current state of the struggle against tuberculosis', *Nobel Lectures, Physiology or Medicine* (1901–1921), Amsterdam, Elsevier Publishing Co., 1967, vol. 1, pp. 169–78.
6 SUTHERLAND, H. G., op. cit., p. 307.
7 Ibid., p. 257.
8 Ibid., p. 379.

H. Attwood
Melbourne (*Australia*)

John William Ballantyne, perinatal pathology and antenatal care

Everyone knows the name, Sir James Young Simpson, and most know something of his achievements. Few know anything about John William Ballantyne. Yet Ballantyne by his advocacy of antenatal care produced as great an impact on the practice of obstetrics as Simpson did with chloroform.

John William Ballantyne was the only son of John Ballantyne, a nurseryman and seedsman in Eskbank, some eight miles from Edinburgh. His mother, Helen Pringle, was the elder daughter of Walter Mercer, a silk mercer in Edinburgh. His schooldays were spent in Peebles at Bonnington Park School and in Edinburgh at George Watson's College. As an undergraduate, at the University of Edinburgh, his early interest in midwifery and gynaecology gained him the Buchanan Scholarship which enabled him to work in the Royal Infirmary as house surgeon to the University Ward for Diseases of Women, under Professor A. R. Simpson, the nephew who succeeded to the Chair of Obstetrics on his uncle's death. After postgraduate work in Berlin, Munich and Gottingen, he returned to Edinburgh in 1885 as Senior Assistant to Professor Simpson at the Royal Maternity Hospital. His teaching association with the University of Edinburgh continued for nearly forty years.

In 1890, he left the main university department for the extramural school in which he was lecturer on diseases of infancy in the school of medicine at the Royal College of Physicians and lecturer on midwifery and gynaecology in both Surgeons' Hall and the Medical College for Women. He lectured earnestly, taking a particular interest in the women students who had recently gained admission. Not surprisingly he returned, in 1916, to the main university department as lecturer in midwifery to women students.

He was a fairly typical, canny Scot. In 1889 he married Emily Rosa Mathews. It is tragic that, despite all the work he did for pregnant women, and the great emphasis that he placed on antenatal care, they had no children. She predeceased him in 1914.

As a young man he played golf and tennis but as the years went by he became more and more engrossed in his books, which eventually were stacked in his bookcases and all around him on the floor. He rose early and by 6 a.m. was in his library, where he worked until ten, when he set out to practise obstetrics. While in his library, he analysed a welter of literary material and wrote many articles. He produced between 300 and 400 articles, but also edited two issues of Green's *Encyclopaedia Medica* and *Dictionary of Medicine* and the second edition of *Encyclopaedia Medica*. Publications made his name familiar to many people throughout the world which was a joy to him. He also gained much delight from his books. Dr. F. J. Browne, his assistant at the Edinburgh Royal Maternity Hospital recalled that during a late visit to the hospital, shortly before Ballantyne died, Browne found him 'hilarious as a Schoolboy, over the parody by Kipling and Graves of the fifth book of the Odes of Horace'. Ballantyne owned at least eight editions of Boswell's *Life of Johnson* and one of his many annotations to the *British Medical Journal* was 'Medical terms in the New English Dictionary'. Because of these qualities, he was an excellent secretary to many societies.

His breadth of knowledge made it difficult for him to be dogmatic and as dogma is beloved by undergraduates, they regarded him as a poor lecturer. While writing in his library, however, he could be Churchillian.

For many years he was an Elder of St. George's United Free Church of Scotland and even found time to act as Session Clerk. On the retirement of his beloved Minister, Dr. Alexander Whyte, Ballantyne, as Session Clerk, wrote a weekly letter telling him about his former church and its congregation. These letters ran to many pages, to the obvious delight of Whyte who called Ballantyne 'the best of correspondents'. He also wrote letters to former women students whose 'confidant' he became when many of them became missionaries.

In several editions of *Who's Who* his recreations are listed as 'Literary research in medicine and addressing Brotherhood meetings'. To clarify the phrase 'addressing Brotherhood meetings' I wrote to Douglas Guthrie. He obviously disliked the phrase, and wrote 'Ballantyne was *never* sectarian, but had the widest Christian outlook'. However, Dr. James Cameron, Professor in Ecclesiastical History in the University of St. Andrews, explains that the Brotherhood referred to was part of the National Brotherhood Movement, one of the many Christian Societies flourishing in the late nineteenth and early twentieth centuries. At least two branches flourished in Edinburgh, one of them in St. George's where a book club and a holiday fund were organized. The main activity seems to have been the Sunday meeting at which Ballantyne so often spoke. This Brotherhood could be looked upon as an evangelical Rotary Club.

Ballantyne wrote many books but his greatest work was done in antenatal pathology, an interest first shown in 1889 in his M.D. thesis – 'Some Anatomical and Pathological Conditions of the Newborn Infant in their relation to Obstetrics', for which he received a gold medal and the Gunning Simpson Prize. In 1892, and 1895 appear the first and second volumes of *The Diseases and Deformities of the Foetus* in the preface to which he gratefully acknowledges access to the libraries of Professor Russell Simpson and the late Sir J. Y. Simpson. During 1894 and 1895 was published the short-lived quarterly journal *Teratologia* which Ballantyne edited and largely wrote.

Teratogenesis: An Inquiry into the Causes of Monstrosities. History of the Theories of the Past was published in 1897. This book is obviously the work of an enthusiast and bibliophile – not content with 381 references it contains notes from Cicero, Galen, Paré, Harvey and Morgagni and quotes from the *Apocrypha*, the *Talmud* and *The Island of Dr. Moreau* by H. G. Wells.

These works were the foundation for his major work, *Manual of Antenatal Pathology and Hygiene* published in two volumes – *The Foetus* in 1902 and *The Embryo* in 1904. These are classics based on careful personal observations of monstrous births, dead born, and babies, mature and premature, dying shortly after birth. His studies made use of the frozen section technique which Berry Hart had introduced to Edinburgh and were embellished by an astonishing review of the literature.

In the preface to Volume I of his *Manual*, he states: 'I began this work in a spirit of something very like active curiosity, I have prosecuted it with an ever-deepening interest and I have brought it thus far with the growing sense that I have been dealing with a subject of tremendous importance for the future of the race and the individual, with, in fact, preventive medicine in its simplest and most hopeful because in its earliest aspect. If we but knew the laws which govern antenatal health and the causes which produce antenatal disease and death, what might we not expect the possibilities of Hygiene to grow to.' (p. vii).

His *Manual* is a treasury for anyone interested in perinatal pathology. Nothing comparable was published until Rupert Willis produced *The Borderland of Embryology and Pathology* in 1958. In Willis's book Ballantyne is referred to frequently and at the end of Chapter IV Willis states 'Ballantyne's is still the most valuable account of teratology in English'.

These volumes should not, however, be considered merely to be curiosa for the curious. An excellent coverage of the history of ideas on monstrosities is joined to a careful, detailed survey of embryology and foetal physiology. On these he bases his study of antenatal pathology and it was from this amalgam that he made his recommendations for antenatal care.

At the time, his approach was new. Of antenatal pathology he says: 'To some extent it may be thought to need a vindication – to be in want of a reason for its existence. Lately unborn among the sciences, it has but recently seen the light, and, like all new-born things, has a hold on life which is uncertain. Full, no one can doubt, of great possibilities, if it be able to reach maturity; but apparently so weak as to suggest to the careless observer little chance of that. Yet, not so long ago was bacteriology – even as antenatal pathology now is – provoking the criticism, that the study of organisms so minute as to need the microscope for their detection was hardly likely, most unlikely indeed, to prove of benefit to the human race, yet pregnant all the while with surgical antisepsis and asepsis, and with the marvels of serum therapeutics. Antenatal pathology, too, deals with small organisms – to wit the little foetus, the tiny embryo, the altogether microscopic ovum and spermatazoon. It thus merits the same condemnation, it may receive a like justification' (vol. 1, pp. 1 and 2). Here, there are pretty plays on words but also much commonsense. Lister was still alive when it was written in 1902, and already the distinction was drawn between antisepsis and asepsis.

How carefully he could analyse a condition is shown by his section on mastitis neonatorum. Quite emphatically he states that the breast secretion is milk, although often referred to in the literature as 'witches' milk'. The current popular treatment of squeezing was dangerous. 'Is it possible, it may be hazarded, that if the foetus from its semi-parasitism shares so intimately in the biochemical changes of the mother, changes which terminate for her in the establishment of lactation, so even after birth the character of the chemistry of the body goes on at first along similar lines and causes activity of the mammary glands in the infant also?' (p. 55). The concept of a hormone had been put forward in the eighteenth century, but the experimental demonstration of such a chemical mediator was announced by Bayliss and Starling in 1902 the very same year that Ballantyne published.

He appreciated the importance of the new bacteriology. This is shown in his coverage of the 'scourge of St. Kilda' (tetanus neonatorum). St. Kilda is an island in the Western Hebrides where, up to the year 1894, nearly 80 per cent of the newborn died. The children were born 'proper bairns' but gave up sucking on the fourth or fifth day and on the seventh 'clenched their gums together so that it was impossible to get anything down their throats' (p. 57). Convulsions preceded death on the eighth day. Among the many theories put forward to explain this disease was eating the fulmar, a particularly oleaginous bird. Sir Arthur Mitchell and other learned authorities, dismissed any possibility of the mismanagement of the umbilical cord. However, it was soon demonstrated that the management of the cord was very important. 'Since the midwifery nurse has secured surgical cleanliness of the umbilical region by cutting the cord with a pair of clean scissors, dusting the stump with iodoform powder, and dressing it with iodoform gauze and sublimate wool the infants of St. Kilda have been practically free from tetanus – . . . along with freedom from the tourist, St. Kilda enjoys immunity, after long years, from tetanus neonatorum. . . . The disease is tetanus, but tetanus modified by the neonatal state, the chief modification being that the bacilli gain access through the umbilical wound' (p. 58).

After a lucid review of erysipelas neonatorum and sepsis neonatorum, Ballantyne emphasized the ubiquity of infective agents. 'The germs are everywhere – in clothes, in baths, in couveuses, in maternal secretions, in the mouth of the infant, round the umbilicus, in the fold of the skin; the newborn is prone to their attack by reasons of the peculiarity of the neonatal physiology, and antenatal pathology and intranatal traumatism; therefore, there is need for an enlightened prophylaxis, which shall not only endeavour to prevent the entrance of microbes along the avenues which have been referred to, but also attempt to strengthen all the defences of the organism against their onslaught when they have entered' (p. 63). This is surely a remarkable understanding of bacteriology and cross-infection.

After a complete review of the anatomical and physiological knowledge of the foetus in utero he classifies the foetal morbid states as:

1. Transmitted diseases.
2. Transmitted toxicological states.
3. Idiopathic diseases.
4. Neoplasms.
5. Traumatic, morbid states.
6. Diseases and morbid conditions of the foetal annexa.
7. 'Pathology of foetal death' (p. 175).

Amongst the transmitted toxicological states is the possible ill effect of chloroform on the foetus. J. Y. Simpson had given evidence of its safety in 1848, but the possibility that jaundice in the newborn might be caused by chloroform was still being discussed. Ballantyne carefully reviewed the literature and, in summary, said: 'There is, therefore, strong evidence in favour of the belief that chloroform gas passes into the foetal blood; and, it may be added, that there is no strong evidence that when there it produces any serious effects.'

Anyone interested in foetal and neonatal pathology must at some time or other consult Ballantyne. Since publication much has been learned but in these volumes there is no faulty reporting and the reasoned analysis of the facts available is astonishingly close to the mark. His greatest error is the use of the term 'manual' to describe each of these volumes. As the reviewer of the first volume in the *British Medical Journal* for 1902 states: 'A standard and an exhaustive work such as this should not be called a manual.'

In 1906, in his inaugural address as President of the Edinburgh Obstetrical Society he mused on what might be achieved in the future. These prognostications were presented as informations received by telephone from 1,9,4,0, a time exchange call from the President of the Society in 1940. 1,9,4,0, tells him that – lectures have been replaced by 'periods of instruction' – not as subtle as may at first be imagined. He postulates, rightly, the increasing use of audio-visual aids and forecasts the use of a time lapse sequence to portray embryological processes. 1,9,4,0 states that one of the greatest advances was made by the production of a 'tocophoric serum' to induce labour. By the use of this tocophoric serum postmaturity had been eliminated. Ballantyne was speaking in 1906 – three years before Dale described the oxytocic effect of the posterior pituitary hormone. Ballantyne suggested that in 1940 a better understanding of infantile death rates would have been obtained through registration of still-births, and often stressed the tragedy of death during birth, 'the infant passing from foetal slumber into the sleep of death, out of the amnios skin of this world into the shroud, the amnios skin of the next'. At the time of his death in 1923, he was working on a survey of still-births for the Medical Research Council. As far as I know, this was never published.

His prognostication that the problem of premature birth would have been solved by 1940 was too optimistic – it still remains a problem.

John William Ballantyne was then a pathologist, a student of disease, who practised obstetrics. From his knowledge of pathology, particularly antenatal pathology he became the strong advocate of antenatal care.

In his successful pleas in the 1901 *British Medical Journal* for a 'promaternity hospital', he stressed that the hospital need not be a separate establishment but on its staff should be a skilled physiological chemist. On 1 November 1901, the Hamilton bed was opened for the care of 'prematernity' patients, for Ballantyne's use of 'pro' as a prefix had been corrected. This bed was named after Professor Alexander Hamilton (1739–1802) who did much to found, in 1791, the Edinburgh Lying-in Hospital 'for the purpose of affording relief to the wives of indigent tradesmen'. The endowment, originally anonymous, had been provided by Dr. Freeland Barbour, a senior colleague of Ballantyne and lecturer in gynaecology in the extramural school. From this beginning grew a ward of twenty-five beds – 'Whilst it would be absurd to contend that these were the first beds set apart for pregnant women, they were the first designed for the specific purpose of the study of the physiology and pathology of pregnancy and of antenatal therapeutics' (Browne, 1951).

In 1915, Ballantyne took over an outpatient service, or antenatal clinic, which Dr. Haig Ferguson had created at the Edinburgh Maternity Hospital following his experience at the Lauriston Prematernity Home where pregnant, unmarried girls were admitted. From 1917 until his death Ballantyne administered this antenatal department the forerunner of all antenatal departments in Britain.

Despite the early start to his day and the arduous life of an obstetrician his activities were not limited by a cardiac malady, almost certainly mitral stenosis. He died at the age of sixty-two, from a ruptured appendix after a short illness.

In his last years Ballantyne believed posterity would remember him for his establishment of antenatal care. Antenatal departments are now universal, but few would connect this work with Ballantyne. On the other hand, his manuals of antenatal pathology and hygiene are classics consulted by all interested in perinatal pathology.

This is a very inadequate coverage of the life and work of John William Ballantyne – a canny Scot, a bookish Scot, a religious Scot. Physically unimpressive and rather a dull lecturer, he was the best of correspondents, a gifted writer and a dogged advocate of antenatal care. Simpson through his knowledge of obstetrics recognized the need for anaesthesia; Ballantyne through his studies of perinatal pathology recognized the need for 'The New Midwifery'. 'With the etymology of obstetrics (latin, ob, over against and sto, I stand) in his thoughts the doctor stands beside his patient during the nine months of her pregnancy as well as in the ten or twelve hours of her labour, and he does not leave her till she is restored and as fit (or fitter) for the next child bearing as she was for the one which is just finished'.

Postscript: Since this paper was written Dr. Helen Russell has published an excellent short biography of J. W. Ballantyne (Royal College of Physicians, 1971).

References

BALLANTYNE'S LIFE AND WORK

Who's Who, 1920 ed., p. 114.

Who was Who, 1916–1928, p. 47.

OBITUARY NOTICES

Br. med. J., 1923, pp. 213–16.

Edinb. med. J., 1923, **30**, 212–14.

Lancet, 1923, p. 258.

Proc. Roy. Soc. Edinb., 1923, **43**, 277–78.

BIOGRAPHICAL NOTES

BARBOUR, G. F., *Life of Dr. Alexander Whyte of St. George's*, 1923.

BROWNE, F. J., *Antenatal and Postnatal Care*, 7th ed., 1951, pp. 6–11.

COMRIE, J. D., *History of Scottish Medicine*, London, 1932.

MILLER, D., 'A Short Record of the Edinburgh Royal Maternity and Simpson Memorial Hospital', *Trans., Edinb. obstet. Soc.*, Session XCVII, 1937, p. 1.

RUSSELL, HELEN, *J. W. Ballantyne, M.D., F.R.C.P. Edin., F.R.S.E.*, The Royal College of Physicians, Edinburgh, 1971.

BALLANTYNE'S PUBLICATIONS (referred to in text)

The Diseases and Deformities of the Foetus, 2 vol., Edinburgh, Oliver & Boyd, 1892 and 1895.

Teratogenesis, Edinburgh, Oliver & Boyd, 1897.

Teratologia (quarterly journal edited by Ballantyne), London and Edinburgh, Williams & Norgate, 1894, 1895.

Manual of Antenatal Pathology and Hygiene – The Foetus, 1902; *The Embryo*, 1904, Edinburgh, W. Green & Son.

ARTICLES

'A plea for a pro-maternity hospital', *Br. med. J.*, 1901, **i**, 813.

'Maternities and prematernities', *Br. med. J.*, 1902, **i**, p. 65.

'The Future of Obstetrics. Inaugural Address as President Edinburgh Obstetrical Society', *Trans. Edinb. obstet. Soc.*, 1906–1907, **3**, 33.

'Sir James Y. Simpson's contributions to antenatal pathology', *Edinb. med. J.*, 1911, **6**, 554.

'Antenatal clinics and prematernity practice at the Edinburgh Royal Maternity Hospital in the years 1909–1915', *Br. med. J.*, 1916, pp. 189, 234, 275.

'The new midwifery', *Br. med. J.*, 1923, 617.

OTHER REFERENCES

BAYLISS, W. M. and STARLING, E. H., 'The chemical regulation of the secretary process', *Proc. roy Soc.*, 1904, Series B, **73**, 310.

DALE, H. H., 'The action of extracts of the pituitary body', *Biochem. J.*, 1909, **4**, 427.

WILLIS, R. A., *The Borderland of Embryology and Pathology*, London, Butterworth, 1959, p. 175

E. Seidler
Freiburg i. Br. (*West Germany*)

Ärzte und Kinder—Motive der neueren Pädiatrie

Es mag auf den ersten Blick befremdend sein, ein offenkundig so wohlumrissenes Fach wie die Pädiatrie nach den Motiven seines Handelns zu befragen. Diese Disziplin, die im Rahmen der Spezialisierung des 19. Jahrhunderts zur Eigenständigkeit gefunden hat, präsentiert sich heute weltweit als ärztliche Wissenschaft vom kranken Kinde, mit eigenen Fachärzten, Kliniken, Forschungszentren und teilweise eigenen Fakultäten. Für den Historiker könnte es daher genügen, den Prozeß der Entfaltung des Faches und seiner Probleme nachzuzeichnen; er trifft dabei intradisziplinär auf ein breites Spektrum imponierender Fakten der medizinischen Fortentwicklung. Dies ist der gängige und von den wenigen Pädiatriehistorikern zumeist und in verdienstvoller Weise eingeschlagene Weg.

Die nähere Beschäftigung mit dem Gegenstand zeigt allerdings sehr bald und sehr deutlich, daß für die Beurteilung der historischen Entwicklung wie auch der aktuellen Aufgabe der Pädiatrie zusätzliche Faktoren in Betracht gezogen werden müssen. Die Probleme umfassen weit mehr als nur den Bereich der Medizin eines bestimmten Lebensabschnittes: sie fordern zwangsläufig die grundsätzliche Überprüfung der jeweiligen Einstellung und Haltung gegenüber dem Kindesalter. Die Heilkunde am Kinde war immer – ähnlich der Psychiatrie – in hohem Maße von der Art und Weise abhängig, wie die Gesellschaft das Kind verstand und auf welche Weise sie es innerhalb dieses Verständnisses dem Arzt präsentiert hat. Es ist daher keinesfalls selbstverständlich, die Pädiatrie einfach als Anwendung medizinischer Erkenntnisse auf das Kindesalter zu interpretieren; das Kind erfordert als zentrales gesellschaftliches Phänomen die ungeteilte Aufmerksamkeit dessen, der sich mit ihm zu beschäftigen hat, bzw. beschäftigen will. Als „infans", als „nicht-sprechendes" Glied der Gemeinschaft war daher seine Begegnung mit der Medizin und dem Arzt stets durch die natürliche Einbindung in die Familie, Gruppe und Gesamtgesellschaft bestimmt. Von daher eröffnet sich ein weites Feld von motivgebenden Elementen, die nach ihrer Tragweite auf die Struktur und Aufgabe der Pädiatrie befragt werden müssen. Die Begegnung mit dem kranken Kind ist somit ein Spiegel des Gesamtproblems des Umganges mit dem Kind und aller ihm innewohnenden Theorien, Tendenzen, Motive und praktischen Konsequenzen.

Dies gilt ganz besonders für die Frage nach den Motiven der neueren Pädiatrie, die seit dem Ende des 18. Jahrhunderts zunehmende Aufmerksamkeit beansprucht. Wenn von der Medizingeschichte dort der Beginn des wissenschaftlichen Interesses am Kinde angesiedelt wird, dann ist dies allerdings nur bedingt richtig. Primär motivgebend ist die allgemeine Zeitsignatur der Aufklärung, in deren Zielvorstellung von der Änderung des allgemeinen Lebens das Kind einen besonderen Platz erhalten musste, weil an ihm als bildungsfähigstem Element der Gesellschaft das Ziel einer allgemeinen Wohlfahrt und Glückseligkeit am besten demonstriert werden konnte. Die Vorboten hierzu waren schon länger vorgeprägt und erhielten durch die Aufklärung, den Rousseauismus und die Philanthropie des späten 18. Jahrhunderts nur ihren endgültigen Impetus: ab dem 15. Jahrhundert erweiterte sich der traditionelle Bereich einer pragmatisch-diätetischen „Practica puerorum" in Dimensionen, welche die Zeit selbst als „Physische Erziehung" bezeichnete. Auf der Basis des alten Topos von der naturgegebenen Schwäche der kindlichen Physis waren schon die antiken Traditionen eher präventiv als curativ ausgerichtet gewesen und wollten mit subtilen Vorsorgeregeln verhindern, dieses fragile Gebäude zum vorzeitigen Einsturz zu bringen. Die alten Regimina hatten sich daher kaum an die Ärzte selbst, sondern an jene gerichtet, die direkt am Kinde beschäftigt sind, an die Mütter, Ammen und Hebammen.

Daran ändert sich nichts, als ab der Renaissance neuere Werke zu kinderheilkundlichen Themen verfaßt werden; sie alle können verallgemeinernd als Reaktion auf das Unvermögen der eigentlich mit dem Kinde betrauten Personen aufgefaßt werden. Neu ist jedoch, daß sich in der Folge die Motive erweitern: der Gesamtkomplex „Physische Erziehung" erforderte in zunehmendem Maße, daß alles, was die Natur zur gesunden Entwicklung des kindlichen Körpers verlangt, gleichzeitig auch seine Rechtfertigung in der Erlangung religiöser, politischer und moralischer Ziele der Kindesentwicklung findet.

Dies meint zunehmend mehr als das Juvenal'sche „mens sana in corpore sano"; dies geht von den Bestrebungen, kräftige (die „Paedotrophia" von Sainte-Marthe 1584), schöne (die „Callipaedia" von Quillet 1656) und gradgewachsene (die „Orthopädia" von Andry 1743) Kinder zu entwickeln – bis hin zu dem aufklärerischen Auftrag an die Ärzte noch des beginnenden 19. Jahrhunderts, die Kinder „zu gesunden Staatsbürgern zu erziehen" (Hecker 1805). Die alten diätetisch-medizinischen Vorsorgebestrebungen der Heilkunde am Kinde trafen sich mit den Konzeptionen der aufgeklärten Pädagogen und überschnitten sich in dem Ziel, „éducation médicinale" und „éducational morale" zusammen zu sehen.

Zur Vertiefung des Gesagten sei daran erinnert, daß dieser Gedanke freilich nicht neu war; die enge Verknüpfung von Pädagogik und Gesunderhaltung des Leibes ist als Motiv seit der „Paideia" des Altertums zu verfolgen. Nunmehr gewinnt dieser Auftrag jedoch eine dezidierte Breitenwirkung in dem neuen Bestreben, einen vernünftigen und nützlichen Erwachsenen aus dem Kinde heranzuziehen. Der Glaube an die Vernunft, an die Bewältigung der Natur und an den damit verbundenen Nutzen wies der alten Präventivtendenz der Kinderheilkunde ein neues, eher sozialpädagogisches als medizinisches Ziel zu. Da Laster, Bosheit und Sittenverfall einem falschen Umgang mit dem Kinde zugeschrieben wurden, erstaunt es nicht, daß auch alle Lehrbücher der Kinderheilkunde am Ausgang des 18. Jahrhunderts – oft schon in der Titelgebung – dieses Motiv des erzieherischen Auftrages der Heilkunde unterstreichen.

Die Zeit, vor allem der nachgerade zur Mode gewordene Rousseauismus, hatte es zusätzlich verstanden, die Kinderliebe fast ins Sentimentale zu wenden. Kindermord und Kindersterblichkeit waren zentrale Themen von der Medizin bis in die dramatische Literatur, allerdings auch handfeste Motivationen der Gesundheits-, Wirtschafts- und Populationspolitik. Diese Bewegung war allgemein und ergriff alle Kulturländer der Epoche; die Ärzte waren hierbei aufgerufen, wiederum weniger sich selbst, als das breite Publikum aufzuklären. Sie wurden angeregt, Pädiatrie erneut mit dem Blick auf die Mütter und Ammen zu betreiben; es entsteht teilweise eine nahezu staatspolitisch motivierte Populärpädiatrie, die ihre Intentionen vornehmlich auf die Selbsterkennung und Selbstbehandlung kindlicher Erkrankungen durch die Familie, die Schule und durch das Kind selbst richtet.

Die gleichwohl parallel zu verzeichnenden Tendenzen einiger Ärzte, das Kind und seine spezielle Physis auch zum Modell der zeitgenössischen, vor allem neuralpathologisch orientierten medizinischen Systeme heranzuziehen, stießen zwar auf breites Interesse, spielten sich jedoch vorwiegend im akademischen Raume ab. Sie waren für die breite Praxis höchstens für einige therapeutische Konsequenzen bestimmend.

Es muß daher konstatiert werden, daß das vielbeschriebene sog. erste neuzeitliche wissenschaftliche Interesse am Kinde im Kontext der Zeitmotive bestenfalls als Sekundärphänomen zu werten ist. Eine Pädiatrie im fachumschreibenden Sinne ist hier nicht entstanden – die impulsgebenden Motive auch für die Medizin kamen dominant aus der Philosophie, der Pädagogik und der Staatsraison. Es kann allerdings nicht deutlich genug gesagt werden, daß der hierdurch gegebene präventive bzw. – modern gesprochen – sozialpädiatrische Impetus als Grundidee des Umganges mit dem kranken Kinde sehr hoch veranschlagt werden muß. Er hat in einigen Ländern, vor allem im philanthropischen Österreich und auch in England dazu geführt, daß die Beschäftigung mit dem Kindesalter bis in die Mitte des 19. Jahrhunderts sich früh und intensiv mit Eigengesetzlichkeiten der Kindheit auseinanderzusetzen begann. Als jedoch neue medizinische Theorien die Möglichkeit boten, das Kind und seine Erkrankungen nunmehr wissenschaftlich zu erfassen, wurde ein deutlicher und sehr brüsker Charakter- und Motivwandel der Pädiatrie eingeleitet. Sie sollte dadurch sehr rasch dieses frühe sozialpädiatrische Motiv wieder verlieren bzw. an andere Instanzen abgeben.

Was sich nunmehr begann, als Spezialzweig der neuen naturwissenschaftlichen Medizin herauszubilden, wurzelte zunächst in der Orientierung der Pariser klinisch-pathologischen Schule. Dort hat Charles-Michel Billard nicht nur eine vorzügliche erste Systematik der kindlichen Pathologie vorgelegt, sondern auch den Weg der vorläufig weiteren Einstellung der Medizin zum Substrat Kind als Objekt naturwissenschaftlicher Betrachtung vorgezeichnet. Da- wie seit altersher betont wurde – das Kind keine Auskunft über seinen Zustand geben kann, sehen wir in der Folge die Medizin bemüht, am Kind objektivierbare Einzelbefunde zu erheben und sie in den wissenschaftlichen Vergleich mit der Erwachsenenpathologie zu bringen. Das dominierende Motiv ist die Gewinnung normierender Erkenntnisse mit der methodischen Prämisse der Quantifizierung der erhobenen Befunde. Die Nosologie unterscheidet z.B. sehr grob in Krankheiten nur am Kinde, vorzugsweise am Kinde und Krankheiten auch am Kinde; oder sie versucht, diejenigen Erscheinungen im Rahmen des neuen Krankheitsbegriffes als Kinderkrankheiten zu klassifizieren, die sich „durch eine überwiegende Frequenz oder durch die Eigenthümlichkeit ihrer Erscheinungen vor den gleichen Affektionen der Erwachsenen auszeichnen" (Henoch 1881). Der Einbau der anatomischen, physiologischen, physikalischen und chemischen Untersuchungsweisen verlief konsequent und parallel zur allgemeinen Entwicklung der Medizin und hat unbestreitbar auch in der Beforschung des Kindesalters zu einer imponierenden Fülle von Einzelerkenntnissen geführt.

Das Kind als Gegenstand dieser neuen Pädiatrie erfuhr jedoch durch diese Entwicklung folgenschwere Umwertungen, wiederum in Richtung auf die Betrachtung der Kindheit als ein zu überwindendes transitorisches Stadium des Menschseins, jetzt aber zusätzlich durch neue Zeitelemente motiviert. Die Neuformulierung des Entwicklungsgedankens durch Charles Darwin führte in seiner letzten Konsequenz zu einer grundsätzlichen Vergleichbarkeit der Erscheinungen auch von Tier und Mensch; was die bürgerliche Gesellschaft nach wie vor mit „Erziehung" ansprach, wurde biologisch zu Problemen der „Aufzucht". Körper und Seele des Kindes standen als vornehmste Substrate der Bildungsfähigkeit zwar weiterhin im Vordergrund der ärztlichen Diskussion, jedoch nur insoweit, als ihre Daten quantitativ zu erfassen waren.

Dies führte zu teilweise grandiosen methodischen Simplifikationen, deren Auswirkungen erst heute langsam, mühevoll und nur noch bedingt durch die Pädiatrie selbst wieder überwunden werden können. Ich erinnere an den Versuch der vergleichenden Psychologie, nur „physiologische Bedingungen der psychischen Vorgänge" erforschen zu wollen, weiterhin an die verhängnisvolle Position des Kindes als quantité négligeable im Sozialdarwinismus, ich erinnere an den problematischen Versuch großer Pädiater wie Adalbert Czerny, das Kind in Ernährung und Nervensystem zu dualisieren (und die Sorge für beides als „Erziehung" zu bezeichnen) und letztlich an die sehr fragwürdige Konsequenz der Reflexlehre Pawlows, Aufzuchtprobleme des Menschenkindes durch die ausschließliche Beeinflussung der kortikalen Mechanismen des Großhirnes lösen zu wollen. Erst in den zwanziger Jahren unseres Jahrhunderts beginnt die Pädiatrie, das wissenschaftliche Bezugssystem Kind-Erwachsener als „schematischen Pauschalbegriff" (Pfaundler) langsam aufzugeben, nicht ohne jedoch – und bis heute – ihre Begründung in der zur Theorie gewordenen Methode ihrer naturwissenschaftlichen Ausrichtung beizubehalten.

Damit hat sich die Kinderheilkunde seit ihrer neuesten Entwicklung als wissenschaftlicher Spezialzweig der naturwissenschaftlichen Medizin in den zwangsläufigen historischen Prozeß zu einer Aspektwissenschaft begeben. Hundert Jahre wissenschaftlicher Pädiatrie haben uns trotz aller wegweisenden Fortschritte einer curativen Kinderheilkunde den Blick auf das Ganze des Problemes Kind zunächst gekostet. Die notwendigen Motive zum Umgang mit dem Kind müssen wir uns heute aus den verschiedensten Disziplinen wieder heraussuchen, die inzwischen ihre eigenen und oft voneinander getrennten Wege gegangen sind. Eine integrierte ärztliche Kinderforschung, welche gleichermaßen vom Anspruch der körperlich, geistig und sozial behinderten Kinder wie auch von der betroffenen Gruppe und Gesellschaft ihren Auftrag erhält, ist ein Desideratum an die Zukunft. Die auf der Basis dieser hier nur global umrissenen Probleme zu leistende Detailarbeit des Historikers kann dazu einen wichtigen und notwendigen anamnestischen Beitrag leisten.

B. Kuhlo
Freiburg i. Br. (*West Germany*)

Der Umgang mit dem kindlichen „Idioten" im 19. Jahrhundert

Der Umgang mit dem sogenannten „Idioten" ist sowohl für die historische, wie auch für die aktuelle Betrachtung ein Problem, welches letzten Endes wenig befriedigend gelöst ist.

Die spezielle Sorge um das geistig schwerbehinderte Kind durchlief seit dem 18. Jahrhundert einen mühevollen, und bisher von der Medizingeschichte eigentlich wenig herausgearbeiteten Weg, an dem Medizin und soziale Institutionen gleichermaßen beteiligt waren.

Das 18. Jahrhundert, so intensiv auch der aufklärerische Impetus in Richtung auf einen humaneren Umgang mit dem Geisteskranken war, hat für den kindlichen Schwachsinnigen dagegen nur weiterhin die Tendenz der Ablehnung, der blossen Bewahrung und allenfalls vereinzelte Erziehungsversuche hinterlassen.

Erst das 19. Jahrhundert hat – aus den verschiedensten Motiven heraus – systematische Überlegungen zum Umgang mit diesen „Verlassensten unter den Unglücklichen" versucht – wie sie Disselhoff noch 1857 bezeichnet hat.

Dabei stellte sich der Schwachsinn als ein juristisches, soziales, medizinisches und pädagogisches Problem dar. Die juristische Seite sei hier ausgeklammert. Erinnert sei nur an die Tatsache, daß Schwachsinnige geringeren Grades – damals wie heute – sich häufig „unter den Bettlerinnen, Vagabondinnen, Diebinnen und liederlichen Frauenzimmern" fanden, und somit durchaus nicht selten auch auf der Anklagebank, sodaß Theorie und Praxis der Blödsinnigkeitserklärung um 1860 Richter und Ärzte beschäftigte.

Die Zusammenhänge zwischen „Idiotie" und sozialer Lage waren – wie ich betonen möchte – im 19. Jahrhundert sehr wohlbekannt.

Brandes hat 1862 darauf hingewiesen, daß 67% der „Idioten" (an anderer Stelle spricht er sogar von 85%) aus ärmsten Verhältnissen stamme. „Idiotismus und Armuth gehen Hand in Hand" sagte er und verwies besonders auf die Zustände in den großen Städten.

Medizinisch gesehen ist es wichtig zunächst hervorzuheben, daß Idiotismus und Geisteskrankheit als zwei grundverschiedene Dinge angesehen wurden. Die Idioten wurden nicht zu den eigentlichen Geisteskranken gezählt.

Der entscheidende Schritt für die Geisteskranken wurde bei Entfaltung der Irrenheilkunde damit getan, daß man sie von den herrschenden Vorurteilen befreite, indem man erkannte, daß es sich nicht um grundsätzlich unheilbare Zustände handelte, sondern daß die Irren als geisteskrank anzusehen seien und damit wie alle

Kranken ein Recht auf therapeutische Bemühung und soziale Anteilnahme haben. Mit der Errichtung von besonderen ,,Heilanstalten" und der Dokumentation therapeutischer Erfolge in diesen Anstalten, änderte sich dann auch zunehmend das öffentliche Bewußtsein.

Jedoch ging – und dies sei herausgestrichen – die Reform des Irrenwesens (ich zitiere Stötzner 1869): ,,an der großen Zahl der unglücklichen Geschöpfe vorbei, die von Geburt an in ihrer geistigen Entwicklung gehemmt sind". Dies ist eine Tatsache, die selten beachtet wird und die in folgendem Zusammenhang gesehen werden kann: Erstens wurde – das haben wir schon erwähnt – klar und grundsätzlich zwischen Irren einerseits und Idioten andererseits unterschieden und diese Unterscheidung schloß gleichzeitig den Idioten von den Bemühungen um den Irren aus. Damerow hat dies zum Ausdruck gebracht, als er 1858 darauf hinwies, daß es sich bei den Insassen der neugegründeten Heil- und Pflegeanstalten um ,,Seelenkranke", d.h. um früher gesunde Menschen handele, dagegen hätten ,,die echten Cretinen und Idioten keine natürliche menschliche Entwicklung, keine persönliche Lebensgeschichte". Er fügt dem noch hinzu, indem er scharf gegen Disselhoff und indirekt gegen die Guggenbühlschen Behauptungen Stellung bezieht: ,,Von eigentlicher Heilung kann bei zahllosen Cretinen und Idioten nicht die Rede sein. Nie seelen- und geistesgesund gewesen, können sie auch nicht seelen- und geisteskrank werden. Es giebt nichts wieder herzustellen, was nie dagewesen ist."

Der zweite Punkt, der Irre und Idioten trennte, ist das Problem, daß es sich bei den Geisteskranken eher um Erwachsene handelt, während die behandlungsbedürftigen Idioten zumeist Kinder sind. Da die Psychiatrie (und damit auch die Psychiatriegeschichte) sich in erster Linie mit dem erwachsenen Seelenkranken befaßt hat, blieb das schwachsinnige Kind weitgehend unbeachtet.

Zwar hat die Frage nach Wesen und Einteilung der Idiotie die Psychiater – insbesondere die der französischen Schule – seit Pinel und Esquirol zunehmend beschäftigt. Die Abgrenzung des Cretinismus gegenüber der Idiotie stellt z.B. den Versuch einer ersten diagnostischen Differenzierung dar; es folgten verschiedenartigste weitere Versuche die Schwachsinnszustände zu definieren oder nach dem Schweregrad einzuteilen und zwar unter Berücksichtigung z.B. von Sprachvermögen oder Aufmerksamkeit, von Gemütszustand oder intellektuellen Fähigkeiten. Sengelmann nennt 1885 in seinem Literaturverzeichnis zahlreiche Titel zu diesem Problem, jedoch hat man den Eindruck, daß er nicht Unrecht hatte, wenn er behauptete, daß – vor allem im deutschsprachigen Raum – die praktische Organisation des Idiotenwesens in der zweiten Hälfte des 19. Jahrhunderts sehr viel weiter fortgeschritten war, als die wissenschaftlichtheoretische Bearbeitung des Problems. Einer nur relativ umfangreichen wissenschaftlichen Literatur standen in Deutschland um 1880 ca. 30 Anstalten gegenüber.

Versucht man sich diese (vor allem für Deutschland charakteristische) Diskrepanz zwischen fehlender medizinischer Theorie bei gleichzeitig in den Anstalten konzentrierter, weitgehend nicht in den Händen von Ärzten befindlicher Praxis zu erklären, so stößt man auf folgende Tatsachen: Es besteht ein enger und alter Zusammenhang zwischen Schwachsinnigenfürsorge und Taubstummenbildungswesen.

Jahrhundertelang hielt man die Taubstummen für bildungsunfähig und zählte sie zu den Idioten. Der ursächliche Zusammenhang zwischen Taubheit und Stummheit blieb lange unentdeckt und wurde von ärztlicher Seite sogar bestritten.

Es war Einzelbemühungen vorbehalten, das Gegenteil zu beweisen. Um 1800 galt es dann als gesicherte Erkenntnis, daß es eine Frage von Unterricht und Methode sei, den Taubstummen zu einer normalen menschlichen Entfaltung zu bringen.

Berücksichtigt man diese Vorgeschichte, so wird verständlich, daß gerade aus der Tradition der Taubstummenbildung heraus die ersten aufsehenerregenden Versuche unternommen wurden, tiefstehende Schwachsinnige systematisch zu fördern. Ich erinnere an die Bemühungen Itards um den sogenannten Wilden vom Aveyron. Itard war 1799 (als das Wildkind in seine Hände kam) als Arzt am Pariser Taubstummeninstitut tätig. Auch in der Folgezeit waren es in Frankreich vorwiegend Ärzte, die sich dem Problem der Idiotie zuwandten, sodaß der Zusammenhang mit der psychiatrischen Schule von Paris gewahrt blieb.

Séguin, der spätere Begründer der Schwachsinnigenfürsorge in den USA fußte auf den Erfahrungen von Itard, und war zeitweise Mitarbeiter von Esquirol, bevor er in Paris um 1845 seine sogenannte physiologische Behandlungsmethode entwarf, eine Methode, die planvoll und systematisch die wenigen Kenntnisse seiner Zeit über die Natur der Idiotie und ihre Erscheinungsformen zu verwerten versuchte.

Über die Methoden, nach welchen man im übrigen in der Schule für Blödsinnige, die der Psychiater Ferrus 1828 in Bicêtre einrichtete, vorging oder wie Voisin in seinem Etablissement orthophrénique in Issy bei Paris arbeitete bzw. nach welchen Gesichtspunkten Falret in der Salpêtrière handelte, darüber ist relativ wenig bekannt. Hervorgehoben sei jedoch noch einmal, daß es hier Ärzte waren, die begannen sich therapeutisch um das idiotische Kind zu bemühen und zwar in Institutionen, die häufig den großen Irrenanstalten angegliedert waren.

Für Deutschland gilt ebenfalls, daß der Anstoß und die ersten praktischen Versuche, sich mit den als unheilbar geltenden Idioten zu befassen, von einzelnen Taubstummenlehrern ausgingen. Diese waren in der Mehrzahl jedoch ausschliesslich Pädagogen, nicht gleichzeitig auch Ärzte. Sie übernahmen die Behandlung der Blödsinnigen an ihren Schulen.

Die Kernsche Anstalt in Möckern (1839) und die Saegertsche Anstalt in Berlin (1843) gelten als die ältesten derartigen Anstalten für blödsinnige Kinder in Deutschland. Sowohl Saegert wie auch Kern hatten zunächst nur Taubstumme unterrichtet. Sie begannen sich mit Schwachsinnigen zu beschäftigen, nachdem – wie Saegert 1843 formulierte – aufgefallen war, „daß unter den vielen wirklich tauben und daher stummen Kindern, auch manches andere stumme Kind vorgestellt wird, dessen Mangel an aller Aufmerksamkeit, dessen thierische Freßgier und unnatürliche Bewegungen oder dessen gänzliche Stumpfheit, Trägheit und Schläfrigkeit" Veranlassung gibt, das Kind als „nicht bildungsfähig" von der Taubstummenanstalt abzuweisen. Das Urteil „nicht bildungsfähig" kam nach Saegerts Aussage einer Verurteilung gleich, da „ein solches Wesen auch in keiner anderen Anstalt Aufnahme und Ausbildung zu gewärtigen hatte."

Diese Festellung steht in Übereinstimmung mit dem Hinweis von Damerow (1858), daß die Irren- resp. Pflegeanstalten nicht Platz für diese Fälle hätten und sie in der Regel gemäß den Statuten nicht aufnehmen dürfen, da es sich einerseits um unheilbare andererseits aber ungefährliche Fälle handele.

Auch Brandes hat 1862 betont, daß Idioten nur dann in den bestehenden Irrenanstalten Aufnahme fänden, wenn sie als gemeingefährlich galten, d.h. in späterem Alter, wenn sie z.B. als Brandstifter, was nicht selten war, oder wegen

Sittlichkeitsdelikten auffielen, aber nicht „in den Kinderjahren, wo die Hülfe gerade für sie am nöthigsten und oft von Erfolg ist". Auch von der Aufnahme in die Waisenhäuser waren sie übrigens ausgeschlossen.

Aus diesen Erfahrungen heraus versuchte nun Saegert ein neues Erziehungskonzept für die Schwachsinnigen zu entwerfen. Er faßte wie Esquirol die Idiotie nicht als Krankheit sondern als einen Zustand auf. Unter Berufung auf Carus spricht er von „Seelenunthätigkeit" und wendet sich entschieden gegen die Kantsche Definition, daß der Blödsinn gleich „Seelenlosigkeit" sei. Indem er sich schließblich ganz auf die Physiologie von Johannes Müller stützt, entwickelte er seine Prinzipien „einer Heilung der Blödsinnigen auf intellectuellem Wege". Er verstand darunter vor allem die Anregung der Sinnesnerven und empfahl systematisch und ganz individuell vorzugehen.

Kern, der im Gegensatz zu Saegert nicht nur Pädagoge, sondern auch Arzt war, verstand unter Blödsinn „denjenigen psychischen Schwächezustand, nach welchem der Mensch nicht vermag innerhalb seiner Lebenssphäre den Anforderungen des gesunden Menschenverstandes gemäß zu denken und zu handeln".

Kern hat viele Probleme bereits sehr deutlich gesehen, z.B. das der Frühdiagnose und Ätiologie, sowie den engen Zusammenhang zwischen kindlicher Entwicklung und sozialen Faktoren. Zu den angeblich so großartigen Heilerfolgen bei Blödsinnigen, speziell Cretinen, an die man überall in Europa mit übertriebenen Hoffnungen aufgrund der Aufrufe und Mitteilungen Guggenbühls glaubte, nimmt er sehr kritisch Stellung und weist – nachdem er den berühmten Abendberg selbst inspiziert hatte – darauf hin, daß sich wo wirklich constatierter und in der ersten Kindheit hervorgetretener Blödsinn auf Krankheit des Gehirns und Nervensystems beruht, sich für Heilung auch nicht ein einziger glaubwürdiger Fall fände. Man könnte nur sagen „die Zöglinge befänden sich in voller Entwicklung".

Kern verlangte daher – um „die Öffentlichkeit nicht weiter irre zu führen" und um „dem Publikum und der Wissenschaft nicht das Unmögliche zu versprechen", daß man in Zukunft nicht mehr von „Heilanstalten für Blödsinnige" sondern schlicht von „Erziehungs-, Unterrichts- und Pflegeanstalten" sprechen möge. Für die Leitung einer solchen Anstalt stellte er klar die noch heute diskutierte Forderung auf, daß der Leiter „als Arzt und Pädagoge gebildet" sein muß. Er teilte somit die Auffassung von Brandes, daß weder der ärztliche noch der pädagogische Stand allein zu dieser Stellung befähige.

Im übrigen betrachtete Kern es als Sache des Staates „der Verkümmerung nach Leib und Seele im Allgemeinen vorzubeugen", und sich aus Gründen der Humanität auch der Idioten anzunehmen. Im Gegensatz zu den Irrenanstalten waren die Schwachsinnigenanstalten jedoch keine staatlichen Einrichtungen. Hubertusburg in Sachsen bildete die einzige Ausnahme.

Disselhoff hat daher 1857 sehr vorwurfsvoll nicht nur an die Kirche sondern auch an den preußischen Staat appelliert.

Damerow hat diesen Vorwurf scharf zurückgewiesen und betont, daß „in der ganzen zivilisierten Welt allein die öffentlichen Irren-Angelegenheiten Staatsangelegenheit" seien und daß die Einrichtung von Idioten- oder Cretinenanstalten vom Staate nicht verlangt werden könne, da – so die Begründung – die „dazu notwendigen Mittel . . . in keinem auch nur einigermaßen berechtigenden Verhältnis zum Erfolg in Betreff Erziehung, Bildung und Heilung" stünden. Entsprechende Anstaltsgründungen empfiehlt er daher als Aufgabe der privaten Wohltätigkeit, „der Barmherzigkeit von Privaten", wie er sagt, sowie Vereinen und Corporationen. Mit dieser Einstellung vertrat Damerow offenbar durchaus die allgemeine Auffassung.

Tatsache ist, daß ein großer Teil der insgesamt 32 Idiotenanstalten, die Sengelmann 1885 namentlich aufzählt und die in der Zeit von 1839–81 in Deutschland gegründet worden waren, sich in den Händen der inneren Mission befand, jener Bewegung zur Tat drängender Nächstenliebe, die – neu angestoßen durch die klassische Stegreifrede Wicherns auf dem Kirchentag in Wittenberg im Revolutions jahr 1848 – versuchte sich der sozialen Schäden aller Art anzunehmen.

Aus der großen Zahl der neuen Anstaltsgründungen nenne ich für Deutschland nur beispielhaft: Hephata, Langenhagen, Alsterdorf und Neuendettelsau.

Die Mehrzahl der Mitarbeiter dieser und anderer Anstalten zeigten eine betont christlich-pietistische Einstellung, geleitet wurden die Anstalten in der Regel von Pfarrern oder Pädagogen. Dies hat für den Umgang mit dem kindlichen Schwachsinnigen erhebliche Konsequenzen gehabt.

Bemerkenswert erscheint z.B. in diesem Zusammenhang, daß ärztliche Erkenntnisse, die in Frankreich oder Amerika die Schwachsinnigenfürsorge entscheidend bestimmten (ich erinnere an Bourneville oder Séguin), in Deutschland offenbar unbekannt, jedenfalls aber ohne nachhaltigen Einfluß blieben.

Dieser kursorische Überblick sollte andeuten, daß man im Laufe der letzten 150 Jahre versucht hat, den Schwachsinn bzw. die Idiotie diagnostisch zu erfassen, therapeutische Konzepte zu entwickeln und institutionelle Voraussetzungen zu schaffen, um dem geistig behinderten Kind eine bestmögliche Entfaltung zu garantieren. Dieser Prozeß ist nur mühsam in Gang gekommen und kann in keiner Weise als abgeschlossen gelten.

Das Problem des Umganges mit dem kindlichen Idioten ist heute so aktuell wie vor hundert Jahren, wenn es sich im Detail auch heute anders präsentiert. Wir möchten jedoch meinen, daß damals wie heute die Art des Umganges mit diesen schwächsten Gliedern der menschlichen Gesellschaft ein Indiz für die Empfindsamkeit des sozialen Gewissens ist.

J. O. Leibowitz
Jerusalem (Israel)

A mental hospital in Bagdad as described by Benjamin of Tudela (twelfth century)

The purpose of this paper is to present and comment upon a twelfth-century description of an Islamic hospital for the insane. The concise report by Benjamin of Tudela has been preserved in the original Hebrew and in numerous translations. The passage sheds some light on the long hospital tradition of the Islamic world, which however, will be only discussed as far as it directly applies to our subject. The most striking features with which we are here confronted are: free admission; supervision by government physicians with responsibility for deciding when patients have regained health and may be released; and the provision of some socio-economic rehabilitation for patients after leaving the hospital.

The second purpose of this paper is concerned with a general point regarding historiography. It should be stressed that medico-historical research into a given topic is intimately connected with the prevailing tendencies of a given time-period: medical, social, and emotional. In general, a writer will be guided in the choice of his topics by his own background, his accumulated knowledge, and an awareness of any gap to be filled in the existing literature. Moreover, the medical historian, will be rewarded in his findings when he himself is stimulated by new medical developments not available to previous writers on the subject. In this way critical interpretation and evaluation become possible, exceeding the satisfaction offered by finding and publishing a certain text or document.

Such was the case with Daremberg (1856) and Cockle (1860) in their French and English translations of Galen when they correctly proposed a diagnosis of mitral stenosis in the famous case history of Antipater. These scholar-translators lived at the time of the newly established science of physical diagnosis inaugurated by Laënnec, and the very beginnings of a modern sphygmology, neither of which was available to previous commentators. My own endeavour to produce a detailed history of coronary disease (1970), was an outflow and consequence of the interest in it and of the growing consciousness of its manifestations, which have penetrated the medical profession, society, and of course the writer of the monograph. The last specimen to be mentioned in this context is an exemplary study, 'Galen on contaminated cereals as a cause of epidemics' (1970), by my collaborator E. Lieber, who has been able to explain a Galenic passage in the light of the recent results of modern mycology and epidemiology.

In accordance with the ideas just proposed, we believe that our subject is topical and in tune with the recently increased interest in the social history of medicine. To this growing branch of knowledge belongs the passage from Benjamin's *Itinerary*, a famous work of medieval Hebrew prose, highlighting some features of the long tradition of Muslim hospital care.

The author, Benjamin, has the title 'Rabbi' (abbreviated to R.) prefixed to his name in all available Hebrew manuscripts, as well as in the numerous translations. However, this does not necessarily imply that he was a rabbi by profession, for the prefixing of an 'R' to a first name as a mark of respect was a well-accepted tradition, similar to the use of 'Esquire' in English. No biographical data on Benjamin are known, not even the dates of his birth and death. The only valid chronological information is the date of his return from his long voyage to his native Spain, which is given as 1173 in the surviving Hebrew manuscripts and in all printed editions. As to the date of commencement of the voyage, scholars differ somewhat in their estimates but are generally agreed upon the period 1160–65. I would add that it could not have been much later, since Benjamin in his description of Egypt and its distinguished Jews, never mentions the name of Maimonides; which proves that Benjamin's notes had been written before Maimonides' fame had been established; in fact, his book contains no less than 248 names of those he knew (see the scholarly entry by W. Bacher in the *Jewish Encyclopedia*, vol. III, pp. 34–35, New York and London, Funk & Wagnall, 1903).

The aim of his long and dangerous voyage may partly have been trade and commerce. However, Benjamin's main desire was an investigation of the status of Jews dispersed in different parts of the world. Therefore, he names all the leaders of the Jewish communities and dwells on the seats of religious education and the holy places of Judaism. Unlike the great traveller Marco Polo, about a hundred years later, who with his father and uncle brought back to Venice 'a great wealth in jewels and gold' (see Olschki, 1944, especially p. 241), nothing of this kind is known of Benjamin. His motto may have been the Biblical: 'I seek my brethren' (Gen. 37: 16). The scope of his observations was, however, very large, from monuments and palaces, through natural phenomena and geography, down to popular folk-tales. The items of medical interest are not very numerous, but are worthy of systematic search; I myself read a paper on his notes on Salerno and the adjacent places at the International Congress at Rome–Salerno, in 1954.

As was the case with Marco Polo, the *Itinerary* was not written down by Benjamin himself. In the preface to the Hebrew manuscript preserved at the British Museum, Benjamin's name is followed by an abbreviation applied only to a deceased person. The 'publishers' of his book testify to having known the author as a trustworthy man, and proceed with the words: 'and such is the commencement of his book'. It seems that the author was deprived of the possibility of revising his work in person. This suggestion is supported by examination of the passage under discussion, where words pertaining to the dismissal of the patients after a period of insanity are twice repeated. Or shall we regard it as analogous to a 'reprise' or 'Leitmotiv' in a musical work? The enthusiasm of the author over the existence of a special house for the insane and over the actual or apparent recovery of a patient, would freely allow for an emotionally dictated repetition, such as we often find in Biblical poetry.

Following the first Hebrew printed edition (Constantinople, 1543), numerous editions have been published both in the original and in translation into Latin, English, Dutch, Judaeo-German, French, German, Spanish and Russian. Some have been included in collections of voyages which were much in demand during the seventeenth and eighteenth centuries (see Bibliography). We refrain from including in this paper a full bibliography with comments on each of the editions, which have been listed in some of the great catalogues and are in part referred to at the end of this paper. Carmoly in 1852, was able to list twenty-six of them and many others have followed since then. For the historian of today, the best is that by M. N. Adler, 1907, where the Hebrew text and English translation have (for the first time!) been established on five Hebrew manuscripts, one of them as early as the thirteenth century, whereas all preceding editions were based on the *editio princeps* and that of Ferrara 1556. One of the translations, that by Baratier, 1734, is here singled out for the curious fact that the translator (1721–40) began work on it when only eleven years old and saw it published when he was thirteen. The first volume contains a richly annotated translation from the Hebrew into French; the second, explanatory essays on Jewish matters, much 'biased against those about whom he was writing' (Moïse Schwab, *Jew. Enc.*, 1903). J. P. Baratier (1721–40), a member of a French Calvinist family living in Germany, is to the best of my knowledge, the only Christian hebraist, who has been able to master the Hebrew language at such a tender age. Of course he was able to draw freely from the first Latin translation (1575) by the famous Spanish Catholic hebraist, Benedictus Arias Montanus, in the same way as the early German and English translators of the Hebrew Bible were helped by the existing Latin translation, the Vulgate, and used it as a guide for their own versions.

In presenting now a translation of the passage into English, I am fully aware of the scarcity of medical details as to therapeutical measures. The absence of a detailed exposition is felt in the whole literature on mental care in the twelfth-century Muslim hospitals. Only in much later descriptions, such as that of a Turkish hospital in Adrianople, about A.D. 1500, have forms of therapy, such as baths and music, been reported (see Staehelin, 1957 on the authority of Ullersperger). As to the translation proper, I have retained that by Adler (1907, pp. 37–38), in spite of its slightly antiquated flavour. Only when another reading, out of the five manuscripts, appeared more appropriate, or when an occasional correction seemed to be indicated, have I changed the translation, as indicated by an asterisk.

He [the Caliph] built, on the other side of the river, on the banks of an arm of the Euphrates which there borders the city, large* houses and hospices for the sick poor who came to be healed. Here there are about sixty physicians' stores which are provided from the Caliph's house with drugs [in Hebrew: spices] and whatever else may be required. Every sick man who comes is maintained at the Caliph's expense and is medically treated. Here is a building [in Hebrew: palace] which is called Dar-al-Maristan, where they keep charge of the demented people who have become insane in the town through the great heat in the summer, and they chain each of them in iron chains until their reason becomes restored to them in winter-time. While they abide there, they are provided with food from the house of the Caliph, and when their reason is restored they are dismissed and each one of them goes to his house and to his dignity* [*kāvod* = honour]. Money is given to those that have stayed in the hospices and the town's* people return each one of them to his house and his respect [Hebrew, again: *kāvod*]. In fact*, every month the officers of the Caliph inquire and investigate whether they have regained their reason, in which case they are unfettered to go* to their houses and on their ways. All this the Caliph does out of charity to those who come to the city of Bagdad, whether they be sick or insane. The Caliph is a righteous man, and all his actions are for good.

Before the final comments and the evaluation of the above passage, we wish to give credit to previous medico-historical writers who have quoted the passage. In chronological order these are: Falk, Ullersperger, Seide, Staehelin, Schipperges and Hes. It has also been twice mentioned, without full quotation: *J. psychol. Med.*, 1850, and Zilboorg, 1941.

It may be noted that the great bibliographer, M. Steinschneider (1841), known for his succinct writing, has devoted a long review of A. Asher's edition of Benjamin's *Itinerary*. He preserved his keen interest in this work and he was the scholar who had given the information to Falk (1866, p. 706) on our passage.

The references to these writers are restricted to publications in the field of medical history only; not included are histories of geography, literature and so on. It was not easy to trace the passage even in the above small list of medico-historical writings and it is possible that one or more quotations of the passage by a previous writer have escaped our scrutiny. Paying due tribute to the research published so far we still feel that a few points remain for us to comment upon.

Most editions and all translations do not contain one crucial word of the description, which is the very backbone of the passage. The British Museum Heb. MS. Add. No. 27,089, reproduced by Adler (1907), has the word *kāvod*, which means honour, dignity, used with reference to the released patients after they had been released after a period of insanity. Thus Benjamin of Tudela stresses a point of the social standing of the patient who, after retention, is restored not only to his home but also to his human dignity. This has always been one of the psychologically most important problems in a post-psychotic medical case-history.

Another item, absent from most editions and from the older translations, is the fact that money was given to those who had 'stayed in the hospices', an act of socio-economic rehabilitation. For the hebraist it may be added, that another translation is also possible; namely that care be given to a regulation that 'their money' should be given to those who had been confined to the hospices [and also to those who had been kept in private houses (?), according to the reading of one manuscript]. 'Their' money would then mean that at the admission, valuables of the in-patients were taken from them to be returned on release as is practised even to the present day. This hebraistic nicety apart, the passage clearly belongs, as already said, to the economical care and aid after the detention.

Benjamin was sagacious enough to note the importance of the Bagdad psychiatric hospital or asylum. Not being a physician himself and covering only the most important items in his brief notes, our traveller apparently considered it a novelty, which he had not come across in his native Spain or elsewhere. Of course, he travelled at a period before the establishment of the mental hospital at Valencia 1409 (see Ullersperger-Peset, pp. 51 ff.); thus, the *bimaristan* of Bagdad was a novelty, which he gladly included in his *Itinerary*.

The last comment concerns the use of manuscript material which is of prime importance. By doing so we have been able to add some words and phrases which are missing in the numerous older editions and thus to increase the significance of the whole passage.

As to the history of Muslim hospitals in general, the medico-historical literature in the West begins with a study by Wüstenfeld, 1846, which deals only with Cairo of the ninth to the end of the thirteenth centuries; two words only refer to our subject: 'imprisoned insane' (p. 31). The most informative work on Islamic hospitals was published by Ahmed Issa Bey (1928). On Bagdad, the pages 175–87 describe nine hospitals, together with brief biographies of physicians, and an extensive bibliography of El Rāzi (pp. 178–80) with no specific reference to mental hospitals. Some mention of a mental hospital *Dair Hizkil* (Ezekiel Convent) is made by Ya'kūbī (died 897 or 905), which in the French translation by Gaston Wiet is found on page 164. Mention must also be made of the works by Le Strange (1934, p. 37) and A. Mez (1922, p. 356), in which the information is limited to a few lines. We have gathered much information on the history of general (as opposed to mental) hospitals in the Islamic world from several modern publications, such as Philipsborn, Hamarneh, Levey and others. This information leads to a high appreciation of the hospital care in Islam (see also Sudhoff, 1929). To that information our paper, we hope, will add a valuable source, which has been philologically enlarged and rectified and historically integrated into the most topical problems of our time when viewed in the light of the new revival of the social history of medicine. In doing so, we feel in agreement with the opinion expressed in the August issue of *Modern Medicine* by Charles E. Newman, an authority on the history of medical education. In a moment of a considerable resurgence of interest in medical history, the latter 'must have a bearing on something going on now to be acceptable to the majority'.

Bibliography

ABRAHAMS, ISRAEL, *Jewish Life in the Middle Ages*, London, Macmillan, 1896.

ADLER, MARCUS NATHAN, *The Itinerary of B. of T.*, critical text, translation and commentary, London, Frowde, 1907.

ASHER, A., *The Itinerary of R. B. of T.*, trans. and ed. by A. Asher, 2 vols., London and Berlin, 1840–41.

ASKENASI, J. 'Quelques reflexions sur B. de T. (1100–1171)', *Rev. Hist. Méd. Hébr.* 1961, **14**, 155–58.

BARATIER, J. P., *Voyages de Rabbi Benjamin fils de Jona de Tudèle, etc.* 2 vols., Amsterdam, 1734.

BERGERON, PIERRE (ed.), in *Recueil de Divers Voyages*, vol. I, pt. 2, *Voyage du celèbre Benjamin au Tour du monde . . .*, trans. from original Hebrew into Latin by Benoît Arian Montan; and from Latin into French, Leyden P. vander Aa, 1729.

BROWNE, E. G., *Arabian Medicine*, Cambridge University Press, 1921, reprinted 1962, cf. pp. 101–2.

CARMOLY, E. and LELEWEL, L., *Notice historique sur B. de T.*, Brussels, 1852.

CASSEL, S., in Ersch und Gruber, *Allg. Encyklopädie*, 2te Section, 27er Theil, pp. 193–95, Leipzig, Brockhaus, 1850.

COCKLE, J., 'Lectures on the historic literature of the pathology of the heart and great vessels', *Br. med. J.*, 1860, 81, 121, 161; cf. p. 123.

DAREMBERG, CH., *Oeuvres . . . de Galien*, 2 vols., Paris, Baillière, 1854–56, cf. vol. 2, pp. 623–24.

DUNLOP, D. M., 'Bimaristan', in *Encyclopedia of Islam*, 1960, pp. 1222–24.

FALK, FRIEDRICH, 'Aelteste Irrenanstalt', in *Miscellen*, p. 706–7. Following his detailed paper 'Studien über Irrenheilkunde der Alten', *Allg. Z. Psychiat.*, 1866, **23**, 429–566, 706–7.

FÜRST, JULIUS, *Bibliotheca Judaica*, Leipzig, Engelmann, 1863, cf. vol. I, pp. 117–19 (*sub voce* Binjamin).

HAMARNEH, S., 'Development of hospitals in Islam', *J. Hist. Med.*, 1962, **17**, 366–84.

HARRIS, JOHN, *Complete Collection of Voyages and Travels, etc.*, 2 vols. in folio, London, Woodward, 1744–48, 1764, 1808, cf. vol. I, pp. 546–55.

HES, JOZEF PH., 'Les soins en psychiatrie à Jérusalem au Cours du Mandat Britannique', *Rev. Hist. Méd. Hébr.*, 1969, **22**, 119–31, cf. note 2a on p. 130.

ISSA, AHMED BEY, *Histoire des bimaristans* (*hôpitaux*), *etc.*, Cairo, Barbey, 1928.

LE STRANGE, G., *Baghdad during the Abbasid Caliphate*, Oxford, Clarendon Press, 1924, (1st ed. 1900).

LEVEY, M., 'Medieval Muslim Hospitals: Administration and Procedures', *J. A. Einstein Med. Center* (Symposium: Hist. Med.), 1962, **10**, 120–27.

LIEBER, E., 'Galen on contaminated cereals as a cause of epidemics', *Bull. Hist. Med.*, 1970, **44**, 332–45.

MEZ, A., *Die Renaissance des Islams*, Heidelberg, C. Winter, 1922, cf. p. 356.

NEWMAN, CHARLES E., 'Medical history in medicine today', [leading article], *Mod. Med.*, 1972, **17**, 474–75.
OLSCHKI, LEONARDO, 'Medical matters in Marco Polo's description of the world', in Supplement no. 3 to *Bull. Hist. Med.* Essays presented to Arturo Castiglioni on the occasion of his 70th birthday, 10 April 1944. Baltimore, Johns Hopkins Press, 1944; cf. pp. 237–59.
PHILIPSBORN, ALEXANDRE, 'Les premiers hôpitaux au Moyen Age (Orient et Occident)', *La nouvelle Clio*, 1954, **6**, 137–63.
PURCHAS, SAMUEL, *Purchas his Pilgrimes etc.*, London, Stanly for Fetherstone, 1625, 4 vols., cf. vol. II, p. 1438. New edition: Glasgow, James Maclehose, 1905, vol. VIII, cf. pp. 523–93.
SEIDE, J., 'Medicine and natural history in the itinerary of Rabbi Benjamin of Tudela (1100–1177)', *Bull. Hist. Med.*, 1954, **28**, 401–7.
SCHIPPERGES, H., 'Der Narr und sein Humanum im islamischen Mittelalter', *Gesnerus*, 1961, **18**, 1–12. Cf. on B. of T., p. 11.
STAEHELIN, J. E., 'Zur Geschichte der Psychiatrie des Islam', *Schweiz. med. Wochenschrift*, 1957, **87**, 1151–57.
STEINSCHNEIDER, M. [Book review, signed M. Sider], 'Asher's Prachtausgabe der Massaot des Rabbi Binjamin von Tudela', *Literaturblatt des Orients*, pp. 335–40, 402–10, 418–23, 437–44, 453–58, Leipzig, 1841.
SUDHOFF, K., 'Aus der Geschichte des Krankenhauswesens im früheren Mittelalter in Morgenland und Abendland' [first published in 1913], *Sudhoff's Archiv*, 1929, **21**, 164–203, cf. pp. 179–81.
ULLERSPERGER, J. B., *Die Geschichte der Psychologie und Psychiatrik in Spanien, von den ältesten Zeiten bis zur Gegenwart*, Würzburg, Stuber, 1871. Used: Translation into Spanish, with introduction, notes and appendices by V. Peset. Madrid, Alhambra, 1954, cf. pp. 58–63.
Unsigned [Forbes Winslow, the editor?] 'The history and present state of lunatic asylums – public and private', *J. psychol. Med. ment. Path.*, 1 October 1850, cf. pp. 450–51.
WRIGHT, THOMAS, *Early Travels in Palestine*, London, Bohn, 1848, cf. Introduction, pp. xxii–xxiv and 63–126.
WÜSTENFELD, D., 'Macrizi's Beschreibung der Hospitäler in el-Câhira', *Janus*, 1846, **1**, 29–39.
YAḲŪBĪ, *Les Pays*; trans. by Gaston Wiet. Tome I, Cairo, Imprimerie de l'institut Français d'archéologie Orientale, 1937.
ZILBOORG, G. and HENRY, G. W., *A History of Medical Psychology*, New York, Norton, 1941, cf. pp. 563–64.

R. G. Hillman
Santa Fe, New Mexico (U.S.A.)

The imprisonment of mentally ill patients in early nineteenth-century provincial France: legal proceedings

The reforms of Pinel in the early nineteenth century heralded the psychiatric revolution that has continued until the present time. In many areas of France, especially the provinces, Pinel's reforms could not be immediately implemented because specialists and special facilities for treating the mentally ill were nonexistent. In Laval, France, the mentally ill were imprisoned in an old chateau which functioned as the departmental prison. Dr. Jean-Baptiste-Denis Bucquet (1771–1841) was the prison physician for the common criminals and the mentally ill imprisoned in the chateau. Bucquet's two manuscripts on the mentally ill male and female inmates provide the only information on the mentally ill inmates during the period 1800–35 when the chateau functioned as an asylum as well as a prison. By 1835, a special psychiatric facility for their treatment existed.

The legal document of the Revolution, the Civil Code of 1804, was a reaction to pre-revolutionary legal injustices and was based on a revolutionary philosophy. Briefly summarized, it was based on the principles of legality (a statute enacted by the legislature for each crime), importance of property rights (which had an anti-feudal flavour), individual liberty and not appealing to a 'higher' (i.e. medical) authority. In addition, early nineteenth-century French judges were ruling on sections of the Civil Code dealing with the mentally ill without either extensive prior legal tradition or a body of supporting psychiatric literature and expert testimony. This paper will examine interdiction proceedings (historically, a declaration of competency; the right to own property and enter into legal contracts) in Laval, France, during the period 1800–35. Where possible, Bucquet's clinical notes will be correlated with the interdiction proceedings in order to ascertain the medico-legal implications of interdiction. Twenty-three of the 208 inmates mentioned in Bucquet's notes were interdicted. The records of only fourteen of these proceedings have survived the socio-political turmoil of early nineteenth-century France. The cases available for examination probably represent the more violent forms of mental illness, thus posing a more difficult problem for the judges.

The specific sections of the French Civil Code of 1804 pertaining to the mentally ill deal exclusively with interdiction. These codes are grouped under sections which include the questions of majority and Court appointed administrators. It must be remembered that in pre-Revolutionary France, the judicial aristocracy failed to distinguish between applying law and making law.[1] They were a specific target of the Revolution. The framers of the French Civil Code forged a document that emphasized the principle of legality: 'no crime without a penalty or a statute enacted by the legislature.'[2] Thus, the judge's function was reduced to finding and applying the correct legislative statute.

Section 489 states that anyone suffering from 'imbecility, dementia or dangerous madness' (*fureur*) must be interdicted 'even if there are lucid intervals'. The interdiction ceased, in the pithy words of the post-Revolutionary period, 'with the causes that made it necessary' (Section 512).[3]

Most commonly, the King's Prosecutor would initiate the proceedings, especially if there were no family or friends to do so. I was able to locate only one case with a physician's examination. The person was diagnosed as suffering from 'dementia'.[4] This man was wealthy, and his family did not want him interdicted in spite of his grossly abnormal behaviour. For the ordinary citizen, a physician's statement was not part of the interdiction proceedings.

The following case is somewhat atypical in that the neighbours of this fifty-seven-year-old disturbed woman attempted to support her but were finally compelled to seek her imprisonment. A letter from the Mayor of Laval to the Prefect stated:

> Anne Bourdin . . . living for eighteen years in this city suffers from mental illness (*aliénation mentale*); . . . this woman who lives in a damp cave has become dangerous (*furieuse*) for several weeks; . . . her neighbours, in spite of being very poor themselves, feel obligated out of charity to feed her and watch her fearing she will set fire to the few decrepit pieces of furniture she still has; . . . during the night they are obligated to lock her in her shack in order to prevent her from wandering and shouting in the streets . . . her neighbours can no longer continue either the attention or the aid she demands . . . and consequently [I] request that this woman be kept in one of the prison's cells. . . .[5]

She was admitted to the prison the same day and she died seven months later. This patient was admitted in 1822, seven years before Bucquet began to keep regular records. If we assume that her neighbours had kept her alive for many years, we can also assume that in prison she languished and died quickly. In Bucquet's notes no information is given as to her diagnosis or course in prison; simply the date of entry and the date of death.

In examining the interdiction proceedings, it is impossible to make specific diagnoses using present-day nosology. I have grouped the examples into three general classes: (1) inmates whose responses are suggestive of a psychotic, organic or mentally deficient etiology, (2) inmates with either a neurotic or character disorder, and (3) a heterogenous group that may have included some individuals who were not insane.

Pierre Loret is an example of the first category of inmates. Biographical information from Bucquet's notes is scanty.[6] He was a thirty-one-year-old married labourer. He first entered the prison at age twenty-five and stayed (as a mentally ill inmate) two months. No observations exist for this two-month period. The next year he had a 'relapse', and he was readmitted to the prison. There are no clinical observations until four years later, when the following examination took place to determine if he should be interdicted: (The questioner is a judge, Bucquet was not present.)

Q. What is your name, age, where do you live, and where were you born?
A. My name is Pierre Loret. I don't know my age. I am a laborer born and raised in Evron.
Q. Do you know why you are . . . [*sic*].
A. But there are many others.
Q. Have you been here a long time?
A. Three hundred thousand years. . . .[7]

Another example, taken from interdiction proceedings, suggests that the inmate, a fifty-four-year-old married man, is very disturbed. He responds in a guarded, angry and at times expansive manner. These tendencies are reinforced by the direct and accusatory tone of the questions posed by the judges. The inmate denies most of the allegations which suggest that he was violent before entering prison. His responses indicate evidence of loose associations. He is delusional, believing people were influencing his wife, calling him a murderer and a bastard. He acted on these delusions by nailing his closet shut and complaining to the city officials on several occasions.

Q. What are your given and proper names, age, occupation, residence and place of birth?
A. I am called Joseph Pottier 'The Gentle,' you are corrupted because I am not corrupted, I am afraid of nothing, I am fifty-four years old, live in Laval and born in Laval.
Q. When you are at home, why do you frequently make noise and why do you insult your neighbours?
A. I don't make noise in my home, and I insult them only when they often say bad things to me. They have no right over me; they've come and said to me: 'Leave this house, you don't live here.' It was Georget and Madame Leclerc who said those bad things to me. . . .
Q. Didn't you put your wife out of the house?
A. I pushed her out of the house one time because I realized that the neighbors were influencing her by signs and cries that they directed towards her.
Q. What do you mean by 'cries that they directed towards her?'
A. Sorcery.
Q. Do you know how to do sorcery?
A. No, I don't know how to do it, but one knows how to realize when it's being done. Moreover, it is not necessary to be a sorcerer in order to do sorcery; they wanted to do it to me but I paid them and I did not become affected, one must be careful; someone directed a '*oui*' on me to kill my wife. But I understood and I didn't act because the '*oui*' didn't come from any person, I have the honour of presenting for the first time to you. . . . You know what I'm telling you.
Q. How does one go about directing a '*oui*?'
A. First of all, it's directed from the mouth, you should realize that. It is Georget who directed it on me. . . .[8]

There are no clinical notes for the first six years Mr. Pottier was in prison. Then there is a brief reference to his 'anxious and irritable' character and his being 'mistrustful'. He is described as being in a 'stationary state' for the last four years (of his eleven-year confinement) before he died.[9]

The final example in the first category is taken from an interrogation of a woman who had been in prison one month because of 'dementia and dangerous madness' and whose childlike and incongruous responses suggest she was either mentally retarded or chronically psychotic. This is more evident towards the end of the interview. This is the woman mentioned earlier in the Mayor's letter.

Q. What is your name, age, occupation, and where do you live?
A. My name is Anne Bourdin, I hope I am fifty-four years old, I'm single, live in Laval, and I was born in Saint-Jean-sur-Mayenne, I don't live here, I work here.
Q. Didn't you try to set fire to your house before coming here?
A. My goodness, I wouldn't think of doing that, what good would that have done me?
Q. Didn't you run through the streets shouting?
A. Yes, because my head was sick. My eyes didn't hurt, but I didn't see very well, and my head was heavy. . . .

Q. Do you know your mother and father?
A. I don't know where my father is, but I know my mother, when I am home in the country she lives with me. It has been a long time since I've seen her.

At that moment she spoke to one of the judges and said: 'Did you get a good wife? Oh, the world has changed.'

Q. Was that the man who married you [indicating someone in the courtroom]?
A. No, that's a small young man who comes from Ermé.
Q. Do you have children?
A. I don't have any now.
Q. How many did you have?
A. I had only one, he was named Nanou like me.
Q. Is it a long time since you've given birth?
A. About fifteen days, don't say anything to Beucher.
Q. What's happened to your child?
A. He's still living, he is with his mother, she took him.
Q. Aren't you his mother?
A. I'm only his mother in a certain way.
The Tribunal stopped the interrogation of Anne Bourdin noting that her physical appearance and her manner of responding denoted a state of complete imbecility. . . .[5]

A search of the departmental archives in Laval produced few cases of what could, today, be termed neuroses or character disorders. This is understandable in that, as a group, these persons were probably either treated as common criminals or were less likely to display enough bizarre behaviour to require their interdiction.

The following interrogation is of a twenty-four-year-old man who was imprisoned for fourteen months. During his confinement, he had epileptic attacks followed by 'fits of fury'.[10] He was combative and had to be put in chains and solitary on several occasions. Bucquet felt that, diagnostically, he resembled a case of mania without delirium. The fact that he requested and obtained his release from prison, as well as the fact that he was arrested as a criminal for shoplifting six months after his release and was never interdicted, suggests that his violence was not a manifestation of a psychotic disturbance. A portion of the interrogation of this man, just after he entered the prison, follows:

Q. . . . Why did the innkeeper kick you?
A. I was tipsy.
Q. Were you not already detained in prison about one year ago for similar causes?
A. Yes, sir, but the gendarmes were wrong.
Q. Didn't you hit the guard Calibourg?
A. Yes, sir, but he started it by socking me. I scratched him.
Q. Are you not often in a state of dementia and fury that causes you to commit acts which are dangerous to public order?
A. Good God, I am flabbergasted. Already I've said more than twenty rosaries. . . .[4]

A number of interrogations seem to defy psychiatric diagnosis. Some of the reasons why this is so are evident in the interrogation which follows: A thirty-year-old-woman had been confined in prison for ten years by the time her interdiction took place. Although the interdiction examination does not specify the circumstances surrounding her being placed in prison, Bucquet's manuscript states that she was arrested for 'mania' in 1827 and released within two months only to be readmitted several days later.[11] Bucquet's notes for this woman diagnose her condition as 'mania and continual tranquil delirium'. There are no clinical notes for the first three years of her confinement. There is a brief mention of her having been 'violent' for a short period when she first entered the prison, but later she is described as being 'sad and perfectly calm'. She must have posed few problems, as Bucquet wrote no notes on her for the last four years of her stay in prison. It is difficult to differentiate how much of her behaviour can be ascribed solely to the effect of confinement. Her interrogation, which took place ten years after she entered prison, suggests that she was a simple and undoubtedly illiterate woman but was not a danger to others. This assumption is supported by the fact that she was ordered to be released from prison several months after the following interrogation:

Q. What is your name?
A. Marie Fouet.
Q. How old are you?
A. About thirty-six to forty years old. I don't know. How old do you think I am?
Q. Why do you spin wool in your room? Why don't you work outside like the others?
A. When someone tells me to go out, I go out. If unfortunate things happen to me, God's grace will lighten my burdens. If I were with others I would perhaps become angry. I like to be alone. . . .
Q. How long have you been here?
A. This is the seventh year. I recall that because it was a holiday like Easter.
Q. Do you get along well?
A. Yes, sir, very well.
Q. Do you sleep well?
A. No, the slightest noise awakens me.
Q. Do you go to Mass?
A. Yes.
Q. Do you know your prayers?
A. She recites several prayers.

They showed her a one-franc piece which she identified as a sou. She identified a twenty-franc piece also as a sou.

Q. Would you like to leave here?
A. No, I feel quite comfortable here. I prefer being here rather than outside . . . than at my father's house. . . .[12]

Several conclusions can be drawn from the examination of the interdiction proceedings. While it is true that, strictly speaking, sections 489–512 of the French Civil Code as written in 1804 deal solely with a person's competency to own property and enter into contracts, it is a mistake to conclude therefore that the application of these sections did not have other goals in mind. Many of the patients interrogated had no property rights to dispose of in the first place. Many of the people examined exhibited such bizarre behaviour that the question of their competency was secondary to the fact that they were seen as being dangerous to themselves or to others. They were imprisoned first (often for several years) and *then* interdicted. It is historically more correct to view the interrogations as psychiatric examinations with a view towards commitment, even though the existing legal structure did not provide for such a goal.

There were no special facilities in Laval for treating mentally ill patients; and up to the point where the mentally ill were sent to prison, the physician exerted little influence. At a later date, the Civil Code was revised to provide for commitment, special psychiatric facilities and expert testimony.

ACKNOWLEDGEMENT

The Bucquet Manuscript was kindly lent to me by Mr. Haskell Norman of San Francisco from the Janus Foundation Collection.

References

1 MERRYMAN, JOHN HENRY, *The Civil Law Tradition*, Stanford, California, Stanford University Press, 1969, p. 17.
2 Ibid., p. 134.
3 TRIPIER, LOUIS, *Les Codes Francais Collationnés sur les Textes Officiels* . . . Paris, Librairie du Conseil d'Etat, 6th ed., 1859, pp. 80–82.
4 *Archives de la Mayenne*, U1028, 1831.
5 Ibid., U1028, 1822.
6 *Buc. Mms. Male*, 13.
7 *Archives de la Mayenne*, U1028, 1830.
8 Ibid., U1028, 1823.
9 *Buc. Mms. Male*, 6.
10 Ibid., 28.
11 Ibid., 11.
12 *Archives de la Mayenne*, U1029.

W. L. Parry-Jones
Oxford (Great Britain)

The role of private madhouses in nineteenth-century England

INTRODUCTION

In psychiatry, as compared with other fields of medicine, I believe that the historical approach has a particularly important contribution to make in allowing a fuller understanding of the background to current problems. This is largely because of the nature of the subject and of the present state of development of the specialty. Although much progress has been made, especially in terms of the application of scientific methodology during the last two decades, and although psychiatry has achieved some degree of re-unification with the mainstream of medicine, it is a field which is still fraught with perplexing problems and areas of uncertainty. Psychiatric nosology and nomenclature, for example, lack standardization; concepts of aetiology in common usage are tentative and often contradictory and treatment techniques remain largely empirical. Whilst the current emphasis is, and will continue to be, on the treatment of the mentally ill without removal from the community, there remains the question of whether those who need residential treatment should continue to be housed separately in mental hospitals. The policy that is being implemented at present is to establish psychiatric units in general hospitals, although one could argue that the underlying philosophy has more to do with decreasing the social stigma and abating the fears associated with mental illness than with furnishing demonstrably better treatment than could be provided in mental hospitals. At a time of such crucial change in the whole direction of psychiatry, there is a need for a thorough understanding both of the here-and-now problems and of the origins and development of our institutional provisions for the mentally ill, in order to provide insight into the reasons for change.

The framework of the mental health services of Britain is still centred largely on asylums, the bulk of which were established from the mid-nineteenth century onwards, with a small number dating from an earlier period. The movement that brought these asylums into being formed a part of the humanitarian reform movement of the early nineteenth century and reflected the growing public concern about the condition of the insane who were confined at this time in gaols, houses of correction, in the small number of lunatic hospitals built with funds raised by voluntary subscription and, above all, in private madhouses. The latter were privately owned establishments for the reception and care of insane persons, conducted as business propositions for the personal profit of the proprietor or proprietors. In view of their obvious importance as predecessors of county and borough asylums, it is of considerable significance to note that the system of institutional care provided by private madhouses has received virtually no serious attention by medical historians. Those few references that have been made to madhouses generally serve to emphasize their notorious reputation. The usual picture is that they were evil, corrupt places where the insane were treated brutally, and confined, frequently, under inhumane and foul conditions. This view is not surprising if the conclusions are based only on the evidence given before parliamentary select committees, and on accounts of popular outcry in contemporary newspapers, journals and novels. But were madhouses really as bad as they were made out to be, or is this yet another of the popular misconceptions with which psychiatric history is fraught? It was partly to answer this question that, several years ago, I embarked on research into the history and role of private madhouses in England and Wales. Some of the general findings of this research are reported very briefly in this paper.

THE PRIVATE MADHOUSE SYSTEM

It is useful to view the history of the madhouse system retrospectively in three, relatively distinct, phases. The first represents the rise of the system and extends from the early seventeenth century up to the latter end of the eighteenth century. Secondly, there is the period covering the last quarter of the eighteenth and the first half of the nineteenth century, which can be regarded as the hey-day of the system. Thirdly, there comes a period of decline, extending up to the present day, when only a handful of registered mental nursing homes, the only surviving descendants of the nineteenth-century madhouses, continue to function.

It was during the second period that madhouses assumed the greatest prominence and fulfilled their most important role. Following an Act of 1774, they had to be licensed by the local magistrates and were subject to regular inspection. The number of houses expanded rapidly and, by 1848, there was a total of 145 houses in England and Wales. This process of expansion was related closely to the rapid increase in the number of pauper lunatics in the country, but the expansive phase was brought to an end by the widespread establishment of county and borough asylums, following the County Asylum Act of 1845. This led to the withdrawal of pauper lunatics from madhouses and, consequently, to a sharp decrease in the number of pauper establishments. This latter decrease was offset, to some extent, by a consolidation in the position of houses receiving private patients, a state of affairs which was maintained until the close of the century. During the third period, these houses catered for the bulk of the insane of the middle and upper classes and, to a lesser extent, for the poorer class of paying patients, who otherwise were not provided for adequately.

ABUSES AND DEFECTS OF THE SYSTEM

The principal public grievance which fostered the notorious reputation of the late eighteenth-century madhouse was the possibility of improper confinement of sane persons as alleged lunatics and their prolonged detention therein for corrupt motives. Accusations of this kind were made frequently and, indeed, it is likely that outrages of this sort did occur. Many factors were responsible for this situation, including the deficiencies of the legislation, the machinations of self-interested and malicious relatives or associates of the alleged lunatic; the reprehensible conduct of unscrupulous, mercenary proprietors and the supporting complicity of ignorant and corrupt medical men, who signed the necessary admission documents. However, there is remarkably little well-documented evidence of such practices and much of the hue and cry seems to have stemmed from the published recollections and sensational accounts of alleged lunatics and ex-inmates of private madhouses. The surviving evidence in this category is often limited and based upon the accounts of persons of somewhat doubtful reliability and, as such, requires cautious assessment. The other area of major concern was the maltreatment of lunatics in madhouses, where they were housed in bad, often appalling, physical conditions. Here the evidence is considerably more substantial and there seems little doubt that the conditions in many madhouses were atrocious, especially in those accommodating pauper lunatics during the first half of the nineteenth century. One must be careful, nevertheless, not to embark on retrospective condemnation without familiarizing oneself with contemporary attitudes towards insanity and social conditions in general. When seen out of context and judged by later standards, in particular those of the era of moral treatment, the prevailing conditions appear disproportionately harsh and brutal, but one must not overlook the fact that daily life in the nineteenth century was coloured, in many aspects, by harshness, squalor and neglect.

THE PUBLIC SERVICE PROVIDED BY MADHOUSES

Whatever their calibre and reputation, however, private madhouses undeniably constituted the principal form of institution catering for the insane in anything approaching a specialized way until the mid-nineteenth century. It is a striking, and virtually unknown, fact that by 1848, one half of the total number of lunatics (approximately 14,000) confined to asylums in England and Wales were accommodated in private madhouses. During the first half of the nineteenth century, the madhouse system catered for pauper lunatics at a time when public provisions, in the form of county and borough asylums, were extremely slow in developing, and it was not until 1845 that the erection of such asylums became compulsory. In the second half of the century, madhouses met a legitimate, if diminishing, demand from the upper and middle classes for facilities that were not widely available elsewhere. Further, there is evidence that their value with regard to paupers continued well into the second half of the century and that they were used in some areas to compensate for the lack of county asylums or for the overcrowding of those which did exist. Moreover, they played a not insignificant part in accommodating both criminal lunatics and idiots. In these ways, I would suggest, private madhouses remained indispensable throughout the nineteenth century, despite the resentment that their continued existence and their prosperity aroused amongst the antagonists of the system.

THE QUALITY OF THE SERVICE PROVIDED

The quality of the service provided, however, is much more difficult to gauge because of the wide variation in the types of establishments and in the calibre of the proprietors and the attendants. The greater number of houses, as far as can be ascertained, contained, or were licensed to receive, up to twenty-five patients. The largest houses, invariably, were those which catered chiefly for paupers and, throughout the nineteenth century, there was a handful of houses, particularly in the London area, which could accommodate several hundred patients. The relative smallness of the bulk of the houses, however, and their frequently close integration with the community which they served generated many of their particular advantages compared with the large asylums that were to follow and which, by the end of the nineteenth century, had developed generally into anonymous, overcrowded and understaffed institutions often completely isolated from the local community. Many of the private madhouses which catered for private patients set out quite explicitly to provide a family-centred, country house atmosphere and it was, perhaps, during the second half of the nineteenth century that private asylums, as they were now called, served their most fitting role by making good provisions for the middle and upper classes in relatively small, well-staffed houses, where privacy and a considerable amount of personal liberty could be enjoyed. Certainly, it was in pauper establishments that the worst conditions prevailed, although it must be added that this was often due to the fact that, frequently, premises quite ill-suited for use as asylums were licensed by the magistrates and allowed to continue in use because of the acuteness of the demand for accommodation.

The proprietors were always a heterogeneous group and, during the first half of the nineteenth century and for the greater part of the second half as well, a considerable proportion were not medically qualified and included a number of women, some of whom were the wives or daughters of former proprietors. Many of these lay proprietors appear to have been ignorant and illiterate persons of low integrity, particularly at the time of expansion in the system when individuals were attracted by the opportunity to exploit the situation to get a good living. Certainly, much of the evidence provided at official inquiries supports this, although when one takes a broader view, I believe that one can be reasonably certain that during the nineteenth century the bulk of proprietors, particularly in the provinces, displayed a responsible attitude towards their duties and recognized that the continued success of their houses depended to a large extent on their personal reputation and on the public confidence which they enjoyed. Not infrequently, individual proprietors displayed humane and charitable attitudes towards their patients over and above the call of duty and expended large sums of money on their pauper departments, even when there was little incentive in terms of financial reward.

Only a small number of proprietors made noteworthy contributions in theoretical and practical terms to the growth of psychiatry and these included such well-known practitioners as Dr. Thomas Arnold (1742–1816), Dr. William Perfect (1737–1809) and Dr. Joseph Mason Cox (1763–1818). During the period of the slow acceptance of the concepts of non-restraint and moral treatment, a small number of private madhouses were in the forefront and establishments like Brislington House, Bristol, and Laverstock House, Salisbury, were in many ways as advanced in their therapeutic regimes as the York Retreat, although they never acquired the same prestige and publicity. The principle of profit on which private madhouses were based always haunted the system. Nevertheless, the successful restoration of the lunatic was clearly the primary objective in many madhouses, and, despite the popular view that patients were retained long beyond their recovery for corrupt motives, there are adequate statistics which point to the fact that fairly short periods of stay were the general rule. Furthermore, it was usual for up to one-third of the admissions to be discharged recovered or improved, particularly amongst the private patients. The figures for paupers were often lower, not necessarily because of bad treatment but because of delayed admission usually due to the parsimony of parish officials, who allowed the disorder to become very acute or intractably chronic before being willing to make the necessary payments for treatment in an asylum.

CONCLUSION

It is hoped that this very brief paper will have succeeded in making a case for a greater recognition of the contribution of the private madhouse system, particularly in its hey-day in the mid-nineteenth century, and will have gone some way towards allaying longstanding prejudices. The limits of time, unfortunately, have meant that conclusions have been stated somewhat baldly, without adequate illustration and corroboration.

The private madhouse system could not compete with the county asylum movement and the clamour of condemnation, the pressures for innovation and for safeguards against abuse won the day. But sporadic outcries of one kind or another continued and the late nineteenth-century asylums have much to answer for in terms of the problems that are still with us today. Reports of scandals and alleged abuses in our mental hospitals over the last few years are so very reminiscent of those which were publicized in relation to private madhouses that one is led to search for some common denominator. Perhaps, after all, it was not the commercialism or the real or fancied corruption in the madhouse system which was at the heart of the matter. Insanity has always aroused particular, intangible fears of its own, and, at the present day, despite extensive education of the general public, misconceptions and mistrust about what goes on in mental hospitals are only too common.

T. Bilikiewicz and M. Lyskanowski
Warsaw (Poland)

Humanitarian traditions of treatment of the mentally ill patients in Poland in the sixteenth and eighteenth centuries

In prehistoric Poland mental diseases were often regarded as linked with religious-demonological concepts. Slavs believed that priests were intermediaries between God and the mentally ill. Apart from prayers, conjurations, and other rites the priests offered remedies that relieved pain and ailments of the sick.

After Christianity had been introduced priests either included old Polish customs and ideas in their rites or treated them with great tolerance. The new church respected old customs. Similarly, public law included situations created by life and strengthened by custom.[1]

As charitable institutions hospitals remained under the protection of the clergy throughout centuries. The king only validated foundations of individual hospitals.[2] Those principles were expressed in decrees of synods which enjoined admission to hospitals for those who were unable to support themselves, disabled or old persons, and those who were affected with incurable diseases. Those who could be cured left hospital as soon as they recovered.[3]

In Poland the first hospitals for mentally ill patients were established in the sixteenth century – in Kraków in 1534 and Gdańsk in 1542.[4]

The first Statute concerned with protection of the poor, the sick, those unable to work, and beggars was issued by King Jan Olbracht in 1496.[5] However, the most important legal act that protected the insane was the Lithuanian Statute issued by King Sigismund the Old in 1529,[6] which constitutes the first act affecting psychiatric patients in the history of Poland. It treated them in a just and objective way as sick, without the slightest trace of demonology. For instance, article 24 of Chapter 7 concerned with manslaughter committed by the insane, stated that the insane or madman should be under the guard of relatives, the poor in towns should be looked after by town councils, and the village poor by landowners or land-stewards. Nevertheless, if the homicidal madman resisted he was to be imprisoned for one year and six weeks. For assault he was to be imprisoned for half a year. Persons instigating or supplying weapons to insane persons were to be punished as malefactors. In case an insane person, after apparent recovery, killed anyone in a subsequent attack of madness, he was to be beheaded.

The first chapter of the third statute, the so-called New Statute of 1588, says that the sovereign had the right to pardon individual follies and blunders.

Undoubtedly, the humanitarianism of the Statute greatly influenced the evolution of ideas of treatment of the mentally ill in Poland during following centuries, particularly in the eighteenth century – a period of tragic decline of the Republic. The eighteenth century in Poland began with natural disasters, which included pestilence, floods, fires, droughts and an invasion of locusts. As a result of numerous wars foreign armies confiscated grain, food, cattle, and imposed heavy taxes and contributions. People died of hunger and poverty.[7]

Even then in the period of the most tragic economic and socio-political decline the mentally ill patients in hospitals were not forgotten. In 1728 an act concerning hospitals run by the Order of St. John of God was published.[8] Chapter 34 of the Act concerned the procedure of visiting the sick by physicians and barber-surgeons: as soon as the physician came bells were to be rung to be heard in the infirmary and hospital. The ward head and apothecary had to record in their books all the physicians' remarks including notes concerning food and drink as well as medicaments and supply of other necessary things. It was the duty of the ward head to report, and the physician would listen. Female patients were carefully examined by the visiting physician. Afterwards the ward head and the physician would go to the gate unless there were more sick persons to be examined and admitted to the hospital.

Chapter 35 was concerned with feeding the sick; mealtimes were to be announced by bell-ringing in the morning as well as in the afternoon. Monks were to bring the meal from the kitchen and the priest gave everybody what had been prescribed for him by the physician. The ward head appointed a Brother who would help those who were unable to feed themselves. Afterwards a Brother of higher rank asked each patient if he had received everything the physician prescribed.

One of the most prominent psychiatrists of this time, a man of great devotion to mentally ill patients, Friar of the Order of St. John of God, Ludwik Perzyna (1742–1812), greatly contributed to popularization of correct and sound ideas concerning mentally ill persons.[9] He wrote *A Physician for Country-Folk*, 1793 – a book meant for country-folk and peasants. He drew his readers' attention to the influence of head injuries and heavy drinking, which was of great significance at that time, as well as various poisons, venoms and animals affected with rabies. He stressed significance of changes in the way of living, food, and use of 'soothing words'. He stressed the role of the brain in mental diseases.[10]

In the Central Archives of Old Acts in Warsaw we found numerous data concerning treatment of mentally ill patients at the end of the eighteenth century. By the terms of a government act of 24 June 1791 the Committee of Security together with the National Education Committee had to keep a watchful eye on all aspects of human health and, consequently, secure physicians, medicaments, surgeons, barber-surgeons, apothecaries, pharmacies, and midwives.

In the light of archival investigations we have found very interesting facts about activities of the committee of Security concerning mentally ill patients.[11] The documents describe treatment of the sick from the moment they became insane to the moment they were cured and allowed to leave the hospital. The proceedings were as follows: (*a*) Notification of the case of psychosis to the Committee of Security. (*b*) Appointment of so-called Inquisitors by the Committee to examine the witnesses. The Inquisitors were handed 'Points to Examine Those Who Witnessed Acts of Madness'. (*c*) Collection of witnesses' accounts and passing them on to physicians. (*d*) Medical examination and physicians' diagnoses. (*e*) Elaboration of acts by the Inquisitors after they had studied the above opinions. (*f*) Sending the patient to a hospital and fixing the fee. (*g*) Medical examination of the patient after treatment and issuing an opinion on the state of his health. (*h*) Permitting the cured patient to leave the hospital.

We would like to stress, that the 'Points to Examine Those Who Witnessed Acts of Madness' constitute an extremely interesting document. We shall now quote an example found in the Central Archives of Old Acts:

Points to Examine Those Who Witnessed Acts of Madness committed by W. Rychtowski; recorded June 12th, 1782.[12]

a. Does the witness know W. Rychtowski, and if so, for how long. Has he observed any differences in his behaviour before and now.
b. Does the witness know W. Rychtowski's diversions, where he goes, where spends his nights, and in what way does he assault people.
c. When and how did he intrude the palace of Prince General of Podolia.
d. Did the witness hear W. Rychtowski threaten Prince General and did he see W. Rychtowski attack the Prince in the street.
e. How does the witness judge deeds, words, and habits of W. Rychtowski if they do not result from madness.

According to the archival documents proceedings concerned not only the upper classes of society, i.e. nobility and aristocracy. The documents mention a 'Charity Fund', 'Fund for the Poor', and a 'Payment from the Government', which manifest help and protection for the sick and poor as well as for the destitute and homeless. Those humanitarian arrangements for the mentally ill patients undoubtedly followed the just ideas of the 1529 Statute and became a basis for the modern school of Polish psychiatry.

References

1 MĘCZKOWSKI, WACŁAW, *Prowizorowie szpitalni w dawnej Polsce*, Warsaw, 1908, pp. 2–3.
2 MĘCZKOWSKI, WACŁAW, *Stan i potrzeby szpitali Królestwa Polskiego*, Warsaw, 1905, p. 3.
3 MĘCZKOWSKI, WACŁAW, *Szpitale dawnej Rzeczypospolitej w uchwałach synodów polskich*, Poznań, 1936, p. 12.
4 BILIKIEWICZ, TADEUSZ, *Jan Gallus. Psychiatria polska na tle dziejowym*, Warsaw, 1962, p. 121.
5 ZAWADZKI, J., 'Dobroczynność w Polsce', *Medycyna i Kronika Lekarska*, R. 3, 1917, p. 133.
6 CZACKI, TADEUSZ, *O litewskich i polskich prawach*, T. 2, Kraków, 1861, pp. 68, 71, 143.
7 GIEROWSKI, JÓZEF, *Między saskim absolutyzmem a złota wolnościa. Z dziejów wewnętrzny ch Rzeczypospolitej w latach 1712–1715*, Wrocław, 1935, pp. 11–12.
8 GIEDROYĆ, FRANCISZEK, *Zapiski do dziejow spitalnictwa w dawnej Polsce*, Warsaw, 1908, pp. 8, 16–17.
9 LYSKANOWSKI, MARCIN, 'Ludwik Perzyna i jego poglady na etiologię oraz leczenie chorób psychicznych', *Neurologia, Neurochirurgia i Psychiatria Polska*, T. XIV, Nr. 2, 1964, pp. 339–41.
10 PERZYNA, LUDWIK, *Lekarz dla Włościan*, Kalisz, 1793, p. 161.
11 ŁYSKANOWSKI, MARCIN, *Postępowanie z psychicznie chorymi w Polsce Centralnej w XVIII w.*, Studia i Materialy z Dziejów Nauki Polskiej, S.B.z. 18, 1970.
12 *Archiwum Główne Akt Dawnych w Warszawie. Tzw. Metryka Litewska*, Dz. IX, Nr. 19, k. 365.

G. N. Grob
New Brunswick, N.J. (U.S.A.)

The mental hospital in nineteenth-century America: an interpretation

Traditionally the history of psychiatry has for all intents and purposes been synonymous with the history of individual psychiatrists and their theories. Whether consciously or unconsciously, the typical history of psychiatry began at a remote point in a dark and distant past when superstition and ignorance predominated and then proceeded to trace the progressive enlightenment of humanity by the heroic figures who contributed to the solution of the puzzles posed by mental illness. The final sections of such works were usually in the form of a peroration: if we are not yet fully enlightened, then certainly we stand on the threshold of an age in which psychiatry – given the necessary support and resources – would play a key role in creating a better and presumably more healthy society. Some historians even divided the history of psychiatry into two general periods: B.F. (Before Freud) and A.F. (After Freud), and then evaluated all psychiatric thinkers in terms of the manner in which they conformed to or deviated from the thought of this epochal and heroic figure.

While I have overdrawn the picture, I do not think that my characterization is inaccurate. Most historians who dealt with this subject were themselves psychiatrists who accepted the assumption that psychiatry was simply a branch of medicine or a semi-autonomous science concerned with certain forms of human behaviour. To understand its development, therefore, required an analysis of its internal logic, assumptions, objectives, and methodology, as well as the sequential pattern of 'discoveries' and 'advances'. Historians of psychiatry were especially concerned with the thought of individual psychiatrists and their noble efforts to resolve the contradictions that usually accompanied the broad theoretical structures that attempted to account for normative and pathological behaviour. Conversely, these historians ignored or neglected those social and environmental determinants that played a significant part in shaping psychiatry. Tacitly, they assumed the existence of a chronic tension between an altruistic profession and a semi-evil social order which resisted enlightenment and refused to provide the resources necessary to combat the ravages of mental illness.

Yet psychiatry did not exist in isolation nor did it remain immune from a variety of external influences that superficially seemed unrelated to the problems posed by mental illness. Indeed, it is impossible to understand fully the history of psychiatry or psychiatric institutions without a full knowledge of the larger society in which both existed. Mental hospitals, for example, performed a variety of functions, some of which were thrust on them by a society that lacked effective means of accomplishing certain ends. They were not only entrusted with the function of caring for sick individuals, but often they accepted old age and indigent persons as well as cases whose behaviour was deemed socially unacceptable by the community or family. The nature of care and treatment, moreover, was also partly a function of individual and group values; psychiatric theory often followed as a rationalization of existing practices. The absence of demonstrable and specific etiological concepts and the vagueness of nosological systems made psychiatric thought especially vulnerable to economic, social, and intellectual influences (although psychiatrists insisted that their theories were scientific and not derived from subjective cultural and personal values). Above all, the fate of the mentally ill was inextricably involved with a series of socio-economic factors, in part because such a high proportion of patients came from lower-class and minority ethnic backgrounds and in part because of the high costs of protracted institutionalization.

Neither American psychiatry nor the mental hospital, then, can be studied in medical and scientific terms alone. On the contrary, both developed out of the interaction of complex social, economic, and intellectual forces, and frequently reflected some of the characteristics of their indigenous environment. The purpose of this paper, then, will be to sketch out in simplified form an interpretive conceptual framework for an understanding of the evolution of nineteenth-century American psychiatry and mental hospitals.

During the seventeenth and eighteenth centuries, mental illness was not recognized in the American colonies as being a major medical problem or a matter of pressing social concern. Population density tended to be low, and most communities were predominantly rural and agricultural. While the family was primarily responsible for the welfare of its members, the community was never able to avoid involvement. Certain behavioural patterns seemed to threaten public safety; in other cases mental illness resulted in a loss of income, which led to the intercession of the community because of its obligation to care for indigent and dependent persons. Since institutionalization was uncommon (if only because a low population density made the establishment of institutions uneconomical), the mentally ill were provided for in a variety of ways, including boarding them out in private homes or providing supplemental grants in order to maintain the household intact. Reliance on familial and community traditions and practices, therefore, made it unnecessary to consider alternative approaches. Consequently, the very concept of social policy – which involved the conscious creation of new public structures or procedures on a regional or national basis to replace traditional means of dealing with distress – was largely absent for most of the seventeenth and eighteenth centuries.

Only in a few of the more urban areas did informal modes of care prove more difficult or impracticable. In these areas, local citizens, often with the aid of the legislature, attempted to found hospitals to deal with problems related in one way or another to disease. Such early efforts, which resulted in the establishment of hospitals in Pennsylvania, New York, and Virginia, were isolated and not part of a more general or systematic attempt to provide medical care and treatment within a comprehensive system. The few institutions founded before 1800 did not reflect the application of new medical knowledge, the energies of informed medical reformers, or the efforts of organized campaigns to improve health conditions or medical treatment. On the contrary, these institutions provided custodial and humane care for sick and dependent persons whose families were unwilling or unable to care for them.

After 1800, however, new circumstances created conditions that stimulated the thrust toward reliance on institutional care of the mentally ill. Demographic changes (including population growth, a sharp increase in immigration of relatively poor and impoverished persons, and urbanization), a growing sensitivity to social and medical problems, a surge in philanthropic giving by elite groups, and knowledge of significant medical and psychiatric developments in France and England, all combined to give rise to a movement to establish both general and mental hospitals. Originating in the more populous Northeast, the movement within a few decades had become national in scope; eventually it transformed the manner in which American society defined and responded to health-related problems.

The hospital movement in its initial phase during the early nineteenth century was a product of private philanthropy. With the financial aid of affluent, elitist groups, psychiatric hospitals were founded in a number of urban areas. Although privately supported, these institutions were nevertheless intended to serve the entire community, including those persons unable to pay for the costs of care and treatment. The relative absence of governmental involvement – especially at the state level – reflected the prevailing localism of American society and the general tendency to deal with social problems in informal ways at the community level. Before 1830 those individuals and groups who played the major role in founding hospitals assumed that private beneficence would prove adequate for existing needs. Therefore, they devoted little or no thought to long-range issues concerning health and dependency. When it became evident that private philanthropy was inadequate to overcome the formidable difficulties that arose out of certain economic and social developments, those mental hospitals already in existence slowly began to redefine their responsibilities. They limited admissions to those individuals who could afford the high costs of protracted treatment, and thereby created the foundations for a system of relatively exclusive private hospitals serving well-to-do groups.

The surge in the founding of corporate institutions by private philanthropy during the first quarter of the nineteenth century, though short-lived in duration, had important consequences. Not the least of them was the stimulation of public awareness of the supposed humanitarian, medical, and economic benefits both to society and the individual of institutional care and treatment of mental illness. At the same time it was becoming increasingly evident that the private sector was unable to provide the resources required for establishing and maintaining a broad network of hospitals that served all groups irrespective of their ability to pay for their confinement. During the second quarter of the nineteenth century, therefore, responsibility for dealing with the problems associated with mental disease slowly shifted away from traditional structures such as the family or hospitals supported by private philanthropy toward public hospitals under state authority and supported by funding from both state and local government sources.

The increasingly important role of the state in providing institutional facilities for the insane, however, did not come about solely because officials and socially-minded individuals and groups recognized that corporate hospitals could not meet the challenges growing out of this malady. The movement to establish public hospitals was also an expression of a growing concern with problems arising out of and related to poverty, pauperism, disease, and crime, which in turn stimulated the emergence of distinct social policies and institutional structures intended to deal with these issues in the early decades of the century. Formation of welfare policies inevitably involved the mentally ill precisely because of the devastating economic impact of mental disease upon family structure and relationships. This impact was especially pronounced among lower-class and immigrant groups. The high incidence of mental illness among such groups merely magnified the economic consequences of the disease. Public mental hospitals, therefore, were from their very inception part of an institutional complex that dealt with problems arising out of and related to welfare and dependency, a fact that was destined to play a major role in shaping both their internal structure and the external legal, administrative, and financial framework within which they functioned.

Between 1830 and 1860 the numbers of mental hospitals in existence increased rapidly. With a few exceptions, most states had at least one (and some more than one) public institution. Larger urban areas had been impelled by circumstances to found their own hospitals, which increased the number of public institutions. Alongside of these public hospitals existed a number of corporate and proprietary institutions that served affluent groups desiring high-cost quality care. Such institutions reflected at least in part an unwillingness of more affluent groups to use a public system that accepted large numbers of persons from poor and minority groups.

For several decades following 1830 the hopes of those active in the drive to found public mental hospitals seemed to be justified by the results of institutionalization. During these years the patient population tended to come from the same background and environment as psychiatrists. Most mental hospitals accepted relatively few lower-class and minority ethnic groups, if only because such groups as late as 1840 constituted a small percentage of the total population. The fact that hospital populations, especially in the 1830s and 1840s, remained relatively small also contributed to the maintenance of an internal therapeutic atmosphere. In addition, many of the early figures prominent in American psychiatry were individuals who had entered the field because of their humanitarian and religious convictions about being of service to those less fortunate than themselves. In their eyes a hospital superintendency was no different than the calling that led some to enter the ministry or others to spend their lives in combating social evils. Many early superintendents brought to their vocation, therefore, a personality-type that often promoted beneficent personal relationships with patients. The recovery rates of this period – even by the best of contemporary standards – were indeed imposing.

Yet the promises of these early mental hospitals were never fulfilled. Indeed, by the 1870s the mental hospital was itself the object of attack by a new generation of individuals who saw it as a dehumanizing receptacle that had few redeeming attributes. The reasons for this transformation, although complex, are not overly difficult to delineate. By the 1850s a variety of circumstances – few of which had been foreseen – had converged to give rise to an institution that deviated sharply from the ideal type. Superintendents had conceived of their institutions in therapeutic terms; from the very beginning they were forced to accept large numbers of chronic insane persons, who came to constitute a significant proportion of the total patient population. Hospitals were intended to remain small in order to promote the type of relationships deemed conducive to recovery; instead they grew in size, thereby hastening the transition from a charismatic-type hospital to one dominated by administrative concerns. In theory all patients received the same quality of care; in practice class, ethnicity, and race played a significant role in promoting differential care. Conceiving of their own role in medical terms, superintendents were nevertheless rapidly transformed into administrators who were concerned with largely managerial problems; considerations of order and efficiency often overshadowed therapeutic concerns.

Regarded as a self-contained medical institution, the mental hospital was unable to retain any significant degree of isolation from the larger society in which it existed. Public policy remained a legislative responsibility, and hospital officials found that their autonomy was limited in significant ways by the general legal, administrative, and financial environment within which they functioned. The decentralized and pre-bureaucratic nature of mid-nineteenth-century American society inhibited the formulation of consistent policies; hospitals were often caught up in the vortex of change and confusion and saw their therapeutic goals transformed by circumstances beyond the control of their officials. Nor did local governments bring any measure of stability or continuity to policy issues; community control and participation – at least as far as the mentally ill were concerned – were inversely related to quality of care and level of funding. The fact that problems arising out of mental illness were inseparable from the broader issues of dependency also had major implications for hospitals. When many states moved to centralize and rationalize their welfare systems during the last third of the nineteenth century, the net result was to enmesh mental hospitals further in an ambiguous welfare system that alternated between compassion and hostility for dependent persons and groups. Under these circumstances the functions of hospitals remained pluralistic rather than unitary; they continued to care for a heterogeneous patient population that included a significant proportion of poor and indigent persons, chronic cases, old-age groups, individuals deemed dangerous to society or who seemed to require a structured environment, in addition to providing care and treatment for acute cases for relatively brief periods.

If the character of mental hospitals was largely determined by more general social and economic determinants, how then shall we view the role of psychiatry in the care and treatment of the mentally ill? Much of the traditional literature on this subject has always placed concepts of mental illness as the central determinant, and assumed that care and treatment was a natural consequence of theory. Yet I do not think that the evidence justifies such a thesis. Indeed, there is considerable evidence that indicates that theory in many respects played at best a minor role in the development of the mental hospital. If this is true, then we must begin to rethink the manner in which the history of psychiatry has been written. Let me, before closing my remarks, sketch out a somewhat different approach to this fascinating historical problem.

One of the byproducts of the founding of mental hospitals was the beginnings of the professionalization of psychiatry. This fact was of major importance; it meant that psychiatric thought and practice had not played the dominant part in shaping the structure and functions of these institutions. Instead the reverse was true. Psychiatry was to a large extent moulded and shaped by the institutional setting within which it was born and grew to maturity. Many dominant characteristics of psychiatric ideology were but rationalizations of existing conditions within mental hospitals as well as popular attitudes. The mental hospital in its formative years was an institution created by society to cope with abnormal behaviour and to provide care and treatment for a variety of dependent groups; the result was that psychiatry – despite its claim about its scientific and medical character – reflected the role assigned to it by society. This was not to imply that psychiatrists *consciously or deliberately* attempted to define their discipline within such a context, or to justify institutionalization on other than medical grounds. It was only to say that psychiatry, as was true of most professions and institutions, was influenced by its peculiar origins. Having developed within an institutional framework created by society in response to its perception of its needs, psychiatrists inevitably absorbed the validity of those needs into their view and understanding of their profession.

The newly-emerging profession in many ways reflected dominant American values. Psychiatric theory and practice, for example, were not only derivatives of European experiences or the results of disinterested scientific knowledge. On the contrary, theory and practice evolved within a much broader context. Although psychiatrists preferred to conceive of the mental hospital as a strictly medical institution, their analysis of the nature and etiology of mental illness as well as modes of care and treatment were not far removed from the values and social structure of American society.

Let me illustrate this point by glancing briefly at the nature of mid-nineteenth-century American psychiatric thought. Before 1880 the absence of demonstrable etiological concepts or the germ theory of disease led most Americans – laymen and physicians – to interpret health as a consequence of a proper and orderly relationship between nature, society, and the individual. Disease followed the violation of the natural laws that governed human behaviour and was indissolubly linked with filth, immorality, and improper living conditions. Health, on the other hand, was synonymous with virtue and order. While such concepts were suitable to sanitary reform and general preventive measures, they offered little guidance when it came to providing treatment for specific diseases. The prevailing emphasis on health, therefore, reflected an inability to deal with disease *per se*. The resulting therapeutic nihilism was further strengthened by the impact of French medicine and the application of the numerical method of Pierre Louis, which demonstrated the ineffectiveness of most traditional remedies.

The specific definition of mental disease was similar in nature; insanity followed the violation of the natural laws that governed human behaviour. Therapy involved the recreation of a healthy and moral environment (i.e. moral management or moral treatment). Yet the theory of moral treatment often tended to be vague and abstract; it meant different things to different psychiatrists. Under these circumstances the mental hospital – precisely because of the diffuse nature of medical theory and its inability to provide firm guidelines – was particularly susceptible to nonmedical influences, including dominant social values as well as changing attitudes and practices toward dependent groups generally.

An analysis of mid-nineteenth-century etiological concepts is revealing in this respect. Most psychiatrists divided the causes of insanity into two distinct classes – physical and moral. The first arose out of organic changes, while the latter grew out of the influence of external environmental influences on the brain (the organ of the mind). Without doubt most psychiatrists were far more interested in the moral causes of mental illness, partly because of their own commitment to prevention and partly because these seemed to account for the largest proportion of cases. As men who were firm believers in the tenets of organized religion, they felt much freer in their discussions of morality than they did in their observations on pathology. The moral causes of insanity included – to cite only a few examples – intemperance, overwork, domestic difficulties, excessive ambition, faulty education, personal disappointments, jealousy, pride, and above all, the pressures of an urban, industrial, and commercial civilization (which was not natural to the human organism). Psychiatrists, in other words, saw mental illness as the inevitable consequence of behaviour that represented a departure from universally accepted social norms. In many ways their beliefs were not fundamentally dissimilar from other critics of American society whose own values were hostile to social and economic changes and who resented the newly-emerging urban-industrial order. A substantial part of psychiatric theory, therefore, was but a reflection of a particular social ideology, but presented as empirical fact.

The character of mid-nineteenth-century American psychiatric thought was not due to accident or chance; it arose rather out of a combination of circumstances. Psychiatrists, it should be noted, tended to share common values because most were from similar backgrounds. Of 81 persons who served as superintendents of insane hospitals before 1875, no less than 34 (42 per cent) were from New England, while an additional 21 (25 per cent) were from Pennsylvania and New York. The overwhelming majority were Protestant, and most had been born and raised in small towns or rural areas; only five came from a major urban centre. Most had grown up in small communities where they imbibed traditional Protestant values and an agrarian and antiurban outlook. It was natural for these men to see mental disease as the inevitable consequence of the violation of the immutable natural laws that governed humanity. Understandably, they defined these laws in terms of the life-style of their own social class.

Nor did their experiences with the mentally ill in any way contradict their own values and beliefs. Insane persons, after all, *did* behave in odd and bizarre ways. Many had been ill for years and had spent extended periods of time in jails and almshouses before being transferred to public hospitals, an experience that undoubtedly influenced their behaviour. Some were filthy; some were violent; some showed little concern either for themselves or others; and most were poor or indigent. A significant proportion after 1850 were from minority ethnic groups; in New England the Irish occupied a disproportionately high percentage of hospital beds. To many superintendents it seemed as though these persons were paying the inevitable price for their strange and aberrant ways and their apparent refusal to follow time-honoured and traditional modes of behaviour. Such attitudes, of course, were by no means unique to psychiatrists, but were rather characteristic of large numbers of their countrymen from similar backgrounds.

The important point to grasp, then, is that the evolution of psychiatric thought and practice did not occur independently of general social and economic forces. The emergence of psychiatry as a profession, as a matter of fact, did not imply a rejection or a questioning of contemporary trends. Indeed, quite the opposite was true. Psychiatrists affirmed many of the dominant features of the developing institutional complex caring for the mentally ill largely because their own training and experience had taken place within the existing structure. The emergence of a psychiatric profession, then, did little to impede and in some respects hastened the trend toward institutional care and the identification of mental illness within the more general framework of welfare and dependency.

The history of the mental hospital in nineteenth-century America offers an illustrative case study of the ironies and ambiguities posed by complex social problems and the reaction of a society to these problems. Convinced of their moral obligation to help those individuals afflicted with mental disease, a group of reformers set to work to found a comprehensive system of public institutions to provide care and therapy and therefore help to eliminate or to contain once and for all this dreaded malady. While they succeeded in their efforts to found hospitals, they were never fully aware of the fact that within a brief period of time the care and treatment of the mentally ill would become inextricably intertwined with broader problems of welfare and dependency as well as conflicting attitudes and values on the part of society, psychiatrists, and patients. The mental hospital in its early years was simply conceived of as an institution that would help all groups; it was not intended in any way to provide differential or discriminatory care. Within a short period of time, however, other factors – most of which could not have been predicted or anticipated – all converged to transform the state mental hospital into more of a welfare-type institution. In this sense the mental hospital reflected the broad dimensions of the larger society in which it existed, with all of the strengths – as well as the weaknesses and shortcomings – of that society.

ACKNOWLEDGEMENT

I wish to thank the National Institute of Mental Health (HEW) for supporting my research on this subject by Grant MH–17859. The first volume of my Mental Institutions in America: Social Policy to 1875 (New York: The Free Press, 1973), covers the subject matter of this paper in detail.

P. J. Dowling and W. K. Tomlinson
New Orleans, Louisiana (U.S.A.)

The role of cultural minorities in the decline of moral treatment – a recurring pattern in American psychiatry

Since 1956, the year in which Bockoven first published those papers which were the precursors to his book (1963) *Moral Treatment in American Psychiatry*, there has been a steady interest in the psychiatry of the early nineteenth century in the United States. Both Grob (1966) and Caplan (1969) have traced the development and decline of that short-lived movement which had successfully wedded the ideals of Tuke and Pinel in the hospital treatment of mental illness.

Although the demise of an apparently successful treatment modality always remains somewhat enigmatic to succeeding generations, all of the writers mentioned have been acutely aware that the decline of moral treatment in psychiatry was in some way related to the waves of poor Irish refugees from the potato famine of the 1840s, refugees who reached American shores barely a quarter of a century after the founding of the Friends' Asylum, the first American hospital modelled on the institution at York. There were of course other factors which contributed to the decline of these hospitals: industrialization, the rise of the cities, changing community attitudes and the breakdown of the small, rural communities on which the early American Republic had been based.

Financial problems had plagued the hospitals from the beginning. The most prestigious of them, the Worcester State Hospital in Massachusetts, was publicly funded, and the ebb and flow of money which was intimately tied to the capricious waves of public opinion profoundly influenced the early history of that institution. Yet, mental hospitals have a way of being ivory towers and it was not inevitable that the system should have collapsed on the basis of those other pressures, so adequately treated by Caplan in her book.

The authors will attempt to show in this paper that the presence of Irish patients in these hospitals, and in particular in the Worcester State Hospital, introduced a situation antithetical to the climate in which moral treatment could be practised and which almost certainly would have led to its downfall, even in the absence of those other outside pressures. Worcester State Hospital, of major importance in the history of this movement because its superintendent, Samuel Woodward, was the acknowledged leader of the profession in his day, will be used as an example of the process which was taking place all over the country as the system declined.

Moral treatment, as it was applied to American psychiatry, was as Bockoven has commented, never clearly defined in the nineteenth century but in a general sense, 'it meant compassionate and understanding treatment . . .'. In its Quaker origins, it was based strongly upon Christian ideals of charity, while, through Pinel, it inherited the French revolutionary notions of the dignity, rights and brotherhood of men.

As it was actually practised in the United States, however, it had a special character all its own. Ideally, it strove for a re-creation within the hospital setting of the compact and interdependent social structure of the early American village, with its emphasis on the extended family. At Worcester, it was the paternalistic, New England family which served as the model of the hospital structure. The enumeration of 'Our Family' which was sent each year by the superintendent as part of the annual report to the trustees, included not only patients and staff but even the children of staff members. Whatever each man's reason was for being at the hospital, and many murderers were admitted in those first years at Worcester, each was treated as humanely as possible. Restraint and seclusion were rare, physical punishment unheard of. Kindness was the order of the day. The attendants were instructed to listen sympathetically to their charges, to condemn little but to divert the patient from morbid and unhealthful topics. Woodward himself, in the years of his tenure as superintendent, met with the patients frequently, listened, advised, and kept records of these meetings which would be the envy of many a modern clinician.

The buildings and grounds of these hospitals reflected the humanistic philosophy. Again, Worcester was typical. Set on a hill in rural Massachusetts, its view of the countryside was spectacular. Spacious grounds were available to the patients for recreation and the sleeping accommodation was designed to be comfortable, although almost from the beginning it was clear that the facilities, as they were designed, would be inadequate to meet the demand for services.

In line with the emphasis on the dignity of each patient, the use of knives and forks was encouraged, a striking innovation at the time; for those patients engaged in manual work, sharp tools were allowed when necessary. Each patient's stay was filled, as far as possible, with diverting activities, not the least of which was the regular attendance at church services. The hospital chaplain, a member of the dominant Protestant sect, was also a leading member of the therapeutic team.

In short, the attempt was made, in the words of Dr. Pliny Earle (1845), '. . . to treat the patients, so far as their condition will possibly admit, as if they were still in the enjoyment of the healthy exercise of their mental faculties . . . make their condition as boarders as comfortable as possible . . . to extend them the privilege or the right, of as much liberty, as much freedom from personal restraint as is compatible with their safety . . . the courtesies of civilized and social life are not to be forgotten . . . as a means of effecting restoration to mental health'.

Such a programme of treatment, as can be readily seen, depends on certain assumptions. First was the assumption of cultural homogeneity. Only a staff which shared the patients' culture could understand that culture and truly recreate it within the hospital setting. Second was the assumption of mutual trust. Although everyone was aware that there were certain situations in which the mentally ill could not be trusted, it was assumed that the dangers they posed were due to their illness, and that in the absence of illness, they would exercise freedom much as the staff itself exercised freedom. Third, there was the assumption of mutual regard. The authors found no mention in the literature for a means of dealing with a genuine dislike for a patient. In short, although a great deal of attention was paid to the patients, their feeling, their pathology and their social backgrounds, little if any attention was paid to the feelings, the short-comings or the biases of the staff.

It was into this setting that the Irish began arriving in the 1840s.

1846 was the year of crisis. For the Irish, it was the beginning of the potato famine. Though there had been a steady trickle of immigration from Ireland since colonial times, by the 1840s they had begun to make a serious impact on the predominantly Anglo-Saxon country, though the number of yearly immigrants had not yet exceeded 100,000, as it was to do in the following year.

Worcester State Hospital received only twelve Irish patients before the beginning of 1846, but in that year, the first of the superintendency of Dr. George Chandler, thirty-four foreign patients were admitted, most of them Irish. The number continued to grow, so that when Chandler identified Irish admissions in 1854, he found that ninety-six had been admitted that year to the hospital. It is difficult to estimate more accurate figures, since the usual term 'foreign born' in the statistical summaries of the hospital years rarely separate Irish from other foreign born. It is known, however, that the numbers continued to grow and that, in addition, a significantly lower discharge rate of the Irish led to a pool of chronic, pauper insane of Irish extraction.

The hospital community reacted almost immediately to the presence of the Irish. The reasons for the reaction, in retrospect, can only be speculated about. In addition to the usual economic and religious explanation usually put forth, we must add the obvious fact that these uneducated paupers with their alien religion and dialect obviously did not fit into the mental hospital 'family' with its Puritan rigidity and narrowness. The forms the response took were multiple, and will form the bulk of the remainder of this paper.

First there was the *ethnic stereotype*. Stereotypes are, of course, a common and necessary part of human society. The flattering stereotype of the middle class New England farmer had given impetus to moral treatment in psychiatry in the first place. By 1846, we begin to see unflattering stereotypes of the Irish patient emerging in the case records. In February of that year, for example, a seventeen-year-old Irish girl named Briget was transferred in chains from an almshouse. She was described on admission as very violent. Two days later Chandler wrote, 'This girl begins to show a little Irish spunk, refuses to take food, and is unwilling to have anything done for her . . . (she has not yet been very troublesome)'. This stereotype is not particularly unfriendly and it should be noted that this girl was discharged five months later, apparently recovered.

With time, these stereotypes became more and more negative, and the phrase 'filthy in personal habits' is frequently seen in the records of patients identified as Irish or Catholic.

More serious than the actual use of the stereotype is its implication for prognosis. In 1847, in his report to the trustees, Chandler was outspoken in his pessimism. 'The want of forethought in them,' he wrote, 'to save their earnings for the day of sickness, the indulgence of their appetite for stimulating drinks which are too easily obtained among us, and their strong love for their native land which is characteristic with them, are the fruitful causes of insanity among them. As a class, we are not so successful with our treatment of them as with the native population of New England.

It is difficult to obtain their confidence, for they seem to be jealous of our motives; and the embarrassment they are under for not clearly comprehending our language, is another obstacle in the way of recovery.'

The message was clearly heard by the trustees, who in the same years reported to the State Legislature that 'the increase of foreigners is an evil the more to be regretted because there is reason to fear it may be, still further, an increase of incurables . . . their misery, their ignorance, and their jealousy stand in the way of their improvement in the hospital'.

So the prejudice was there, and was clearly stated in both the case records and the annual reports. Ignorance, nostalgia and intemperance, widely believed to be predispositions to insanity, were part of the Irish stereotype, yet no observation was probably so damning to the frugal New Englander as the comment in the Seventeenth Annual Report, 'the expenses here of the Irish are never, I believe, paid by themselves'. In the end, this was to be the undoing of the Irish and of moral treatment.

Yet the ethnic prejudice, as blatant as it was, was not something with which Chandler and the board of trustees were ever very comfortable. In the first place, as Chandler said in his first report, 'to afford an asylum for the destitute and insane was among the designs of the founders of this hospital'. In 1848, apparently as an answer to criticism of his outspoken comments the year before, he stated that 'in this hospital, no distinction to their prejudice is made between them [the Irish] and those who are more favored in their place of nativity'.

Second there was staff *insensitivity*. As the ethnic bias against the Irish became increasingly hostile with the passage of time, it became apparent that no provisions would be made for their special needs. Despite the staff turnover of nearly one-third per year, there is no indication during the period of Chandler's administration, that is the period of the decline of moral treatment, that Irish were recruited as attendants.

More importantly, one searches in vain for any sign of empathy with the religious position of the Irish. Attendance at Chapel was a compulsory part of the hospital routine. The hospital chaplain was a Unitarian, and the forms of worship were distinctly Protestant. For the rigidly Catholic Irish immigrant, this must have posed a particular hardship, not only because he was cast into a situation totally unfamiliar to him, perhaps personally offensive, but also because at that period of the nineteenth century taking part in Protestant worship services carried with it serious ecclesiastical penalties, and might even entail excommunication. Among the mentally ill, often already tortured by feelings of guilt, this was certainly antitherapeutic. In addition, the religion of the Irish was often regarded as in itself a possible cause of mental illness. Thus, their religious feelings were not only ignored, but were viewed as positively harmful.

In addition, family ties of the Irish patient were largely ignored. In the early reports, repeated mention is made of the absence of stable families in whose care they could be discharged. This was undoubtedly true of some, perhaps most, but there is no mention in the patient records of attempts to contact relatives. The Catholic Church, which might have served as a resource in this regard, was never called upon.

The ignorance, poverty and deprivation of the Irish patients was ascribed to the fact that they had, in the words of Edward Jarvis, a commissioner who reported to the Legislature in 1854, 'less sensibility and fewer wants to be ratified to than the Americans, and that they more commonly failed to supply them. There is also a greater irritability; they are more readily disturbed when they find themselves at variance with the circumstances about them, and less easily reconciled to difficulties they cannot overcome.' This attitude which confused deprivation with lack of sensibility reflected the common feeling of the hospital establishment.

The corollary was not long in being acted upon. When it was understood that the Irish could not appreciate, because of their insensitivity, the humane treatment central to moral psychiatry, then that humane treatment was abandoned. Crowding, neglect and finally the common use of restraint replaced the patient understanding which had been Woodward's ideal. For the Irish, moral psychiatry ended almost as soon as it had begun.

Third there was *rejection*. The economic dependency of the Irish was their most damning attribute in the eyes of the Anglo-Saxon American. Many had been admitted from almshouses, while others were '. . . found wandering about either accidentally or with the assistance of others in the immediate vicinity of the institution, in a state of violent insanity and great destitution . . .', as Chandler wrote in 1846. Since they had no money for their own support, the State assumed liability for the non-resident patients, and since about two-thirds of the pauper insane were foreign born and therefore not the responsibility of an individual community, the cost had to be borne by the State Legislature.

As the antipathy toward the Irish grew within Massachusetts state politics, it was generally expressed in economic terms. Cheaper ways were sought to deal with pauper insane, particularly the Irish. Theoretically, the hospital had acquired at an early date the right to transfer patients back to jails and houses of correction. It was not until the establishment of the state almshouses in 1852, and later the Act of 1856 permitting the transfer of pauper insane to the state almshouses, that the Irish were expelled from the hospital in large numbers, after being given 'a fair trial of treatment'. Examining the patient records of the 1850s, one finds such notations as 'transferred by executive order', or 'discharged for want of room', appearing repeatedly in the records of patients identified as Irish. At the same time, middle class, native-born patients were kept in the hospitals for years at a time, often in a state of incurable illness. The records, which became increasingly sparse during the early 1850s, sometimes completely failed to note the progress of the Irish patient. Thus, for economic reasons, the Irish were systematically removed from the hospital, and an attempt was made to stabilize the ratio of Irish to native-born patients within the hospital.

The final response of the hospital community to the Irish patient was *segregation*. In addition to the economic reasons for getting rid of the Irish, there was from the beginning uneasiness about the possible effect their presence might have on the native-born insane. As the annual report of 1854 stated, 'Among the insane of this State are wives and daughters, widows and orphans, farmers, mechanics, ministers, schoolmasters and the like. These women were taught in our public schools, trained in our proverbial neat and orderly households, and accustomed to cultivated society . . . now, they do not lose their sensibilities by becoming insane, and they ought not to have them wounded by being herded together in the same apartment with persons whose language, whose habits, and whose manners, offend and shock them. Besides, such associations do not promote the good of any patient, but may retard, and perhaps prevent, the cure of some.'

As early as 1848, serious consideration was given to Dr. Luther Bell's suggestion of a separate hospital for Irish patients, administered by an Irish superintendent, but the suggestion was finally dropped, presumably because the legislative committee investigating the problems at Worcester felt it to be in conflict with the national ideal of a 'melting pot'. The pressure for separation continued, patients became increasingly classified according to their ethnic background and socio-economic standing, and finally, shortly after Dr. Merritt Beemus succeeded Chandler in 1856, he initiated a system of separation of those '. . . of low and degraded propensities and filthy habits' from those of 'neat and orderly habits'. This was an economic decision, in that the actual separation was of state paupers, overwhelmingly Irish, from those who were economically not clearly stated, '. . . segregation at Worcester was really based on unconscious class antipathies and feelings.'

With segregation, there is no question that the Irish were finally reduced to the status of custodial patients and what therapeutic skills the hospitals had left were directed at the native born. By this time, the hospital had, however, clearly become demoralized and ideals on which moral treatment had been built were shattered.

This paper is both a record of historical fact and a modern parable. The Irish found themselves in a new land, and when they became mentally ill, they were sent to a mental hospital as effective as any that had ever been built, and yet the meeting, far from being therapeutic, was destructive both to the Irish and to the system from which they sought help, not because of what the Irish were, or because of what they needed, but because of what they were thought to be. The distortions and biases, the loss of enthusiasm, the displacement of class antipathies to hard questions of finances, and the rationalization used to cover irrational bias, all combined to destroy the climate in which good psychiatric treatment could take place.

In the United States, we are faced with a similar problem today. In the late 1940s and early 1950s, the system of state mental hospitals underwent a series of reforms that rescued them from being nearly custodial institutions. The early experiences of Woodward and his colleagues were influential in these reforms. They resembled moral psychiatry and emphasis on the humane treatment of patients. With the discovery of major tranquillizers, further systems of mental health clinics was established, initially an excellent system which combined the use of medication with various forms of psychotherapy in order to provide aftercare and support for many newly discharged hospital patients, and to provide an alternative to hospitalization for others of the mentally ill.

And then came the blacks. The reforms of the 1940s and 1950s had been largely oriented to middle class white America, as had the community mental health clinic movement of the 1960s. The blacks just didn't fit. Many of the clinics made a good start in accommodating them. Fewer actually succeeded, but as recent reports now show, mental hospital population is again rising and the system, still managed largely by the white middle class, is showing serious signs of deficiency.

Perhaps a review of the parallel situation of the Irish in the mental hospitals in the 1840s and 1850s with the added objectivity of the historical, casts light on what is happening today.

Bibliography

BOCKOVEN, J. S., *Moral Treatment in American Psychiatry*, New York, Springer, 1963.
CAPLAN, RUTH B., *Psychiatry and the Community in Nineteenth Century America*, New York, London, Basic Books, 1969.
GROB, GERALD, *The State and the Mentally Ill*, Durham, The University of North Carolina Press, 1966.
Case Records of the Worcester State Hospital.
Annual Reports to the Trustees, Worcester State Hospital.
Annual Reports of the Trustees to the State Legislature, Worcester State Hospital.

R. A. Chase
Baltimore, Maryland (U.S.A.)

A new programme of undergraduate instruction in psychiatry

During the 1969–70 academic year, the Department of Psychiatry and Behavioral Sciences, under the direction of Professor Joel Elkes, revised the Introductory Program in Psychiatry and Behavioral Sciences required of all medical students in their first year of full-time studies at the Johns Hopkins University School of Medicine. It is the purpose of this paper to review the character of the revisions undertaken, and, in so doing, to identify some of the concerns that moved us to effect these revisions.

The concerns that underly the design of this teaching programme are very broad. We are concerned about man – his normal processes of growth and development – of competent and adaptive behaviours – and the failures and misfortunes that produce pain and suffering, physical and psychological, alone and in groups. And so, in addition to the traditional objectives of developing skills in the diagnosis and treatment of patients with disordered behaviour, we are increasingly concerned with the growth of skills relevant to the understanding and repair of pathology in human groups, including large social systems. Concerns about war and peace have prompted the design of classes intended to enlarge our understanding of the conditions under which men fight, and the conditions under which aggression can be brought under constructive control. Concerns about the fragility of the earth and its unique life systems have prompted the design of classes dealing with population dynamics, pollution ecology, the evolution of urban settlements, and human behaviour and environmental design. Concerns about the growing inventory of ethical dilemmas that confront late twentieth-century man have led us to consideration of the conditions that enlarge opportunities for social justice and social equality; the conditions that, for our time, enhance the quality and character of the lives of communities as well as individuals.

It is now clear that students of human biology are under great pressure to develop increasing competence in dealing with the special problems of human survival and human welfare that have been given urgent definition during the past few decades. A considerable effort is made to achieve clarification of the responsibilities and opportunities that present to students of human biology in general, and human behaviour in particular, as a result of the accelerated pattern of social change that increasingly characterizes our time.

The programme is organized around the following major topic or problem areas:

1. Introduction to Psychiatry and the Behavioral Sciences. Designers: Dr. Richard Allen Chase and Dr. Joel Elkes.
2. Ontogeny of Behavior. Designer: Dr. Richard Allen Chase.
3. Principles of Behavior Analysis and Behavior Modification. Designer: Dr. Joseph V. Brady.
4. Human Sexual Behavior. Designer: Dr. John Money.
5. Conflict, Violence and Aggression. Designer: Dr. Jerome D. Frank.
6. Human Ecology. Designer: Dr. Bruce L. Welch.
7. Topics in Clinical Psychiatry. Designer: Dr. Jerome D. Frank.

A. ONTOGENY OF BEHAVIOUR

The first section of the programme deals with the development of behaviour, and is designed to make clear that behaviour changes over time, and that, at each stage in the historical development of an individual, behaviour has multiple determinants.

The section begins with a series of lectures on behaviour genetics, developmental neurology and developmental neuropsychology. These presentations make clear the essential inseparability of the biological and psychological determinants of the structure of human behaviour. Speech and language acquisition and the development of gender identity constitute cases that are examined in some depth in order to reinforce the point that the student of human behaviour must constantly deal with a critical synthesis of biological and psychological data.

Efforts to achieve skill in the observation of human behaviour have resulted in a large-scale exercise that allows students to observe parallel demonstrations of the behaviour repertoires of infants and young children through the age range of several months to five years. Each examination station provides opportunities to observe the behaviours of children in different age groups. As the students move from one examination station to the next they observe the sequential growth in the repertoire of human behaviour through the first five years of life.

The crucial importance of the supporting social environment for the growth and development of the human infant is considered through study of the organization and activities of a comprehensive parent-child centre programme involving day care, parent education, and home visit activities.

Finally, the problems and methods of child psychiatry are outlined against the broad background of information about normal growth and development outlined above. We feel that the heavy emphasis that has been placed on the vulnerability of the human organism during the early years of life has not been sufficiently complemented by an appreciation of the far reaches of human behavioural potential and the significance of early experience in the realization of that potential.

B. PRINCIPLES OF BEHAVIOUR ANALYSIS AND BEHAVIOUR MODIFICATION

This section places emphasis upon the observable interaction between organism and environment. Objective definition of the characteristics of such interaction provides the basis for distinguishing major classes of behavioural events and for differentiating relationships between behavioural events and their controlling influences. This approach to the analysis of the conditions under which specific behaviours occur provides an opportunity to construct an enlarging inventory of relationships between environmental events and observable behaviours. Skill in this type of observation is clearly relevant to the diagnostic and therapeutic mission in psychiatry. Observation of the conditions under which specific behaviours occur is facilitated by acquisition of the technical language that has been developed by students of human operant behaviour. Principles related to behaviour acquisition, strengthening, weakening, maintenance, and control are presented and illustrated through film presentations and animal experiments conducted in the lecture hall. The applications of information derived from the experimental analysis of behaviour to problems of behaviour modification in man are given close attention. Clinical case presentations are used to supplement the teaching of behaviour modification techniques.

In recent years there has been a growing concern about the ethics of behaviour control. This concern has, quite properly, influenced thinking and action in psychiatry. To date, the medical students have been more concerned about the ethics of behaviour modification than the faculty has been and, as a result, this question has frequently been on a 'hidden agenda' that influences discussion in the classroom. We have decided to place the question on the formal agenda. Accordingly, a panel consisting of members of the faculty and students will address itself as a body, and in conversation with the entire class, to broad questions of ethics as they apply to judgments about behaviour modification and the selection of methods for behaviour modification.

C. HUMAN SEXUAL BEHAVIOUR

This section has as its major objectives the development of an attitude of nonjudgmentalism on the part of the student as he approaches the study of human sexual behaviour coupled with an enlarged understanding of the biological and psychological determinants of individual patterns of gender identity and sexual behaviour. We have found that the examination of the full-spectrum of visual images of sex, through use of slides and motion picture films, assists the development of an attitude of nonjudgmentalism. We attempt to develop a broad appreciation of normal behaviour development as a background against which pathology can be studied more objectively and more critically. Genetic, prenatal hormonal and experiential determinants of gender identity are explored, and clinical cases in which gender identity is ambiguous are studied in support of that exploration. The natural history of love relationships is explored for our own dominant culture and subcultures, as well as other sharply contrasting cultures. Principles of sexual interviewing are reviewed, and homosexual behaviour is studied from the vantage point of genetics, hormonal influences on sexual behaviour, cultural influences on sexual behaviour, as well as sociological and political thought.

We have invited advocates of special interest groups, and adversaries of some traditional medical positions concerning human sexual behaviour to address the class. Groups representing the Women's Liberation Movement and the Gay Liberation Movement have addressed students in the programme. Both presentations resulted in substantial, and most welcomed controversy.

D. CONFLICT, VIOLENCE AND AGGRESSION

Dr. Jerome Frank notes in his introductory statement to this section of the programme:

Programs of violent behavior, with accompanying states of emotional arousal that are triggered by specific environmental stimuli are built into the nervous systems of all living creatures, including man. Humans are the only creatures, however, that indulge in cruelty – the infliction of suffering for its own sake; commit premeditated murder; and wage war on their own kind. These behaviors have high survival value for both the individual and the group in some circumstances. The unique instrumental capacities and symbolic powers of humans, however have enabled them to create genocidal weapons and use them on each other in quarrels over values and ideals as well as territories and resources. As a result, the human propensity toward violence now endangers the continuance of the species.
Prevention of certain forms of violence in individuals and treatment of their consequences have always been legitimate concerns of physicians. Prominent examples are suicide (self-directed violence), epileptic furors, paranoid panics and man-inflicted injuries. Although physicians have assumed responsibility for combatting threats to the public's health such as pestilence and famine, they have ignored collective violence such as war as a health menace for many reasons. Among them may be that although war has always been an important cause of injury and death to circumscribed groups over short periods of time, as a general cause of mortality it has never even approached epidemics and starvation. Now, for the first time, man has become by far the greatest menace to his own survival. Does this have implications for the physician's responsibilities?[1]

The section on human aggression begins with a lecture on aggressive behaviour in animal societies. Aggression in human societies is then explored, and the roles of group expectations and relative deprivations are examined as determinants of collective violence. Determinants of normal patterns of individual violence such as child-rearing practices, imitation and obedience provide a background for the study of pathological violence in the individual. Psychopathic behaviour patterns are examined in detail. A panel of prisoners and ex-prisoners discusses with the class experiences within the prison system, as well as relevant aspects of preceding individual life histories.

The section is completed with a lecture on sources of international conflict that seeks to identify psychological instigators and exacerbators of international conflict.

E. HUMAN ECOLOGY

Students of biology have joined with students of social behaviour and social institutions in showing increasing concern about enlarging our understanding of interactions in life systems. The section on human ecology begins with lectures outlining, in evolutionary perspective, the natural history of human populations in relationship with their environments. Specific effects of social and physical environments on patterns of psychophysiological response are examined next. Emphasis is placed on alterations in neuroendocrine, neurochemical, and neuropharmacological responses.

Population ecology constitutes a case study that is developed in depth, including consideration of the dynamics of human population growth, and the prospects for the control of human population numbers. The section concludes with a series of case studies on the design of physical environments intended to support specific patterns of behaviour. Applications of information about human behaviour to the design of inner city neighbourhoods are explored in collaboration with members of the research division of the Department of Planning for the City of Baltimore.

F. TOPICS IN CLINICAL PSYCHIATRY

A series of topics in clinical psychiatry is introduced by broad consideration of the ways in which mental illness is defined, both within medicine, and by culture and society. We consider it essential that medical students gain, from the start, an appreciation of the diversity of human behaviour repertoires and the importance of viewing the behaviour of an individual within a social context. The same topography of behaviour may be maladaptive in one social context, and adaptive in another, even for the same individual. The growth of sensitivity to the diversity of human behaviour and adaptational models for viewing mental illness can produce considerable discomfort in students seeking explicit and unalterable criteria for the diagnosis of disorders of behaviour. It is helpful to remind these students that we are not without anchor points for evaluation of mental health and mental illness, even in the context of the changing social fields within which human behaviour expresses itself. Introducing the concept of 'freedom' has been useful in this regard. The concept of freedom is expressed in just this manner by Dr. Lawrence S. Kubie in the following quotation.

> The measure of health is flexibility, the freedom to learn through experience, the freedom to change with changing internal and external circumstances, to be influenced by reasonable argument, admonitions, exhortation, and the appeal to emotions; the freedom to respond appropriately to the stimulus of reward and punishment, and especially the freedom to cease when sated. The essence of normality is flexibility in all of these vital ways. The essence of illness is the freezing of behavior into unalterable and insatiable patterns. It is this which characterizes every manifestation of psychopathology. . . .[2]

The following topics define the series of classes on clinical psychiatry: introduction to mental illness, psychodynamics of neuroses, family therapy, drug abuse and alcoholism, the dying patient, suicide, crisis intervention, the mental status examination, interdisciplinary approaches to the diagnosis and treatment of children with multiple handicaps, behavioural effects of focal brain disease, behavioural effects of diffuse brain disease, epilepsy, schizophrenia, the affective disorders, the organization of health care services, and the role of the humanities in the practice of medicine.

At the present time, medical students in the United States are very concerned about the delivery of high-quality medical care. Accordingly, they are intent upon developing practical skills and knowledge relevant to clearly-identified clinical responsibilities. At the same time, we have found students and faculty to be tolerant and supportive of the innovative components of the programme, that have been largely shaped by a growing concern about the integration of Medicine and Biology with the Social Sciences.

References

1 FRANK, J. D., 'Introduction to aggression and violence', in Richard A. Chase, Linda J. Ryan and Peggy S. Baker (eds.), *Course Outline: Year II Program in Psychiatry and Behavioural Sciences*, Baltimore, Maryland, Department of Psychiatry and Behavioural Sciences, The Johns Hopkins University School of Medicine, 1972.

2 KUBIE, L. S., *Neurotic Distortion of the Creative Process*, New York, Noonday Press, 1965.

W. K. Tomlinson and P. J. Dowling
New Orleans, Louisiana (U.S.A.)

The 'medical model' concept in psychiatry: a classical heritage

Recently there has been growing interest in the history of the evolution of psychiatric thought. Ellenberger's[1] study of the development of the concept of the unconscious, as well as other recent publications, reflect the shift of interest from the history of the practice of psychiatry to the history of its theory. Such a shift is not surprising in view of the fact that psychiatry, perhaps more than any other specialty, remains under the domination of its theoretical systems. Such studies as we have mentioned provide a valuable service, in as much as historical perspectives may be of considerable assistance in helping to clarify and define those conceptual and methodological conflicts which have their roots within the theoretical development of the specialty.

I. PURPOSE

The purpose of this paper is essentially two-fold. First, it focuses attention on the Hellenistic period in medicine, when Alexandrian medicine dominated the thinking of the Roman world. Many of the basic assumptions still prevailing in Western psychiatric thought have their origins firmly rooted in that era. Secondly, the authors hope to demonstrate that a study of the medical authorship of the period demonstrates the implicit existence of the 'medical model' for psychiatric illness, a model in which mental disorders are defined as being a definite morbid process having a characteristic group of symptoms with specific etiology, clinical course, and prognosis. This model, which has been widely criticized and has been under attack for several decades since the beginning of the psychoanalytic movement, will be shown to be intimately related not only to concepts of mental disease that we have inherited from the Hellenistic physicians, but also to conventions of diagnosis which are still widely used.

II. METHOD

Fortunately, for the modern historian the compositions of the era under consideration have provided us with textbooks which are strikingly parallel in their form and clinical data. Although these works have not survived intact, it is possible, by collating them and collecting the available clinical data, to reconstruct the conclusions drawn from that data. This is true even when the works being collated represent antagonistic points of medical view.

The authors who we will be primarily interested in will be Soranus of Ephesus and Aretaeus of Cappodocia. Both studied at Alexandria, and both travelled to Rome where they had highly successful medical practices. Both wrote medical works on *Acute and Chronic Diseases*,[2,3] parallel works which reflect the opposing schools of thought. We have passed over other authors of the general era, such as Celsus[4] and Galen, because they are either foreign to the medical traditions of the time, as in the case of Celsus, or, as with Galen, too confusing theoretically to be of much value to us today.

III. ETIOLOGY AND PATHOGENESIS

Rational medicine, as opposed to folk medicine and magic, is based on the concept that illnesses are caused, that they have a specific etiology, and that they develop in a specific pattern. The concepts of causation, presuppose, in their turn, underlying assumptions about the nature of the universe.

Both Soranus, who was a Methodist, and Aretaeus who was a Pneumatist, shared deep roots in the philosophical system of Democritus, the early Greek philosopher, who had answered the age-old problem of change by theorizing that nothing ever essentially changes, but that the universe is made up of unchanging atoms of infinitesimal size, which are constantly being rearranged. This system was passed down almost intact to the Epicureans of the Hellenistic period, and consequently the Methodist School of Medicine, which was related philosophically to Epicureanism. It was also adopted in a somewhat modified form by the Stoics, strongly influencing the Pneumatist School of which Aretaeus was an adherent.

The system of Democritus and its Hellenistic expression were thoroughly materialistic. Anything real was made up of atoms. For the Stoics even quality consisted in collections of atomic particles. The soul, including the entire mental apparatus, was thought of as exquisitely subtle atoms of fire joining together the other atoms of the body. The Pneuma of the Stoics was also a 'firey substance' rather than a breath of ordinary air as the name would suggest.

This materialism was highly useful from the psychiatric point of view, because it eliminated the need for the duality of body and mind which has plagued psychiatric theory through the centuries. Thus, when we read in Aretaeus that, 'in certain of these cases, there is neither flatulence nor black bile, but mere anger and grief, and sad dejection of mind; these were called melancholics, because the term "bile" (*chole*) and "anger" (*arge*) are synonymous in import and likewise "black" (*melanina*), with "much" (*polle*) and "furious" (*theriodes*)', this must be taken to read literally, and not to mean, as some recent writers have claimed, that he was aware of both psychological and physical causes of the illness, but rather that he was unable to discern any differences between the two, and that anger and bile refer to identical substances.

As representatives of opposing schools of medicine, Aretaeus and Soranus could disagree over whether the etiology of the illnesses they saw was due to constriction and relaxation of the pores or to an incorrect mixture of heat and cold, but they shared a number of assumptions about etiology and pathogenesis which were direct corollaries of the philosophical system they also shared. These assumptions can be summarized as follows: (1) Mental illness is a physical condition with physical causes.

(2) Etiology represents the addition, subtraction or dislocation of discreet and unchanging physical particles. Because no change takes place in the particles themselves, pathogenesis is always reversible, at least in theory. (3) Because mental illness and its causes are physical entities, they must have locations somewhere within the body.

These assumptions, so modern in their implications, though arising from the general philosophical milieu, place mental illness totally within the province of medicine. They represent the epitome of the medical model of etiology in Western medicine.

IV. DIAGNOSIS

Veith[5] has correctly observed that the Greco-Roman physicians had no terms such as 'nosology' or 'nosography' for the description and classification of disease. They did, however, inherit from Greek philosophy a well-developed logic of categories. The idea, crudely stated, is to divide the universe into discreet packages with nothing left over. The four elements are such categories.

If we disregard sexual disorders, we find that the Hellenistic physicians had four major diagnostic categories referring to disordered states of consciousness: phrenitis, lethargy, mania, and melancholia. Aretaeus was of the opinion that mania and melancholia were two manifestations of the same illness.

The two acute states described in the literature are *phrenitis* and *lethargy*.

Phrenitis is an acute delirious state invariably associated with fever. The clinical signs necessary for the diagnosis are, according to Soranus, 'acute fever, mental derangement, small and rapid pulse, and the plucking at straws and hairs'. Many other clinical signs, commonly associated with phrenitis are mentioned by Soranus, (Aretaeus's chapter on phrenitis being lost), but clinical symptoms, i.e. the subjective reports of his patients, are virtually non-existent. Thus, while Soranus reports that the patient talks to those who are not present, and even to the dead, he ignores Celsus' symptom of 'vain images' or visual hallucinations. There was a brisk controversy among previous writers as to whether phrenitis was a direct affliction of the brain (Asclepiades) or was the secondary symptom of fever itself (Aurelianus) but this debate is dismissed by Soranus, who writes that, since the fever is an invariable part of the disease the disease must be located in the entire body, with particular reference to the head and the senses. Phrenitis is clearly a unitary disease, and he dismisses those deliria caused by fevers clearly associated with other illnesses such as pneumonia.

Lethargy, the other acute febrile illness associated with the disordered states of consciousness, is generally ignored by psychiatric writers, possibly because this symptom no longer falls within the province of psychiatry. The name refers to the loss of memory associated with the illness. It is regarded by Soranus as related to, but more serious than, phrenitis. The necessary clinical signs include 'impairment and dulling of the senses, stupor, acute fever either continuous or remittant, and large, slow, empty inflated pulse.' Like phrenitis, lethargy is a disease of the whole body, though the head is felt to be more affected than the other organs.

Mania is a unitary diagnostic entity which embraced a wide variety of deranged and disordered behaviour. As Aretaeus observes, 'the modes of mania are infinite in specie, but one alone in genus'. The single clinical feature which seems to consistently distinguish mania from other categories of mental illness is loss of reason or judgment in the absence of fever and without the ingestion of toxic drugs. Delusions, erratic behaviour, and instability of mood are agreed upon as common elements of the illness. Hallucinations, which in Alexandrian medicine implicate the special senses, are not reported by Aretaeus to be found in mania. He distinguishes hallucinations from illusions, and ascribes the former to phrenitis alone.

Although some individuals suffering from mania are elated and may 'laugh, play, dance night and day, and sometimes go openly to the market crowned, as if victors in some contest of skill', others are 'unreasonably despondent when the disease tends to bloom' (Aretaeus). The observation that a patient suffering from mania may be either elated or depressed is also made by Soranus, who reports that '. . . the patient's madness is manifested by dejection . . . or . . . playful childishness'.

Melancholia is defined by Aretaeus as a 'lowness of spirits from a single fantasy without fever'. Unlike those individuals suffering from mania, the melancholic turns 'to sorrow and despondency only'. Although these are consistent features in melancholia, Aretaeus observes that there is considerable variation of the symptoms, 'so that some patients were suspicious of poisoning . . . (and others) . . . contracted a hatred for life'. He further notes that if the condition becomes more serious there are 'vain lamentations; they complain of life, and desire to die'. Soranus leaves us a similar description, defining the symptoms of melancholia as 'mental anguish and distress, dejection, silence, animosity toward members of the household, sometimes the desire to live and at other times a longing for death'.

The physical signs associated with melancholia, particularly flatulance and the vomiting of black bile, are extremely important, since it is on this basis that according to Soranus the differential diagnosis with mania is made. Soranus ridicules Aretaeus' view that these are two expressions of a single illness. For him mania is clearly a disease of the head, while the physical symptoms of melancholia are just as clearly located in the oesophagus. Aretaeus on the other hand sees them as two aspects of a single pathological process, in both cases originating in the bowels. If the bile passes upwards and downwards from the diaphragm where it collects, melancholia results. He maintains, however, that '. . . it also affects the head from sympathy', and 'these become mad rather from the increase of the disease than from change of the affection'. Thus, seeming to differ, both men reassert their common supposition of localization.

V. PROGNOSIS

Prognosis in ancient medicine refers to two major questions: How long will the illness last? Will the patient survive?

The first of these questions could be answered in terms of the diagnosis. Each diagnostic category was classified either as acute or chronic. These categories were purely predictive of the rapidity and the duration of the pathological process. 'Chronic' certainly did not imply a malignant, irreversible or incurable process, as it sometimes does in modern usage.

The second, the question of survival, depended in the Hellenistic system principally upon whether the patient's body, with the aid of a physician, was able to reverse the pathological process. As was mentioned earlier in the section on etiology, the philosophical system eliminated any true concept of corruption, so that only the simple mechanical operations of addition, subtraction, and displacement of atoms were recognized as part of the pathological process. Theoretically, these were always recognized as reversible processes. But practically speaking, as Aretaeus states, 'it is impossible, indeed, to make all the sick well, for a physician would thus be superior to a god; but the physician can produce respite from pain, intervals in diseases, and render them latent'. Many illnesses were recognized, therefore, as practically incurable, and mania engendered by melancholia is put in this class by Aretaeus. The chances for complete recovery depended largely on the chronicity of the disease since the slower the disease process, the more time was available for therapeutic intervention.

VI. TREATMENT

Rational treatment is, of course, the ultimate goal of the medical model. The particular therapy employed should follow logically from the diagnosis but the underlying suppositions about etiology will always in fact be the determining factor.

Both the Methodist and Pneumatist schools of medicine were based upon the 'polarity between opposite qualities'. The task of therapy, as seen by the Hellenistic physicians, was to cure by provoking the quality opposite to that which was responsible for the illness. If a part of the body was too hot, it should be cooled; if too moist, it should be dried. The same therapeutic principles apply to psychiatry as applied to all other branches of medicine. Purging, cupping, venesection, and the use of drugs were the common and direct treatment modalities, along with rest, diet, and exercise.

Of particular interest to the modern historians has been the evidence of some form of 'psychotherapy' among the ancients. Soranus, for example, prescribed stage performances, giving speeches to a small audience, and even playing checkers. Although suggestive of modern milieu techniques, and undoubtedly having the same effects on patients, these measures were conceived in the Hellenistic medicine as having much the same effect as physical exercise and were not meant merely as a diversion. The same criteria were employed in prescribing them as might be employed for prescribing exercise on a mended leg.

VII. CONCLUSIONS

The authors believe that on the basis of the review of the historical evidence we have presented, as it is contained in the writing of two of the major physicians of the Hellenistic era and collated in this paper, one of the fundamental propositions of Greco-Roman medical thought was that grossly aberrant behaviour was an *illness*, the study and treatment of which was within the purview of the medical profession. Although Aretaeus mentioned that there was a form of mania which was of divine origin, and then excluded this from consideration, the consensus of the time was in the Hippocratic tradition that mental illness had a *natural cause*, a *natural history* and was amenable to a regime of treatment which utilized *rational therapy*. This approach was justified largely by the prevailing philosophy of the time, a thoroughly materialistic atomism. The mind-body problem was resolved by reducing the mind to a material substance.

Modern psychiatry has been shaped by many of the assumptions which had their genesis in the clinical writings of this period. In recent decades, however, psychoanalysis, the development of anthropology and the growing interest in transcultural psychiatry have advanced a provocative challenge to these assumptions. The new and sharply divergent views of mental illness which they have provided, devoid of satisfactory solutions to the mind-body problem, have opened the door for the criticisms of Thomas Szasz,[6] R. D. Laing[7] and others, who reject the medical model of mental illness as merely an unjustified metaphor.

As this paper demonstrates, the medical model was, in its inception, no metaphor, but the logical corollary of a thoroughly materialistic cosmology. If, today, we again view man as a material being, and mental illness as a natural process, then the medical model is as valid today as it was in Hellenistic time as the ideal of sound psychiatry.

Bibliography

1 ELLENBERGER, H. F., *The Discovery of the Unconscious: The History and Evolution of Dynamic Psychiatry*, New York, Basic Books, 1970.

2 AURELIANUS, *On Acute Diseases and on Chronic Diseases*, ed. and translated by I. E. Drabkin, Chicago, University of Chicago Press, 1950.

3 *The Extant Works of Aretaeus, the Cappodocian*, ed. and trans. by Francis Adams, London, Sydenham Society, 1856.

4 STEGALL, JOHN, *The First Four Books of Aur. Corn. Celsus, 'De re medica'; with an ordo verborum and literal translation*, London, Churchill, 1837.

5 VEITH, I., 'Psychiatric nosology: from Hippocrates to Kraeplin', *Amer. J. Psych.*, 1957, **114**, 385.

6 SZASZ, T. S., *The Myth of Mental Illness*, Harper & Row, New York, 1961.

7 LAING, R. D., *The Divided Self*, Tavistock Publications, London, 1959.

K. T. Barkley
Cincinnati, Ohio (U.S.A.)

The history of the ambulance

'An ambulance', according to Webster's Dictionary, 'is a temporary field hospital, organized to follow an army in its movements; hence, in civil life, an organization for rendering first aid; also a wagon or other conveyance fitted for carrying wounded or sick persons.'

Although litters for transporting the sick and wounded probably were in use even before A.D. 900, wounded soldiers were usually left unattended until after the battle when they were cared for where they lay; or they were carried to the field hospital by their companions.

The following dates highlight the use of the ambulance as an organized service:

1792 Baron Dominique Jean Larrey's 'flying ambulance' during the Napoleonic Wars.

1862 Jonathan Letterman initiated the use of an Ambulance Corps at Antietam in the War between the States.

1865 First civilian ambulance service in connexion with a hospital – Cincinnati General Hospital, Cincinnati, Ohio.

1869 First New York City ambulance service – Bellevue Hospital Ambulance service in New York City.

1870 British Ambulance Association was founded – a first aid association which originated in 1048 during the Crusades.

1918 Airplane ambulance service during World War I.

1950 Helicopter ambulance came into use.

1960 Specialized ambulances for specific illnesses – such as Coronary Care Mobile Units and those vehicles equipped to care for the Newborn In Distress.

Future Operating Room On Wheels – the ambulance of the future.

THE HAMMOCK WAGON

The Anglo-Saxon hammock wagon was used about A.D. 900. It was in common use for transporting invalids at that time. When the wagon was travelling downhill, the horses could not hold the wagon back, so the rear wheels were snubbed with chains to keep them from turning. The braking was dependent on the strength of the attendants to hold the snubbing chains.

THE HORSE LITTER

When the Normans came to England in 1066 they brought the idea of the litter supported by horses. A bed was suspended on poles which extended to special horse harnesses at each end. There was considerable bouncing but less than those beds with wheels on the ground. The use of the horse litter was the best way of moving the sick and wounded from 1066 until 1640.[44]

LARREY'S FLYING AMBULANCE

Dominique Jean Larrey, Napoleon's surgeon, is credited with the first ambulance designed to remove the wounded during the battle. Up to that time the wounded were left on the field until after the battle when the ambulance came to pick them up and transport them to the field hospitals. Many died for want of care during that time of waiting. Larrey then conceived the idea of constructing an ambulance which could remove the wounded during the battle. The ambulance was to follow the advanced guard in the same way as the flying artillery. It was called the 'flying ambulance'. Napoleon called Larrey 'the most virtuous man that I have ever known' in recognition of his accomplishments in bettering the welfare of the troops and the introduction of skilful management of the wounded.

Although the 'flying ambulance' was constructed in 1792, the medical organization for battlefield care was not used again until the battle of Antietam in 1862 during the Civil War.[42,43,69]

GENEVA CONVENTION OF 1864 FOR THE AMELIORATION OF THE CONDITION OF THE WOUNDED IN ARMIES IN THE FIELD

Jean Henri Dunant (1828–1910) had two inspirations to set about forming the humanitarian movement we know today as the Red Cross. Florence Nightingale's service in the Crimean War (1854–56) and his own experience on the battlefield of Solferino in 1859. French and Italian troops had been victorious over the Austrians but at a terrible price in lives.

In a book entitled *Un Souvenir de Solferino*, Dunant told of the preventable suffering of the soldiers left on the battlefield. There were 40,000 dead and wounded still lying uncared for the day after the battle. He suggested an international conference for consideration of the formation of volunteer units to aid the sick and wounded. These units became the Red Cross societies of today.

Several articles adopted at the Geneva Convention related to ambulance services, establishing the personnel to be neutral and thus to be protected by both sides.

A uniform flag was adopted – the red cross on a white background. This insignia reversed the Swiss flag honouring Jean Dunant who was a native of Switzerland.[7,42]

THE AVALANCHE

During the Civil War in the United States, the matter of transportation of the wounded to the base hospitals demanded some sort of ambulance service. Slightly wounded men had to walk to the primary stations. The badly injuried were at the mercy of stretchermen who loaded them into ambulances for a bumpy ride to the field hospital.

The two Bull Run engagements were disastrous for the Union. Ambulances were too few, too far between and too late, and driven by civilian drunks and thieves who ran when they heard the guns. The Quartermaster Corps decided to use two-wheeled ambulances thinking they would ride better. Not a few were jarred to death and the wagon became known as the 'avalanche'. Fortunately, these were abandoned after the first year of the war. Most of them had broken down and were beyond repair by that time.

When Jonathan Letterman became the Medical Director of the Army of the Potomac, the Union ambulance system began to improve. McClellan gave him a free hand to do what was needed to improve the care of the sick and wounded. Letterman took the ambulance away from the Quartermaster Corps and made this his own responsibility. By 1864 Congress had created an Ambulance Corps for the entire Union forces. Ambulance wagons were aided by the railroad hospital trains, some coaches being equipped with beds, surgeries, etc. By the autumn of 1862, a regular daily hospital train service was in effect between Washington and New York.

The South was at a definite disadvantage because of lack of ambulance wagons and horses, as well as adequate train cars.[8]

THE 'RUCKER' AMBULANCE

The Rucker ambulance wagon was constructed under the direction of Major General Rucker of the United States Quartermaster's Department. It was recommended for adoption as the regulation ambulance wagon of the United States Army. It accommodated both ambulatory and recumbent patients (4 recumbent or 8 to 10 ambulatory patients).[42,43]

STEAMBOAT HOSPITAL TRANSPORTS AS PART OF THE AMBULANCE SYSTEM

At the outbreak of the Civil War there was not a single Army General Hospital. The staff consisted of the Surgeon General, thirty surgeons and eighty-three assistant surgeons. Some of these resigned to serve the Confederacy.

Although an ambulance service was suggested to the Army in 1861, nothing was done about it. However, on 31 June 1861, Lincoln approved an order creating the United States Sanitary Commission. The Reverend Henry Bellows, Unitarian minister, was president of the Commission which became the Red Cross of the Civil War. Hospital transports were maintained and directed by the Sanitary Commission.

In 1862, Fort Donelson fell to Union forces. Severe injuries were treated on the spot. Others went to the rear of the fighting via ambulance where they stayed until further arrangements were made. Usually the next move was by steamer down the Cumberland River to hospitals along the Ohio River.

The Cincinnati branch of the U.S. Sanitary Commission chartered the steamboat *Allen Collier*, a 133-ton stern-wheel vessel built in Cincinnati. The ship was stocked with hospital supplies and staffed with surgeons and nurses. There was such confusion and resentment on the part of the state equipped transports that the hospital ship almost returned home from Fort Donelson without any passengers. However, the staff insisted in helping the wounded and managed to take eighty-one to a military hospital in Cincinnati. This was the first recorded trip of a United States Sanitary Commission hospital steamer in the west.

Many other boats were used for transporting the wounded to hospitals. Unfortunately, military officers were not responsible to a private system of transports and therefore did not have to obey orders which came from the volunteers serving on the ships. Eventually the United States Government took over the Sanitary Commission's boats including the doctors and male nurses.[6,19,55]

CINCINNATI COMMERCIAL HOSPITAL FIRST

Although Bellevue Hospital in New York claimed to have the first ambulance service which served the whole city in 1869, the record shows that hospital ambulance service was introduced by the Commercial Hospital (now the Cincinnati General) in Cincinnati, Ohio, before 1865. The list of employees for the year ending 28 February 1866 names James R. Jackson, employee No. 27 as 'driver of ambulance' at an annual salary of $360.[36]

THE HAMMOCK VAN

Richard Davy, Surgeon to the Westminster Hospital, in 1876 wrote some *Remarks on the Transit of Invalids*. He began his discourse by comment, 'The British public have practically evinced a far higher regard for the removal of valuable furniture than for the transit of delicate Christians'. Because of this situation, Mr. Davy introduced a hammock van for the convenience of invalids. The carriage could be drawn by one or two horses and permitted two hammocks to be swung, one above the other. It was furnished with strong springs, India rubber tyres, seats for attendants, lavatory and its accompaniments. By employing this type of van, Dr. Davy, claimed the patient was subjected to the least amount of inconvenience. The van may be placed on a railway truck at the station, and on reaching the end of the journey can be taken off the railway truck and again attached to horses for the trip to its destination.

The van was made only by Messrs, Seydel and Co. of Birmingham, England. In 1882, six years after his first article was published, Dr. Davy again directed his attention to the absolute necessity of improvement in carriage for the comfort of the patient and for the convenience of the surgeon in charge. This time he advocated the use of a three-wheeled van, length 9 ft. breadth $4\frac{1}{2}$ ft. and height $4\frac{1}{2}$ ft. This van was large enough to receive the patient's own bed if this seemed practical. He offered to exhibit the van to anyone interested.[13]

HORSE AMBULANCES IN CONNEXION WITH HOSPITALS

Captain William Joynson, Chairman of the Northern Hospital, Liverpool, England, reported to a Hospitals Association meeting held on 15 April 1885, the following information: At the close of 1882, he had made a voyage to America via the Cunard ship *Gallia*. Upon arriving in New York, an invalid aboard ship was removed from the ship by means of an ambulance carriage and taken with every comfort to the hospital. This service was rendered upon the receipt of a telephone call to the hospital from the captain of the ship. Captain Joynson was so impressed with this experience in New York that he had then established the perfect ambulance service in connexion with the Liverpool Northern Hospital. He explained that the ambulances were really moving hospitals with a surgeon on the spot to render those services which might mean the difference between life and death.

Rapidity of action was ensured by the use of a patent American clip-harness. The harness was suspended from the ceiling, the saddle and collar were hung ready to be dropped into place. When the bell sounded the horse was placed under the shafts and the harness, saddle and collar were immediately snapped on. The driver took the ambulance to the front of the hospital and picked up the surgeon and according to Captain Joynson, the moving hospital was on its way in two minutes.

The Liverpool ambulance was designed by Mr. John Furley of the St. John Ambulance Association and was built of English oak and American ash and birch. There were two stretchers in each carriage, both provided with telescopic handles. Medical appliances, splints, bandages and other requisites were ready for use in each ambulance.

The ambulance in use was called about three times every two days. The time from call to departure was 2·14 minutes by day, and 4 minutes by night. Each journey from call to return, was 18 minutes and 30 seconds.[35]

RED CROSS AMBULANCE OF 1898

Ambulances marked with a red cross were furnished by the German Army Quartermaster Corps as early as 1870, in the Franco-Prussian War. However, the first effort of a civilian corps to provide ambulances at any battle-front was during the period of the Spanish–American War. Six ambulances were sent to Cuba in 1898. Although Clara Barton had become interested in the Cuban revolt in 1897, she avoided provoking international complications which might lead to war between the United States and Spain. After the declaration of war against Spain on 25 April 1898, the U.S. Government officially accepted the aid of the American Red Cross. A committee was formed under the title of 'First New York Ambulance Equipment Society'. Its purpose was to purchase and equip ambulances. The Society raised money and purchased the vehicles from the Studebaker Brothers Manufacturing Co. of South Bend, Indiana.

Miss Barton travelled to Cuba to survey the needs there. Six ambulances were shipped to Havana by Stephen Barton, Clara's nephew, who was chairman of the 'President's Committee for Cuban Relief'. Later the Committee sent forty mules to Miss Barton, with fodder and harnesses. Owing to the delay in unloading, the six ambulances could be put to no use in Cuba, and they were returned to New York after the signing of the armistice on 24 October 1898. In November 1898, official protest was made by the Red Cross to the U.S. Government for its delayed delivery of the ambulances and for having seized ten thousand dollars worth of supplies.

On 23 July 1898, two ambulances and mules were shipped from Tampa, Florida, to Puerto Rico. These proved of great value in emergency cases requiring quick transportation of soldiers and supplies. When the station closed in Puerto Rico, the vehicles were sold to a Mr. Hersey for $200.[7,12]

VELOCIPEDE AMBULANCE

An ambulance velocipede was patented in the United States and used at the Royal Charité Hospital, Berlin, in the late 1800s. Many of the disadvantages of the horse-drawn vehicle were thought to be overcome. The litter had a canvas covering, adjustable head rest and mattress. The bed rested on springs supported by bearings, the vehicle ran on five wheels with pneumatic tyres. The four rear wheels supported the body of the ambulance. The front wheel was the guiding one. It was propelled by two persons, the one in front being the driver. The one in the rear watched the patient through the rear window. There were two side windows which admitted light and air. The inside was lighted by electric lights. A box beneath the bed held medicine, bandages and instruments. The vehicle could be widened for two litters.[61]

STREET CAR AMBULANCE

The street car ambulance was used in Bahia, Brazil. There were five compartments. The one in the centre was a fumigating compartment and nurse's room. Two iron beds were supplied with rubber-tyred rollers, springs and regular mattresses.

In 1894, St. Louis, Missouri, had a street car ambulance which was able to travel to all sixteen infirmaries in the city.[63]

ST. JOHN AMBULANCE ASSOCIATION

In 1877, the Order of St. John decided to form the St. John Ambulance Association to train personnel in First Aid to minister to the sick and wounded in war, as well as in peacetime. The principle objective of this Association was first, 'the instruction of pupils in first treatment of injured persons' and second, 'spread of useful ambulance material'.

The Association was ridiculed at first but this attitude changed when the Grand Prior of the Order, Edward, Prince of Wales (later, King Edward VII), asked for a guard of honour of men in St. John uniform. Facing members of the press, he said, 'Gentlemen, this is a good uniform. I believe much good will come of it'.

In 1883, the Invalid Transport Corps was established. In 1898, a permanent Ambulance Station was established in the churchyard of St. Clement Danes, later removed to Uxbridge.

In 1887, the St. John Ambulance Brigade was created. This brigade has given innumerable services to the public. They have also published books and set up training classes.[21,30]

THE AEROPLANE AMBULANCE

During the First World War aviation rapidly passed from the experimental stage to that of a powerful arm of the military service, without having had the opportunity of being applied to commercial uses. The war surplus of airplanes after the war easily met the demand and no new designing took place for several years.

The actual designing of airplanes as ambulances did not take place until the late 1920s or early 1930s. In 1929 the Air Corps had three Cox-Klemin planes which were designed for ambulance service. These planes had a speed of 100 miles an hour, carried six hours of fuel, and transported two litter patients, pilot and attendant.[67]

THE HEARTMOBILE

It is a well-known fact that most deaths from myocardial infarction occur before the patient can be admitted to the hospital. Use of a mobile coronary unit would therefore improve greatly the chances of survival. The cost, both initial and operational, of maintaining a 'heart ambulance' is prohibitive to most communities.

However, in San Francisco, California, a system has been found which is fairly efficient. Mount Zion Hospital in co-operation with Electro-Biometrics of Lancaster, California, and the San Francisco Ambulance Service, a private ambulance company, are providing a valuable service to heart disease patients.

The operation of the telemetry system occurs as follows: the physician calls the ambulance company and instructs it to take the patient to the hospital and monitor the patient. When the ambulance attendants arrive and take the patient into the ambulance, disposable ECG electrodes are taped to the chest. The attendants radio the ambulance base dispatcher who then telephones the hospital coronary care unit. The demodulator and tape recorder are turned on in the coronary care unit. The ambulance dispatcher connects the phone patch which permits the hospital personnel to speak directly to the ambulance. Data transmission and voice communication use the same line, the sound of the voice automatically shutting off the data transmission. Under these circumstances the telemetry serves to put the physician's skills in the ambulance with the trained ambulance attendant acting as his hands.

The concept of a mobile coronary unit developed from the pioneering work of Dr. J. F. Pantridge in Belfast, Ireland, where a unit was first used in January 1966.

Many communities are now finding it justifiable to establish mobile coronary units because so many lives can be saved by this service.[50,51,54,71,72]

MEDICOPTER

Helicopter evacuation of men wounded in combat in Korea and Vietnam with emergency medical care before and during flight to the hospital has shown that the helicopter can be a major factor in saving lives.

The Ohio Army National Guard, the highway patrol, and the university hospitals co-operate to save lives in Ohio. A National Guard UH–19D helicopter has been adapted for emergency use. This is in Columbus, Ohio. The helicopter has walk-around space for two or three medical workers and room for two stretchers and medical equipment. A longitudinal pole with hooks is placed along the ceiling to hold bottles for intravenous fluid administration.

Lessons learned after experimenting with the use of the Medicopter were: (1) The need for an integrated team effort; (2) the importance of keeping intravenous fluids warm; (3) the need to change state laws so qualified physician's assistants may administer fluids and drugs and perform intubations.[18,40,56]

HESS AND EISENHARDT, AMBULANCE BUILDERS

The Hess and Eisenhardt Co. near Cincinnati, Ohio, is known the world over for its ambulances, hearses, and custom cars. It is the world's oldest builder of ambulances and funeral cars. In 1937, the company sold the first air-conditioned ambulance built in America. Ambulances are now built in three sizes, for one, two and four patients.

The firm began building carriages in 1876 as the Sayers and Scovill Co., using the trademark S&S, which is still being used. In 1891, two office boys were hired, Emil Hess and Charles A. Eisenhardt, Sr. Today the sons of these men are Willard Hess, president of the company and Charles A. Eisenhardt, Jr., chairman of the board.

Custom cars are less and less in demand but the market for ambulances is growing rapidly. Using Cadillac chassis, ambulances and hearses take about three months to build. They are noted for their individualized trim and high quality of finish. The first ambulance was built in 1890, it had one lantern, a stretcher and two crude attendant seats which were padded boards let down from the wall.

Today's ambulance is a closed car with a commercial size oxygen tank that has a seven- to eight-hour supply. There is plenty of space for the attendant to move about with ease. There is air conditioning, full medicine cabinets, roof lights and a two-way radio. H&E officials believe that an ambulance should be a pre-hospital emergency room. Mr. Eisenhardt comments that the police and fire departments are up to date. But, is not a human life more important to save than a building? Buildings can be replaced – human beings cannot.

However, it is difficult to persuade communities to see the importance of having a good ambulance service. People always have the idea that accidents happen to the other person and his family.

Emergency Medical Service is an issue which needs updating in every community. It requires the co-operation of medical centres, ambulance companies, municipal and county and state governments.

The University of Cincinnati's College of Medicine has just graduated the first resident in the world in Emergency Medicine. It is a step in the right direction but we need to go a lot further. There is no completely adequate system of emergency care anywhere. Which community will be the first to consider human lives the most important?[27]

COMMITTEE ON TRAUMA RESPONSIBLE FOR IMPROVED AMBULANCE SERVICE

The Committee on Trauma of the American College of Surgeons was established fifty years ago in 1922. Although the name was changed several times, the original objective has been unchanged – improvement in the care of the injured. Regional committees, state/provincial and local committees have been acting extensions of the Committee on Trauma. There are 58 state committees. Several major metropolitan areas have been given state status because of the large population represented. All but one of these committees have projects underway designed to improve ambulance service. Their voices were usually unheard by local government officials. When the National Highway Safety Bureau was created, the trauma committees were there to promote the use of Federal funds to support state improvements in emergency ambulance service.

Regional committees have provided continuing education courses in emergency procedures. Several books have been published which are guides for emergency care.

Annually, a symposium on trauma has been a Trauma Committee responsibility. Dr. Robert Kennedy, long-time active member of the committee, has presented a trauma field programme panel every year since 1961.

In 1957, the Trauma Committee of the ACS, the American Association for the Surgery of Trauma, and the National Safety Council formed a joint action programme which sponsored a nationwide survey of emergency services.

Three grants from the John A. Hartford Foundation established the Trauma Field Program with Dr. Robert Kennedy as the Director. The survey of ambulance equipment and service shocked those who read the results. Almost immediately, the committee developed a list of 'Minimum Equipment for Ambulances'. The list was updated in 1969 by J. D. Farrington. 'Essential Equipment for Ambulances' is now the nationally accepted standard. In 1970, Dr. Farrington published a *Curriculum for Training for Emergency Medical Technicians-Ambulance*. Dr. Kennedy has been the leader in promoting and providing educational materials on emergency care and services for the last decade.[20,45,48]

DEVELOPMENT OF AMBULANCE SERVICES IN THE UNITED KINGDOM

In 1970, John H. Daykin, Chief Ambulance Officer in Leeds, commented that he knew of only two communities in the United Kingdom that had set up separate accident services within their ambulance service – Liverpool and London. Most ambulance services handle what is known as 'sitting cases'. In other words, the vehicles transport people from home to hospital out-patient treatment units. He said that emergency calls are quite unpredictable and if no ambulances are set aside for emergencies, the calls could come in when there are no conveyances available.

Ambulance design has improved greatly in the last several years. Each year the companies building ambulances are adding features to make the patient more comfortable with better means of treatment during transportation. Helicopters are also being improved as air ambulances. Stretchers and wheelchairs have become more sophisticated making it easier for the attendants as well as the patients. However, Dr. Daykin says, 'Despite all the equipment improvement, none of it is any use unless the operators are trained to use the devices and can recognize the circumstances which call for their use'.

Ambulancemen are now required to have physical and mental examinations. They must also take an aptitude test and a driver's test in an ambulance. The Millar Report, Part I, a report by the Working Party on Ambulance Training and Equipment, made detailed recommendations on the method of training and standard to be achieved. The National Joint Council for Manual Workers in Local Authority Services set up standards for pay and working conditions for ambulance attendants. The Department of Health and Social Security set up the Ambulance Services Advisory Committee which advises the Ministers of Health on Ambulance services.

The attitude toward ambulance services varies from those who are proud of them and spend a great deal for efficient services – to those who begrudge any funds spent on good ambulance service.

The United Kingdom hopes to be the best in the world in ambulance services, eventually. If all the nations would concentrate on this objective, think how many lives would be saved.[15]

ACKNOWLEDGEMENTS

This history of the ambulance was initiated by Dr. Cecil Striker of Cincinnati. I would like to thank all those who helped me in this compilation. The list is very long. Much aid was also received from the National Library of Medicine and Cincinnati General Hospital Library.

References

(*Note*: This bibliography is for a more extensive paper, from which these excerpts were taken.)

1 American Society of Anesthesiologists: 'Community-wide emergency medical services. Recommendations by the Committee on Acute Medicine of the American Society of Anesthesiologists', *J. Amer. med. Ass.*, 1968, **204**, 595–602.

2 ARP, L. J. *et al.*, 'An emergency air-ground transport system for newborn infants with respiratory distress', *Penn. Med.*, 1969, **72**, 74–76.

3 ASH, R. V., 'Transport of sick and wounded in countries, bearing especially on the late Kaffir campaigns', *Trans. Internat. med. Cong.*, 1881, **2**, 501–4.

4 BAKER, G. L., 'Design and operation of a van for the transport of sick infants', *Amer. J. Dis. Child.*, 1969, **18**, 743.

5 BARNSLEY, R. E., 'A search rewarded – discovery of horse drawn ambulance wagon', *Lancet*, 1958, **ii**, 1372.

6 BARNES, JOSEPH K., *The Medical and Surgical History of the War of the Rebellion (1861–65)*, Washington, D.C., U.S. Government Printing Office, 1870, pt. 1, vol. 1.

7 BARTON, CLARA, *The Red Cross*, Washington, D.C., American National Red Cross, 1898.

8 BROOKS, STEWART, *Civil War Medicine*, Springfield, Illinois, C. C. Thomas, 1966.

9 BROWN, H., 'Camel stretcher carrier; method of carrying casualties on a stretcher for use with camels', *J. R. Army Med. Corps.*, 1938, **71**, 48–49.

10 CARLISLE, R. J., *An Account of Bellvue Hospital*, New York, Society of the Alumni of Bellevue Hospital, 1893.

11 CLARKE, J. T., 'Canada's first ambulance train', *Mil. Surg.*, 1931, **68**, 649–50.

12 COLLINS, H. R., *Red Cross Ambulance of 1898 in the Museum of History and Technology*, Paper 50, Bulletin 241 (Contributions from the Museum of History and Technology, Smithsonian Institution), 1965.

13 DAVY, R., 'On invalid transit', *Br. med. J.*, 1882, **ii**, 1142.

14 DAVY, R., 'Remarks on the transit of invalids', *Br. med. J.*, 1876, **ii**, 553.

15 DAYKIN, J. H., 'The development of ambulance services in the United Kingdom', *R. Soc. Hlth J.*, 1970, **90**, 5.

16 'Directory of emergency physicians', *Med. Opinion*, 29 August 1972.

17 DRUM, W. F., 'Ambulance train in 1864', *Mil. Surg.*, 1932, **70**, 607–11.

18 EDWARDS, A. G., 'Helicopter rescue service', *Lancet*, 1958, **i**, 470–72.

19 EVANS, J., 'Motor barge as ambulance ship', *Br. med. J.*, 1941, **ii**, 59–60.

20 FARRINGTON, J. D., 'Transportation of the injured', *Postgrad. Med.*, 1970, **48**, 139–43.

21 FLETCHER, N. CORBET, *St. John Ambulance Association, its History and its Part in the Ambulance Movement*, London, St. John's Ambulance Association, 1930.

22 GEARTY, G. F. *et al.*, 'Pre-hospital coronary services', *Br. med. J.*, 1971, **iii**, 33.

23 GRACE, W. J., 'The mobile coronary care unit and the intermediate coronary care unit in the total systems approach to coronary care', *Chest*, 1970, **58**, 363–68.

24 GRACE, W. J., 'The mobile coronary care unit', *Dis. Chest*, 1969, **55**, 425.

25 GRAF, W. S., 'Problems in establishing a mobile coronary care unit', *Med. Opinion*, December 1970, 72–78.

26 HENDERSON, P. H., 'Ambulance transport in undeveloped countries', *Proc. R. Soc. Med.*, 1931, **24**, 35–51.

27 HESS and EISENHARDT, 'A history of achievement since 1876', *Cincinnati Mag.*, June 1968.

28 HORNER, W. E., 'Ambulance', *Amer. Cycl. Pract. Med.*, 1834, **1**, 338–41.

29 HORNUNG, C. P., *Wheels Across America*, New York, Dover, 1959.

30 HUME, EDGAR E., *Medical Work of the Knights Hospitallers of St. John of Jerusalem*, Baltimore, Johns Hopkins Press, 1940.

31 HUNTLEY, HENRY, C., 'Emergency health services for the nation', *Public Health Rep.*, 1970, **85**, 517.

32 HUNTLEY, HENRY C., 'Emergency-care system for national political conventions in Miami Beach', *Med. Opinion*, 20 August 1972, vol. 1.

33 HUNTLEY, HENRY C., 'How is emergency care in your communityè', *Emergency Med.*, April 1972, pp. 51–55.

34 ISLER, CHARLOTTE, 'Dial 911 for the coronary ambulance', RN 32, August 1969, pp. 48–51.

35 JOYNSON, WILLIAM, 'Horse ambulances in connection with hospitals', *Br. med. J.*, 1885, **i**, 909–10.

36 KANE, JOSEPH N., *Famous First Facts*, 3rd ed., New York, Wilson, 1964.

37 KEGGI, K. J., 'Yale confronts urban trauma', *Roche Med. Image & Com.*, 1968.

38 KIRSCHNER, M., 'Surgical ambulance with roentgen service, operating room and car for seriously wounded, for use during campaign and in time of public calamities', *Chirurg.*, 1938, **10**, 713–17.

39 KNAPP, J., 'Carriage for cholera patients', *Lond. med. Gaz.*, 1832, 825.

40 LEWIS, RICHARD P., 'A town that does. Columbus, Ohio, mobile coronary care unit', *Emergency Med.*, July 1971, **3**, 57.

41 'Lives saved vs. dollars spent transporting emergency patients', *Perspective*, 1971, **6**, 9–17.

42 LONGMORE, T., *A Treatise on the Transport of Sick and Wounded Troops*, London, Her Majesty's Stationery Office, 1869.

43 MCKENNY, ELLEN M., 'History of the motorized ambulance transport', *Mil. Med.*, 1967, **132**, 819–22.

44 MARTEN, E. T., 'Modern ambulances have developed from rude beginnings', *Mod. Hosp.*, 1934, **42**, 43–46.

45 *Medical Requirements for Ambulance Design and Equipment*, National Academy of Sciences National Research Council Task Force, Washington D.C., September 1968.

46 'Medical World News Staff: The crisis in emergency care', *Med. World News*, 4 December 1970, pp. 24–32 and 16 April 1970, pp. 41–48.

47 MILES, A. B., 'The Charity Hospital ambulance service', *New Orl. med. surg. J.*, 1885–6, **13**, 51–56.

48 'Minimal equipment for ambulances. American College of Surgeons Committee on Trauma', *Bul. Amer. Coll. Surg.*, 1967, **52**, 92–96.

49 'Modified coronary ambulance', *Med. J. Aust.*, 1969, **2**, 1182.

50 MURPHY, STEPHEN P., 'San Diego plan for emergency services', *Amer. J. Nursing*, 1972, **72**, 1615–19.

51 NAGEL, EUGENE, and HIRSCHMAN, J., 'Pre-hospital care: time for decision', *Med. Opinion*, December 1971, **7**, 28.

52 NEWHOUSE, N. H., 'Alligator ambulance', *U.S. Navy med. Bull.*, 1942, **40**, 719–20.

53 PACKARD, FRANCIS R., *History of Medicine in the United States*, vol. 1, New York, Hafner, 1963.

54 PANTRIDGE, J. F., and GEDDES J. S., 'A mobile intensive care unit in the management of myocardial infarction', *Lancet*, 1967, **ii**, 271–73.

55 PRESTON, ROBERT H., 'Hospital transports with special reference to the steamboat Allen Collier and the Cincinnati branch of the U.S. Sanitary Commission', *Ohio State med. J.*, 1957, **53**, 1037–38, 1165–66.

56 ROBERTS, STUART, *et al.*, 'Medicopter: an airborne intensive care unit', *Ann. Surg.*, 1970, **172**, 325.

57 SAFAR, PETER, 'Ambulance design and equipment for mobile intensive care', *Arch. Surg.*, 1971, **102**, 163–71.

58 SAFAR, PETER and BROSE, R. A., 'Ambulance design and equipment for resuscitation', *Arch. Surg.*, 1965, **90**, 343–48.

59 SAFAR, PETER, 'Community concern sparks ambulance service', *Mod. Hosp.*, 1969, **13**, 93–98.

60 SCHWARTZ, MORTIMER, 'Mobile coronary care unit', *Med. Opinion*, 1970, **6**, 52.

61 *Scientific Amer.*, 1896, **75**, 284, Velocipede.

62 Ibid., 1900, **82**, 148 – Electric automobile.

63 Ibid., 1913, **108**, 316 – Streetcar ambulance.

64 SCOTT, T. E., 'New pack saddle litter for Panama jungle', *Mil. Surg.*, 1936, **79**, 203.

65 SEWALL, C. A., 'A new extemporaneous litter, copied after the Mojave Indian method of carrying the wounded', *Med. Rec.*, 1890, **38**, 461.

66 SHEPARD, K. S., 'Air transportation of high risk infants utilizing a flying intensive-care nursery' *J. Pediat.*, 1970, **77**, 148.

67 SIMPSON, R. K., 'Airplane ambulance: its use in war', *Mil. Surg.*, 1929, **64**, 35–48.

68 SMELLIE, HUGH M., 'An ambulance chair', *Br. med. J.*, 1891, **i**, 1133.

69 TALBOTT, JOHN H., *A Biographical History of Medicine*, New York, Grune & Stratton, 1970.

70 TUNIS, EDWIN, *Wheels: a Pictorial History*, New York, World Publications, 1955.

71 UHLEY, HERMAN, 'Ambulance hot line for coronary care', *Roche Med. Image & Com.*, 1971, pp. 6–9.

72 UALEY, HERMAN, 'Electrocardiographic telemetry from ambulances – a practical approach to mobile coronary units', *Amer. Heart J.*, 1970, **80**, 838.

73 WARM, H., 'Tomorrow's ambulance: an emergency room on wheels', *Amer. J. Surg.*, 1970, **120**, 780.

74 WARREN, JAMES V., 'Mobile coronary care in the logistics of surviving a heart attack', *Med. Opinion*, 1970, **6**, **14**.

Y. Nagatoya
Osaka (Japan)

Florence Nightingale's influence on the science of nursing in Japan

It is well known that Florence Nightingale, who was born in 1820 and died in 1910, had a great influence on the science of nursing and the training of nurses in many countries all over the world. Though Japan is quite far from England, her methods were accepted there relatively rapidly and faithfully. In Japan she has gained high esteem and her name is known to all of the people. So, I would like to tell you about the early history of the Nightingale System in Japan.

HISTORICAL BACKGROUND

Japan had adopted a national isolation policy for 200 years or so, but immediately after the opening of the country in 1854 and the Meiji Restoration in 1868, she suddenly turned into a modern state. In 1869, the decision was made to adopt the medical science practised in Germany, and for this purpose German lecturers in medicine were invited. Medical science, however, had already been introduced from England and the United States, and even after this policy was adopted, the English and American system partially remained. In Japan feudalism had long been predominant and there was still a tendency to regard women as inferior to men. And, therefore, nurses were not highly regarded. The relief and protection of those wounded during the war was mainly performed by men. The nation put emphasis on medical education, but nurses received little training.

EARLY TRAINING SCHOOLS FOR NURSES

(1) *Tokyo Yushi Kyoritsu Hospital Training School for Nurses*

Kanehiro Takagi, who was born in 1849 and died in 1920, was one of the very few doctors who studied medicine in England. He founded the Jikei University, one of the most famous private medical colleges in Japan, in 1882. From 1875 to 1880 he studied at St. Thomas's Hospital Medical School, where Florence Nightingale had her training school. While studying there, he must have become interested in Florence Nightingale and her training school. On returning to Japan, he established Tokyo Yushi Kyoritsu Hospital, the predecessor of the present Jikei University Hospital, but he also felt the need for a nurses' training school. He searched for a nurse from abroad to teach at his school and engaged M. E. Reed from the United States in 1884. She is thought to have been a graduate of the Nightingale Training

School, but we cannot be sure of this. The school was named Tokyo Yushi Kyoritsu Hospital Training School for Nurses and Reed began to give lessons to the nurses twice a week in April 1885. In 1886 students were accepted and a regular course of instruction was started, and five nurses graduated in 1888. They were the first nurses trained in Japan. Reed went back to the United States in 1887, but the school continued and after many changes is known today as Jikei School of Nursing.

(2) *Kyoto Training School for Nurses*

The second training school for nurses in Japan was founded in April 1886 and was called Kyoto Training School for Nurses. This school was established by Jo Neejima, who was born in 1843 and died in 1890 and is famous for founding Doshisha, Christian university. After consultations with a missionary doctor, John C. Berry, sent to Japan by the American Board of Commissioners for Foreign Missions, he decided to invite a training instructor for nurses from the United States. The very famous Linda Richards, who was born in 1841 and died in 1930, answered this invitation. She is said to be America's first trained nurse. She met Nightingale in 1877 and is regarded as a person of her mettle. The school started in 1886 with five students and four of them graduated in 1888. Linda Richards left Japan in 1890.

(3) *Sakurai Girls' Training School for Nurses*

The third training school for nurses in Japan was established by an American lady missionary, M. T. P. True, at Sakurai Girls' School in November 1886. Sakurai Girls' School was a private mission high school directed by Kajiko Yajima, and the training school was called Sakurai Girls' Training School for Nurses.

A British nurse Agnes Vetch visited Japan for sightseeing in 1886, and was asked to stay and teach. She remained in Japan till 1888. She is thought to have been a graduate of the Nightingale Training School. This school started with eight students, and as there was no hospital to practise in, they spent the latter half of their two-year course at the First Medical College Hospital, the predecessor of the present Tokyo University Hospital, and six out of the eight students graduated in 1888.

(4) *The Japan Red Cross Central Hospital Nurses' Training School*

At the Japan Red Cross Central Hospital, nurses' training was heavily emphasized and the director Tsunatsune Hashimoto wanted to employ an instructor from Europe, a graduate of the Nightingale Training School if possible, but he was unable to find anyone. The school started in 1890 with a training principle very similar to that of the Nightingale System. The first ten students had three-year courses at the school and all graduated in 1893. This school is now known as the Japan Red Cross Central Junior College for Nursing.

Thus, the modern nursing education in Japan started in 1885 and the Nightingale System was brought in mainly by nurses from abroad during the period from 1885 to 1890. Its introduction is to be regarded as an innovation not only for Asia, but also for the whole world. The Nightingale System was adopted in Japan by the doctors who studied medicine in England or in the United States and both the Japanese and foreign Christians. They made extraordinary efforts and society recognized their usefulness so their ideas and methods won wide acclaim. All these schools are now regarded as the origin of nursing education in Japan, and some of their graduates became the leaders of the following generation and advanced nursing in Japan.

INTEREST IN FLORENCE NIGHTINGALE IN JAPAN

Japanese people were very much interested in Florence Nightingale even while she was alive. Two doctors (T. Ishiguro and R. Saiki) and two lady instructors (U. Tsuda and T. Yasui) met her in person and her first biography was printed in 1901. Since then, fourteen biographies, a total of eighteen volumes, have been published, some of them translated from other languages. A magnificent statue of her was erected in Kawanishi City, Hyogo Prefecture, and there is a statue or portrait of her in every nurses' training school. Her birthday, 12 May, is celebrated as the Nightingale Day every year. When she died in 1910, the Japan Red Cross Central Hospital held memorial services for her and decided to award a medal with her name on to nurses with exceptional ability. It was some years before the Florence Nightingale Medal was instituted by the International Committee of the Red Cross in 1912. The Japan Red Cross Central Junior College for Nursing keeps a record of her voice.

LATER DEVELOPMENTS OF NURSING

The nursing education in Japan was therefore of quite high standard and later the American system of education was introduced by the St. Luke's International Hospital Nursing School. However, generally speaking, the training of nurses did not develop satisfactorily because the administrators did not fully understand the essence of the Nightingale System and took it for granted that nurses should work under unfavourable conditions with low wages. The government emphasized only the nursing of those wounded during the war and of those high in the social scale. In addition women had a low status in Japan before World War II and did not try to emancipate themselves. When the war ended in 1945 the American nursing method came into Japan on a large scale and the nurses' training system made rapid progress. Nowadays the status of a nurse has been well established and nursing is honoured as a profession. Nurses have also increased in number, but in general there is still a great lack of them.

Nightingale is very much revered in Japan, but up to now she has been a little superficially idealized and deified. Full-scale studies on her have been rather neglected. However, the time is rapidly getting ripe for recognition of her work.

Mihai Popoviciu and Mariana Popoviciu
Braila (Romania)

L'activité sanitaire de la Commission Européenne du Danube

Le Danube, qui prend sa source au coeur de l'Europe, pour se jeter dans la Mer Noire, en faisant de telle manière la liaison avec l'Orient, a constitué depuis les temps les plus reculés une importante voie de navigation commerciale.

D'innombrables états étaient intéressés à l'exploitation de ce fleuve, ce qui a conduit au déclenchement de conflits militaires et diplomatiques concretisés dans de divers traités et conventions.

Dès le XVème siècle le Danube fut transformé dans un véritable fleuve ottoman. Cette période dura jusqu'au XVIIe siècle quand à raison de la stagnation économique, l'empire ottoman se vit forcé d'accorder une série des privilèges de navigation aux marchands grecs, arméniens, et petit à petit à ceux de la France, l'Angleterre, les Pays Bas, la Russie et l'Autriche.

Par le traité de Passarovitz de 1718 (tractatus commercii et navigationis) sont réglementées les relations entre l'Autriche et la Turquie en ce qui concerne la navigation sur le Danube, et en 1774 par la paix de Kuciuk-Kainargi, la Russie aussi put obtenir le même régime de navigation.

A Vienne en 1815 on a mis les bases du régime de navigation sur les fleuves internationaux. En 1829 par le traité d'Adrianople, la Russie réussit à compléter l'occupation sur les embouchures du Danube, et on établit dans l'article 3 de ce traité que la Turquie, quoique maîtresse du bras St. Georges, ne pouvait construire dans cette zone que des bâtisses destinées aux opérations de quarantaine.

La convention russo-autrichienne signée à St. Petersbourg en 1840 est le premier document de droit international qui s'occupe exclusivement du Danube – les autres se réfèrent seulement incidemment à la navigation sur ce fleuve.

La plupart des épidémies de peste et de choléra ont leur origine dans l'Orient. Le Danube constitue, par les navires qui remontent le fleuve, une voie de pénétration de ces épidémies et en même temps un grand danger pour l'Europe Occidentale. A l'époque où l'Etat souverain des embouchures du Danube était la Turquie, les mesures sanitaires relatives au Danube étaient appliquées à Soulina par les services sanitaires des embouchures qui dépendaient du Conseil supérieur de Santé de Constantinople créé en 1838 par le sultan Makhmoud II le Réformateur. Ainsi à Soulina fait son apparition un service sanitaire de quarantaine avec du personnel turc qui contrôlait du point de vue sanitaire tous les navires qui passaient par ce port en percevant une taxe sanitaire qui constituait également le fond d'entretien des autres services sanitaires des ports turcs danubiens jusqu'à la frontière serbe.

Or, parmi les mesures de défense établies par le Réglement Sanitaire Ottoman, la manière d'application apportait des obstacles considérables à la navigation et au commerce des pays coïntéressés, de sorte que cette question de la quarantaine avait déclenché l'ouverture en 1852 à Paris de la première Conférence sanitaire internationale à laquelle ont participé les représentants de 12 pays.

A cette occasion on proposa que dans le Conseil supérieur de Santé de Constantinople devaient se trouver tous les états qui avaient des représentants diplomatiques dans la Capitale Ottomane.

Le régime des quarantaines de Soulina est devenu une source permanente des malentendus parce que la Turquie ne voulait pas céder sa suprématie sur cette région importante du Danube.

Le 28 Décembre 1854, les ambassadeurs des grandes puissances accrédités auprès de la Cour Imperiale de Vienne, ont adressé un mémorandum au prince Gortchakov – le représentant de la Russie – dans lequel on réclamait la liberté de navigation sur le Bas Danube. A la fin des débats où s'affrontèrent les points de vue de l'Autriche, l'Angleterre, la France d'une part, et de la Russie d'autre part, on élabora un protocole le 23 Mars 1855 dans lequel on prévoyait selon la proposition de l'Angleterre la fondation d'une Commission Européenne. De ce jour-là les quarantaines établies autrefois sur le bras de Solina, furent abolies.

Par le traité de Paris de 30 Mars 1856 on fonda la Commission Européenne du Danube avec la stipulation dans l'article 15, que les réglements de police et de quarantaines à établir pour la sûreté des Etats séparés ou traversés par ce fleuve seront conçus de manière à favoriser autant que faire se pourra la circulation des navires.

Art. 16: Dans le but de réaliser les dispositions de l'article précédent, une Commission (dans laquelle la France, l'Autriche, la Grande-Bretagne, la Prusse, la Russie, la Sardaigne, et la Turquie seront chacune représentées par un délégué – on remarque l'absence des Principautés Roumaines) sera chargée de désigner et de faire exécuter les travaux nécessaires pour dégager les embouchures du Danube en aval d'Issaktcha et les parties avoisinantes de la mer dans les meilleures conditions possibles de navigabilité.

Au début les Turcs ont renoncé à leur service sanitaire de quarantaine mais seulement pour un court temps, en revenant avec des mesures excessives en les considérant comme des actes d'administration intérieure. Après plusieures années de discussion entre la C.E.D. et le Conseil supérieur de Santé de Constantinople ayant trait au régime des quarantaines des embouchures du Danube, tout juste quand on prévoyait des conditions bilaterales, – surtout après une nouvelle conférence sanitaire internationale faite à Paris, – une épidémie de choléra fit irruption en Europe arrivant aussi à Soulina en 1865. Alors le gouvernement ottoman prit des mesures sanitaires si rigoureuses, que la navigation fut presque interrompue et l'exercice de la police fluviale totalement suspendu. C'est pourquoi l'Acte public de 1865 de la C.E.D. consacrait aux quarantaines les dispositions de ses articles 18, 19 et 20.

Il reconnaissait au Conseil supérieur de Santé de Constantinople le droit de régler les mesures sanitaires applicables aux embouchures du Danube, en précisant qu'elles devaient être conçues de manière à concilier dans une juste mesure les garanties sanitaires et les besoins du commerce maritime.

Alarmés des ravages du choléra, les états-membres de la C.E.D. convoquèrent en 1866 une conférence sanitaire internationale à Constantinople et on élabora un projet de réglement spécial pour les épidémies auquel la C.E.D. fait en 1868 une série d'amendements.

Les nouvelles épidémies de choléra de 1871 à Constantinople et en Russie, ont imposé aux gouvernements ottoman et roumain l'obligation de prendre des mesures sévères de quarantaine sur le Danube, et la C.E.D. élabora en 1873 un mémorandum auquel adhèrent aussi les Principautés Roumaines, surtout que dans la même année le choléra avait fait son apparition à Galatz.

A la suite du changement de souveraineté résultant du Traité de Berlin 1878, le Gouvernement roumain transforma l'Office de Santé de Soulina en une institution roumaine, conserva le personnel nommé par la Sublime Porte et appliqua le Réglement sanitaire ottoman. A partir de cette date, le gouvernement roumain avait son délégué dans la C.E.D. Puis, en 1879, le 26 Octobre/7 Novembre, il publia dans le Moniteur Officiel un Réglement sanitaire pour les ports roumains du delta du Danube préparé par le Conseil sanitaire supérieur, et nomma comme directeur du Service sanitaire des embouchures du Danube, le Directeur des hôpitaux de la Commission Européenne.

Dans cette année-là on fait des propositions par un Acte additionnel de constituer un Conseil international de Santé à Bucarest, mais qui ne fut jamais fondé, à raison de l'opposition de la Roumanie qui le considérait comme une immixtion dans ses travaux administratifs internes.

Par l'article 7 de l'Acte additionnel à l'Acte public, par les Réglements du 16 Novembre 1882 de la C.E.D. et le Réglement roumain du 26 Juillet/7 Août 1884, en ce qui concerne la perception des taxes, ainsi que par un modus vivendi établi entre le Gouvernement roumain et la C.E.D., résulte le fait que le Conseil international de Santé de Bucarest n'a jamais été constitué et que c'est la puissance territoriale qui exerce les droits reconnus au Conseil International de Santé.

L'office de Santé de Soulina dépendait exclusivément de la Direction générale du Service de Santé de Bucarest conformément au Réglement sanitaire des embouchures du Danube, et son personnel était nommé par le Gouvernement roumain. Il convient de faire remarquer que le Directeur du Service sanitaire des embouchures du Danube se trouvait être en même temps un des directeurs des services de l'hôpital de la C.E.D. à Soulina.

La nécessité d'organiser un service hôpitalier fut reconnue et affirmée par la Commission dès ses premières séances. A cet effet le Comité administratif avait été chargé de faire des démarches auprès du Gouvernement ottoman «afin d'obtenir un vieux vaisseau qui aurait dû servir à la fois de logement des ouvriers employés aux travaux des embouchures du Bas Danube et d'hôpital».

En 1857 la Commission a créé deux hôpitaux, l'un à Toultcha et l'autre à Soulina, destinés exclusivement au traitement des ouvriers employés aux travaux des embouchures et qui ont fonctionné jusqu'en 1860 quand fut prise la décision de transformer ces deux institutions en un hôpital de la Marine à Soulina, destiné à l'hospitalisation des matelots de tous les pavillons, des pilotes et du personnel des services fluviaux.

L'hôpital de Toultcha a été fermé en 1865 lorsque la Commission a supprimé les chantiers qu'elle avait dans cette ville.

A raison de l'augmentation progressive du nombre des matelots soignés dans l'hôpital de Soulina, et en tenant compte de l'experience acquise pendant les épidémies de choléra de 1865 et de 1866, l'hôpital fut reconstruit entre 1867–69, en fonctionnant sous cette forme jusqu'en 1893. C'est ainsi qu'au mois d'Août 1893 pendant l'épidémie de choléra qui s'était déclarée à Soulina, l'hôpital fut largement ouvert à tous les matelots quelles que fussent leur maladie et leur nationalité.

Le Directeur de l'hôpital de ce temps, le docteur Petresco, attira l'attention de la Commission sur les inconvénients de ce fait, que pendant l'épidémie toutes les salles étaient occupées par les contagieux au détriment des marins pour lesquels l'hôpital avait été créé.

Ainsi la C.E.D. a construit un autre hôpital spécialement destiné au traitement des maladies épidémiques et qui entra en fonction le 15 Juin 1894.

Les établissements hospitaliers créés par la Commission en 1869 et en 1894 et augmentés par la suite d'annexes et de services auxiliaires, ont correspondu au point de vue de l'hygiène et du comfort aux besoins des malades et étaient prêts à toutes les éventualités pour le traitement des maladies de toute nature en temps normal comme en temps d'épidémie; ils pouvaient hospitaliser 40 malades non-contagieux et 110 contagieux.

On fonde aussi une section d'obstétrique – gynécologie pour les femmes du personnel et de la population et une section de traumatologie pour les soins spéciaux à donner aux ouvriers de la Commission en cas d'accidents de travail. En dehors des deux hôpitaux de Soulina, la C.E. se préoccupant d'assurer également les soins médicaux de ses fonctionnaires et ouvriers des autres ports du Bas Danube ainsi que des marins étrangers, a organisé à Toultcha, à Galatz et à Brăila un service médical qui fut confié dans chaque de ces villes à un médecin agréé par elle; elle disposait en outre – par suite d'un contrat avec l'hôpital Elisabeta Doamna de Galatz – de quatre lits mis à sa disposition.

La C.E. a accordé certains avantages à la ville de Soulina en ayant en vue qu'ici vivaient la plupart de ses employés, et qu'ici étaient installées la plupart de ses services.

Ainsi en 1864 la C.E. a installé un cimetière commun à toutes les confessions chrétiennes et en 1871, un cimetière mussulman.

La C.E. a contribué à l'hygiène de la ville. Déjà dès les premières années, elle a assaini cette région insalubre par des canaux d'écoulement des eaux des marais. La conséquence de travaux d'assainissement de la ville n'a d'ailleurs pas tardé à se faire sentir. Ainsi, tandis que pendant la période de 1868 à 1870 on comptait parmi les malades entrés dans l'hôpital 31,20 p. 100 des malades atteints de malaria, ce pourcentage tombait progressivement jusqu'à 2,35 p. 100 dans la période 1921–30.

Les conférences sanitaires internationales de Dresde en 1893 et de Venise en 1897, ainsi que la C.E. elle-même, avaient depuis longtemps recommandé d'assurer aux navires qui s'arrêtaient à Soulina, aussi bien qu'à la population de la ville, l'eau potable, – dont l'absence aurait pu, en temps d'épidémie, avoir des conséquences graves. Les installations furent terminées vers la fin du siècle dernier, mais elles se sont révélées par la suite insuffisantes; le Gouvernement roumain décida en 1929 de procéder à leur réfection totale et il s'adressa à la C.E. qui aussi était intéressée dans ces travaux en contribuant à leur exécution avec la somme de 100.000 francs-or.

Entre 1920–21 eut lieu à Paris la Conférence internationale pour arrêter le statut définitif du Danube qui fut promulgué le 1 Octobre 1922.

A cette occasion la délégation roumaine démontra que la C.E. fut instituée et maintenue par des traités qui ont réglementé sa composition, ses droits et ses pouvoirs. Les conditions qui ont déterminé sa création sont disparues et la Roumanie supporte, mais n'accepte pas son existence, de sorte qu'on réclame la suppression de la C.E.D. A peine par l'arrangement de Sinaia de 1938, la C.E. cessait l'exercice de sa compétence concernant la navigation sur le Bas Danube.

A partir de cette date, les taxes sanitaires sont perçues par l'Etat roumain et les hôpitaux de la Commission passent avec leur patrimoine à l'état roumain.

De ce court coup d'oeil sur l'existence d'un organisme international, il résulte qu'indifféremment des aspects diplomatiques insérés dans les divers traités ou conventions, les problèmes hygièniques et sanitaires ont constitué un côté important, étant dictés tout d'abord par l'existence des épidémies qui périclitaient les intérêts de plusieurs états. L'efficacité de l'organisation du réseau sanitaire aux embouchures du Danube ne pouvait être assurée sans la collaboration des autorités sanitaires de l'Etat souverain, qui est le plus intéressé à la sauvegarde de la santé intacte de la population sur son territoire.

Bibliographie

RĂDULESCU, L. GH. and CANJA, E. GLASER, *Contribuţii la studiul istoriei regimului internaţional de navigaţie pe Dunăre,* ed. Stiinţifică, Bucureşti, 1957, vol. I.

BANU, A. C. and RĂDULESCU, L., *Delta Dunării,* Bucuresti, 1959.

BERCUŞ, I. C., Serviciile sanitare de carantină la gurile Dunării în sec. XIX (manuscris), 1971.

BLARAMBERG, NICOLAS, 'Essai comparé sur les institutions et les lois de la Roumanie – depuis les temps les plus reculés jusqu'à nos jours', Bucarest, 1885, Imprimerie du *Peuple Roumain.*

BOTEZ, E. P., *Dunărea şi comisiile ei,* Bucureşti, 1925.

DEMORGNY, G., *Service sanitaire et gestion du fonds sanitaire à Soulina,* Galatz, J. Schenk-Burbea, 1909.

Dobrogea – cincizeci de ani de vieaţă românească 1878–1928, Bucureşti, Cultura Românească, 1928.

Documents officiels relatifs à la Commission Européenne du Danube, Traités Acte public, Acte additionnel, Réglement intérieur, Galatz, J. Schenk, 1890.

GOGEANU, PAUL, *Dumărea în relaţiile internaţionale,* ed. Politică, Bucureşti, 1970.

GRECEANU, N. ing., *Comisia europeană a Dunării şi gurile Dunării,* Bucureşti, 1938.

La Commission européenne du Danube et son oeuvre de 1856 à 1931, Paris, Imprimerie Nationale, 1931.

Monitorul Oficial – Bucureşti (colecţia 1889–1891).

Protocoles des séances de la Commission Européenne du Danube (depuis 1856).

D. B. Weiner
Purchase, N.Y. (U.S.A.)

Napoleon and the nation's health

Under the Old Régime, until the reign of Louis XVI, the nation's health was of marginal concern to the government. The medical profession treated the rich as well as it knew how, the Church cared for the poor owing to the charitable exertions of the nursing orders, and the king decreed emergency measures in case of epidemics and similar disasters.[1] But when, during the French Revolution a constitutional committee under the presidency of the Duc de la Rochefoucauld-Liancourt proposed that the state owes the ailing poor 'prompt, complete, guaranteed, and free medical care', it outlined a programme that democratic governments have yet fully to implement.[2]

The importance of the nation's health to a well-functioning government had been widely recognized by the French Encyclopedists,[3] publicized in John Howard's famous surveys[4] and in Johann Peter Frank's *System einer vollständigen medizinischen Polizei.*[5] In revolutionary France, civil upheaval and foreign war had interrupted and postponed active concern with medical care and public health. Therefore historic accounts of the 'advance to social medicine'[6] often jump from the eighteenth century to Lister and Sir John Simon, to Pettenkofer and Semmelweis, indeed to Virchow and Pasteur.[7]

In this connexion, I have long been puzzled by an assertion Erwin H. Ackerknecht made twenty-five years ago when he wrote that: 'The hygiene movement . . . reached an all-time peak in France in the years between the Napoleonic Wars and 1848; and France . . . might well be credited with leadership in . . . preventive medicine for the period under discussion.'[8] There must be a bridge that connects the philosophy and legislation of the late eighteenth century with the sanitary and preventive excellence of Restoration France and this bridge must be sought in the Napoleonic era.

Napoleon's interest in national health care may be said to have centred on 'airs, waters, and places'. He favoured preventive medicine and sanitation, and all those health measures easily co-ordinated with 'law and order'. Though he scorned physicians and remedies, he had the professional general's concern for a healthy population – especially of strong young men. One might say that he contributed to France's progress toward national health care – in spite of himself.

Legislation was a major aspect of his contribution. As in the case of the Civil Code of 1804, he neither initiated this permanent modern medical legislation nor did he carry it out singlehanded. But he saw it through to completion, and he enforced it.

The need for these laws was urgent. Indeed, the Revolution, after abolishing the medical faculties, created Health Schools without examinations or diplomas. From 1794 on, France had therefore fallen victim to hundreds of medics whose schooling was scant, whose experience had often been garnered on the battlefield only, and whose main purpose was financial gain. Legislation and control were imperative.[9]

The sale of remedies was also in urgent need of regulation, so that published patents could be protected and proprietary medicines controlled.[10] Owing to the advances in chemistry and its application to pharmacy, a new scientific field, toxicology, emerged, and a new specialty, legal medicine, was born during this era.[11]

To implement his legislation, Napoleon chose administrators of outstanding quality. Either he was extremely lucky, or he was an excellent judge of men, or the Revolution had indeed brought to the fore a brand of talented individuals for whom careers were now opening up. This is not to say that personalities as effective as Chaptal, Froschot, Thouret, Parmentier, or Camus did not leave their imprint on late eighteenth-century France – which boasted its Turgot, Necker, or Vicq d'Azyr. But under the Old Régime neither the well-intentioned Louis XVI nor these talented administrators were able to overcome the vested interests of privileged groups and corporations. A recent remarkable study by Marcel Candille of the failure to decentralize the Hôtel-Dieu in the 1770s and 1780s is a case in point.[12]

With the backing of the First Consul and Emperor, these administrators achieved remarkable feats of modernization in French health care. In Paris, this was brought about with the help of a new agency, the Conseil général d'Administration des Hôpitaux et Hospices de Paris, created by Napoleon's Minister of Interior, the physician and chemist Jean-Antoine Chaptal[13] and presided over by the Préfet de la Seine, Nicolas Froschot.[14] This Council, created in 1801, was responsible for the administration of hospitals, old-age homes, welfare centres, home care, baby nursing and foster homes.[15]

The original and modern aspects of the Council's work can be summarized as follows:

A central diagnostic service. An Admitting Office at the Hôtel-Dieu now sorted applicants in need of mere relief from the genuine medical cases. For some of these an instant consultation with the doctor would suffice, or else referral to the outpatient clinic at one of the city's forty-eight Welfare Bureaux[16] that also administered home care, with the help of local doctors and pharmacists paid by the city, and the free services of the Sisters of Charity.[17] During the first eighteen months of its existence, the Bureau d'Admission saw almost 35,000 applicants of whom it rechannelled or rejected about one-third. And the 'faux-malades' stopped coming.[18]

The specialization of hospitals was encouraged. With the opening of the Maternité, its use as a teaching hospital and its school for midwives, a new attitude toward mothers and infants was adopted by the administration. Illegitimate and unwanted babies had been brought to Paris in increasing numbers during the preceding two centuries. Together with those abandoned at the Maison de la Couche and those born at the Hôtel-Dieu and rejected by their mothers, they had all been taken to the Enfants-Trouvés and then farmed out to the countryside. About nine-tenths died.

It was Mesdames Dugès and Lachapelle (her daughter), head-midwives at the Hôtel-Dieu, who first proposed the *novel* scheme of keeping babies with their mothers. And the confiscated monastery of Port-Royal, transformed into the Maternité, opened in 1797. But not until the adoption of the commonsense modern notions of M. Hombron (the astute though uneducated lay administrator, as important to the modernization of the Maternité as his contemporary, M. Pussin, was to Pinel at Bicêtre) did the first French lying-in hospital emerge.[19]

The first Children's Hospital in Europe was opened in what had been a school for young ladies owned by the Sisters of St. Thomas de Villeneuve, transformed, under the Revolution, into an orphanage. In April 1802 it became the Hôpital des Enfants Malades, thus ending the objectionable practice of hospitalizing children with adults. Boys and girls were segregated and, after 1808, contagious and chronic patients were admitted, but housed in special wings. The architect Clavareau welcomed the innovation, and so did Napoleon's personal physician, Baron Corvisart.[20]

Nothing original seems to have been added to help the handicapped for whom truly creative concern had blossomed in the late eighteenth century. The Revolution merely nationalized the recently founded institutions for blind children[21] and for the deaf-and-dumb,[22] the ancient hospital for the blind[23] and the first paying insane asylum, the Maison nationale de Charenton, which then housed its most famous tenant, the Marquis de Sade.[24]

The specialization of services was also introduced at this time, including a central bakery (Hôtel Scipion), central slaughterhouses and wine-cellar, and – most important – the central pharmacy (Hôtel des Miramiones) whose creation owes much to the celebrated Antoine-Auguste Parmentier (1737–1813) of potato fame.[25]

Architectural changes were needed and accomplished. One can read about them in a panegyric to Bonaparte, the *Mémoires sur les hospices civils de Paris* by Nicolas-Etienne Clavareau (1757–1815), the municipal architect.[26] The changes he wrought in the distribution of light, air, and space in the old hospital structures are the visual embodiment of the new relationship between religion, health care, and the government. Large, airy wards for single beds only, convalescents' quarters, operating rooms with spectators' benches, often took the place of altars, chapels, or the living quarters of monks and nuns. Clavareau rebuilt much of the Hôtel-Dieu, constructed a women's ward at the Charité and a clinical school in its former chapel, while his colleague Charles-François Viel (1745–1819) modernized the Pitié and Cochin, built the central pharmacy in the Hôtel des Miramiones, and the great amphitheatre at the Hôtel-Dieu. Their style was functional, monumental, neo-classic, as befitted the emerging empire.[27]

While the Conseil des Hôpitaux was thus streamlining procedures, personnel, and buildings, it left untouched the vast area of sanitary and preventive care. (What *really* happened was that Paris had two prefects, and the Préfet de la Seine, Froschot, had manoeuvred to monopolize the entire health budget.) Therefore, when the famous pharmacist Cadet de Gassicourt proposed the creation of a Paris Health Council, the other prefect, the Préfet de Police Dubois, responded with surprising speed. The four original members of this Council (first meeting, 6 July 1802: Deyeux, Parmentier, Cadet, all chemists; Huzard, Sr., veterinarian) soon grew to seven (by 29 October 1807), including Dr. Michel-Augustin Thouret, the Director of the Paris Faculty of Medicine who was also a member of the Conseil des Hôpitaux, which soon co-opted Parmentier. The channels of communication were now open.

The Health Council's work was as impressive as its purview was vast. For years, it turned out some three hundred reports annually. Everything affecting public health was considered a germane task. The Council made regular inspection tours of prisons, four times a year, and twice a year it checked the first aid equipment for rescuing drowning persons – jumping into the Seine being the favoured means of suicide for Parisians before the Eiffel Tower was built. The Council conducted chemical tests of the drinking water consumed by Parisians and analysed mineral and medicinal waters for which curative powers were claimed; it examined the varieties of flour used by bakers, inspected the cattle in the slaughterhouses and the meat sold in the markets. It investigated cases of mushroom poisoning and tested a suspect synthetic lemonade (in 1809 the British blockade had cut off the supply of lemons). It tasted wines to decide whether they had been diluted, chose the vegetables for soup kitchens, and the location for cemeteries outside city limits. It often referred problems to the Faculty of Medicine or the National Institute in order to obtain the best expert opinion.

Did the Health Council's reports lead to action? Yes! Factories that emptied poisonous waste products into the Seine were forced to move downstream, the sale of dangerous products was forbidden, two cemeteries – Père Lachaise (1803), Montparnasse (1826) – were established out of town. Inspectors would check on offenders and the police would punish infractions of the health laws.

True, none of these actions was wholly original. The Lieutenant de Police had pursued similar goals under the Old Régime, and so had the Société royale de Médecine from 1776 on. The new aspect was the existence of a municipal council and of governmental backing – with powerful inspectors and even with funds.[28]

A unique opportunity arose with the discovery of vaccination. Jenner's *Inquiry into the Causes and Effects of the Variolae Vaccinae*, published in June 1798, was immediately translated into French by the Geneva physician Antoine Aubert.[29] Interest among the medical and scientific community in France was instant and acute.

France and England had been at war for seven years. But the scientific establishments of the two countries managed to maintain friendly contacts and a fitful correspondence.[30] This civilized relationship enabled Dr. William Woodville, the assistant to Dr. Jenner, Director of the Smallpox and Inoculation Hospital in London who, by May 1800, had vaccinated nearly 4,000 persons, to bring cowpox vaccine to France. His was the fourth attempt to do so;[31] what had previously reached Paris turned out to be 'false' or 'bastard' vaccine. Dr. Woodville succeeded only because he vaccinated several children on his way through Boulogne. They had been 'bien envachinés'[32] (as one journal put it) so that the 'malady special to English cows' could now be given to French children. Eventually that great humanitarian, the Duc de la Rochefoucauld-Liancourt, proposed the founding of a vaccination institute.[33] It was to be financed – in the 'Anglo-Saxon' manner – by public subscription. The sum needed was soon raised. Among the subscribers were Froschot, the Préfet de la Seine, Lebrun, one of the three Consuls, Talleyrand, the Minister of Foreign Affairs, and Lucien Bonaparte, the Minister of Interior. Napoleon favoured vaccination.

The subscribers organized what later became known as the Comité central de Vaccine whose medical committee of nine included Drs. Philippe Pinel, Thouret, Joseph-Ignace Guillotin, and a François Colon, who put his country house in Vaugirard at the Committee's disposal. There thirty young orphans were successfully vaccinated. Addressing the First Consul in October 1803, the President of the Paris

Vaccination Committee, Dr. Guillotin, declared: 'There is no doubt, Citizen First Consul, smallpox will be eliminated. . . . Your government will support vaccination, since they both entered our happy land together.'[34] And when Pope Pius VII visited Paris in March 1805, he received Guillotin and his Committee in a special audience and praised their work. Vaccination had arrived.

When limited, reachable objectives were in view, such as controlling food and drugs, or preventing smallpox, and reliable medical means were at hand to attain these objectives, Napoleon would lend his prestige and power to his doctors and public officials. These were experiments that he controlled. At the same time he missed three major opportunities for creative innovation: in 1800, by a stroke of the pen, he could have granted his army doctors the status they were being denied by the regular officers: he could have created a French Army Medical Corps. Instead, he subordinated his doctors to the Supply Corps, degrading them, it was said, to the rank of 'bakers and butchers'.[35] French military medicine rankled with discontent until the situation was remedied, in 1876.[36]

In 1807, at a national nursing conference held in Paris under the auspices of Madame Mère, Napoleon tried to form a national professional nursing association, but failed to breach the consistent refusal of the nursing orders to abandon their own, religious, rule.[37]

His most harmful measure was the creation of the 'officiers de santé' in 1803, in many ways a revival of the barber-surgeons of the Old Régime.[38] Napoleon would have done better to institute a network of public health officials, those well-paid public servants envisaged by Vicq d'Azyr and the Société royale in the 1780s. Ironically, such a network of cantonal physicians existed at that very time, in Napoleon's very Empire, namely in Alsace. While it is unlikely that this French monarch would have been eager to learn from his German neighbours, the fact remains that the poorly trained second-rate medical practitioners whom he legalized in 1803 were deplored and despised by the French medical profession until their abolition in 1892.

The negative side of the balance sheet also shows that Napoleon slowed the advance toward national health care. He drained France of young men, one million of whom died in his wars. And he flooded her with cripples and invalids. Censorship and government control hampered the medical profession's freedom of inquiry, thus retarding progress. His disinterest in popular education precluded the training of the key persons in dispensing family hygiene, proper diet, and home nursing – namely women. Owing to his vast military expenditures, funds for health, education, and welfare were scarce.

It would seem that a professional soldier can champion his nation's health only at the expense of his martial designs. But to give medical needs priority over military purposes was inconceivable for a general like Napoleon Bonaparte.

ACKNOWLEDGEMENTS

Research for this paper was undertaken while the author was a Senior Fellow of the National Endowment for the Humanities, and travel to London was made possible by a grant from the American Council of Learned Societies. The support of these institutions is here gratefully acknowledged, as is the hospitality of the Center for

Advanced Study in the Behavioral Sciences, Stanford, California, where the paper was completed.

References

1 The problem of medical help to the indigent in late eighteenth-century France is explored in BLOCH, C., *L'assistance et l'état en France à la veille de la révolution 1764–1790* (Paris Law Thesis, 1908); DREYFUS, F., *L'assistance sous la Législative et la Convention 1791–1795*, Paris, Bellais, 1905; LALLEMAND, L., *La révolution et les pauvres*, Paris, Picard, 1898; MCCLOY, S. T., *Government Assistance in Eighteenth-Century France*, Durham, N.C., Duke University Press, 1946.

The role of hospitals in providing medical assistance to indigents is discussed in IMBERT, J., *Le droit hospitalier de la révolution et de l'empire*, Paris, Sirey, 1954; FOSSEYEUX, M., 'L'Hôtel-Dieu de Paris sous la révolution, 1789–1802', *La révolution française*, 1913, **66**, 40–85.

For an excellent historical overview of the problem, see CANDILLE, M., 'L'évolution des principes d'assistance hospitalière', *Revue d'Assistance publique*, 1958, pp. 43–51; see also LEPOINTE, G., 'De la charité à la sécurité sociale', *Revue des Sciences humaines*, nlle série, no. 54, 1949, pp. 83–95.

2 The basic documents pertaining to the Poverty Committee of the Constituent Assembly, presided over by Liancourt, are to be found in BLOCH, C. and TUETEY, A. (eds.), *Procès-verbaux et rapports du Comité de mendicité de la Constituante, 1790–1791*, Paris, Imprimerie nationale, 1911; the above quotation is from this source, p. 391. The only thorough work on the Health Committee of the Constituent Assembly is INGRAND, H., *Le Comité de Salubrité de l'Assemblée nationale constituante: Un essai de réforme de l'enseignement médical, des services d'hygiène, et de la protection de la santé publique*, Paris Medical Thesis, 1934.

For more general and recent discussions, see ROSEN, G., 'Hospitals, medical care and social policy in the French Revolution', *Bull. Hist. Med.*, 1956, **30**, 124–49, and WEINER, D. B., 'Le droit de l'homme à la santé – Une belle idée devant l'Assemblée constituante: 1790–1791', *Clio Médica*, 1970, **5**, 209–23.

The whole problem of the relationship between the medical profession and the ailing poor at the time of the French Revolution has recently been re-examined in a brilliant and provocative manner by Michel Foucault in *Naissance de la clinique: Une archéologie du regard médical*, Paris, Presses Universitaires de France, 1963; recent work inspired by Foucault and, it would seem, Claude Lévi-Straus, includes PETER, J.-P., 'Malades et maladies à la fin du 18ème siècle', *Annales E.S.C.*, 1967, pp. 711–51, and the same author's 'Les mots et les objets de la maladie', *Revue historique*, no. 499, July–September 1971, pp. 13–38.

3 See, e.g. ROUSSEAU, J.-J., 'Discourse on the Origin and Foundations of Inequality Among Men', *The First and Second Discourses*, ed. by R. D. Masters, New York, St. Martin's Press, 1964, esp. pp. 108–11; MONTESQUIEU, CH. DE SECONDAT, BARON DE, *L'Espirit des lois*, bk. XXIII, ch. XXIX; DIDEROT, D., article 'Hôtel-Dieu', TURGOT, A. R. G., article 'Fondation', DURIVAL, M., article 'Infirmier', all in *Encylopédie ou Dictionnaire raisonné des Sciences, des Arts et des Métiers*, Lausanne and Berne, 1782.

4 HOWARD, J., *The State of the Prisons in England and Wales with Preliminary Observations and an Account of some Foreign Prisons*, Warrington, 1777–80, and HOWARD, J., *An Account of the Principal Lazarettos in Europe with Various Papers Relative to the Plague, Together with Further Observations on Some Foreign Prisons and Hospitals and Additional Remarks on the Present State of those in Great Britain and Ireland*, London, 1789.

5 Vienna, Schwann, Cotta & Schaumburg, 1779–1819, 6 vols.

6 SAND, R., *The Advance to Social Medicine*, London and New York, Staples Press, 1952.

7 The view that 'social medicine' is a nineteenth-century concept, closely related to the effects of the Industrial Revolution, is most thoroughly documented by George Rosen in 'What is social medicine? A genetic analysis of the concept', *Bull. Hist. Med.*, 1947, **21**, 674–733. Rosen is, however, well aware of antecedent French thought, witness his article cited above, n. 2.

8 ACKERKNECHT, E. H., 'Hygiene in France, 1815–1848', *Bull. Hist. Med.*, 1948, **22**, 118.

9 The Law of 19 Ventôse, Year XI (11 March 1803) regulated the training of doctors, and the Law of Germinal, Year XI (30 March 1803) that of pharmacists and midwives.

On the main architect of this legislation, A.-F. Fourcroy, see SMEATON, W. A., *Fourcroy, Chemist and Revolutionary, 1755–1809*, Cambridge, Heffer, 1962; on the general problem, see ACKERKNECHT, E. H., *Medicine at the Paris Hospital, 1794–1848*, Baltimore, Johns Hopkins Press, 1967, and HUARD, P., *Sciences, Médecine, Pharmacie*, 1789–1815, Paris, Dacosta, 1970.

10 The classic study of French pharmacy during this era is BOUVET, M., *La pharmacie hospitalière à Paris de 1789 à 1815*, Paris, Société d'histoire de la pharmacie, 1943, see also the same author's *Histoire de la pharmacie en France des origines à nos jours*, Paris, Occitania, 1937.

11 On legal medicine, see BASS, G., *Die Gerichtsmedizin als Spezialfach in Paris von 1800 bis 1850*, Zürich, Juris, 1964; background information can be found in BALTHAZAR et DÉROBERT,

'Histoire de la médecine légale' in LAIGNEL-LAVASTINE, M. (ed.), *Histoire générale de la Médecine, de la Pharmacie, de l'Art dentaire et de l'Art vétérinaire*, Paris, Albin Michel, 1948, vol. 2, pp. 457–74.

12 CANDILLE, M., 'Les projets de translation de l'Hôtel-Dieu de Paris hors de la Cité', *Revue de l'Assistance publique*, 1956, **44**, 743–52; 1957, **46**, 239–63; 1957, **47**, 343–59, 1957, **48**, 433–49.

13 On Chaptal, see PIGEIRE, J., *La vie et l'oeuvre de Chaptal* (1756–1832), Paris, Domat-Montchrétien, 1932, and Chaptal's own memoirs, *Mes souvenirs sur Napoléon*. Paris, Plon Nourrit, 1893.

14 Froschot may well have been the initiator of this reform: see IMBERT, J., op. cit., pp. 234–41. On Froschot, see PASSY, L., *Froschot, Préfet de la Seine*, Evreux, Hérissey, 1867; CANDILLE, M., 'Un grand commis de l'administration française, Nicolas Froschot (1761–1828)', *L'Hôpital et l'aide sociale à Paris*, 1961, **2**, 605–9, as well as the much less substantial RICHE, J., 'Froschot, préfet de la Seine sous le premier empire, sa carrière, pendant l'époque révolutionnaire', Société pour l'histoire du droit et des institutions des anciens pays bourguignons, comtais et romands, *Mémoires*, 1960, **21**, 43–62.

15 Paris. Conseil général d'administration des hôpitaux et hospices de Paris. *Rapports au Conseil général des hospices sur les hôpitaux, les secours à domicile, la direction des nourrices*, Paris, Imprimerie des hospices civils, AN XI [1803], and *Rapport fait au Conseil général des hospices par un de ses membres sur l'état des hôpitaux, des hospices, et des secours à domicile, à Paris, depuis le 1er janvier 1804 jusqu'au 1er janvier 1814*, Paris, Imprimerie de Mme Huzard, 1816; also *Inventaire analytique des délibérations*, now being undertaken at the Archives de l'Assistance Publique. The work has been completed for the period under discussion.

16 The original 'bureaux de charité' had, under the Old Régime, been organized by the parish priests and financed with charitable contributions. They emerged, after the Revolution, as 'bureaux de bienfaisance', under the mayors of the Paris arondissements. They deserve serious study. The best work to date, on these welfare centres and on medical home care, seems to be: FOSSEYEUX, M., 'Les Ecoles de charité à Paris sous l'ancien régime et dans la première partie du 19ème siècle', *Société de l'histoire de Paris et de l'Ile de France. Mémoires*, 1912, **39**, 225–366; GILLE, F., *Le Traitement des Malades a Domicile, son histoire et ses rapports avec les bureaux de bienfaisance de la Ville de Paris*, Paris, Baillière, 1879; ORSEL, J., *Essai sur les hopitaux et sur les Secours à Domicile distribués aux indigents malades*, Paris, Le Normant, 1821; SOVICHE, J., *Des Hopitaux et des Secours à Domicile*, Paris, Gabon, 1822.

17 On the religious nursing orders during this era, see WEINER, D. B., 'The French Revolution, Napoleon and the nursing profession', *Bull. Hist. Med.*, 1972, **46**, 274–305.

18 The Admitting Office was created by the decree of 4 December 1801 and began functioning on 22 March 1802. Two physicians and two surgeons were now on duty from 9-4 every day (Paris, Conseil général d'administration . . ., *Rapport . . . 1804 . . . 1814*, pp. 221–38). In contrast, under the Old Régime, admission was handled by an Augustinian nurse and a surgeon, one of those practitioners without a general knowledge of medicine, unable to thwart the religious nurse whose charitable purpose was to admit all the suffering poor. This attitude was the chief source of overcrowding at the Hôtel-Dieu.

19 CARRIER, H., *Origines de la Maternité de Paris. Les maitresses sages-femmes et l'Office des accouchées à l'ancien Hôtel-Dieu, 1378–1796*, Paris, Steinheil, 1888; DELAUNAY, P., *La Maternité de Paris* (*Port-Royal de Paris – Port-Libre – L'Hospice de la Maternité – L'école des sages-femmes et ses origines*), *1625–1907*, Paris, Rousset, 1909; Paris, Conseil général d'administration des hôpitaux et hospices de Paris. *Mémoire historique et instructif sur l'hospice de la Maternité*, Paris, Imprimerie des hospices civils, 1808.

20 LAMBEAU, L., *Le couvent des Hospitalières de St. Thomas de Villeneuve, rue de Sèvres 25–27* (1698–1907), Ville de Paris, Commission du Vieux Paris. Annexe au procès-verbal de la séance du 25 mai 1907; LAMBEAU, L., *La Maison royale de l'Enfant-Jésus, actuellement Hôpital des Enfants Malades, rue de Sèvres 149* (*1694–1908*), Ville de Paris, Commission du Vieux Paris. Annexe au procès-verbal de la séance du 16 novembre 1907; SIGURET, G. R., *Histoire de l'hospitalisation des enfants malades de Paris*, Paris, Medical Thesis, 1907; VALLÉRY-RADOT, P., 'L'Hôpital des Enfants Malades', *Paris d'autrefois, ses vieux hôpitaux. Deux siècles d'histoire hospitalière*, Paris, Paul Dupont, 1947, pp. 217–24.

21 Valentin Haüy (1743–1822), the champion of blind children, adopted a system of writing later to be superceded by Louis Braille (1829). Haüy's *Essay on the Education of the Blind* (1786) led to the founding of a small school, financed by the Paris Philanthropic Society. This school was transformed on 21 July 1791, into the 'Institution nationale des jeunes aveugles' who were adopted as 'wards of the nation'; see GUILLIÉ, *Rapport fait à S. Exc. le Ministre Secrétaire d'Etat au Département de l'Intérieur sur l'état de l'Institution royale des jeunes aveugles, pendant les exercices 1815 et 1816*, Paris, Chanson, 1818, and GUADET, J., *L'Institution des jeunes aveugles de Paris, son histoire et ses procédes d'enseignement*, Paris, Thunot, 1849; also PEAN DE ST. GILLES, M. P., *La Maison philanthropique de Paris*, Paris, Lemerre, 1892.

22 The Abbé Charles Michel de l'Epée (1712–1789), author of *The True Manner of Teaching the Deaf-Mute Confirmed by Experience* (1784) founded a small school (1755) that his successor, the Abbé Ambroise Sicard (1742–1822) induced the government to finance (1778). Again the Revolution merely nationalized a going concern (Decree of 24 August 1790), founding the 'Institution nationale des sourds-muets'. See, GERANDO, BARON J.-M. DE, *De l'éducation des sourds-muets de naissance*, Paris, Méquignon l'aîné, 1827, 2 vols.; SAUREL, E., *Un bienfaiteur de l'humanité: L'abbé Sicard, 1742–1822*, Toulouse, 1958.

23 On the Hôpital des Quinze-Vingt, see RIFFARD-ST. MARTIN, F. G., *Rapport sur l'Hôpital des Quinze-Vingt*, Paris, Imprimerie nationale, 1792, and BATTELLE, H., *Notice historique et statistique sur l'Hospice des Quinze-Vingt*, Paris, Crapelet, 1867.

24 The Hospice de la Charité de Charenton had been founded by a layman, Le Blanc, in 1641 and was, since its inception, staffed by the Brothers of Charity. Nationalized on 27 Prairial, Year V, and dubbed 'Maison nationale de Charenton', it was to become world famous when J. E. D. Esquirol was appointed psychiatrist-in-chief in 1826, and introduced novel architectural and therapeutic concepts.

25 BOUVET, M., *La pharmacie hospitalière à Paris. . . .*

26 Paris, Prault, 1805.

27 Clavareau spoke of 'the monumental impression that every public building should convey', and stated his intention of 'giving the very form of the establishment a moral purpose', *Mémoires . . .*, p. 112. See also VIEL, CH.-F., *Des anciennes études de l'architecture; de la nécessité de les remettre en vigueur, et de leur utilité pour l'administration des bâtiments civils*, Paris, Tilliard, 1807.

28 On the Conseil de Salubrité de la Ville de Paris, and the problem of municipal health councils in other French cities, see MOLÉON, V. DE, *Rapports généraux sur la salubrité publique . . . 1802 à 1826*, Paris, Au bureau du Recueil industriel, 1828; PÂRENT-DUCHATELET, A. J. B., 'Quelques considérations sur le conseil de salubrité de Paris', *Ann. Hyg. publ. Med. leg., Paris*, 1933, **9**, 243–56; TRÉBUCHET, A., 'Rapports géneraux des travaux du conseil de salubrité, 1829–1839', ibid., 1841, **25**, 61–99.

Discussions regarding all conceivable aspects of this problem by highly qualified professional men fill the pages of the above-quoted journal which was founded in 1829.

29 AUBERT, A. (tr.), *Rapport sur le cowpox ou la petite vérole des vaches et sur l'inoculation de cette maladie*, Paris, An VIII; see also AUBERT, A., *Rapport sur la vaccine, ou Traité dans lequel on trouve la Réponse aux questions rédigées par les commissaires de l'Ecole de médecine de Paris sur la pratique et les résultats de cette nouvelle inoculation en Angleterre. Nouvelle édition augmentée du Traité de la vaccine chez la vache*, Paris, Richard, Caille et Ravier, An IX [1800–1801].

30 In a fascinating book called *The Sciences Were Never At War*, London, Thomas Nelson, 1960, Sir Gavin de Beer, the distinguished British embryologist, has documented this relationship with new archival material. A British ship would hijack a French vessel on the ocean, imprison the crew, confiscate the supplies and appropriate the ship – but the captain would take special care of that heavy box filled with seeds, stuffed birds, sketches of natives and exotic fauna and flora collected by the naturalist on board the French vessel. And the precious box would often find its way to its original destination in France.

31 The difficulty, of course, arose from the fact that knowledge of the cowpox vaccine was entirely empirical. No one had ever seen the cowpox virus or knew how to transport it over long distances. The first three times virus was sent on cloth soaked in vaccine, either via Geneva or directly from London, once in a 'vial filled with hydrogen gas over mercury and covered with a bladder.' Rapport du comité médical, *Recueil périodique de la société de médecine de Paris*, 1799, **8**, 239. For a good account of this story in English, see DUNBAR, R. G., 'The Introduction of the Practice of Vaccination into Napoleonic France', *Bull. Hist. Med.*, 1941, **10**, 635–50; in French, see COLON, F., *Histoire de l'introduction et des progrès de la vaccine en France*, Paris, Le Normant, 1801.

32 Quoted in Colon, op. cit., p. 39.

33 In Paris, the Society of Medicine had been the first to act. It appointed Philippe Pinel, the celebrated clinician and psychiatrist, to investigate Jenner's procedure. In early 1800 both the Faculty of Medicine and the Institut de France set up additional committees to study Jenner's vaccine.

34 *Le Moniteur universel*, 14 Brumaire, Am XII (8 November 1803).

35 CHEVALIER, A. G., 'Physicians of the French Revolution', *Ciba Symp.*, 1946, **7**, 250.

36 WEINER, D. B., 'French Doctors Face War: 1792–1815', in *From the Ancien Régime to the Popular Front: Essays in the History of Modern France in Honor of Shepard B. Clough*, C. K. Warner (ed.), New York, Columbia University Press, 1969, pp. 51–73.

37 WEINER, D. B., 'The French Revolution, Napoleon, and the nursing profession', *Bull. Hist. Med.* 1972, **46**, 274–305.

38 HUARD, P., 'L'officiat de santé, 1794–1892', *Concours médical*, 83ème année, no. 22, 1961, 3231–39.

J. H. Sypkens Smit
Hattem, Gelderse Dÿk 3 (Holland)

Cornelis de Mooy, Arzt und Erfinder (1834–1926)

In der Ruhmeshalle von Chicago prangt unter den Ärzten, deren Namen als erwähnenswert angesehen werden, auch der von Cornelis de Mooy.

Trotz dieser Huldigung, trotz Ehrungen in vielerlei Form: Ernennungen, Medaillen, Orden, ist dieser typische ,,Soldatendoktor", sowohl national wie international gesehen, eine auffallend wenig bekannte Persönlichkeit geblieben.

Gerade weil viele seiner Erfindungen-durch kein Patent geschützt-namenlos durch andere in den Handel gebracht, die Grenzen passierten, schien es berechtigt, auf einem Kongress wie diesem, für diesen ,,Berufserfinder", dessen einzige Triebfeder war, seinem Nächsten zu helfen, einen Augenblick Ihre Aufmerksamkeit zu erbitten bei dem Thema ,,Medizin und Gesellschaft".

Die mir zugestandene Zeit erlaubt nur einen flüchtigen Hinweis ohne Einzelheiten.

Fragt man sich nun, rund 50 Jahre nach seinem Tod, worin die Bedeutung dieses Sanitätsoffiziers bestanden hat, dann sehe ich das in seiner ständigen Bemühung, eine Reihe von Dingen, die ein Militärarzt täglich gebraucht: Nahtmaterial, Verbandsmaterial, Transportmöglichkeiten und Unterkünfte derartig zu verbessern, dass sie unter Kriegs- und andere Notzuständen völlig den Anforderungen des Arztes entsprachen. Stets stand ihm vor Augen Zeit, Raum, Material, Geld und Personal zu sparen. So entwickelte er ein System von Apparaten zur schnellen und erfolgreichen Durchführung sowohl der konservativen als auch der operativen Chirurgie unter schwierigen Umständen. De Mooy lieferte hiermit einen wesentlichen Beitrag zur Geschichte der Ersten-Hilfe-Leistung.

In verschiedenen Rot-Kreuz-Ambulanzen in Indonesien, im französisch-deutschen Krieg, im ersten Weltkrieg haben seine Erfindungen bewiesen, dass sie völlig den damals zu stellenden Erwartungen entsprachen.

Heutzutage scheint vieles veraltet, wichtig ist aber, dass seine Ausgangspunkte noch heute gültig sind und dass seine Prinzipien in modernerer Form bis heute angewandt werden.

Herkunft und Lebenslauf bestimmten deutlich den Verlauf seiner Kreativität. Sein Vater war auch Sanitätsoffizier. Cornelis de Mooy wurde 1834 in Middelburg geboren, aber bereits mit 3 Jahren lebte er in Niederländisch Ost-Indien. Schon in sehr jungem Alter begleitete der unternehmungslustige Junge dort seinen Vater bei Krankenbesuchen. Die empfangenen Eindrücke brachten ihn zu dem Entschluss, wie sein Vater Sanitätsoffizier zu werden. Dieser unwandelbare Entschluss zwang seine Eltern, ihren Sohn nach Holland zu schicken. Als nach mehr als halbjähriger (abenteuerlicher) Fahrt die Bark „Louise“ in den Niederlanden Anker warf, brach eine harte Studienzeit an: Internatsschule in Breda, Lateinschule, zuletzt die staatliche Akademie für Militärärzte in Utrecht. An der gleichen Schule wurden Ant. Mathijsen, der Erfinder des Gipsverbandes, Cornelis Donders, der begabte Physiologe und Augenarzt und später Zwaardemaker ausgebildet.

Interessant ist, wie C. de Mooy, 1866 nach Maastricht abkommandiert, dort ein Ophthalmophantom konstruierte, das die Beweglichkeit des lebenden Auges nachahmte, um hieran die Durchführung von Augenoperationen zu lehren. Dieses Phantom erlangte die Billigung von Donders.

1878 veröffentlichte de Mooy seine Experimente mit Gipsverbänden nach Ant. Mathijsen. Er riet, sie mit Leinöl aufzuweichen, wodurch man sie leichter öffnen und daraus Schienen und auch Moullagen von pathologischen Objekten machen konnte.

Das alles war lange nach seiner Studienzeit (1853–57) und seiner Ernennung zum Sanitätsoffizier.

An einem seiner ersten Standorte, Haarlem, war er genötigt, seinem Vater ärztlichen Beistand zu leisten bei einem verengendem Prozess in Oesophagus und Magen. Das gab ihm Veranlassung, Speiseröhrensonden und auch Knopfsonden für Urethrastrikturen zu konstruieren, die er später in Indien noch verbesserte.

Zur gleichen Zeit verfertigte er eine neue Art von Kugelzange, die Vorteile gegenüber den üblichen Modellen besass, weil die Ein-und Ausschussöffnung nicht erweitert werden müsste und wobei ein klug ausgedachter Satz anschraubbarer Einzelteile in vielseitiges Instrument mit kleinem Umfang schuf. Die Zange blieb von 1864 bis 1912 in Gebrauch und verlor erst ihre Bedeutung, als die Beschaffenheit der Kugeln sich stark änderte.

1866 verzog er nach Maastricht. Obwohl er dort wegen familiärer geldlicher Schwierigkeiten äusserst ärmlich leben musste, gehörte die dort verbrachte Zeit zu einer der glücklichsten seines Lebens Er arbeitete mit grosser Hingabe und war sehr erfinderisch. Abgesehen von kleinere Sachen, wie einem Fomentationsapparat, womit man jemand Kälte oder Wärme verabfolgen kann und ein Stiefelmesser, entwarf er 1872 eine Feld-Zahnzange. Es wurde ein fester Arm und ein anderer mit verstellbaren losen Haken.

Auch fertigte er Trepanationsbohrer an, wobei das Instrument automatisch anzeigte, wenn der Schedelknochen durchbohrt war. Diese Instrumente wurden schnell in Lüttich, Berlin, London und Paris gebraucht, und Veranlassung, dass er zum Mitglied der Société de Chirurgie de Paris ernannt wurde.

Sehr wichtig war auch de Mooy's Konstruktion von Operations-nadeln und Einfädlern, die, insoweit sie unter seiner persönlichen Aufsicht angefertigt waren, vortrefflich arbeiteten. 1870 wurden sie als das Beste auf diesem Gebiet angesehen. Erst nach Deutschland, später auch nach England, Frankreich, Belgien und der Schweiz fanden sie ihren Weg. Die Vettern Jacques und Auguste Reverdin fanden sie besser als ihre eigenen Instrumente und nahmen sie in Gebrauch.

de Mooy gebrauchte eine Einkerbung im schneidenden Teil der Nadel statt des federnden Ohrs der Englischen Nadeln. Die originelle Konstruktion machte Pinzetten usw. überflüssig.

In de Mooy's Zeit war der Krankentransport höchst mangelhaft und verlangte für den Ambulanzwagen 4 Pferde, womit dann 8 sitzende oder 2 liegende Patienten transportiert werden konnten. Überdies gab es noch einen begleitenden Tornisterträger.

1867 opferte de Mooy seine letzten Pfennige, um die Weltausstellung in Paris zu besuchen; denn Gauvin sollte eine neue Räderbahre erfunden und ausgestellt haben. Sie war dort tatsächlich, aber welche Enttäuschung, sie war nichts besser als die vorhandenen Modelle: viel Personal erforderlich, keine Bremsschuhe, unbrauchbar für unebenes Gelände, ausserdem konnte der Patient herausfallen.

Bereits auf der Rückreise von Paris hat de Mooy seine eigene Erfindung konzipiert. Sechs Monate später standen Räderbahre mit zugehöriger Trage zur Erprobung bereit. In Den Haag bei der Gründung des Niederländischen Roten Kreuzes erwarb sie eine Goldmedaille. De Mooy hatte die Lehre von Solferino begriffen! Der Entwurf war grossartig. Die Einsparung der Körperkräfte war derartig, dass *ein* Krankenträger imstande war, während $2\frac{1}{2}$ Stunden 2 kranken Soldaten mit ihrer Bagage, zusammen 200 kg, der Kolonne über unebenes Gelände nachzubringen.

De Mooy schrieb darüber in verschiedenen Zeitschriften. Es wurden zahlreiche Versuche mit allerlei Modifikationen unternommen. Immer wieder ergab sich, dass de Mooy's Räderbahre hervorragend befriedigte. Eine einfache Federung bewirkte, dass sie über derbe Querbalken gefahren werden konnte. Er wählte sehr lange Federn. Ferner musste das Transportmittel leicht sein. Der Verletzte musste auf derselben Trage liegen bleiben können. Die Trage musste bequem zu befestigen und in Gänze aus-und einzuhaken sein.

Nun kam auch de Mooy's Vorliebe für Boerhaave's Anschauung zum Ausdruck, dass es dem Arzt nützlich ist, die Mechanik zu verstehen, auf dass er ,,um die Ecke sehen" kann. Er sah, dass bei zweirädrigen Wagen eine Kraft nötig ist, um sie waagerecht zu halten und eine, um sie vorwärts zu schieben. Je niedriger die Last in Bezug auf die Achse placiert ist, desto kleiner wird die erste Kraft. Ferner muss man die Bahre soweit möglich in beständigem Gleichgewicht halten. Um die schiebende Kraft nun auch so gering wie möglich zu machen, sind sehr hohe Räder nötig. De Mooy liess seine Räderbahren, von ihm anfangs ,,Lechophoren" genannt, selbst durch Kinder ausprobieren, um ihre Leichtigkeit zu beweisen.

De Mooy liess seine Instrumente und Räderbahren in Metz, Strassburg, Sedan und Brüssel auch in der täglichen Praxis erproben. Seine militärischen Chefs zeigten sich leider sehr abweisend. Jalousie de métier? Im Urlaub und bei seiner Hochzeitsreise fuhr er nach Aachen und anderswohin, um mit eigenen Augen zu sehen, inwieweit seine Erfindungen Erfolg hatten. Der kinderlose de Mooy pflegte seine Räderbahre später sein ältestes Kind zu nennen.

Ein Erfinder wird in seinem eigenen Land selten gewürdigt, sagt man wohl. So ging es auch de Mooy. Derweilen wurde in Frankreich die Räderbahre als ,,porteur universel parachoc" nachgemacht.

De Mooy beantragte Versetzung nach Niederländisch Indien um zu versuchen für seine Erfindung dort Eingang zu finden. Aber er musste erfahren, dass er dort nicht nur wenig Beistand fand, sondern dass sogar Sabotage gegen seine Erfindung geübt wurde: man setzte die Räderbahre falsch ineinander, um zu zeigen, dass sie nichts taugte. Aber de Mooy liess sich nicht schlagen.

In Indien bietet die Natur von selbst an, mit Bambus und Rotang zu arbeiten. De Mooy liess kleine Matten davon flechten, die geeignet waren, als Schienen um die verschiedenen Körperteille gewickelt zu werden, wie heute die Plastikschienen.

Die Schnelligkeit dieser Verbandweise hat denn auch Herren Dr. Van Hasselt, Generalstabsarzt der holländischen Armee, veranlasst den Rotangverband unter den Namen ,,Schnellverband" im Gegensatz zum ,,Schnellfeuer" der Combattanten bei der Ambulance einzuführen.

Auch entwarf er einfache ,,vliegende kampementen" mit Bambusbaracken und bahren.

Die grosse Chance alle seine Fähigkeiten zu entfalten und den wirklichen Wert seiner Erfindungen zu beweisen, ergab sich zwischen dem 6. und 24. Mai 1878. Der Gouverneur von Atjeh, General K. van der Heyden, rüstete auf Grund von wiederholten überfällen auf einen niederländischen Stutzpunkt eine Strafexpedition aus. Die Expedition erwies sich als unerwartet schwierig. Die feindlichen Angriffe waren zahlreich. Bei dieser Gelegenheit zeigte de Mooy einen beinah übermenschlichen Mut und Geschicklichkeit. Bei der Rückkehr wagte er, sich selbst dem höchsten Befehlshaber, General van der Heyden, zu widersetzen, als dieser dieselbe Truppe noch einmal zurückführen wollte. Er machte ihm klar, dass daran mit diesen verseuchten, erschöpften Mannschaften nicht zu denken sei. Für seine hervorragende Haltung im Jahr 1878 erhielt er erst 1905 den höchsten Militär-Willemsorden.

1878 begann de Mooy mit den Entwurf eines Rahmengestells für Kranke, das den Transport von Schwerverwundeten unter schwierigsten Bedingungen, über steile Treppen, in engen Gangen und Laufgraben, in Schiffsräumen und Gruben ermöglichte. Schliesslich wurde es ein Rahmen, auf dem man als Mumie verpackt, in allen Stellungen transportierbar war und *unangetastet* auf das Bett gelegt werden konnte.

Aus Gesundheitsgründen musste de Mooy in die Niederlande zurückkehren. Nach einer scharfen Kritik an einer ungeeignet gebauten Kaserne, die gerade durch die Autoritäten als beispielhaft hingestellt wurde, quittierte de Mooy 1891 den Militärdienst.

Als Zivilist suchte er voller Energie neue Aufgaben. Hieraus ergaben sich ein praktisches antiseptisches Verbandspäckchen (in der Nachfolge von Lister), die Idee, Hunde zum Aufspüren von Verwundeten abzurichten, der Entwurf von einer ganzen Reihe von Zelten. Er nannte sie tragbare Pyramide, Buckel-oder Harmonika- und Reifenzelte. Sie waren aus einem Stück gefertigt und aussergewöhnlich leicht. Die quadratischen Zelte hatten innen einen Ständer, der bei Regen sich senken konnte, wodurch das Ausspannen von Tauen ausserhalb der Zelte überflüssig wurde. Auch konstruierte er Doppelzelte.

Diese zusammenlegbare Zelte kamen überall in Gebrauch, zum Beispiel in Südafrika im Burenkrieg. Über diesen Weg kamen die Modelle wahrscheinlich wieder nach England; auch nach Bulgarien, Japan und Italien. (Expeditionen von Scott und Shackleton.)

1895 experimentierte de Mooy mit einer Art vergrösserter Diebslaterne, dem ,,Paralux", womit er nachts Teile eines Schlachtfeldes hoffte erleuchten zu können, um Verwundete ungesehen durch die Feinde zu finden.

1898, als Titular-Colonel, machte er eine interessante Zeichnung, in der er Verwundetentransport *schnell* und *schockfrei*, mit Ballons, vorschlug, eine Vorstellung, auf die er dann als Titular-General-major 1910 zurückkommt und nun das Flugzeug einbezieht. Als in Frankreich der erste Verwundetentransport mit dem Flugzeug startet, bezeichnen die Franzosen de Mooy höflich als den ,,Jules Verne" des Krankentransportes durch die Luft.

So steckte de Mooy voller Ideen: Specialpanzer, um Verwundete aus dem Kampfgeschehen zu schaffen (1917), die Konstruktion eines Beatmungsballons lange vor Ruben (1868), er sagte die Schaukelmethode nach Eve voraus, überlegte, wie Feuerraketen vielleicht gebraucht werden konnten, um einen Kontakt mit dem festen Ufer zustande zu bringen (1896) und konstruierte eine Grubenschleppbahre aus Aluminium, die 1909 in Washington prämiert wurde.

Ohne Zweifel war der freundliche, enthusiastische und unerschrockene Generalarzt Cornelis de Mooy ein gleichsam kindlich eitler Mann. Er war von solch leidenschaftlichem Ehrgeiz für sein erwähltes Arbeitsgebiet erfüllt, dass es ihn völlig in Beschlag nahm, all seine Zeit und sein ganzes Denken erfüllte.

Liebe zum kranken Menschen und Pflichtgefühl als Offizier trieben dabei immer seinen Eifer an (Amoret). ,,Labor improbus omnia vincit" war sein Wahlspruch. Zahlreich waren die Modelle, verkleinert oder im Masstab, die er anfertigte. Finanziellen Vorteil suchte er niemals. Ja, manchmal schenkte er den Ertrag seiner Erfindungen invaliden Soldaten. Wohl stritt er sein Leben lang für das geistige Eigentumsrecht an seinen Ideen.

Wer sich mit der ganzen Sammlung – C. de Mooy – Schriften und Modellen-befasst, wie sie jetzt in der ,,Juliana van Stolberg" kaserne in Amersfoort bewahrt wird, begreift, dass auf dem Kaminsims seiner Haager Wohnung nicht ohne Grund die Statuen von Forschung (Studium) und Arbeit prangten.

A. Beck
University of Hartford, Connecticut (U.S.A.)

The state and medical research. British government policy toward tropical medicine in East Africa

Since the start of modern science in the seventeenth century the relationship between government and the promoters of science has been close. When the Royal Society was established under the patronage of the Crown in 1662, it was the start of a new era in which the state would sponsor the development of science for utilitarian reasons and for the sake of pure research. Although the Royal Society did not provide a living for those it encouraged to investigate the empirical basis of science, its patronage gave them prestige in their unpaid efforts to find solutions to problems of mechanics, physics and astronomy. From the very start it was understood that inventions, experiments and new theories which were not immediately useful to society must be supported in the public interest.

In the nineteenth century when medicine emerged as a science and when the beginnings of industrialization attracted attention to the health of the people, it was the state that was called upon to promote public health. Throughout the nineteenth- and early twentieth-century debates on the role of government in medicine, the question was not whether the state should concern itself with the growth of medicine, but how much it could do. Medical training, hospital construction, the licensing of physicians, the promotion of public health and the sponsorship of research were considered the legitimate concern of the Crown and Parliament. The establishment of the Medical Council in 1858, the appointment of a Medical Officer to the Local Government Board and the founding of boards of health illustrate this trend. Parliamentary investigating committees reflect the public demand for protection from the evils of the new industrial society. This was natural considering that the changes of the new urbanized society were so puzzling to the observers and analysts of the time, that they asked for the state to control and preserve their health and their environment. The Duke of Northumberland said at the opening of the Sanitary Institute in 1876 that new manufactories and new communities had created 'a state of things unknown since the creation of the world'.[1] New concepts like the 'right' to live in happiness and health or the new 'sanitary idea' led to a critical spirit of investigation and an almost fanatic and relentless drive to improve the society of modern man. Research was the best answer to the new demands, and controlling legislation was the next best thing. Both were practised by England from the middle of the nineteenth century on. England, therefore, seemed well prepared for its new role as promoter of public health and curative medicine when she embarked on her career as a colonial power in East Africa after 1880.

It was logical, therefore, that at the start of the medical services in Kenya and Uganda in 1895, it was the British government which became the guardian of health through its Foreign Office. The missions, it is true, had been engaged in medical work for at least a decade before the Foreign Office assumed control of the East African protectorates. But their work had to be limited to the local perimeter of their settlements and their funds were too restricted to permit them experimentation and expansion. They continued their excellent work after the establishment of the protectorates and did not interfere with the government services. Wherever possible in the outlying districts, they supplemented them.

Tropical East Africa presented an ideal field for the state to protect the lives of millions of people and to set up research in the battle against tropical diseases. For several reasons, however, this did not happen immediately after the British established colonial government in East Africa. While the protectorates were under the authority of the Foreign Office, long-range plans were not made and large appropriations were not available. Before the protectorates came under the control of the Colonial Office in 1905, however, external circumstances forced the British government to take action and changed its role in medical matters. Malaria and sleeping sickness required experimentation after 1901 and the Royal Society was asked for help. The first commission of investigation which it sent out arrived in 1903. It set up a laboratory and brought along a bacteriologist, an entomologist and a naturalist. The second commission of the Royal Society arrived late in 1903 and returned after having definitely confirmed the trypanosome as the protozoa responsible for the epidemic, and the tsetse fly as the carrier of the trypanosoma. However, research was not properly co-ordinated and did not lead to substantial results as far as the spread of trypanosomiasis was concerned.

Purely medical and biological research did not have priority between 1904 and 1914. Dr. Moffat, the Senior Medical Officer in Uganda in 1905, did not assign priority to what he called the pursuit of 'abstruse scientific research' although he admitted that continued investigations into the life cycle of the trypanosoma within the fly might lead to interesting insights. But he thought that the reality of vanishing life in the bush and near Lake Victoria was not necessarily helped by these esoteric experiments.[2] He was wrong, however, since the continued research into the habits of the fly led to an exact knowledge of the mode of transmission.

The attacks by some of the administrators in Uganda on the Royal Society in London and the incompatibility of the philosophies of the administrator and the scientist are classic examples of two widely separated points of view. Without the support by the Colonial Office and the Royal Society the attack on sleeping sickness would not have led to decisive results even though the knowledge of trypanosoma and tsetse was only the first step in the control of the disease. The second step was in the hands of the governor, the Principal Medical Officer and the departments of agriculture and forestry in devising fly-free zones in which the fisherman and the peasants could safely live and work. Practical considerations, the difficulty of funding resettlement, and the unwillingness of peasants to leave their old homes required a pragmatic policy during this stage. But research into the social conditions of the people and their ability to absorb new agricultural methods remained a continuing factor which required further research.

Research was introduced into tropical Africa by the force of circumstances. It was not planned in anticipation of the unknown forces of nature which bred disease, famine and poverty in the protectorates. It was not systematically pursued during the years before World War I, a fact which is partly accounted for by a general absence of planning during this period. The medical directors had a difficult task and were forced to limit their goals to the fulfilment of their annual programmes allowing them to keep epidemics under control, reporting the death rates on the basis of incomplete statistics and trying to distribute their always inadequate staff in the most strategic positions near government stations. They could not even attempt to investigate the sanitary conditions in the reserves more systematically or to trace the causes of disease and physical disabilities. They recorded commonly known diseases such as tuberculosis, blackwater fever, smallpox and bilharzia. They acknowledged that sanitary conditions in the reserves were generally poor.

A Tropical Diseases Research Fund existed and its Advisory Committee was set up in London in 1904 but, as its report for 1907 acknowledged, there was no link between scientific research and medical training as yet. The Committee tried to have an influence on the training of colonial officers in the London and Liverpool Schools of Tropical Medicine but they had to admit that this was impractical.

During World War I such medical shortcomings as malnutrition, chronic disease, and untreated malaria were found prevalent among many Africans when medical examinations were given to male recruits. Of those examined in the province of Kikuyu in 1917 33·99 per cent were rejected on medical grounds.[3] Probably an even larger number was medically unfit since the district officers sent only the healthy looking men to the examinations. In 1918 the health of the people was described as generally bad. High prices, famine, an influenza epidemic, and tuberculosis were responsible. By 1920 an improvement was noted and the start of new medical policies was recorded. In Kenya government began to establish medical centres in the Reserves. Tangible evidence was thereby given to the African that government assumed a personal interest in his well-being. In 1921 the medical departments increased their personnel and became in fact government agencies entrusted with the maintenance of health for the entire population. Twenty-five years after the first health services had been set up in the East African protectorates, the British government assumed a policy toward health in the colonies which it had practised in England since the middle of the nineteenth century.

With planning for better health, there came an added incentive for the medical personnel to systematize measures against disease and to undertake research into their etiology. Officials investigated the habits of people in areas where malnutrition prevailed and tried to ascertain the relationship between malaria and low standards of living. Research projects of this type had been undertaken before 1920 but they operated on special budgets and for a limited time only. There was no organization to collect data and information systematically.[4]

After the comeback from general retrenchment in 1933, medical research on a permanent basis was finally given consideration by the colonial administrators. At the annual governors' conference in 1933 a joint research organization for Kenya, Tanganyika and Uganda was proposed and in 1936, a standing medical research committee met for the first time. The outbreak of World War II interrupted further planning and in 1942 the medical director of Kenya expressed disappointment that research into problems of health and medicine were not given the place in East

Africa which they ought to occupy in order to solve very elementary social problems. The time for reflection before action had not yet arrived.[5] After the end of World War II a new orientation towards development in the interest of the African had evolved but a newly formed development committee did not list medical research as a major project. There was still a general feeling that academic research should be kept to a minimum in deference to fundamental psychological and socio-preventive investigations into the African community.

In spite of such hesitations an East African Bureau of Research in Medicine and Hygiene was finally established in 1948. At a time when East Africa was changing rapidly and when science and medicine exercised a great influence on every aspect of traditional patterns of African society, colonial governments could no longer ignore the urgency of modernizing agricultural production and of supporting the trend toward higher standards of living. And for this reason a permanent research organization in East Africa had become a necessity.

A particularly strong request for change came from political organizations in colonial East Africa such as the Kenya African Union and the Tanganyika African National Union. In their programme they gave priority to the improvement of the standard of life of the African. The colonial government responded to the demand for better health and more education and investigated the means by which the African level of living could be improved. The task was undertaken by the departments of agriculture, education and medical services. E. B. Worthington, the first scientific research secretary of the East African High Commission was appalled that prior to World War II scientific considerations had been ignored in the development of East Africa. But still worse, he found that a great deal of development in the past had taken place in the wrong way. He recommended that government give assistance to development in three areas. They were (1) the productive services like mining, fisheries, agriculture and forestry; (2) the social services including medicine, education, social welfare and labour; and (3) the common services which are rendered by modern government.[6]

The special services, especially the impact of medicine on the standard of living, were given increased attention in the 1950s. After a bureau of medical research had been set up under the governors of East Africa in 1948, further development of research needed only an organizational expansion of the basic structure. The High Commission which replaced the Governors' Conference in 1948 became the administrator of all medical research services. Other advisory bodies were added but the most important steps toward the creation of an autonomous research organization came in 1955 when the East African Council for Medical Research was founded and an ancillary Scientific Advisory Committee was created at the same time to carry out the research planned by the Council.[7] The Council had its own budget and was a policymaking body that set priorities for research considered relevant to the raising of the standard of living.

The trend which began in 1920 had finally reached its ultimate goal. In a report by a parliamentary committee appointed in 1920 to inquire into the colonial medical services, there seemed to be agreement that there could be 'no better investment for the money of any Colony than scientific research, both medical and economic' and the setting up of 'such a department' was recommended.[8] In 1951 E. B. Worthington, the scientific research secretary of the High Commission, was aware of objections to research on the ground that science cost money. He did not share this view, but in order to make research acceptable he emphasized the usefulness of properly selected research projects such as agricultural production, the social improvement of the peasant, and the control of disease which, unchecked, would cost the government dearly and reduce the capacity of the labourer. The new Medical Research Council got on its feet when it was placed under the East African Common Services Organization which replaced the High Commission after Tanganyika became independent in 1961. In 1967 the East Africa Medical Research Council changed masters again when it became a part of the newly established East African Community, a new interterritorial body which served Kenya, Uganda and Tanganyika in the administration of common technical, economic, and agricultural services. From now on the East African Community provided a portion of the financing of research but even the combined treasuries of the three countries were not sufficient and foreign aid was needed to continue the programmes begun in 1948.

Though still struggling for survival, even under the East African Community, medical research has become a full-fledged partner in government programmes carried on in the interest of the public. Political instability has affected the Community but research activities have maintained their priorities, and, as D. M. Wako, Deputy Secretary for Social and Research Services, said in 1967, the progress of science and the benefit of health, education, and national institutions will to an increasing extent depend on research.

The research undertaken since independence follows the lines laid down before. Pure research has been continued although its applicability to practical problems cannot always be determined. Public health is supported by an intensive programme which searches for the factors and causes of greatest social loss in terms of human lives. In 1966 A. S. Msangi of the Medical School in Dar es Salaam, assigned priority in the field of public health to malaria, bilharzia and kwashiorkor.[9] In the planning of other projects agricultural research, biological aspects of the soil and the diseases of livestock were given continued attention. The shortage of trained personnel and the continued inadequacy of financial support have been an obstacle to medical research in the last years. But the new interterritorial organization of scientific research has proved the vulnerability of research. It has shown that development should follow, rather than precede, long-range planning which depends on a thorough knowledge of usable resources. It has shown that obstacles to growth in East Africa have often been due to the unpreparedness of an untrained population. It has revealed the formidable factor of risk caused by natural forces in tropical climates. And it has confirmed the old experience of the colonial period that research in tropical East Africa depends on public funds in spite of the frustrating and bureaucratic delays which such sponsorship may involve, a fact which has been proved in the history of research in East Africa. When the Crown and Parliament applied their nineteenth century experiences to the colonial scene in East Africa, they were sidetracked in their efforts by the uncertainty of the political and economic prospects of the colonies and by conflicting interest groups that influenced policies. Under present conditions national political considerations will again be obstacles to the inter-territorial approach for practical as well as ideological reasons. But the governments of the East African Community are aware of the dependence of development on research and are attempting to balance political factors with developmental necessities.

References

1 *The Times*, 14 July 1876.
2 Moffat to Bruce, 25 January 1905. Bruce Letters, Library of the Royal Society of Tropical Medicine, London.
3 *A Short History of Kikuyu Province*, Nairobi, Kenya National Archives, PC/CP1/1/2 p. 18.
4 *Annual Medical Report*, Kenya, 1929, p.17.
5 PATERSON, A. R., *Annual Medical Report*, Kenya, 1942, p. 4.
6 WORTHINGTON, E. B., *A Survey of Research and Scientific Services in East Africa, 1947–56*, Dar es Salaam, Tanganyika National Archives, File 34057, p. 1.
7 *Annual Report of the East African Council for Medical Research, 1954–1955*, Nairobi, 1955, p. 3.
8 *Report of the Departmental Committee, appointed by the Secretary of State for the Colonies to Enquire into the Colonial Medical Services*, London, 1920, Parliamentary Papers, vol. XIII, p. 11.
9 MSANGI, A. S., 'Research Goals in Public Health', *Research Priorities for East Africa*, Nairobi, The East African Institute of Social and Cultural Affairs, 1966, pp. 32–35.

B. D. Petrov
Moscow (U.S.S.R.)

Deontology in the history of Russian medicine

The problems of deontology have always attracted the attention of medical people in Russia. The English philosopher J. Bentham is known to have developed in 1839 the doctrine of duty in connexion with representatives of various professions. Bentham's idea was eagerly taken up by medical people. There appeared many works dealing with the doctor's duty and several other particular questions of this profession.

The term 'deontology' emerges in Russian medical literature relatively late, but relevant problems have always interested medical men in this country.

The first Russian clinicians, S. Zybelin, D. Samoylovitch, M. Mudrov, and J. Djadkovsky, have already written on the problems of the doctor's duty and obligations, and given lectures on the theme. N. Pirogov, V. Manassein, S. Botkin, and a number of other outstanding physicians often told what a doctor must be, how he must work, and what obligations his profession places upon him.

The reference to medical deontology covers over five hundred titles in Russian.

To be a doctor is not only a profession, it is a mission, a devoted service to people. Deontology was understood by our medical men not as a code of rules determining professional behaviour of doctors, but as a teaching on a doctor's duty, on his obligations as a citizen, his duty not only in front of patients, but in front of other people as well.

Russian doctors interpreted deontology widely, they included in it both personal and civic morality. This interpretation of doctor's duty was expressed in a most vivid and complete manner by I. Pavlov: 'Whatever I am doing, I am always thinking to serve thereby as far as I can my country for all.'

Deontology is most closely connected with the very heart of the medical profession, with its contents, with the philosophy of medical art, with the sense of doctors' work. The activity of a physician has been ever interpreted in Russian medicine as a duty, as the matter of his whole life; there has been always present an element of sacrifice and self-sacrifice, it has been virtually incorporated in the very meaning of medical work.

Medical people in this country were greatly influenced by progressive public men and philosophers, for instance A. Herzen, revolutionary democrats such as D. Pisarev, N. Tchernyshevsky. The latter wrote: 'The work of a doctor is virtually most effective work – by preventing illness, by rehabilitating the health, doctor returns to society all the strengths which would otherwise perish.'

Deontology was expressed not in speeches or declarations of Russian physicians, but in their behaviour and actions. Meaningful is not the discussion but the real example set by the doctor in the course of many years of his whole life.

Heroic actions, self-sacrifice was not only a compulsory demand, it was the norm of conduct for Russian doctors. There are many examples testifying this concept: H. Gamaleja proved on himself the effectiveness of antihydrophobia vaccine in 1886. In 1902 V. Favr intoxicated himself by a bite of a malaria-mosquito to check its role in malaria dissemination. G. Gabritchevsky injected in the same year into his own body the vaccine of scarlet fever in order to prove its harmlessness for human beings. C. Dzershgovsky proved on himself that active anti-diphtheria immunization would bear no harm. N. Sacharov inoculated himself with tropical malaria.

Soviet doctors and scientists continued this old glorious tradition of Russian medicine. M. Pokrovskaja and N. Shukov-Vereshnikov tried on themselves Soviet anti-plague vaccine. The anti-encephalitis vaccine was demonstrated on himself by M. Tchumakov. Experiments with cholera germs were carried out on her own organism by Z. Ermoljeva.

The lives of many Russian doctors are vivid examples of service to people. Dr. F. Gaas (1780–1853) did not leave any scientific works but for a line on his tombstone 'Be quick to make good' – that was the motto of his life. He devoted it to most unfortunate and destitute people – to the convicts. For twenty-five years there was no group of convicts which would leave Moscow deportation jail without the goodwill parting words of the 'Sanct Doctor'. When F. Gaas died, in all Russian jails from St. Petersburg to Akatuj there were lighted icon-lamps bought for pennies gathered by convicts.

A rather small scientific inheritance – *Manual for Psychiatry* – was left behind by Professor I. Belinsky (1827–1902), the founder of the first Russian psychiatric clinic, but of uppermost value is the sentence he had inscribed on his gravestone: 'A friend and servant to insanes.' These words stuck in memory, they expressed the meaning of doctor's duty in a most distinct way.

The interpretation of physician's duty by Russian medical public was greatly shaped by the editor of the *Vratch* magazine, V. Manassein (1827–1902). He was called 'doctor's conscience', 'knight of medical ethics'. This outstanding clinician and public man upheld always a characteristic opinion, revealing the very nature of medical activity: 'A good doctor is always an explorer. He always investigates when not in the laboratory, then at the patient's side.'

Our medical public was characterized by high requirements for those who were going to become doctors. In deontologic concepts the main principle was the following: to become a doctor one must have a calling for it. It has been precisely expressed by A. Tchekhov: 'The profession of a doctor is a feat. It requires sacrifice, pure soul and pure intentions. Not everybody is able to do so.'

The first requirement for success is to deserve the patient's confidence, the first task – to encourage the patient, to uphold him in a struggle against illness. As V. Bechterev said: 'If after a talk with a doctor the patient did not feel his illness to subside, it has not been a doctor.'

In Russia there happened once an accident which agitated all the medical audience, exposing the high level of responsibility imposed by the doctor on himself. Professor S. Kolomin (1842–86) committed suicide after a patient's death due to his negligence.

His action cannot be accepted, but it clearly indicates how highly the doctor appreciates the confidence of his patient.

Deontology was understood by our medical people also as a requirement to build a collaborative collective in the clinic or hospital encompassing, on the principle of equal rights, representatives of various groups of medical people, of different qualifications. The rise of the role of ancillary medical personnel was regarded as important.

Here is an example showing how important this problem was to the famous gynaecologist, Professor V. Snegirev. There hung in the conference room of his clinic portraits of outstanding clinicians and scientists – N. Pirogov, Ch. Darwin, etc. And Snegirev once hung also an oak-framed portrait of the nurse Makarova. The legend tells that he has nursed a thousand post-operative patients.

Always bear in mind the patient, his mood – of this our clinicians never tired to remind themselves. G. Zachatjin emphasized: 'We must remember that patients in general are being with rare exception, in depressed mood. To succeed the doctor has to cheer him up, to give him hope for convalescence. Such motivated promotion provides the patient sometimes with sleep which he so badly needs for recovery of the nervous system and accordingly for the organism as a whole.'

Disease prevention is the most important task of a doctor. Already M. Mudrov wrote that 'the doctor has not to cure illness but to prevent it, to teach to spare the organism'. V. Manassein even said that 'Hygiene is just a part of treatment, it is separated in a special discipline only for convenience of teaching and better development of certain questions'. F. Erisman emphasized: 'Each doctor must be a hygienist.'

This tradition is now continued by Soviet physicians – prophylaxis is known to be a leading principle of Soviet medicine. Z. Solovjev wrote about the unity and fusion of prophylaxis and treatment.

Deontology as understood by family doctors strictly demands continuous self-education, never ceasing improvement of knowledge and skill. 'There is no doctor who can boast to have completed his education', M. Mudrov wrote. A. Ostroumov underlined: 'To learn his whole life for the public benefit – this is the destiny of a physician.' N. Tchistovitch added: 'One must work continuously and indefatigably to be a good doctor; only the physician doing everything possible to be on the heights of contemporary medical level can regard himself as a conscientious man accomplishing his duty.'

The views of many generations of physicians were shaped under the influence of N. Pirogov and his concepts on the doctor's behaviour, doctor's destiny, his obligations, his duty. N. Pirogov demanded that the physician would see his own mistakes and, what is even more important, admit his guilt, show it to others in order to enrich their experience, to draw appropriate conclusions, to armour physicians with new knowledge. Famous are his words: 'From the very beginning of my medical career I took for the rule: never conceal my errors, my failures. I have proved it by publicly exposing them, I am innocent before the court of my conscience, I can challenge everybody to reproach me of at least one of my faults, one of my errors which I had tried to conceal.'

Physician's Notes by V. Veressajev gives an image of the doctor's duty as understood by Russian medical men. This book is as a matter of fact a real treatise, an encyclopaedia on deontology, encircling a vast field of problems. In lectures, scientific works, memoirs of each great Russian physician we can find ideas about the doctor's destiny, and about the requirements of the doctor's profession.

It is interesting to note that all these concepts are flowing in a mutual stream, they keep in general the line of deontology characteristic of home medicine, but at the same time each physician contributes his own original ideas. The clinician N. Borovsky, who described leishmaniasis, used to say: 'I have not so much time at my disposal as to perform medical examination in a hurry.'

M. Mudrov advised: 'Do not sit over a blank form in front of the patient.' The great Ukrainian physician F. Janovsky repeatedly told: 'Do not forget to doubt.'

A thorough acquaintance with the history of Russian deontology, with the history of the emerging and developing of deontologic requirements shows immense scientific and moral values incorporated in the deontologic inheritance of home medicine. The education of future doctors and teaching in medical institutes carried out under this aspect would open wide possibilities.

We can most resolutely attribute to deontology also everything called recently a curative-preventive regime in the work of polyclinics and hospitals. During the joint session of the Academy of Sciences and Academy of Medical Sciences of the U.S.S.R., Professor A. Mjasnikov said: 'A bond between medicine and physiology – that is Pavlov's very idea, which requires putting into practice not isolated examples by splendid scientists but general organization principle as a mass-phenomenon, as a real base for our scientific and in some regards also clinical work.'

M. Levit
Moscow (U.S.S.R.)

Les sources de la médecine d'initiative commune en Russie

Les initiatives sociales des médecins russes progressistes qui avaient opportunément évalué l'importance de la situation révolutionnaire, créée dans le pays à la suite de la défaite de la Russie féodale dans la guerre de Crimée de 1853–56, ont changé la physionomie de la médecine, fixé ses objectifs et défini les voies de son développement ultérieur, élaboré les procédés de travail dans des conditions historiques concrètes, les méthodes de lutte pour la santé des paysans qui constituaient alors la majorité de la population.

Etant donné qu'au cours des transformations révolutionnaires les événements historiques se mesurent en de très brefs laps de temps, en quelques années seulement (1856–64) toutes les idées concernant les voies de développement de la médecine d'initiative commune en Russie, ainsi que ses buts, ont subi une révision. Des formes et méthodes nouvelles de lutte et de travail ont fait leur apparition. Des sociétés médicales se distinguant foncièrement des sociétés d'autrefois, ont été fondées. Ont commencé à paraître des périodiques médicaux, coordonnant et dirigeant les activités des médecins. Les médecins pouvaient désormais se communiquer par l'intermédiaire de la presse, au sein de leurs sociétés et, un peu plus tard, à leurs congrès.

C'est au moment culminant de la situation révolutionnaire des années 1859–61 qu'ont été mis au point les principes et les objectifs fondamentaux de l'activité des médecins des zemstvos.

Le terme de la «médecine d'initiative commune» n'avait pas encore de définition précise, ni de place à part parmi les termes déjà connus, à savoir: police médicale, médecine légale, hygiène commune, hygiène publique, protection de la santé populaire, organisation de la santé publique, hygiène sociale, médecine sociale.

Les conceptions actuelles identifient tous les termes mentionnés. Cependant, le terme de la «médecine d'initiative commune» comporte un sens différent. Il correspond directement aux phénomènes nouveaux dans l'histoire de la médecine russe (et non seulement russe, d'ailleurs) qui jusqu'à présent ne sont pas appréciés à leur juste valeur, ils n'ont même pas de désignation autonome.

Fait partie de ces phénomènes l'activité des médecins progressistes (et souvent non seulement des médecins) qui cherchaient, de leurs propres forces, à améliorer l'assistance médicale au peuple, à attirer l'attention de la société sur l'état insatisfaisant de la médecine nationale, – activité que personne ne réglementait ni encourageait (matériellement ou moralement), et qui souvent était même réprimée.

Inlassables fondateurs de revues et de journaux spéciaux, animateurs des sociétés de médecins, organisateurs des congrès de naturalistes et de médecins, ils formulaient et examinaient à leurs risques et périls les questions de la plus brûlante actualité dans le domaine qui leur était le plus familier, celui de la protection de la santé du peuple.

A notre avis ces manifestations spécifiques d'un service volontaire et plein d'abnégation à son peuple se résument bien par le terme de la «médecine d'initiative commune» qui doit être mis en lumière à côté des autres termes susmentionnés.

L'évolution de la médecine en Russie durant la période de la situation révolutionnaire fut liée avec tous les changements socio-économiques qui avaient eu lieu dans le pays à la fin des années 50 et au début des années 60.

Il se trouve qu'un grand nombre de médecins avaient participé au mouvement révolutionnaire de l'époque. C'est là un fait de prime importance, puisqu'il nous permet de parler non seulement de l'influence de caractère général que des démocrates révolutionnaires avaient exercée sur la propagation des idées sociales parmi les médecins, non seulement des liens idéologiques qui avaient uni Tchernychevsky, Pissarev et les médecins progressistes. Il s'agit d'une coopération étroite, d'une activité révolutionnaire énergique, d'une lutte dans un même camp, dans un même réseau ramifié de cercles et d'actions révolutionnaires.

Des facteurs objectifs importants, tels que la santé du peuple et de l'état de l'assistance médicale, ont également beaucoup influencé les médecins professionnels, témoins oculaires et permanents de la souffrance populaire. C'est aussi dans cette optique que les personnels médicaux voyaient les faits. C'est pourquoi il importe d'avoir une idée nette sur la santé populaire et l'état de l'assistance médicale à la population de Russie entre la fin des années 50 et le début des années 60, du XIXe siècle. Il fut établi par la suite que les 23 millions de paysans du département des biens de l'Etat et les 23 autres millions de paysans, libérés par l'abolition du servage, soit plus de deux tiers de la population russe en 1863, se trouvaient pratiquement en marge de l'assistance médicale.

Il en ressort que l'activité des médecins en vue de créer un système d'assistance médicale au peuple, ainsi que la médecine dite «des zemstvos», avec ses particularités en ce qui concerne les services rendus à la population rurale, ont vu le jour avant tout en raison d'une nécessité historique, d'un impératif social.

La presse médicale d'avant-garde fut le premier porte-parole des tendances nouvelles de son époque.

Les meilleures revues de ce temps représentent un phénomène parfaitement inédit dans le journalisme médical, puisqu'elles traitaient non seulement des problèmes spéciaux délimités, non seulement des problèmes de la science médicale, ce qui, en soi, est d'une incontestable importance. Mais non moins important et propre à cette période fut le besoin de verser de la lumière sur des problèmes socio-médicaux, de mettre au point des formes nouvelles de contacts entre médecins, de fonder des sociétés de médecins de type nouveau en convoquant des congrès de médecins.

Parmi les 25 périodiques médicaux fondés entre 1856–64, les plus influents en matière de développement de la médecine d'initiative commune en Russie, furent la «Gazette médicale de Moscou», la «Médecine contemporaine» et le «Messager médical». Des journaux étroitement académiques et professionnels, ces trois périodiques sont devenus organes nationaux de la presse médicale, qui reflétaient les faits de l'époque dans le domaine de médecine et agissaient sur leur évolution.

D'importants changements d'ordre quantitatif et qualitatif se sont opérés au sein des Sociétés de médecins russes. Entre la fin des années 50 et le début des années 60, on vit apparaître des dizaines de nouvelles Sociétés de médecins russes de «goubernie» départementales. Nous avons pu trouver les documents confirmant l'existence de 28 sociétés de ce genre, fondées de 1858 à 1864. Or, des preuves indirectes nous indiquent qu'il y en eut même plus dans cette période. C'est là un fait significatif en soi-même, témoignant de l'éveil des masses médicales russes à l'activité pour le bien du peuple.

Dans le fond, les nouvelles sociétés se distinguaient sérieusement des sociétés précédemment créées. Les sociétés de médecins se mirent à s'assigner des missions consistant à modifier et à améliorer l'assistance médicale au peuple, et en premier lieu aux paysans.

Formulée au sein de la «Société des médecins russes à Moscou», la question de convocation des congrès de naturalistes et de médecins russes a bénéficié d'un ample appui aussi bien parmi les périodiques médicaux progressistes, que parmi les multiples sociétés de médecins. Cependant, ces congrès ne furent pas autorisés. Fait marquant, signifiant que l'opinion médicale prenait des forces et que le gouvernement s'attendait à des manifestations indésirables de sa part. Le premier congrès ne fut réuni qu'en 1867.

Les initiatives communes des médecins russes s'avérèrent beaucoup plus vitales et conformes aux besoins du moment, que celles de l'opinion dite «administrative», constituée par les comités de la santé publique des départements et des districts et par les comités des hôpitaux.

Les revues médicales et les Sociétés des médecins ont tracé une série de mesures propres à être immédiatement mises en oeuvre, et ceci en dépit de la pénurie de fonds et des possibilités minimes. Les médecins ont mis sur pied des infirmeries gratuites, alors que la formation du personnel paramédical se voyait améliorer et élargir. Un intérêt nouveau se précisa pour la médecine populaire, pour l'implantation de ses procédés dans la pratique médicale.

C'est justement à cette époque qu'est né parmi les médecins un mouvement d'immense portée pratique qu'avait pour but l'organisation des infirmeries gratuites pour malades ambulants. Nous avons établi l'existence de 20 établissements de ce type, mis en place rien qu'entre 1861 et 1865.

Ainsi donc, les médecins prenaient eux-mêmes quelques mesures, sans solliciter le concours des organismes officiels. Ces actions ne furent ni simples, ni faciles. Elles demandaient un travail opiniâtre, de l'obstination, de l'abnégation, du travail non-rémunéré, et, souvent, le sacrifice des fonds particuliers des médecins. Or, sans que leur vie soit facile, ni aisée, les médecins l'acceptaient consciemment. C'est bien pour cette raison que nous sommes en droit de parler d'un phénomène nouveau, propre à la plupart des médecins et pour cela distinctif et significatif.

Les médecins progressistes ne pouvaient ne pas constater la presque nullité des mesures que les pouvoirs mettaient en oeuvre pour améliorer la situation désespérée en matière d'organisation de l'assistance médicale.

La totalité des facteurs socio-politiques et spéciaux poussait objectivement les médecins à formuler, discuter, analyser et, si possible, à résoudre les problèmes étroitement liés à la protection de la santé populaire.

On dégagera parmi les autres les problèmes primordiaux, qui sont d'égale importance et indissolublement diés les uns aux autres. Il y a en trois: (1) qui doit payer l'assistance médicale au peuple; (2) qui doit dispenser les services médicaux aux paysans: un médecin, un feldsher, un prêtre ou bien tout simplement une personne instruite; (3) quelle sera la forme de secours à la population – médecine ambulante ou stationnaire.

La résolution de ces problèmes a suivi un chemin tortueux, barré de vives polémiques, obstrué par la confrontation des tendances démocratiques, libérales et réactionnaires.

L'essence de chaque problème cardinal relatif à l'élaboration du système d'assistance médicale au peuple se résume comme suit:

(1) Il fallait des moyens pour mettre ce système en application. Les pouvoirs publics allouaient des sommes misérables à l'assistance médicale. Le traitement à l'hôpital (5 à 7 roubles par mois), les médicaments (40–50 copecks une ordonnance), les consultations de médecin (30 à 50 copecks), – tout cela était absolument inaccessible aux paysans. C'est évident compte tenu de leur situation économique, des gains qu'ils pouvaient escompter.

Ce n'est pas seulement à cause du faible nombre des médecins et de la distance qui les séparait des campagnes, que les paysans ne pouvaient point compter sur l'assistance médicale, mais encore parce que, en règle générale, les hobereaux ne disposaient d'aucun secours médical dans leurs domaines et que, après la «libération des paysans», même l'assistance médicale en présence cessait d'être subsidiée par les hobereaux et s'anéantissait.

La plupart des hobereaux avaient un minimum de serfs dans leurs propriétés. C'est à dire que leurs idées sur la nécessité de l'assistance médicale aux paysans avaient à l'origine les indices économiques de la petite exploitation agricole. En général, ils ne pouvaient pas se permettre de construire un hôpital pour paysans, d'inviter un médecin ni même d'engager un feldsher.

Les hobereaux avaient un règlement rigoureux pour les malades et établissaient eux-mêmes la rétribution des paysans: 12 copecks-argent par jour fut le maximum de rémunération du travail d'un paysan à la corvée. D'après les calculs effectués par les hobereaux eux-mêmes, le revenu annuel d'une famille de fermiers de six personnes se chiffrait à 37 roubles 50 copecks. Ce sont précisément ces chiffres qui doivent servir de point de départ à toute évaluation des propositions concernant la réorganisation de l'assistance médicale à la campagne.

D'une façon générale, les propositions relatives des hobereaux se résumaient à ce que les paysans supportant eux-mêmes le poids économique de l'assistance médicale.

(2) C'est justement à partir des conditions économiques que nombre de projets des hobereaux ont vu le jour; on préconisait le point de vue prétendument exprimé par les paysans, selon lequel le médecin serait le «docteur des seigneurs», alors que le feldsher serait le «docteur des moujiks».

(3) C'est également à cette époque que fut proposé le principe des «outchastoks» (secteurs) pour l'assistance médicale à la campagne; peu à peu, il s'est cristallisé au point d'avoir la primauté parmi les autres propositions. Il est entendu qu'il n'a pas été appliqué en pratique; d'ailleurs, il n'était pas susceptible de l'être. Toutefois, au moment de la réforme des «zemstvos» (1864) il était tout à fait achevé sur le plan théorique.

Il se trouve que la plupart des propositions émanant des médecins consistaient à dispenser l'assistance médicale à la population rurale par l'entremise des médecins de secteurs, de ceux, par exemple, qui étaient à la tête de l'hôpital d'un village. C'est notamment ce principe «stationnaire» qui constituait l'élément tout à fait nouveau qui assurait, ainsi que la pratique historique l'a confirmé par la suite, le développement de la médecine rurale à l'avenir, qui fournissait une base solide à la bonne organisation de cette oeuvre, qui fut à l'origine de la médecine des «zemstvos». Le principe des secteurs élaboré en Russie, fut mondialement reconnu par la suite.

Nées à la crête de la vague révolutionnaire de la fin des années 50 – début des années 60 du XIXe siècle, les idées et les initiatives communes des médecins russes représentent en fin de compte un effet des actions populaires de masse, alors que les changements vers l'amélioration de l'assistance médicale sont un résultat accessoire de la lutte du peuple pour ses droits politiques.

Aussi insignifiantes et isolées qu'elles puissent paraître, tantôt entreprises, tantôt abandonnées dans divers points du pays, les initiatives communes des médecins russes dans leur ensemble n'avaient cessé de faire pression sur l'appareil d'Etat tout en préparant l'opinion publique à l'assimilation de cette vérité absolue qu'il est nécessaire de subvenir aux besoins du peuple en assistance médicale.

Les problèmes essentiels que les médecins russes progressistes avaient volontairement formulés et étudiés à la fin des années 50 et au début des 60 années ont été repris par les générations postérieures et se sont incarnés avec le plus d'éclat dans la médecine des zemstvos. Cependant, ils n'ont pas trouvé de solutions tant soit peu complètes avant la Grande révolution Socialiste d'Octobre. Ils ont été résolus au cours de l'édification de l'Etat des Soviets et de la mise en place de la santé publique soviétique dont nombre de pays imitent aujourd'hui l'exemple.

M. K. Kuzmin
Moscow (U.S.S.R.)

Main trends in the Socialist society's medical development

Soviet medicine, which has come into being after the victorious Great October Socialist Revolution in Russia, is a new stage in world medical development. Prevention is one of the most important features of the socialist state's medicine.

The sources of prevention are found in the works written by scientists in the previous epoch. In 1703 Bernardico Ramazzini, a prominent Italian scientist, said that the 'prevention of diseases is a greater service than the treatment of them'. In 1820 M. Ya. Mudrov, a well-known therapeutist in Russia, said that the 'prevention of diseases is easier than the treatment of them'. M. I. Pirogov, a prominent Russian surgeon, held that the 'future belongs to preventive medicine'. In the capitalist epoch, these progressive ideas did not become very popular. In Russia, prevention became part and parcel of medicine only after the establishment of a new, socialist system.

The Communist Party Programme of 1919 said: 'The Russian Communist Party intends above all to carry out wide-scale health-improvement and sanitary measures to prevent the development of diseases as the basis of its activities in the field of public health.'[1] That is when prophylaxis came into being and became a leading trend in Soviet medicine.

N. A. Semashko, a prominent Soviet scientist and an organizer of public health, believed that prophylaxis should be regarded as measures taken by the Soviet state to improve the people's health, and that it should 'permeate' the entire organization of medical treatment.

Soviet medicine is preventive medicine. This is evident at all the stages of a doctor's practical activities. In the Soviet Union, most medical establishments are called therapeutic-preventive establishments, because, apart from treating the sick, they take part in carrying out general measures to prevent diseases and create healthier working and living conditions.

The method of dispensarization and the *uchastok* principle of giving medical treatment to the population are now the most important methods and principles in the therapeutic-preventive establishments' activities. The method helps to synthesize therapeutic and preventive medicine.

In the Soviet Union, mass medical check-ups are made for early case finding. In 1966, 11,000,000 workers, 36,300,000 students and 9,200,000 persons working at food, children's and therapeutic-preventive establishments were checked up. As many as 118,200,000 persons were examined in the country for early case finding of tuberculosis. That same year, over 14,500,000 patients suffering from hypertension, rheumatism, stomach and duodenal ulcers and other diseases received dispensary treatment from doctors working at therapeutic-preventive establishments.[2] About 32,000,000 persons were checked up for malaria during the trying years of the Great Patriotic War. Moreover, 2,500,000 patients were treated for malaria in 1944.

A strong technical basis makes Soviet medicine preventive. In 1958, the Soviet Union had 25,975 hospitals and hospital establishments and 15,529 dispensaries and dispensary departments. A streamlined system of sanitary and epidemic control has been set up. In 1964, the Soviet Union had 4,470 sanitary and epidemiological centres. By their current and preventive sanitary supervision, these establishments are a connecting link between therapeutic and preventive medicine. The new five-year plan for Soviet medical development sets the task of switching over to 'complete dispensarization' for therapeutic and preventive purposes.

The main problems of clinical medicine – etiology, diagnostics, treatments and prevention – are developing on the basis of the main preventive trend. I. P. Pavlov said: 'A cause can be fought only when it is known. But what is more important is to prevent it from coming into action, that is, from penetrating into the body.'

The Soviet doctor must know the causes of a disease not only to set a diagnosis and treat for it, but also mainly to prevent one disease or another. The doctor's main task is to set a diagnosis as early as possible. This has given rise to a new 'teaching of pre-disease' in Soviet medicine. M. P. Konchalovski, the founder of this teaching, believed that a clinical doctor's most important task is to 'see' the initial forms of disease, holding that this will make therapeutic and preventive aid effective.

Prevention also plays a part in the therapeutic service. Doctors have treated patients for diseases quite well in the past, and they successfully treat them for disease today. The Soviet Union has a new trend called 'pathogenetic therapy'. The doctors widely use sclerosis control treatment, vaccine therapy, iodining, treatment of pre-infarct cases, and so on.

In the Soviet Union, diseases are prevented by eradicating their causes and by making a person non-susceptible to them. The state plays a big part in the eradication of diseases. The public health bodies make people non-susceptible to diseases by carrying out wide-scale vaccinations. In the Soviet Union, sera and vaccines are being mass produced. The number of sera and vaccine institutes increased to ten in 1955–56. Soviet medicine has twenty types of live vaccines: fourteen are virus vaccines and six are vaccines for bacterial infections.[3] In the Soviet Union, over 190,000,000 vaccinations of live poliomyelitis vaccine were made in 1963 alone.

Such diseases as the plague, smallpox, cholera, malaria and dracunculosis have been eradicated in the Soviet Union owing to wide-scale social and preventive measures. The Soviet scientists must continue to look for new ways and means of preventing, reducing and eradicating various diseases.

The preventive trend in Soviet medicine is clearly expressed in medical science. The Soviet Union has many schools of theoretical, clinical and preventive medicine. Although they have their own distinguishing features, they develop on the basis of the main preventive trend. Scientists have made many discoveries in this respect. K. M. Bykov and G. I. Kurtsyn have worked out a cortico-visceral theory of ulcers. Ye. N. Pavlovski and his school have worked out the theory of the natural focus of diseases. B. A. Kudryashov and others have worked out the teaching of the anticoagulation system in a body, A. L. Myasnikov has advanced a new concept of the nature of hypertension, and V. P. Filatov has advanced the method of seraplastics (the giving back of eyesight to patients). Soviet hygienists have worked out the problem of collective and individual protection against radioactivity, and so on.

In the epoch of scientific and technological progress, Soviet hygienists are working out not only the means of protecting a person from harmful effects, but are also taking part, together with engineers, in making equipment that would prevent industrial accidents and other harmful effects on man.

The medics are successfully tackling the main task of Soviet medicine, which is to ensure a high level of people's health. In several socialist countries, many persons support the preventive trend as the main trend in modern medicine. In the foreseeable future, medicine will become hygienic in the broad sense of the word, and the preventive trend will be established more firmly in the doctor's practical activities.

References

1 *CPSU in the Resolutions and Decisions of Congresses, Conferences and Plenums of the Central Committee* (in Russian), part I, seventh printing, Moscow, 1953, p. 429.
2 PETROVSKI, B. V., '50 Years of Soviet Public Health' [Speech], Moscow, 1967, p. 17.
3 SOKOLOV, M. I., *Prevention of Infections by Live Vaccines*, Moscow, 1960, p. 14.

A. R. Chokin and K. B. Tsmogulova
Chekin (U.S.S.R.)

Medical education in Kazakhstan

In the very middle of the Eurasian Continent lies the ancient land of the Kazakhs. The territory of this republic is 3,000 km from east to west, from the Kaspian to the Altai mountains, and 1,800 km from north to south, from the Siberian taiga to the hot sands of Kizil-Kum.

The Kazakhs were one of the backward peoples of Tsarist Russia. The October Revolution has radically changed the lives of all peoples of our country – including the Kazakhs. During the years of Socialist construction Kazakhstan was turned into an advanced republic with a strong industry, mechanized agriculture and high cultural level.

Before the revolution there was no higher or secondary education in Kazakhstan. Kazakh children were forbidden to be educated. The establishment of Tomsk University in 1888 was of great importance for the training of physicians for Kazakhstan. In 1889, in accordance with the requests of the town authorities of Petropavlovsk, Semipalatinsk, Pavlodar and others, special stipends were introduced for citizens of these towns. In 1894 Kazakh children were given permission to be educated in Kazan University. According to pre-revolutionary data there were only twenty-three Kazakh physicians. These were mainly children of the rich, who had graduated from Saratov, Omsk, Moscow, Kiev and Tomsk Universities as well as from the Military Medical Academy.

Medium grade medical personnel were trained from 1872 in Orenburg feldsher school. Altogether, there were 200 physicians and about 300 medium grade medical workers in pre-revolutionary Kazakhstan.

It was only after the establishment of Soviet power in Kazakhstan that the training of Kazakh medical personnel became possible. The services of the physicians themselves in helping to establish Soviet power are worthy of mention. They saved many wounded Red Army officers and soldiers.

After Lenin signed the decree on the creation of the Autonomous Kazakh Republic in August 1920, the first Kazakh Commissars of Public Health, M. S. Shamov, M. M. Tshumbalov and A. B. Abdrachmanov became initiators of special courses and schools to train medical personnel amongst the native population. This was a very difficult task. The Russian Federal Republic offered its help. Its Commissariat of public health sent medical personnel to Kazakhstan and invited Kazakhs to study in Russian schools. In 1920, 213 people were sent to be educated in Russia, forty-four of them to the medical faculty.

In 1923, in the town of Orenburg (the former administrative centre of Kazakhstan) a medical medium grade school was opened. This was followed by similar schools in other towns. By 1950 there were already seventeen medium grade schools, whilst at the present there are twenty-five. Besides this there are 130 affiliated schools where 2,500 students are trained.

Especially great was the role played by the Medical Institute opened in Alma Ata in the training of native physicians. Special buildings were founded for the Institute, the teachers and professors were invited from other republics. The first school year began in April 1931. 134 students were registered, including fifty-four Kazakhs. In September 1931 the second recruitment of students took place – 168 persons including ninety-one Kazakhs.

Great help was offered during these years by the Leningrad Military Medical Academy. As a result, by the end of 1931 five professors, and thirteen assistant professors taught at the Institute. Only two of them, however, were Kazakhs.

To facilitate the recruitment of students, to make it possible for young people to enter the Institute, special courses, called 'workers' faculty courses' were established. These functioned for eleven years.

In 1934 the Institute was enlarged by the addition of a new building and students' quarters. By 1940 the Alma Ata Medical Institute had 1,402 students and 120 professors and teachers.

However, a great shortage of paediatricians made imperative the establishment of a paediatric faculty. This was opened in 1938 and since that time 3,718 paediatricians have been trained – 1,175 of them Kazakhs.

During the war the Institute changed its programme in order to pay more attention to military medical training. Many graduates of the Institute fought at the front. Eighty-four professors and teachers of the Institute and 262 students were enlisted as volunteers to the front. One of these students, a girl – Manshuk Mametova – was posthumously given the title of Hero of the Soviet Union. During the war years 2,000 physicians graduated from the Institute. Nearly 74 per cent of them joined the fighting troops. In 1943, a new sanitary hygienic faculty was established at the Institute to provide for the great masses of people moving to the Middle Asian Republics. These were partly workers and partly evacuees.

In 1954 a pharmaceutical faculty was established and 1961 witnessed the addition of a stomatological faculty. Thus, during the years of its existence, the Alma Ata Medical Institute has trained 16,360 physicians and 1,620 pharmacists amongst whom 4,755 were Kazakhs.

At present the Institute consists of four faculties. There are 5,630 students, 50 per cent of which are Kazakhs. There are 540 teachers and professors many of whom are engaged in research.

The Alma Ata Medical Institute was followed by many others in various towns of the Kazakh Republic – in Kazaganda in 1951, Semipalatinsk in 1953, and Tselinograd in 1964. Altogether, 2,000 physicians graduate annually from the medical institutes of the Republic. At present in Kazakhstan there are 28,670 physicians, which equals twenty-two physicians for 10,000 people. There are also more than 104,816 medium grade workers.

Thus, we are able to assess the great changes which have taken place in Kazakhstan during the years of socialist Soviet power.

V. N. Emeliyanov
Yaroslavl (U.S.S.R.)

On the history of public health in three regions of the Upper Volga

The development of public health in pre-revolutionary Russia synchronizes with the rise of social enthusiasm in the 1860s, with the abolition of serfdom and with the development of capitalism. A number of reforms were introduced by the Russian government during this period. One of them was the 'Zemstvo' reform of 1864 according to which zemstvo system of local government was created over part of the territory of Russia. Progressive representatives in the zemstvo councils fought for improvement of medical services for the rural population. In the second half of the nineteenth century these doctors promoted the development of public health services. A system of organization of medical care was proposed, the most important links in which were the district hospital and rural medical districts. Parallel to this, so-called urban and factory medicine began to develop as a result of other reforms. The history of zemstvo, factory and urban medicine is one of the most striking pages of Russian pre-revolutionary public health.

Our paper deals with Vologda, Kostroma and Yaroslavl regions, denominated as guberniyas in pre-revolutionary Russia. In the nineteenth century the territory of these guberniyas was 459,000 square versts (1 verst = 1·0668 kilometre) and the population – 4,149·5 thousands. At present the territory of these oblasts is 242·3 thousand square kilometres and the population – 3,567 thousand according to the census of 1970.

The low sanitary and cultural level of the population, the patriarchal tenor of life, underdeveloped industry and agriculture, and wide extension of migratory labour were characteristic of all these guberniyas. However, by 1913 thirty zemstvo hospitals were established in Vologda, sixty in Kostroma and thirty-five in Yaroslavl guberniya. The radius of the zemstvo medical districts was reduced from 40 kilometres in previous years to 14.

Zemstvo and factory forms of medical care were based mainly on the so-called travelling-doctor principle. Only by the 1870s did the largest enterprises began to establish special hospitals (for instance in textile fabrics in Yaroslavl, Gavrilov-Yam, Kosroma) and some smaller ones organized posts of medical aid.

A certain role in organizing public health service in these guberniyas was played by meetings of zemstvo doctors. The agenda of these meetings included different questions of organization of medical care for the population, such as: the sanitary and epidemiological condition of guberniyas, morbidity, medical care for children, pharmaceutical and dental services and so on. Most serious attention was paid to establishing the network of zemstvo medical units and especially rural district hospitals, to the development of sanitary services of guberniyas, to the creation of smallpox calf-sheds, to the training of medium grade medical workers. To the latter end all the guberniyan hospitals opened schools for training doctors' assistants. A considerable role in the organization of medical services in guberniyas was also played by medical associations. For example, The Yaroslavl medical association, founded in 1861, was one of the first provincial medical societies. The members of this association aspired to scientific work as well as to the organization of free medical care for the population. It was not by chance that in 1861 the Association opened the public Volga hospital, giving free medical attention, which incorporated a maternity ward with six beds and a midwifery school. This public hospital was the first in the Russian provinces, followed by the Maximilian public hospital in Petersburg. Since the Yaroslavl and later on the Vologda and Kostroma medical associations published their records, the results of their activities became known to all guberniyan doctors.

One of the peculiar features of Russian public medicine was the activity of progressive social-minded physicians who fought for the development of public and preventive medicine. Such were N. V. Golosov, G. I. Kurochkin, P. P. Voskresensky, I. I. Tryasunov and other physicians, working in the above-mentioned guberniyas. One of their achievements was abolition by 1914 of private medical attention in Yaroslavl and Kostroma guberniyas.

However, in spite of the fact that public medicine in pre-revolutionary Russia was an unprecedented example of a system of public health service, it was unable to make any essential change in promoting the health of the Russian people. The number of public health establishments was quite insufficient, sanitary services were practically non-existent, factories had posts of medical aid instead of hospitals, specialist medical care was almost lacking. All this determined a low level of sanitary condition for the population. The mortality of the population of Yaroslavl guberniya in 1913 was more than 33 per 1,000, and infant mortality more than 400 per 1,000 births. In Kostroma guberniya in 1910 the mortality was 34 per 1,000, and infant mortality more than 340 per 1,000 births. Infectious disease was very high in all three guberniyas.

On the eve of the Great October Socialist Revolution in Yaroslavl guberniya there were only fifty hospitals with 1,678 beds in which 142 physicians worked. In Kostroma guberniya eighty-four hospitals had 2,864 beds or 2·1 beds per 1,000, and the number of physicians was 125, or one per 10,000 population. Still worse, in Vologda guberniya there was less than one bed per 1,000 population. Not without reason Vologda guberniya was a place of exile for progressive men and revolutionaries.

After the Great October Socialist Revolution construction of the new life began fully in keeping with the interests of the working people, including their interests in regard to public health. A new system of public health services was established based on the following main principles: the State control of the system, including its planning on a State basis and the fact that it is free of charge, universally accessible and provides a high standard of medical care; its emphasis on prophylaxis; close links between medical research and practice, and broad participation of the people themselves in developing the public health system.

The guberniyas of the Upper Volga passed through a period of construction of Soviet public health. At first special medico-sanitary departments were set up by guberniyan soviet authorities. For instance, in Yaroslavl a collegia of three persons and after that a medico-sanitary department were established. In the process of searching for new unified forms of public health authorities, the activity of the Supreme Soviet Inspection, created in 1918 with M. S. Kedrov as the head, played a certain role. It had carried out much organizing work in Arkhangelsk, Vologda, and Kostroma regions with the aim of reorganization of the old authorities, setting up of new ones, and selection of medical personnel. The Inspection came across many difficulties: hospitals were ruined, there were no drugs in the stores, and unco-operative medical personnel. In order to train new medical personnel the medical faculty of the Yaroslavl university was opened in 1919.

On 11 July 1918 the People's Komissariat of Health of the Russian Soviet Federal Socialist Republic was established as the central public health authority of the country, which was followed by organization of guberniyan and uyezd public health departments. These new authorities were to solve three main problems: the control of infectious diseases, the fight for preserving and promoting children's health, and the centralization of medico-sanitary services. The broad participation of the people themselves in public health and sanitary work was especially characteristic of the first years of the Soviet power. It was manifested in different ways: 'weeks of fight for cleanness and sanitary well-being', 'bath and laundry weeks', 'workers' fighting for cleanness councils', and so on. On 7 November 1920 one of the first houses for health education in the country was established in Yaroslavl.

Of great significance for the determination of the future paths of public health in the U.S.S.R. was the Eighth Congress of the Russian Communist Party (Bolsheviks) in March 1919, which adopted a new Party programme, including a special section dealing with public health services, and defined the basic principles of the Soviet public health system. Declaring the right for health the Soviet state took the responsibility by law to provide the people all kinds of medical attention. The main emphasis in the programme was laid on prophylaxis. V. I. Lenin himself contributed greatly to the construction and promotion of Soviet public health. He signed more than one hundred decrees dealing with public health.

Summing up the achievements of the ten-year development of Soviet medicine, we may say that by 1927 the period of formation of Soviet public health services ended. By this year Yaroslavl region had seventy-one hospitals with 2,685 beds, twenty-two anti-tuberculosis establishments with 329 beds, eighty-two rural medical districts, forty of which had hospitals, forty-eight midwife posts, eight women's consulting clinics, 396 doctors and so on. Similar developments occurred in the Vologda and Kostroma regions. In the latter there were 245 doctors and in Vologda, 111, which means more than one doctor per 10,000 population.

By the end of the 1920s during the period of industrialization and the collectivization of agriculture, public health services were faced with new tasks, particularly with the protection of the health of the workers in the leading branches of industry and of those taking part in the establishment of collective and State farms. Most important at this time became the establishment of what was known as the 'health posts' in industrial undertakings instead of previous 'posts of first aid'. The strengthening of the prophylactic foundations of the public health services was reflected in the ever-growing application of the 'dispensarization' method, which means a synthesis of therapeutic and preventive medicine. Naturally the carrying out of a combination of medical and social measures, essential for this method, required the establishment of a powerful material and technical base for the health services, a considerable increase in medical staff and other conditions. That is why it was only later that dispensarization on a large scale became possible.

The unified State system of public health protection established during the years of Soviet power was subjected to a very severe test during the Second World War. In the Yaroslavl, Vologda, and Kostroma regions as well as in many other parts of the country besides the provision of medical aid to hospitalized soldiers, the health authorities faced the urgent task of providing medical care for the civilian population, particularly workers in the defence industries.

After the war much attention was paid to further developing the material and technical basis of the public health system, raising the standard of medical care, extending its specialization and increasing the number of medical workers. As a result of this work, by 1971 public health services of, for instance, Vologda district, had 13,940 hospital beds and 1,875 doctors, Kostroma district had over 9,500 beds and over 1,200 doctors; in Yaroslavl district the number of hospital beds was 16,000 and doctors, 2,500.

Thus, during the years of Soviet power Vologda, Kostroma and Yaroslavl oblasts from backward guberniyas of the tsarist Russia were converted into regions with high levels of culture and economy. Besides old textile factories new branches of industry were developed in these regions, such as metallurgy, chemistry, machine-tool construction, oil-refining and electrotechnical industries. In all the centres there are higher and medium grade schools including Yaroslavl university and higher medical school.

In recent years big specialized medical departments were established in the three districts, such as neurosurgery, thoracic surgery, anaethesiology, resuscitation, rheumatology, occupational pathology, haematology, and so on. In the hospitals all the modern methods of diagnosis and cure are used.

The results of this development are manifested in the following indices: mean expectation of life is over seventy years, overall mortality is 8 per 1,000 population, infantile mortality is 21–23 per 1,000 births. The indices of physical development of children became considerably better. Almost 100 per cent of expectant mothers are kept under medical observation up till childbirth.

As a result of the realization of the resolutions of the XXIV Congress of the Communist Party of the U.S.S.R., dealing with improvement of the material and technical basis of public health, the Vologda, Kostroma and Yaroslavl regions by 1975 will provide over twelve hospital beds per 1,000 population and one physician per 300. All these measures will contribute to further promotion of the health of the population of the three regions of the Upper Volga.

F. S. Haddad
Beirut (*Lebanon*)

Organized medicine in relation to Arab society

INTRODUCTION

I shall try to trace the picture of organized Arab medicine in relation to Arab Society, including systems of medical care, medical institutions, medical education and hospitals between A.D. 700 and 1400.

HOSPITALS

Although the idea of a hospital as an institution for the treatment of the sick is as old as civilization itself, it is generally conceded that the Arabs were the first to establish well-organized and well-administered hospitals. History has recorded the existence of hospitals in at least thirty-one Arab cities, a few of which like Baghdad, Cairo, Damascus and Aleppo had more than one hospital each.

Arab hospitals, as the remains of some of them show, were well constructed on carefully chosen sites. The hospital medical staff and administrative personnel were well diversified, specialized, capable, responsible and well qualified. The hospital pharmacy and stores were well stocked. Medical libraries and conference rooms formed an integral part of the hospital and thus made it easy for the hospital to become the centre of medical education and instruction.

Arab hospitals were not only non-profit-making organizations founded by the rich, but were invariably sufficiently well endowed to be able to offer their services on a wholly and totally benevolent basis without any charge or fee; they continued to function for long periods; some, for as long as 1,229 years, like the Walid Hospital in Damascus (707–1936).

THE SITE OF THE HOSPITAL AND ITS CONSTRUCTION

The site of the hospital was chosen after careful consideration and depended not only on the need of the neighbourhood, but also on the hygienic, climatic and sanitary conditions prevailing in the various sections of the town.

The hospital was usually constructed around a central courtyard and consisted of separate pavilions for male and female patients, a psychiatric ward, a pharmacy, an out-patient clinic, a library, a lecture hall and a public bath. The hospital building was not only functional in its construction but was also artistically decorated.

THE STAFF

The hospital staff was usually appointed after thorough deliberation and careful examination. The staff was usually diversified and of a highly specialized nature. It generally included the chief physician, the physicians, the assistant physicians, the superintendent, the oculist, the resident physician, the chaplain or his equivalent, the pharmacist, the maintenance man, male nurses, female nurses, the bursar and the musicians.[7]

THE PHARMACY

Each hospital had a pharmacy well stocked with medicines, syrups, drugs, ointments and all kinds of useful and valuable medicine that could not be found elsewhere. The hospital pharmacy also contained valuable pharmaceutical instruments such as Chinese porcelain jars and jugs and the like that could not be afforded elsewhere (10, p. 20). A competent and licensed pharmacist was in charge of the hospital pharmacy. He had under him several assistants (10, p. 21).

LIBRARIES

In a culture and a land where so many libraries both public and private existed, it is no wonder that every hospital had its own medical library. It usually contained manuscripts of the medical works of Hindu, Persian, Greek and Arab authors. The Tulun Hospital Library founded in Cairo in 872, for example, contained 100,000 volumes (10, p. 39).

MEDICAL EDUCATION

Two kinds of medical education existed side by side: the first was provided for in the various hospitals and included both theoretical and clinical instruction, while the second was conducted in special medical schools where the instruction was solely theoretical. It was common for a prospective physician to follow simultaneously the two kinds of medical education provided for, and also to travel in search of further knowledge in the big medical centres of the times.

In hospitals, medical students attended the clinics and followed the physicians on their daily hospital rounds. After the morning rounds, the attending physicians and the medical students would gather around the chief physician in the large auditorium, which was very nicely furnished. The chief physician would then conduct discussions concerning medical subjects and difficult cases for about three hours; this would also include formal lectures and tutorial instruction (8, vol. 2, p. 155).

HOSPITAL ADMINISTRATION

The administration of the hospitals was entrusted to high dignitaries and was the subject of the most careful supervision.

The position of director of a hospital was considered one of the highest in the government and was generally placed in the hands of one of the princes or one of the nobles. The hospital director was a man of ability, highly cultured and well respected; he had access to the Caliph's palace on the same footing as the ministers.

He had entire charge of the administration, supervision and custody of all supplies, medications and furniture; he also had sometimes to administer the endowment. Under the director were the supervisors; and under these worked the orderlies and the servants.

The director was installed in office in a ceremonious inauguration that included an official parade and a colourful procession whereby the director was accompanied to the hospital by high governmental officials mounted on horses and in flowing robes (10, p. 23).

The director administered all hospital activities except the medical functions which were under the control of the chief physician or dean who was ably assisted by the different heads of departments and these in turn were helped by their assistants and apprentices.

THE HOSPITALS WERE WELL ENDOWED AND BENEVOLENT

All Arab hospitals were of the endowed benevolent category. They were supported by wakf (property entailed in perpetuity). In every instance legal documentary evidence was put through the proper courts entailing the property for the specific purpose of building, running and operating the hospital. The whole order of things and the general atmosphere centred around the principle that the people should be able to get free medical services.

A few excerpts from the endowment document of Qalawun, Sultan of Cairo, will be most revealing and will give us a pathway into the thoughts and aims of those responsible for the foundation of Arab hospitals. Sultan Qalawun states in his document (A.D. 1281) that his hospital 'shall be open to groups of people as well as to individuals, to the old, to the young and to adolescents, to children, to women and to infants, it shall be open to the admission of poor patients, male or female, in order that they may be treated and cared for until they are cured. The medications prepared in the hospital shall be dispensed to patients coming from far as well as those living in the neighbourhood, to the citizens as well as the foreigners, to the strong and the weak, to all without any condition, reservation, objection or rejection whatsoever but for the plenty of God' (10, p. 138).

In the same document (line 404) the Sultan further says: 'The responsible executive of this testament shall not favour the dignitaries over the meek nor the powerful over the weak, nor the townsfolks over the foreigners . . .' (10, p. 147). The Sultan also states (lines 40–42): 'The great Chair in the Hospital shall be reserved for a wise physician-teacher who shall be knowledgeable in medicine and its various aspects, expert in its scope and one with a wide practice and large experience' (10, p. 152). Amazing words for the thirteenth century and well ahead of their times!

In drinking a toast to his hospital, during its dedication ceremony, the Sultan said: 'I dedicate this hospital to my peers and my inferiors, and constitute this wakf for the benefit of the king and the subject, the soldier and the prince, the great and the small, the freemen and the slave, for men and for women' (11, p. 406 and 6, p. 175).

Every patient, when cured and discharged received a suit of clothes and a certain sum of money to defray necessary expenses until he became self-supporting (9, 6, p. 173 and 10, p. 281).

The testament of endowment of several hospitals did not forget those who were sick and remained home: 'Those that are sick at home and poor shall receive what they need in the form of medicines and shall receive other necessary home services' (10, p. 152).

Free benefits did not stop with death, for the endowment provided for interment costs including the cleaning of the dead body, the embalming, the coffin, the digging of the grave and all other expenses (10, p. 152).

All these benefits sound so modern that one is amazed at their existence so many centuries ago.

HOSPITAL DEPARTMENTS

The Arab hospitals were very well organized. There were two separate sections completely independent of one another: one for males and the second for females. Each of the two sections was well equipped with all the necessary furniture, equipment and instruments and had the necessary personnel including servants, maids, orderlies and supervisors (8, vol. 1, p. 310).

In each of the two sections, there were different wards for the different medical conditions: a ward for internal diseases, a ward for surgical diseases, a ward for eye cases, a ward for orthopaedics (8, vol. 2, p. 242), a ward for patients with dysentery, a ward for psychiatry (8, vol. 2, p. 260), a special ward for fever cases (8, vol. 1, p. 254 and vol. 2, p. 243) and a ward for those patients who were convalescing (10, p. 102).

The wards were spacious and were provided with running water (8, vol. 2, p. 260); they were heated in winter with perfumed incense and were ventilated in summer (10, p. 102).

Musico-therapy and entertainment were very highly developed; special choirs and music bands entertained the patients daily by providing singing and musical performances on the various instruments. There were also special story tellers, dancers and comic performers as well (10, p. 102).

SPECIAL HOSPITALS AND SPECIAL CLINICS

The vast majority of Arab hospitals were of the general hospital type; only a few were special hospitals reserved for the treatment of one kind of disease only. There were, for example, psychiatric hospitals, ophthalmic hospitals and military hospitals. We encounter also certain special clinics, like the mobile clinics for rural areas, the prison clinics and the school clinics.

MEDICAL LICENSURE

Sinan was the Official Chief Medical Examiner of the Caliph al-Muqtadir. In the year A.D. 931 he examined over 860 physicians in Baghdad, not including the very famous physicians, nor those in the service of the Sultan (8, vol. 1, p. 222). These examinations formed the beginnings of the system of medical examination and licensure which 200 years later found their way to Sicily and were emulated for the first time in Europe (1140) by Roger, the founder of the Christian Kingdom of Sicily.[1]

In seeking hospital appointments, physicians had to pass an examination in their specialty. This is interesting, as even today we are still arguing about whether a physician should pass an examination and be licensed to practise a specialty.

CONCLUSION

Although some of the reported facts seem to have been embellished by the chroniclers and some of the figures seem to have been blown up, these are, in relation to the actual historical context, what the caricature is to the photograph; they tend to define more clearly certain salient aspects of the picture. Nonetheless, after *all* the recorded facts are reviewed, it becomes apparent that the Arabs had a coherent, well organized and comprehensive system of medicine with the following characteristics:

1. An advanced state of justice, benevolence and social conscience revealed by free treatment of the poor, non-discrimination in admitting patients to hospitals and equality between the sexes and between the social classes before the health services and the medical profession.
2. A relatively well-qualified medical profession with advanced specialization, supported by an efficient para-medical staff organized on the principle of division of labour.
3. Two complementary systems of medical education: didactic instruction in special medical schools and clinical instruction in the hospitals.
4. A system of supervised medical examination, licensure and specialty certification.
5. An overall quality of the hospitals, their buildings, their equipment and their management, with an organized and co-ordinated medical staff.
6. A vast medical literature including translations of all major Greek and Hindu medical works and an extensive library of original Arabic medical texts.
7. A comprehensive and benevolent system of free medical care. This included home visits, clinic visits, hospitalization, medications and death and interment expenses, as well as army mobile hospitals, school and prison clinics and ambulatory clinics for the outlying districts.

ACKNOWLEDGEMENTS

I am grateful to Dr. Robert Audi, my wife Huda and my son Sami for their valuable suggestions.

References

1 ELGOOD, C., *Medical History of Persia*, Cambridge, 1957.
2 HADDAD, FARID SAMI, 'Spain', *Ann. Rep. Orient Hosp.*, 1961, **14**, 71.
3 HADDAD, FARID SAMI, 'Pioneers of Arabian Medicine', *Leb. med. J.*, 1968, **21**, 67–80.
4 HADDAD, FARID SAMI, 'The permanent contributions of the Arabs to medicine' (unpublished).
5 HADDAD, FARID SAMI and BITAR, EMILE, 'Les principes déontologiques dans la Médecine Arabe', *Congrès International d'histoire de la Médecine*, Bucarest, 1970, 1972, pp. 65–66.
6 HADDAD, SAMI *et al.*, 'A study of Arab Hospitals in the light of present day standardization'. *Bull. A.C.S.*, 1936, **21**, 173–77.
7 HADDAD, SAMI, 'The Arab physician', *Ann. Rep. Orient Hosp.*, 1961, **14**, 28–33.
8 IBN ABI USAYBI'A (in Arabic).
9 BALAWI quoted by 10.
10 ISA, *L'histoire des Bimaristans dans l'Islam*, 1939 (in Arabic).
11 MAQRIZI (in Arabic).

D. W. Amundsen
Bellingham, Washington (U.S.A.)

The medical legislation of the Assizes of Jerusalem

After Jerusalem was conquered by the crusaders in 1099, Godfrey of Bouillon, as Baron and Defender of the Holy Sepulchre, created two courts: the high court (*Haute Cour*) and the lower court (*Cour des Bourgeois*).[1] Cases between members of the nobility were judged in the high court and those between the free non-nobles in the lower court.[2] Litigation between noble and non-noble was held in the lower court.[3] Local tradition in the Latin Kingdom of Jerusalem holds that Godfrey had also ordered a compilation of the existing usages of his day, the so-called *Lettres du Sépulcre*. These were not a formal code of laws but consisted of provisions drawn up to meet the immediate contingencies of the newly created kingdom. They were revised, amended and added to as the occasion arose but the entire code was lost when Jerusalem fell to Saladin in 1187.[4] Oral tradition based on familiarity with the *Lettres du Sépulcre* was that upon which the customary law was founded that governed the kingdom until the compilation of the two major divisions of law of the kingdom that are extant: the *Assises de la Haute Cour* and the *Assises de la Cour des Bourgeois*.[5] It is upon the latter that I wish to concentrate for therein are contained various regulations governing the medical profession.[6]

There has been considerable debate as to the date of the writing of the Assizes of the lower court. Suffice it to say that they were compiled during the first half of the thirteenth century.[7] Many parts of the Assizes of the lower court seem to be basically case law, that is specific law based upon precedent. Whether any particular section was based on the transcript of an actual adjudication or on oral tradition is difficult if not usually impossible to determine with certainty. Nor can we assume that this code gives a picture of conditions in the Latin Kingdom of Jerusalem for any specific period. These were not rigid laws that were not subject to change. Accordingly, the extent to which any part represents customary law and procedure of the early Latin Kingdom of Jerusalem is highly debatable.

Chapters 236 and 238 of the *Assises de la Cour des Bourgeois* are devoted to medical regulations.[8] Although the text does not divide the chapters into individual rubrics, chapter 236 contains eleven different laws and chapter 238, twelve. Eighteen of these twenty-three laws are concerned with the liability of the physician for what we would term negligent or ignorant malpractice.

The distinction between negligent and ignorant malpractice can be rather nebulous[9] and, in the broadest sense of the word, the definition of what constitutes ignorant malpractice presents a problem of some magnitude. In an attempt to protect society from the incompetent physician, legislators periodically have attempted to impose standards of medical practice and have promulgated punitive legislation designed to punish the guilty physician and to deter his colleagues from similar malpractice. Providing a means for redress to the victim of the incompetent physician or to his relatives has also been a goal of such legislation.[10]

There are instances where the prohibitive measures directed against the members of the medical profession forbid or limit the use of one specific mode of treatment. An example of this is found in the *Lex Visigothorum* where a physician who killed a man by excessive blood-letting would be turned over to the relatives of the deceased to be dealt with as they should see fit. Weighed against the other laws in the *Lex Visigothorum* that regulated medical practice, it becomes evident that it was enacted for the protection of the patient against a specific type of treatment excessively engaged in primarily by those members of the medical profession whose level of competence was low.[11]

The making of a physician's liability dependent upon the unfavourable results of specific types of treatment was employed extensively by the *Cour des Bourgeois*. In chapter 236 there are three laws dealing with the improper treatment of wounds, one with the improper treatment of a boil, all resulting in the death of the patient. In each of these the patient was a slave. In all of these instances the physician is ordered to pay to the slave's owner as much as the slave was worth while in good health. In chapter 238 there are eight cases of improper treatment of ailments resulting in the death of a slave. These range from administering laxatives to a patient with dysentery to burning out the intestine in an attempt to cauterize haemorrhoids with a hot iron. In these also the physician must indemnify the owner for the death of his slave. There is in chapter 236 one case where a physician poorly set a slave's broken arm or leg causing him to be crippled. The court ordered the physician to buy the slave for the sum he was worth before his injury or, if he lacked the means, to pay to the slave's owner the amount of the slave's diminution of value.

Roman law indirectly provided the basis for a great part of the *Assises de la Cour des Bourgeois*.[12] Jurists in the Latin Kingdom of Jerusalem could easily have found legal precedents in Roman law for making the physician, who by negligence or incompetence caused the injury or death of a slave, responsible for indemnification of the slave's owner.[13] Not so, however, when the patient who was injured or killed by the negligent or incompetent physician happened to be a free man or a free woman. There was no penalty in Roman law for the negligent injuring or killing of a free man. Intent was a necessary factor in homicide. Also, since there was in Roman law no defined concept of tortious liability, at the most the negligent or incompetent physician would be liable only for expenses. The *Cour des Bourgeois*, in dealing with the killing or injuring of a free man or a free woman by a negligent or incompetent physician, made the matter of intent irrelevant. In chapter 236 there are three laws dealing with the treatment of wounds, one with the treatment of a boil, all resulting in the death of the slave-patient. After these is the following provision: 'And if this physician has thus, as is stated above, badly treated any free man or free woman and he dies from it, reason judges that this physician ought to be hanged and as much as he owns ought to be the lord's by right. But if the physician has received something from the dead man, this ought to be given to the relatives of the diseased from the possessions of the physician for this is right and reason'.[14] Also in chapter 236 it is ordered that, if a physician so badly sets a free person's broken arm or leg that he is crippled on that account, he ought to have his right hand cut off and be compelled to return any fee that he had received. In chapter 238, following those treatments listed that had proved fatal to patients who were slaves, appears this stipulation: 'Likewise, if any physician has thus treated any free man or free woman, reason judges and commands that this physician ought to be hanged and that all that he owns be given to the lord. But before he is hanged, he ought to be whipped through the city with a urinal in his hand, for this is right and reason to frighten the others from this malpractice, for this is right and reason by the assizes.'[15] The concern of the court here was not directed toward the compensation of the victim or his relatives seeking redress. Nor is this an instance of the application of the *lex talionis* as was the case in the example given from Visigothic law. The severity of the punishment of physicians in cases such as these, indeed the very necessity of judgments of this nature, listing a wide variety of specific treatments considered improper for specific ailments, is surely an indication that a fairly sizeable segment of the medical profession was of a low calibre. This was not an attempt on the part of the promulgators of law to establish a fixed body of proper and improper medical procedures. The *Assises de la Cour des Bourgeois* are, after all, case law. As individual cases were judged, precedents would be established based on the peculiarities of the case at hand.

The responsibility of the promulgators of law to protect the general public from the quacks, charlatans and pseudophysicians reaches its highest realization in the establishment of an enforceable system of medical licensure. And the *Assises de la Cour des Bourgeois* did create a system of medical licensure. No foreign physician, whether he came from Christian Europe or from pagan countries[16] was allowed to practise medicine by means of urine until he had been tested by other physicians, the best in the land, in the presence of the bishop.[17] If found competent, he would be given letters from the bishop certifying that he could legally doctor by means of urine.[18] The law goes on to say that if he is not found to be a good physician, the bishop and court must command that he leave the city or remain in the city without practising medicine. It does not state, however, that he would be allowed to continue practising medicine but without the right to use urine analysis as a diagnostic method. Further, it says that if any physician practises medicine in the city without leave of the court and the bishop, he must be seized and thrown out of the city.[19] Once again there is no mention of practising medicine by means of urine. Accordingly, it seems that any physician who wished to engage in any type of medical practice would first have to submit to an examination of his ability to diagnose through urine analysis. There is no evidence to indicate that there was any dichotomy between the practice of medicine and surgery. Initially there might seem to be evidence to support such a contention: The cases in chapter 236 deal primarily with what would be under the purvue of the surgeon and those in chapter 238 for the most part involve medicine. In the punishment ordered for the guilty physician, the major difference between the two chapters is that in chapter 238 there is the additional stipulation that the physician, before being hanged, is to be whipped through the city carrying a urinal in his hand. The same word, however, is used to designate the medical practitioner in both instances.

What was the source of their policy of medical licensure? During the time of the existence of the Latin Kingdom of Jerusalem, systems of medical licensure were being brought into force in Europe. The first instance comes from Sicily. In 1140 King Roger II issued an order that anyone wishing to practise medicine should present himself to the royal officials and judges and undergo their examination. His explanation was that 'in this way we are taking care that our subjects are not endangered by the incompetence of physicians'.[20] Not only the right to grant the medical licence but also the examination of the candidate's ability were reserved for the king and his officials.[21] In 1231 Frederick II, as King of Sicily, promulgated his *Constitutiones Imperiales* containing laws specifying procedure for granting a licence to practise medicine and surgery.[22] Improving upon the procedure employed by Roger II, Frederick made a fixed course of study followed by examination before the masters of the medical school of Salerno prerequisites for licensure.[23] To know the date of the initiation of the system of medical licensure in the Latin Kingdom of Jerusalem might prove helpful in determining whether or not any relationship existed between its institution and the developments in Sicily during the twelfth and thirteenth centuries. It is very possible that the medical licensure provisions of the Assizes antedate the legislation of Roger II. It would then be the first known provision for medical licensure in the western world.[24]

Since the arrangement of the *Assises de la Cour des Bourgeois* is topical and not chronological, the fact that the provisions for licensure occupy the last part of the sections devoted to medical practice does not mean, *ipso facto*, that they were drawn up later than the rest of the same section. But the provisions for licensure surely are not a product of case law and would not have been based on specific precedent as the other cases at which we have looked were. One motivating force behind instituting a system of medical licensure is the desire to protect the public from the incompetent medical practitioner. That was the express concern of Roger II of Sicily. Similar to but probably not in any way dependent upon the Sicilian legislation, the medical licensure provisions of the Latin Kingdom of Jerusalem were a logical development of case law. The attempt to define, punish and curtail medical malpractice led to the creation of a primitive system of medical licensure not designed with the intent of their superseding the malpractice laws but with the hope that need of application of the malpractice laws would be substantially diminished.

ACKNOWLEDGEMENTS

I wish to acknowledge my appreciation to Professor Arthur Kimmel for his philological assistance, to Professor LeRoy Dresbeck for his historical guidance and to Professor Gary Ferngren for his general help and advice.

References

1 *Livre de Jean d'Ibelin*, I, 2, in M. Beugot, *Les Assises de Jerusalem, Recueil des Historiens des Croisades, Lois*, Paris, 1841–43, vol. I, p. 23.

2 It should be noted that the high court did not stand in appellate relation to the lower court.

3 LAMONTE, J. L., *Feudal Monarchy in the Latin Kingdom of Jerusalem 1100–1291*, Cambridge, Mass., 1932, p. 106.

4 It has become fashionable to deny the very existence of the *Lettres du Sépulcre*; however, for a defence of their historicity, see J. L. LaMonte 'Three questions concerning the Assises de Jerusalem', *Byzantina-Metabyzantina*, 1946, 1, 204 ff.

5 These are published in Beugnot, op. cit., vols. I and II respectively.

6 There are in the *Assises de la Haute Cour* a few references pertaining to forensic medicine. For these see BRITTAIN, R. P., 'The history of legal medicine: the Assizes of Jerusalem', *Medico-*

Legal J., 1966, **34**, 72 f. Brittain's concern here is strictly limited to forensic medicine in the *Haute Cour*.

7 GRANDCLAUDE, M., in his excellent study of the Assizes (*Étude Critique sur les Livres des Assises de Jerusalem*, Paris, 1923, 66 ff.), sets the date of composition between 1229 and 1244; PRAWER, J. ('L'établissement des coutumes du marché a Saint-Jean d'Acre et la date de composition du livre des Assises des Bourgeois', *Rev. hist. Droit Français et Etranger*, 1951, **28**, 346 ff.) argues for a more limited period, 1240–1244.

8 These are printed in Beugnot, op. cit., vol. II, pp. 164–69.

9 In none of the laws under our perusal is the negligence of the physician mentioned except as a possible contributing factor. Accordingly, it is to ignorant malpractice that the *Cour des Bourgeois* directed its attention.

10 SPECTOR, B., 'The growth of medicine and the letter of the law', *Bull. Hist. Med.*, 1952, **26**, 499–525; OPPENHEIMER, H., 'Liability for Malapraxis in ancient law', *Trans. Medico-Legal Soc.*, 1910, **7**, 98–107; TWEEDY, J., 'The deterrent influence of social and legal restrictions on the medical thought and practice', ibid., 1911, **8**, 1–8; SIGERIST, H. E., 'The history of medical licensure', *J. Amer. med. Ass.*, 1935, **104**, 1057–60.

11 For a discussion of the medical regulations in Visigothic law, see AMUNDSEN, DARREL W., 'Visigothic medical legislation', *Bull. Hist. Med.*, 1971, **45**, 553–69.

12 LAMONTE, *Feudal Monarchy . . .*, op. cit., p. 101, note 5. According to PRAWER, J., 'Etude preliminaire sur les sources et la composition du "Livre des Assises de Bourgeois" ', *Rev. hist. Droit Français et Etranger*, 1954, **31**, the section in which the medical regulations appear was not influenced extensively by Roman legal principles nor is there any indication in that section of borrowing from earlier or contemporary codes (p. 210 f.).

13 The law that detailed procedure for claims resulting from damage to property was the Lex Aquilia, for which see LAWSON, F. H., *Negligence in the Civil Law*, Oxford, 1950.

14 Et se celuy miege avet enci malement megé, come est dit desus, aucun franc home ou aucune franche feme, et elle en moret, la raison juge que celuy miege det estre pendus, et can que il a det estre dou seignor, par dreit. Mais ce il avet riens receu dou mort, si det estre rendu as parens dou mort des choses dou miege, car ce est raison et dreit.

15 Encement se aucun miege avoit enci megé aucun franc home, ou aucune franche feme, la raison juge et coumande que celuy miege devra estre pendus, et can que il a det estre dou signor de la tere. Mais avant c'on le pende, det estre menés frustant par la vile, un orinal en sa main, car ce est dreit et raison, por espaventer les autres de ce maufaire, car ce est droit et raison par l'assise.

16 William of Tyre asserts that the nobility of the Latin Kingdom, through the influence of their women, preferred the services of Jewish, Samaritan, Syrian and Saracen physicians to Latin physicians (*Rerum in Partibus Transmarinis Gestarum*, XVIII, 34). The *Synodicum Nicosiense* in March 1252, under Hugh of Fagiano, Archbishop of Nicosia, whose area of jurisdiction included the Latin Kingdom, included the following prohibition: 'Prohibemus etiam districte, ne quis Christianus sanus aut infirmus medicum advocet infidelem, Judaeum videlicet aut Saracenum: sed nec ab eo, vel de eius consilio medicinam aliquam recipiat, quia hoc pia confideratione in sacris canonibus prohibetur. Nam ex hoc contingit nostram fidem haberi despectui: cum ipsi Judaei vel Saraceni, huiusmodi Christianorum uti ministerio dedignentur, et reputent propter hoc offendere suam legem' (in MANSI, J. D., *Sacrorum Conciliorum Nova, et Amplissima Collectio*, vol. XXVI, col. 314). This prohibition is repeated in the *Constitutio Instruens Graecos, ibid.*, col. 328 f. This apparently was ignored: e.g. shortly after this, Hugh III, King of Jerusalem and Cyprus, is known to have had a Jewish court physician.

17 Woodings, A. F., 'The medical resources and practice of the Crusader States in Syria and Palestine 1096–1193', *Med. Hist.*, 1971, **15**, 269, errs in ascribing to the bishop, on the basis of this law, either the right or the ability to judge the competence of the candidate.

18 Chapter 238, Beugnot, op. cit., vol. II, p. 169.

19 Ibid.

20 'Hoc enim prospectum est, ne in Regno nostro subiecti periclitentur ex imperitia medicorum.' Quoted from GAROFANO-VENOSTA, F. and DE ROSA, E., 'Le Leggi Sanitarie nelle Augustali Federiciane', *Pag. Stor. Med.*, 1970, **14**, 63.

21 Contrary to the assertion made by Sigerist (op. cit., 1058), no mention is made of the school of Salerno in Roger's medical regulations. See KRISTELLER, P. O., 'The School of Salerno, its development and its contribution to the history of learning', *Bull. Hist. Med.*, 1945, **17**, 164 f.

22 The Latin text of his medical legislation can be found in Garofano-Venosta and de Rosa, op. cit., pp. 63 ff. An English translation has been published by HARTUNG, E. F., 'Medical regulations of Frederick the Second of Hohenstaufen', *Med. Life*, 1934, **41**, 592 ff.

23 Since Frederick II was also King of Jerusalem in name for eighteen years, although in person for only a few stormy months, it is tempting to seek evidence of his able hand's involvement in the formulation of the Latin Kingdom's medical licensure policies. However, in light of the feudal structure of the kingdom and the court system in force, such is virtually impossible. See LAMONTE, *Feudal Monarchy . . .* (op. cit.), p. 101.

24 Unfortunately, the evidence is scanty and inconclusive for dating these provisions. William of Tyre's story of the fear-motivated refusal of physicians to treat the feverish King Amalric with a purgative in the year 1174 could point to the existence of a precedent for one of the laws found in chapter 238 (op. cit., xx, 31). Although the *Assises de la Cour des Bourgeois* were not written down in present form until the first half of the thirteenth century, many of their provisions are from the twelfth century. The medical regulations, of course, could be included among them.

J. B. de C. M. Saunders
San Francisco, California (U.S.A.)

The influence of Alexander von Humboldt on the medicine of Western America

The single most powerful and influential personality in the science of the first half of the nineteenth century undoubtedly was Alexander von Humboldt (1769–1859). He not only contributed to the substance of science but, in co-ordinating political, economic, educational, scientific and public thinking, he created a holistic intellectual climate all his own on the interconnectedness of all the features of a limited earth. He was the last of the great generalists who, since the time of Aristotle, rested their beliefs upon the unity and harmony of nature. However, Humboldt's views were quickly overshadowed by the rise of specialization in science which began in the year of his death with the publication of Charles Darwin's *Origin of Species*, followed almost immediately by the birth of the germ theory of disease. Nevertheless, Humboldt's environmentalism was the dominating influence upon many of the physicians of America who, conditioned by the Hippocratic treatise *Airs, Waters and Places*, were seeking a universal theory of medicine.

Alexander von Humboldt's famous explorations in Central and South America over the five year period 1799–1804 were being followed in North America with the greatest interest through articles and letters in the press. He had scarcely arrived in Cuba on his return voyage to Europe when he received an invitation from President Thomas Jefferson to come to Philadelphia and discuss his observations. The invitation was promptly accepted and Humboldt's arrival in the United States was announced on 24 May 1804.

Philadelphia was the centre of the scientific activity of the American republic and its Philosophical Society the gathering place of the new nation's intellectuals. Philadelphia was also the medical centre of the country, the first medical school in America having been established there in 1765. Humboldt took the opportunity while in Philadelphia of talking with the leading physicians of the age such as Benjamin Rush (1745–1813), Caspar Wister (1760–1853), Benjamin Smith Barton (1766–1815), Philip Syng Physick (1768–1837), and Anthony Fothergill (*c.* 1732–1813) on topics ranging from Indian culture to the botany and materia medica of the new continent. At meetings of the Philosophical Society, of which a substantial portion of the membership consisted of the medical profession, Humboldt gave an account of his journey and statistical data in support of his well-known doctrine of the isothermal zodiac. It will be recalled that Humboldt's aims in undertaking his journeys were not only to study the geography and geology of the earth but 'to analyse the atmosphere, to measure with sensitive instruments its pressure, humidity, the electric and magnetic charge, to observe the influence of the climate on the distribution of plants and animals, [and] to relate chemistry to the physiology of organised beings . . .'.

The visit of Humboldt to Philadelphia in 1804 came at a most propitious time for both political and medical reasons. He was accepted as a major figure in European science and his charm of manner and grace of figure conquered all. His ideas on the isothermal zodiac and progress of civilization provided a quasi-scientific basis for the westward progress of empire and consequently fitted Thomas Jefferson's policy of Western expansionism. Indeed discussions were held between Humboldt and Jefferson on the division of the two American continents into three empires with the examination of possible sites for a canal to connect the Pacific to the Atlantic coast so as to provide an economic base for the new nations by draining Oriental trade to the Americas.

Senators Thomas H. Benton (1782–1858), Jefferson's son-in-law, and William Gilpin (1813–98) were the inheritors of the ideas of Humboldt and the Jeffersonian circle in Philadelphia. Gilpin in particular absorbed and popularized the new geopolitics with their special meaning for the West. He wrote, 'This mission of civic empire has for its oracular principle the physical characteristics and configuration of our continent, wherein the *Basin of the Mississippi* predominates as supremely as the sun among the planets.'[1]

The new scientific rationalization added a new dimension to discussions on agrarianism and the primacy of Asiatic trade in Western expansionism. The new interpretation appealed not only to Western sectionalism but especially to emigrant physicians ready by training to accept the thesis of the biological adjustment of man to his milieu in health and disease. These physicians, often financed by the Philadelphia circle, became the spearhead of expansionism policy, providing scientific information on the new lands of the West as well as attending to their medical duties.

The first fruit of Humboldt's visit was the establishment of America's first meteorological service, strangely enough under the auspices of the Medical Department of the United States Army. Although observations on temperature, pressure and other aspects of the weather had been made by individuals such as Thomas Jefferson and simultaneously by James Madison at their homes in Virginia from 1772 to 1777, the first official meteorological records began with the order of Dr. James Tilton (1745–1822), Surgeon General of the Army, dated 2 May 1814.[2] Humboldt in his writings repeatedly refers to this development and his influence on it is apparent. The official order, renewed by Dr. Joseph Lovell (1788–1836) reads in part: 'Every physician who makes a science of his profession or arrives at eminence in it will keep a journal of this nature, as the influence of weather and climate on diseases, especially epidemic, is perfectly well known.'

The renewed emphasis on climatology greatly favoured the anti-contagionist position of the Philadelphia physician Benjamin Rush who had refused to accept the popular view held since the days of Girolamo Fracastoro (1478–1553). His erroneous generalizations were based upon his experience with malaria and yellow fever, vector diseases, which prompted his dogmatically advanced idea of the epidemic constitution of the atmosphere created by decaying vegetable and other organic matter polluting the air. The views, bitterly contested elsewhere, became characteristic of Western physicians trained in Philadelphia and Cincinnati. Humboldt's influence passed from his teachers Rush, Wistar and Benjamin Barton to Daniel Drake (1785–1852) who regarded himself as a scientist applying the Humboldtian method by systematically observing and collecting data on the operation of nature upon a diverse population occupying a relatively unexplored and unchartered land. In 1810, soon after he left Philadelphia, Drake began his *Notices Concerning Cincinnati*, an assessment of the consequences of physical environment upon social organization and development. These essays were but prelude to his more sophisticated two-volume work, *Treatise on the Principal Diseases of the Interior Valley of North America* (Cincinnati, 1850–54). Fielding Garrison called it 'a wonderful encyclopaedia of the topography, hydrography, climate and meteorology, plants and animals, population . . . of the Mississippi Valley',[3] and Henry Sigerist dubbed it 'a magnificent fresco, one of the greatest masterpieces of medico-geographic research'.[4] Drake's debt to Humboldt in every phase of his works is profound.

American physicians, for the most part trained in the medical schools of Pennsylvania and Ohio, were associated with the progressive penetration of the far West to enter Upper California, then the region extending from the Rocky Mountains to the Pacific coast. Many of these physicians such as Victor Fourgeaud (1816–75), Felix Wierzbicki (1815–60) and George Lyman (fl. 1850) were associated with Senator Benton, William Gilpin and General John C. Frémont (1813–90) in the Western expansions carrying forward the Jeffersonian agrarian traditions. It was Frémont who, in his *Geographical Memoir upon Upper California* (1848), named the Humboldt River and the Humboldt Mountains 'as a small mark of respect to the *Nestor of Scientific travellers*', from whence the name spread in the West alone to five counties, eight townships, a marsh, glacier, sink, fort, national forest and a state park, to become the most honoured geographical name in the region.

Even prior to the American occupation and take over of Upper California from Mexico, Dr. George Lyman had provided estimates on the agricultural potential of California to Thomas J. Farnham (1804–48), Senator Benton's intermediary. But these physicians were also the vanguard of Humboldtian ideas on the isothermal zodiac and on the importance of climatic conditions for the control of health and the development of a new civilization. Dr. Fourgeaud, who had been assisted by Senator Benton in 1846 to immigrate to California, wrote in a special edition of the *California Star* of 1 April 1848, issued at the occupation, in fulsome praise of the new land, 'the most healthful territories on the continent with a climate unrivalled in purity and equability. . . .', and further that, 'The surgeons of San Francisco have remarked that wounds heal here with astonishing rapidity, owing, it is supposed, in a great measure, to the extreme purity of the atmosphere'. In the same issue, two thousand copies of which were dispatched by pony express Eastwards, he wrote a note on the gold find in the American river, on which he had made the initial assay. This note set in motion the great 'Gold Rush' of California. Thus the pursuit of health and wealth became the two most important factors in populating California.

The most remarkable of the physicians dominated by the Humboldtian dicta on climatology and its extension into a science of health was Thomas Muldrop Logan (1808–76),[5] first president of the California Medical Association, first secretary of the State Board of Health, and first California resident to become president of the American Medical Association. After graduation in 1832, Logan proceeded to London and Paris when Humboldt was resident in the latter city and had reached the height of his fame and influence. On his return to America Logan eventually migrated to California where he promptly established a meteorological and hydrographic station to measure climatic conditions and the annual floods of the great Sacramento River. From his pen emerged a remarkable series of articles on disease and climate published in the Smithsonian reports and in medical journals in which epidemic conditions were related to Humboldt's isothermal lines and with extensive references to the scientific methods of Humboldt and his followers Arnold Guyot, Louis Agassiz, and Matthew Maury. In addition, Logan was instrumental in establishing a special committee of the California Medical Association – the 'Committee on Medical Topography, Meteorology, Endemics and Epidemics'.

Dr. Logan's organization had fantastic repercussions. Dr. David Hoffman (1827–88), founder of the San Diego Medical Society, contributed a typical Humboldtian report on the geography, geology, anthropology, mammals, birds, reptiles, fish, flora, climate and diseases of the southern end of California. Articles exhibiting the same influence were contributed by the leaders of medicine in the state, Doctors George Graves (1832–90), M. H. Briggs (fl. 1858), Frederick Hatch (b. 1822), and Henry Gibbons (1808–84),[6] among others.

The reciprocal to the dictum that climate and environment are causes of disease is the view that climate and environment can lead to good health. By the time California joined the Union, in 1850, the notion that the state possessed some special healing climate was well established, serving to attract a steady stream of patients suffering from tuberculosis into the state. In his report of the state board of health for 1874–75 to Governor Romualdo Pacheco, Dr. Logan stated that California had already been given the title of the 'Sanitarium of the World',[7] and that Los Angeles was so flooded with consumptives that its hospitals were scarcely able to take care of the case load and the city fathers were forced to petition the Legislature for financial support. At Santa Barbara there were more consumptives than healthy inhabitants. Tuberculosis became the major cause of death and Dr. Henry Gibbons in 1871 reported that one in five deaths in Los Angeles and one in three at San Diego, San Luis Obispo and Santa Barbara were due to this disease. Physicians who failed to find wealth in the gold mines began to return to their profession and were now attracted by the consumptives to Southern California in such numbers as to establish the fantastic ratio of one physician to 200 of the population. Although it may be argued that this mass migration of consumptives and of others seeking relief from chronic diseases was related to the contemporary state of medical opinion which recommended a change of climate as standard therapy, the climatic health myth became the hallmark of Western physicians inspired by Humboldt and his pupils. The most extravagant of medical writers promulgating climatology was Dr. Peter Remondino (1847–1926), author of the quaint volume entitled *The Mediterranean Shores of America* (1892), inspired by Louis Agassiz who had come to America on Humboldt's recommendation.

The influence of Alexander von Humboldt on medicine reached the Pacific slope of America from another direction. In 1829 at the invitation of the Czar, Humboldt made his famous journey through Russia to Siberia.[8] He carried with him special thermometers calibrated by Guy-Lussac and Bessel and, in addition, a special non-magnetic tent to house a Gambey magnetometer to observe the dip and declination in various regions. On his return in November a special meeting of the Imperial Academy of Science was convened at St. Petersburg to hear a report on his discoveries. It was a brilliant occasion of pageantry and fulsome oratory during which Humboldt made a special plea for the establishment under the auspices of the Academy of a network of scientific stations across the vast domain of Imperial Russia. He referred to the meteorological stations and publications of the Medical Department of the United States Army and his relationship to their establishment following his visit to President Jefferson. The plea was successful, leading to the immediate formation of a special committee under the direction of Count Cancrin and Academician Kupffer of the University of Kazan with whom Humboldt had corresponded. With extraordinary alacrity for Czarist Russia a chain of such stations extending across Russia to her colony in Alaska was established and staffed.

By 1835 Professor Kupffer's meteorological and magnetic station was operating in New Archangel (now Sitka), the capital of the Russian North American colony. The population of the settlement had grown to around a thousand persons and was in need of a resident physician rather than relying upon, as in former years, the services of some naval surgeon whose ship happened to be in port. The physician appointed was Edward Blaschke, a member of the Imperial Russian Medical Society and of the Geological Society of St. Petersburg.

Inspired by the familiar Humboldtian principles on the unity and harmony of nature and their relationship to health, Dr. Blaschke immediately began a geographical and meteorological survey of the region.[9] He received the co-operation and assistance of the governor of the colony, Admiral Kuprianof, who provided maps and access to the accounts of various expeditions exploring the coast. Professor Postel's report on the geology of Alaska, Unalaska, the Pribilof Islands and the northern coast, compiled during the exploration of 1826–28, was made available. Dr. Blaschke analysed the mineral content of the water and investigated the therapeutic value of the numerous hot sulphurous springs of this volcanic region. He established a herbarium at the hospital and forwarded specimens to the celebrated botanist C. A. Meyer for identification and publication in the *Actae* of the Academy of Science. Assisted by Bongard's *Observations sur la Végétation de l'Ile de Sitcha*, he identified some 227 plants from forty-six different genera, wrote, on marine biology, on the birds and other fauna. He examined the population, its internal structure, crafts and skills, food, habits, manner of dress and sexual life. He described the social life and recreations of the various ethnic groups, studied the incidence of disease in relationship to the seasons, and observed the native methods of therapy. Besides all these, he provided detailed and complete vital statistics on the various peoples of the region.

Of special interest are the epidemics. Dr. Blaschke was present during the first recorded epidemic of smallpox which appeared among the Tlingit tribes from the south and spread northwards to the Arctic where it ceased in 1840. The mortality from this epidemic among the Tlingit (Kolosh) was appalling – 50–60 per cent of the population died. The Russian fur traders escaped, doubtless because they had been vaccinated by members of Otto von Kotzebué's expedition in 1823–26. Dr. Blaschke organized a vaccination service, trained medical assistants, and sent field parties to the remote villages of the interior. In 1838 he followed the epidemic to Unalaska and thence to the Arctic. He reported[10] that in this region more than 3,000 died before vaccination could be initiated due to the difficulties in overcoming the superstitious beliefs of the Aleuts and Tlingit. With Blaschke, Humboldt's influence had encircled the world to meet itself on the Pacific coast.

Alexander von Humboldt, generous by nature, was quick to acknowledge good work and to incorporate it into his broad scheme of natural history, geophysics and geopolitics. On his visit to Mexico in 1803 he encountered a remarkable manuscript written by a young physician José Mariano Moziño Suárez de Figueroa (1757–1820), born of Spanish parents but educated in Mexico City. Moziño was co-opted by his classmate José Maldonado to accompany Juan Francisco de la Bodega y Quadra's expedition to Nootka Sound on Vancouver Island in 1792 at a time when Nootka had become an object of great international moment between Great Britain and Spain and, to a lesser extent, the United States and Russia.

Moziño, on returning to Mexico, wrote an account of extraordinary comprehensiveness entitled *Noticias de Nutka.*[11] In twelve articles he described the discovery of Nootka, its geography, climate, natural products and the social organization of its inhabitants, with chapters on their houses, furniture, food and drink and with an examination of their religious beliefs and system of government. The fertility of the women, childbirth, customs, health, diseases and occupations were examined in detail and followed by a discourse on the language. Several chapters were devoted to the exploration and trade of Nootka and a catalogue of animals and plants classified in the Linnean system with illustrations of distinction.

This astonishing document was not published until 1913 although the famous Swiss scientist Augustin-Pyramus de Candolle, who saw the illustrations in 1816, wished to do so. However, Humboldt, as related in his *Political Essay on the Kingdom of New Spain* (1811), made copious notes from the *Noticias de Nutka.* The work was undoubtedly the prototype that Humboldt had in mind when he inspired the extraordinary environmentalist position taken by the physicians associated with the opening of the far West. His particular contribution to medicine deserves to be remembered as we pass in our own age to a new appreciation of the interdependence between man and his surroundings for the maintenance of a healthy society.

References

1 GILPIN, WILLIAM, *The Central Gold Region. The Grain, Pastoral and Gold Regions of North America*, Philadelphia and St. Louis, 1860, p. 103.
2 SMART, CHARLES, *U.S.D.A.*, *Weather Bureau, Bulletin No. 11*, 1894–96, pp. 207–8.
3 GARRISON, FIELDING H., *An Introduction to the History of Medicine*, Philadelphia and London, 1929, p. 442.
4 SIGERIST, HENRY E., *American Medicine*, New York, 1934, p. 95.
5 SAUNDERS, J. B. DE C. M., *Humboldtian Physicians in California*, University of California, Davis, 1971, p. 14.
6 Ibid., p. 16.
7 *Third Biennial Report of the State Board of Health of California, 1874 and 1875*, Sacramento, 1875, p. 3.
8 BECK, HANNO, *Alexander von Humboldt*, Wiesbaden, 1961, vol. II, cap. 2.
9 BLASCHKE, E., *Topographia Medica Portus Novi-Archangelscensis*, Petropoli, 1842.
10 BLASCHKE, E., *Morskoi Sbornik*, St. Petersburg, 1848, pp. 115–24.
11 MOZIÑO, JOSÉ MARIANO, *Noticias de Nutka* (tr. and ed. Iris H. Wilson), University of Washington Press, Seattle and London, 1970.

M. Maragi
Bologna (Italy)

Temi di medicina sociale in Ulisse Aldrovandi

Ulisse Aldrovandi (1522–1605) è stato, dal 1568 fino alla sua morte, capo dell'amministrazione sanitaria di Bologna, con giurisdizione territoriale che – secondo l'ordinamento dello Stato Pontificio del tempo – si estendeva alla Romagna e a parte delle Marche.

In tale veste, egli – sostenuto particolarmente dalle sue qualità di studioso attivissimo e di rigoroso ricercatore sperimentale – ha promosso una vasta serie di iniziative pratiche e legislative, che rivelano una concezione tipicamente sociale della medicina e una impostazione organica di politica sanitaria.

Questo settore di attività dell'Aldrovandi è ancor quasi del tutto inesplorato.[1] Gli scritti in materia – sparsi per il vastissimo 'corpus' delle documentazioni da lui lasciate e conservate, com'è noto, presso l'Università di Bologna – sono ancora quasi del tutto inéditi: in gran parte, veramente, non erano destinati alla pubblicazione, benchè il livello letterario della stesura in cui ci sono pervenuti potrebbe, in diversi casi, consentirla.

Oltre ad una lunga lettera al medico Gian Vincenzo Pinelli,[2] che costituisce un piccolo trattato di problemi sanitari collegati con l'urbanistica, ci sono studi e lavori preparatori di progetti legislativi, testi di questi progetti (in parte poi effettivamente emanati), relazioni al Senato bolognese e al Governo centrale, alcune prolusioni a corsi universitari, corrispondenze con colleghi e personalità italiane e straniere e appunti vari.[3]

Questa mia comunicazione vuol essere un tentativo di schematizzare il contenuto di tali scritti e di contribuire così da far conoscere l'opera aldrovandiana anche in questo settore.

Secondo l'Aldrovandi, è compito preciso e tassativo dello stato tutelare la salute dei singoli e della collettività, operando anche sul piano della collaborazione internazionale, promuovendo direttamente le istituzioni e le iniziative idonee a tale scopo e vigilando sulle istituzioni e sulle iniziative di origine privata.

Questa azione dello stato si deve orientare in quattro direzioni fondamentali:

(1) accertamento e controllo delle condizioni naturali dei luoghi dove sorgono o si vogliono far sorgere centri abitati, affinchè tali condizioni siano confacenti alla salute umana;

(2) formazione di una classe medica non solo tecnicamente preparata, ma anche deontologicamente sensibilizzata ai problemi umani e sociali connessi con lo sviluppo scientifico della medicina e con l'esercizio della professione medica;

(3) educazione igienico-sanitaria per tutte le categorie sociali (specialmente dei ceti popolari) e per determinate categorie professionali (per le quali ci sia motivo di dover vigilare sull'idoneità fisica dei lavoratori e sui contatti fra questi e le altre persone); (4) promozione di tutte le iniziative che possano rendere accessibile a tutti – specialmente ai ceti meno abbienti – un'adeguata assistenza sanitaria, con uguali possibilità e garanzie.

Nell''Epistola' al Pinelli, l'Aldrovandi costruisce anzitutto un prototipo urbanistico, con caratteristiche ottimali sotto l'aspetto igienico-sanitario e con riferimento sia alla salubrità naturale del luogo, sia alla struttura e ai tipi delle opere d'insediamento costruite dall'uomo. In base a questo prototipo egli esamina poi la situazione di Bologna[4] deducendone pregi e difetti.

In sostanza, il prototipo è concepito come base di una politica urbanistica organica, da realizzarsi mediante piani generali e parziali di tutela, di conservazione e di sviluppo.

Fra le condizioni naturali che rendono ottimale l'insediamento umano sotto l'aspetto igienico-sanitario, l'Aldrovandi considera principalmente i fattori climatologici e metereologici, nonchè la natura del suolo in quanto condiziona lo scorrimento delle acque e la scelta delle colture. Si tratta, in definitiva, dei fattori che influiscono sulla salubrità dell'aria: l'aria 'corrotta', afferma l'Aldrovandi sulle orme del Fracastoro e in accordo con l'Ingrassia e con l'Alpino, è la causa prima di tutte le manifestazioni morbose, specialmente di quelle epidemiche, diffusive, contagiose.[5]

Le opere dell'uomo debbono quindi preservare l'aria dalla 'corruzione', mirando particolarmente ad impedire lo stagnare delle acque, la formazione di depositi di sostanze putrescenti (come immondizie, scorie di processi produttivi, rifiuti in genere) e il diffondersi, da taluni tipi di stabilimenti artigiani o industriali, di esalazioni miasmatiche e di quei 'corpuscoli', 'fuliggini' o 'polveri', la cui presenza nell'atmostera respirabile è spesso subdola e che fa pensare all'odierno problema dello 'smog'.

All'interno del sistema urbano è significativa la netta distinzione che l'Aldrovandi delinea fra zone residenziali e zone industriali, nonchè la classificazione di queste ultime a seconda che vi siano esercitate industrie nocive o meno. Le attività produttive che danno luogo ad esalazioni miasmatiche e fuligginose debbono svolgersi fuori della cerchia urbana, a conveniente distanza da questa, ubicate ed orientate in modo che le correnti atmosferiche allontanino lo smog dalla città. Fra il circuito delle mura e l'insediamento industriale dovranno inoltre costituirsi cortine di verde arborato, preferibilmente di piante resinose e odorifere, come le più idonee – secondo la concezione corrente del tempo – a 'risanare l'aria corrotta'. Fascie di verde, e possibilmente anche spazi prativi, dovranno però circoncare anche gli opifici tollerabili entro le mura.

Sia i centri urbani che quelli rurali debbono avere un organico regolamento sanitario.

Per la campagna, l'Aldrovandi accenna alle strutture della 'corte' come centro dell'azienda agraria, distinguendo norme igienico-sanitarie per le abitazioni, le stalle, le concimaie e i magazzini.

Per la città, l'Aldrovandi formula una serie di provvedimenti normativi ancora esemplari per organicità e saggezza. Il regolamento per il Comune di Bologna contiene infatti separate disposizioni per la tutela delle condizioni igienico-sanitarie di abitabilità del territorio, per l'igiene delle persone, delle abitazioni, delle fabbriche e dei luoghi pubblici.

Particolare rilievo hanno le disposizioni sulla costruzione e manutenzione delle fognature (che debbono essere tutte coperte e dotate di pozzi di decantazione) e sul servizio della nettezza urbana (che prevede anche l'incenerimento dei rifiuti).

Per le abitazioni popolari, ogni edificio – il cui standard a Bologna pare che comprendesse allora 4–5 appartamenti – dovrà essere dotato di un sufficiente pozzo per l'approvvigionamento potabile, di scarichi collegati con la rete urbana delle fognature, di servizi igienici. L'Aldrovandi ha calcolato degli standard per il fabbisogno pro capite di acqua potabile, per le dimensioni dei tubi di scarico e di scorrimento delle acque nere, per la cubatura dei vani in rapporto al numero degli abitanti. Ha inoltre prescritto che gli edifici siano cinti alla base da marciapiede, a protezione contro l'umidità naturale del suolo (che a Bologna è notevole).

Interessanti anche le norme igieniche sui luoghi pubblici, che distinguono fra luoghi aperti e luoghi chiusi e prendono in particolare considerazione i mercati e i magazzini alimentari. Pei luoghi chiusi sono previsti divienti e limitazioni contro l'eccessivo affollamento e accorgimenti per l'aereazione.

Per le fabbriche, si dovranno considerare – in rapporto alla natura del processo produttivo – le condizioni di affollamento, di luce, di temperatura e di ventilazione, alle quali gli operai debbono sottostare. Per determinate attività – corrispondenti a quelle che oggi ancora diciamo 'pesanti' e 'nocive' – sono previsti accertamenti preventivi e periodici sulla idoneità fisica, specifica e generica, dei lavoratori.

La tutela della salute pubblica dev'essere affidata ad una classe medica formata attraverso studi scientifico-naturalistici[6] ma anche attraverso la sensibilizzazione alla funzione sociale della medicina. La componente deontologica ha, per l'Aldrovandi, una importanza non minore di quella scientifica, pratica e sperimentale. La medicina, come scienza e come professione, è per lui missione di umanità, quindi di civiltà, che si rivolge all'intero corpo sociale: non ci possono essere distinzioni di classe fra i suoi destinatari perchè salute del singolo e salute collettiva si condizionano a vicenda. E' un corollario del principio secondo cui, per l'Aldrovandi, la scienza deve servire al benessere di tutta l'umanità, con esclusione di qualsiasi scopo di distruzione, di sopraffazione, di violenza fra gli uomini o fra i popoli.

Per quanto riguarda l'educazione igienico-sanitaria, specialmente dei ceti popolari e di determinate categorie di lavoratori, appare da molti scritti – specialmente da lezioni universitarie e da relazioni al Senato – che l'Aldrovandi sentiva fortemente il problema e si rendeva conto che eventuali provvedimenti, semplicemente imposti dall'autorità, avrebbero trovato oppositori ed evasori se non avessero incontrato la convinzione dei destinatari sulla loro necessità e utilità.

Egli si preoccupava soprattutto che la gente del popolo, per la sua generale ignoranza, non incorresse in pericoli di salute per sé e non si facesse involontario fòmite e veicolo di processi contagiosi. Alle classi popolari egli si rivolge in vari modi: stimolando l'azione capillare dei medici e agendo attraverso la scuola e i luoghi di lavoro. Ai medici, raccomanda di considerare il loro rapporto col malato come un rapporto eminentemente umano. Per quanto riguarda le scuole, non è a caso che, proprio nell'epoca aldrovandiana, si verifichi in Bologna una notevole fioritura di scuole primarie, anche ad opera di ordini religiosi, ove l'insegnamento e la pratica di norme igienico-sanitarie ebbe adeguato rilievo. Se non è dimostrabile, in ciò, l'intervento diretto dell'Aldrovandi, non se ne può escludere l'influenza, in rapporto, ad esempio, alla legislazione da lui promossa per la sanità e l'igiene nelle istituzioni comunitarie, negli ospizi e dovunque si svolgesse vita collettiva o di gruppo: e sappiamo anche quanto sollecita e intensa fosse l'attività ispettiva dell'Ufficio protomedicale.

Non c'è dubbio che la frequenza e la diffusione di tali accertamenti sanitari e la frequenza, altresì, di bandi non solo imperativi ma anche esplicativi, contribuissero a formare nella popolazione una certa consapevolezza dei problemi dell'igiene e della salute. Si può dare atto che la sistematicità e la serietà di questa azione educativa è diventata tradizionale a Bologna, dove anche in seguito (come nella stressa grande epidemia del 1630) non si ebbero mai moti contrari o elusivi alle leggi sanitarie, nè cacce alle 'streghe' o ad 'untori' di manzoniana memoria.

Per assicurare a tutti, in perfetta parità di condizioni e di sicurezza, l'assistenza sanitaria, l'Aldrovandi promosse vari provvedimenti, che in questa sede mi limiterò ad elencare:

(1) gratuità di tutte le misure profilattiche e di quelle, in genere, che la legge rende obbligatorie;
(2) costituzione di un orto dei semplici a gestione comunale, come il solo autorizzato a produrre, importare e commerciare i semplici, ritenuti materia prima dell'industria farmaceutica; potranno esserci altri orti solo presso gli ospedali, per il servizio dei rispettivi degenti;
(3) mentre è lo stato che produce e provvede le materie prime, la produzione dei farmaci è lasciata all'industria privata, la cui attività è però soggetta ad ispezione da parte dell'Ufficio protomedicale e deve tassativamente uniformarsi alle norme contenute nella farmacopea;
(4) questa farmacopea è 'ufficiale', cioè formata dal Collegio medico, ma approvata dall'autorità governativa con forza di legge: ricordo che l'Aldrovandi, nell'attesa che si formasse questa farmacopea (emanata poi nel 1575) rese obbligatoria la Farmacopea di Edimburgo; da notare altresì che nella farmacopea promossa dall'Aldrovandi si trovano compresi solo i farmaci preventivamente sottoposti ad esame sperimentale;
(5) l'autorità sanitaria prescrive i tipi e i quantitativi di semplici e di farmaci di cui in ogni momento ciascuna farmacia dev'essere provvista, in base alle più correnti esigenze; stabilisce pure i prezzi di vendita dei medicinali;
(6) divieto ai medici di possedere e gestire officine farmaceutiche.

Nel concetto di municipalizzazione della produzione dei semplici, c'è un interessante risvolto economico-sociale. Lo stato fornisce alle farmacie la materia prima a prezzo politico, sostanzialmente pari al costo: così ha una base per poter stabilire anche il prezzo di vendita dei medicinali al pubblico e per contenere questo prezzo al livello delle possibilità anche più modeste. L'Aldrovandi si preoccupava, a tal fine, dei ceti piccolo-artigianali, che costituivano l'ossatura della società e dell'economia bolognesi del tempo. Questi ceti, mentre avevano titolo per l'assistenza ospedaliera, per l'assistenza medico-ambulatoriale e domiciliare fruivano solo di parziali prestazioni mediante la corporazione cui appartenevano e nessuna provvidenza esisteva per l'assistenza farmaceutica (se non in rari casi, da parte delle corporazioni medesime).

Di tutte queste carenze l'Aldrovandi tende a far carico al Comune. Ma in questo modo l'assistenza stessa può esser erogata a tutti, e non più soltanto agli iscritti a corporazioni o a confraternità religiose. Ed è a questo risultato che mira la politica sanitaria aldrovandiana, come il solo che possa assicurare uguali possibilità di prestazioni per tutti i cittadini.

Sembrano, ancor oggi, aperture avveniristiche, e tali furono effettivamente a quei tempi, anche se siamo nella dòtta Bologna e in clima umanistico-rinascimentale. Ed erano, anche allora, le intuizioni di una mente elevata ed aperta, e soprattutto disinteressata, spesso in contrasto con la mediocrità neghittosa di molti e con l'interesse partigiano di oligarchi. L'Aldrovandi dovette lottare vari anni, ad esempio, per ottenere l'orto pubblico e la farmacopea ufficiale; sostenere dure polemiche con le categorie industriali i cui opifici, per ragioni sanitarie, dovevano essere trasferite in zone extra-urbane; battersi per far approvare dallo stesso Senato – non immune da interessi di parte – quel regolamento sanitario che avrebbe posto il Comune di Bologna all'avanguardia; e subire addirittura l'espulsione dal Collegio medico per aver preteso di sottoporre ad esame sperimentale un farmaco inverosimile come la teriaca.

Ma non è consolante pensare che battaglie di questo tipo non sono ancora scomparse.

References

1 L'Aldrovandi, com'è noto, cominciò a pubblicare le sue opere all'età di ottant'anni; morì dopo l'uscita del 3°; volume dell' 'Ornitologia'; poi fu pubblicata un'altra decina di volumi di zoologia e di botanica. Gli scritti di medicina e d'interesse medico sono quasi interamente inéditi. Cf. SAMOGGIA, L., *U.A. medico e igienista*, Bologna, 1962; MARAGI, M., 'Ricerche medico-farmacologiche di U.A. nell'Italia meridionale', in *Atti XIX Congresso Nazionale di Storia della Medicina, L'Aquila, 1963*; id., 'L'idrologia medico-termalistica nel Corpus Aldrovandiano', in *Atti I Congresso Italiano di studi storici termali*, Salsomaggiore, 1963; id., 'L'igiene industriale in U.A.', *in Atti XXIII Congresso Nazionale di Storia della Medicina*, Modena, 1967; id., 'Corrispondenze mediche di U.A. coi paesi germanici', in *Atti XXI Congresso Internationazionale di Storia della Medicina*, Siena, 1968; id., 'Motivi deontologici nelle norme protomedicali di U.A., in *Atti XXII Congresso internazionale di Storia della Medicina*, Bucarest, 1970.

2 'Ulyssis Aldrovandi Epistola de aëre et situ civitatis Bononiae Perillustri viro D. Joanni Vincentio Pinello', datata 'Bononiae, pridie kal. Aprilis 1583 (Segnatura: 5).

3 Cf. *Catalogo dei manoscritti di U.A. a cura di Lodovico Frati*, Bologna, 1907.

4 Su questo, l'A. ritornò nello scritto 'De situ, ventis, aquis, aëre ac morbis quibus Bononia subiacet' (Segnatura: 21, vol. IV, c. 248).

5 'Avvertimenti necessari per prohibire la corrottione dell'aria' (Segnatura: 6, vol. II, cc. 28v–37v); 'Avvertimenti necessarii per obviare alla corruzione dell'aria' (Segnatura: 21, vol. III, cc. 499–502r).

6 'Trattato dell'utilità ed eccellenza . . . dell'historia naturale' (Segnatura: 21, vol. IV, cc. 36–72): è una relazione al Senato di Bologna; 'Intorno all'utilità della scienze . . .' (Segnatura: 66, cc. 262–73 e 355–67): lettera al Cardinale protettore del Collegio di Spagna, in Bologna, datata Bologna, 12 novembre 1567.

J. Spielmann
Tg. Mureş (Romania)

Différenciation et intégration dans l'histoire de la médecine

(À la mémoire de mon Maître le Professeur V. L. Bologa)

Notre époque a été appelée tour à tour en partant des critéria quelquefois opposés: l'époque atomique, de la révolution technico-scientifique, de l'explosion des informations, des révolutions sociales, de l'effondrement du système colonial etc. Idyllique, notre époque ne l'a point été et ne saurait l'être. Nous vivons dans un monde en pleine effervescence sociale. Nous sommes les témoins d'un progrès prodigieux de la science, l'homme contemporain, qui ne se veut pas seulement un contemplateur passif de la société, mais un être lucide, participant aux événements contemporains, ne pouvant éviter les grands problèmes de conscience, de responsabilité morale générés justement par le progrès de la connaissance.

Nous voilà dans le domaine de la médecine. Le processus de différentiation, de spécialisation à outrance, la prépondérance de l'esprit scientifique et même scientiste, quantitativement et analytiquement, parfois au détriment d'une vision synthétique sur l'homme et l'esprit clinique traditionnel, est une réalité incontestable. Contre l'esprit analytique et contre le scientisme localiciste dans la médecine, qui continuent même de nous jours, de vives réactions ont apparu dès les premières décennies de notre siècle. Cela a représenté un phénomène naturel, un mécanisme d'auto-défence de la science. On pourrait l'appeler avec un terme à la mode, un mécanisme «feedback», apparaissant dans l'histoire de la médecine chaque fois que les tendances de différentiation excessive d'analyse atomisante, d'émiettement d'une vision unique ont réussi à prévaloir.

Les textes hippocratiques ne parlent-ils pas d'une «ancienne» médecine, en combattant son unilatéralité? La grande synthèse intégrative de Galien, en dépit de ses limites dogmatiques, n'est-elle pas parue à la suite des tendances analytiques de la médecine alexandrine et à l'atomisme méthodiste romain? La différentiation analytique de la science médicale aux XVIe et XVIIe siècles, n'a-t-elle pas été substituée par les efforts synthétiques de la médecine du XVIIIe siècle? La nécessité de rétablir la vision unique sur l'homme bien portant et malade n'a-t-elle pas inspiré tant de systèmes du XVIIIe siècle parmi lesquels la grande synthèse boerhavienne d'inspiration hippocratique?

Le problème de l'unité de la science médicale a pris un nouvel aspect, lors de l'apparition du courant étiologique bactériologique et de la cristallisation des tendances morphologiques de la pathologie cellulaire virchovienne. La médecine moderne doit énormément à ces nouveaux courants. C'est uniquement le romantisme historique qui pourrait contester les découvertes que la médecine doit à la bactériologie et à la pathologie cellulaire.

L'application dogmatique de l'esprit analytique a donné quant même naissance par le même mécanisme de «feed-back», dès la deuxième moitié du XIXe siècle, à des vives réactions parmi lesquelles la médecine expérimentale de Claude Bernard, opposée par sa vision aux conceptions technico-analytiques sur l'homme.

Dans la première moitié de notre siècle, la surestimation des résultats de laboratoires et techniques, la substitution de «la médecine des organes et de la cellule» à la «médecine de l'organisme» a donné naissance à de nouveaux et répétés essais d'intégration dans le but de rétablir l'unité de la vision médicale. Le conditionalisme, le constitutionalisme, le nervisme, l'endocrinologie, le psychosomatisme, la théorie du stress etc., ne sont-ils pas autant d'essais d'opposer l'organisme comme un tout à ses parties disjointes, aux efforts «atomisants» dans la médecine?

Le mouvement néohippocratique est né lui aussi de la même nostalgie de l'unité perdue, mais toujours guérie de la science médicale. Au début, variété de la «médecine romantique» (H. Sigerist), le néohippocratisme de nos jours a réussi à se séparer d'une série de courants médicaux hétérodoxes qui s'y étaient cramponnés et à déclarer par ses adeptes autorisés, qu'il ne cherchent pas à s'opposer au progrès de la médecine, qu'il n'était pas une tentative de restauration d'une doctrine forcément ancienne de nos jours, mais qu'il conservait de la pensée hippocratique tout ce qui n'avait pas certainement changé tout ce qu'il y avait d'humain dans son essence, en cherchant la synthèse entre la médecine hippocratique et les données de la médecine moderne.[1]

Cet aspect du néohippocratisme, la mise en évidence de l'importance du moment de la continuité dans le devenir historique de la médecine, des éléments unanimement valables des données, de la méthode et des conceptions médicales du passé, revêt une importance particulière, car elle met en relief le rôle de l'histoire de la médecine dans la cristallisation d'une vision médicale intégrative. La connaissance du passé nous épargne certaines fautes à présent et nous donne la perspective de l'avenir, en mettant en évidence les possibilités intrinsèques de la science médicale, fait intégrer la médecine actuelle dans le processus de son devenir historique.

La reconnaissance ci-dessus explique aussi l'attention dont jouit de nos jours l'histoire de la science en général auprès des savants de prestige. La véritable histoire de la science n'est pas une simple énumération de faits, mais l'élaboration des directions futures de la science, en tenant compte de l'expérience du passé. Ou, aussi que dit le savant français de réputation mondiale Louis de Broglie: «L'histoire de la science ne saurait pas ne pas intéresser les chercheurs des sciences de la nature. Le savant y trouvera de nombreux renseignements et, enrichi de sa propre expérience, pourra mieux les interpréter en connaissance de cause.»[2]

Cette assertion est liée organiquement aux affirmations de Littré dans sa célèbre introduction à l'édition commentée des textes hippocratiques: «Moins que jamais, il est permis à la médecine d'oublier son passé, de s'enfermer exclusivement dans le domaine de l'observation contemporaine, de sacrifier au présent les expériences qui ont été faites, les pensées générales qui ont été disséminées . . . de renoncer à l'intelligence de la loi qui a présidé au développement intérieur d'une science aussi ancienne et aussi vaste. . . . En science, comme en tout autre chose, rien n'est qui n'ait été en germe.»[3]

Pour rétablir la vision intégrative de la médecine à côté d'autres savants, les médecins roumains ont apporté aussi leur contribution. Dès l'époque classique de la bactériologie, Victor Babes (1854–1926) a accentué l'importance du terrain et du rôle causal de la bactérie, en manifestant un intérêt particulier à la réactivité de l'organisme. Babes a montré le rôle des associations bactériennes et de l'antagonisme bactérien, en combattant la vision simpliste qui mettait le signe d'égalité entre la bactérie et la maladie.

Le physiopathologiste Daniel Danielopolu (1884–1955) a contribué en grande mesure à la connaissance du rôle intégratif du système nerveux sympathique-parasympathique, en distinguant les types constitutionnels: vagal, sympathique, amphotrope et en enrichissant, entre autres, la médecine de la notion de pharmacodynamique non spécifique.

Une remarquable contribution à la cristallisation d'une vision philosophique intégrative de la médecine a eu le regreté iatro-historiographe V. L. Bologa[4] (1892–1971), récemment disparu. V. L. Bologa a répondu par écrit (4) parmi les premiers, avec un grand enthousiasme, «à la proclamation des néohippocratiques» comme on pourrait appeler le travail de Arturo Castiglioni «L'orientamento neohippocratico del pensiero medico-contemporane» (1933). Au fil des années, en poursuivant une évolution propre, V. L. Bologa passe du néohippocratisme à une conception intégrative personnelle qu'il a fait connaître dans une série de travaux qui ont suscité un grand intérêt. Le savant roumain revendique une nouvelle conception dynamique de la médecine, le passage de l'analyse à la synthèse, d'une vision mécaniciste basée sur le jugement du fait particulier à une vision de synthèse, fondée sur le jugement du «fait complet». Il condamne la mise en opposition forcée du laboratoire à la clinique et exige l'assimilation des éléments valables des tendances morphologiques et analytiques. Toutefois, il exige une hiérarchie équitable «entre le localicisme et le constitutionnalisme de combattre le technicisme étroit et de l'effort «pour que le moyen ne se transforme en fin».[5]

«Le médecin doit connaître l'histoire de la médecine, doit savoir ce qu'on a connu jusqu'à lui s'il ne veut pas se tromper ni tromper les autres» accentue Bologa.[6] Les renseignements de l'histoire de la médecine sont donc d'une réelle valeur pratique pour la cristallisation d'une conception intégrative moderne.

Aux tendances purement analytiques il reproche «de ne plus voir le malade dans son intégrité somato-psychique, en s'arrêtant sur l'organe avec ses modifications pathologiques visibles, sur le symptôme, sur la maladie en tant qu'entité ontologique».[7] Le médecin «n'a plus l'horizon large, il se perd en détails, il devient impersonnel devant le malade, qu'il ne voit plus dans sa personnalité, mais dans ses organes».[8]

Dans la vision intégraliste du prof. Bologa, dans la genèse de la maladie, on doit prendre en considération non seulement les microbes mais en même temps, l'état psychique, les réactions paradoxales de l'organisme, le milieu ambiant, les facteurs climatiques, les facteurs sociaux etc., en un mot, il faut comprendre la bio-psychologie du malade, qui n'est pas une machine extrêmement compliquée, mais un être social.[9] En mettant en valeur ces critéria, «le médecin d'aujourd'hui ne cherche plus la maladie, mais il reprend le contact avec l'homme malade».[10]

Au médecin analytique qui ne voit dans le malade qu'un cas scientifique, il oppose le médecin humaniste qui s'intéresse d'abord au destin de l'homme.

En brossant de main de maître un tableau de l'évolution de l'histoire de la médecine, Bologa montre qu'à la suite des tendances analytiques, la dissolution de l'unité de la vision médicale, il y a toujours eu, avec nécessité, des tendances intégratives, d'où la conclusion capitale: «le grand renseignement que l'histoire nous donne est que seulement une vision intégraliste offre pour la pensée médicale la perspective juste, que la méthode analytique étroite mène à une impasse . . . que l'intégralisme ne saurait s'épanouir que sur une base conséquemment matérialiste.»[11]

En intégrant les connaissances présentes à celles du passé de la médecine, l'histoire de la médecine devient une science intégrative de première importance, une discipline de synthèse de l'enseignement médical. La connaissance «doit conduire le médecin d'esprit mûr à une issue du fractionnement de ses préoccupations (nécessaires mais non idéales du point de vue d'une vision médicale intégrative) vers une platforme élevée d'où il puisse contempler sa mission dans une perspective philosophique et morale».[12]

La vision intégraliste, l'idée de l'organisme humain comme un tout harmonieux, a été soutenue par le prof. Francisc Josif Rainer (1874–1944), humaniste de culture encyclopédique, professeur d'anatomie et d'anthropologie à l'Université de Bucarest. Fondateur de l'école d'anatomie fonctionnelle et biologique roumaine, Rainer a introduit une nouvelle conception dans l'anatomie qu'il définit comme la science «de la forme vivante». Dans sa vision anatomique large, cette science est: «l'étude de l'ontogenèse, l'ontogenèse étant pourtant une partie infime de la philogenèse, de la vie de la substance vivante depuis le début de son existence sur notre planète».[13] Cette vision cosmique de l'anatomie biologique et fonctionnelle conduira Rainer à une conception unitaire évolutioniste apparenté à celle de W. Roux. Pour l'anatomiste et l'anthropologue roumain la conception intégraliste est la base même de la médecine. Il notera cette idée comme aphorisme dans son journal: «Idée commune qui relie les connaissances de toutes sortes qui donnent les disciplines médicales; la représentation du corps humain.»[14]

Rainer appelera cette idée unitaire une culture scientifique. Il posera cette question «Qu'est-ce que la culture scientifique? Elle n'est égale ni à l'information ni à l'orientation. Les conceptions plus larges brisent à la fin toutes les résistances ostensibles ou sourdes. . . . Quelle est la nécessité des idées générales? Elles servent à la modification ininterrompue des notions. . . . Nécessité absolue des idées générales. Tu dois demeurer en état de suivre la pensée de ceux qui ont créé la science médicale et de ceux qui la font progresser»,[15] écrit Rainer.

Et plus loin: «Il est indispensable de faire sortir notre solidarité avec le passé, même le plus éloigné. . . . Ce qui était humain en eux et qui l'est aussi en nous demeure.»[16]

Cet ancrage dans le passé ne représente pas chez Rainer, en aucune façon, une immobilité scientifique. A côté de la continuité, il fait ressortir avec force l'évolution, le vieillissement des conceptions caduques. «La science est une victoire ininterrompue sur les connaissances acquises» – écrit-il. «Quand une théorie est consolidée, c'est alors qu'on s'approche du moment de son insuffisance. Apparaissent alors des faits et des conceptions de plus en plus difficiles à encadrer en elle, et sa modification ou son remplacement va alors s'imposer. Une partie de cette théorie consolidée subsistera toujours, sous une forme ou sous une autre.»[17]

Dans cette dialectique de la connaissance, le présent s'allie au passé d'une manière organique. Rainer est réservé quant au caractère unilatéral de certaines théories médicales. C'est pourquoi il affirmera: «La banalité n'existe pas dans la nature, elle réside seulement dans l'esprit de l'observateur.»[18]

En effet, quoi de plus banal que le fait solitaire aspirant à la prétention de théorie générale? Le caractère unilatéral est encore plus clairement condamné par Rainer lorsqu'il écrit: «Toute conception de la vie découlant seulement de la biologie est subhumaine. Par contre une conception de la vie ne doit pas être en contradiction avec la biologie.»[19] Rainer délimite sa pensée des conceptions biologisantes qui cherchent à serrer les phénomènes sociaux dans une camisole de force, en les expliquant par des lois purement biologiques, mais en même temps il condamne les tentatives pseudo-scientifiques qui tendaient à priver la médecine de sa base biologique. Très proche de la conception de Sigerist, Rainer mettait la médecine à la frontière qui sépare les sciences naturelles et les sciences sociales. Sa vision anthropologique représente un témoignage dans ce sens.

Il faut nous demander si pendant les deux dernières decennies de notre siècle, la pensée intégrative, pour laquelle ont milité Bologa et Rainer, aux côtés d'autres savants, s'est définitivement imposée.

L'apparition de quelques sciences intégratives comme l'informatique, la cybernétique, nouvelles sciences interdisciplinaires, a beaucoup fait, sans doute, pour homogénéiser et unifier la science.

Mais ces efforts, particulièrement méritoires, ont conduit assez souvent à certaines exagérations qui – disait Rainer – cherchaient à substituer l'information et l'orientation à la vision unitaire et à la culture scientifique, tout comme le développement encourageant de la technique de laboratoire a donné plusieurs fois naissance au danger d'une transformation techniciste antihumaniste de la science, ainsi que montrait Bologa.

L'informatique représente un auxiliaire de grande valeur pour toutes les sciences. La prétention de certains de ses adeptes d'élaborer un «language mathématique unique de la science» est pourtant aussi exagérée et vouée à l'échec que la prétention des savants des XVIIe et XVIIIe siècles de donner un langage géometrique unique à toutes les sciences. Les formules mathématico-cibernetiques élargissent la possibilité d'exprimer certains problèmes médicaux. Mais dans la médecine tout ne peut être exprimé en termes mathématiques. Parler de valeurs significantes pour l'amour de la mode mathématisante, là où ce terme est une pure formalité, ne fera que reproduire la faute du pseudo-savant, ironisé à son temps par Claude Bernard qui, en cherchant à tout prix des valeurs moyennes, croyait pouvoir effectuer l'analyse «des urines moyennes européennes» en prélevant son matériel «expérimental» dans la vespasienne d'une gare où passaient les voyageurs de toutes les nationalités.

On a beaucoup parlé du remplacement total du jugement du médecin par les résultats obtenus au «cerveau électronique», en attendant de celui-ci le miracle d'analyser toutes les données de laboratoire et d'individualiser le diagnostic et le traitement. En abordant le problème de telle manière on risque de déshumaniser la médecine dans un sens technique.

Sans sous-estimer les services que les machines à diagnostiquer peuvent rendre à la médecine, il faut rappeler que l'être humain est plus que la somme des ses fonctions qui pourraient être transcrites en résultats de laboratoire. L'être humain est un tout. Après les premières années d'enthousiasme, on est arrivé d'ailleurs à la conclusion que les cerveaux électroniques ne peuvent pas être considérés des copies fidèles du cerveau naturel. Ils sont plutôt des «modèles de la pensée» que du cerveau. W. R. Ashby, l'un des plus compétents connaisseurs du problème arrive à la conclusion que, par rapport au cerveau artificiel, le cerveau naturel est incomparablement plus complexe et irremplaçable. Celui-là peut uniquement être considéré utile pour étudier la raison de l'homme, tout comme le télescope nous permet de connaître les secrets du ciel. Il ne peut pas s'agir donc d'une substitution du cerveau humain par celui artificiel.[20]

On a aussi beaucoup parlé de l'application de la théorie de l'information en biologie moléculaire. En réalité, la découverte du code génétique a été faite sans l'aide d'une formule mathématique quelconque. Il s'agit seulement du fait que les nouvelles notions de la biologie moléculaire peuvent être plus facilement exprimées dans le langage de l'informatique. Les mathématiques et l'informatique ont eu un rôle catalytique et non générateur dans la naissance de la biologie moléculaire, comme on a affirmé à juste titre.[21]

Certains adeptes de la biologie moléculaire tendent à rompre, à isoler cette branche de la science de la biologie générale, la base de la physiologie de l'organisme. La biologie moléculaire est seulement une partie subordonnée à la biologie génerale. C'est pourquoi des savants de prestige comme le biologiste Albert Szent Györgyi, lauréat du Prix Nobel, s'élèvent contre de telles conceptions atomisantes, au nom d'une conception intégrative «Je ne veux aucunement dire, écrit-il, que les résultats de la biologie moléculaire soient à mépriser. Il est nécessaire de connaître le plus possible les molécules, les quantas et arriver ainsi plus près de comprendre la vie. N'oublions pas pourtant que le niveau moléculaire est une étape seulement dans l'ensemble de la structure de l'organisme, mais que la vie est la totalité de toutes ses fonctions et réactions. La vie est caractéristique pour l'organisme entier. L'organisme indivisible à ce niveau met devant le chercheur certaines tâches particulièrement compliquées et difficiles, mais il y découvre à la fois toute la beauté et tous les caprices de la vie. Pour comprendre toutes ces liaisons intimes il ne suffit pas de faire attention aux mouvements des aiguilles de nos instruments de recherche, mais avoir aussi des contacts personnels avec l'organisme vivant. J'ose affirmer que l'organisme ne peut être compris que si nous aimons la vie et si nous avons le désir de pénétrer dans ses profondeurs. Dans ce but, deux anciens instruments sont toujours nécessaires: notre oeil et le cerveau. Il n'est pas exagéré de dire que la vie peut être comprise uniquement par celui qui a dans son âme des qualités de poète.»[22]

On a beaucoup écrit ces derniers temps de l'angoisse que les perspectives ouvertes par le progrès de la science et surtout les possibilités créées par le développement spectaculaire de la technique font naître dans la conscience de l'homme moderne. Serait-il un peu du hasard que I. Neumann, le créateur des machines à calcul digital précisément ait montré, parmi les premiers, les dangers qui menacent l'humanité par la technique, en formulant la question dramatique: «Pourrons-nous survivre à la technique moderne?»

D'où provient cette sombre perspective? La science, dans son essence, est neutre. Elle peut non seulement laisser naître l'espoir que par ses moyens l'humanité sera épargnée à l'avenir des dangers mais aussi les craintes justifiées que les résultats de la science pourraient être utilisés dans le but de détruire l'humanité, d'où le sentiment du danger et de l'instabilité de l'avenir. A cette tendance il faut opposer l'espoir certain que la science apportera à l'humanité uniquement des «nouvelles heureuses» dont parlait Frédérique Joliot Curie, quant à l'éradication des maladies, au prolongement de la vie, à la liquidation de la sous-alimentation chronique.[23] Ce but peut être atteint, montrait Neumann, avec «patience, élasticité et intelligence».

Ce n'est pas incidentellement que A. Szent Györgyi parlait de la nécessité d'être poète pour comprendre la vie. Pour contrebalancer les effets négatifs possibles du développement de la technique on a besoin de la chaleur humaine de l'art. La technique est neutre, l'art est, par contre, engagé en défendant l'homme.

La science et la technique médicales sont arrivées de nos jours à un épanouissement impressionant. Leurs données pourront être coordonnées dans une vision unitaire seulement à l'aide d'une conception de synthèse intégrative. La technique médicale doit être subordonnée au but général de la prophylaxie, du diagnostic, du traitement. Mais seulement l'humanisme du médecin, l'art médical dont parlait Hippocrate, l'art engagé au service de l'homme pourront dissiper tous les nuages qui couvrent encore le ciel de la science et de la technique. L'art médical engagé, animé d'un idéal «Kalokagatonique» de la beauté et de la morale, servira à l'avenir d'étoile polaire qui conduira à bon port le vaisseau de la médecine moderne assaillie par des vagues fortes. Et au cours de ce long voyage, l'histoire de la médecine, science intégrative, mémoire collective du passé millénaire, sera pour les Aesculape de l'avenir la boussole d'orientation de la plus grande importance.

Bibliographie

1 PALOFAX, S., Discours tenu au Congrès International Néohippocratique, 1965, Madrid, cf. BRĂTESCU, G., *Hipocratismul de-a lungul secolelor*, Editura ştiinţifică, Bucuresti, 1968, pp. 288–89.

2 DE BROGILE, L., cf. Scînteia, 1971, 22 august.

3 LITTRÉ, E., *Introduction aux oeuvres complètes d'Hippocrate*, vol. I, Paris, 1839, p. 4 et p. 223.

4 BOLOGA, V. L. and MATEESCU, V. G., 'Noul hipocratism', *Clujul medical*, 1934, nr. 7 (tiré à part).

5 BOLOGA, V. L., *Analiză şi spiritualitate în medicină*, Cartea Romãneasca, Bucuresti, 1943, nr. 8, seria III, p. 8.

6 BOLOGA, V. L., 'Cîteva puncte de vedere cu privire la rostul gîndirii istorice în medicină', *Clujul medical*, 1957, nr. 2, p. 10.

7 BOLOGA, V. L., Ibid., p. 8.

8 BOLOGA, V. L., 'Perspectiva istorică în medicina', *Ardealul medical*, 1948, nr. 5, p. 285.

9 BOLOGA, V. L., 'Cîteva puncte de vedere cu privire la rostul gîndirii istorice în medicină', *Clujul medical*, 1957, nr. 2, pp. 5–15.

10 BOLOGA, V. L., *Voir Bibliographie*, no. 8.

11 BOLOGA, V. L., *Voir Bibliographie*, no. 9.

12 BOLOGA, V. L., Memoriu în problema învătămîntului de istoria medicinei (manuscrit).

13 RAINER, FR. I., 'Jurnalul de la Iaşi', în *Revistele Fundaţiilor regale*, 1945, anul XIII, nr. 3, p. 503.

14 RAINER, FR. I., *L'oeuvre scientifique*, Editura Academiei Române, Bucureşti, 1947, vol. IV, p. 20.

15 Ibid., p. 15.

16 Ibid., p. 16.

17 Ibid., p. 17.

18 Ibid., p. 17.

19 Ibid., p. 15.

20 ASHBY, W. R., cf. VEKERDY, L., *Kalandozások a tudomany történetében*, Budapest, 1969, Magvetö, pp. 300–15.

21 VEKERDY, L., op. cit., pp. 306–7.

22 SZENTGYÖRGYI, A., *Introduction a l'oeuvre de Hans Selye: 'In vivo'*, Akadémiai kiado, Budapest, 1970, pp. 9–10.

23 JOLIOT-CURIE, FR., *Ştiinţa şi viitorul omenirii*, Editura ştiinţifică, Bucureşti, 1963, pp. 226–27.

R. Dupuis
Levallois (France)

L'adaptation du médecin aux aspects nouveaux de la littérature médicale

C'est une constatation bien banale, notre civilisation se transforme rapidement; jamais la médecine n'a fait autant de progrès, jamais il n'y eut autant de connaissances à transmettre. Les publications médicales: livres, brochures, revues, journaux, subissent des modifications profondes que les lecteurs médecins observent avec surprise et embarras. Parallèlement, la formation médicale devient un problème difficile, médical et social, d'intérêt mondial. Ce problème intéresse la communication du savoir médical et, notamment, le rôle et la valeur pédagogique de la littérature médicale. C'est donc étudier un des aspects de «La Médecine et la Société» que d'essayer de décrire, sommairement, ces transformations, chercher à en comprendre les causes, les mécanismes, les conséquences et les possibilités d'adaptation.

Les transformations de la littérature médicale actuelle portent sur la quantité et la qualité, la forme et le contenu; elles sont caractérisées par la surabondance, la nouveauté et la complexité.

La Chambre syndicale de la presse médicale française comprend 200 titres environ. Le nombre de pages, de textes et de rubriques de cette presse traditionnelle a très nettement augmenté au cours de ces dernières années. Mais il existe aussi des publications plus ou moins publicitaires, périodiques ou non, que chaque médecin reçoit quotidiennement à titre gratuit, même sans demande, même sans préoccupation de recherche documentaire. Le nombre de ces publications croît sans cesse et il est très difficile de les dénombrer toutes avec certitude.

Quelles sont les raisons d'une telle profusion? Les progrès de la médecine, la complication croissante de la vie professionnelle, créent des besoins qui correspondent à deux nécessités principales:

(1°) Nécessité d'une formation universitaire et post-universitaire renouvelée par l'extension des sciences fondamentales, des techniques d'investigation et l'évolution thérapeutique rapide.
(2°) Nécessité, aussi, d'une formation et d'une information psychologique et sociologique plus étendue, en raison des relations plus étroites entre la médecine et la société. Le médecin est de plus en plus souvent consulté en tant que conseiller psychologique. Les rôles et les fonctions se modifient fréquemment dans la vie professionnelle. Chaque jour apparaissent de nouveaux problèmes qui obligent à chercher une information appropriée.

Or, il n'est pas possible de tout lire, de tout retenir et assimiler. Pour le médecin encombré le risque de dispersion ou de désintérêt grandit avec le temps. La nécessité d'une information accrue s'oppose à une exigence intime: le besoin d'approfondissement, l'obligation du choix, la critique des valeurs et des significations. La pratique de la lecture est ainsi remise en question et devient un objet d'étude et de réflexion, différent des problèmes de bibliographie, de recherche documentaire et d'information automatisée.

Les nouveautés portent sur la forme et sur l'esprit. Les formats sont maintenant presque tous les mêmes. Des résumés en tête des principaux articles permettent, d'un rapide coup d'oeil, de choisir le sujet d'intérêt. La mise en page fait apparaître une présentation typographique plus claire, plus ordonnée. La combinaison subtile des titres, des textes complémentaires dans les marges, la variété des caractères typographiques et des couleurs rendent la lecture plus facile. L'illustration s'enrichit; les graphiques deviennent plus variés et savants, tandis que les tableaux placent, sous les yeux du lecteur, la rigueur des faits chiffrés, ordonnés en colonnes. Les images, plus souvent en couleur: schémas, dessins, photographies, donnent en revanche une information plus globale, plus suggestive, parfois accompagnée d'un réel plaisir visuel. L'évolution accélérée des connaissances entraîne la création de mots nouveaux, souvent empruntés à une langue étrangère. Le sens n'en est pas toujours fixe ni bien défini. Ce qui explique l'apparition de nombreux dictionnaires, glossaires du langage médical d'actualité et index des abréviations. L'actualité est introduite massivement: actualité scientifique, clinique, thérapeutique mais aussi professionnelle, régionale, nationale, internationale; nouvelles brèves, résumés d'articles, de livres, comptes-rendus de réunions, de congrès. Pour ne pas être en retard sur l'actualité, éphémère et «périssable», certaines revues publient même des numéros séparés. Une autre tendance c'est la recherche de nouvelles formes de communication par la sollicitation du public médical pour un dialogue et une collaboration, c'est aussi la recherche d'une éducation plus active, renouvelée par la variété et les questions à choix multiple.

Mais toute innovation, tout changement, a pour conséquence de supprimer ce qui était une habitude, un rite, des liens affectifs. Les présentations actuelles mettent en jeu des modes de perception et de pensée souvent différents de ceux qui furent utilisés au moment de l'apprentissage. A la tradition d'ordre, de méthode, de réflexion, d'austérité, s'oppose une tendance plus journalistique, plus sensible à l'effet immédiat, à l'événement et à l'exploit. Au savoir constitué, plus abstrait, s'oppose le savoir «naissant», plus mobile et dispersé. Ces tendances contraires ne sont pas sans produire quelques remous, des résistances et des querelles.

Les progrès des connaissances médicales et l'extension du champ médical sont à l'origine d'une complexité croissante des informations et des communications. Chaque nouveau domaine s'individualise par son objet, ses moyens, ses méthodes et son langage particulier. Les communications deviennent ainsi plus difficiles, mais aussi plus nécessaires, car aucune spécialité ne peut vivre et se développer isolément, séparée du reste de la médecine. Cette complexité se retrouve dans le corps médical qui doit assurer de nouvelles fonctions et de nouveaux rôles. Plus encore, la médecine cesse d'être le domaine exclusif du médecin: elle devient un lieu de rencontre pour de nombreux spécialistes qui interviennent, à titres divers, dans la Santé publique: qu'il s'agisse de psychologues, de sociologues, ou encore de techniciens des communications de masse, de la Presse, de la Publicité, qu'il s'agisse enfin de spécialistes des recherches pédagogiques, notamment par les méthodes audio-visuelles.

Les publications de l'Industrie pharmaceutique ont pris, dans la dernière décennie, une place de premier rang dans la littérature médicale. La métamorphose de la publicité médicale en information didactique a une double origine: économique d'abord, par le jeu de la concurrence internationale, du regroupement et la nécessité de l'innovation et de la diffusion de produits nouveaux, administrative ensuite, du fait des réglements qui, en France, obligent les laboratoires pharmaceutiques à consacrer une grande partie de leur publicité à la diffusion des connaissances médicales. Les publications de l'Industrie pharmaceutique ont pour caractères:

(1⁰) leur extrême diversité de forme, de contenu, de niveau et de qualité.
(2⁰) leur large distribution, sans demande, et gratuite.
(3⁰) leur adaptation, rapide et souple, à l'évolution des connaissances et aux besoins du médecin.
(4⁰) l'utilisation généreuse des ressources graphiques permettant, en particulier, la publication d'atlas photographiques de qualité.

Les réalisations principales comprennent: d'une part, la diffusion de renseignements bibliographiques, index, fiches signalétiques, résumés d'articles, couvrant la littérature mondiale, des mises au point et des monographies d'actualité;
d'autre part, l'organisation de réunions, source d'idées, d'informations originales et d'esprit de communication.

La lecture des publications médicales, tout au long d'une carrière, demeure pour le médecin la voie la plus utilisée de la formation continue. Longue pratique, constamment enrichie, cette connaissance livresque et théorique, accompagne, soutient, réfléchit l'expérience personnelle. Elle permet la mise à jour des données fondamentales, elle contribue aussi à former notre conception générale de l'homme malade et notre sentiment de la relation thérapeutique. Ce lent et laborieux mûrissement risque d'être altéré par les difficultés actuelles. L'information surabondante, parcellaire, dispersée, multipliant les particularismes, ne se suffit jamais à elle-même. Elle n'est jamais pure et immaculée, mais toujours porteuse, plus ou moins directement, d'intentions et d'esprit de système. Elle tend à modifier notre vue, notre conception du monde et à diriger notre action. Le médecin lecteur est soumis à deux tendances opposées: acquérir de nouvelles connaissances en s'enrichissant de la culture générale, mais, en même temps, garder sa personnalité, son identité et son histoire, préserver ses valeurs et ses connaissances anciennes, sa culture personnelle. Autrefois, la formation continue du médecin par la lecture des publications médicales était une activité de caractère essentiellement individuel. Aujourd'hui, l'information du médecin dépend, pour une part grandissante, de conditions sociales et économiques.

La diffusion des connaissances et des informations médicales intéresse les enseignants, préoccupés par les méthodes et les moyens pédagogiques nouveaux, les éditeurs, soucieux d'adapter leur production aux besoins et aux goûts du public médical, les journalistes et les publicitaires, désireux d'obtenir la meilleure forme de communication. Tous s'engagent sur la voie de la recherche et multiplient les études, les enquêtes et les sondages. Ce qui apparaît ou réapparaît dans ces démarches c'est la complexité des mécanismes psychologiques de la lecture. Il y a d'abord le rôle de la perception visuelle, de l'attention, des voies déductives ou inductives de l'intelligence, des différentes qualités de mémoire. Il y a aussi, plus obscurément, le rôle des éléments affectifs: désir, plaisir, demande, capacité adaptative de la personnalité. Deux difficultés paraissent particulières à notre époque: l'insuffisance théorique et pratique des relations interdisciplinaires et le défaut de conception d'ensemble des différents moyens pédagogiques dont l'activité complémentaire n'est pas encore réalisée de façon satisfaisante.

La lecture des publications médicales apparaît donc comme une rencontre entre le savoir personnel et le savoir collectif, comme une relation entre l'individu et la société, comme une conduite personnelle. Mais c'est aussi, à notre époque, une activité médicale et sociale, qui ne peut prendre de véritable valeur créatrice sans être, pour chacun, objet d'informations et de formation continue.

Bibliographie

AMSLER, R., 'Sur quelques aspects de la littérature médicale', *Le Concours médical*, 1964, **86**, 43.

AMSLER, R., 'De l'honnêteté fondamentale des publications médicales', *Le Concours médical*, 1971, **93**, 5.

ALBOU, P., 'Formation et perfectionnement', *Humanisme et Entreprise*, Paris, 1965, vol. 8.

BALLET, M., 'La communication, forme achevée de l'information', *Humanisme et Entreprise*, Paris, 1970, vol. 10.

BOBON, J., 'Psychopathologie de l'expression', Rapport de psychiatrie présenté au Congrès de Psychiatrie et de Neurologie de langue francaise, Anvers, 1962. Paris, Masson editeur, 1963.

BOURGUIGNON, A., 'Enseignement et initiation', *La Semaine des Hôpitaux*, 1963, vol. 27.

BOURGUIGNON, A., 'Une nouvelle réforme des études médicales', *La Semaine des Hôpitaux*, 1967, vol. 14.

CHAVEZ, I., 'Grandeur et misère de la spécialisation médicale, aspiration à un nouvel humanisme', 3ème Congrès Mondial de Cardiologie. Bruxelles, 1958; Paris, Santé Publique, 10 Octobre 1958.

EDITORIAL, 'Vers nos lecteurs', *Le Concours médical*, 21 November 1970.

EDITORIAL, 'Les problèmes d'avenir de la presse médicale', *Le Concours médical*, 10 April 1971.

EDITORIAL, 'Ce que sera La Nouvelle Presse Médicale', *La Nouvelle Presse médicale*, 1972, vol. I.

ESCARPIT, R., 'Le retour de l'information. Table-ronde', *Santé mentale*, 1970, vol. I.

L'Information Medicale, 'Compte-rendu d'une table-ronde', *Médecine mondiale*, 10 March 1970.

MAILLARD, J. N. et BENHAMOU, J. P., 'L'article médical', *L'Expansion éditeur*, Paris, 1970.

PELICIER, Y., 'La culture et le désir', *Le Concours médical*, 25 December 1971.

PELICIER, Y., *Intégration des données sociologiques à la psychiatrie clinique*, Paris, Masson éditeur, 1965.

RICHAUDEAU, F., *La lisibilité*, Paris, Denoël éditeur, 1969.

SIVADON, P., 'Psychopathologie de la communication', *Médecine mondiale*, 1971.

Editions de L'Industrie Pharmaceutique

ALBOU, E. et LANFRANCHI, J., *Atlas d'angiocardiographie des cardiopathies congénitales*, Paris, Laboratoires, Geigy, 1971.

ARCHIMBAUD, J., *Bibliographie et recherche documentaire en médecine et en pharmacie*, Paris, Laboratoires, Sandoz, 1970.

CALAZEL, P., DUBOUCHER, G., et MIGNON, J. P., *L'Angiocardiographie*, Paris, Laboratoires, Sandoz, 1968.

HIMBERT, J. et LENEGRE, J., *L'infarctus du myocarde*, Paris, Laboratoires, Sandoz, 1967.

LABADIE, P., *Le métabolisme du myocarde*, Bordeaux, Laboratories, Labaz, 1970.

ROUILLER, C., FORSMANN, W. G. and SIEGRIST, G., 'La microscopie électronique et ses applications', *Acta Clinica*, Basle, Laboratores, Geigy, 1968.

TRICOT, R. et RAGOT, M., *Anatomie du coeur*, Paris, Laboratoires, Sandoz.

TRICOT, R., NOGRETTE, P. et VISSUZAINE, C., *Les endocardites*, Paris, Laboratoires, Sandoz, 1970 et 1971.

SOULAIRAC, A., *Les mécanismes de la douleur*, Paris, Laboratoires, Roussel, 1971.

Ö. Larsen
Oslo (Norway)

Medical theory and clinical practice in eighteenth-century Scandinavian medicine – quantitative analyses of medical text materials. A computerized method for evaluation of verbal sources

INTRODUCTION

Quantitative studies of medical source material from periods prior to the development of medical statistics are rather scarce. So are also text analyses performed by means of computerized methods which are in relatively frequent use within, e.g. linguistics and music research, although a lot of medical material existing apparently may reveal new historical information when treated in this penetrating way.

At the section for medical history at the University of Oslo we therefore try to develop a method suitable for computerized comparisons of different types of medical text material.

We have started with sources describing medical theory and medical practice of the eighteenth century. Our object is to study the medical recommendations from the contemporary scientific thinking and its relationship to the medical service really offered patients and society. The history of 'first line medicine', i.e. the medical care for the majority of a population calls for special attention, because of the vast human and social implications of this aspect of medicine.

VERBAL SOURCES

We may assume that the personal notes of the physician must form the most reliable and the closest of material to the medicine really practised. However, records from individual doctors are seldom available for research purposes, and the material occasionally at hand as a rule only gives scattered glimpses into the professional activity. Therefore, hospital records generally remain as the best and most suitable sources in this connexion.

Systematic collections of hospital records as a rule will not be found from periods earlier than the later half of the eighteenth century. Thus the desire to apply quantitative methods on first-hand case reports encounters this age limit. The main obstacle in an attempt to approach medical history at this level in the first decades from which records are preserved, is the scarcity or even absence of source material for comparison and control. This fact raises the demand for a special method which allows extensive and exhaustive evaluation of the existing sources; thus justifying extrapolations and generalizations of historical interest.

The theoretical counterpart of the case records are the medical concepts as presented to the first-line doctor, the student of medicine, the barber-surgeon's apprentice or the layman seeking medical advice. Our sources in this field are primarily the textbooks and handwritten manuscripts. In contrast to the records, we here find material in abundance from almost any age, from which verbal sources of history are preserved.

Researchers familiar with old medical textbooks will agree, however, that especially the rules for medical treatment and the use of the 'materia medica' show a diversity to such a degree that the logical patterns and the mutual relationships sometimes remain concealed, when different texts are compared.

On the other hand, the same extent of variations may present itself in the handwritten case reports, e.g. from the medical departments of the eighteenth-century hospitals. We must admit that for both sorts of material, a quantitative approach can extend our present knowledge; for instance to reveal how medical theory has penetrated into medical practice at various times.

METHODS

We have chosen a computer-based method, which permits mutual comparisons of text fractions to a considerable degree. Our aim is to apply and adjust methods already in use, e.g. in humanistic disciplines, for the special needs of the medical historian.

The basic principle is to transform our texts into a fully computer-readable version, so that an extensive indexing and key-word searching with subsequent information retrieval may be performed automatically.

With the technical equipment at our disposal, the first step in the process is to re-write the complete text on an input device. We have chosen paper tape for practical reasons. The information is then transferred to magnetic tape or computer discs when the necessary corrections of the unavoidable punching errors have been made.

At the computer centre of the University of Oslo, a series of computer programmes are prepared to perform linguistic analyses of text material. The medical historian may treat his texts just in the same way as the researcher of linguistics, only with the difference that the object is the contents of the sentences, not the language itself.

When the tapes or discs are ready for use, a complete listing of the text may be printed out. However, it is more useful for our purpose to split it up, and to write out the text in the form of a vocabulary with annotations of the frequencies of the occurrence of the different words. This vocabulary will increase with the length of the text, but as the text increases, the percentage of new words gradually diminishes. The number of different words approaches the medical vocabulary of the author and his professional language, and therefore always has overseeable extents. The words from the dictionary may be used as key-words for the contents of the book or manuscript. By means of a key-word, the contexts where the word occurs in the original text can be printed out by the computer.

Therefore, when we have the computer-readable editions of a series of books, manuscripts or other verbal sources, the descriptions of a specific item may be compared and printed out without difficulties. This method can be used for any text. When dealing with handwritten medical case reports which are unsystematic and hard to read, a manual method with edge notched cards may be advantageous in some cases as pre-treatment for punching, or even as the only means, if the material is limited in amount and complexity.

ANALYSES OF THEORY AND PRACTICE IN EIGHTEENTH-CENTURY MEDICINE

To illustrate one of the many ways this method may be used in medical history, our current project comparing theory and practice in Danish hospital medicine of the later half of the eighteenth century can be mentioned.

(a) *Textbooks transferred to computer-readable form*

In Copenhagen, Frederik Ludvig Bang (1747–1820) was one of the leading medical professors at the end of the eighteenth century. He taught medical students in the Royal Frederiks Hospital, and he wrote a textbook *Praxis medica systematice exposita* (1789), which formed a standard reference book together with a printed collection of case histories from the Hospital: *Selecta diarii* (1789). These works were translated into German, and the *Medicinische Praxis* (1791) was chosen for computer transformation.

Further texts are necessary for control and comparison. As we have some experience in quantitative research in eighteenth-century naval medicine, we selected a manual written by Urban Bruun Aaskow (1742–1806), a prominent physician within contemporary Danish naval medicine. His book *Anviisning til den rette og bestemte Brug af de Lægemidler, hvormed de Kongelige Krigsskibe paa deres Söetog forsynes*, Copenhagen, 1778, is a pragmatic handbook for naval surgeons, based on the use of the contents of the medicine chest.

For comparison and supplement we chose a Swedish medical manual with a popular form: S. A. Hedin's *Handbok för pracktiska Läkare-Vetenskapen*, Stockholm, 1796.

(b) *Medical records*

In the State Archive of Copenhagen (Rigsarkivet), a unique collection of medical records from the Royal Frederiks Hospital is preserved. This hospital was designed as a university hospital at the foundation in 1757, and must be regarded as the most important hospital in Denmark until it closed its gates and was replaced in 1910. The files of the archive contain an almost unbroken line of case records from these 153 years, carefully stored and safely bound.

For our analysis, we selected a number of case reports from different periods of the last half of the eighteenth century. These were microfilmed, and the negatives later enlarged, so that the records of individual cases could be attached separately to edge notched cards.

Admittedly, a university hospital cannot be regarded as representative for the medical service offered to the population of a country. Supplementing sources pertaining to first-line medicine at this time are scarce. However, the State Archive in Copenhagen also preserves a collection of naval surgeons' records. Earlier analyses of these show that general conclusions to a certain degree may emerge from sources of naval medicine.[1]

(c) *Analysis*

The key-word searching and retrieval is very useful for the evaluation of the records. For practical reasons, we classify the case reports as far as possible by means of the edge notched cards. We then select our items from the diagnostic or curative principles which seem to exist in the reports, and try to verify them by printing out from the books the contexts of the appropriate key words. More textbooks for comparison are desired, but the cost of the computer-readable editions and the time-consuming preparation at the moment give certain limitations.

A presentation of the results of our study lies beyond the scope of this communication, and will be published separately.

FURTHER RESEARCH

The experience gathered indicates that our method renders several advantages in medical historical research. When the computer-readable material is prepared, a series of different questions may be answered. Therefore, our aim is to build up a 'library' of texts, which may be used for analyses in different connexions.

Mutual comparison of old medical textbooks is of obvious interest. E.g. the origin and the ideas of the medical recommendations in the abundant herbal ('Kräuterbücher') literature may be investigated far more thoroughly than with conventional methods.

We have tried the method in somewhat newer hospital history. In Norway, the development of a modern hospital system is comparatively young, due to political events. As late as in the later half of the nineteenth century we only find humble and scarce medical institutions serving the first-line medicine for most of the Norwegian population. Some archive material from hospitals of this category is preserved. In this case we have tried a fully computerized record analysis without pre-classification.

CONCLUSIONS

Within medical history, we find that there exists a need for quantitative research based on primary sources. In addition to pure numerical evaluations, our computerized method allows almost unlimited comparisons of text fractions. When the library of computer-readable texts increases, the number of problems which possibly may be solved within medical history also is enlarged.

In addition to the strictly medicohistorical research, the text-material may be used for e.g. linguistic investigations. The development of the professional language in medicine is in this respect a field of interest.

Last, but not least, the computer-tapes allow printing of cheap editions of the old texts.

Because the usefulness of a computer-readable library of handwritten and printed texts increases with the amount of material accessible, the cumbersome transformation of texts must have the utmost priority. When done on a fee-base by technical aides, this investment rapidly exhausts the generally limited funds available for medical historical research. Therefore, a solution of the financial problem is the first need for this approach to medical history.

On the technical side, the development of devices for optical reading of letters may be a help in future. However, as so much of the material is handwritten or printed with gothic types of various kinds, it seems unwise to expect too much.

ACKNOWLEDGEMENTS

Mr. Ivar Fonnes, Institute of History, University of Oslo, is responsible for the computer programmes used.

The Norwegian Research Council has provided funds for the investigations.

Reference

1 LARSEN, Ö., 'Historische Forschungsaufgaben in der dänisch-norwegischen Marinemedizin', *Jahrbuch der Universität Düsseldorf, 1970/71*, Düsseldorf, Michael Triltsch Verlag, 1972, pp. 309–22.

J. O. Baylen
Atlanta, Georgia (U.S.A.)

Gerald J. Macaura: Anglo-American quack

Stewart Holbrook has described the first two decades of the twentieth century as 'The Golden Age of Quackery' and more specifically the year 1906 as the 'High Noon of Quackery'.[1] In Britain and the United States, patent medicines and mechanical nostrums flourished and a major feature of the patent medicines was still the 'Universal Pill' which claimed to cure everything.[2] But technological progress and increasing reverence for the machine as a means of resolving all human problems proved to be a great boon to the medical quacks and charlatans. Thus, Dr. Hercules Sanche marketed in 1893 the 'Electropoise' – a three and a half inch cylinder sealed at both ends with an insulated electric cord attached to one end – which, when attached to wrist and ankle, claimed to cure 'all forms of disease' and especially all fevers in a few hours. Sanche soon issued an improved 'Electropoise', which was now called the 'Oxydonor', a device purporting to 'vitalize' the blood by feeding oxygen to the blood through 'myriad pores of the skin'.[3] By clever high-powered advertising and a barrage of pamphlets, Sanche achieved enormous success for the 'Oxydonor'. Indeed, its success inspired the development of a battery of imitations which included the 'Oxygenor King', the 'Oxygenator', the 'Oxytonor', and 'Oxybon'.[4] Holbrook is convinced that 'The Oxydonor ushered in an era of mechanical therapy which reputable physicians and makers of patent medicines alike were to ridicule as the wire-and-gaspipe lunacy'.[5]

What Hercules Sanche created was emulated by the 'Dean of all twentieth century charlatans', Dr. Albert Abrams. A physician with a medical degree from the University of Heidelberg, Abrams had become chief of the medical clinic at Cooper Medical College in San Francisco before he left traditional medicine in 1910 to practise a blend of osteopathy and chiropractic which he called 'Spondylotherapy'. Proceeding to the 'discovery' of what he termed 'Electronic Reactions' – a variant on the old notion that disease causes changes in the 'electrical skin potential' – Abrams developed an electronic device for diagnosis and an instrument known as the 'Oscilloclast' to cure a wide variety of illnesses.[6] Abrams' financial success with these 'inventions' inspired others to develop such cure-all machines as the 'Animator', the 'Novora', the 'Vocorbis', and Dr. Gaylord Wilshire's 'magnetic life buoy', the 'Ionaco'. Like Abrams, the Hollywood entrepreneur, Wilshire (who claimed the friendships and endorsements of William Morris, H. G. Wells, Havelock Ellis, James Bryce, and Bernard Shaw), parlayed the 'Ionaco' into a comfortable fortune. The 'Ionaco' was a coil of insulated wire, eighteen inches in diameter, which cost $5.75

to produce and was marketed for $58.50 cash, or $65.00 on the hire-purchase plan.[7] It was the example of Sanche, Abrams, and that superb confidence man, Wilshire, which provided a pattern of operation for Gerald J. Macaura.

Macaura's early and later years are shrouded in mystery. Of Irish parentage, he was apparently born in the late 1870s or early 1880s in either the United States or Ireland and educated in Middle Western United States. Macaura claimed to have graduated with a degree in medicine from the National Medical University in Chicago, but the official roster of the University's alumni did not list his name. Even if he had received the degree from the National Medical University, it would have been bogus because the University was a notorious degree-mill described by the American Medical Association as 'an institution of the sun-down variety whose reputation was so unsavory that it was not recognized by the authorities of the very state in which it did business'.[8]

In 1904, Macaura was known to have provided 'electric treatment' in Baltimore. A year later, he was in Dublin where, in partnership with another quack, Dick Sorelle, he briefly conducted a medical 'institute' entitled the 'American Doctors' which offered relief for all illnesses 'with costly and elaborate apparatus'. In 1906, he was practising medicine in Liverpool and Manchester, advertising himself as a licensed physician and surgeon, a member of the 'Physicians Association of America', the 'British Pharmaceutical Conference', the 'Royal Society of Arts', and the 'Royal Institute of Public Health', as a 'Fellow of the Royal Medical Society', and as an 'Honorary Physician to the Actors Association'.[9] Macaura's advertisement claimed that not only were his inventions 'endorsed by His Majesty's Royal Letters Patent', but his treatments were recommended by 'numerous physicians'. He offered free consultations and examinations by 'Edison X-Light, . . . [to tell with] . . . certainty what . . . [the] . . . ailment is', and produced testimonials from former patients as proof of 'what science can do with disease'. These testimonials included letters from the Rector of Ebchester, the President of the New Church Conference in Manchester, the Chairman of the Leeds Consumption Hospital, a Newcastle physician, a Liverpool stationmaster, and a grateful mother attesting to the success of the 'Macaura vibration treatment' of rheumatism and paralysis. 'He has cured hundreds of hopeless cases [proclaimed the advertisement]. Perhaps he can cure you. At all events it will not cost you a penny to find out. If he can't benefit you he will tell you so in plain English. If he accepts you as a patient you will be treated for a moderate fee. He does not claim to perform miracles. His cures are all natural and without any unpleasant sensations. Physicians who investigate Dr. Macaura's methods are astounded by the magnitude of his costly and elaborate electrical apparatus.'[10]

During his stay in Liverpool and Manchester, Macaura began to use the 'blood circulator', which was at first called the 'Pulsator', but later its name was changed to the 'Pulsocon'. After achieving considerable success in the Mersey area, Macaura moved on to greater things in London during spring 1910, and it was here that he demonstrated 'his advertising genius'.[11] He spent hundreds of pounds on clever sensational advertisements in such tabloid newspapers as Alfred Harmsworth's *Daily Mirror*. The advertisements were published as if they were regular news stories, with an almost imperceptible mention at the close of the stories that they were advertisements.

In London, Macaura established an office and 'Demonstrating and Consulting

Rooms' at Clavier Hall, 12 Princes Street, Hanover Square, and in April 1910, launched his career in the capital with a well-publicized 'demonstration' for two nights at the Royal Albert Hall. It was not long before the *Daily Mirror* printed a story-advertisement under the headline, 'This Doctor's Wonderful Work is the Talk of London. He Daily Relieves over 100 Persons with Rheumatism, Sciatica, Lumbago, Paralysis, Rheumatoid Arthritis, and Deafness', which invited the public 'to see and try the Doctor's treatment' free of charge in 'public and private demonstrations daily from 10 to 1 and 3 to 7'. The 'wonderful healing-work of . . . [this] . . . clever young doctor now in London on a short visit . . .' was declared the 'talk of the town' – all the more so because he 'renounced drugs' for 'something far better than any pill, potion, or powder ever compounded . . .'. In fact, 'As proof of his remarkable theories, the Doctor . . . demonstrates how it is possible within 5 to 15 minutes to enable a goodly percentage of the deaf, lame, and halt to hear, walk, and run almost as well as if they had never been afflicted with Deafness, Rheumatism, Rheumatoid Arthritis, Sciatica, Lumbago, Paralysis, or Locomotor Ataxia. . . . *And the Doctor is doing his good work without pay.*'[12] To the audience in Clavier Hall, Macaura stated: 'don't pay me a penny. Come and see my treatment. Try it, too, if you like. I will charge you no fee. . . . I will try to prove to you that your trouble is not so hopelessly chronic or incurable as the failure of your medicines must . . . have led you to believe. I am here in London for a short while – just to prove by ocular and sensory demonstration how my "Pulsometer" treatment does do all that no mere drug can ever do. . . . In my "Pulsatory" treatment I use a mechanical invention of mine . . . [which] . . . pulsates the affected joint, part, or organ at the rate of 3,000 to 5,000 or more pulsations per minute. . . .'[13]

The 'Pulsometer', as applied directly on or near the organ 'afflicted' with rheumatic stiffness or 'deformities', explained Macaura, is 'purely and simply a mechanical means of stimulating the circulation of the blood, thereby creating health-normal conditions in any part affected by Rheumatism, Rheumatoid Arthritis, Sciatica, Lumbago, Paralysis, and Deafness'. He disclaimed being a 'miracle-worker' and 'the altogether too magnificent titles that some of the poorer or less well-informed of my patients are pleased to bestow upon me in the exuberance of their gratitude for what I have been able to do for them'. All that he sought to do, averred Macaura, was 'deliberately . . . to deal more or less publicly with . . . difficult chronic – and so-called incurable – complaints . . . because the evidences of the success of . . . [the] . . . "Pulsometer" treatment in these would . . . more quickly establish that . . . [the] . . . blood-circulating invention is a thoroughly practical and vastly superior method of relieving and curing many different diseases and disorders of the human system . . .'. He would not demand fees, declared Macaura, because he was not 'dependent' on such revenues. 'Everyone is welcome to all the good to be obtained from my daily free treatments.'[14]

The advertisement assured the reader that London had never before seen so many of the 'afflicted' (100 to 200 per day) come to and leave Macaura with 'so marked a difference in their condition as the reward of their five to fifteen minutes' treatment'. The nature of Macaura's treatment was described as merely the application of the 'Pulsometer' to the 'afflicted' part 'without the removal of clothing' and 'in the privacy of a cubicle' with ladies attended by a female nurse. Every visitor and patient would receive a copy of Macaura's book, *The Cure of Disease by Vibration and Hygiene*,[15] which explained and illustrated 'the Doctor's treatment, its principle, its successes, the diseases or disorders which it relieves or cures, and the testimony of many well-known people who have tried and found in . . . [the] . . . Pulsometer treatment the relief or cure they desired'.[16]

On 18 June another story-advertisement told of Macaura giving daily 'public demonstrations of a wonderful invention' which in five to fifteen minutes time enabled 'many sufferers . . . to hear, walk and use their limbs as well as though they had never been . . . afflicted'. In fact, the 'Doctor' was so convinced of the efficacy of his 'simple drugless method', that he was offering 'public demonstrations' free of charge. All he asked was for people to let him prove that their ailment was not 'so hopelessly chronic or incurable as . . . past unfortunate experiences with various remedies . . . have led . . . [them] . . . to believe'. What drugs can never do, declared Macaura, 'I can prove that my invention does'. The 'Pulsometer' stimulates the flood of blood to the afflicted part of the body and washes away all 'obstructive deposits' just as a downpour of rain washes the streets clean. 'As a consequence, the pain is immediately relieved, and the treatment being continued, the disorder itself is banished from the system.' In the case of deafness, it can be cured by the 'Pulsometer's' vibrations unclogging the catarrhal accumulated in the middle ear.' Because of Macaura's anticipated 'short stay in London', his public demonstrations and treatments would be given daily between 10 a.m. and 6 p.m.[17]

As Macaura's 'short stay' extended into September, he arranged for a two-night show at Royal Albert Hall to demonstrate his 'Massotherapeutic invention' to the London public and continued to publish the two-column story-advertisements in the *Daily Mirror*. On 3 September, an article told of the wonders of the 'Macaura Machine' and its 'remarkable powers' to free the joints of sufferers from rheumatism, gout, arthritis, and sciatica and, for the first time, published testimonials from the cured ('a well-known London City Missionary' and a genteel lady in Kensington).[18] During the week before Christmas 1910, the *Daily Mirror* published a photograph of Macaura demonstrating the use of the 'Pulsometer' – now called the 'Pulsocon' – at Clavier Hall with the announcement that he was discontinuing public demonstrations during the week and would devote the remaining few days before Christmas to giving free treatments to the poor.[19]

After Christmas, Macaura announced that on 1 January, the price of the 'Pulsocon Blood Circulator' would be increased from 38s. to 50s. 'Further, that owing to the proposed co-operation of his medical friends he was placed in a quandary as to . . . whether he should continue to sell his machine, or instead, as was urged upon him by his medical friends, to lend the machine . . . and have the suffering public come to him for a course of treatment, and . . . [to conduct] . . . a private practice as any other specialist would.' This, averred Macaura, would be more beneficial to him from a financial point of view 'as well as a point of dignity', which, Macaura sarcastically added, is 'the all-important factor of the Medical Profession'.[20] This remark was an acknowledgement of the medical profession's increasing criticism of his extravagant claims. That it had caused Macaura to restrict his public and private treatment of patients was apparent in his emphasis on the use of the 'Pulsocon' by patients 'to treat and cure themselves at home . . . at a most nominal cost'. When he had announced that the sale of the 'Pulsocon' would cease on 1 February 1911, explained Macaura, he was 'inundated with letters from all sources requesting that he should not discontinue the sale of his machine . . .' and, therefore, he had decided to continue to market the device. Indeed, 'facing the serious opposition of the medical profession, and that section of the Press that supported it, . . . [Macaura] . . . started on a bold and elaborate campaign of . . . convincing the world of the benefit and curative power of the Mechanical Vibratory Massage as . . . administered by his "Pulsocon" machine'. He was confident of victory because already 'one by one the medical practitioners who have investigated or watched chronic cases known to them . . . [which] . . . have stubbornly refused to yield to medicine, . . . have in every instance yielded almost miraculously to a single treatment of . . . [the] . . . "Pulsocon" machine'. In reply to the medical profession's criticism of his advertising the 'Pulsocon' like 'a pill merchant' and selling the device 'as a grocer sells his wares', Macaura declared: '. . . how would I have brought my invention to the attention of the public . . ., unless by advertising its merits and actually demonstrating its immediate curative powers by treating and curing any and every sufferer. . . .' Whatever his final decision might be in regard to the sale of the 'Pulsocon' and to providing free treatment, Macaura pledged not to ignore 'the claims of the poor' and declared himself ready to co-operate with 'charitably-disposed persons – including physicians' – in establishing 'small institutes' where the 'suffering poor' could be treated free or for a nominal charge.[21]

In his conflict with the British Medical and American Medical Associations, Macaura found a temporary ally in W. T. Stead, the editor of *The Review of Reviews*. Stead was a veteran journalist who had achieved renown during the last two decades of the nineteenth century as the most controversial editor and publicist in Britain. After a very successful career as editor of the Darlington *Northern Echo* in the 1870s, Stead moved to London where, during the 1880s, he revolutionized the British press with the sensationalist 'New Journalism'. As editor of the *Pall Mall Gazette*, Stead conducted successful campaigns which compelled the government to dispatch 'Chinese' Gordon to the Sudan, to modernize the Royal Navy, to raise the age of consent for young girls, and to repeal the Contagious Diseases Acts. As an ardent supporter of Mrs. Josephine Butler's crusade against the Contagious Diseases Acts and as a result of the negative attitude of the medical profession to the methods he used in his campaign against child prostitution, Stead had acquired an intense dislike for the medical profession.

On leaving the *Pall Mall Gazette* in 1890, Stead founded the monthly *The Review of Reviews*, and edited the periodical until his death on the *Titanic* in 1912. As editor-publisher of *The Review of Reviews*, Stead advocated most of the policies and causes which he had espoused in the *Pall Mall Gazette* and campaigned for international arbitration, the limitation of armaments, a better understanding of psychic phenomena, and 'reform' of the medical profession. He was basically an honest and generous man who was intensely loyal to friends and inordinately sympathetic to the underdog. Egalitarian in outlook, open-minded, and imaginative, Stead disliked dogmatism and exclusiveness, especially as he thought they existed in religion, science, and medicine.[22]

From 1890 through 1896, Stead had championed the notorious 'cancer cure' of the Italian homeopath, Count Cesare Mattei, and stoutly defended Mattei against the medical profession and the British Medical Association.[23] Stead's major accusation against the doctors was that they were a tight, 'closed-minded' oligarchy which monopolized health care in Britain. Thus, in October 1910, Stead publicized the work of the London osteopath, H. A. Barker, as 'a brilliantly successful explorer of the Hinterland of Surgery', and defended Barker's 'manipulative surgery' against the strictures of the British Medical Association. The medical profession, charged Stead, 'bellows . . . anathemas upon all undiplomaed persons who venture to stray beyond the constituted boundaries which have confined from days immemorial the too adventurous spirits of the profession . . .'.[24] When, during Macaura's stay in London, the health insurance provision of David Lloyd George's National Insurance Bill of 1911 provoked the British Medical Association to lead the so-called 'Doctors' Revolt' of 1911–13 against the bill,[25] Stead rallied to the defence of Lloyd George and the Asquith Government. In an editorial on the 'Despotism of the Doctor', Stead recalled that Mrs. Josephine Butler had prophesied 'the threatened advent of a new heirarchy of priests who would build upon their alleged capacity to heal the body a despotism far more intolerable than that exercised by the hierarchy that claimed an exclusive monopoly of the right to save the soul . . .'. Since Mrs. Butler's time, wrote Stead, 'the pretensions of the new priesthood have become more arrogant than ever. The intolerance of the chiefs of the medical Sanhedrin could not be exceeded in the days of Torquemada. . . . To oppose the prejudices of their professional trades union, even when . . . you . . . relieve pain and remove disease is "infamous conduct", justifying the pitiless . . . sentence of major excommunication, even when it entails the ruin of the outcast. Admirable as doctors are individually, collectively they . . . seem to lose all perception of justice or of humanity. . . . The Contagious Diseases Acts, Compulsory Vaccination, Vivisection, and the application of the stigma of "infamous conduct" to all those who dare to heal diseases by unorthodox methods – these are but symptoms . . . of the spirit in which the new despotism would be exercised. . . .'[26]

Because of his antipathy towards the British medical profession[27] and his great sympathy for anyone who claimed to alleviate human suffering, Stead was attracted to, and for a brief period was exploited by, Macaura. In late November 1910, Stead read one of Macaura's two-column advertisements and was persuaded by a friend to view Macaura's demonstration at Clavier Hall to obtain 'clear and incontrovertible proof' of what Macaura claimed to accomplish. 'I will take anyone who claims to benefit humanity . . .,' Stead told his friend. 'But before I can speak favourably of Dr. Macaura I must have . . . proof. . . . All that I want is that . . . Macaura should cure, or perceptively relieve, subjects of my selection . . . suffering from chronic rheumatism . . . and . . . after a fair test, . . . I would report the results . . .' to the public. At Clavier Hall, Stead heard Macaura describe his treatment and saw him illustrate his lecture with 'radiographs' showing the various joints liable to be immobilized by 'chalky deposits' and 'tortured by rheumatism'. The treatment was effected by the 'Pulsocon's' mechanical message. 'You turn a handle, and the indiarubber plunger taps thousands of times a minute on the surface of . . . where the . . . [chalky] . . . deposit has accumulated. The penetration of the massage and the tapping cause a flow of blood to the . . . organ . . . and the patient obtains relief.' Stead, however, observed that there was nothing new in the principle because 'Massage is one of the earliest forms of treatment which man has devised to rid himself of pain'.[28]

During Macaura's demonstration, Stead viewed a young and an old patient suffering from rheumatism treated with the 'Pulsocon' and proclaim that they had obtained immediate relief from the treatment. Stead was impressed, but still sceptical and, when told that Macaura had cured Field Marshal Lord Roberts' wife of sciatica, he later obtained a statement from the Countess Roberts confirming what he had been told.[29] At the close of the demonstration, Stead spoke to Macaura who agreed to treat and cure 'absolutely' any three persons suffering from rheumatism or sciatica, which Stead would bring to him, and to undertake 'to pay for the publication of . . . [Stead's] . . . report of the result . . .'. Stead was determined to proceed with the experiment. Thus he wrote that 'The man who can relieve the tortures of the unfortunate sufferer is a benefactor, but the man who claims to do it without being able to make good his words is a scoundrel. Everything depends upon the proof . . .'.[30]

Macaura immediately made the most of Stead's proposal by blatant use of Stead's name as a huge advertising asset. In two-column advertisements in the *Daily Mirror* on 16 and 18 January 1911, Macaura announced that Stead would test the 'Pulsocon' and that he would publicly treat Stead's patients 'under observation of physicians appointed by the Editor of the "Review of Reviews" ' on 19 and 20 January. Macaura stated that it was his intention to discontinue 'Public Demonstrations', but would give two more demonstrations to accommodate Stead's challenge. At the close of these demonstrations, he planned to move to larger premises from Clavier Hall. To assist those who could not purchase a 'Pulsocon' until after the Christmas holidays, Macaura pledged to continue to sell the machine at 'the reduced price' of 38s. until the end of January, when it would be increased to 50s. The advertisement concluded with the assertion that Macaura's 'campaign' for vibro-therapy, 'though as bold and daring as it was startling and convincing, is one that few would dare undertake in the face of the scepticism of the Press and public, and the almost complete ostracism from the medical profession of . . . Britain, on account of the necessary advertising which he employed attracting the attention of the public, which, as he says, "Are the real judges of the benefits of his invention, and its power to cure . . .". *There will be . . . thousands awaiting the judgement of Mr. Stead – which, to a great extent, constitutes the judgement of the Press. . . .*'[31]

On 21 January, a three-column advertisement in the *Daily Mirror* told of the treatment of Stead's patients before an 'enormous crowd of the fashionable type' and many physicians and clergymen in Clavier Hall and proclaimed in a headline that 'Mr. Stead Expresses Delight at Results'. Shortly after 2 p.m. on 19 January, Macaura mounted the platform with Stead and, after explaining Stead's 'challenge', expressed 'his high appreciation of . . . Stead's bluntness and straight-forward manner of investigation'. Stead then explained the nature of his challenge and declared that it was made 'with an earnest determination to probe the merits of Dr. Macaura's "Pulsocon" to the very bottom . . .'. After presenting his four 'cases', each of which had been given a certificate describing the nature of their illness by Stead's physician, the experiment began. All four patients suffered from chronic rheumatism and, according to Macaura's advertisement, following fifteen minutes of treatment by the 'Pulsocon', declared themselves free of pain and walked where they had heretofore hobbled. Three other cases were treated in the second test on 20 January, 'with the same unfailing beneficial results'. Stead was reported to have told the audience that 'he was completely satisfied with the results' and 'could not do less than compliment

Dr. Macaura most highly . . . [for] . . . the immediate and remarkable relief of the Pulsocon. . . .'[32]

Stead was so astonished by Macaura's misrepresentation of the facts that he immediately published a letter in the *Daily News* on 23 January, deprecating the statements in Macaura's advertisements and stating that nothing was witnessed in the experiment beyond the fact that 'the . . . treatment produced considerable immediate relief from pain'. He declared that it was unjust to his professional medical adviser and himself to suggest that they were completely satisfied that the Macaura treatment could effect a permanent cure for rheumatism.[33]

In spite of Stead's denial, Macaura's remarks and Stead's alleged statements elicited an editorial in *The Medical Press* on 'Stead and the Macaura Treatment' which accused Macaura of using a title 'unrecognized medically in the United Kingdom' and declared that Stead's opinion on the effectiveness of the Macaura treatment was 'From the scientific point of view . . . absolutely worthless'. It challenged Stead to produce the names of physicians who had provided reports on the patients treated in the experiment and suggested that 'before he accepts the serious responsibility of advocating the treatment of diseased conditions by any person, he should first satisfy himself as to . . . what is the diploma or degree upon which Macaura styles himself "Dr." . . .'. *The Medical Press* reminded Stead that the fact that he had previously shown 'a leaning . . . in the direction of various forms of unqualified medical practice', did not strengthen the credibility of his statements on the Macaura treatment.[34]

Nevertheless, Macaura continued to make the most of his association with Stead. Thus, in a two-column 'story' in the *Daily Mirror* on 30 January, he stated: 'Of course, Mr. Stead's opinion, which he expressed in favour of Dr. Macaura's treatment, and which has been published in most of the London . . . papers, is no doubt also responsible for the immediate and unusual increase in the number of sufferers now daily visiting Clavier Hall, for, naturally, Mr. Stead is a well-recognized analytical man, whose opinion is weighty in the minds of the British Public. . . . The fact that the "Pulsocon" is capable of accomplishing what its inventor claims . . . has therefore been driven home, with the result that Dr. Macaura's friends have during the past week multiplied by leaps and bounds throughout the British Isles. . . .'[35]

Macaura's exploitation of Stead again provoked *The Medical Press* to attack Stead for his support of unlicensed medical practitioners. While acknowledging Stead's 'candour and sincerity of purpose', especially in his letter to the *Daily News* rejecting Macaura's extravagant claims, *The Medical Press* again criticized Stead for his credulity. 'For a man who has shown himself a master of modern journalism to pose on that account as an authority upon medical matters, [wrote *The Medical Press*] is to assume a ridiculous and untenable position of intellectual arrogance. Had the incident rested at that point it is unlikely that any further notice would have been taken of it. . . . [But] now that he comes forward once again in support of another unlicensed practitioner to "cure" various diseases, his credibility as a serious witness is naturally discounted considerably by previous fiascoes in the deadly role of amateur physician. . . .' It challenged Stead to publish 'the names of any qualified medical practitioners who had . . . cooperated with him in the public investigations of the so-called "cures" . . .', and to reply to the criticisms of his conduct.[36]

In the February 1911, issue of *The Review of Reviews*, Stead attempted to clarify his statements on the Macaura treatment and to reply to his critics in the medical profession. 'My own impression from the two days I attended at Clavier Hall,' wrote Stead, 'is that Dr. Macaura's instrument, and the way in which it was used . . ., undoubtedly did produce an immediate relief from pain, and . . ., if only temporary, loosening of the joints. . . .' But he denied having stated, as alleged in Macaura's advertisements, that Macaura could cure all of the seven test cases in one month. He presented his physician's report on the cases twelve days after their first 'Pulsocon' treatment and pledged to publish reports on the progress of the patients at the close of a month and again after a lapse of six months.[37] In reply to the doctors' criticism of his conduct, Stead declared that he had experienced great difficulty in enlisting the assistance of any physician in testing Macaura's claims because of the physicians' fear of risking 'the kind of insult and attack to which medical men are liable if they venture to assist anyone in exploring the Hinterland of Surgery or the undeveloped land of medicine'. How is it possible, asked Stead, 'that a profession which elsewhere is so wideawake and keen to test the value of every new discovery should be so obstinately conservative as to refuse even to examine into the truth or falsehood of alleged cures made by irregular methods . . .'.[38] The attitude of the medical profession towards all such experiments, he declared, is 'aptly illustrated by the comments of the *Medical Press* and if this journal thinks he would be provoked by its "challenge" to fling his doctor into the arena to be worried by the wolves as a reward for giving . . . [him] . . . a scientific opinion upon specific cases submitted to him for diagnosis, the *Medical Press* makes a mistake. . . .'[39]

Nor was this all. On 6 February, *The Times* published a letter from Stead in which he referred back to the case of the osteopath, H. A. Barker, and his 'challenge' to the medical profession 'in the name of humanity and common sense, either to disprove . . . [Barker's] . . . statements, or to insist upon a professional inquiry into the merits of his case . . .'. The passivity and lack of response of the medical profession to his challenge, wrote Stead, had convinced him of its 'professional inertia and . . . prejudice. . . . They refuse even to make inquiry into the facts, appearing to prefer that their patients should continue to suffer, . . . rather than they should be cured by . . . [Barker's] . . . system at their own hands. Is this reasonable? Is it fair to their patients? Why should professional etiquette be allowed to afford a shelter to ignorance that refuses to be enlightened, to incapacity that refuses instruction?'[40]

Stead's letter in *The Times* and Macaura's advertisements reporting 'The Remarkable Improvement of Mr. Stead's Crippled Patients' had increased the public demand for the 'Pulsocon',[41] inspired a physician to write to *The Medical Press* assailing Stead for his credulity and 'medical meddling'. 'A few hours a week for a few months devoted to a study of human physiology and pathology would surely render Mr. Stead more diffident in accepting stories of miraculous . . . cures in medical and surgical diseases, and in charging the profession with almost criminal conduct in neglecting, or conspiring to persecute the discoverers of these marvellous processes. . . . A little scientific learning of this kind in Mr. Stead's case could not be a dangerous thing. He would soon have forced upon him the fact that medical quackery constitutes one of the greatest evils at present afflicting society. . . . And he would surely find out that in his blind quixotic zeal on behalf of suffering humanity he is doing more than most journalists . . . to promote and aggravate abuses. . . .'[42]

In the meantime, Macaura had announced on 6 February, that he was moving to more permanent and commodious quarters, with a private Lecture Theatre, at Pembroke House in Oxford and Wardour Streets and that, as advised by his medical friends, he would terminate the sale of the 'Pulsocon' and provide it only to 'sufferers' who had completed a course of treatment and had been partially cured at his 'Institute'. Those who could not come for treatments personally might arrange for courses of treatment by 'correspondence'. Macaura also stated that he would retain a part of Clavier Hall, where he would provide 'Pulsocon' treatment and, 'when necessary, suitable nourishment to the needy patients of London . . .'.[43] Again, Macaura stated that 'A brilliant and convincing climax to his initial educative campaign was doubtless the public treatment of . . . Stead's crippled patients . . .'.[44]

In the March issue of *The Review of Reviews*, Stead attempted to refute Macaura's statements by stating that he had given 'no warrant' to Macaura to make the assertions which he had published in the various advertisements. 'I most emphatically assure my readers that I do not think that Dr. Macaura, or any living man, with any machine in the world, can achieve results which Dr. Macaura claim in every case. . . . Macaura . . . says that he can do these things, and I have challenged him to do it in seven specific cases which are still under trial. He has not cured one of them yet, although he seems to have done all of them more or less good. Two months have now elapsed, and I see that Dr. Macaura announces in his advertisement that some of my cases are cured. . . . I have no knowledge of any such result being achieved. . . .'[45] But in the same issue, Stead defended 'The Virtue of Mechanical Massage' and averred that his experiment with the 'Pulsocon' treatment was not 'a test of the well-known and established principle of vibratory massage, but a test of the ability of Dr. Macaura to cure rheumatism by the use of the Pulsocon . . .'.[46] In April, Stead again stated that he would not express any judgment on the efficacy of Macaura's treatment until six months had elapsed and he had received a report on each of the seven cases from his personal physician. However, added Stead, judging from the reports he had received on the condition of the patients, there seemed to be 'little doubt' that Macaura had done them some good.[47]

By mid-1911, Macaura's 'pitch' was beginning to pall. A lecture and demonstration at Royal Albert Hall during the evening of 11 May, in which Macaura announced that he would produce Stead's patients *before* the expiration of the six months' trial period as proof that they were completely cured,[48] were disrupted by a large group of medical students from several London hospitals who heckled and shouted down Macaura with 'approbious epithets'. As the students left the hall, 'they burst a large number of bladders of foul gas . . . and strewed chemicals on the seats'.[49] When order was restored, Macaura introduced some of Stead's patients and asserted that he had cured three absolutely and that the remaining four were already partially cured. In his report of the test in June, Stead published letters from the patients stating that they had experienced decided improvement as a result of the Macaura treatment.[50] A month later, Stead reported that although each patient had received a half-hour treatment every day for six months from Macaura's 'skilled operators' and had used the 'Pulsocon' at home for thirty minutes each day, only two had achieved a 'half cure'. Therefore, wrote Stead, on the basis of the facts,

Macaura's claim that the 'Pulsocon' would cure all cases of rheumatism seemed exaggerated.[51]

In late August, as he was preparing his final report on the experiment with the Macaura treatment, Stead confided to a friend in Chicago: 'Dr. Macaura made certain claims which I subjected to a test, and the result has not been to justify the assertions which he made.'[52] Stead confirmed this statement in his 'Final Report on the Merits of the Pulsocon' in the September 1911 issue of *The Review of Reviews* when he wrote: 'The conclusion which I draw . . . is that while vibratory treatment applied by the Pulsocon will in some cases effect an immediate relief, there is no basis in the results of this particular experiment to justify the confident claims put forward by Dr. Macaura.'[53]

But Stead's rejection of Macaura's claims did not improve his relations with the medical profession in Britain and the United States. Thus, the *Journal of the American Medical Association*, in warning that Macaura, having reaped a harvest in Britain, was planning to return to the United States, blamed Stead for facilitating Macaura's 'quackery'. 'Mr. Stead's advocacy of anything medical', wrote the editor of the *Journal*, 'is . . . *prima facie* evidence of its unscientific and bizarre character. . . .'[54] More specifically, the editor, Dr. George H. Simmons, told a correspondent who had presumed to defend Stead that 'Stead is sincere and is anxious to do what is right. It is for this reason that his championship of a notorious quack is all the more to be regretted. It is true, as Mr. Stead says, that Macaura failed to make good his bluff, but *Mr. Stead's interest in the matter invested Macaura with an air of respectability that he would not otherwise have had*. . . .'[55] Similarly, a physician in Ireland wrote to *The Medical Press* deriding Stead for having constituted himself as 'critic-in-chief of medical men' and 'Lord of Appeal on medical matters' and observed that 'It is indeed hard to blame poor, simple country folk for being fooled and quizzed by quacks when men of the calibre of . . . Stead can be found to come forward to take cognisance of their challenges'.[56]

Meanwhile, as Macaura's 'blatant and mendacious' advertising began to fade and Stead's rejection of his claims diminished his clientele and the sales of the 'Pulsocon', the American Medical Association learned from 'an authoritative source' that Macaura was planning to return to the United States with the 'tainted money' he had 'wrung from the ignorant sick and the gullible suffering of the British Isles . . .'. The *Journal of the American Medical Association* opined in August 1911: 'The most we can do is to felicitate the people of London on being rid of a most undesirable citizen. Their gain is our loss.'[57] But before he left Britain in early 1912, for greener pasture on the Continent, Macaura became involved in a damaging legal action in the courts.

In mid-November 1911, a former resident and marble works manager from Durban, Arthur Wade, sued Macaura for 'wrongful dismissal'. Wade charged that Macaura had brought him from South Africa in January 1911, with an advance of £100 and the promise of employing him for a year at £15 per week as business manager of the Macaura enterprise and as a writer of advertising copy. But shortly after Wade's arrival in London, Macaura asked Wade to lecture on the 'Pulsocon' at £10 per week. After working for four months, Wade refused to continue as a lecturer and as a composer of advertising copy and on 10 April 1911, was dismissed by Macaura. Wade testified that Macaura had trained him to see patients, to hear their complaints, and to prescribe treatments. For his part, Macaura denied having promised Wade £15 per week and asserted that Wade had been employed only for lecturing and writing advertisements. Since the advertisements written by Wade were unsatisfactory and Wade had refused to go to Belfast to present in a lecture a mere 'description' of the 'Pulsocon', he was dismissed. However, the court rendered a verdict in favour of Wade and ordered Macaura to pay £262 and costs.[58] In reporting the court action, *The British Medical Journal* described the 'Pulsocon' as a compact version of the French 'Vedee Vibrator' which was available for sale in chemists' shops throughout London.[59]

Contrary to the expectations of the American Medical Association, Macaura did not return to the United States and instead went to Paris in early 1912. In mid-May, the Paris correspondent of the ever-vigilant *Journal of the American Medical Association* reported that Macaura (listing himself as M.D., F.R.S.A., and former member of the Royal Commission on Hygiene in London) had during the past few months been attracting large numbers of patients by advertisements in the Parisian daily press asserting that the 'Pulsocon' *guaranteed* a cure for rheumatism, sciatica, locomotor ataxia, paralysis, and deafness 'in ninety-nine cases out of a hundred . . .'.[60] In late June, the public prosecutor moved against Macaura and his associates on the complaints (1) of the medical profession in Paris that they were illegally practising medicine and (2) of several clients that he had defrauded them. After protesting that he did not practise medicine and merely confined himself 'to extending the use of the "Pulsocon" ',[61] Macaura secured a delay in the court action and left France.

In autumn 1912, Macaura appeared in Berlin and within a short time was in trouble with the German authorities. As in Britain and France, Macaura sought to introduce the 'Pulsocon' through a series of free demonstrations at the Wintergarten. *The New York Times* reported that so many of the 'afflicted' came that 'the police had to intervene to prevent them from blocking the traffic in the street outside' the hall.[62] Macaura then proceeded to announce in the press that 'anybody who could not afford to buy his apparatus would receive one free'. According to the information which *The New York Times* obtained from Macaura, among those he rid of sciatica was a young stable boy who mentioned his cure to the Kaiser's Master of the Horse and 'respectfully' suggested to his supervisor that his daughter, bedridden with rheumatism, might also benefit from the Macaura treatment. The young lady was treated by Macaura and, for the first time in three years, was able to leave her bed and walk. But the doctors of Berlin were not convinced and the Berlin medical society induced the Police President of Berlin 'to declare . . . Macaura an obnoxious foreigner' on the grounds of illegal medical practice and fraud.[63] On being given three days to quit Prussia, Macaura secured the intervention of the Master of the Horse who had the expulsion decree nullified. When the Berlin doctors repeated the charge of fraud and accused Macaura of having violated the law relating to 'unfair competition by giving away medical goods', Macaura saw that his position was untenable and, after according the franchise for the sale of the 'Pulsocon' to a Berlin firm, quit Germany in mid-December 1912.[64]

After a relatively dormant year in Britain, punctuated by a libel suit which he had initiated and withdrawn, Macaura inexplicably returned to Paris in 1914 to face the long delayed trial with his British and French confederates for illegally practising medicine and for fraud in connexion with the sale of the 'Pulsocon'. On 14 May, Macaura was sentenced to three years imprisonment and fined £120. Nine of the others who had assisted Macaura in France received sentences varying from two to twelve months and fined sums ranging from £4 to £20. Three were accorded the benefit of the first offenders act and the tenth was acquitted. While the Parisian medical societies concerned in the case as 'interveners' were awarded damages, the court set aside the charge of illegally practising medicine against Macaura and convicted him on the charge of fraud.[65]

The American Medical Association exulted that Macaura had been put away, but noted that 'After Macaura had served "time" he will probably return to the United States . . .' and that 'the device by which he has swindled so many thousands, has come to the United States ahead of its self-styled inventor' where it was being marketed as the 'Cirkulon'. 'We may expect three years hence,' declared the Association, 'when its "inventor" is able to put aside his convict's suit and again don civilian garb that an energetic campaign will be started . . .'.[66]

But on the completion of his sentence in 1917, Macaura did not return to resume his pitch in the United States. In August 1920, the American Medical Association received a query from H. L. Glasgow, a director of the *Mid-Ulster Mail* in Cookstown, concerning the career of Macaura in which Glasgow stated that Macaura had purchased 'a castle and wooded demesne' near Cookstown and was denuding the woods to produce timber for sale.[67] This was the last news of the existence of Macaura; he appears to have subsided into obscurity in Ireland. A fitting epitaph for the career of Macaura is the thought that 'So long as gullibility remains rampant – so long will swindlers of the Macaura type flourish'.[68] One might also add that just as 'The savage trusts to his amulet; [so] the civilised man, . . . submits himself with childish . . . simplicity to the pretences of the quack . . .'.[69]

References

1 HOLBROOK, STEWART H., *The Golden Age of Quackery*, New York, 1959, pp. 3–6.
2 Remarks of the reviewer of Elizabeth Burton, *The Early Victorians at Home, 1837–1861*, London, 1972, in *Times lit. Suppl.*, no. 3, 673, 21 July 1972, p. 841.
3 HOLBROOK, op. cit., pp. 123–24.
4 Ibid., p. 125.
5 Ibid., p. 123.
6 Ibid., pp. 129–34.
7 On the career of Gaylord Wilshire, see ibid., pp. 135–45.
8 'Gerald Macaura – international quack', *J. Amer. med. Ass.*, 1914, **62**, 174. Hereafter cited as 'Gerald Macaura', *JAMA* (1914).
9 See *Liverpool Echo*, 16 October 1906.
10 Ibid.
11 'Gerald Macaura', *JAMA* (1914), 1742.
12 *Daily Mirror*, 4 June 1910. [My italics].
13 Ibid.
14 Ibid.
15 MACAURA, G. J., *The Cure of Disease by Vibration and Hygiene. The Book of Health*, Leeds, [n.d.].
16 *Daily Mirror*, 4 June 1910.
17 Ibid., 18 June 1910.
18 Ibid., 3 September 1910. See also 'Gerald Macaura', *JAMA* (1914), 1742.
19 *Daily Mirror*, 19 December, 1910.
20 Ibid., 10 January, 1911.
21 Ibid.
22 On the life and career of W. T. Stead (1849–1912), see WHYTE, FREDERIC, *The Life of W. T. Stead*, New York, 1925, 2 vols.; STEAD, ESTELLE W., *My Father: Personal and Spiritual Reminiscences*, London, 1913; ROBERTSON SCOTT, J. W., *The Life and Death of a Newspaper:*

An Account of the . . . Editors of the 'Pall Mall Gazette', London, 1952, pp. 72 ff.; and BAYLEN, JOSEPH O., 'W. T. Stead and Boer War: the irony of idealism', *Canad. hist. Rev.*, 1959, **11**, 304–14; 'W. T. Stead's *History of the Mystery* and the Jameson Raid', *J. Br. Stud.*, 1964, **4**, 104–32; 'W. T. Stead and the Russian Revolution of 1905', *Canad. J. Hist.*, 1967, **2**, 45–66; 'W. T. Stead and the "New Journalism" ', *Emory Univ. Quart.*, 1965, **21**, 196–206; 'A Victorian's "Crusade" in Chicago, 1893–1894', *J. Amer. Hist.*, 1964, **51**, 418–34.

23 On Stead and the Mattei controversy see BAYLEN, JOSEPH O. 'The Mattei cancer cure: a Victorian nostrum', *Proc. Amer. phil. Soc.*, 1969, **113**, 149–76.

24 STEAD, W. T., 'The hinterland of surgery. The strange true story of a pioneer in Park Lane', *The Review of Reviews*, 1910, **42**, 340–41. See also [W. T. Stead], 'The Bonesetter and the Doctors', ibid., November 1910, pp. 513–14.

25 For information on Stead and the 'Doctors' Revolt', I am indebted to James S. Herndon's excellent unpublished paper on 'The British Medical Association and the "Doctors' Revolt" of 1911–13'.

26 STEAD, W. T., 'The progress of the world', *The Review of Reviews*, 1911, **43**, 538–39.

27 Stead bitterly disliked what he called the 'intermeddling fingers' of the doctors. Stead to John Naylor, 26 June [1909?], W. T. Stead Papers.

28 STEAD, W. T., 'What about Macaura and his Pulsocon. My challenge: how it was accepted', *The Review of Reviews*, 1910, **42**, 617–18.

29 Ibid.

30 Ibid., p. 618.

31 *Daily Mirror*, 16 January 1911. [My italics.]

32 Ibid., 21 January 1911.

33 *Daily News* (London), 23 January 1911.

34 'Mr. W. T. Stead and the Macaura treatment', *Med. Press Circ.*, 25 January 1911, p. 79.

35 'Mr. W. T. Stead. Rapid improvement of his crippled patients', *Daily Mirror*, 30 January 1911.

36 'Mr. W. T. Stead and Unlicensed Medical Practice', *Med. Press Circ.*, 1 February 1911, p. 106.

37 STEAD, W. T., 'Can Dr. Macaura cure rheumatism? Mr. Stead's report on the response to the challenge', *The Review of Reviews*, 1911, **43**, 208.

38 Ibid., p. 203.

39 Ibid.

40 Stead's letter of 4 February, to the Editor of *The Times*, 6 February 1911.

41 See *Daily Mirror*, 4 and 6 February 1911.

42 'Mr. Stead and the profession', *Med. Press Circ.*, 15 February, 1911, p. 181.

43 *Daily Mirror*, 6 and 15 February 1911.

44 Ibid., 15 February 1911.

45 STEAD, W. T., 'Dr. Macaura and the Pulsocon. Further report on the test cases', *The Review of Reviews*, 1911, **43**, 316.

46 STEAD, W. T., 'The virtue of mechanical massage', ibid., p. 320.

47 STEAD, W. T., 'Dr. Macaura's Pulsocon. My test cases', ibid., p. 424.

48 STEAD, W. T., 'Dr. Macaura and the Pulsocon. Within a month of the close of the test', ibid., 1911, p. 648.

49 'Disturbance at the Albert Hall. Medical students' demonstration', *The Times*, 12 May 1911. See also ibid., 13 May 1911.

50 STEAD, W. T., 'Dr. Macaura and the Pulsocon . . .', *The Review of Reviews*, 1911, **43**, 648.

51 STEAD, W. T., 'Can Dr. Macaura cure rheumatism? Report on result of six months' treatment', ibid., 1911, **44**, 108–9.

52 Stead to Dr. Daniel S. Hager, 24 August 1911, Department of Investigation Files, American Medical Association (hereafter cited as AMA), Chicago, Illinois.

53 STEAD, W. T., 'Dr. Macaura's challenge. Final report on the merits of the Pulsocon', *The Review of Reviews*, 1911, **44**, 318.

54 'Macaura Comes Back', *J. Amer. med. Ass.*, 1911, **57**, 485.

55 Dr. George H. Simmons to Dr. Daniel S. Hager, 18 September 1911, copy, Department of Investigation Files, AMA. [My italics.]

56 See letter of Cecil J. Corby to the Editor on 'Quackery', *Med. Press Circ.*, 18 October 1911, p. 432.

57 'Macaura comes back', *J. Amer. med. Ass.*, 1911, **57**, 486.

58 'Wrongful dismissal. Wade v. Macaura', *The Times*, 21 November 1911; see also 'The ways of platform healers', *Br. med. J.*, 1911, **ii**, 1448.

59 *Br. med. J.*, 1911, **ii**, 1448.

60 'Paris letter. The impunity of a charlatan', *J. Amer. med. Ass.*, 1912, **58**, 1767.

61 'Paris letter. The arrest of Macaura', ibid., 1912, **59**, 130.

62 *New York Times*, 1 December 1912.

63 Ibid.

64 Ibid., *Berliner Borsen-Courier*, 5 December 1912.
65 *Chicago Daily News*, 14 and 15 May, 1914; *Br. med. J.*, 1914, **i**, 1146.
66 'Gerald Macaura', *JAMA*, 1914, **62**, 1743.
67 H. L. Glasgow to the American Medical Association, 13 August, 1920, Department of Investigation Files, AMA.
68 'Gerald Macaura', *JAMA*, 1914, **62**, 1743.
69 POTTER, G. W., 'Matteism: an exposure', *Br. med. J.*, 1892, **ii**, 370.

S. Izsak
Cluj (Romania)

La vaccination jénnerienne dans la vie médico-sanitaire roumaine à l'époque des lumières

L'un des aspects majeurs du développement de la médecine roumaine à l'époque des lumières est constitué sans doute, par l'assimilation de la médecine et la santé publique moderne.

Le contact pris par les médecins roumains avec les progrès de la médecine des lumières dans les pays de l'Europe occidentale et centrale, avait porté fruit dans l'évolution de l'activité médicale et sanitaire roumaine.

Dès la première décennie du XIXe siècle une amélioration sensible se fait déjà sentir dans l'enrichissement de la médecine roumaine avec les nouvelles acquisitions de la médecine clinique de même qu'avec les progrès réalisés dans le domaine de la santé publique.

Quant aux derniers, une place à part est tenue par la vaccination antivariolique, élaborée par Edward Jenner (1749–1823). La particulière importance présentée par celle-ci, l'effet vraiment révolutionnaire exercé sur la pratique et la pensée médicale de cette époque, reste indiscutable. Cependant, le grand retentissement qu'elle avait produit dans les cercles de médecine européens avait bientôt entraîné l'apparition des opinions et des courants pro et contra.

Si on veut prendre en vue la réceptivité de la médecine roumaine envers la méthode de la vaccination antivariolique, il faut mentionner qu'elle l'avait saluée dès son apparition, l'avait mis en oeuvre le plus tôt possible et avait confirmé son efficacité.

C'est dans un délai très court (à peine deux ans) à partir de la date où l'oeuvre classique de Jenner fut publié (London, 1798), que les premières vaccinations antivarioliques furent appliquées dans la Valachie (Bucarest, 1800).

Ce mérite revient au médecin roumain Constantin Caracas (1773–1828), qui, en 1800 procède à la vaccination des enfants appartenant à un quartier de Bucarest. A propos de cet événement significatif, il faut rappeler que le jeune Caracas était récemment revenu, même cette année-là, de Vienne, où, lors des dernières années du XVIIIe siècle, avaient eu lieu les célèbres expériences de contrôle, ayant démontré d'une manière incontestable l'efficacité de la vaccination jénerienne antivariolique.

En 1801, on procède, avec succès, aux premières vaccinations en Transylvanie.

L'initiative du docteur Constantin Caracas ne resta pas sans écho; les documents d'histoire de la médecine roumaine mentionnent qu'en Moldavie, les médecins G. K. Hesse et Frölich ont également pratiqué avec succès, durant les années (1803–4), la vaccination antivariolique.

Ces débuts couronnés de succès, la méthode de vaccination jénnerienne est devenue de plus en plus connue et son aire de mise en pratique élargie. Le même docteur Caracas mentionne qu'en 1802 la vaccination est devenue générale dans la ville de Bucarest, tout comme dans les autres localités.

Les intellectuels roumains illuministes, préoccupés pour le progrès social et culturel du peuple, s'efforcent de favoriser la diffusion de la vaccination de Jenner et de mettre ses fruits à la portée de tout le monde.

À partir de 1803, des ouvrages et des publications en roumain, des traductions aussi bien que des travaux originaux vont paraître dans toutes les provinces roumaines; grâce à ceux-ci, la vaccination est définitivement entrée dans la culture médico-sanitaire roumaine.

Il s'en ajoute des lettres publiques adressées aux fidèles, dont l'objectif était d'instruire le clergé, afin de conseiller et stimuler le peuple d'accepter la vaccination jénnerienne.

La série de publications roumaines qui propageaient la vaccination avait été inaugurée par la traduction en roumain du travail du protomédecin de Transylvanie, Michael Neustädter (1736–1806), publié sous le titre d'«Abrégé sur l'inoculation de la vaccine, pour le renforcement du coeur, destiné à tous les parents de Transylvanie» (Sibiu, 1803; 63 pages).

Le livre connut un tirage considérable pour ce temps-là (4.600 exemplaires), et par suite fut diffusé non seulement en Transylvanie, mais également au-delà des Carpathes, dans la Valachie et la Moldavie.

Ce livre fut suivi par la brochure *Invăţătura de bubatul de vacă pentru dezrădăcinarea şi istbovirea bubatului firesc* (Buda, 1804). Suivant toutes les probabilités, il s'agit d'une traduction (d'après un modèle autrichien), dont l'auteur semble avoir été le remarquable érudit roumain Gheorghe Sincai (1754–1816) qui, à cette époque, se trouvait comme correcteur à Buda. Il faut remarquer la comparaison qu'on y fait entre la variolisation et la vaccination élaborée par Jenner, cela, bien entendu, en faveur de la dernière.

La même imprimerie fait paraître *L'Abrégé pour la variole salvatrice* (Buda, 1817), qui n'est pas autre chose que la traduction abrégée du travail portant le même titre du médecin Iosif Bene, professeur à la Faculté de Médecine de Pesta. Le livre fut imprimé et distribué par les autorités officielles.

Tout en rendant hommage à Edward Jenner, les médecins illuministes, convaincus des fruits et des résultats de cette méthode à réprimer les épidemies varioliques, instituent la vaccination *de facto*, à une échelle toujours plus grande dans toutes le provinces roumaines. L'institution *de facto* de la vaccination est peu après devenue *de jure* dans le cadre le la législation sanitaire.

L'introduction législative de la vaccination antivariolique dans la Valachie, la Moldavie ainsi que dans la Transylvanie avait été précédée par des ordonnances et des dispositions qui la recommandait, mentionnant ses avantages.

Pendant les années où l'on procéda à une nouvelle organisation administrative et juridique de la vie d'état publique dans les Principautés Roumaines autonomes (après la paix d'Adrianopol, 1829) par les *Réglements Organiques* (l'un pour la Valachie, introduit en 1831 et son similaire pour la Moldavie, introduit en 1832), la vaccination antivariolique est devenue un acte officiel. Chaque médecin de district était obligé de vacciner «tous les enfants et les adultes qu'il comptait être nécessaire, et cela sous une particulière surveillance».

Une loi parue en 1842 complétait les dispositions du *Réglement Organique*, attribuant au médecin de district la tâche de nommer des personnes destinées à effectuer les vaccinations au sein de la population «. . . et de les laisser procéder seules à cette besogne», son rôle se bornant uniquement à surveiller la périodicité de ces vaccinations. Pour que tout enfant soit vacciné, le médecin du district pouvait recourir aux autorités locales.

Peu après la promulgation des *Réglements Organiques*, on fait imprimer à nouveau des publications d'éducation sanitaire sur la vaccination antivariolique ainsi que d'autres publications destinées aux médecins. Dans la première catégorie se situe le petit livre du médecin *Zisu Conofan*, imprimé à Bucarest en 1833, dont le titre était «*Description de la maladie de la variole, son étendue et ses périls de même que l'usage sauveur de la vaccination ou de la greffe avec du pus de vache*».

Dans ce travail destiné à l'information des masses à propos de la vaccination antivariolique, l'auteur porte un grand éloge «à monsieur Edward Jenner», qui, en 1798 avait publié son livre sur la vaccination, «après s'en être convaincu, à la suite de plusieurs années d'essais, qu'elle ne trouble que peu l'organisme humain et ne cause que très rarement d'ennuis».

Les mêmes efforts de vulgarisation et de diffusion de la vaccination jennerienne sont déployés par les médecins de Transylvanie.

De la sorte, l'illustre médecin *Pavel Vasici Ungureanu* (1806–81), lorsqu'il traduit et publie la fameuse oeuvre de Christian Wilhelm Hufeland, à laquelle il avait donné le titre roumain de *Macrobiotique ou l'art de prolonger la vie* (Brasov, 1844–45), fait insérer une annotation personnelle sur la vie et l'activité de Jenner, respectivement l'importance de la vaccination antivariolique.

C'est le plus profond et sincère hommage écrit que la médecine illuministe roumaine avait porté à l'oeuvre médicale de Jenner.

«Le mérite de Jenner est resté immortel», écrivait *Pavel Vasici-Ungureanu*, «aussi bien dans l'histoire de la médecine que dans l'histoire de la culture humaine.»

Soulignant la valeur prophylactique de la vaccination antivariolique, l'auteur roumain conclut que dans le cas où «quelqu'un n'use pas de ce moyen léger et sans aucun endommagement pour soi et ses enfants, pèche contre soi-même et contre l'humanité» . . . (Vasici-Ungureanu, IIe volume, p. 80).

Grâce au prestige dont jouissait *Vasici-Ungureanu* comme médecin et comme homme de culture, son apport dans le domaine de la propagation du vaccin de *Jenner* a été considérable. La «Macrobiotique», traduite en roumain par Vasici Ungureanu, avait été l'un des livres d'éducation sanitaire les plus lus et répandus dans tous les pays roumains.

À propos des préoccupations occasionnées par la vaccination antivariolique, il faut mentionner aussi la publication avec le titre *Legiuirea pentru hultuire* (Législation pour la vaccination) rédigée par le protomédecin de la Moldavie, le docteur Gheorghe Cuciureanu (1814–86), inspirée également des prévoyances générales comprises dans les *Réglements Organiques sur la vaccination*. Celle-ci comprend une description détaillée de la technique de vaccination, offre des conseils aux médecins, de même qu'aux chirurgiens vaccinateurs tout en consignant de manière comparative, dans un tableau, le développement des symptômes chez les personnes non vaccinées (ou malades de la petite vérole) et respectivement vaccinnées (ou malades de varioloïde).

Grâce à ses qualités particulières, cette publication avait joui d'une large diffusion dans les Principautés Roumaines, étant d'une grande utilité pour les médecins et les chirurgiens vaccinateurs.

VI CONGRESS THEME

Relations between British Medicine and Medicine in Other Countries

D. G. de Freitas
São Paulo (Brazil)

Médecins britanniques au Brésil

JUSTIFICATION

Lors de la réalisation du «XXII Congrès International de l'Histoire de la Médecine», qui eut lieu en Roumanie et auquel j'étais présent, il fut convenu que le prochain Congrès se tiendrait en Angleterre. En apprenant cette décision, j'eu l'idée d'écrire «Médecins Britanniques au Brésil», que je destinerai au Congrès de 1972. De retour à mon pays je commençai la recherche bibliographique et ne trouvai que deux «informateurs»: Licurgo de Castro Santos Filho, professeur d'Histoire de la Médecine à la Faculté de Médecine de Campinas (Etat de São Paulo) et Gilberto Freyre, sociologue de rénommée internationale.

Licurgo de Castro Santos Filho, dans son *Histoire de la Médecine au Brésil* (1947), dans l'Appendice III du 2e tome, *Relation de quelques médecins étrangers qui visitèrent le Brésil ou s'y installèrent pour exercer leur profession* dédie quatre pages aux «médecins anglais», relationnant 20 noms, accompagnés, pour quelques uns, de petites informations biographiques. Sachant que cet Auteur préparait la 2e. édition de cette oeuvre méritoire (la plus complète publiée à ce jour au Brésil), je l'ai consulté à ce sujet. Il me reçut fort aimablement, me fournit quelques informations supplémentaires . . . et me conseilla de faire des «recherches avec patience, car ce thème l'intéressait vivement».[1]

Gilberto Freyre publia, en 1949, *Anglais au Brésil.* Dans le chapitre «Les Anglais dans les annonces des journaux brésiliens de la première moitié du XIX siècle» il informe que «les annonces de médecins anglais n'étaient pas rares». Après avoir indiqué une demi-douzaine de noms, il s'exprime ainsi à ce sujet: «Les médecins anglais au Brésil constituent une étude à part. Ils furent une institution.» Dans un «avis» qui précède la préface de ce livre, Gilberto Freyre avise qu'au volume *Anglais au Brésil* suivront deux autres: *Autres Anglais au Brésil,* dont le Ve chapitre sera consacré a *Autres Anglais dans les annonces des journaux brésiliens* (XIX siècle), et *Encore les Anglais au Brésil,* abordant au I chapitre, *Quelques Médecins.* Cet «avis» est de 1948!

Ces deux ouvrages ne figurant pas dans la bibliographie de Gilberto Freyre après plus de vingt ans, je décidai de lui écrire et lui demander des informations. La réponse m'arriva rapidement, malgré sa grande activité culturelle: «Je vous informe qu'aucun des livres en projet et annoncé sur les Anglais au Brésil n'a été écrit ou publié par moi.» Et le Maitre Gilberto me donne ce conseil: «Je crois que ce sujet des Médecins Anglais au Brésil est digne de votre attention et étude. Ne manquez pas de la faire.»[2]

Muni de telles informations et flatté par les paroles d'encouragement de ces deux auteurs, je commençai mes recherches (consultant livres et publications qui pourraient me fournir de nouvelles données). Je fis aussi des enquêtes auprès de personnes portant les mêmes noms et sollicitai la collaboration des historiens de la Médecine de diverses cités brésiliennes. Le résultat ne fut pas brillant, mais quelque chose de «nouveau» apparut qui possibilita une petite augmentation de la relation de Licurgo Santos Filho, ainsi qu'une amélioration (par elimination de quelques inexactitudes) et amplification de quelques biographies. Je présenterai donc la relation que j'ai préparé, par ordre alphabétique de noms. Cela me parait plus à conseiller et même plus didactique. Je ne relaterai pas les détails de chaque biographie, comme j'en avais l'intention, étant limité par l'espace d'accord avec le «Réglement» du Congrès. Je reserve le travail complet pour une autre occasion, et n'indiquerai dans ce travail que de légers «traits biographiques» (lieu de naissance, école où ils se formèrent, date d'arrivée au Brésil, ville où ils exercèrent leur profession, etc.) sous une forme synthétique. Toutefois, avant de présenter cette liste, je ferai une petite «introduction», relatant comment les Anglais débarquèrent au Brésil le long des siècles; les uns comme simples aventuriers ou négociants, les autres avec un esprit scientifique pour étudier certains aspects du Brésil, surtout la flore brésilienne et la nature humaine, la grande majorité, enfin, pour se fixer dans notre territoire adonnée aux emplois les plus divers.

INTRODUCTION

Des citoyens britanniques commencèrent à visiter les terres brésiliennes, quoique sporadiquement, peu après leur découverte par le capitaine-chef portugais Pedro Álvares Cabral, le 22 Avril 1500. Corsaires, aventuriers, trafiquants, négociants en «pau Brasil», etc. débarquèrent ici pour tenter la réalisation de leurs objectifs, emportant le fruit de leur travail ailleurs, pour le transformer en argent. Rares furent ceux qui fixèrent domicile ici.

Ce ne fut qu'au dernier quart du XVIe siècle que l'Angleterre parait avoir pris connaissance de l'existence du Brésil, quand cette possession portugaise passa sous la domination espagnole (1580). A partir de cette époque les eaux territoriales brésiliennes furent infestées de corsaires anglais, protégés par la propre reine Elizabeth (fille de Henri VIII, 1533–1603), qui encourageait avec sa protection les expéditions des grands aventuriers de l'Atlantique contre les possessions du monarque espagnol. De ces corsaires je citerai:

Edward Fenton (mort en 1603), marin et aventurier qui, à la tête d'une expédition commerciale, tenta de prendre d'assaut le port de Santos mais fut repoussé, vers 1582;

Thomas Cavendish, en 1591, se trouvant dans une mauvaise situation financière, organisa une nouvelle aventure américaine (il avait déjà passé par Cabo Frio en 1586), envahissant la ville de Santos où il resta deux mois, pratiquant toute sorte de dévastation et pillage, mais qui se termina par un échec. Son compatriote Anthony Knivet, qui faisait parti de cette expédition, fut abandonné à terre et se mit par la suite au service de Martim de Sá (fils du gouverneur Salvador Correia). Il écrivit

«Vária fortuna e estranhos feitos». A Santos, Knivet rencontra John King, qui résidait en cette ville depuis 15 ans et qui parait être le premier citoyen britannique à élire domicile au Brésil. Ce même Thomas Cavendish revint l'année suivante au Brésil, et n'obtint pas plus de succès que la première fois. Il fut obligé de se retirer et mourut pendant le voyage de retour.

Richard Hawkins Knight passa aussi au Brésil en 1593;

James Lancaster, en 1595, entra à Recife avec une flotte de sept navires et pendant un mois mit à sac la ville, mais il dut l'abandonner à la suite d'une attaque qui fit plusieurs morts.

Toutes ces expéditions, qui comptaient des centaines d'hommes, devaient inclure dans leurs équipages des personnes ayant des connaissances de Médecine, voire des médecins et chirurgiens pour assister les marins, comme le prouve la présence de «Mestre João», «chirurgien du Roi» dans l'expédition de Pedro Álvares Cabral, et celle du grand médecin Garcia de Orta, dans l'expédition de Martim Afonso de Souza (1534) qui voguait en direction de l'Inde. Toutefois, à ce jour les Archives n'ont pas dévoilé les noms de ces esculapes. Je citerai, à peine de passage, que Knivet, qui fit part de l'expédition de Cavendish en 1591, se réfère légèrement à un certain Andrew Tower, marin du navire *Desire*, qui «avait connaissance de l'art de guérir»[3] et informe que dans le navire *Admiral Leicester* existait le «lit du chirurgien»[4]; sujet auquel je donnerai plus d'emphase quand je traiterai spécifiquement des *Médecins Britanniques au Brésil.*

Aux XVIIe et XVIIIe siècles, la Grande Bretagne ne manifesta pas un grand intérêt pour le Brésil, malgré les privilèges acquis par le «Traité de paix et d'alliance avec le Portugal», signé le 23 juin 1661, qui lui donnait le droit de maintenir quatre familles britanniques dans chaque ville d'importance capitale: Pernambuco, Bahia et Rio de Janeiro. Toutefois, au début du XIXe siècle, surtout après «l'ouverture des ports» (1808) qui permit l'entrée de ses citoyens au Brésil, plusieurs d'entre eux se fixèrent ici, s'intégrant à la population autochtone et s'occupant des activités professionelles les plus diverses. Mais auparavant, en 1805, une escadre anglaise, commandée par l'amiral Home Papham, comptant 60 voiles et conduisant une troupe expéditionnaire sous les ordres du général David Baird, mouilla à Bahia, sur son chemin pour le Cap de Bonne Espérance. Il reçut des negociants de Bahia, y compris du colonel Felisberto Caldeira Brant, les secours les plus urgents et des provisions fraiches.[5] Une telle escadre de cinq douzaines de bateaux devait forcément avoir un «corps médical» à bord qui, certainement, prêta ses services cliniques à quelques habitants de Bahia, ville qui ne comptait pas un grand nombre d'esculapes.

Comme dit Octávio Tarquínio de Souza, «avec l'acte d'ouverture de nos ports en 1808 au commerce avec les nations amies, commence l'histoire proprement dite des relations anglo-brésiliennes. Sans hésitation, les Anglais se convainquirent qu'ils trouveraient au Brésil une excellente opportunité pour l'expansion de leur industrie et de leur commerce. Profitant, en bons réalistes, des circonstances favorables, ils continuèrent la même politique pratiquée au Portugal: obtenir le maximum de faveurs et le maximum de bénéfices.»[6]

Gilberto Freyre fait observer que «Les Anglais, comme les Français, apparurent d'abord sous la forme de pirates, aventuriers et négociants, sur les côtes de l'Amérique tropicale. Se distanciant des Français, leurs rivaux de longue date, les Anglais finirent par atteindre chez nous une prépondérance économique, basée sur leurs négociants et techniciens, qui – ostensive sous D. João VI quand cette prépondérance prit un aspect franchement impérialiste et non seulement impériale – s'accentua entre 1835 et 1912, pour décliner lentement par la suite, vaincue par l'expansion Nord-Américaine et minée par l'allemande.»[7]

Les Anglais qui vinrent au Brésil appartenaient aux professions les plus diverses: commerçants, ingénieurs, techniciens, aventuriers, missionnaires, traducteurs, consuls, magiciens, commissaires priseurs, mécaniciens, marins, gérants de Banque et d'entreprises, fabriques de gaz et de sucre, superintendants de compagnies de chemins de fer et de télégraphe, machinistes, chauffeurs et aussi dentistes et médecins. Ils choisissaient le Brésil pour leur champ d'action, amenant avec eux leurs us et coutumes et «anglicisant» le milieu brésilien à tel point qu'on pouvait dire, avec juste raison, que le XIXe siècle au Brésil «fut le siècle anglais par excellence».[8]

Cette observation de Richard Burton au sujet de l'arrivée d'un Anglais au Brésil est vraiment intéressante: «Dès que nous débarquons à Pernambuco les questions qu'on nous pose sont les suivantes: Vous êtes commerçant? Ingénieur? Naturaliste? Docteur? Non! Alors vous devez être dentiste! C'est que le brésilien s'est tellement habitué à considérer les britanniques comme appartenant à une de ces professions, que la demande est faite spontanément. . . .»[9]

Quel était le principal motif qui poussait l'Anglais, à partir d'une certaine époque, à rechercher le Brésil? Il n'y avait pas une raison unique, mais plusieurs, d'accord avec l'activité professionnelle:

(*a*) Le commerçant voyait un excellent marché pour la vente des produits anglais et pour l'exportation de certaines matières premières, principalement le coton, qui existait en quantité appréciable et à bas prix.
(*b*) Les naturalistes se laissèrent séduire par l'immense variété de la flore et de la faune brésilienne.
(*c*) Les ingénieurs étaient sollicités par les puissantes firmes chargées de construire les routes, les chemins de fer, les usines à sucre, etc.
(*d*) Les médecins venaient prêter leurs services aux firmes qui exploitaient les richesses du sol, et dont l'hégémonie allait appartenir à Mina de Morro Velho. Il y en avait, toutefois, qui venaient recherchant un climat différent, plus favorable à leurs maux et souffrances. Se sentant bien ici, ils élirent domicile.
(*e*) Quant aux dentistes, pour compléter la citation de Richard Burton, je dois dire que mes recherches n'ont pas dévoilé un nombre appreciable qui justifierai la question entendue au débarquement à Pernambuco.

Outres ces professionels, beaucoup d'autres vinrent au Brésil, y voyant un champ propice à leur activité qui serait naturellement mieux rémunérée; d'autres, encore, se rendirent compte de l'excellence du climat, typiquement tropical, un des plus sain du monde; les prêtres et missionnaires voulaient disséminer les postulats de la religion anglicaine aux sujets anglais domiciliés ici; et les représentants diplomatiques s'installaient dans les principales villes du littoral pour servir S.M.B.

On ne peut préciser, même approximativement, le nombre de britanniques qui s'établirent au Brésil durant le XIXe siècle. On ne peut même pas présenter des chiffres exactes pour la population brésilienne! Avant 1872 il y eut diverses tentatives pour recenser la population au Brésil; mais tous les travaux furent incomplets. Le premier en date est de 1776. Sans aucun doute, le contingent britannique était appréciable, localisé surtout le long de la côte, dans les villes les plus importantes et accessibles à la navigation: Recife, Salvador, Rio de Janeiro, São Luiz do Maranhão et, plus tard, Santos. Pour l'intérieur du Brésil ils donnèrent la préférence à Minas Gerais et à São Paulo, à cause des conditions exceptionelles du sol (mineraux et pierres précieuses à Minas, café à São Paulo). Ils avaient une certaine «attraction» les uns pour les autres, comme c'est naturel d'ailleurs, car toutes les colonies étrangères menaient une vie sociale à part, motivée par la diversité des coutumes et la difficulté de comprendre le portugais, sans compter que la religion qu'ils professaient et voulaient garder, les éloignaient de la population brésilienne. Malgré tout ils se sentaient bien sur le sol brésilien, et beaucoup d'entre eux (ingénieurs, négociants, missionaires et médecins) restèrent pour toujours. A leur mort, ils étaient ensevelis au cimetière anglais, presque toujours après une cérémonie présidée par un prêtre ou pasteur anglais, dans une chapelle anglicaine ou protestante. Plusieurs constituèrent ici une famille: Dodsworth, Studart, Mac Daurel, Drumond, Speers, Simonsen, etc., y compris des médecins: Abbot, Ellis, Whately, Hall, Cochrane et d'autres encore. Certains épousèrent des brésiliennes. Des enfants, il y en eut qui se «brasilienisaient» de suite, d'autres, comme le fait remarquer Gilberto Freyre, «se conservèrent *Anglais d'eau douce* pour une ou deux générations, conservant les habitudes de l'île, parlant mal le portugais ou avec accent, exagérant la réserve, le flegme et le silence des Anglais».[10]

Intrinséquement «negociants» par nature et tempérament, les Anglais qui s'établirent ici furent utiles au Brésil. Ils contribuèrent à son développement et progrès, et méritent notre estime et gratitude.

MÉDECINS BRITANNIQUES AU BRÉSIL

Gilberto Freyre et Licurgo de Castro Santos Filho avaient raison quand ils attirèrent mon attention sur la pénurie des sources d'information, et la nécessité de rechercher patiemment pour ammener à bon terme la tâche que je m'étais imposée. Cet effort était compensateur, vu l'importance du sujet, inexistant dans la bibliographie médicale, historique ou sociale du Brésil.

Acceptant le conseil ami de ces deux Maîtres, je n'économisai pas mes efforts pour dénicher dans les livres et publications, page pour page, de petites «notes» ayant rapport avec le thème en question. Je reconnais que la recherche n'a pas été aussi complète que l'aurait voulu l'importance du sujet, mais l'approximation de la date du Congrès m'oblige à interrompre la lecture d'autres oeuvres pour commencer la rédaction de ce travail en me servant des informations recueillies à ce jour.

Le thème est séduisant, mais vaste et difficile à traiter. Il devrait être confié à une «équipe de travail» à plein rendement pendant une longue période de temps. Cette «communication» au «XXIIIe Congrès International d'Histoire de la Médecine» ne sera pas une «dissertation», mais une modeste contribution à l'Histoire des «Médecins Britanniques au Brésil»; «l'Ouvrage Original» sera probablement publié ultérieurement dans la *Revista de História*, organe du Département d'Histoire de la Faculté de Philosophie, Lettres et Sciences Sociales de l'Université de São Paulo, et contiendra tous les éléments informatifs recueillis durant de longs mois de consultations et patientes recherches.

J'emploi le terme «britannique» pour tous ceux issus de n'importe quelle parcelle de «territoire anglais»: Angleterre (proprement dite), Ecosse, Irlande, Pays de Galles, Afrique du Sud, etc.

Pour l'instant je présenterai une relation des médecins originaires de Grande Bretagne qui vécurent au Brésil jusqu'à la fin du XIXe siècle, les uns exerçant leur profession pendant quelque temps, les autres de passage seulement sur la terre brésilienne, mais avec la possibilité d'avoir mis à la disposition des populations qu'ils contactèrent leurs connaissances de «l'Art de Guérir». Je ne peux garantir que tous les noms qui seront cités possédaient réellement un diplôme d'une Faculté ou d'une Ecole de Médecine; car a cette époque il y avait des personnes qui obtenaient des titres de «chirurgien approuvé» voire une «autorisation» pour soigner les malades; conditions qui pouvaient être mises à profit au Brésil, face à la pénurie de professionels authentiques aux premiers siècles de notre histoire. De plus, les sources d'informations ne nous fournissent pas avec la clarté désirable de tels détails, qui seraient la condition «sine qua non» pour justifier le titre de cette «contribution»: «Médecins Britanniques au Brésil».

Une fois faites de telles réserves et pondérations, je passe à la présentation de la liste que j'ai réussi à organiser, indiquant quelques traits biographiques, subordonnés à un nombre déterminé d'articles pour réduire l'extension de ce travail:

(A) Local e date de naissance.
(B) Filiation.
(C) Faculté où il obtint son diplôme et à quelle date.
(D) Raisons de leur venue au Brésil et date d'arrivée.
(E) Temps de permanence au Brésil et lieux où ils exercèrent leur profession.
(F) Spécialité.
(G) Principaux travaux médicaux publiés.
(H) Etat civil (si marié, nom et nationalité de l'épouse, nombre d'enfants brésiliens en spécifiant si quelques-uns suivirent la carrière médicale).
(I) Lieu et date de décès.

Pour simplifier l'exposition, j'indiquerai les éléments informatifs que j'ai réussi d'obtenir pour chacun des alineas cités plus haut:

Abbott, Jonathas

(A) Lambeth (Londres); 6 août 1796.
(C) Collège de Médecine et Chirurgie de Bahia, 1821.
(D) Il vint comme «groom», en compagnie du Dr. José Álvares do Amaral – 1812.
(E) Jusqu'à sa mort en 1868.
(F) Anatomie; Professeur au Collège de Bahia de 1828 à 1861.
(G) *Collection de dix discours consecutifs pour l'inauguration du cours d'Anatomie* (1845); *Formulaire de chirurgie de l'Hôpital de la Santa Casa de Bahia* (1838).
(H) Marié avec Cecília Valters (Bahia); trois enfants «naturels», mais reconnus, dont Jonathas Abbott Filho, diplomé en Médecine en 1848 et qu'il exerçat à Rio Grande do Sul, surtout à São Gabriel.
(I) São Gabriel; 8 mars 1868.

Adams, João Henrique

(A) Colonie du Cap (Afrique du Sud); 1822.
(C) Marbourg (Hesse) – Allemagne.

(D) 1841 ou 1842.
(E) Jusqu'à sa mort en 1901. Sorocaba (1844–86); connu comme le «Docteur Anglais», Rio de Janeiro.
(H) Marié avec la fille du Baron de Mogi-Mirim (Manuel Claudiano de Oliveira) et de Balbina de Toledo en 1869.
(I) Rio de Janeiro; 2 novembre 1901.

Bill, Carlos
(A) Angleterre.
(D) Il passa par Bahia vers la fin de 1832, sur le paquebot *Lady Mary Pelhom*. Il fut arrêté avec d'autres membres de l'équipage et passa quelque temps en prison.

Birt,
(A) Angleterre.
(D) Prêter ses services à la Mine de Morro Velho; 1848.
(E) En 1865 il était à Bahia.
(F) Il se dédiait, à des «services de statistique» (taux de mortalité, température, etc.).

Black, Elias
(C) Docteur en Médecine.
(D) Vint de l'Ile Maurice (Océan Indien), pour s'établir à Rio de Janeiro; 24 novembre 1811.

Blumberg, David
(A) Anglais.
(C) Il y a des doutes quant à sa profession; il doit s'agir d'un «guerisseur», comme on dit.
(E) En 1896 il exerçait la profession à Barra Mansa (Etat de Rio de Janeiro).

Campbel, Colen
(A) Anglais(?)
(D) Se présenta à la «Police» de Rio de Janeiro, pour la «legitimation d'étrangers» le 4 août 1813.
(F) Chirurgien.

Coates, Daniel
(A) Ecossais.
(D) Se présenta à la Police le 28 juin et 2 juillet 1841, en provenance de Liverpool.
(F) Médecin (Dr.).

Cochrane, Tomás
(A) A Madras (Inde); 16 mai 1805.
(B) L'Honorable Basil Cochrane et Lucy Sutton.
(D) 1829.
(E) Jusqu'à sa mort en 1873. Rio de Janeiro.

(F) Homéopathie.
(G) *Medicina Doméstica Homeopáthica*, Rio, 1849.
(H) Marié avec Helena Augusta Velasco Nogueira da Gama (de Ouro Preto, veuve du médecin anglais Robert Wallace Mac Farlane).
(I) Rio de Janeiro; 26 janvier 1873.

Cormick, Henry M.
(A) Anglais.
(D) Le 1 février 1821 parti pour Ilha Grande.
(F) Chirurgien.

Cramfordt, Diogo
(A) Anglais.
(D) Le 17 mai 1833 parti pour Ubatuba.
(F) Chirurgien (Dr.).

Crawford, James
(A) Anglais.
(D) Le 14 avril 1837 parti pour l'Angleterre; le 13 mai 1837 Londres.
(F) Chirurgien (Dr.).

Crump, John
(A) Anglais.
(D) Arriva d'Angleterre le 14 mars 1833.
(F) Chirurgien (Dr.).

Darney, Tomás
(A) Anglais.
(D) Parti pour Ilha Grande le 1 decembre 1832.
(F) Médecin (Dr.).

Daunt, Ricardo O'Connor Gumbleton
(A) Chateau de Kilcascan (Irlande); 30 août 1818.
(C) Edimbourg.
(D) Vint de la Colonie du Cap, où il cliniqua, révalidant son diplôme à la Faculté de Médecine de Rio de Janeiro (1843).
(E) Jusqu'à sa mort en 1893; il cliniqua à Macaé, Campinas et Itu.
(H) Marié avec Francelina de Camargo; neuf enfants.
(I) Campinas (Etat de São Paulo); 7 juin 1893.

Dayrel, John Mortimer
(A) Ecosse.
(D) Première moitié du XIXe siècle.
(E) Jusqu'à sa mort. Diamantina (Minas Gerais). «Médecin habile et humanitaire.»
(H) Marié; nombreuse descendance.

Dundas, Roberto

(A) Anglais.
(E) Le 27 septembre 1817, était à Rio de Janeiro; le 22 juin 1819 «part pour Bahia». En octobre 1821 il était chirurgien de l'hôpital des Anglais, annexe de la Chapelle Anglaise de Salvador (Bahia).
De 1840 à 1854 il collabora à l'organisation de la Bibliothèque de la Faculté de Médecine de Bahia.
(F) Chirurgien.

Dunlop, Carlos

(A) Anglais.
(E) Exerça sa profession au Brésil, à Rio de Janeiro semble-t-il.

Elincoe, Guilherme

(E) São Paulo (avant 1809). Guarapuava. Curitiba.
(F) Chirurgien.

Ellis, William

(A) Londres; 1807.
(B) Richard Ellis et Sophia Harvey.
(D) Raisons de santé; décembre 1832.
(E) Jusqu'à sa mort en 1873. São Paulo.
(H) Marié avec Maria do Carmo da Cunha Bueno (pauliste); quatre enfants dont deux médecins: Guilherme (formé en 1873) et Alfredo (formé en 1869).
(I) São Paulo; 1873.

Fairbanks, Jorge Eduardo

(A) Anglais
(D) En 1838 fut nommé membre du «Conseil de Salubrité» de Bahia.
(H) Au «Cimetière des Anglais», à Salvador (Bahia), il y a une tombe de John Edward Fairbanks, mort le 12 decembre 1853, à l'âge de 26 ans, fils de George Edwards Fairbanks et Joaquina Silveira Fairbanks.

Farlane, Robert Wallace Mac

(A) Ecossais(?); 1797.
(B) Daniel et Elisa Mac Farlane.
(D) Au début de la décade 1830–40.
(E) Valença (Etat de Rio) et Rio de Janeiro.
(F) Homéopathie.
(H) Épousa Helena Augusta Velasco Nogueira da Gama (1835); deux enfants.
(I) Rio de Janeiro, 9 novembre 1844.

Gagarty, André

(A) Anglais.
(D) Le 29 août 1839; Falmouth.
(F) Médecin.

Gardner, Daniel
(A) Anglais.
(D) Ant. à 27 juin 1810.
(E) Rio de Janeiro.
(F) «Docteur en Médecine».
(G) *Silabus ou Compêndio de lições de Quîmica*, Rio, 1810.

Gardner, Jorge
(A) Anglais.
(D) 1836.
(E) 1836–41.
(F) Médecin et Chirurgien.
(G) *Travels in Brazil* (Londres, 1846).

Geald, Hugh
(A) Anglais.
(D) Parti pour Le Havre, le 24 juin 1838.
(F) Médecin (Dr.).

Glass, Alexandre
(A) Anglais.
(D) Le 19 decembre 1834 «en provenance de Santos»; le 26 octobre 1835 Santos.
(F) Médecin (Dr.).

Goodridge, Augustus Frederich
(A) Grande Bretagne.
(D) Vint pour cliniquer à la «colonie» anglaise de Mato Dentro. Le 30 mai 1835; Falmouth.
(F) «Docteur».
(I) Itabira, 1 novembre 1839.

Gordon, Charles
(A) D'origine écossaise.
(C) Université d'Edimbourg.

Hall, James
(A) Anglais.
(C) Université de St. Andrews (Ecosse).
(D) 1812.
(E) Maranhão, jusqu'à sa mort.
(F) Médecin.
(H) Marié, un fils: Thomas Wright Hall, médecin, de l'Université d'Edimbourg (Brésilien, naturalisé Anglais).
(I) Maranhão, janvier 1832.

Hardy, Arthur Mac
(A) Anglais.
(C) «Fit vérifier son diplôme» par la Faculté de Médecine de Bahia, en 1836.
(F) Médecin.

Hartshorne, Carlos
(A) Anglais.
(D) Le 26 juillet 1839, «venu de Santos».
(F) Médecin (Dr.).

Jones, Arthur Meyrick
(A) Anglais.
(C) «Bachelor of Medicine» de Durham et «Fellow of the Royal College of Surgeons» d'Angleterre.

Kenzie, João
(A) Anglais.
(D) Le 22 janvier 1841, part avec sa femme et deux enfants pour Setubal; le 3 juin 1841 part avec sa femme et ses enfants pour Lisbonne.

Landell, Roberto
(A) Edron (Comté de Berwick); 1768.
(B) Guilherme Landell et Isabel Masen (Ecossaise).
(C) En Ecosse; revalida son diplôme à Porto Alegre en 1833.
(D) 1827.
(E) Porto Alegre jusqu'à sa mort.
(F) Médecin (Dr.).
(H) Marié avec Sara Thompson Graham (de Berwick); il eut un fils, João, né à Porto Alegre en 1827, qui se forma en médecine en Angleterre.
(I) Porto Alegre; 12 janvier 1878.

Lindsay, George
(A) Anglais.
(D) Recife (Pernambuco); 9 juin 1858.
(E) En 1859 «était membre de la Southern Cross» à Recife.
(F) Chirurgien.

Loudon (ou London), João
(A) Ecossais.
(D) 1821(?)
(E) Recife, enregistra son diplôme en 1833.
(F) Médecin et naturaliste.
(G) *Observations météorologiques* . . . (1842–43).
(I) Recife; 1843.

Malet, Christofer F. L.
(A) Anglais(?); Irlandais(?)
(E) 1847 à 1850 (au moins), Rio de Janeiro.
(C) Trinity College (Dublin).
(F) Chirurgien.

May (ou Mayer), Guilherme
(A) Anglais.
(D) 4e décade du XIX siècle.

(E) Recife; un des fondateurs de la «Sociedade de Medicina de Pernambuco».
(F) Médecin.

M'Intire,
(A) Anglais(?)
(E) Mines de Morro Velho; 1867.
(F) Médecin.

Monach, Roberto
(A) Anglais.
(E) Mines de Morro Velho (1843).
(F) Médecin.
(G) *Rapport sur la santé des Nègres.*

Moojen, João Jorge
(A) Anglais.
(E) 2 juin 1840 «vint de Angra dos Reis»; le 1 juillet 1840 «part pour Santos».
(F) Médecin (Dr.).

Murray, Pedro Paulo
(A) Anglais.
(E) Le 20 mai et 12 juin 1838; Santos.
(F) Chirurgien.

Paterson, John Ligertwood
(A) Comté d'Aberdeen (Ecosse); 14 septembre 1820.
(C) Aberdeen; 23 avril 1841.
(E) Paraíba (1841); Bahia (1842 jusqu'à sa mort).
(F) Un des trois savants et fondateurs de l'«Escola Tropicalista Bahiana».
(G) Divers travaux publiés dans la *Gazeta Médica da Bahia.*
(I) Salvador; 9 decembre 1882.

Ramsay,
(A) Ecossais(?)
(E) Recife; ant. à 1821.

Reid, Jorge
(A) Anglais.
(D) Le 19 avril 1839, déclarant «venir de Londres».
(F) Médecin (Dr.).

Richardson, Arthur
(A) Anglais.
(E) Le 3 juin 1868 «il commença» à la «Southern Cross» (Recife) et y resta jusqu'à 1872 au moins.
(F) Chirurgien.

Sampayo (ou S. Payo), José Maria Floriano de
(A) Londres.
(E) En 1812 il quitta Bahia pour s'établir à Vila Santo Amaro das Grotas.
(F) Chirurgien.

Smith, William
(A) Anglais.
(D) Arriva de Liverpool le 25 août 1839 et de Londres le 11 août et 16 août 1839.
(F) Médecin (Dr.).

Speer,
(A) Anglais.
(E) Cliniqua de nombreuses années dans les Mines de Morro Velho (Vila Nova de Lima).
(F) Chirurgien (Doutor Speer).

Strain, William Loudon
(A) Anglais.
(E) Sao Paulo; il fut le ler. directeur-médecin de l'Hôpital Samaritano (inauguré en 1894). Un des fondateurs de la «Société de Médecine et Chirurgie de São Paulo».
(F) Chirurgien.
(I) Angleterre.

Tower, André
(A) Anglais(?)
(D) 1593 (emprisonné à Ilha Grande).
(F) Avait des connaissances de «l'Art de Guérir» (Sorcier).

Tyndall, John
(A) Anglais.
(E) Le 4 octobre 1808; Buenos Aires; le 6 avril 1809; Chili.
(F) Médecin.

Walker, Thomas
(A) Anglais.
(E) En 1855 était dans les Mines de Morro Velho.
(F) Docteur en Médecine.
(I) Vers 1858.

Walsh, Robert
(A) Waterford (Irlande); 1772.
(C) Aberdeen (1820).
(D) Accompagna Lord Strangford (1828), retourna en Angleterre en 1829.
(I) Finglas (Dublin); 1852.

Wey (ou Weir),
(A) Ecossais.
(E) Mines de Morro Velho (à partir de 1866).

White, John

(A) Anglais(?)

(D) 1787, comme chirurgien d'une expédition qui cherchait l'Australie.

(E) Peu de temps (quelques jours): Rio de Janeiro, où il pratica quelques interventions chirurgicales.

Williams, Eduardo

(A) Anglais.

(E) Vint d'Angleterre le 21 janvier 1836.

(F) Médecin (Dr.).

Wile, Guilherme

(A) Anglais.

(E) Pernambuco (1839).

(F) Médecin (Dr.).

(I) 2e. semestre de 1844 – Paranaguá.

Wylie, William

(A) Anglais.

(D) Le 26 mars 1831; Granada.

(F) Médecin-chirurgien.

Voici la liste que j'ai pu établir, fruit de patientes consultations et recherches. Il s'agit de 60 «professionels» de la médecine, de nationalité britannique, qui vécurent au Brésil; les uns sporadiquement et de passage, les autres en se fixant ici pour exercer leur métier.

On peu affirmer, sans crainte de démenti, que ces médecins britanniques n'ont pas eu une grande influence sur l'évolution de la Médecine Brésilienne, qui commença réellement avec la fondation des Collèges Médico-Chirurgicaux de Bahia et Rio de Janeiro, en 1808. Nous devons, toutefois, en toute justice, mettre en évidence les figures de Jonathas Abbott (professeur d'anatomie à Bahia), de John Ligertwood Paterson, le véritable créateur de l'école de médecine tropicale de Bahia (école qui au XIXe siècle modernisa les études médicales à Bahia, et par influence au reste du Brésil, employant la méthode expérimentale dans l'étude de nos endémies) et de William Ellis, qui eut sous sa responsabilité les soins d'une grande partie de la population de São Paulo, ayant été Directeur du principal hôpital qui existait en cette ville, l'Hôtel Dieu. A tous ces médecins, qui obtinrent une renommée ou se limitèrent à prendre soin de la santé des brésiliens, l'expression de notre gratitude.

Références bibliographiques

1 Lettre du 2 février 1971.
2 Lettre du 11 mars 1971.
3 'Notavel viagem que, no ano de 1591 e seguintes, fez Antonio Knivet, da Inglaterra ao mar do sul, em companhia de Thomaz Candish', in *Rev. Inst. Hist. Geog. Bras.*, 1878, **41**, part. ler, p. 191.
4 Loc. cit., p. 200.
5 'Annotation' de Américo Jacobina Lacombe, in GRAHAM, MARIA, *Notas de uma viagem ao Brasil*, p. 160.
6 In FREYRE, GILBERTO, *Ingleses no Brasil*, préface, p. 15.
7 FREYRE, GILBERTO, *Ingleses no Brasil*, p. 35.

8 PANTALEÃO, OLGA, in *História Geral da Civilização Brasileira* (dirigée par Sérgio Buarque de Holanda), tome II, vol. Ier, *A presença inglesa*, p. 65.
9 BURTON, RICHARD F., *Viagens aos planaltos do Brasil*, tome I: *Do Rio de Janeiro a Morro Velho*, p. 19.
10 FREYRE, GILBERTO, loc. cit., p. 111.

Bibliographie

Arquivos do Instituto Bahiano de História da Medicina, vol. I, 1949.
AZEVEDO, AROLDO DE, *Cochranes do Brasil*, S. Paulo, Comp. Edit. Nacional, 1965.
BLAKE, AUGUSTO VICTORINO ALVES SACRAMENTO, *Diccionario Bibliográfico Brasileiro*, vol. 4e, Rio, Impr. Nacional, 1898.
British Medical Journal, 10 March 1883.
BURTON, RICHARD F., *Viagens aos Planaltos do Brasil*, tome I: *Do Rio de Janeiro a Morro Velho* (trad. de Américo Jacobina Lacombe), S. Paulo, Comp. Edit. Nacional, 1941.
CALMON, PEDRO, *História da Literatura Bahiana*, Salvador, Prefeitura Municipal, 1949.
CASTRO, OSCAR OLIVEIRA, *Medicina na Paraíba*, João Pessoa, A União Editora, 1945.
CONI, ANTÔNIO CALDAS, *A escola tropicalista bahiana*, Bahia, Tip. Beneditina, 1952.
COSTA, AFONSO, 'Diccionário de Intelectuais Bahianos', in *Rev. Inst. G. H. Bahia*, no. 55, 1929.
ELLIS JUNIOR, ALFREDO, *Um parlamentar da República*, S. Paulo, 1949.
FAZENDA, VIEIRA, 'Antiqualhas e memórias do Rio de Janeiro', in *Rev. Inst. H. G. Bras.*, **95**, 149.
FORTES, JOÃO BORGES, 'Em torno da personalidade do Prof. Jonathas Abbott', in *Rev. Inst. G. H. da Bahia*, no. 59, 1933.
FREYRE, GILBERTO, *Ingleses no Brasil*, Rio, Livr. José Olímpio Edit., 1948.
Gazeta Médica da Bahia, Divers numéros.
GRAHAM, MARIA, *Diário de uma viagem ao Brasil* (trad. e annotations de Américo Jacobina Lacombe), S. Paulo, Biblioteca Pedagógica Brasileira, vol. 8, 1956.
KOSTER, HENRY, *Viagens ao Nordeste do Brasil* (trad. e annotations de Luís Câmara Cascudo), S. Paulo, Comp. Edit. Nacional, 1942.
LACAZ, CARLOS DA SILVA, Vultos da Medicina Brasileira (vol. II), São Paulo, 1966.
LEÃO, ERMELINO AGOSTINHO DE, *Dicionário Histórico e Geográfico do Paraná*.
LEITÃO, C. DE MELO, *O Brasil visto pelos ingleses*, S. Paulo, Comp. Edit. Nacional, 1937.
LUCCOCK, JOHN, *Notas sobre o Rio de Janeiro e pontos meridionais do Brasil* (trad. de Milton da Silva Rodrigues), S. Paulo, Livr. Martins, 1942.
MARTINS FILHO, ENEAS, 'O cirurgião João Adolfo Schram', in *Rev. Inst. H. G. Bras.*, vol. 271, avril/june 1966, Rio, 1967.
MEIRA, RUBIÃO, *Médicos de outrora*, S. Paulo, 1937.
MOREIRA, JÚLIO, *História da Medicina no Paraná*, Curitiba, Impr. Oficial do Estado, 1953.
MOORE, JOSEPH WILLIAM, *The revolution of 1831* (with notes by J. M. Harvey).
NOBRE, ANTÔNIO DE GOES, *Esboço Histórico da Real e Benemérita Sociedade Portuguesa de Beneficência em São Paulo* (Ier. vol.: *1859–1894*), S. Paulo, Cia. Paul, Papéis e Artes Gráficas, 1919.
PANTALEÃO, OLGA, 'A presença inglesa', in *História Geral da Civilização Brasileira* (dirigée par Sérgio Buarque de Holanda), tome II, S. Paulo, 1962.
PEREIRA, ANTÔNIO PACÍFICO, *Memória sobre a Medicina na Bahia*, Bahia, Impr. Oficial do Estado, 1923.
Registro de Estrangeiros (*1808–1822*), Rio, Arch. Natl., 1960.
Registro de Estrangeiros (*1823–1830*), Rio, Arch. Natl., 1961.
Registro de Estrangeiros (*1831–1839*), Rio, Arch. Natl., 1962.
Registro de Estrangeiros (*1840–1842*), Rio, Arch. Natl., 1964.
Registro de Estrangeiros nas Capitanias (*1777–1819*), Rio, Arch. Natl., 1963.
ROCHA, LEDUAR DE ASSIS, *História da Medicina em Pernambuco* (siècle XIX), Recife, Arquivo Público Estadual, 1962.
SANTOS, ANTÔNIO VIEIRA DOS, *Memória Histórica da cidade de Paranaguá e seus Municípios*, Curitiba, Secção de História do Museu Paranaense, 1952.
SANTOS FILHO, LICURGO DE CASTRO, *História da Medicina no Brasil*, tome II, S. Paulo, Editora Brasiliense, 1947.
Sociedade Hospital Samaritano, Folheto informativo, São Paulo, s/d.
TAUNAY, VISCONDE DE, *Estrangeiros ilustres e prestimosos do Brasil*, S. Paulo, Comp. Melhoramentos, 1932 et in *Rev. Inst. H. G. Bras.*, tome 58, part II, 1895, pp. 225 à 248.
VOTTA, RAUL, *A Irmandade da Santa Casa de Misericordia de São Paulo nos primórdios de sua existência*, S. Paulo, Tip. Irmãos Dupont, 1951.

N. Riad
Cairo (Egypt)

L'influence de la médecine égyptienne sur la médecine britannique

L'influence de la médecine égyptienne sur la médecine britannique a commencé depuis l'aube de l'histoire de l'Angleterre jusqu'au 19e siècle de notre ère. En plus, nous avons pu révéler des traces de la civilisation égyptienne antique (pharaonique) en Angleterre d'après plusieurs facteurs: habitudes sociales, mythes, certains fleuves et villes d'Angleterre qui portent des noms hieroglyphiques. Horus sur les crocodiles, tenant des serpents, est à l'origine de Saint Georges sur un cheval, tuant le dragon. La «vache sacrée» est transportée d'Egypte aux Indes à l'Est, et à l'Europe greco-romaine et l'Angleterre à l'Ouest. Le mot Oxford est dérivé du nom égyptien qui signifie lieu de taureaux.

Pour Rendel Harris, les égyptiens sont entrés dans le sud et le sud-ouest de l'Angleterre par Dover, en traversant la France, ou par l'Espagne. Je vois dans le mot «Stonehenge» une dérivation du mot égyptien Tobe = pierres. A Dorset, où on coupe les pierres, nous trouvons «Yourbel» qui est un nom égyptien qui veut dire lieu du travail. Une école d'ethnographes a été jusqu'à montrer que toutes les constructions de pierre faites dans n'importe quel pays du monde devaient s'expliquer par des migrations des égyptiens. A Stonehenge avec son Hinkit (qui veut dire offrande en égyptien) nous trouvons des tombeaux comme en Egypte, contenant des mastabas et une ouverture par laquelle le mort reçoit sa nourriture à l'intérieur de son tombeau.

En entrant en Angleterre par Dover nous trouvons Kent, qui est Khent en égyptien et qui signifie «traverser» ou «marcher sur l'eau». Tanit, au sud-est de Kent, porte le nom de la ville égyptienne Tanis. Puis nous trouvons Thotens (de Thomos l'égyptien) et Ramlet bera (de Ra et «bera» qui veut dire «pharaon»).

En arrivant à l'Ile de Wight nous trouvons aussi des noms égyptiens: l'église de Maker (de Makareos qui veut dire le triomphant). Nous trouvons aussi des tombeaux comme à Stonehenge.

Avant de vous parler des apports dans la médecine et la pharmacie transportés en Angleterre par les Grecs et les Romains, je vous signale d'abord comment la civilisation égyptienne est arrivée en Europe. Les recherches modernes ont prouvé les erreurs commises par les écrivains européens jusqu'au 19e siècle, qui disaient que la civilisation européenne est venue des civilisations asiatique et grecque, sans chercher plus loin comment sont venues ces civilisations. Il a été prouvé à présent qu'il est faux de dire que la civilisation européenne est venue par l'invasion du peuple asiatique avant l'époque historique. L'influence de la culture pharaonique sur l'Europe existait avant cette invasion asiatique. L'enquête médicale récente nous a dévoilé que les crânes et les os anciens des habitants de l'Egypte avant l'époque historique et avant l'invasion asiatique sont de la même catégorie que celle des habitants de l'Afrique du Nord et du Sud de l'Europe à l'âge de la pierre (Sarguy et Eliot Smith cités par H. Kamal). L'Egypte fut la seule nation qui améliora sa civilisation en s'éloignant de l'époque de l'âge de pierre pour arriver «seule» à l'âge du cuivre, puis à l'âge du bronze. La méthode d'enterrement en Egypte à l'époque précédent l'Histoire, est la même que celle qui fut employée en Europe vers la fin de l'âge de la pierre. Avant l'Histoire, on posait le mort sur le côté gauche en lui pliant les jambes et les pieds. A l'époque des Pyramides (de la 4e à la 6e Dynastie) les Egyptiens posèrent leurs morts en position de membres étendus. Le Professeur Orsi a découvert que ce changement dans la méthode d'enterrement s'est opéré aussi au Sud de l'Europe et en Sicile (2.750 ans av. J.C.).

Les Asiatiques n'ont envahi l'Europe que grâce aux instruments métalliques qu'inventèrent les Egyptiens. De celà nous voyons que la civilisation égyptienne est entrée en Europe par deux voies: l'une directe, celle par le Sud, et l'autre indirecte: l'agression asiatique: celle de l'Est. L'Egypte a donc le privilège d'avoir donné la civilisation à l'Ouest et à l'Est, c'est-à-dire au monde entier. J'ai remarqué pendant mon séjour à Sienne, en Italie, lors du précédent Congrès International de l'Histoire de la Médecine, que beaucoup de drapeaux Siennois portent des dessins égyptiens, comme le faucon et le «Knoum» des pharaons, ainsi que des signes hiéroglyphiques. Ceci ne nous étonne pas car les Siennois sont des descendants des Etrusques qui sont d'origine asiatique et ont pris leur civilisation des Egyptiens avant de venir en Europe. Leur art présente des analogies certaines avec celui des égyptiens: l'aile d'Isis, le Sphinx etc., car leurs divinités et leurs personnages mythologiques sont les descendants directs des dieux égyptiens qui sont devenus des héros des autres peuples, comme en Crète et à Mycènes. La langue étrusque dérivée apparemment d'un dialecte asiatique dérive des hiéroglyphes égyptiens. Les lettres dérivées de l'alphabet grec archaïque sont dérivées de l'alphabet égyptien. Le texte étrusque d'Agram est rédigé sur des bandelettes qui entouraient la momie d'une princesse égyptienne. Ce texte qui comprend un total de 1500 mots est une énumération de prescriptions rituelles. Certains mots étrusques sont par ailleurs passés dans le latin. On prétend même que le nom «Rome» est dérivé d'un terme étrusque. Comme les Pharaons, les Etrusques bâtissaient sur le bord d'une rivière, ils réservaient la rive opposée pour y établir la nécropole. Villes des morts et des vivants se faisaient face (comme Sakhara et Memphis en Egypte) C'est le cas à Vulci, à Cerveteri et à Tarquinia en Italie. Entourées de puissantes murailles, ces cités étaient groupées autour d'un temple; un puits creusé à proximité était censé assurer la communication avec le monde souterrain, celui des défunts comme on en a trouvé aux tombeaux (Mastaba) de Sakhara en Egypte. L'existence étrusque était tournée vers l'au-delà; la mort était inséparable de la vie. Comme en Egypte, un clergé tout puissant exerçait une influence déterminante sur les destinées de la Nation. Rues, temples, portes et places publiques étaient dédiés aux principales divinités; les funérailles donnaient lieu à des fêtes et à des cérémonies en l'honneur du défunt. Comme à Louxor en Egypte, les tombes étrusques des nécropoles de Cerveteri et de Tarquinia sont de véritables maisons souterraines. Ces lieux contenaient des trésors; orfèvrerie, poteries, bijoux, fresques et sculptures. L'apport étrusque dans la civilisation romaine est considérable. Les étrusques ont appris aux Romains à construire des voûtes et des ponts et à créer des statues colossales comme en Egypte. En effet, l'Egypte est la partie des arts et on y conserve des monuments innombrables. Ses principaux temples et les palais subsistent encore, quoique les moins anciens de ces édifices aient été construits avant la guerre de Troie. Homère, Lycurgue, Solon Pythagore et Platon se rendirent en Egypte pour y étudier les sciences, la religion et les lois. Alexandre y fonda une ville opulente qui jouit longtemps de l'empire du commerce et qui vit Pompée, César, Marc Antoine et Auguste décider entre eux du sort de Rome et de celui du monde entier.

Le Professeur Pierre Gilbert nous dit que le Panthéon répond, par l'appel intérieur du sommet, à l'effet extérieur de la pyramide égyptienne, et il y a quantité d'autres indices d'une influence de l'Egypte sur la Grèce et sur Rome. La salle basilicale, caractérisée par une nef centrale éclairée latéralement au-dessus du niveau des bas côtés, fut créée dans la salle hypostyle du Karnak égyptien de 1300, et passa de l'Egypte alexandrine à tout le monde hellénistique pour établir à Rome le prototype de toutes les grandes églises de la Chrétienté.

Les grecs avaient l'habitude depuis l'époque de Hérodote de représenter les dieux égyptiens comme leurs dieux grecs. Ils ont donné des noms grecs aux dieux égyptiens. Ils ont aussi vénéré certains dieux égyptiens même sans leur avoir donné des noms grecs comme les dieux Bes Taurt et Sobek.

Ils ont ainsi adopté la croyance égyptienne.

Parmi les bas-reliefs égyptiens nous citerons celui du Temple «Kom-Ombo» en haute Egypte où *Dollfus* voit des pinces, des ciseaux, des sondes ou cautères et des bistouris, des ventouses et une balance. Cet étage d'instruments est absolument semblable à celui des instruments réels, ceux-là trouvés dans la trousse d'un oculiste gallo-romain exposée au Musée des Antiquités Nationales. En outre, les bistouris sont exactement de la même forme que ceux conservés au Louvre et qui datent de la fin de l'époque pharaonique.

Les pharaons connaissaient il y a 5000 ans l'antimoine dans le traitement de l'hématurie parasitaire d'Egypte.

On a trouvé en Egypte des flacons à collyre qui sont constitués par 2 tubes ou 4 tubes jumelés, certains sans couvercle, d'autres avec un couvercle tournant en ivoire le flacon étant en bois ou en terre émaillée. Leur usage médical est prouvé par la peinture de la tombe d'Ipy oculiste (No. 219 de la Nécropole de Deir-el-Medinah de Luxor Egypte) mais aussi par des inscriptions gravées sur le flacon tel celui, quadruple, conservé au Louvre portant: «Bon antimoine, bon pour la vue, repousse le sang (décongestionne), repousse la douleur» et sur un flacon double du British Museum conservé avec trousse de toilette: «Poudre pour enduire les yeux, pendant la période de l'inondation». Loret analysant des restes de poudre pris dans ces flacons, y a retrouvé des sels de cuivre et d'antimoine. Ces sels sont souvent mentionnés dans des papyrus médicaux – Les égyptiens opéraient la cataracte par la technique de l'abaissement, comme le firent les Romains et les Gallo-Romains.

La pharmacopée égyptienne est très riche et s'adresse à tous les règnes, végétaux, animaux, minéraux. Pour les végétaux nous en trouvons qui ont été utilisés pendant des millénaires: la myrrhe, l'encens, la sciure de cèdre, du sycomore, les gommes d'acacia, la cendre de dattes, d'oignon, la rose et le safran. *Nous les retrouvons tous sur les cachets d'oculistes gallo-romains.* Les matières animales servaient souvent d'excipient pour des pommades ou onguents, comme la graisse d'oie ou de porc, le miel, mais nous trouvons aussi le foie que les égyptiens conseillaient dans le traitement d'une mauvaise vision nocturne. Aujourd'hui nous connaissons que le foie est riche de Vitamine A (2 gr. donnent 1000 u. I) qu'on donne pour cette maladie. Beaucoup des matières minérales de l'Egypte sont encore utilisées avec succès actuellement dans tous les pays tels le sulfate de cuivre (utilisé dans le trachome maintenant encore), l'oxyde de cuivre, le sel marin (notre sérum) l'antimoine, le nitrate de potasse, les sels de plomb (ils sont la base de la pommade au précipité blanc et de la pommade jaune), l'oxyde de zinc, l'hématite et, comme astringent l'alun, la poudre de Lapis-Lazuli et même le naphte (notre vaseline s'extrait bien du pétrole).

En 1937 le danois B. Ebbel effectua la première véritable traduction du Papyrus Ebers- Puis l'allemand Hermann Grapow et ses collaborateurs Hildegard von Deines et Wolfhart Westendorf en publièrent une seconde. La variété de la *pharmacopée égyptienne* que Ebbell a trouvé dans ce Papyrus est étonnante. Le Papyrus indiquait, a lui seul, la composition de 900 remèdes. Il s'agissait de médicaments véritables et non d'exorcismes ou de formules incantatoires. Le nombre et la nature des drogues que le déchiffrement des hiéroglyphes a permis de situer confirme, en effet, l'hypothèse selon laquelle un 1/3 au moins des ingrédients qui figurent au Codex officinalis aurait déja figuré dans la pharmacopée égyptienne. Nous en citerons quelques-uns à titre d'exemple: Genièvre, coloquinte, grenade, graines de lin, fenouil, érable, cardamome, cumin, ail, laitue, résine de pin, térébenthine, feuilles de séné, lis, bryone, ricin, rose de Noel, thym, térébinthe, chélidoine, potentille, rampante, céleri, tamaris, salsifis sauvage, joncet lotus. *Et un remède égyptien surtout spn qui veut dire pavot.* Pour la première fois dans l'histoire de la médecine l'Egyptien mentionne le pavot qui fournit l'opium, la morphine, la codéine, la narcotine et la papavérine. Sans le pavot dont le pouvoir analgesique et antispasmodique est connu et utilisé depuis des millénaires il n'y aurait probablement pas de médecine moderne. Homère, qui célèbre la richesse en plantes médicinales de l'Egypte, fait sans doute allusion au pavot dans le passage de l'Odyssée ou il raconte qu'Hélène offre a Ulysse attristé par le souvenir de Télémaque un «breuvage d'oubli». Il décrit d'une manière très claire pour des spécialistes l'action soporifique de jus de pavot et conclut: «La fille du dieu possedait diverses drogues magiques et efficaces dont lui avait fait présent Polydamne, une égyptienne, épouse de Thot.»

Le Papyrus Ebers parle aussi d'un ingrédient sous forme de poudre qui fait disparaître les douleurs «Causées par les vers dans l'intestin c'est la jusquiame dont le nom Scientifique est Hyoscyamus».

La jusquiame, elle aussi, joua un rôle important dans l'histoire de la médecine égyptienne en tant que narcotique «qui abaisse les paupières avec une puissance invisible» employé en décoction; son action provoque des phénomènes hallucinatoires. En dehors de la narcose, la jusquiame était également génératrice d'hallucinations véritables et de troubles du système nerveux qui, dans certains cas, pouvaient aller jusqu'à la démence. Dans la jusquiame les chimistes modernes ont également découvert de la scopolamisse, alcaloîde dont l'effet sur certains centres nerveux est mis à profit pour le traitement des troubles du système neurovégétatif.

Aussi la pharmacopée égyptienne mentionne *le datura*; on crut longtemps que la première mention connue du datura figurait dans la relation des campagnes d'Antoine contre les Parthes qui avaient envahi l'Asie Mineure (36 av J.C.) Le passage en question précise: «Les soldats durent se rebattre sur les racines et sur des herbes dont ils ignoraient tout. Ils en trouvèrent une qui tuait après avoir troublé l'esprit. Quiconque en mange oubliait ce qu'il avait fait jusqu'alors et ne se rendait plus compte de rien» En fait, les Egyptiens utilisaient depuis fort longtemps une variété de datura, la *stramoine*, renfermant de l'hyoscyamine et de l'atropine pour calmer la douleur.

Les Egyptiens avaient parfaitement conscience de la toxicité des ces plantes. Les médecins s'efforçaient de les doser et ne les administraient qu'après avoir soigneusemant pesé et mesuré les ingrédients entrant dans la fabrication des potions et des médicaments. Ceci permet d'affirmer que la préscription et l'ordonnance furent inventées par des Egyptiens. D'alleurs le *Rp* par lequel les médecins commencent leurs ordonnances est originaire d'Egypte – Les anciens avaient l'habitude d'invoquer le Dieu. Le dieu égyptien Horus avait perdu son oeil dans une lutte contre Seth. Cet *oeil de Horus* qui *ressemble à un R* est devenu une convention médicale depuis l'Antiquité jusqu'aujourd'hui.

Aussi les égyptiens se servaient-ils des différentes parties de cet oeil *Oudjet* (c'est à dire de l'oeil de Horus mis en morceaux par Seth) comme symbole de fractions d'une mesure de capacité tant pour les grains que pour les liquides. Cette mesure est le hequat, boisseau, unité de mesure correspondant à une capacité de 4,785 l. qui jouait, dans la vie quotidienne, un rôle beaucoup plus important que la balance; l'unité de mesure pour la composition des remèdes était le «ro» (320e partie du boisseau qui équivalait *grosso modo* au contenu d'une cuiller à soupe (15 cc). Le henou = 0.478. Les Anglais ont employé ces différentes parties de l'oeil de Horus aussi comme signes de mesures minutieuses dans leur médecine.

Iwti, médecin à la cour, contemporain de Ramsis 1er et de Selhi I., possédait dans son laborataire un riche assortiment de drogues, d'onguents, de végétaux et de substances diverses «produits» d'une tradition qui comprenait plusieurs dizaines de générations de médecins. Ce n'était qu'une partie de son «arsenal», de plus la bibliothèque d'Iwti renfermait plusieurs traités permettant de préparer plusieurs centaines de remèdes. Chose plus importante, les traités indiquaient quand il convenait de prescrire tel ou tel médicament compte tenu d'un ou de plusieurs symptômes, et ils énuméraient les signes spécifiques de la plupart des affections, ils signalaient, entre autres, que les maladies étaient la conséquence du mauvais fonctionnement des organes et non pas celle d'interventions d'esprits malins et de créatures démoniaques. Parmi ces traités figurait, en bonne place, le Papyrus Ebers comme nous l'avons montré.

Au Moyen Age le rôle des médecins arabes comme Avicenne dans la transmission de la médecine et la pharmacie en Europe était très grand. Beaucoup de mots et termes égyptiens et arabes sont introduits dans les langues européennes.

Par exemple: Le mot *girofle* vient du mot arabe: «Kironfel». Le mot *Carmin* (qui signifie rouge foncé) vient du mot arabe «Kormosi». Le mot *Safran* (Zaffrano en italien) vient du mot arabe «Zaafran». Le mot *Lilas* (qui signifie couleur violette) vient du mot arabe «Lila». Le mot épinard (Espinach en ancien français et spinaci en italien) vient du mot arabe «Spanich». Le mot *gala* (qui signifie fête ou cérémonie) vient du mot égyptien «gala» (qui signifie «la chose qui brille» de gala on a eu les mots de familles nobles: galante en français, galanti en italien, d'où est dérivé le mot galanterie. Le mot *nitrate* vient du mot égyptien «natrou» endroit qui existe en

Egypte depuis le temps des Pharaons, où l'on extrayait les sels du Natron nécessaires à la momification. Après avoir sorti la cervelle par les narines et les organes abdominaux, on mettait le corps, à sec, dans ces sels, durant quarante jours. Sous l'action de ces sels l'eau est imbibée, l'effet destructeur des bactéries supprimé, et ainsi le corps se conserve durant des milliers d'années. Le mot *jupe* vient du mot arabe «gibba». Le mot blouse dérivé du nom d'une ville égyptienne «Blouseum» connue pour la fabrication des blouses de couleur bleue que les européens portaient depuis le moyen âge. Le mot *coupe* (coppa en Italien) vient du mot indo-européen et arabe «kouba» désignant la construction en coupole. De ce mot on a cup en anglais, kopf en allemand, etc. Le mot *banane* est dérivé du mot arabe «banane» qui est le doigt au milieu de la main.

Outre qu'en Egypte, en Italie, en France, en Allemagne et aux pays arabes, des manuscrits arabes sur la médecine et la pharmacie se trouvent dans le magnifique *Catalogue of Arabic Manuscripts on Medicine and Science in the Wellcome Historical Medical Library*, de A. Z. Iskandar.

Bibliographie

ALLEN, G. F., 'Bilharzia, hoematobia & Circumcision', *The Lancet*, May 1909.

BERLIN PAPYRUS: W. Wressinski, *Der Grosse medizinische Papyrus der Berliner Museum*, Leipzig, 1909.

DOLLFUS, M. A., 'l'ophtalmologie dans l'ancienne Egypte', *Bulletin de la Société française d'Egyptologie*, no. 49, juillet 1967.

MADDEN, FRANK COLE, *The Surgery of Egypt*, Cairo, The Nile Mission Press, 1919.

EBBEL, 'Die ägyptische Krankheitsnamen', *Z.A.S.*, 1927, **62**, 16.

EBBEL, *The Ebers Papyrus*, Copenhagen: Levin and Minkagaard, 1937.

EBERS PAPYRÜS, G., *Ebers und L. Stern, Papyrus Ebers: Das hermetische Buch über die Arzneimettel der alten Aegypter*, Leipzig, 1875, 2 vols. Transcription, W. Wreszinski, Der Papyrus Ebers, Leipzig, 1912.

GRAPOW, *Untersuchungen über die altaegyptische medizinischen Papyri*, 1935 and 1936, tome 11, p. 101.

GILBERT, PIERRE, *La valeur de la civilisation égyptienne*, extrait du no. 9 de la Revue Internationnale Synthèses, Bruxelles, 1948.

GILBERT, P., *La poésie égyptienne*, Bruxelles.

Hearst Papyrus, REISNER, G. A., *The Hearst medical Papyrus*, Leipzig, 1905, transcription, W. Wreszinski, *Der Londoner Medizinische Papyrus und der Papyrus Hearst*, Leipzig, 1912, pp. 1–133.

JONCKHERRE, *Une maladie égyptienne: l'Ematurie parasitaire*, Bruxelles, 1944.

LEFEBVRE, C., *Essai sur le Médécine Egyptienne de l'époque Pharaonique*, Presse Universitaire de France, 1956.

LONDON PAPYRUS (see Hearst Papyrus above), transcription Wreszinski.

PFISTER und UEBER, 'das Penisfutteral des agyptischen gottes Bes' (Ein Bertrag zur Feschachte des Kondoms), *Arch. F. Gesch d. Med. Leipzig*, **6**, 59–64.

RIAD, NAGUIB, Comment prédire le sexe de l'enfant avant sa naissance, etc., thèse de doctorat en médecine, Genève, 1945.

RIAD, NAGUIB, *La médecine au temps des Pharaons*, Edition Maloine, Paris, 1955.

RIAD, NAGUIB, Parasitic Hoematuria in Ancient Egypt', Proceeding of the 1st International Symposium of Bilharziasis, part 1, pp. 171–74, Scientific and Technical Documentation Divisions of National Research Centre of Egypt, Dokki Cairo.

RIAD, NAGUIB, *History of Medicine in Ancient Egypt and its influence on Greco-Roman and European thought*, 'sous presse'.

WALKER, K, *Histoire de la Médecine*, Marabout université.

M. Bihan
Paris (*France*)

Episode des relations de la médecine britannique avec la médecine française; à propos de Jenner et de la vaccine

Un certain nationalisme scientifique et notamment quelques chauvinismes médicaux sont la manifestation la plus internationale . . . du sentiment patriotique: il n'est guère de grande découverte qui n'ait été revendiquée par plusieurs autres que celui à qui elle avait été initialement attribuée: plusieurs Européens et plusieurs Asiatiques auraient inventé la boussole avant le marin d'Amalfi, découvert l'Amérique avant Christophe Colomb, l'imprimerie avant Gutemberg ou expliqué la circulation du sang avant Harvey. . . . Chaque pays veut absolument s'honorer de posséder parmi ses grands hommes tel ou tel chercheur qui avait découvert la microbiologie avant Louis Pasteur ou avant Robert Koch et le phénomène antibiotique avant que Fleming trouvât la penicilline.

La différence entre le véritable inventeur et les inventeurs supposés ou prétendus est le plus souvent la trouvaille de celui qui, grimpé dans l'Arbre de Science, cherche et découvre le fruit mur et le cueille à celui qui le voit tombé à terre, écarte l'herbe et le ramasse.

Nous avions adopté, en France, sans discussion, la version classique chez nous, et même populaire qui veut que, sans partage, Edward Jenner soit le découvreur de la vaccine. J'avais récemment relu dans une traduction française, *publiée en 1811*, d'un Eloge de Jenner par le docteur Lettsom, à la Société de médecine de Londres, éloge prononcé de son vivant et, peut être, en sa présence:

qu'il avait observé vers 1775, en inoculant la variole (smallpox) que ceux qui avaient contracté l'éruption des trayeurs de vaches (cowpox) résistaient à l'épreuve;
qu'il avait été frappé et bientôt convaincu de l'idée que l'inoculation «artificielle» du pus prélevé sur des vaches ou sur des individus *spontanément vaccinés*, préservait l'homme de la petite vérole;
Nous croyions aussi que la «Recherche sur les causes et les effets de la vaccine variolique» était la conclusion de 23 ans d'observations menées par un génial empirique avec une rigueur scientifique voisine de la perfection et, donc, que Jenner était «seul, l'architecte qui avait édifié, depuis la base, le temple glorieux».
Nous croyions savoir par ailleurs que la vaccination jennérienne avait diffusé en France (et du vivant même de Jenner) mieux et plus vite qu'en son pays.

C'est ainsi que dans une collection de vieux documents, nous avons lu le texte d'une lettre pastorale de l'archevêque de Paris autorisant, en 1822, ses prêtres à contraindre leurs paroissiens à se faire vacciner sous la menace de se voir refuser les sacrements . . . ainsi que de nombreuses et très officielles *Instructions sur la Vaccine* imprimées par ordre des autorités nationales et départementales françaises.

Or, soudain dans le texte de l'une de ces instructions, la phrase suivante nous a fait sursauter: «Il parait certain que la découverte de la vaccine est due (sous entendu: non pas à Jenner mais) à un français, Mr. Rabaut-Pomier, Ministre du culte réformé. . . .» Et la plupart des dictionnaires encyclopédiques français aussitôt consultés reprenaient cette affirmation avec plus ou moins de vigueur.

Ce bouleversement de notions universellement acquises nous a amenés à consulter l'encyclopédie médicale de Panckoucke – monument scientifique, critique et polémique en 60 volumes, publié entre 1812 et 1821, c'est à dire du vivant de Jenner – à l'article «vaccine». Nous avons lu ceci (je résume): «la propriété antivariolique de la maladie des vaches était connue aux Indes, en Chine, en Amérique du Sud, dans de nombreux comtés d'Angleterre, en Allemagne et ailleurs, bien avant que le docteur Jenner publiât ses travaux; le docteur Sutton, célèbre inoculateur anglais de la variole dès 1768, avait constaté que la vaccine accidentelle prévenait de la petite vérole aussi bien inoculée qu'épidémique; mais ce fut en France, entre 1781 et 1784, qu'on eut l'idée première du transport immunisant pour l'homme de l'éruption purulente (la picotte) des pis des vaches; cette idée fut émise par le pasteur Rabaut-Pomier à deux anglais qui passaient l'hiver de 1784 à Montpellier: un industriel de Bristol, Mr. James Ireland et un médecin, le docteur Pugh, lequel promit d'en aviser Jenner dont il connaissait la personnalité et les travaux.»

Le ton de l'article du Panckoucke était non seulement affirmatif, mais revendicatif et même agressif: à l'époque, entre la France et l'Angleterre, ce n'était pas l'Entente cordiale, ni les prémices du Marché Commun et, pendant qu'il y était, l'auteur de l'article, le médecin Husson, n'hésitait pas à accuser les Anglais d'avoir, pêle-mêle «emprunté» à la France, avec la vaccine, le principe de la presse hydraulique, celui de la machine à vapeur, celui de la lampe à gaz d'éclairage, ceux des affûts de marine et des moyens de désinfection des bateaux par fumigations, la théorie du chlore et une méthode d'enseignement mutuel dite «méthode de Lancastre. . . .»

Inquiet pour l'honneur national de chacun de nos deux pays et pour l'éthique de ce qui, un peu moins de deux siècles plus tard, allait devenir le Marché Commun de la science, nous avons scrupuleusement analysé la correspondance autographe de Rabaut-Pomier ainsi que son personnage:

Il était d'une famille de pasteurs protestants, les Rabaut, dont le rôle et l'activité, considérables pendant les premières années de la révolution française, se sont traduits par l'introduction de la tolérance religieuse, de la liberté de conscience et de l'égalité des droits dans nos constitutions.

(Dans un autre ordre d'idées, c'était, peut être, aussi important que d'avoir inventé la vaccine.)

Il me semble certain qu'il eut la nette intuition entre 1781 et 1784 – mais pas plus que l'intuition – de la possibilité de substituer la vaccination (cowpox) à la variolisation (smallpox).

Mais il n'était pas médecin, et ne consigna pas par écrit son observation; il semble hors de doute qu'il en fit part, mais verbalement, à plusieurs médecins compatriotes à Montpellier, et notamment, ensuite, en 1784, au médecin anglais Pugh; mais en quels termes? . . . et rien ne prouve qu'il fut écouté et encore moins suivi;

rien ne prouve non plus que le Dr. Pugh connaissait Jenner et ses collaborateurs ou ses correspondants et lui transmit les idées de Rabaut-Pomier.

Toujours est-il qu'entre 1784 et 1799 – pendant quinze ans, les quinze années essentielles des travaux de Jenner – il n'y eut ni ne put guère y avoir de rapports entre celui-ci et Rabaut-Pomier.

Du reste, ce dernier faisait alors une carrière politique agitée à l'extrême qui ne lui laissait guère le temps de se livrer à des travaux d'amateur en matière de pathologie infectieuse. . . .

Ce n'est qu'en 1800, à l'occasion d'une trêve franco-anglaise, et des préliminaires de la Paix d'Amiens, lorsque la vaccination jennerienne eut passé la Manche et «fait un triomphe» comme on dit, dans notre pays, que Rabaut-Pomier eut l'idée de réclamer sa part de gloire.

Il écrivit à son ami anglais Ireland qui convint volontiers et confirma (en français),

qu'il se rappelait la conversation avec le docteur Pugh (sur l'hypothèse d'inoculer à l'homme la picote ou petite vérole des vaches (ou cowpox) pour adoucir les effets de l'autre), mais qui ajoutait: «Ce que vous avez constaté au docteur Pugh l'an 1784 à Montpellier a été éprouvé ici *avant* l'an 1784 et confirmé par l'indéfatigable recherche de Monsieur Jenner. . . .»
Rien de plus, dans la lettre de M. Ireland sinon que le docteur Pugh était mort depuis 6 ans; rien sur le fait qu'il eut ou non rapporté à Jenner ou à d'autres médecins anglais les dires de Rabaut-Pomier.
Celui-ci obtint cependant du Comité central de vaccine de Paris, qu'il fut fait mention dans son rapport annuel de 1810, de son observation de 1784.
Objectivement, c'est tout. Il ne semble pas non plus qu'il existe dans les archives ou dans les bibliothèques anglaises la moindre trace de l'intervention de Rabaut.
En 1811, Napoléon faisait vacciner le Roi de Rome et nommait Jenner membre étranger de l'Institut de France («cela lui est bien dû»). Pas question de Rabaut-Pomier à ce moment là. Pourtant, il était bien vivant. Député à la convention, il avait voté la mort du Roi, mais sans intention de la donner et fut exilé quelques années de 1816 à 1823 comme régicide, puis pardonné. On peut dire, de même – sous réserve de l'existence de documents plus probants que ceux que nous avons consultés – qu'il avait imaginé la Vaccine sans intention de l'inventer et encore moins de la pratiquer. . . .

Quelles conclusions tirer de ces épisodes? Rien de plus et rien de moins pour ce qui concerne l'immense gloire de Jenner, consacrée par des milliards de vies humaines sauvés.

En revanche, une preuve de plus de l'absolue internationalité des Sciences et surtout médicales et de la merveilleuse perméabilité aux notions humanitaires de frontières apparemment fermées par l'état de guerre, l'état de haine ou l'état de blocus.

La preuve aussi peut-être, d'un état de faits qui n'est institutionnalisé que depuis peu: à savoir, que les grandes découvertes ne sont et n'ont été pas plus le fait d'un seul hasard que d'un seul homme mais d'une étude, d'une recherche plus ou moins rapide, plus ou moins concentrée et cohérente et d'une équipe plus ou moins dispersée, constituée ou géniale.

Enfin, et en revanche, que le titre de bienfaiteur de l'humanité ne se partage pas comme un prix Nobel.

N.B. Mes sources ont été essentiellement l'article «Vaccine» du Panckouke et le dossier Rabaut-Pomier àla Bibliothèque du protestantisme français, Rue des Saints Pères.

J. Brossollet
Paris (France)

Expansion européenne de la suette anglaise

La Guerre des Deux Roses déchirait l'Angleterre depuis 35 ans lorsque la bataille de Bosworth Fields donna la victoire aux Tudors en août 1485 et le pays espéra connaître enfin une période de paix et de prospérité. Mais les armes ne sont pas le seul fléau redoutable et, à l'automne, une maladie épidémique d'une nature inconnue décima l'Angleterre jusqu'au printemps de 1486, dont Thomas Le Forestier, médecin français de passage à Londres, donna la première description.

La maladie reparut ensuite dans la capitale en 1507 puis, en 1517–18 à Londres et à Chester d'abord avant d'envahir le reste du pays, tuant si vite qu'elle fut surnommée l' «Ephémère».

Dix ans plus tard Londres et le Pays de Galles en subirent à nouveau les assauts mais, cette fois la maladie ne limita pas à l'Angleterre le privilège de ses ravages et, en 1529, le nord de l'Europe occidentale apprit à la redouter: France, Suisse, Belgique, Hollande, Danemark, Allemagne, Suède, Norvège, Pologne, Lithuanie et Russie d'Europe maudirent la «suette anglaise» (*sudor anglicus*), que les français nommèrent «trousse-galant» d'après le sens «enlever rapidement» du verbe trousser.

La maladie sembla avoir trouvé sur le continent un milieu lui convenant davantage et elle quitta définitivement l'Angleterre après une dernière apparition en 1551. John Caiüs, médecin à Shrewsbury, publia l'année suivante *A Boke of Counsell against the Disease Commonly called the Sweate or Sweatyng Sickness*, qui est la plus importance source de renseignements sur les épidémies anglaises de suette; c'est également le premier livre médical imprimé en Angleterre consacré à une seule maladie.

Caiüs décrit l'attaque brutale avec sensation d'appréhension, rappelant le mal cardiaque de Celse et Galien, frissons glacés, vertiges, maux de tête, douleurs dans le cou, les épaules, les poumons, prostration; cette phase glacée (allant d'une ½ heure à trois heures), est suivie de la période avec sueurs qui donne son nom à la maladie: sueurs profuses et malodorantes, venant subitement et accompagnant la montée de la fièvre (pouvant dépasser 40°C comme on le vérifiera plus tard), délire, soif intense, pouls rapide et collapsus final. Le cours de la maladie est extrêmement rapide et le malade, angoissé et souvent lucide, meurt en quelques heures. Ceux qui survivent à la 24° heure sont considérés comme hors de danger.

Caiüs insiste sur l'aspect strictement britannique de l'affection, rapportant que les étrangers visitant l'Angleterre n'en furent jamais atteints et que l'épidémie de 1529 n'avait touché, sur le continent, que les anglais en voyage.

Pourtant cette même année 1551, d'authentiques allemands de Stuttgart, Marburg, Strasbourg et de véritables hollandais succombèrent à la suette anglaise, dont personne n'entendit plus parler durant un siècle et demi.

Elle reparut en 1712 à Montbéliard et en 1718 le nord de l'Italie, la Normandie, l'Ile de France et l'Orléanais la subirent, ainsi que la Picardie où elle fut particulièrement intense. Mais son aspect s'était modifié et si elle fut moins meutrière que sur le sol britannique, elle ajouta à ses symptomes une éruption papulaire et vésiculaire et son cours fut plus long. Elle cessa du reste d'être qualifiée d'anglaise et devint la «suette picarde» ou «suette miliaire».

La France, l'Allemagne et l'Italie du Nord virent apparaître des épidémies de suette avec des intervalles silencieux sur l'origine desquels il n'est pas possible, actuellement, de porter un jugement: la maladie disparaissait-elle totalement pour resurgir brutalement, ou bien était-elle devenue tellement banale que seuls en étaient rapportés les épisodes particulièrement graves?

L'Italie souffrit de la suette principalement en 1755 et 1774 à Novare, en 1790 à Vérone, en 1817 (Novare et Vicence), 1823 (Novare), 1835 (Vénétie et Frioul), 1836 (Toscane); mais il semble qu'elle ait été endémique dans tout le nord du pays.

L'Allemagne et l'Autriche en reconnurent aussi la fréquence et elle fut assez répandue à la fin du XVIIIe siècle pour figurer sur l'acte de décès de Mozart (bien que les symptomes de la suette ne se rapportent pas aux circonstances de la mort du compositeur). Signalons la gravité des épidémies de 1801 (Bade, Bavière et Wurtemberg), 1830, 1835 et 1844.

Mais c'est en France qu'elle s'implanta le plus fermenent et, après avoir hésité entre le Nord (épidémie de Guise en 1759), la Normandie (Louviers en 1770, dont Lepecq de La Clôture donne une importante étude), la Provence (Forcalquier en 1772), la Picardie (1774 et 1832), le Languedoc (1781–82), l'Oise (1821) et la Seine et Oise (1839), elle choisit dans l'ouest de la France trois foyers principaux: Dordogne, Poitou et Charentes, qu'elle marqua profondément jusqu'au début du XXe siècle Après l'épisode de 1906 dans les Charentes, la suette n'a jamais repris, en France, les allures d'une grave épidémie. Cependant elle apparaît, presque chaque année, dans les relevés épidémiologiques départementaux, avec la déclaration d'un cas isolé (maladie à déclaration obligatoire no. 7).

Durant l'épidémie poitevine de 1887, M. M. Roux et Chantemesse se rendirent sur place pour tenter de découvrir le microbe responsable, mais leur recherche fut vaine, tout comme celles de leurs successeurs et les traités de médecine, reflétant l'incertitude et la diversité des opinions émises sur l'origine de la maladie, qualifient souvent la suette de «mystérieuse».

Pourtant la bibliographie la concernant est relativement abondante et chaque grande apparition de la maladie a été décrite soigneusement par les témoins.

Le Pecq de La Clôture, dans ses *Observations sur les Maladies épidémiques, année 1770*, étudia la suette de Louviers et considéra:

le climat: «après un été humide, il tombait de grandes pluies . . .» cette humidité sera remarquée par tous les auteurs anciens, à l'exception de Caiüs qui qualifie d'hiver sec la saison qui précéda la suette de 1551.

le site: «sol plat et fertile . . . petite chaîne de collines, la ville ouverte au nord, au nord, au midi et au sud où se trouvent les marais. . . .»

les habitants: «des centaines d'ouvriers employés dans les filatures habitant des cabanes humides où les familles sont entassées». Il remarque que tous les âges et les deux sexes sont également atteints.

le cours de la maladie: débute avec un «mal de tête violent, l'horreur fébrile, l'oppression avec anxiété dans les parties précordiales»; ces signes s'affirment jusqu'au 10e jour où apparaissent des taches pourpres à la poitrine, aux poignets et au cou: «quelques pustules semblables à de la rougeole boutonnée, avec des sueurs d'odeur aigre pourri et un resserrement des hypocondres augmentant la gêne précordiale.» Il indique une guérison dans plus de la moitié des cas. Cependant «si la nature devait succomber, les accidents devenaient effrayants, délire, convulsions, pouls petit et irrégulier; le ventre coulait abondamment». Il nota aussi une surdité vers le 7e jour, une toux douloureuse et la particularité de certains éléments cutanés «gros comme une fraise, d'autres lieu sombre ou noir, d'autres s'ulcèrent ou se gangrennent».

La description de Le Pecq de La Clôture est précise au point de remarquer «des pétéchies ressemblant à des piqûres de cousins», détail que les épidémiologistes du XXe siècle retiendront pour y voir la trace d'un vecteur.

L'épidémie de Louviers fut si tristement célèbre, en France, que onze ans plus tard, lorsque la suette miliaire reparut en Languedoc, la peur s'empara des habitants au point d'inciter les médecins à se soucier surtout de rassurer les esprits en atténuant les effets du fléau. L'Intendant de Toulouse écrivait: «Cette maladie n'est rien en elle-même . . . elle n'a fait de bruit que par la terreur que quelques uns se sont plus à inspirer. . . . C'est une fièvre miliaire très bénigne, mais que la frayeur aggrave à tel point que les malades et ceux qui les entourent s'étouffent pour se faire suer et qu'il en résulte de grands inconvénients.» Entre cette négation de la gravité et le chiffre de 30.000 morts avancé par la rumeur publique, il est malaisé d'estimer l'épidémie du Languedoc que les praticiens traitèrent par des saignées, de l'ipecachuana, de la pâte d'écrevisses et de la corne de cerf calcinée.

Celle qui frappa la Dordogne en 1841 a été décrite par Parrot qui, après une étude topographique du département, un aperçu sur les habitants et leur mode de vie, aborda l'invasion et la marche de la suette qualifiée par lui de «périgourdine». Il précisa d'abord la persistance des fièvres éruptives qui, deux ans auparavant, n'avaient pas quitté la région: scarlatine, variole, mais surtout rougeole et ces affections, généralement bénignes avaient eu souvent une fin brutale si rapide que parfois ½ heure ne s'écoulait pas entre l'état le plus satisfaisant et la mort.

«Et soudain, raconte Parrot, à la suite d'un orage, le vendredi 7 mai et les jours suivants, il se manifesta une maladie bien différente de la rougeole, mais difficile à reconnaître . . . tant elle était . . . sous la dépendance de la maladie qu'elle venait brusquement remplacer.» L'une après l'autre les communes souffrant de la rougeole sont atteintes par la suette qui étonne et surprend les praticiens: elle enlève une grande partie des malades et disparait une semaine plus tard pour reparaître un mois après ailleurs, toujours aussi rapide et aussi néfaste. Elle fut parfois si violente et de si courte durée que lorsque les médecins, officiellement requis par l'administration, arrivaient pour inspecter le nouveau foyer, elle en avait déjà disparu.

Parrot chercha à en comprendre la marche et rapporta, lui aussi, les sites atteints, les habitants frappés, sans trouver de lien entre les apparitions. Dans sa description clinique de la suette «périgourdine» il insista sur deux aspects de la maladie: des cas si légers que les malades ne s'alitaient pas ou très peu et, inondés de sueurs et couverts de pustules, vaquaient néanmoins à leurs occupations; par contre d'autres cas tuaient en quelques heures des malades qui paraissaient légèrement atteints; ceux qui survivaient à l'aggravation brusque des symptômes restaient longtemps affaiblis.

Il ordonna surtout le sulfate de quinine et avait une telle confiance dans cette thérapeutique qu'il indiqua plusieurs fois que tel ou telle malade mourut «de n'avoir pas pris le sulfate de quinine que je lui avais ordonné». Il conseilla aussi la saignée et la purgation, mais déconseilla de provoquer les sueurs en couvrant exagérément les malades.

Après avoir rapporté l'inoculation qu'il pratiqua sur lui-même d'un peu de sang de cadavre, qui lui provoqua le lendemain une plaque rouge semée de vésicules, tombant en farine le 3e jour, il rappella que la suette de 1841 fut, après sa disparition de la Dordogne, suivie d'une véritable épidémie de jaunisse.

Mais, après l'apparition de la maladie dans l'île d'Oléron en 1880, au cours de laquelle sont appliquées avec succès les frictions à l'eau froide aux malades ayant une fièvre à 40°C, c'est la grave épidémie du Poitou en 1887 qui a suscité un très grand nombre d'études, tant locales que dues aux éminents praticiens envoyés de Paris par le Ministère du Commerce et de l'Industrie (dont dépendaient à l'époque les services d'hygiène). Brouardel et Thoinot l'étudièrent, guidés par les découvertes bactériologiques récentes, mais ne purent en découvrir l'agent, pas plus que Roux et Chantemesse, venus du laboratoire pasteurien de la rue d'Ulm (Chantemesse tentera vainement encore d'en isoler l'agent, avec Marchoux et Haury, dans les Charentes en 1906). Les auteurs réaffirmèrent la simultanéité de la suette et de la rougeole, celle-ci apparaissant d'abord et celle-là survenant brusquement, soit de façon franche, soit sous la forme d'une «rougeole miliairée» ou d'une «suette rougeoleuse»; ils rattachèrent aussi la suette à la scarlatine.

Peu après cette épidémie du Poitou, Colin, rédigeant l'article «Suette» du *Dictionnaire Encylopédique des Sciences Médicales de Dechambre*, donna une large étude des maladies passées et discuta les théories contemporaines: il insista sur la tendance de la maladie à se perpétuer comme une endémie tenace en certains foyers très circonscrits, remarqua la haute léthalité de certains épisodes, comparables par leur densité à ceux du choléra ou de la grippe, et son extrême rapidité puisqu'en certaines communes elle disparaissait en 48 heures; mais le cours normal semble être d'une semaine et cette brièveté s'oppose au temps nécessaire à la convalescence. Il admit la non-contagion interhumaine: «la suette parait indépendante des communications humaines, la soudaineté de ses apparitions, sur des points éloignés, l'immunité des localités interposées entre les centres atteints, témoignent de la réalité d'un autre procédé de diffusion.» S'il rappela combien la saignée, recommandée encore par Broussais, a été néfaste, il vante les avantages des émétocathartiques et les heureux résultats des affusions froides dans les cas d'hyperthermie. Mais il resta très évasif quant à la nature de l'affection.

En 1906, les Charentes souffrirent de la suette miliaire que Haury décrivit, l'ayant étudiée sur place avec Chantemesse déjà témoin de celle du Poitou en 1887. Après avoir rappelé les précédentes apparitions de la maladie dans cette région (1841, 1855 en même temps que le choléra, 1858, 1887), Haury rappela une fois encore la présence de la rougeole précédant la suette; l'invasion est toujours la même: brusque et souvent nocturne, avec sueurs abondantes et, après une courte période de frissons glacés, fièvre, état gastrique, angoisse thoracique et apparition de l'éruption au 3e ou 4e jour; rarement localisée à la face, elle survient sur le cou, les membres supérieurs le dos et la poitrine; les vésicules coniques, rouges ou blanches, ressemblent à un grain de mil mais l'aspect n'en est pas uniforme et les médecins locaux disent que les malades ont «la rougeole d'un côté du corps et la scarlatine de l'autre». L'éruption est généralisée en 48 heures, amenant une baisse rapide de la température et des phénomènes nerveux. La desquamation se produit vers le 8e jour, en grands lambeaux, parfois en poussière et peut durer plusieurs semaines; la convalescence, longue et lente, voit les malades encore très affaiblis après plusieurs semaines ou plusieurs mois.

Haury observa aussi les différentes formes de la suette, graves, mortelles, légères et frustes. Dans les formes hyperthermiques (où les fièvres à 42°–43°C ne sont pas rares), les bains froids ont permis une baisse rapide de la température.

Dans son rapport statistique, géographique et épidémiologique de la maladie, Haury insista sur l'hygiène précaire des paysans et sur les mesures élémentaires à instaurer: aérer les chambres, changer le linge, couvrir moins chaudement les malades. Puis il chercha, lui aussi, l'origine de la suette et il chercha une clé à l'inexplicable survenue et disparition de la maladie dans la localisation essentiellement rurale qui, au XIXe et au XXe (et à l'inverse de ce qui s'était produit au cours des siècles précédents) a toujours épargné les villes et les communautés humaines (couvents, pensions, casernes), pour frapper électivement les campagnes, d'une façon désordonnée, discontinue, illogique du point de vue humain. Il confirma la notion importante de non-contagion interhumaine.

Avec Chantemesse et Marchoux, il étudia l'extension en tache d'huile autour d'un premier cas et, conscient de la non-contagion (et de l'expression populaire «la suette est un venin de terre»), ils avancèrent l'hypothèse selon laquelle «la suette est une maladie d'un rat, probablement le rat des champs ou campagnol, transmissible à l'homme par les puces» et les auteurs appuyèrent leur démonstration sur l'envahissement des Charentes par les campagnols, peu avant le déclenchement de l'épidémie.

Cette hypothèse s'ajoutait à la longue liste des étiologies proposées pour expliquer la suette. Elle a été en effet jugée:

consécutive à la variole, la scarlatine, la fièvre typhoide, la jaunisse, le choléra et la rougeole.
et surtout identifiable à ces affections, ainsi qu'à: une forme grave de la fièvre récurrente, un empoisonnement par les végétaux ou l'arsenic, l'influenza, le paludisme, la peste, une maladie infectieuse dont le germe est localisé dans le système nerveux central, une fièvre inflammatoire rhumatismale. Mais c'est avec la rougeole que la suette miliaire fut le plus souvent confondue.

Mais jusqu'ici la suette miliaire continentale garde, tout comme la suette anglaise, le mystère de son origine, de son évolution et de sa disparition. L'identité de l'une avec l'autre fut, longtemps, un sujet de controverses: pour certains auteurs, la suette anglaise fut une maladie nouvelle apparaissant en 1485 pour disparaître définitivement en 1551 et qui doit être classée dans les maladies éteintes. Mais pour nombre d'autres, les différences apparentes entre l'une et l'autre ne doivent pas faire sous-estimer les liens profonds qui les rattachent et l'histoire des maladies épidémiques propose bien des exemples de maladies qui, suivant leurs déplacements, affectaient ici ou là une forme modifiée. Mais dans cette quête d'une origine déroutante, l'aide du laboratoire, précieuse dans un si grand nombre de maladies infectieuses, a été infructueuse pour la suette dont le germe n'est toujours pas isolé. Cependant les approches d'une identification sont entreprises dès que l'histoire clinique d'un cas le permet: ainsi en 1960, en France, Melnotte et Foliguet ont proposé, lors d'une observation à Nancy, un rapprochement avec la fièvre Q et, sans rien conclure, interrogèrent: «La suette miliaire est-elle une rickettsiose?»

D'autre part, l'implantation et l'extension d'une maladie nouvelle arrivée en France après la dernière guerre et dont les foyers bordent les zones atteintes au siècle dernier par la suette, incitent à étudier, à propos de la tularémie (dont cependant les manifestations ne peuvent être rapprochées de la suette) le rôle des populations de rongeurs et de leurs parasites dans ces deux affections.

Les quelques cas actuellement rares sont-ils les dernières traces de la suette miliaire, premier avatar de la suette anglaise et celle-ci, se modifiant une seconde fois, prépare-t-elle un retour imprévisible?

Bien que vaines jusqu'ici, toutes les recherches que l'étiologie de la suette a suscitées depuis 5 siècles se trouvent justifiées par l'auteur anonyme qui, dans l'*Edinburgh Medical & Scientific Journal* de 1808 réfutant une hypothèse donnant pour origine à la suette anglaise la consommation de blé corrompu, commençait son article par cet encouragement: «Every attempt to investigate the nature and causes of an epidemical disease, although unsuccessful, is still meritorious.»

P. Dumaître
Paris (France)

Quelques livres des imprimeries anglaises dans le fonds ancien de la Bibliothèque de la Faculté de Médecine de Paris

Cet exposé a surtout pour but de faire connaître aux spécialistes de l'histoire de la médecine – à travers quelques livres anglais – le fonds ancien de la Bibliothèque de la Faculté de Médecine de Paris [12, rue de l'Ecole de Médecine, Paris (VIe).] Nous nous sommes en effet maintes fois aperçus en consultant divers ouvrages d'histoire de la médecine, et non des moindres, que leurs auteurs, faisant le recensement de quelques livres rares ou précieux, orgueil des Bibliothèques, omettent de signaler la Bibliothèque de la Faculté de Médecine de Paris. Ils semblent ignorer que son fonds ancien est un des plus riches du monde. Quel est ce fonds? Comment a-t-il été constitué? Voilà les questions auxquelles nous essaierons de répondre. Cependant dans cet ensemble si riche, non seulement en ouvrages sortis des presses françaises mais en ouvrages édités en Allemagne, en Angleterre, en Hollande, en Italie, en Espagne, il nous a paru utile de signaler au public quelques productions des ateliers anglais qu'il n'aurait peut-être pas eu l'idée d'y venir chercher.

Il y a près de six siècles, en 1395, une petite Bibliothèque existait déjà à la Faculté de Médecine de Paris et il est probable qu'elle existait depuis le XIIIe siècle, depuis cette année 1200 où commencèrent à se réunir dans l'île de la Cité, autour de Notre-Dame, les quatre groupes des «théologiens», des «décrétistes», des «physiciens» et des «artistes», qui vont former l'Université de Paris. Pendant longtemps, près de trois siècles, les «physiciens» c'est-à-dire les médecins, n'eurent pas de domicile fixe. Ils tenaient leurs réunions la plupart du temps chez le doyen, aussi est-ce tout naturellement celui-ci qui fut choisi pour garder le bien le plus précieux de la Faculté, ses manuscrits, que le doyen sortant faisait transporter chez son successeur élu et responsable. Nous en avons la preuve dans le tome 1 des Commentaires, collection d'archives conservée à la Bibliothèque, écrite de la main des doyens et retraçant l'histoire de la Faculté de 1395 jusqu'à la Révolution. En effet, le 6 novembre 1395, le doyen Pierre des Vallées, dressant l'inventaire des biens qui allaient lui être confiés, ainsi qu'il était d'usage à chaque nouveau décanat, déclare avoir reçu treize livres dont il donne l'énumération: Averroès, Avicenne, Albucasis, Rhazès, Mesué le Jeune, Nicolas Myrepse, Galien. On reconnaît bien là toute la littérature médicale du temps.

Treize livres! Ce nombre peut nous paraître bien infime, mais c'était pourtant déjà une bibliothèque honorable. La Faculté considérait ses livres comme un véritable trésor. Quand ses coffres étaient vides, elle les engageait contre de fortes sommes et le roi Louis XI lui-même, fort féru de médecine, dut payer cent écus d'or lorsqu'il voulut emprunter les deux volumes du Continens de Rhazès. Pour précieux qu'ils fussent, il y a loin pourtant de ces treize volumes aux neuf cent mille environ que la Bibliothèque de la Faculté possède actuellement et qui font d'elle une des premières bibliothèques médicales du monde.

Cette Faculté errante, un jour vint où le nombre des élèves s'étant multiplié, elle sentit le besoin d'avoir une maison à elle pour y abriter ses Ecoles. En 1470, grâce à un legs du chanoine Jacques Despars, médecin de Charles VII, elle achetait une maison sise non loin de la Seine rue de la Bûcherie, où tout naturellement, et selon le voeu même du légateur, la «librairie» comme on disait alors, trouva sa place. A vrai dire, dans les siècles suivants, les médecins semblent s'être quelque peu désintéressés de leur Bibliothèque. De 1395 à 1516 les Commentaires ne mentionnent guère qu'une quarantaine de volumes. Cette indifférence continua pendant tout le XVIe et le XVIIe siècle. La Faculté s'agrandissait, achetait de nouvelles maisons, faisait construire en 1620 le théâtre anatomique dit de Riolan, mais elle achetait peu de livres, si bien que le Père Jacob disait en 1642 de la Bibliothèque: «Il n'en reste à présent que la mémoire dans les autheurs.» Au début du XVIIIe siècle elle ne comptait pas plus de trente-deux volumes, dans l'abandon le plus complet.

En vérité, la naissance réelle de la Bibliothèque, telle que nous la voyons aujourd'hui, date de 1732, année où mourut le docteur François Picoté de Belestre, savant homme qui possédait une très précieuse collection de livres qu'il légua à sa mort à la Faculté de Médecine. «Je lègue, écrivait-il dans son testament du 10 mars 1732 . . . ma bibliothèque . . . pour estre . . . établie, en mon nom, au service public dans l'Université de Paris d'où je suis docteur». Les 3456 volumes de cette bibliothèque auxquels se joignirent quelques dons, constituent donc le premier fonds de la Bibliothèque actuelle de la Faculté de Médecine de Paris.

La Faculté prenant son rôle très au sérieux, après tant d'années de négligence, installa ses volumes dans la sacristie de la chapelle de ses Ecoles, rue de la Bûcherie; le doyen Baron lui-même en rédigea un catalogue, les dons affluèrent, un bibliothécaire fut nommé, enfin on travailla si bien que le 3 mars 1746, sous le décanat de G. J. de l'Epine, la Bibliothèque était solennellement ouverte et le public y était admis tous les jeudis à 2 heures et demie jusqu'au soir.

La Révolution de 1789 qui devait tant bouleverser le monde allait se révéler favorable à la Bibliothèque. Depuis quelques années déjà elle avait dû quitter son antique demeure. Au début du règne de Louis XVI, la Faculté avait en effet abandonné ses locaux vétustes de la rue de la Bûcherie et les livres avaient suivi son sort. Ils étaient maintenant abrités dans les anciennes écoles de Droit, rue Saint Jean de Beauvais. Pendant ce temps, les chirurgiens si longtemps humiliés et qui avaient retrouvé en ce siècle leurs droits, honneurs et privilèges, s'installaient dans les nouveaux bâtiments que Jacques Gondoin, architecte du roi, avait entrepris pour eux dès l'année 1769, en face du couvent des Cordeliers, bâtiments que l'on peut toujours voir rue de l'Ecole de Médecine. Destiné à recevoir à la fois l'Académie royale de chirurgie et le Collège des chirurgiens-jurés, ce monument fut inauguré en octobre 1774 par le jeune roi Louis XVI. L'Académie royale de chirurgie y transportait alors sa bibliothèque dont le fonds principal était formé essentiellement par les 1392 volumes dus au legs généreux en 1747 de son fondateur François Gigot de la Peyronie à laquelle vinrent se joindre les 800 volumes des maîtres-chirurgiens jurés.

Les chirurgiens ne devaient jouir que peu de temps de leur magnifique demeure. La tourmente révolutionnaire survint qui atteignit en même temps la médecine et la chirurgie. Un décret de la Convention le 8 août 1793, supprime Académies, Sociétés littéraires et Bibliothèques. Un autre décret, le 13 septembre, décide la suppression des Facultés. De leur côté, les biens ecclésiastiques ayant été confisqués ainsi que ceux des princes et des émigrés, les livres précieux des couvents et des grands seigneurs étaient devenus le bien de la Nation. Soucieuse de conserver toutes ces bibliothèques enlevées à leurs propriétaires, l'Assemblée législative, qui avait pris en 1791 le décret contre les émigrés, les avait fait transporter dans huit grands dépôts littéraires établis dans d'anciens collèges ou des églises désaffectées. Le patrimoine littéraire et scientifique de la France était maintenant hors d'atteinte.

Après avoir démoli, il fallut bien reconstruire et le 14 frimaire an 3 (4 décembre 1794) la Convention prit un nouveau décret. Celui-ci établissait trois Ecoles de santé, à Paris, Montpellier et Strasbourg, abolissant du même coup la séparation entre la médecine et la chirurgie. Par ce même décret l'Ecole de Paris se voyait attribuer le local occupé par l'Académie de Chirurgie, ainsi que le couvent des Cordeliers. Il était stipulé en outre que chaque Ecole devait avoir une bibliothèque et celle de Paris un bibliothécaire.

Le local trouvé -celui où fut la Faculté de Médecine de Paris jusqu'en 1970, celui où se trouve notre Bibliothèque, celui-là même qui avait été construit pour les chirurgiens rue de l'Ecole de Médecine,- il fallait trouver l'homme. Le choix se porta sur Pierre Süe, savant chirurgien, descendant d'illustres chirurgiens, esprit fort distingué, qui fut nommé le 3 janvier 1795 «professeur-bibliothécaire» avec la lourde tâche de reconstituer et d'organiser la Bibliothèque.

La chance de la Bibliothèque, c'est d'avoir rencontré Pierre Süe. Cet homme infatigable ne recula pas devant un labeur immense auquel il consacra toute sa vie. Tout d'abord il eut à réunir les livres des Bibliothèques de l'Académie royale de chirurgie et des chirurgiens-jurés avec ceux de la Faculté de Médecine. Si les premiers étaient restés sur place, les seconds avaient été transportés de la rue Saint-Jean de Beauvais dans le grand dépôt littéraire installé rue des Cordeliers. Pierre Süe ne devait pas se contenter de les récupérer. Soucieux d'accroître ses collections, il profita d'un décret du Comité d'Instruction publique l'autorisant à choisir dans les divers dépôts littéraires les livres relatifs à la médecine, et il en profita largement. Pendant quatre ans, aidé d'un seul aide-bibliothécaire, Pariset, «élève de la Patrie», il passa, dit-il, «presque tous les jours l'hiver comme l'été un temps considérable dans tous les dépôts littéraires pour y choisir sur à peu près un million de volumes, ceux qui pouvaient convenir à la Bibliothèque de l'Ecole».

Telle donc a été l'origine du magnifique fonds ancien de la Bibliothèque de la Faculté de Médecine de Paris. Près de 25.000 volumes le composent – car il y eut aussi des achats du XIXe siècle – et si ce fonds ne comporte qu'une centaine d'incunables, les livres au XVIe siècle abondent, et les XVIIe et XVIIIe siècles ne sont pas moins représentés. Une Réserve a été constituée en octobre 1960 où, sous l'œil de maîtres anciens, figés dans leurs peintures, Avicenne, Galien, Jean Fernel, Dalechamps, Garengot et bien d'autres, les lecteurs peuvent travailler en paix. Parmi tous ces livres, nous voudrions détacher quelques livres anglais, dont il est difficile de démêler l'origine, mais qui témoignent du caractère universel de nos collections.

Deux livres rares, datant tous deux du début du XVIe siècle, s'imposent tout d'abord à nous: le *Judycyall of uryns* (F.M.P. 9009) dont nous ne connaissons ni l'auteur, ni l'éditeur, mais qui sortit probablement des presses de Treveris à Londres vers 1527. Une gravure délicieusement archaïque orne la page de titre de ce livre qui, avec ses lettres gothiques, semble encore un incunable. L'autre livre, celui du chirurgien Hieronymus Brunschwig, paru en 1523 dans les mêmes ateliers, n'est pas un ouvrage inédit. Il est déjà célèbre par l'édition en allemand: *Dis ist das Buch der Cirurgia*, imprimée par Grüninger à Strasbourg en 1497, avec les jolies gravures sur bois si connues du public, l'apothicaire, l'homme percé de flèches, le médecin au chevet du malade, les réductions de fractures. Mais les gravures de l'édition anglaise parue sous le titre: *The noble experience of the vertuous handy warke of surgery* (F.M.P. 6526) ces gravures là nous les reconnaissons bien, mais ce ne sont plus celles de Brunschwig jugées sans doute désuètes, mais celles d'un autre chirurgien éminent, lui aussi de Strasbourg, Hans Von Gersdorf. Celui-ci venait en effet de publier dans cette ville en 1517, sous le titre *Feldtbuch der Wundartzney*, un des premiers livres de chirurgie écrit en langue vulgaire où les opérations nous sont présentées d'une manière beaucoup plus réaliste et précise que dans le dogmatique traité de Brunschwig. Sans doute les éditeurs anglais ont-ils pensé qu'il n'était plus possible, après avoir eu connaissance des gravures de Gersdorf, de rééditer celles de Brunschwig, et selon les coutumes de ce temps là où les illustrations étaient copiées sans vergogne d'un livre à l'autre, ils ont emprunté pour illustrer le vieux traité de Brunschwig les toutes nouvelles planches du récent traité de Gersdorf. Sur la page de titre nous reconnaissons les trépanations faites avec le trépan perforatif, le «triploïde», inventé par Gersdorf, qui n'est autre que la «tarière» de Galien munie ici d'un dispositif spécial permettant de la manœuvrer sans danger: ce trépan est garni d'un bouton en forme de manche que l'opérateur fait tourner avec la main seule, les trois pieds de l'instrument appuyant sur le crâne d'un homme dont le visage tourmenté porte très exactement les marques de la paralysie consécutive au violent traumatisme qu'il a subi. Si nous feuilletons le livre, nous retrouvons au passage toutes les gravures de Gersdorf à peine modifiées: les célèbres planches montrant une extraction de flèche sur le champ de bataille, l'amputation d'une jambe, l'extension de membres grâce à un appareil perfectionné par Gersdorf, et bien d'autres encore, mais de petites gravures charmantes, qui ne sont pas de Gersdorf, apportent une note archaïque, tel ce savant tenant une rose entre les doigts. Une mention manuscrite sur une page de ce livre nous apprend le nom de son propriétaire avant qu'il n'entrât dans nos collections: *James Bardvell owe this Book*. A la dernière page la magnifique marque de Petrus Treveris: deux Sauvages, un homme et une femme, soutiennent l'écusson aux initiales P.T. suspendu à un arbre. A leurs pieds, une arbalète et sur un ruban le nom: Petrus Treveris, d'où certains ont conclu que l'éditeur était originaire de Trèves.

Un livre, un autre très grand livre anglais est aussi l'honneur de notre Bibliothèque. Il s'agit de cette première contrefaçon de Vesale, parue en 1545, deux ans seulement après la Fabrica, à Londres chez J. Herfordie et due, selon certains, à Pierre Coeck, selon d'autres à Thomas Gemini. Quoiqu'il en soit, ce dernier, un Flamand qui se disait chirurgien, fut l'éditeur de l'ouvrage qu'il dédia au roi Henri VIII sour le titre: *Compendiosa totius anatomiae delineatio aere exarata*, inscrit au bas d'un grand frontispice portant les armes d'Angleterre (F.M.P. 300). Ce bel in-folio reproduit trente-neuf planches exactement copiées sur celles de la Fabrica, avec les mêmes explications, mais cette fois gravées sur cuivre probablement par Gemini lui-même d'après les bois magnifiques dus au Titien ou à son élève Calcar, ce qui était une grande nouveauté, les livres étant jusqu'alors décorés de bois. A l' «Epitome» de Vesale, Gemini avait aussi emprunté les deux figures nues de l'homme et de la femme, gravées également sur cuivre mais son esprit imaginatif les avait transformées en Adam et Eve en substituant au crâne que l'homme de Vesale tenait dans la main gauche une énorme pomme, sans doute cadeau d'Eve. Le serpent tentateur avait abandonné l'arbre traditionnel pour sortir d'un crâne posé à terre. Cette gravure inspirera deux siècles plus tard François Michel Disdier dans son «Exposition exacte, ou Tableaux anatomiques» parue à Paris chez Charpentier, l'année 1758 (F.M.P. 2174). Toutes ces planches de Gemini sont si parfaitement belles qu'elles font de ce livre un monument dans l'histoire de l'art graphique en Angleterre.

Mathieu de Lobel fut un médecin français, né à Lille en 1538, docteur de Montpellier, qui après avoir beaucoup voyagé en Allemagne, en Suisse, dans le Nord de l'Italie, après avoir pratiqué la médecine à Anvers, à Delft, se rendit en Angleterre où il herborisa, car il était un botaniste distingué, fut honoré de l'amitié du roi Jacques et mourut à Highgate en 1626. S'il a laissé son nom à une charmante plante de la famille des Campanulacées, appelée Lobelia, il a aussi laissé des ouvrages, encore recherchés aujourd'hui. La première édition en collaboration avec Pierre Pena, de son ouvrage *Stirpium adversaria nova*, dédié à la reine Elisabeth d'Angleterre et paru à Londres en 1570 chez Thomas Purfoot (F.M.P. 959), porte sur la page de titre une jolie carte de l'Europe des frontières de la Moscovie jusqu'à celles de la Barbarie. En 1605, il fit imprimer à Londres chez le même Purfoot un autre ouvrage: *In F. Rondeletii methodicam pharmaceuticam officinam ad animadversiones* (F.M.P. 970) où nous reconnaissons sur la page de titre, à côté des armes d'Angleterre, le cachet *Jacobins R. S. Honoré* indiquant que ce livre fut la propriété à Paris du couvent des Jacobins.

Deux colonnes encadrant une mer où flottent des navires, tel est le majestueux frontispice de l'ouvrage capital de François Bacon, chancelier d'Angleterre, qui, après avoir été un homme politique, consacra exclusivement ses dernières années à la science et à la philosophie. Sous le titre général: *Instauratio magna*, il publiait, l'année 1620, avec de nouveaux développements, une version latine de son livre sur l'avancement des sciences qu'il liait à son célèbre traité: *Novum organum* (Londres, apud Joannem Bilium) (F.M.P. 1477). Dans son œuvre la médecine devait trouver les bases d'une nouvelle méthodologie. Au-dessous de ce noble frontispice, convenant bien à un livre qui contenait toute la pensée de Bacon, une devise «Multi pertransibunt et angebitur scientia», «Beaucoup traverseront et la science avancera». Et sous nos yeux, les navires semblent progresser sur la mer de la Connaissance.

Au XVIIe siècle nous nous étonnons un peu de trouver les Oeuvres complètes d'Ambroise Paré publiées à Londres l'année 1634 chez Ph. Cotes and R. Young sous le titre *The workes of that famous chirurgion Ambroise Parey* (F.M.P. 9037), dans une traduction de Th. Johnson faite d'après l'édition latine de 1582 et non d'après le texte français, ce qui est assez surprenant, Paré ayant écrit toutes ses œuvres en français. Si presque toutes les figures sont celles des éditions françaises, le frontispice, lui, est entièrement différent. Dû au réputé graveur Thomas Cecill, il montre des scènes de chirurgie avec les instruments, de pharmacie, d'anatomie, de distillation, et aussi les monstres chers à Paré avec tout en haut le portrait de l'auteur, déjà âgé, que nous reconnaissons comme étant celui de la 4e édition des Oeuvres complètes de 1585, celui de Vallée ou de Horbeck.

A côté de Paré, nous voulons citer un autre chirurgien, Thomas Gale, surnommé le Paré de l'Angleterre, qui est représenté dans nos collections par un seul petit livre, rare, et dont nous n'avons pas trouvé mention dans le catalogue de la Bibliothèque Nationale. Ce livre *Certain workes of chirurgerie newlie compiled and published by Thomas Gale, master in chirurgerie* (London, printed by Thomas East, 1586) (F.M.P. 6308) ne se signale d'ailleurs par aucune illustration.

L'ouvrage du médecin anglais Francis Glisson: *Tractatus de natura substantiae energetica seu de vita natura*, paru à Londres, sur les presses de E. Flesher en 1672, est, croyons-nous, assez rare, aussi notre Bibliothèque s'honore-t-elle d'en posséder deux exemplaires (F.M.P. 6249 et 6249 A). Glisson publia ce livre quand il était déjà âgé et le succès ne dut pas en être très grand puisque ses contemporains n'en parlent pas et qu'il ne fut pas réimprimé.

A la fin du XVIIe siècle, l'anglais William Cowper avait causé quelque scandale dans son ouvrage: *The anatomy of human bodies* (Oxford, 1698, printed at the Theater, for S. Smith and B. Walford) (F.M.P. 2042) par ses emprunts à l'*Anatomia humani corporis* du Hollandais Bidloo paru à Amsterdam en 1685, dont les planches, au nombre de cent cinq, avaient été gravées par A. Blooteling et les frères Van Gunst d'après les dessins originaux du peintre Gérard de Lairesse. Cowper, chirurgien de Londres de grand talent, avait acheté à un libraire d'Amsterdam les 105 planches de Bidloo et les avait publiées sous son nom, accompagnées d'un texte anglais entièrement nouveau et d'ailleurs plus complet et plus précis que celui de Bidloo. Celui-ci, bien qu'il fût nommé dans la préface, se fâcha et ce fut le début d'une célèbre controverse entre Bidloo et Cowper. Il faut reconnaître que Bidloo avait ses raisons: le frontispice de l'ouvrage de Cowper en est la preuve évidente. Ce frontispice, qui d'ailleurs n'est pas dû au talent de Gérard de Lairesse, est le même que celui de Bidloo: dans un décor théâtral, encadrée par des draperies, l'Anatomie, un livre d'une main, un scalpel de l'autre, est assise sur un piédestal au centre duquel un cartouche porte le titre de l'ouvrage. Examinons l'écusson du livre de Cowper à travers la lumière: nous y voyons apparaître le titre de l'édition hollandaise de Bidloo, en dessous de l'inscription actuelle. A un examen plus étroit, nous découvrons que la nouvelle inscription est en effet gravée sur un morceau de papier grossièrement collé et que l'inscription qui est effacée est celle que l'on voit sur la planche de l'édition hollandaise de Bidloo *Ontleding des Menschelyken Lichaam Godaan door Govard Bidloo Anat. et Chirurg. Professor* de 1690. Tel quel, l'ouvrage de Cowper, par la beauté de ses gravures sur cuivre, reste le plus remarquable atlas anglais d'anatomie de son siècle. William Cowper devait publier en 1724, sous les auspices du Docteur Meade, un bel in folio, la *Myotomia reformata* (F.M.P. 1892) avec de très belles planches dessinées les unes d'après Ruben, Raphaël, et d'autres d'après nature. Nous ne sommes pas près d'oublier ces écorchés, souvent réunis à plusieurs sur la même planche, dont les attitudes pleines de vie ne manquent pas cependant d'un certain pathétique.

Au XVIIIe siècle, c'est à un autre Anglais, à William Cheselden, premier chirurgien de la reine Caroline, que la Bibliothèque doit de posséder un autre magnifique ouvrage d'anatomie: *l'Osteographia or the Anatomy of the bones*, paru à

Londres en 1733 (F.M.P. 1897) dont le solennel frontispice découvre Galien en contemplation devant un squelette. Cinquante-six splendides gravures sur cuivre montrent les os en grandeur naturelle ainsi que des squelettes d'animaux et des figures d'os malades. Ces planches, faites la plupart par Gérard Vandergucht, d'autres par l'artiste hollandais Shinevert, ont été exécutées dans une chambre noire permettant un dessin plus précis et plus rapide. Cette «caméra obscura» est représentée en sanguine sur la page de titre avec la manière de s'en servir. On y voit Vandergucht devant la chambre noire dessinant un thorax qu'un des assistants de Cheselden tient suspendu, pendant qu'un autre, à côté, prend des notes. Quelques années plus tard, en 1749, l'éditeur Knapton publiait à Londres une édition anglaise du chef-d'œuvre d'Albinus *Tabulae sceleti et musculorum humani corporis* (F.M.P. 1676), déjà paru à Leyde en 1747, édition à la vérité moins belle que l'édition hollandaise, car, si les planches étaient les mêmes, l'exécution avait été confiée à C. Grignon, artiste moins heureux que Wandelaer qui avait su, dans les planches de Leyde, porter la représentation picturale à sa perfection.

Une découverte aussi importante que celle de la vaccination se devait d'être marquée dans nos collections par le livre de l'Anglais Edward Jenner: *An inquiry into the causes and effects of the variolae vaccinae* (Londres, 1789) (F.M.P. 6484) livre qui, croyons-nous, est d'une excessive rareté.

Au début du XIXe siècle, les livres des frères Bell, chirurgiens réputés en même temps qu'artistes de grands talents, seront les derniers livres anglais que nous signalerons, avant que le livre n'entre dans la grisaille des temps modernes. De John Bell, la Bibliothèque possède la 3e édition parue en 1811: *The anatomy of the human body* (F.M.P. 38116) avec d'admirables dessins des deux frères, et de Charles Bell: *A series of engravings explaining the course of the nerves* (London, Longman, 1803) (F.M.P. 6493) et l'on retrouve ce merveilleux crayon de Charles Bell dans les *Illustrations of the great operations of surgery*, paru à Londres en 1821 (F.M.P. 680), qui reproduisent admirablement les opérations de ce chirurgien réputé: trépanations, lithotomies, hernies, anévrysmes, et particulièrement une belle amputation de l'épaule à sa jonction.

Nous allons maintenant revenir trois siècles en arrière pour rappeler que, si notre Bibliothèque possède deux ouvrages rares, c'est à deux Anglais que nous les devons. Les *Tabulae anatomicae sex* d'André Vesale, publiées à Venise en 1538, cinq ans avant la *Fabrica*, sont aujourd'hui si rares qu'il n'en existe que deux exemplaires connus, l'un à la Bibliothèque de San Marco à Venise, l'autre en la possession de la Famille Stirling-Maxwell. En 1874, une réimpression tirée seulement à cent exemplaires fut faite, à titre privé, par les soins de Sir William Stirling-Maxwell; son fils, en 1909 devait offrir un de ces très rares exemplaires à la Bibliothèques de la Faculté de Médecine de Paris (F.M.P. 2012).

Plus émouvant est pour nous l'autre livre, un petit in octavo, rare lui aussi, puisqu'il n'en existe que trois exemplaires dans les bibliothèques françaises. Il s'agit du seul livre d'Ambroise Paré qui manquait dans nos collections: l'*Anatomie universelle du corps humain*, sorti à Paris des presses de Jean Le Royer l'année 1561 (F.M.P. 82, 949). Sir William Osler, le distingué professeur de médecine de l'Université d'Oxford, avait eu la chance de l'acheter en 1916 pour la somme de 250 francs – somme considérable pour l'époque – au libraire Lucien Gougy, lequel ne put lui en indiquer la provenance, l'ayant acquis dans un lot de livres non reliés. Lucien

Gougy fit habiller le livre par Chambolle-Duru d'une belle reliure de maroquin rouge et le vendit à Osler. Celui-ci écrivait en 1917 *La justice des choses demande que cet exemplaire finisse par retourner en France, à la grande collection de l'Ecole de Médecine* et il eut le beau geste, bien que ce livre n'existât pas au British Museum, de le léguer à notre Bibliothèque qui entra en possession de l'ouvrage en 1924, cinq ans après la mort d'Osler, survenue en 1919. Nous sommes heureux d'avoir ici à Londres l'occasion de l'en remercier publiquement. L'évocation de ce livre français donné par un Anglais nous semble la meilleure conclusion à notre étude du fonds ancien de la Bibliothèque de la Faculté de Médecine de Paris.

N.B. Lescotes indiquées entre parenthèses sont celles de la Bibliothèque.

Bibliographie

CHEREAU, ACHILLE, 'Notice sur les origines de la Bibliothèque de la Faculté de Médecine de Paris', in *Union médicale*, 3e série, 1878, **25**, 545–47, 597–602, 745–51, 777–82, 829–35.

FRANKLIN, ALFRED, *Recherches sur la Bibliothèque de la Faculté de Médecine de Paris*, Paris, Aubry, 1864.

GONDOIN, JACQUES, *Description des Ecoles de Chirurgie*, Paris, Pienes, 1780.

HAHN, ANDRÉ, *La Bibliothèque de la Faculté de Médecine de Paris*, Paris, Le François, 1929 (Thèse Méd. Paris, 1929, no. 417).

HAHN, ANDRÉ et DUMAITRE, PAULE, 'A propos de l'histoire de la Faculté de Médecine de Paris. Les Commentaires (1395–1792)', in *Annales de l'Université de Paris*, 1949, **19**, 498–507.

HAHN, ANDRÉ, DUMAITRE, PAULE et SAMION-CONTET, JANINE, *Histoire de la médecine et du livre médical à la lumière des collections de la Bibliothèque de la Faculté de Médecine de Paris*, Paris, Olivier Perrin, 1963.

HIND, ARTHUR M., *Engraving in England in the sixteenth and seventeenth centuries*, Cambridge, 1952.

LOWNDES, WILLIAM THOMAS, *The bibliographer's manual of English literature*, London, H. G. Bohn, 1858–1864, 10 vols.

OSLER, WILLIAM, 'The "Anatomie universelle" of Ambroise Paré', in *Annals of medical history*, 1917, **1**, 424–25.

POLLARD, A. W. et REDGRAVE, G. R., *A short title catalogue of books printed in England, Scotland and Ireland and of English books printed abroad 1475–1640*, Londres, the Bibliographical society, 1950 (continué par WING, DONALD, 1641–1700, New Haven, Conn.).

RUSSELL, KENNETH FITZPATRICK, 'A check list of medical books published in England before 1600', in *Bulletin of the history of medicine*, 1947, 21, 922–58.

P. Huard and M. J. Imbault-Huart
Paris (France)

Le voyage de Jacques Tenon (1724–1816) en Grande Bretagne (1787) et ses conséquences

Nous étudierons successivement les motifs, les acquisitions et les conséquences de ce voyage. Nous avions[1] depuis longtemps signalé l'intérêt des notes manuscrites prises par Tenon dont une étude récente de L. S. Greenbaum a montré toute la valeur.[2]

I. LES MOTIFS DU VOYAGE

Ce voyage se place d'abord dans un contexte général très développé en Grande-Bretagne et en France, mais aussi aux Pays-Bas et en Autriche: c'est l'émergence de la philanthropie et de la médecine sociale à laquelle nous avons déjà fait allusion.[3] Au début, ce voyage devait se dérouler dans plusieurs pays d'Europe mais sa durée aurait été trop longue. Il fut donc limité à l'Angleterre.

Agé déjà de soixante trois ans, Tenon «passa» la Manche, accompagné de Coulomb. Ce fut pour de multiples raisons: ses recherches personnelles sur la réforme des hôpitaux qui était à l'étude depuis un mémoire célèbre lu en 1773 à l'Académie des Sciences par le physicien J. B. Le Roy (1720–1800); la confiance qu'il inspirait à ses confrères de l'Académie des Sciences et au baron de Breteuil (1730–1807), ministre de la Maison du Roi; enfin, le dessein du gouvernement français de prolonger le traité de commerce Vergennes-Eden (1786–87) par un rapprochement sur le plan culturel, un *commercial treaty of Humanity* (un traité de commerce d'humanité). Le voyage de Tenon était donc autre chose qu'un simple voyage d'études scientifiques. C'était aussi une mission officielle dont l'Académie des Sciences avait informé la Royal Society et dont la réussite donnerait la température des relations franco-britanniques. Elle intéressait Vergennes aussi bien que Breteuil. S'il n'est pas directement en rapport avec notre ambassadeur à Londres, le comte d'Adhémar, Tenon est constamment pris en charge par son premier secrétaire Fr. Barthélémy (1747–1830), par le marquis d'Herbouville et le chevalier Quesnay de Beaurepaire petit-fils du chirurgien-économiste Fr. Quesnay (1694–1774).

Tenon ne fréquentait ni les salons anglophiles, ni les cercles aristocratiques devenus anglomanes à la suite du duc Philippe d'Orléans. Il avait la plus grande estime pour Howard et d'autres philanthropes d'Outre-Manche mais en bon sujet de Louis XVI, ni voltairien, ni rousseauiste, il admirait autant St-Vincent de Paul que Louise de Marillac dont il adressait les biographies à ses amis anglais, ainsi que des exemplaires de *De Vita Cartusiana*. Il leur conseillait aussi la lecture du «Voyage du jeune Anacharsis» par l'abbé Barthélémy.

Il ne parlait pas l'anglais (lacune qu'il regrettera plus tard) et il aurait été incapable de faire des cours dans cette langue comme certains professeurs libres parisiens, par exemple son collègue R. B. Sabatier (1732–1811). Il n'employait pas les techniques des chirurgiens britanniques comme le firent A. Louis et Desault.

En outre, il n'avait jamais passé la Manche comme l'avaient fait avant lui plusieurs chirurgiens français: J. Méry, J. S. Morand, Chopart et Antoine Dubois. Il ne connaissait donc pas la Grande-Bretagne et il y était totalement inconnu, aucune de ses publications n'ayant été traduite en Anglais. Il savait cependant le goût des insulaires pour les vins français et il débarqua avec 36 bouteilles de «Bordeaux» qui furent, d'ailleurs, saisies.

II. LE VOYAGE

Avant son départ de France, Tenon avait consulté le récit du voyage que le chirurgien tchèque J. Hunczovsky[4] (1752–98) avait exécuté en Angleterre et en France, sur l'ordre de l'empereur Joseph II. Une traduction incomplète du texte allemand existe dans les papiers de Tenon et a été publié avec des notes par J. Mounier. Ce voyage avait été effectué en 1777, mais la relation n'en fut imprimé à Vienne qu'en 1783.

La méthode suivie par les deux chirurgiens diffère fondamentalement. Malgré la longueur de son séjour en Grande Bretagne (13 mois), l'envoyé de l'empereur Joseph II (probablement moins bien introduit que Tenon) dans les milieux britanniques ramena dans son pays une documentation sérieuse mais certainement moins importante que celle de son collègue français. Par contre, beaucoup plus chirurgien qu'hygiéniste, il nous donne de nombreux détails sur les chirurgiens anglais qu'il a rencontrés, sur leur instrumentation et sur leur technique. Malgré cet aspect positif, son travail passa à tort, inaperçu alors que celui de Tenon fut l'objet des commentaires les plus élogieux des médecins britanniques.

Le voyage d'études de Tenon se situe du Ier juin au 3 août 1787. Compte tenu de la lenteur des moyens de communication de l'époque, on est étonné du grand nombre d'établissements étudiés, des nombreuses visites faites et de l'importance de la documentation déposée sur le bureau de l'Académie des Sciences et sur celui de Breteuil. Les notes personnelles de Tenon qui voyageait toise à la main sont d'une précision et d'une minutie extraordinaires, tant sur le plan architectural que sur le plan sanitaire et financier. Elles sont complétées par de nombreux croquis dont aucun ne parait avoir été publié jusqu'ici.[5]

Le programme qui lui avait probablement été en partie imposé lui facilitait des rencontres avec des naturalistes comme Sir Joseph Banks et avec des astronomes comme Nevil Maskelyne et Sir William Herschel. Pour le reste, tout fut sacrifié à l'assistance sociale, à la philanthropie et à l'hygiène hospitalière et Tenon dut rester sur sa faim en ce qui concerne deux disciplines qui lui étaient particulièrement chères, l'anatomie et la chirurgie.

S'il a pu visiter le musée de William Hunter, sous la conduite de son neveu W. Baillie, le 24 juin, il n'a pas été reçu dans la grande école anatomique de Windmill Street et il n'a pas vu, semble-t-il, le grand musée de John Hunter.[6] Il n'a pu s'entretenir qu'avec un petit nombre de chirurgiens britanniques.[7]

Néanmoins les contraintes de sa mission ne font pas oublier à Tenon qu'il est un praticien. Il note les maladies les plus couramment observées dans chaque hôpital et le traitement employé. Il n'oublie ni les femmes enceintes ni les nouveaux-nés dont le sclérème le préoccupe. La mortalité des accouchées varie de 1/54 (*British Lying-in Hospital*) à 1/100 (*London Lying-in Hospital*). La position obstétricale est le décubitus latéral avec accouchement postérieur. La mortalité néo-natale est de 1/60. A l'hôpital de Birmingham il apprend que «la digitale à fleurs rouges est employée avantageusement contre l'hydropisie»[8] et que l'arsenic est un fébrifuge.[9]

Le 30 juin, il visite l'hôpital français de Londres, fondé en 1716. Le directeur est un homme d'affaires, M. Gaussin. Sa capacité est de 200 personnes, nées en Angleterre mais d'origine française et de religion protestante. «Tout le monde parle français dans l'établissement. Notre présence attendrit ceux que nous y vîmes». Il ajoute que l'ambassadeur de France étant administrateur du *Guy's Hospital* (moyennant cinq guinées par an), des français indigents peuvent y être admis.

III. LES CONSÉQUENCES DU VOYAGE DE TENON

Si le contexte socio-politique français était resté à son retour d'Angleterre, le même qu'à son départ, il est probable que l'opinion publique aurait stimulé très fortement l'action gouvernementale en faveur des hôpitaux. Malheureusement ce thème fut largement dépassé dès 1789 par des problèmes d'une importance beaucoup plus grande pour le peuple français et pour ses dirigeants.

Dès son retour, Tenon fit la synthèse de la documentation énorme qu'il avait accumulée depuis longtemps. Il rédigea deux mémoires sur les hôpitaux anglais et leurs différences avec les hôpitaux français et contribua à la rédaction du troisième mémoire sur les hôpitaux, déposé sur le bureau de l'Académie des Sciences (1788).

Pendant ce temps, son confrère J. B. Le Roy faisait paraitre le travail qu'il avait lu à l'Académie des Sciences en 1773, avant que l'Imprimerie Royale n'édite le fameux *Mémoire sur les Hopitaux*. Tenon l'envoya par priorité à ses amis anglais et à leur roi Georges III, accompagné d'une lettre où il définissait la position que les gouvernements devaient adopter face aux deux grands maux sociaux qu'étaient le paupérisme et la maladie. Selon lui, il s'agissait d'un problème international qui ne pourrait être résolu que par la collaboration pacifique de toutes les nations européennes.

Dès la convocation de l'Assemblée Constituante, ses Commissions de Mendicité et de Santé firent appel à un grand nombre de spécialistes consultants dont certains envisagèrent la suppression de toute l'infrastructure médicale française et par conséquent celle des hôpitaux.[10] Cette attitude négative ne dura pas et la philanthropie de Tenon n'a pas été sans influencer celle du duc de La Rochefoucauld-Liancourt lorsque le Comité qu'il présidait proclama le droit de l'homme à la santé et la responsabilité gouvernementale en matière de paupérisme et de maladie.[11]

En 1791, Tenon rappelle aux assemblées révolutionnaires sa doctrine socio-hospitalière et il essaie de lui donner une consécration pratique, en tant que président du Comité des Secours Publics de l'Assemblée Législative. Mais effrayé par les massacres de Septembre 1792, il abandonne la vie politique pour se réfugier dans sa propriété de Massy et y continuer ses études d'anatomie comparée. Il en sort, en 1793, pour participer à une étude tendant à transformer le monastère du Val de Grâce en une maternité et en une école de sage-femmes. La participation de Tenon est très importante, mais le rapport remis à la Convention est seulement signé de Raphaël Bienvenu Sabatier, et de J. B. Le Roy, le physicien-hygiéniste dont nous avons déjà parlé. Ce rapport, demandé à trois savants éminents (dont deux étaient des spécialistes de l'hygiène hospitalière) montre le souci des gouvernements révolutionnaires d'être à la fois populaires et scientifiques. Il est le résultat de quatre séances de travail, au cours desquelles les capacités hospitalières du monastère sont étudiées étage par étage ainsi que le cubage des locaux et les mesures nécessaires pour obtenir une bonne aération des locaux.[12]

Malgré l'état de guerre, l'exemple des hôpitaux anglais est très souvent rappelé pour proposer des réunions et des concerts dans l'Eglise; approvisionner les réserves d'eau, avec l'eau de pluie ruisselant sur les toits et en particulier celui du dôme; assurer l'hiver la fluidité de l'eau contenue dans les réservoirs au moyen d'un poêle; installer des latrines, telles que chaque ouverture ou fermeture de la porte fasse jaillir automatiquement l'eau dans la cuvette; brancher sur les poêles des tuyaux permettant d'avoir toujours du linge chaud dans les salles.

Par contre, le plancher de la salle de travail, susceptible de pourriture, doit être remplacé par un dallage à la française, la jointure des dalles étant réalisée avec du plomb au lieu du mastic.

Ce rapport resta sans effet puisque le Val de Grâce devint finalement un hôpital militaire, la Maternité et le service des nouveaux-nés de l'Hôtel-Dieu étant installés dans les bâtiments de l'Oratoire et dans le monastère de Port-Royal. Telle est, du moins, la dernière participation de Tenon. Il ne semble pas s'être intéressé à l'introduction de la vaccination en France grâce aux efforts conjugés du gouvernement consulaire et d'émigrés comme le duc de La Rochefoucauld-Liancourt.

Quoiqu'il en soit, il n'en continua pas moins, plus qu'octogénaire à servir de trait d'union culturel entre l'Angleterre et la France en entretenant une importante correspondance avec ses partenaires britanniques, en favorisant leur élection dans les sociétés savantes parisiennes, en répondant à leurs demandes de renseignements avec diligence et bonne grâce, en les mettant en rapport avec leurs homologues français et en les recevant lui-même.

Pendant tout le XIXe siècle, les directives de Tenon en matière hospitalière sont souvent citées et ont eu une grande importance théorique en France et en Angleterre.

Dans une première période qui s'arrête vers 1795, les suggestions de Tenon (lit à une place, lit métallique, salles d'opérations isolées, désinfection des habits des malades, normes en matière de cubage d'air, de renouvellement d'air, de propreté, etc. . . .) firent l'objet de nombreux textes administratifs dont l'exécution ne pouvait être que partielle. A partir de 1795, il en fut de moins en moins question; la salubrité des hôpitaux cessa d'être un objectif gouvernemental et fut abandonnée aux cadres subalternes. Par contre, dès le Consulat, la gestion des hôpitaux parisiens fut totalement remaniée, tant sur le plan du personnel administratif que sur le plan du personnel médico-chirurgical (externat, internat, clinicat, médecins et chirurgiens des hôpitaux) et fut, en grande partie, purgée des erreurs de l'Ancien Régime.[13]

L'Hôtel-Dieu dont la démolition était prévue, dès 1787, ne fut que partiellement renové par Clavareau[14] en 1802 et resta une des formations sanitaires «les plus insalubres d'Europe». D'autres hôpitaux installés dans d'anciens couvents ne furent pas davantage l'expression des idées de Tenon dont deux directives furent pourtant retenues: le remplacement des chapelles affectées à chaque service par une chapelle centrale et la création d'amphithéâtres d'anatomie et de chirurgie dans l'enceinte des hôpitaux. Cependant, dès 1787 (et d'ailleurs indépendamment de Tenon) Desault[15] avait créé en dehors de toute aide officielle sa grande école anatomo-chirurgicale en assignant aux hôpitaux une finalité différente de celle de Tenon. Celle-ci, essentiellement philanthropique pense l'hôpital uniquement en fonction du malade. Dans la conception de Desault (et surtout de la génération suivante), l'hôpital devient, avant tout, un lieu d'enseignement et le laboratoire de la science. Dès lors, le malade-sujet des philanthropes se transforme pour la médecine nouvelle, à base d'autopsies en un malade-objet. Il constitue un indispensable matériel d'enseignement pendant sa vie et après sa mort, et le substrat obligatoire de la nouvelle école anatomo-clinique.

En terminant, notons que longtemps après Tenon, la médecine anglaise continuera à fasciner la France.[16] Le nom prestigieux de Lister ne doit pas faire oublier tous les praticiens britanniques qui avant et après lui ont reçu leurs nombreux collègues français curieux de visiter les hôpitaux britanniques.

References

1 HUARD, P., 'Les papiers de Jacques Tenon', *Congrès int. Hist. Méd.*, Bâle, 1964; TENON, 'chirurgien, anatomiste, philanthrope et pionnier des techniques hospitalières', *L'Hôpital et l'Aide Sociale à Paris*, 1966, no. 41, pp. 627–33; Nous avons consulté les manuscrits NAF 22744 et NAF 11354 et 11360 du fond Tenon (B.N.). Il contient un répertoire alphabétique et une table des matières.

2 GREENBAUM, LOUIS S., *The Commercial Treaty of Humanity*. 'La tournée des hôpitaux anglais par Jacques Tenon en 1787', *Revue d'Histoire des Sciences*, **24**, no. 4, October/December 1971, 317–50.

3 HUARD, P., 'L'émergence de la médecine sociale au XVIIIe siècle', *Concours Médical*, 1958, pp. 780–83.

4 Consulter MOUNIER, D., 'Journal du voyage médico-chirurgical de Jean Hunczovsky (1752–1798) en Europe occidentale', *Thèse de Méd. de Rennes*, 1968, no. 697.

5 Tenon était un dessinateur médiocre mais ses papiers contiennent d'assez nombreux croquis représentant le *Guy's Hospital*, un plan de Londres localisant les hôpitaux, des dispositifs de water-closets permettant de remplir et de vider la cuvette en ouvrant la porte etc. . . . Le Duc d'Orléans avait fait installer une de ces 'lunettes de commodité' au Palais Royal par des ouvriers anglais, Tenon écrit à l'architecte Dance: 'Je ne m'érige pas en architecte mais je me borne à faire des calculs de la longueur des lits, des salles, leur hauteur, la quantité d'air nécessaire à chaque malade, l'escalier pour les hommes faibles et boiteux, la longueur des brancards, les ouvertures des croisées, l'éclairage, etc.'

6 Consulter HUARD, P., William Hunter (1728–93) et John Hunter (1728–93), *Histoire de la Médecine*, 1958, no. VIII, pp. 3–40.

7 Les chirurgiens londoniens avec lesquels Tenon a été en contact sont: Poignant, Thomlison, Adair, Blizand, Baril. Il a eu des rapports particulièrement amicaux avec S. F. Simmons (1750–1813) de Londres, son correspondant favori. Il l'interroge sur les plus petits détails. 'Je vois que l'on éclaire vos hôpitaux avec l'huile de baleine. J'ai perdu de vue les moyens qu'on emploie pour la rectifier, je vous prierais de me le mander' (lettre du 13 novembre 1788). Il lui fait porter une lettre par une relation commune, le chirurgien prussien Goercke (1750–1822). Il le fait nommer son correspondant à l'Académie des Sciences en 1787, le jour même où Sir Joseph Banks est nommé associé étranger. En 1804, Simmons devient correspondant de l'Institut. De son côté, il recommande à Tenon deux étudiants qui viennent à Paris en aout 1788. Le 23 juin 1789 il lui demande des éclaircissements sur une technique urologique française, la taille vésicale en deux temps. Consulter à ce sujet, HUARD, P. et IMBAULT HUART, M. J., 'La cytostomie en deux temps', *Episteme*, 1970, no. 1, pp. 91–98.

8 Employée immémorialement par la médecine populaire britannique dans les hydropysies, la digitale fut introduite dans la matière médicale par W. Withering (1741–99) en 1785.

9 Tenon fait ici allusion à la pratique de Thomas Fowler (1736–1801) qui a donné son nom a une solution arsenicale (*liquor potassi arsenitis*). Il avait montré son intérêt en particulier dans les fièvres remittentes (depuis 1786).

10 Consulter HUARD, P., *Sciences, Médecine et Pharmacie de la Révolution a l'Empire*, Paris, Dacosta, 1970, p. 380.

11 Cf. WEINER, DORA B., 'Le Droit de l'Homme à la Santé. Une belle idée devant l'Assemblée Constituante, 1790–1791', *Clio Medica*, 1970, **5**, 209–23.

12 Tenon fut invité à se rendre à la maison du Val de Grâce pour y constater l'état de salubrité par la Commission de secours public. La lettre rédigée le 19 Vendémiaire an III est signée Roland (B.N. N.A.F. 22746); cf. HUARD, P., 'Eléments d'un rapport tendant à transformer le

monastère du Val de Grâce en Maternité' in *Clio Medica*, 1967, **2**, 249–54; TENON, FONDS, B.N. N.A. no. 22, 743, *Hôpitaux de Paris*, fols. 231–39; Consulter aussi, SERVIER, *Le Val de Grâce*, Paris, G. Masson, 1888; *Le Val de Grâce et l'Ecole d'application du Service de Santé militaire*, Paris, S.P.E.I., 1957; Le 23 Brumaire, il avait reçu de Levasseur, Thouret et Cousin, les directives du groupe de travail de la Commission des secours publics concernant la médicalisation du Val de Grâce et une lettre documentée de Hombron. Il avait lui même rédigé un mémoire pour savoir dans quelles conditions le monastère pourrait recevoir les femmes enceintes, les accouchées, les nourrices, les sevreuses et les enfants de la Patrie (B.N. N.A.F. 22746).

13 Cf. HUARD, P., op. cit., pp. 128 à 135.

14 Clavareau (1757–1804) construisit la nouvelle entrée de l'Hôtel-Dieu en l'an XII et apporta quelques améliorations au vieil hôpital sans beaucoup se soucier des observations de Tenon. (Cf. HUARD, op. cit., pp. 132 à 136.)

15 HUARD, P. et IMBAULT HUART, M. J., 'Pierre Desault (1738–1795)' in *Biographies médicales et scientifiques*, Paris, Dacosta, 1972, pp. 119–80; HUARD, P., 'Desault (1738–1795)', *Concours Médical*, 1970, **14**, no. 11, 8407–10.

16 Tenon ne sera pas d'ailleurs oublié en Angleterre. Voir MONAT, F. J. and SNELL, H. S., 'Tenon's proposed hospital', *Hosp. Const. . . . Londres, 1884*, pp. 264–70.

G. Legée
Paris (France)

Un concept né en Angleterre et son évolution aux XVIIIe et XIXe siècles: le concept d'irritabilité

Si on peut faire remonter la doctrine de l'irritation à Galien,[1] si le mot *irritatio* est utilisé par Vésale, en 1543, dans sa Fabrica (1 v, ch. VIII), et par Harvey qui explique la systole cardiaque par une irritation (1628), le concept d'irritabilité prend véritablement naissance chez Glisson (1596–1677), où il s'insère dans une théorie générale de la vie. A la suite de Glisson, le problème de l'irritabilité sera souvent lié à celui de la vie, mais il subira de nombreuses fluctuations.

Francis Glisson né en 1596 (la même année que Descartes), dans la province où vivait la famille de Locke, fit ses études à Cambridge et Oxford. Docteur en médecine en 1634, il fut nommé, en 1639, professeur d'anatomie à Londres. Ses principaux ouvrages sont:

l'*Anatomia hepatis*, paru en 1654, qui eut plusieurs éditions, et fut louée par Haller;
Le *Traité de la nature énergétique de la substance*, ou de la vie de la nature et de ses trois facultés originelles: perception, appetition, mouvement (1672).[2]
Le *Tractatus de ventriculo et intestinis*, paru l'année de sa mort, en 1677.

La théorie de Glisson apparaît dans l'Anatomie du foie sous un aspect anthropomorphique. Glisson explique une propriété physiologique à partir de concepts psychologiques. La vésicule et les canaux biliaires secrètent abondamment la bile quand ils sont irrités, c'est-à-dire provoqués. On trouve dans cet ouvrage les mots: *irritare, incitare, exstimulare, vigorare*, utilisés comme synonymes. Nous verrons aussi, dans l'évolution du concept d'irritabilité, les termes inciter ou exciter se substituer à celui d'irriter.

Toute irritation suppose et révèle une perception. L'être provoqué, irrité réagit pour se soustraire à l'offense parce qu'il perçoit ce qui le blesse (une morsure, une piqûre, par exemple). Le mouvement de rétraction, dû à une contraction musculaire, est soumis à une finalité. C'est pourquoi Glisson distingue trois facultés mises en jeu dans l'irritabilité:

perceptio sive sensatio,
appetitus,
motus musculorum,

la perception montrant la voie aux deux autres.

C'est la présence de filets nerveux dans la paroi des cavités contractiles qui induit Glisson à penser qu'elle est sensible, capable de perception, et de réaction ou contraction grâce à ses fibres musculaires. A cette époque, l'innervation est considérée nécessaire à toute réaction sensitive et motrice.

Dans le Traité de l'Estomac et de l'Intestin, un long développement est consacré à l'irritabilité de la fibre (cap. 7 et 8). Haller en fait mention dans l'histoire abrégée de l'irritabilité qui termine sa Dissertation sur les parties irritables et sensibles des animaux.[4] Glisson y montre que l'irritabilité n'est pas toujours accompagnée de sentiment; ainsi, après la mort les chairs se contractent quand on les touche avec des liqueurs âcres et piquantes. Il pense que l'irritabilité des fibres cardiaques est soustraite à l'action des nerfs. Il étend cette propriété à toutes les parties de l'organisme, et l'accorde même aux os et aux différents sucs. Il reconnaît des degrés d'irritabilité et son excès pathologique. Toutes ces notions trouveront divers développements chez les auteurs des 18e et 19e siècles.

C'est dans le traité de la nature énergétique de la substance que Glisson donne le plus de généralité à sa doctrine, en l'étendant à l'Univers entier. Pour lui, tout ce qui est, est de nature vitale. Il existe une force immanente à la matière, il y a identité de la substance et de la vie, d'une vie primitive, originelle et simple qui ne meurt jamais. La matière n'est pas une chose inerte et stupide, quelque chose de passif dont la raison d'être est de remplir l'espace. Créée par Dieu, elle est douée des attributs de l'esprit perception et appetition. C'est pourquoi Glisson va distinguer trois sortes de perception:

la perception naturelle, commune à toute substance, qui préexiste à l'organisation,
la perception animale, liée à la présence d'organes des sens,
la perception intellectuelle ou réfléchie qui «perçoit sa perception»; et de même trois sortes d'appetition (naturelle, sensitive et réfléchie), et trois sortes de mouvements (naturels, animaux et libres). Il existe donc trois vies superposées: naturelle, animale, humaine, douées de degrés différents de perception, d'appetition et de mouvement.

Cette doctrine, qui a pu influencer Leibniz dans sa Mondologie, est une philosophie de la Nature qui rappelle surtout celle de Spinoza. Le silence s'est d'ailleurs fait assez longtemps autour de la doctrine de Glisson, comme il s'était fait autour de celle de Spinoza, à cause de leur résonnance matérialiste, et l'animisme de Stahl (1660–1734) qui attribuait l'irritabilité à l'âme se développa.

Haller fut un des premiers à lire, avec intérêt, l'œuvre de Glisson et à lui donner des bases expérimentales, mais il n'en vit pas toute l'étendue. Il reprit le concept d'irritabilité pour le limiter à la fibre musculaire. Il établit l'indépendance de l'irritabilité et de la sensibilité et les définit ainsi:

J'appelle partie irritable du corps humain, celle qui devient plus courte quand quelque corps étranger la touche un peu fortement.

J'appelle fibre sensible dans l'homme, celle qui étant touchée transmet à l'âme l'impression de ce contact . . . dans les animaux . . . celle dont l'irritation occasionne chez eux des signes évidents de douleur et d'incommodité (op. cit. p. 5).

Il montre qu'un nerf irrité reste parfaitement immobile (pas de force d'oscillation due aux nerfs), et qu'un muscle est capable d'irritabilité même après section de son nerf. Il conclut: «Les parties sensibles du corps sont celles qui reçoivent des nerfs, et les nerfs eux-mêmes» (p. 39). «(De toutes ces expériences réunies), il paraît qu'il n'y a d'irritable dans le corps humain, que la fibre musculaire» (p. 72).

Il pense que l'âme n'est pas le principe de l'irritabilité, comme l'affirme Whytt (1714–66). Le système des animistes conduit à des contradictions. Puisque l'irritabilité subsiste après la destruction des nerfs, elle ne peut dépendre de l'âme; de plus, elle s'exerce sans que l'âme sente et n'est point soumise à la volonté.

Dans ses *Elementa physiologiae* (1755–66), tome IV, il montre cependant que la puissance nerveuse qui émane uniquement du cerveau, met en jeu l'irritabilité musculaire, dans les mouvements volontaires, où elle agit comme excitant.

Pour Haller, l'irritabilité est une propriété des parties gélatineuses souples ou gluten, non des parties sèches et friables. Nous retrouvons chez Lamarck la même idée. Poursuivant son analyse, Haller pense que l'irritabilité «a une cause physique sans doute, qui dépend de l'arrangement des dernières parties, mais que nous ne pouvons pas connaître, parce qu'il ne peut pas être saisi par des expériences aussi grossières, que celles auxquelles nous sommes bornés» (op. cit. p. 77).

Cette réflexion trouve un développement chez les solidistes de l'Ecole d'Edimbourg: Cullen (1712–90), élève de Monro (1697–1767), et J. Brown (1735–88) mais également, plus tard, chez Lamarck (1744–1828). Chez ces auteurs, elle va retrouver, pour le vivant, le caractère de généralité qu'elle avait chez Glisson, et donner naissance à de nouvelles théories de la vie.

Le solidisme, opposé à l'humorisme d'Hippocrate, considère le corps composé d'atomes en mouvement. Les différents états du corps traduisent les rapports respectifs des atomes: le *strictum* correspond au resserrement des atomes, le *laxum* à leur relachement, une position moyenne représente l'état de santé. L'état pathologique relevera donc soit d'une médication stimulante ou excitante, soit d'une médication sédative.

L'ouvrage le plus important à considérer, à ce point de vue, est celui de John Brown; ses *Eléments de médecine*, parus en latin en 1780, qui eurent trois traductions françaises la même année, en 1805, dont une dédiée à Corvisart (1755–1821).

Chez Brown, les termes d'*incitabilité* ou d'*excitabilité* se substituent à celui d'irritabilité. La vie, qu'elle soit animale ou végétale, est caractérisée par un certain degré d'incitabilité, c'est-à-dire par la propriété de ressentir l'action de certains agents extérieurs, et d'être affecté par certaines fonctions (op. cit., p. 3). Ces agents extérieurs et ces fonctions constituent les *forces* ou *puissances incitantes* (ou excitantes). Le résultat de l'action de ces forces sur l'incitabilité s'appelle *incitement*, qui correspond au degré de fonctionnement de l'organisme, à son énergie. Brown peut donc dire: «L'incitement, effet des puissances incitantes, est cause prochaine de la vie.» «L'incitement est cause de la maladie et de la santé.» Un degré moyen d'incitabilité et d'incitement traduit l'état de santé. L'épuisement de l'incitabilité qui correspond au maximum d'incitement, comme l'excès d'incitabilité qui correspond à un incitement trop faible ou nul, conduisent à la mort. La vie, la santé et la maladie dépendent donc exclusivement des puissances incitantes. Brown distingue deux états pathologiques: la *sthénie* ou état d'excitation (excès d'énergie) et l'*asthénie* ou état de faiblesse directe (défaut d'énergie), et de faiblesse indirecte (énergie extrême). Il explique que 97 pour-cent des maladies sont asthéniques; la plupart des remèdes doivent donc être des stimulants (vin, spiritueux, opium) dont il affirme les propriétés excitantes.[5]

Haller avait isolé irritabilité et sensibilité et leur avait assigné deux sièges différents. Brown ne distingue plus qu'une seule propriété et déclare: «Le siège de l'excitabilité, dans les corps vivants est la substance médullaire nerveuse et le tissu musculaire. Je désigne cet ensemble par le nom de système nerveux. L'excitabilité qui y réside ne diffère pas selon les diverses parties, c'est une propriété simple, une et indivisible dans tout le corps comme le prouve la production subite et instantanée du sentiment, du mouvement, des idées et des affections morales, par les puissances excitantes» (op. cit. pp. 31–32).

L'originalité de la doctrine de Brown réside:

(1) dans sa généralité: il l'applique au règne végétal comme au règne animal (pp. 264–70),

(2) dans l'importance qu'il attribue au milieu extérieur, source de stimulus (p. 609),

(3) et dans la définition qu'il donne de la vie, état permanent d'excitation: «La vie est un état forcé, dirigé et maintenu par une application convenable des puissances excitantes, dont l'action nous conduit naturellement et nécessairement à la mort. La vie, la santé, la maladie et la mort, sont donc également l'effet des mêmes forces stimulantes» (§ 327) (cf. aussi § 72).

Cette définition s'oppose à celle donnée par Bichat au début de ses Recherches physiologiques sur la vie et la mort: «La vie est l'ensemble des fonctions qui résistent à la mort.» Dans le vitalisme de Bichat, les lois vitales qui régissent la vie s'opposent aux lois physiques génératrices de la mort. J. B. Lamarck (1744–1829), dans ses *Recherches sur l'organisation des corps vivants*, commence par réfuter cette idée: «Je dois m'opposer à la propagation de quelques erreurs qui empêchent qu'on ne saisisse en quoi consiste réellement le phénomène de la vie.» «Il n'est pas vrai, comme on l'a dit,[6] que tout ce qui entoure les corps vivants tende à les détruire, en sorte que si ces corps ne possédaient pas en eux un principe de réaction, ils succomberaient bientôt par les suites de l'action qu'exercent sur eux les corps inorganiques qui les environnent.»

En réalité, la cause qui amène la mort de chaque corps vivant est en lui, et non hors de lui. Lamarck envisage une cause chimique: la tendance qu'ont les éléments constitutifs des composés à se dégager de l'état de combinaison; et deux causes physiologiques: la rupture de l'équilibre entre matières assimilées et rejetées, et l'indurescence progressive des organes qui cessent d'être irritables.

L'étude de l'irritabilité tient une grande place dans l'œuvre de Lamarck, et l'article irritabilité du Nouveau Dictionnaire des Sciences Naturelles, édité par Deterville, lui fut confié (tome XVI, 1817).

Ses conceptions présentent des points communs avec celles de Glisson, de Haller et de Brown. Il définit ainsi l'irritabilité: «Cette faculté est le propre de la nature animale, elle prend sa source dans l'*orgasme*, et elle est nécessaire à l'exercice du sentiment, dont elle est néanmoins toujours distincte» (*org. Corps vivants*, p. 209).

Il avait dit, quelques pages auparavant (186): «La nature animale exige pour exister dans un corps vivant, la faculté d'être irritable dans ses parties. Ainsi, la présence seule de l'irritabilité subsistante dans les parties d'un corps vivant, décide et constitue la nature animale.»

Par la notion d'orgasme et par l'importance attribuée au milieu environnant, Lamarck se rapproche de Brown: «J'appelle orgasme vital, dit-il, dans les animaux, une tension particulière dans tous les points des parties molles des corps vivants qui tient leurs molécules dans un certain écartement entre elles, et qu'elles sont susceptibles de perdre, par le simple effet de l'attraction, lorsque la cause qui l'entretient cesse d'agir» (op. cit. p. 79).

La variation d'intensité de cette tension ou orgasme rend possible les contractions et distensions subites des parties. «C'est la cause première de l'irritabilité.»

Toute excitation est susceptible de modifier l'orgasme. Une excessive tension, dit Lamarck, est connue sous le nom d'*éréthisme* dont le maximum produit l'inflammation, une excessive diminution de l'orgasme est en général désignée par le nom d'*atonie*. Si l'orgasme, et par suite l'irritabilité, s'éteignent, l'animal meurt. Comme chez Brown, la santé, la maladie et la mort, sont l'expression du tonus ou de l'état énergétique des solides organiques.

La cause qui entretient l'orgasme est un fluide subtil et expansif qui émane continuellement du sang artériel, mais dont l'origine est un fluide de même nature répandu dans les milieux environnants. Ce dernier fluide est la cause unique de l'orgasme des animaux qui manquent de système circulatoire. Ainsi l'influence extérieure, loin de les détruire, est au contraire la seule cause de leur conservation.

Une excitation peut agir en dissipant le fluide qui maintient l'orgasme. Les molécules peuvent alors se rapprocher, c'est l'origine d'une contraction. Comme Haller, Lamarck distingue l'irritabilité de la sensibilité. L'irritabilité n'a pas besoin d'organe spécial, c'est une propriété générale à tous les animaux et qui subsiste quelque temps encore après la mort. La sensibilité, qui cesse avec la vie, nécessite la présence d'un système nerveux, d'un «centre de rapport», dans lequel la sensation prend naissance. Il s'agit là de la *sensibilité physique*, que Lamarck distingue de la *sensibilité morale*, consciente. Son analyse, sans être expérimentale, est beaucoup plus fine que celle de Haller. Il reproche à Cabinis (1757–1808) de confondre irritabilité et sensibilité en voulant attribuer cette dernière à tous les animaux.[7] Enfin, la théorie de Lamarck s'étend à l'échelle cosmologique et, par certains points, se rapproche du naturalisme de Glisson. Mais Lamarck peut donner plus de précision et d'étendue à ses idées, car il bénéficie des nouvelles recherches sur l'électricité et le galvanisme,[8] ainsi que des progrès de la biologie.[9] Il insiste sur le fait que l'état des parties, et la cause qui le provoque ou orgasme, suffisent seuls à la production de l'irritabilité qui caractérise la vie animale. L'orgasme ne peut exister que dans les parties molles souples, où le mouvement moléculaire reste possible. C'est pourquoi la vie a dû naître dans un état gélatineux: «C'est un fait généralement vrai que tout corps qui reçoit la vie, ou qui reçoit les premiers traits de l'organisation qui prépare à la possession de la vie, est alors nécessairement dans un état gélatineux, en sorte que ses solides, c'est à dire, les plus solides de ses parties, ont la plus faible consistance et la plus grande flexibilité, et sont par conséquent dans le plus grand état de souplesse possible» (*Org. Corps viv.*, p. 95).[10]

Comme pour Glisson, la nature crée elle-même les premiers traits de l'organisation dans les masses où elle n'existait pas (p. 92). Mais chez Lamarck la nature ne crée pas les organes, c'est l'usage de la vie qui les développe et les compose, car il distingue vie et nature, alors que pour Glisson la vie est inhérente à la nature.

Lamarck analyse la façon dont la nature crée la disposition des parties ou premiers traits de l'organisation, et par suite l'orgasme, et l'irritabilité qui permet le mouvement organique vital. C'est un fluide cosmique qui agit, émané de la lumière du soleil. La lumière est source d'un fluide calorique très subtil ou feu éthéré, fluide tranquille réparti partout. Il montre que tous les fluides subtils ont cette origine cosmique.

Envisageant toute la série animale, il constate que l'irritabilité est plus grande et plus durable quand l'organisation animale est la plus simple possible. Il s'appuie sur des faits expérimentaux: une chenille complétement vidée de ses organes et recousue, continue à se promener (op. cit., pp. 86–88).

Il établit un parallèle avec les phénomènes de régénération et de multiplication, si actifs chez les animaux les plus inférieurs. Un fluide fécondant, une flamme invisible, une vapeur subtile, crée l'organisation première, l'irritabilité et la vie, dans l'œuf fécondé.

Dans les animaux possédant un système nerveux, le fluide nerveux éteint l'orgasme et détermine la contraction. Il agit en dissipant le fluide calorique apporté sans cesse par le sang artériel, et qui maintient l'orgasme à un certain niveau. Ce fluide nerveux a lui même une origine cosmique: le feu fixé des aliments s'est transformé en feu calorique véhiculé par le sang, puis en fluide nerveux ou feu éthéré animalisé par les circonstances où il se trouve (op. cit., p. 163).[11]

Ainsi Lamarck peut citer le mot de Lavoisier: «Dieu en apportant la lumière a répandu sur la terre le principe de l'organisation, du sentiment et de la pensée» (p. 102). C'est ainsi un vaste tableau de la vie animale en relation avec le milieu cosmique que nous trace Lamarck, et qui témoigne de la richesse de sa pensée. Bien que ses études médicales aient été fugitives et incomplètes, il était nécessaire de lui réserver ici une place importante pour ses conceptions profondes sur l'irritabilité.

Le système de Brown se répandit surtout en Allemagne, en Italie (Rasori et Tommasini), et jusqu'en Amérique. En France, parmi les médecins, il n'eut pas le même succès. Le vitalisme de Montpellier [Bordeu (1722–76) et surtout Barthez (1734–1806)] et celui de Paris avec Bichat (1771–1802), dominaient. Ils n'admettaient pas l'excitabilité abstraite de Brown comme principe unique de vie.

Bichat loue Stahl (1660–1734) qui fit le premier pas vers la découverte des *propriétés vitales* en reconnaissant la discordance des lois physiques avec les fonctions des animaux. Mais en attribuant, dit-il, tous les phénomènes vitaux à un principe unique, à l'âme, la vérité lui échappa. Le principe vital de Barthez n'a pas plus de réalité.

Pour Bichat, les propriétés vitales sont les mobiles premiers des phénomènes physiologiques. Dieu doua les corps vivants de sensibilité et de contractibilité, comme il doua tous les corps de gravité, élasticité etc. . . . (Anatomie générale, tome I, pp. 1–4). Il subdivise ces deux propriétés selon la distinction qu'il établit entre les deux vies, animale et organique, et précise ce qu'on doit désigner par le terme irritabilité: «Si vous comprenez, dit-il, sous le nom d'irritabilité, et les mouvements des muscles qui se contractent par les stimulans, et ceux des muscles que l'influence cérébrale met en jeu, il est impossible que vous vous entendiez.»

Toutes les disputes, pour savoir si la sensibilité est la même que la contractibilité ou si les deux propriétés peuvent se séparer, disparaissent en admettant la distinction suivante dans les propriétés vitales:

(1) dans la vie animale: sensibilité et contractilité animales ne sont pas nécessairement liées;
(2) dans la vie organique, les deux propriétés sont toujours liées; exemples:
(*a*) mouvements du cœur: sensibilité organique suivie de contractilité organique sensible;
(*b*) sécrétions: sensibilité organique suivie de contractilité organique insensible (op. cit., pp. 76 et sv.).

La contractilité organique sensible, seule, constitue pour Bichat l'irritabilité.[12]

La théorie de Bichat présente quelques points communs avec celle de Lamarck: – les propriétés vitales siègent dans les solides, et les fluides ne servent que d'excitants; mais les fluides considérés par Bichat sont seulement les «fluides de composition», comme le sang ou le chyle (op. cit., p. 29).

—les propriétés vitales appartiennent à l'arrangement organique des molécules (p. 48), mais pour Bichat cet arrangement n'est pas lui-même le résultat de la vie. Il est originel, donné avec les différents organes et tissus. Cette notion de tissu lui appartient.[13]

—la sensibilité animale nécessite le rapport à un centre commun situé dans le cerveau d'où la contractilité animale tire son principe. La sensibilité organique de Bichat et la sensibilité physique de Lamarck sont très voisines.

Les maladies sont des altérations des propriétés vitales, le but des médicaments est de les ramener à leur type naturel. Chaque force vitale a ses médicaments qui lui conviennnent.[14] Les symptômes des maladies portent sur les solides mais leur cause peut être dans les fluides et les solides, donc: «Une théorie exclusive de solidisme ou d'humorime est un contre-sens pathologique» (p. 36). Le défaut trop généraliser nuit à la science.

Broussais (1772–1838) est à la fois disciple de Bichat et de Brown. Dans son ouvrage sur l'*Irritation et la folie* (1828), il déclare: «Nous professons d'abord avec Brown, que la vie ne s'entretient que par l'excitation.»

Mais il abandonna la voie de l'abstraction utilisée par Brown dans son étude de l'excitabilité, et préfère étudier ce phénomène dans les organes et les tissus, à la manière de Bichat, dont il adopte le vitalisme. Dans le chapitre III de son Traité de physiologie appliquée à la médecine (1822), il parle de propriétés vitales de tissus, de forces et de lois vitales, irréductibles à de simples concepts physiques. Broussais reprend le terme d'irritabilité en lui restituant toute sa généralité, c'est la propriété commune à tous les tissus, à tous les êtres vivants, depuis les végétaux jusqu'à l'homme (Irr. et fol. p. 2).

La sensibilité est une conséquence de l'irritabilité, et non l'inverse comme chez Glisson. Mais cette sensibilité nécessite toujours la présence d'un «appareil nerveux muni d'un centre, c'est à dire d'un cerveau», apte à réagir et la sensibilité organique de Bichat n'est qu'une abstraction superflue, puisqu'elle se confond avec la contractilité (Irr. fol. p. 3). Les excitants ou stimulants sont appelés *modificateurs*, l'excitation correspond à l'excitement de Brown. L'excitation normale cause l'éréthisme vital, l'excitation excessive, pathologique, cause l'irritation, base de la doctrine «physiologique» de Broussais.

Au point de vue thérapeutique, cette doctrine, qui considère au fond les maladies comme sthéniques (à l'inverse de Brown) conduisit à l'abus des saignées et à l'échec. En réalité, la «physiologie» de Broussais n'est qu'empirique et spéculative, c'est une *idéologie médicale* (Georges Canguilhem). La médecine deviendra physiologique grâce à la physiologie expérimentale qui commence à se développer avec Magendie (1783–1855), Legallois (1770–1814) et Flourens (1794–1867). Une ère nouvelle s'ouvre pour le concept d'irritabilité, sa compréhension sera liée à l'expérience sur l'animal.

Legallois, en démontrant expérimentalement que la puissance nerveuse n'est pas due seulement au cerveau, mais appartient aussi à la moelle épinière, modifie le sens du mot irritabilité. Il faut distinguer, dit-il, les mouvements d'une grenouille décapitée qui dépendent du principe «duquel dépend la faculté de sentir et de se mouvoir», c'est à dire du principe de la vie, des mouvements provoqués dans une cuisse de grenouille isolée, qui sont des phénomènes d'irritabilité. L'irritabilité, suivant Legallois, est donc indépendante de la puissance nerveuse, indépendante de la vie. Les résultats de ses expériences le conduisent à cette définition de la vie: «La vie est due à une impression du sang artériel sur le cerveau et la moelle épinière, ou à un principe résultant de cette impression» (*Expériences sur le Principe de la vie*, 1812, pp. 46 et 135).

En 1822, Flourens présente un mémoire à l'Académie des Sciences, dont la première partie s'intitule: Détermination des propriétés du système nerveux ou recherches physiologiques sur l'irritabilité et la sensibilité.

Il cherche à délimiter expérimentalement les parties du système nerveux sensibles, c'est à dire capables de faire naître des contractions et les parties irritables, capables de faire naître des contractions. Avant de commencer le compte-rendu de ses expériences, il éprouve le besoin de préciser le sens des termes: *sensibilité*, *contractilité*, *irritabilité*. Le nerf n'est ni contractile, ni sensible, ces propriétés n'appartiennent qu'au muscle et à certaines parties du système nerveux, il est irritable. Ainsi, avec Flourens, l'irritabilité redevient une propriété nerveuse. Cuvier (1769–1832), dans son rapport, lui reproche de n'avoir pas gardé le sens attribué par Haller. Il lui conseille d'utiliser, pour la propriété du nerf la périphrase: «conducteur de l'irritabilité et de la sensibilité», expression critiquée dans le *Journal de médecine et de chirurgie d'Edimbourg*, en 1824. Lordat (1773–1862), dont Flourens avait été l'élève, voit dans le reproche de Cuvier l'occasion d'une attaque contre l'Ecole de Montpellier, et donne une réponse fort judicieuse, montrant que Cuvier n'est pas physiologiste.

Il fait un long développement sur la naissance du vocabulaire physiologique à partir du vocabulaire psychologique déjà existant, qui rappelle quelques reflexions de Bichat par rapport au vocabulaire physique (*Vie et mort*, p. 104).

A la suite des remarques de Cuvier, Flourens utilisa le mot *excitabilité*, qui remplace, dans l'ouvrage imprimé en 1824, celui d'irritabilité du manuscrit. Mais ces termes n'avaient-ils pas déjà été synonymes au cours de l'évolution que nous étudions? Il le seront encore au cours de la période suivante, période de la physiologie générale inaugurée en France par Claude Bernard (1813–78), et déjà en Allemagne avec Virchow (1821–61). «Toute activité vitale suppose une excitation, ou, si vous le préférez, une irritation. L'excitabilité des diverses parties est le seul criterium qui nous permette de juger si la partie est ou non vivante» (*Path. cell.*, p. 240).

L'irritabilité ou excitabilité devient, après l'établissement de la théorie cellulaire, la propriété vitale de l'élément histologique (Cl. Bernard, *Tissus vivants*, p. 60), la propriété du protoplasme. Elle nécessite, pour se manifester, une organisation due à une disposition particulière des molécules, et un milieu qui fournit les irritants, conditions déjà si bien explicitées par Lamarck, et qui gardent toute leur vérité jusqu'à l'époque actuelle de la biologie moléculaire.

References

1 Cf. TEMKIN, OWSEI, 'Les racines classiques de la doctrine de Glisson', in *Bulletin d'histoire de la médecine*, juillet-août 1964.

2 Ouvrage écrit en latin, très rare en France. Henri Marion, professeur d'histoire de la philosophie à Paris, dans sa thèse sur Glisson (thèse latine traduite en français dans la *Revue philosophique*,

en 1882), en cite cinq exemplaires; mais il ignore l'existence des deux exemplaires de la Bibliothèque de la faculté de Médecine de Paris.

4 HALLER, *Dissertation sur les parties irritables et sensibles des animaux*, Trad. Tissot, Lausanne, Bousquet, 1755, pp. 78–85.

5 Avant Brown, tous les médecins considéraient l'opium comme un sédatif. Haller explique cette action par une diminution de l'irritabilité.

6 LAMARCK cite: BICHAT, *Recherches sur la vie et la mort*; CUVIER, *Leçons d'anatomie comparée* tome I, p. 3. *Dans sa Philosophie zoologique* (tome II, p. 87); il cite encore RICHERAND (*Physiologie*, tome I, p. 82), qui considère les affinités électives comme des forces de destruction.

7 *Philosophie zoologique*, ed. Martins, Paris, 1873, tome II, p. 40.

8 Galvani (1737–98) et Volta (1745–1827).

9 Lamarck, lui-même, crée le mot biologie en 1802, la même année que Treviranus. En 1800, on le trouve déjà chez Burdach, mais avec un sens différent.

10 Chez Haller, l'irritabilité était déjà une propriété des parties gélatineuse ou gluten (cf. plus haut).

11 Lamarck insiste sur cette notion de circonstances. Il dit ailleurs (*philozoo*, tome II, p. 89): 'Il n'y a nulle différence dans les lois physiques par les quelles tous les corps qui existent se trouvent régis, mais il s'en trouve une considérable dans les circonstances où ces lois agissent.'

12 Il remarque que certains auteurs désignent par ce terme la sensibilité et la contractilité organique toujours liées. La contractilité organique insensible est, pour lui, la tonicité (*Vie et mort*, 4e ed., 1822, p. 140).

13 Bichat distingue à côté des propriétés vitales, des propriétés de tissus: l'extensibilité et la contractilité de tissus, de degré variable selon les tissus. Magendie fait remarquer, à juste titre, que ces propriétés ne sont que l'élasticité (op. cit., pp. 169–81).

14 La doctrine médicale de Rolando (1772–1831), s'éloigne de celle de Brown et se rapproche de celle de Bichat, par la multiplicité des excitabilités qu'il distingue.

Bibliographie

BICHAT, X., *Recherches physiologiques sur la vie et la mort*, 4e ed., augmentée de notes par F. Magendie, Paris, Béchet, 1822; *Anatomie générale*, tome I, nouvelle édition, Paris, Brosson, 1821.

BERNARD, CLAUDE, *Leçons sur les propriétés des tissus vivants*, Paris, Germer Baillière, 1866; *Leçons sur les phénomènes de la vie, communs aux animaux et aux végétaux*, Paris, Baillière, 1878.

BROUSSAIS, F. J. V., *Traité de physiologie appliquée à la pathologie*, tome I, Paris, Delaunay, 1822; *De l'irritation et le la folie*, Paris, Delaunay, 1828; *Examen des doctrines médicales et des systèmes de nosologie*, 3e éd., tome II, Paris, Delaunay, 1829.

BROWN, J., *Eléments de Médecine*, tr. R. J. Bertin, Paris, Th. Barrois, an XIV–1805.

CABANIS, P. J. G., *Rapports du physique et du moral de l'homme*, 3e éd., Paris, Caille et Ravier, 1815.

FLOURENS, P., *Recherches expérimentales sur les propriétés et les fonctions du système nerveux dans les animaux vertébrés*, Paris, Crevot, 1824; *De la vie et de l'intelligence*, 2e éd, Paris, Garnier, 1858.

GLEY, E., *Essais de philosophie et d'histoire de la biologie*, Paris, Masson, 1900.

GLISSON, F., *Anatomie hepatis*, Londini, Du Gardian, 1654; *Tractatus de natura substantia energetica*, London, H. Brome, 1672; *Tractatus de ventriculo et intestinis*, Amstelodami, ap. Jacobum Juniorum, 1677.

HALLER, A. VON, *Dissertation sur les parties irritables et sensibles des animaux*, trad. Tissot, Lausanne, Francisci Grasset, 1762.

LAMARCK, J. B., *Recherches sur l'organisation des corps vivants*, Paris, chez l'Auteur, an X; *Philosophie zoologique*, ed. Charles Martins, tome I, Paris, Savy, 1873; *Inédits de Lamarck présentés par M. Vachon, G. Rousseau, Y. Laissus*, Paris, Masson, 1972.

LEGALLOIS, C., *Expériences sur le principe de la vie*, Paris, d'Hautel, 1872.

LORDAT, *Douze leçons de physiologie sur les fonctions privées du système musculaire de l'homme*, Montpellier, 1 jullien 1835.

ROLANDO, L., *Inductions physiologiques et pathologiques sur les différentes espèces d'excitabilité et d'excitement*, trad. Jourdan-Boisseau, Paris, Caille et Ravier, 1822.

TOMMASINI, *Exposition précise de la nouvelle doctrine italienne*, trad., Paris, Béchet, 1821.

VIRCHOW, R., *La pathologie cellulaire*, trad. P. Picard, Paris, Baillière, 1861.

P. Huard and M. J. Imbault-Huart
Paris (France)

Médecine française et médecine anglaise au XIXe siècle

Après un rappel des relations de tous ordres entre la France et l'Angleterre, nous étudierons successivement:

(1) les médecins français ayant voyagé ou séjourné en Angleterre,
(2) Les médecins anglais ayant voyagé ou séjourné en France,
(3) Les contacts médicaux franco-anglais.

I. FRANCE ET ANGLETERRE AU XIXe SIÈCLE

A la charnière du XVIII et du XIXe siècle, le temps de Georges III (1760–1820) c'est à dire la révolution industrielle et les grands mouvements économiques et sociaux concomitants font de la Grande Bretagne une nation pilote de l'Europe occidentale au point que l'on a pu parler d'une «Europe anglaise».[1] Elle attire de nombreux français. Après les guerres de la Révolution et de l'Empire, les deux pays ne cessent de se rapprocher, sur le plan de la science, de la technique, de la littérature, de la mode et de la politique, des sports (boxe, trot, carrossine anglaise, courses de chevaux). De nombreux mots anglais entrent dans notre langue: club (le Jockey Club est fondé en 1828) *dandy*,[2] *water-closet, punch, groom, etc. . . .*). Il y a des unions franco-anglaises[3] et des français anglophiles. Réciproquement, de nombreux anglais viennent en France où s'ouvrent de nombreux «Hôtels d'Angleterre».

II. LES MÉDECINS FRANÇAIS EN ANGLETERRE

Il est impossible de faire un dénombrement même approximatif des nombreux médecins français venus en Angleterre, soit comme prisonniers de guerre, soit pour faire un voyage d'études, soit pour s'y installer. Nous retiendrons particulièrement ceux qui ont laissé des publications.

A la première catégorie appartiennent notamment Pierre Lefort (1767–1843) ultérieurement inspecteur général permanent des prisonniers français en Angleterre, Récamier, Bollon, M. H. Benoist (1754–1840), Mabit (1781–1846), Legris-Duval (1780–1841), Bouchet, Brunet, Lavort (1778–1858).

Dans la seconde catégorie, on peut également citer, Bertin (1801), Valentin (1803),[1] Roux (1814),[4] Cadet de Gassicourt (1817),[5] Pichot (1822),[6] Ferrus (1826), Billard (1828),[7] Foullioy (1829),[8] Magendie (1831),[9] Mabit (1832), D. Larrey,[10] Bourjot

Saint Hilaire (1836),[11] Dupuytren et Caffe (1837),[12] Bureaud-Riofrey (1839),[13a] Marjolin (1840),[13b] Pointe (1844),[14] Duval (1847), Tourdes et Aronsohn (1847), Sédillot (1847),[15] Daremberg (1848),[16] Topinard (1860),[17] Le Fort (1858 et 60),[17] Nélaton (1861), Rayer (1862), Liégard (1862), Gayet (1862), Demarquay (1862), Blondel-Ser (1862), Courty (1863),[18] Morel et Fabret (1864), Ch. Sarrazin (1866),[19] Lucas-Championnière (1867), Perrier, Nicaise et Terrier (1868),[20] Robin (1869), Bonnafont (1870),[21] Brochin (1870),[22] Budin (1875),[23] Guéneau de Mussy (1875) (1879 et 1886), Lucas-Championnière et Pozzi (1876),[25] Manoury (1876).[26] On pourrait encore ajouter les noms de Bretonneau, de L. F. Sanson, Prunelle, Anselmier, Jalade-Lafond, Daniel Mollière, Ricord,[27] Giraldès, Civiale,[28] Péan,[29] Husson,[17] L. Legouest, P. Broca,[30] Ant. Muron,[31] A. Poncet, Théodore et Eugène Boeckel (1831–1900), Charcot. . . . Ant. Cros (1833–1903) lit un mémoire sur la plessométrie à la Soc. médicale de Londres, 9 avril 1883. La troisième catégorie, assez restreinte, est disparate. Il y a d'abord les réfugiés politiques: Landel,[32] qui épouse une nièce du Lord Chancelier; Deligny, J. P. Durand (1826–1900), Brouse, A. Deville (+1879) (qui soigna Victor Hugo en 1863[33]) et bien d'autres exilés à la suite du coup d'état de 1852; Bernard Simon qui fournit les explosifs et l'argent dont Orsini avait besoin pour préparer son attentat; Paul Lafargue (1842–1912) gendre de Karl Marx, exclu des facultés françaises en 1865,[34] V. Jaclard (1843–1903) ancien communard collaborateur de Clémenceau; Lucien Corvisart (1824–82) médecin de Napoléon III, exilé, Pierre Leroux[33] etc. . . .

Viennent ensuite les praticiens installés à Londres: Meric, Fellow du R.C.S., Heurteloup[36] l'urologiste qui exerce tantôt à Paris, tantôt en Angleterre; Et. Bertin (1780–1874) médecin de l'ambassade française à Londres pendant vingt ans, Bureaud-Riofray (+1880) fondateur d'une revue médicale franco-anglaise; Paul Simon (1839–1900), Victor Regnier (1822–88) qui servit plus tard d'intermédiaire entre Bismarck et Bazaine, Paul Curie, grand-père de Pierre Curie; Achille Vinitras (+1904), fondateur de l'hôpital français de Londres, dont l'un des médecins fut A. Lutaud (1847–1925).

L'abondance des amphithéâtres publics et privés d'anatomie attira à Paris de nombreux anglais, parmi lesquels Alex Thomson (1802–38) fils de Anthony Todd Thomson, professeur de jurisprudence médicale à l'Université de Londres. Il a été quelquefois confondu avec Allen Thomson (1809–84), lecteur de physiologie à Edinburgh (1842–48) et professeur d'anatomie à Glasgow (1848–77). Etudiant à Saint-John à Cambridge, il travaille à Paris sous la conduite de J. Coste (1807–73) et d'autres maîtres. Il a laissé d'importantes publications avant de se suicider. Il expliqua son suicide dans une brochure lithographique devenue introuvable.[53]

Les médecins anglais installés en France sont assez nombreux pour avoir fait l'objet d'une étude de Liveing et constituer une société médicale.[54]

Edward Rayner (1814–74) marié avec la veuve de Thomson eut une très grosse clientèle parisienne qui le rémunérait non d'après le nombre de ses visites mais après un forfait basé sur la durée probable de la maladie. Boggs (+1890) fut correspondant du *Lancet* et le doyen des médecins anglais de Paris. George Wickham (+1900) fonda la chambre professionnelle d'orthopédie.

Sir Joseph Oliffe soigna le duc de Morny tandis que Napoléon III consulta Sir W. Fergusson (1856) et se fit plus tard opérer par Sir Henry Thompson (1820–1904).

W. B. Costello (1800–67), mort à Saint-Mandé fit ses études médicales à Dublin et à Paris. Elève de Heurteloup, il l'assista dans ses lithotrities à Londres (1832). Il traduisit les articles de Rayer en anglais. Il édita, en anglais, une encyclopédie chirurgicale dont les collaborateurs furent Bouvier, Broca, Désormeaux, Follin, Fouché, Gallard.

Les noms de quelques médecins d'origine anglaise sont également à retenir: Stuart-Cooper (+1850), ancien interne des Hôpitaux de Paris; W. Turner; Ch. Campbell (1820–79), agrégé à la Faculté de médecine de Paris, assistant de Paul Dubois quelquefois confondu avec son collègue obstétricien W. Campbell (1788–1848) d'Edimbourg: E. Turner (1826–92), ancien interne des Hôpitaux de Paris; Edwards Milne-Edwards: Benjamin Ball (1834–93), médecin des Hôpitaux et agrégé à la Faculté de Médecine de Paris, issu d'un père anglais et d'une mère suisse; Brown-Sequard (1818–94), métis franço-anglais comme David Ferrier (1843–1928) et Aug. Desiré Waller (1856–1922), né à Paris, élève de Magendie. On pourrait enfin citer un certain nombre de thèses de Paris soutenues par des britanniques (Stormont, Conwell, Bennett, Good, etc.).[55]

Pendant la guerre de 1870, John Wyat (+1874), chirurgien major du régiment des Coldstream-Guards est délégué par le gouvernement anglais en qualité de commissaire médical auprès du grand quartier général français. Enfermé à Paris pendant toute la durée du siège, il prodigue ses soins aux malades et aux blessés. Sir William MacCormac (1836–1901) dirige une ambulance et en publie, plus tard, le journal.[56]

Dans le Sud-Ouest de la France, Breen (+1903), irlandais, fonde à Bordeaux un cabinet réservé, en principe, à la clientèle britannique. Daniel Hack Take (1827–95), visite, en 1879, les «cagots» pyrénéens.

Dès la Restauration existe à Pau un cercle anglais. Mais c'est le Midi méditerranéen qui attire le plus les Anglais.

Le philosophe John Stuart Mill (1806–73) mourra à Avignon.

Dès le XVIIIe siècle, le chirurgien Tobias Smollett (1721–71) découvre la Côte d'Azur où naîtra Henri Cavendish (1731–1810), à Nice, et où sera enterré Spencer Wells (1818–97) dans le cimetière anglais de Cannes. Un de ces découvreurs est le docteur James Henry Bennett (1816–91) qui fit connaître Menton vers 1860; tandis que Douglas Duke (+1900) fondait un hôpital anglais à Cannes.

III. LES MÉDECINS ANGLAIS EN FRANCE

Si nous mettons à part les nombreux élèves anglais de Laennec,[38] étudiés ailleurs, nous retiendrons la venue sur le Continent[39] de Gr. Watt (1801)[40]; Carpue[41]; H. Matthews,[42] (1817–19); John Bell[43] (1817); Hickman[44] (1828); John Cross[45] (1820); Th. Alcock (1823); Benjamin Philipps[46] (1830), James Hope[47]; Sir Astley Cooper[48] (1834), Alex. Stewart[49] (1839, 1840); Sir Ch. Bell[50] (1840); C. Kidd (1848). Sir James Paget[51] (1867), Sir Th. Spencer Wells et Keith (1866); J. Samson Gamgee[52] (1867); Sir Rutherford Alcock (1816–97), Sir Henry Thompson (1820–1904), grand admirateur de Civiale et de Mercier,[40] Teale, élève de Lisfranc, W. Ireland, etc. . . .

IV. LES POINTS DE CONTACT MÉDICAUX FRANCO–ANGLAIS

1. Au début du siècle, l'adoption de la vaccination jennerienne fut l'œuvre du Premier Consul, d'émigrés comme le duc de La Rochefoucauld-Liancourt et de

l'Ecole de Médecine de Paris qui imposèrent à une France réticente le «poison anglais».[42]

2. Un second pôle d'attraction est constitué par les premiers essais d'antisepsie avec la liqueur de Labarraque. Ils font l'objet, en 1827, d'une étude de Thomas Alscock (1784–1833).

3. Un peu plus tard, les Anglais sont attirés par la clinique médico-chirurgicale française enseignée par Laënnec, Andral, Louis, Dupuytren, Lisfranc, etc. Quelques rares Français, dont Foullioy,[57] s'intéressent à la propreté des hôpitaux anglais, aux pansements sans cérat ni charpie, à la suture primitive des plaies, aux ligatures des grosses artères, aux résections articulaires, inconnus chez nous.

L'anesthésie chirurgicale par inhalation est démontrée, dès 1824, par Henry Hill Hickman. Méconnu dans son pays, il vint en France pour demander la protection de Charles X (1828). Ultérieurement, le «chloroforme à la reine» fut introduit en France et Sédillot apprendra de Hancock l'anesthésie à l'éther (1847).

Mackenzie et Gendron eurent, en même temps (1825), l'idée de traiter les laryngites pseudo-membraneuses par le nitrate d'argent.

Les épidémies de choléra furent aussi l'occasion d'un trait d'union franco-anglais.[45]

Au milieu du siècle, le bandage herniaire anglais s'oppose au bandage français; la jambe de bois à genou mobile aux pilons. La dentisterie anglaise crée avec Thomes un nouveau type de davier adapté à chaque dent dont le mérite revient, en partie, à un Français émigré à Londres, Evrard.[58]

Mais ce sont les succès des ovariotomistes anglais qui font réfléchir nos chirurgiens,[59] encore que Spencer-Wells et Keith viennent voir opérer Koeberlé à Strasbourg dont le monde entier adoptera la pince à forci-pressure.

Avant Koeberlé,[60] les Anglais connaissaient déjà le clampage des pédicules, les ligatures perdues, l'aspiration des liquides par des siphons de caoutchouc et la toilette du péritoine.

Pendant la guerre de Crimée, 19,5 pour cent des blessés français sont amputés avec une mortalité de 60 pour cent. Les chiffres correspondants de l'armée anglaise sont de 4,6 pour cent et de 27,5 pour cent (Chenu). Le *nursing* (Florence Nightingale), la propreté et la bonne nourriture expliquent cette différence.

La fin du siècle, est dominée par la lutte contre l'infection et l'émergence d'une neurologie active.

Inutile de revenir sur l'antisepsie[47] listérienne (1867) et l'asepsie pasteurienne, «qui a fait pénétrer l'esprit bactériologique dans les salles d'opérations» suivant le mot de Félix Ferrier (1882). On connait aussi l'amitié de Lister et de Pasteur[61] dont le point culminant se situe le 27 décembre 1892, lors du jubilé de Pasteur dans le grand amphithéâtre de la Sorbonne où les deux savants se donnent l'accolade. Si l'antisepsie eut des partisans français enthousiastes comme Antoine Hoseph Gilbin (1833–1903) qui l'introduisit à l'hôpital de Metz, en 1872, et Lucas-Championnière[62] qui exposa la méthode plus clairement et plus complètement que Lister, elle eut aussi des détracteurs. C'étaient d'abord les laparotomistes, comme Koeberlé ou Péan qui savaient que Lister n'était pas un chirurgien abdominal et qui redoutaient l'action de l'acide phénique dans le péritoine. C'était aussi Léon Le Fort[63] (1829–93) qui, de 1865 à 1871 avait combattu la vieille théorie de l'air nocif ou du germe ferment, chère à Lister, pour lui opposer la théorie du germe-contage que les mains, les instruments, les éponges et les objets de pansement propagent d'un sujet infecté à un sujet sain. Fidèle à sa doctrine de la contagion et de l'asepsie, qui lui avait donné de beaux succès, il repoussait l'acide phénique «plus coagulant qu'antiseptique» et il pansait ses plaies non pas avec de la charpie, mais avec des compresses trempées dans une solution d'alcool camphré, recouverte d'un morceau de taffetas gommé. On sait que l'alcool[64] avait été réintroduit en chirurgie par Batailhé (1817–75) vers 1850, méthode reprise par A. Nélaton (1863). Un moment, le pansement ouaté d'Alphonse Guérin, concurrença celui de Lister (1871). Enfin, certains partisans de Lister trouvant sa méthode trop compliquée la simplifièrent en supprimant le spray (Pozzi, 1876). Parmi les listériens de la première heure, se placent F. Terrier qui traduisit en français (1873) *The System of Surgery* de Lister (1871).

Beaucoup de chirurgiens ne se rendaient d'ailleurs pas compte que ce qu'ils attribuaient au topique (acide phénique) était dû à la méthode et que la technique de Lister avait un caractère général lui permettant de s'accommoder de n'importe quel antiseptique, comme le comprit Tarnier.

Or, on s'était aperçu que les antiseptiques lèsent les tissus et provoquent des exsudations dont il faut assurer le drainage. Pour obtenir une réunion *per primun* sans drainage, il fallait donc s'en tenir à l'asepsie stricte. Le premier moignon suturé hermétiquement dans ces conditions à Paris sortit des mains de Pierre Delbet (1888).[65]

La neurologie fut un second pôle d'attraction entre la France et l'Angleterre. La clinique neurologique de Ch. Bell, dont on sait les démélés avec Magendie, fut connue en France par les traductions d'Amédée Pichot.[52] Il en fut de même pour la dégénérescence wallerienne du nerf sectionné, étudiée par Cruveilhier (1850) et pour l'épilepsie corticale localisée appelée par Charcot jacksonienne, en hommage à John Hughlings Jackson (1834–1911). Inversement David Ferrier (1843–1928) proposa de donner le nom de Paul Broca à la 3e circonvolution frontale ascendante.

En médecine tropicale, la pratique de la ponction des abcès du foie est rapportée des Indes par un chirurgien de la marine, Brossard. Le drainage chirurgical des abcès tropicaux du foie mis au point par Louis Stromeyer Little (1840–1911) au *Shangai Hospital General* (1869–99) fut adopté par les chirurgiens de la marine française et perfectionné en 1895 par Jules Ant. Fontan (1849–1931).

Un dernier problème est celui de la grande chirurgie digestive dont les pionniers furent Billroth et une brillante équipe de chirurgiens germaniques. Après avoir été à l'avant garde de la chirurgie moyenne, vasculaire et gynécologique, les britanniques se tinrent en retrait sur ce point, estimant que la mortalité et la morbidité enregistrées ne justifiait pas ces grandes opérations, abdomino-pelviennes, malgré leurs bases scientifiques. Les Français, bien revenus de leur *prurigo secandi*, plus cliniciens qu'opérateurs, partagèrent cette attitude.

En chirurgie urinaire la prostatectomie transvésicale de Sir Peter Johnson Freyer (1852–1921) attira de nombreux urologues français à Londres à partir de 1900.

In fine, signalons qu'en physiologie l'influence de Cl. Bernard fut considérable chez les savants anglo-saxons (Olmsted).[67]

Notes

Une bibliographie importante se trouve déjà dans la thèse de F. Prigent, Contribution à l'étude des rapports médicaux franco-anglais du XVIe au XIXe siède (*Thèse de Méd. de Rennes*, 1964, no. 411).

1 Pour les généralités, consulter Pierre Reboul. Le mythe anglais dans la littérature française sous la Restauration. *Travaux et Mémoires de l'Université de Lille, 1962* et André Parreaux, professeur à la Sorbonne. *La Société Anglaise de 1760 à 1810. Introduction a une étude de la civilisation anglaise au temps de Georges III*, 132 pp. (Publications de la Faculté des Lettres et Sciences humaines de Paris–Sorbonne, Série 'Etudes et Méthodes', tome 15). Sur les voyages des Français en Angleterre, lire: SAY, J. B. (1767–1832), *De l'Angleterre et des Anglais*, Paris, A. Bertrand, 1815, 56 pp.

TRISTAN, FLORA (1803–44), *Promenades dans Londres*, Paris, H. L. Dellaye, 1840, lxv+412 pp. (3 éditions en 2 ans).

ESTOR, H., 'Voyage en Angleterre du doyen V. Broussonnet', *Monspeliensis Hippocrates, 1966*, no. 31, p. 1720.

BOUCHER DE PERTHES, J., *Voyages en Angleterre, Ecosse et Irlande en 1860*, Paris, Jung-Treuttel, 1868, 318 pp.

DREYFUS, F., *Une philanthrope d'autrefois. La Rochefoucauld-Liancourt* (1747–1827), Paris, Plon, 1903, xvi+547 pp. port.

LA ROCHEFOUCAULD, FR. DE, *La vie en Angleterre au 18e siècle*, Paris, de Prat, 1945.

SOUDAN DE PIERREFITTE, J., *Petite histoire méconnue de l'entente cordiale*, 1953.

LANESSAN, J. L. DE, *Histoire de l'entente cordiale Franco-Anglaise: Les relations de la France et de l'Angleterre depuis le XVIe siècle jusqu'a nos jours*, Paris, Alcan, 1916, xii+312 pp.

A propos des prisonniers français en Angleterre, voir: HUARD, P., ROUSSEAU, A. et WONG, M., 'Les prisonniers de guerre aux XVIII et XIX° siècles', in *Comptes Rendus du 91ème Congrès National des Sociétés Savantes*, Rennes, 1966, tome I, pp. 87–91.

BERTIN, RENÉ-JOSEPH HYACINTHE, *Quelques observations, critiques, philosophiques et médicales sur l'Angleterre, les Anglais et les Français, détenus dans les prisons de Plymouth*, Paris, Barrois Jeune, 1801, xxiv+135 pp.

Lorsque la Société de médecine et de chimie de Londres, fondée en 1805 à l'imitation de la Société de Médecine de Paris, commença à publier ses *Transactions*, Deschamps fils se chargea de les traduire et d'en rendre compte à la Société de Médecine.

Voir aussi, FILVEE, *Lettres sur l'Angleterre*, Paris, 1802.

VALENTIN, L., 'Deuxième fragment d'un voyage médical en Angleterre fait au printemps de 1803', *Journal général de médecine . . . Paris*, 1805, **24** an **14**, 297–318.

Description des pièces remarquables des musées de John et William Hunter (enfant à deux têtes, tumeur osseuse du col du fémur).

Description du jardin botanique de Kew avec les kangouroux. Visite de Bath, Bristol, Gloucester, Cheltenham, Oxford, Windsor. Visite à l'astronome Herschel à Slough.

DEMOLINS (Ed.), *A quoi tient la supériorité des Anglo-Saxons?* Paris, Firmin Didot, 1897, iv+412 pp.

Sur la vie des Anglais en France, consulter, MOORE, THOMAS (1779–1852), *The Troge family in Paris (1818)*.

TROLLOPE, FRANCES (1780–1863), *Paris and the Parisians in 1835*, Paris, Baudry, 1836.

Signalons la fin lamentable à Calais de Lady Hamilton (1765–1815) maitresse de l'amiral Lord Nelson.

2 Le dandysme est un humanisme rajeuni et rénové, une sorte de stoicisme égotiste, fondé sur le culte de soi-même, sur une certaine élégance personnelle. Le premier dandysme est byronien. Le second s'attache à Georges Bryan Brummel (1778–1840) qui mourut désargenté à Caen, laissant à Barbey d'Aurevilly le soin de défendre sa mémoire (1845). Parmi les dandystes français on pourrait citer: Chateaubriand, Stendhal, Delacroix, Vigny, Custine, Molènes, Th. Gautier, Mérimée, Baudelaire, etc.

Stendhal s'intéressait beaucoup à son 'Courrier anglais'. Il avait des amies américaines, les dames Garnett et Fanny Wright, l'émancipatrice des Noirs. D'Alton Shee fut, un temps, le compagnon d'Alfred de Musset. Marie Clarke avait ouvert un salon, rue des Petits Augustins à Paris, fréquenté par Fauriel.

Mérimée connaissait l'Angleterre par les élèves anglaises de sa mère et par le salon de Georges Cuvier où il avait connu sa belle fille Sophie Duvancel, l'amie de l'avocat Sutton Sharpe, peinte par Lawrence. Il était aussi entré en rapport avec la veuve de Shelley. Toute sa vie, Fanny Layden (1796–1879) et sa sœur Mrs. Eiven lui témoignèrent un parfait dévouement. Fanny fut enterrée au cimetière anglais de Cannes à côté de son vieil ami. Ajoutons que dans son âge mur, Mérimée passait volontier le pas de Calais pour se délasser «entre les bras blancs et un peu mollasses des belles de Covent Garden et de Drury Lane».

Cf. BARBEY D'AUREVILLY, J., *Du Dandysme et de Georges Brummel*, Caen, B. Mancel, 1845, 1861, 1879, vii+118 pp.

Cf. HUYGHE, RENÉ, 'Delacroix et le Dandysme', *Revue des Deux mondes*, 1er mai 1963.

D'Orsay fut l'ami de Macreadry, Thackeray, Disraeli, P. Maclise, Lord Lindhurst, et Dickens. Le Comte de Franqueville (+1919) membre à l'Institut, se remaria en 1903 avec Lady Sophia

Palmer. Il a laissé des Mémoires inédites (*Revue des Deux Mondes*, 15 juillet 1965) dans lesquels il parle de l'Exposition Universelle de Londre (1862).
Hariett Howard fut la maitresse du prince Louis Napoléon futur Napoléon III.

3 Notre premier couple sera celui Edouard Auguste, futur duc de Kent, amant de Julie de Montgenet de St. Laurent baronne de Fortisson, rencontrée au Canada en 1791. Il quitte au bout de 28 ans (1791–1818) la 'dame Française' pour épouser Victoria de Saxe-Cobourg, future mère de Victoria.
Vient ensuite le cas de Lord Seymour (+1859) dit milord l'Arsouille, fils naturel de la marquise de Hertford et de Montrond, l'ami de Talleyrand.
Il s'interessa aux hôpitaux de Londres et de Paris. Alfred d'Orsay (1800–52), beau-frère du duc de Guiche fut l'amant de la comtesse de Blessington et le mari (1827) de lady Hariett Gardiner, plus tard maitresse du duc d'Orléans.
Nous terminerons par les grands mariages franco-anglais, Cambronne, Lamartine, Vigny, Davaine, etc.
Lamartine assista en 1838 à une rencontre entre Bretons et Gallois à Abergavenny et y prit la parole.
Consulter Jean Stem, Lord Seymour. Paris, La Palatine, 1963.
Cf. Eliane Engel, Une amitié profonde, Dickens et d'Orsay. *Revue de Paris*, novembre 1968.

4 ROUX, PHILIBERT-JOSEPH, *Relation d'un voyage fait à Londres en 1814. Du parallèle de la chirurgie anglaise avec la chirurgie française*, Paris, Méquignon-Marvis, 1815.
FLEURENT, C. H., 'Philibert Joseph Roux's account of his own visit on 21 August 1814', *Annals of Royal College of Surgeons*, 1958, **23**, 47–52.
En 1814 après la paix, quelques chirurgiens anglais vinrent à Paris et manifestèrent publiquement en maintes circonstances le sentiment intime de leur supériorité chirurgicale. Il en résulta un étonnement parmi les chirurgiens français et Roux décida d'aller se faire une opinion sur place. Il se rendit donc à Londres en août 1814 pour y passer un mois. Il conclut: 'à côté des traits les plus brillants, la chirurgie anglaise offre les plus grandes imperfections, la chirurgie française est plus généralement bonne'. Il introduisit en France, en 1816, l'usage du pansement au diachylon dans les ulcères des jambes. C'était la pratique de Hunter, Cooper, Bell et Baynton. En septembre 1819, il opéra un étudiant anglais suivant la clinique de la Charité, nommé John Stephenson, d'une division congénitale du voile du palais. Il donna le nom de staphyloraphie à cette opération, qui fut suivie d'un succès rapide et dont il reste le créateur.
Voir à ce sujet, BUSQUET, PAUL ROUX, PHILIBERT-JOSEPH, in *Bibliographies médicales*, Paris, J. B. Baillière, 1929, no. 25, pp. 297–308.

5 CADET DE GASSICOURT, CH. L., 'De l'état de la médecine et de la pharmacie en Angleterre, *J. de Ph.*, 1817, **3**, 321–34. Article Charlatans, in *Dictionnaire des Sciences Médicales*, Paris, Panckoucke, 1812–22, pp. 543–53.

6 Amédée Pichot, grand érudit et écrivain (1795–1877) a publié de nombreux livres sur l'histoire et les grands hommes de l'Angleterre: Histoire de Charles-Edouard, précédée d'une histoire de la rivalité de l'Angleterre et de l'Ecosse. Voyage historique et littéraire de la Grande-Bretagne, L'Irlande et le pays de Galles. Voyage pittoresque d'Ecosse. Il a traduit également de nombreux ouvrages anglais: Byron, Shakespeare, quoique médecin. Il fut envoyé par Roux à Londres où il rencontra Sir Astley Cooper, qui après l'avoir invité à déjeuner et à diner, le fit assister à une de ses opérations chirurgicales. Lors de l'intervention, Pichot ne put se prévenir d'un malaise et comme le lendemain il allait s'en excuser et maudissait son 'système nerveux': 'Non, non, lui dit Sir Astley, vous en triompherez; je peux vous adresser à Charles Bell qui vous dira ce qu'il lui a fallu de courage pour faire sa première saignée'. Il fut très bien reçu et c'est à la suite de ce voyage que Pichot écrivit une première esquisse sur Charles Bell avant de publier en 1858 'La vie et les œuvres de Sir Charles Bell' (œuvre dans laquelle nous avons trouvé de nombreux renseignements au sujet de la querelle qui l'opposa à Magendie). Sur un autre plan, Amédée Pichot, DM en 1817, était rédacteur en chef de la 'Revue Britannique' tandis que Guerland de Beaumont (1845) était rédacteur au *Times Médical*.

7 BILLARD, C., 'Coup d'œil sur les hôpitaux, les établissements de charité, et l'instruction médicale en Angleterre', in *Archives Générales de Médecine*, 1828, **16**, 40–61.
Ch. Michel Billard (1800–32), interne des Hôpitaux de Paris aux Enfants Trouvés, rédigea un 'traité des maladies des enfants nouveaux-nés', voyagea en Suisse et en Angleterre. Il fut très bien reçu à Londres.

8 Voir note 43.

9 Magendie et Nathalis Guillot vont étudier le choléra en Irlande en 1831 et deux membres de l'Académie de Médecine avec Mabit vont à Londres en 1846, lors d'une épidémie de choléra. Magendie faillit se faire expulser comme tête de Turc des antivivisectionnistes.
Cf. OZER, M. N., The British vivisection controversy, BHM 1966, no. 2, pp. 158–67.

10 D. Larrey était très lié avec l'amiral Sir Sydney Smith, fixé à Paris, président de la *Société antipirate des chevaliers libérateurs des esclaves blancs* (1839) qui fit partie du nouvel ordre du

Temple ressuscité par Fabré Palapret. Il fit également un voyage en Angleterre après la chute de l'Empire.

11 BOURJOT SAINT HILAIRE, A., *Lettre à un médecin de province sur les établissements médicaux et particulièrement sur les dispensaires ophtalmiques de Londres*, Paris, l'auteur, 1836, 31 pp.

12 'En septembre 1826, Dupuytren se rendit en Angleterre pour y étudier les progrès et les audaces de la chirurgie anglaise. Dès la chute de l'empire, les relations s'étaient renouées entre les chirurgiens anglais et leurs confrères français. Le voyage de Roux en Angleterre au mois d'août 1814, dont il publia la relation en 1815, révéla la chirurgie anglaise au public médical français. Peu à peu, s'établirent des rapports intimes entre les savants des deux pays et le 20 août 1817 la Société de Médecine conféra le titre de correspondants étrangers à dix chirurgiens anglais: Brodie, Abernethy qui le premier avait osé lier l'artère iliaque externe (1796), A. Cooper, Home, Ch. Bell, Hey William, Carpue, Adams, Willoch et Baynton.

La chirurgie anglaise brillait surtout par les audacieuses innovations de ses chirurgiens dans les ligatures des troncs artériels et les résections osseuses. Dupuytren qui, dès 1810, avait voulu tenter la ligature de l'artère sous-clavière et en avait été empêché par son chef Pelletan, pouvait mesurer alors tout le chemin parcouru. En matière de résection, il pouvait au moins revendiquer le mérite d'avoir reséqué le premier avec succès tout le corps de la mâchoire inférieure et quelques années plus tard, le maxillaire supérieur.

Dupuytren fut accueilli à Londres comme le prince de la chirurgie. Astley Cooper l'invita chez lui plusieurs fois, dans la maison qu'il habitait à la campagne où il s'était retiré. Un jour que Dupuytren lui faisait compliment sur cette maison toute princière et admirait surtout la beauté des arbres gigantesques du parc: 'Oui, dit le chirurgien anglais, ils sont fort beaux. Tous les matins, je les examine pour voir celui où je me pendrai. A Londres, je serai mort de fatigue. Ici, je mourrai d'ennui'. 'A votre place, je retournerais à Londres.' répliqua Dupuytren.

Cooper reprit en effet l'exercice de sa profession qu'il continua jusqu'à sa mort (1841). Ce fait impressionna beaucoup Dupuytren qui répétait souvent 'J'exercerai ma profession jusqu'à la fin. Quand je ne pourrai plus visiter mes malades, je me ferai porter près d'eux.'

Dupuytren fut traduit en anglais. Cf. BARON DUPUYTREN, *On lesions of the vascular system diseases of the rectum and other surgical complaints, being selections from the collected edition of the clinical lectures*, translated by F. Le Gros Clark, London, Sydenham Society, 1854, 8, 378 pp.

13a BUREAUD-RIOTREY, A. M., *Londres. Ancien et Moderne ou recherches sur l'état physique et social de cette métropole*, Paris–Londres, Baillière, 1839. 138 pp. Cette étude comprend: (1) Un précis de l'histoire médicale de Londres jusqu'au XVIIIe siècle (étude des maladies et de la salubrité. Rapport entre les deux). (2) Etude de Londres au XVIIIe siècle où les fléaux les plus meurtriers disparaissent. (3) Londres contemporain. Seule la première partie est vraiment développée.

Il a fait plusieurs publications en français et en anglais et a eu l'idée d'une revue médicale anglaise, publiée à Paris, chez Crochard.

Bureaud-Riofrey habitait en 1836 Newmor street et Oxford street 22.

13b René Marjolin (1818–95) fit un voyage en Angleterre avant de se présenter au bureau central (1840). Il fut admirablement reçu par Sir Astley Cooper, Lawrence, Ch. Bell, Syme et Benjamin Brodie (Paul Reclus, *Revue Scientifique*, 1895, p. 100).

14 POINTE, J. P., 'Notice sur l'Hôpital Guy à Londres', *Loisirs médicaux et littéraires*, Lyon, 1844.

15 TOURDES, G., 'Excursion médicale à Londres', in *Gazette Médicale de Strasbourg*, no. 11, 20 novembre 1847, pp. 350–76.

'Londres sous bien des rapports est inférieur à Paris mais il y a dans la capitale anglaise une grandeur sérieuse et forte que la nôtre ne présente pas.' Il ajoute: 'à la différence de la France, fortement centralisée, l'instruction médicale en Angleterre s'est créée et organisée d'elle même. Le corps enseignant est distinct de celui qui donne les grades et seule la corporation accorde le droit de pratiquer.'

D'autres strasbourgeois ont passé la Manche: Jacques Léon Aronsohn (1793–1861) professeur agrégé à Strasbourg, fut cordialement accueilli à Londres par Astley Cooper, Lawrence, Brodie, Tynell. Sedillot (1847) va voir Hancock et rapporte à Strasbourg la pratique de l'anesthésie générale à l'ether.

16 DAREMBERG, CHARLES, 'Résumé d'un voyage médico-littéraire en Angleterre', *Gazette Médicale de Paris*, 4 novembre 1848, no. 45, pp. 863–76.

Le but de ce voyage était d'étudier les manuscrits de médecine contenus dans la bibliothèque de Londres, d'Oxford et de Middlehill. Il constata que la plus riche collection de manuscrits grecs et latins est à Bodley (Oxford) ensuite à Middlehill, puis à la Société de Médecine.

17 Lorsque les succès des ovariotomistes anglais ont été connus en France, nombreux sont les chirurgiens français qui sont allés en Angleterre. Quelques noms doivent être signalés: Topinard, *Thèse de Méd. Paris (1860)*. Blondel-Ser: *Rapport sur les hopitaux civils de la ville de Londres, au point de vue de la comparaison de ces établissements avec les hopitaux de la ville de Paris*, Paris, 1862, in 4°, 238 pp. Gayet va voir opérer à Londres Spencer Wells et Baker Brown. Il assiste

à la première ovariotomie lyonnaise suivie de succès exécutée par Desgranges, chirurgien chef de l'Hôtel Dieu, le 10 septembre 1862.
La malade fut opérée à son domicile, alors qu'elle avait été hospitalisée dans son service. Demarquay perd à Paris une opérée et va s'informer à Londres en 1862. Il est suivi par A. Nélaton qui va voir opérer Spencer Wells et Baker Brown. Ce dernier reçoit également la visite de Giraldès, Péan et A. Liégard. (Cf. LIEGARD, A., 'Une visite à l'hôpital Ste Marie à Londres et à la maison de santé du Dr Baker-Brown', *Gazette des Hôpitaux*, 1862, pp. 349–51).

17 TOPINARD, P., 'Quelques aperçus sur la chirurgie anglaise' (*Thèse de médecine de Paris, 1860*). Topinard fut reçu en 1860 par Lawrence, Syme, Thomson et Deville.
Il visita notamment le *California*, dreadnought de 120 canons, à l'ancre sur la Tamise et transformé en hôpital pour tous les marins du monde. Voici ses conclusions: (1) La mortalité des opérations sanglantes en général parait plus élevée à Paris qu'à Londres. (2) La mortalité dans les grandes amputations des membres est considérablement plus élevée à Paris qu'à Londres. (3) La pyémie est plus fréquente à Paris qu'à Londres. (4) Le procédé opératoire de Teale et la simplicité du traitement ultérieur diminuent la mortalité des amputations.
Un peu avant lui, Léon Le Fort s'était rendu en Angleterre en 1858 avec le désir d'étudier quelques points de la chirurgie anglaise et surtout la question des résections articulaires. Par son mémoire sur les résections du genou (1859) il fut amené à étudier la statistique d'amputation de la cuisse dans les hôpitaux britanniques et constata dans la mortalité consécutive à ces amputations une grande différence à l'avantage de l'Angleterre. Les mémoires de Le Fort étaient les premiers où les résections de la hanche et du genou faisaient l'objet d'un examen complet où toute la littérature mondiale était commentée après une enquête faite en Angleterre, où, pendant cinq mois, la technique opératoire, les soins post-opératoires, les conditions hospitalières et les résultats définitifs avaient été passés en revue. Le Fort voulut rechercher la cause des meilleurs résultats obtenus en Angleterre et retourna en 1860 visiter les principaux hôpitaux en Angleterre, Ecosse, Irlande, Hollande et Belgique. De retour à Paris, il rassembla ses observations et conclusions dans un travail intitulé *Notes sur quelques points de l'hygiène hospitalière en France et en Angleterre*, Paris, Masson, 1862, 48 pp.
Une comparaison entre les hôpitaux de Paris et de Londres est faite plus tard par Le Fort, Malgaigne, Topinard, Husson et Verneuil. Husson, haut fonctionnaire de l'Assistance Publique, considère que le niveau parisien est acceptable. Par contre, en 1823 il y a à Londres 200.000 lieux d'aisance (dont 10.000 W.C.). Paris n'en compte que 70.000.

18 COURTY, AMÉDÉE, *Excursion chirurgicale en Angleterre, Lettres adressées à Mr le Professeur Bouisson*, Paris, P. Asselin, 1863, 96 pp.
Dans ce travail dédié à J. V. Simpson, sont signalées comme des nouveautés l'usage des pinces à pression continue sur les veines (Spencer Wells); l'aspiration avec un siphon de caoutchouc des liquides kystiques; la toilette du péritoine et les ligatures perdues intrapéritonéales (Tyler Smith).

19 SARRAZIN, CHARLES, 'Essai sur les hôpitaux de Londres', *Annales d'hygiène publique et de médecine légale*, 1866, **25**, 45–72.
'Essai sur les hôpitaux', *Annales d'hygiène publique et de médecine légale*, 1865, **24**, 295–374.

20 1888, Ch. Penier, Nicaise et Tenier vont voir Lister à Glasgow et Spencer Wells à Londres. Tenier voit aussi Lawson Tait et plus tard Horsley.

21 BONNAFONT, 'Souvenirs de voyage en Ecosse. Une journée passée à Edimbourg avec le Dr Simpson', *Union médicale*, 1870.

22 Cf. BROCHIN, *Gazette des Hôpitaux*, 22 novembre 1872, pp. 281–83, 290–91.

23 Pierre Budin fut opéré par Lawson-Tait.

24 Guéneau de Mussy était bien connu en Angleterre et s'y plaisait beaucoup. L'un de ses voyages coincide avec ceux de la jeune école de chirurgie française chez Lister. Il considère ce dernier comme le premier chirurgien qui ait osé (sous le couvert de l'antisepsie) faire de grandes incisions; lier de grosses veines au catgut; ouvrir les hydarthroses chroniques, les explorer au doigt et suturer la rotule fracturée. Personne ne l'avait fait avant lui.
Cf. GUÉNEAU DE MUSSY, NOËL, 'Notes et impressions de voyage dans les trois royaumes écrites au courant du crayon', *France médicale*, 1875, nos. 82, 84, 88, 92, 96, 98, 100 et 101 bis. Voir aussi, 'Souvenirs et impression du meeting de l'association médicale britannique à Cork (1879)', *Union Médicale*, 1886, 6, 8, 15, 22, 29 janvier, 12, 19 février, 2, 3, 4, 9 mars.

25 POZZI, S., 'Quelques observations à propos du pansement de Lister', *Progrès Médical*, 1876, pp. 813–15, 835–36, 857–59, 878–81. Pozzi avait traduit Darwin en français.

26 MANOURY, G., 'La chirurgie antiseptique à Edimbourg', *Progrès Médical*, 1876, no. 42, pp. 701–4, no. 43, pp. 714–15.

27 Ricord traduisit plusieurs ouvrages anglais d'histoire naturelle, tandis que son frère Jean-Baptiste, Docteur en Médecine de New York, est l'auteur d'une grammaire anglaise longtemps classique dans les collèges d'Amérique. Au cours d'un voyage à Londres, assistant à une séance du Collège Royal des Chirurgiens de Londres, il fut complimenté par le Président comme fils du savant traducteur de John Hunter et l'auteur de nombreux travaux. Et Ricord répondit: 'Je

vous remercie, Monsieur le Président, du haut témoignage d'admiration que vous venez de donner à mon père, mais mon père, c'est moi!'

28 HUARD, P. et VETTER, TH., 'Le docteur Jean Civiale et la lithotritie', *Episteme*, 1967, no. 3, pp. 239–54.

29 DIDIER, R., *Vie et souvenirs du Dr Albert Brochin* (*1844–1932*), Paris, Pierre André, 1935.
DIDIER, R., *Péan*, Paris, Maloine, 1948, 242 pp., 24 pl.

30 VOIR LE GAUBICHON, J. H., 'Bio-Bibliographie de Pierre Paul Broca', *Thèse de Méd.*, Rennes, 1962, no. 286.

31 Muron (+1874) ancien interne des Hôpitaux de Paris, préparateur de Ranvier et collaborateur de la Gazette médicale de Paris voyagea en Angleterre (*Progrès médical*, 1912, pp. 27–29).

32 VOIR MÉLOT, H., 'Contribution à l'étude du développement de la Médecine et de la Pharmacie à Rennes et dans la région rennoise', *Thèse de médecine*, Rennes, 1963.

33 Amédée Deville (+1879) fut interne des hôpitaux en 1841, puis aide d'anatomie en 1843 et prosecteur des hôpitaux en 1846. Malgré sa valeur il échoua à l'agrégation (1847) et au bureau central (1850). Républicain, il s'abstint de toute activité politique lors du coup d'Etat de 1851. Néanmoins, il fut arrêté et condammé à la déportation à Cayenne. Ses amis dont Paul Broca purent intervenir à temps pour que Deville soit arrêté à Brest et que sa déportation soit commuée en exil. Il débarqua à Londres en 1852 et essaya d'abord d'y avoir une activité scientifique. Il rédigea une série d'articles sur la chirurgie anglaise. A la suite d'un incident où les torts ne paraissent pas être de son côté, il fut expulsé du *Guy's Hospital* en 1854, dans des conditions stigmatisées par Paul Broca. Il ouvrit alors un cabinet qui lui rapporta 25.000 francs par an. En quelques années, il avait fait 125.000 francs d'économies. Il signa la protestation de 1855 contre l'expulsion des proscrits de Jersey. Il eut comme client Victor Hugo, envoyé à sa consultation de Londres par le Dr. Corbin de Jersey. Il était écrit que la malchance le poursuivrait toujours. En 1861, il présenta des troubles mentaux et dut être hospitalisé jusqu'à la fin de la vie dans une maison de santé d'Ivry. Caffe et Paul Broca ont rédigé sa nécrologie. Cf. BROCA, PAUL, 'Armand Deville', *Gaz. hebd. Méd. chir.*, 1879, no. 92, pp. 675–76 et *Progrès Médical*, 1879, p. 841.
Armand Deville a donné ses impressions sur la médecine londonienne dans deux séries d'articles: (1) 'Coup d'œil sur la chirurgie anglaise', *Mon. hop.*, 1853, pp. 25, 36, 42, 50, 57, 74, 90, 97, 107, 114, 130, 162, 170, 186, 195, 213, 228, 253, 267, 276, 283, 300, 305, 389, 396, 419, 473, 650, 674, 683, 692, 702, 706. (2) 'Revue clinique des hôpitaux anglais', *Mon. hop.*, 1853, pp. 1205–430. 'Sur les médecins de Victor Hugo, voir Maurice Genty', *Progrès médical*, 1935, no. 6, pp. 41–48.

34 Paul Lafargue (1842–1912) né à Santiago de Cuba, fut exclu des Facultés françaises pour avoir pris part au Congrès de Liège (1865). Docteur en médecine de Londres, gendre de Karl Marx, il se suicida avec sa femme.

35 Pierre Leroux (1797–1871) exilé à Jersey a ensuite enseigné la phrenologie à Londres en 1863. Il créa le mot socialisme. Cf. GRIFFITHS, DAVID A., 'Un ouvrage inconnu de Pierre Leroux. Cours de Phrénologie, 1853', *RHES*, 1962, no. 2.

36 Heurteloup employa son instrumentation de lithotritie huit fois en Angleterre et deux fois en France avant de recevoir un prix de 5.000 francs de l'Institut (1828). Il résida plusieurs années à Londres et fit plusieurs démonstrations de son procédé auxquels s'intéressèrent Costallat, A. Cooper et Crampton. Leston et Brodie y furent opposés, tout au moins au début.

37 A. Lutaud (1847–1925), ancien mousse, exerça au Pérou de 1862 à 1866 avant de se fixer à Londres. Anglophile et antipastorien, il devint médecin de l'Hôpital français de Londres en 1874 et collabora au *British Medical Journal*. Il fonda le *Journal de Médecine de Paris* en 1881. Il édita sous le pseudonyme de Dr. Minime, *La médecine anecdotique, historique et littéraire*, 3 vols., Paris, 1901–4.

38 Laennec n'est jamais allé en Angleterre comme son oncle mais a eu de nombreux élèves britanniques parmi ses trois cents élèves étrangers. Cf. HUARD, P. et GRMEK, M., 'Les élèves étrangers de Laennec', *Congrès des Sociétés Savantes Nantes*, 1972. Voir aussi, Laennec et M. Baillie (*Ann. Roy. Coll. Surg. England*, 1965, **36**, 67).
et l'autobiographie de Matthew Baillie (*Practitioner*, juillet 1896, pp. 51–65).

39 Sur les rapports entre savants anglais et français et sur les anglais internés en France sous le Consulat et l'Empire, voir LANZAC DE LABORIE, L. DE, *Paris sous Napoléon*, Paris Plon, 1905–13, 8 tomes.
PAUL, SIR JOHN DEAN, *Journal d'un voyage à Paris au mois d'août 1802*, Paris, A. Picard, 1913, traduit et annoté par Paul Lacombe, 162 pp., pl.
YORKE, H. REDHEARD, *Paris et la France sous le Consulat*, Trad. Lerole, Paris, Perrin, 1896.
LAWRENCE, J. H., *A picture of Verdun*, 2 vols. 1810.
FORBES, JAMES, *Letters from France written in the years 1803–1804*, Londres, 1806, 2 vol.
BATTEAU, ALBERT, *Les Anglais en France après la paix d'Amiens. Impressions de voyage de Sir John Can*, Paris, Plon, 1898, 300 pp., pl.
BEER, SIR GAVIN DE, *The Sciences were never at war*, Londres, Thomas Nelson, 1960, xv+

279 pp. Rapports entre savants français et anglais entre 1650 et 1815: inédits de Néamur, Banks, Delambre, Jenner, etc.

39 Watt (père et fils) correspondent avec Monge en 1791 et en 1793 (AMRF juillet–septembre 1963). Davy débarqua à Morlaix en 1813 et passa deux mois à Paris avant d'aller en Italie. Il assista à une séance solennelle de l'Institut, assis à droite du Président. Il fut reçu par Ampère, Laplace, Gay Lussac, Thénard, Berthollet, Cuvier etc. Cl. Niepce passa en Angleterre pour essayer de vendre un navire propulsé par un système de fusée. Il y meurt dans la misère.

40 Gregory Watt (1777–1804), 'Tour on the continent 1801, presented by Sir Gavin de Beer', *Annals of Science*, 1957, no. 3, pp. 127–36. Sir Rutherford Alcock (1809–97), étudiant en médecine à Paris, chirurgien militaire en Espagne et au Portugal (1832–36), consul à Foutcheou, puis à Changaï, soigna gracieusement son collègue français Montigny en Angleterre.

41a Carpue vint à Paris et assista avec Percy à une cystostomie sus-pubienne faite par Soubervielle sur M. Walwille administrateur de l'hôtel des Invalides, en août 1817.

41b Sur Jenner, voir LE FANU, W. R., *A bio-Bibliographie of Ed. Jenner*, Londres, 1950.

42 MATTHEWS, HENRY, *The diary of an Invalid, being the journal of a Tour in Portugal, Italy, Switzerland and France in years 1817–1819*, Londres, 1819.

43 AVERY, HAROLD, 'John Bell's last tour', *Medical History*, janvier 1964, pp. 69–77. Il débarqua à Paris en juin 1817 et vit son ami D. Larrey. Il partit ensuite pour Lyon et Rome où il sera enterré au cimetière des Anglais en 1820. Consulter aussi WALLS, E. W., 'John Bell (1763–1820)', *Med. History*, janvier 1964, pp. 63–69.

44 Hickman vient à Paris en 1828 à l'Hôtel des Ambassades, 11, rue Notre Dam des Victoires.

45 CROSS, J. G., *Paris et Montpellier ou Tableau de la Médecine dans ces deux écoles*, Paris, Montpellier, 1820.

ESTOR, H., 'Quelques maitres de la Faculté de Médecine de Montpellier vus par un Anglais', *Monspeliensis Hippocrates*, 1959, no. 4, pp. 22–29.

CLARK, SIR JAMES (1788–1870), *Medical notes on climate, diseases, hospitals, and medical schools in France, Italy and Switzerland*, Londres, 1820.

46 Benjamin Phillips témoin des expériences de Velpeau (1830) les répète à Londres (1831).

47 James Hope (1801–41), est l'élève de G. Andral (1797–1876).

48 Sir Astley Cooper vint à Paris en 1834 avec Diettenbach et Heine qui faisait la démonstration de son ostéotome.

49 Alexandre Stewart, ami de Guéneau de Mussy suit la clinique de Chomel en 1839. L'année suivante il étudie le diagnostic différentiel du typhus et de la fièvre typhoide.

50 Sir Charles Bell fut l'hôte de Roux à Paris (1840); KIDD, C., 'A letter to the editor on the present appearances the hospitals of Paris', *Dublin G.J.M. Soc.*, 1848, **6**, 216–22.

51 Sir James Paget visite le service de Larrey où aucun décès n'avait jamais eu lieu après une désarticulation de l'épaule. Or un sujet de cet ordre était à la morgue mais mort de pneumonie (1862). Cf. *British Medical Journal*, 1862, **2**, 157.

52a SPENCER WELLS, THOMAS, 'Some causes of excessive mortality after surgical operations', *Brit. Med. J.*, 1864, no. 2, pp. 384–88.

Wells a été le premier chirurgien à noter l'importance des travaux de Pasteur sur la mortalité post opératoire.

Spencer Wells et Keith viennent voir opérer Koeberlé à Strasbourg. Koeberlé leur donna (1866) des drains en verre de sa fabrication que les chirurgiens anglais employèrent avec succès. Consulter aussi SIMMS, F., *A winter in Paris. A few experiences of French medical and sanitary matters during the season of 1865*, Londres, 1866.

52b GAMGEE, SAMSON, 'The present state of surgery in Paris', *Lancet*, 1867, **2**, 393.

53 E. Ackerknecht (*Medicine at the Paris Hospital 1794–1848*, Baltimore (1967)) donne une liste très représentative des maîtres français et de leurs visiteurs anglais: Malgaigne, Spencer Wells; P. Louis; Forbes, Badd, Farr, W. H. Walshe, Carswell, Marshall Hall; Andral; Hope; Piorry, A. V. Waller; Doné; J. H. Bennett; Equirol; W. A. F. Brown et A. Morison. Il ajoute aussi les noms de E. H. Sieve-king et W. Bowman.

54 J. H. Bennett et Oliffe fondent la *Paris Medical Society* commune aux Anglo-saxons et aux médecins de langue allemande (E. Ackerknecht).

55 Cf. LIVEING, EDWARD, 'English medical practitioners in France', *Lancet*, 1889, **ii**, 1144. Sur les controverses franco anglaises sur l'exercice de la médecine, voir LUTAUD, 'L'exercice de la médecine en France par les médecins étrangers', *Rev. Méd. Leg. Paris*, 1896, pp. 137–39; et Roger Mauvaise qui fit un article sur la loi sur l'exercice de la médecine et sur les réactions désagréables du *Lancet* en 1879 (*Gaz. heb. med. chir.* 1879, p. 177).

56 VAULTIER, R., 'La médecine militaire en 1870', *Presse Médicale*, 1957, no. 94, pp. 2203–7.

Voici quelques thèses soutenues à Paris par des Anglais: STORMONT, CH., 'Essai sur la topographie médicale de la Côte occidentale d'Afrique', *Thèse de Med. Paris*, 1822, no. 72, 69 pp.

CONWELL, WILLIAM E. E., 'Recherches sur les propriétés médicinales et l'emploi en médecine

de l'huile de Croton iglium et quelques propositions sur les maladies de l'Inde', *Thèse de méd. de Paris*, 1824, no. 19, 25 pp.
Il a probablement introduit le stéthoscope en Inde: *Observations chiefly on pulmonary disease in India and an essay on use of the stethoscope*, Malacca, Mission Press, 1829.
BENNET, J. H., 'Sur les ulcérations et les engorgements du col utérin', *Thèse méd. de Paris*, 1843, no. 206. Il écrit en anglais. A practical treatise of inflammation of the uterus, Londres. J. Churchill, 1849, traduit en français par F. A. Aran sous le titre: Traité pratique de l'inflammation de l'utérus, de son col et de ses annexes. Paris-Labé, 1850, 429 pp.
GOOD, R. R., 'De la résection coxo-fémorale pour carie', *Thèse méd.*, Paris, 1869, no. 37.

57 Foullioy, chirurgien de la marine française fut envoyé en Angleterre en 1829 pour étudier le procédé de salaison des viandes de la Marine Anglaise. Il introduisit à Brest la propreté et l'aération britannique. Il épouse Mademoiselle Blunt, fille d'un général adjoint de Wellington au Portugal et venu se fixer à Lorient.
Bien d'autres médecins français firent le voyage d'Angleterre. Par exemple, DUVAL, H., d'Argentan publie 'Deux mots sur l'hôpital de Jersey' (*J. des con. Méd. Pratiques*, mai 1847), pp. 281–83 où il déclare n'avoir vu aucune mort pour amputation en deux ans, mais des guérisons en 15 à 20 jours. Cf. BERGUES, C., 'La supériorité de la chirurgie anglaise au milieu du XIXe siècle et l'essor de la chirurgie moderne', *Thèse de méd.*, Lyon, 1966, no. 214.

58 J. M. Evrard (1808–82), ancien employé de Charrière à Paris, devint le collaborateur de Sir John Tomes (1815–95) en émigrant à Londres.

59 C'est Nelaton qui introduisit l'ovariotomie à Paris à la suite d'un voyage en Angleterre. Quand l'ovariotomie nous vint pour la première fois d'Angleterre vers 1840, il y avait pourtant plus de 20 ans qu'on la pratiquait aux Etats-Unis. Mais il faut dire que les premières tentatives faites en France n'avaient pas été heureuses, et qu'en Angleterre même les chirurgiens les plus éminents l'avaient condamnée. Ce sont les succès répétés de Spencer Wells et Baker Brown qui fixèrent de nouveau tous les regards sur cette opération. Au mois de novembre 1861, voulant juger les choses par lui-même, Nelaton se rendit en Angleterre. Cinq opérations pratiquées sous ses yeux par Baker Brown levèrent tous ses scrupules: il revint convaincu.

60 HUARD, P., 'Eugène Koeberlé pionnier de l'asepsie, de l'hemostase, de la gynécologie et de la chirurgie moderne', *Epistème*, 1968, no. 3, pp. 219–43.

61 En août 1881, Pasteur est délégué de la France au Congrès médical international de Londres. Il y reçoit un accueil triomphal. L'entrée de Pasteur dans la salle du Congrès, qui groupait trois mille médecins, présidé par le Prince de Galles et le Prince de Prusse, est racontée dans la 'Vie de Pasteur' par son gendre René Vallery-Radot: 'pendant qu'il (Pasteur) se dirigeait vers les marches de cette estrade, les applaudissements éclatèrent. De toutes parts, on poussait des vivats, des hurrahs. Pasteur se retourna vers ses deux compagnons qui étaient son fils et son gendre et leur dit avec un mouvement d'inquiétude 'c'est sans doute le Prince de Galles qui arrive, j'aurais dû venir plus tôt'. 'Mais c'est vous que tout le monde acclame!', dit avec son grave et affectueux sourire, le Président du Congrès Sir James Paget'. A la suite de Paget, de Lister, toute la médecine anglaise réserva un accueil triomphal à Pasteur, le distinguant seul parmi tous les savants réunis, chacun connaissant ses travaux et ses recherches. Après avoir fait des communications, en particulier sur la vaccination contre le choléra des poules et le charbon, Pasteur remercia les membres du Congrès en ces termes 'Permettez-moi, Messieurs, de ne pas terminer sans vous témoigner la joie que j'éprouve en pensant que je vous ai parlé vaccine et vaccination d'une maladie plus terrible peut-être pour les animaux domestiques que la variole pour l'homme, et que je l'ai fait à titre de membre d'un congrès international siégeant en Angleterre. La science, je l'espère, consacrera, à l'avenir, l'extension que j'ai donnée à l'expression de vaccination, par hommage pour le mérite et les immenses services rendus par un des plus grands hommes de l'Angleterre, votre Jenner. Quel bonheur pour moi de glorifier ce nom immortel sur le sol même de la noble et hospitalière cité de Londres!' Pour terminer ce voyage, Pasteur visita une laiterie fondée sur ses travaux. La visite de Pasteur à Londres eut un tel retentissement que son discours fut imprimé et distribué à tous les membres de la Chambre des Communes.
Tout au long des recherches de Pasteur qui s'acharne contre la rage, biologistes et médecins anglais seront ceux qui, avec les Russes, feront tout de suite confiance à la vaccination pasteurienne. Au milieu d'Avril 1886, le gouvernement anglais avait nommé une commission pour vérifier les faits relatifs à la vaccination anti-rabique. Sir James Paget en était le président, mais c'est surtout avec le secrétaire de ce comité, le Docteur Victor Horsley, que Pasteur nouera des relations étroites. Horsley vint lui même à Paris, avec Burdon Sanderson, pour voir appliquer la méthode. Il envoya des malades à Pasteur.
Le comité fera son rapport en 1886: 'Report of the committee of inquiry into Mr. Pasteur's treatment of hydrophobia.' Ce document est le sujet de toutes les conversations aussi bien à Londres qu'à Paris. Il est pour Pasteur une arme contre ses ennemis français, Peter et Lutaud qui l'attaquent aux séances de l'Académie de médecine.

En 1889, Pasteur est invité à Londres par Sir James Paget pour y prendre la parole au cours d'un meeting tenu à Londres contre les antivivisectionnistes, mais il est encore très gêné par l'hémiplégie qui l'a atteint en octobre 1887 et ne peut prendre la parole en public. Il envoie alors à Londres Roux et Yersin, qui viennent de publier leurs travaux sur la diphtérie.

62 Lucas-Championniere fonda le *Journal de Médecine* en 1830. Propagandiste du pansement 'Listérien' il était allé l'étudier en 1869 à Glasgow. Il fit à la suite de ce voyage un article qui resta sans écho. C'est en mars 1875 seulement que, pour la première fois, il fut question à la *Société de chirurgie de Paris* du pansement de Lister. En 1876, il fit paraître sa *Chirurgie antiseptique* tellement claire et didactique qu'elle fut traduite en anglais.

63 PROVOST, E., *Bio-bibliographie de Léon Le Fort (1829–1893)*', *Thèse de med.*, Rennes, 1959.

64 Sur l'amélioration des statistiques opératoires de Nélaton par l'emploi de l'alcool voir Wangensteen, OWEN, H., 'Préludes to Lister and the interdependence of the sciences', *Surgery*, 1965, **58**, no. 5, 931–34; 'Some highlights in the history of amputations reflecting lessons in wound healing', *Bull. Hist. Med.*, 1967, **41**, no. 2, 97–131; 'Military surgeons and surgery old and new. An instructive chapter in management of contaminated wounds', *Surgery*, 1967, **62**, no. 6, 1102–24.

65 La suture primitive des moignons avait été introduite dans les hôpitaux de Paris par Ph. Roux. En 1832 il suturait d'élégants moignons au prix d'une mortalité énorme. Son beau-père, le baron Boyer, vieux et goutteux, laissait ses moignons béants et les remplissait de bourdonnets de charpie. Les guérisons étaient nombreuses mais au prix d'un moignon conique.
Dans les hôpitaux de la Marine (beaucoup plus propres que ceux de Paris) J. Arland par la suture sur drainage préventif avait désarticulé vingt deux membres sans un seul décès en 1866. Mais il n'avait pas été suivi. Si bien que peu après la guerre de 1870, trois pansements avaient leurs partisans. En Allemagne, Billroth retroussait les manchettes de ses moignons et les laissait plusieurs jours exposés à l'air, sans les suturer. A Paris, Alphonse Guérin maintenait les parties molles en contact à l'aide de son énorme pansement ouaté, A Londres, Lister suturait, drainait et appliquait son pansement phéniqué.

66 PELLET, L., 'La médecine navale française au XIXe siècle, *Thèse med. de Rennes*, 1966.

67 OLMSTED, I. M. D., 'The influence of Claude Bernard on medicine in the United States and England', *California A. West. Med.* (*San Francisco*), fév.-mars 1935, **42**, nos. 2 et 3, 111–74.

Th. Vetter
Paris (France)

Histoire naturelle et médecine à travers les relations entre la Grande-Bretagne et Strasbourg, du XVIe siècle à la Révolution

Trois ordres de faits jalonnent les communications intellectuelles, peu connues dans leur ensemble, entre la Grande-Bretagne et la cité de Strasbourg. Une première étape s'inscrit en un destin historique commun qui est celui de la turbulence religieuse. Malgré sa situation géographique plaçant l'Alsace en deçà des itinéraires habituels ayant pour but Paris, la Provence et l'Italie, comme le fait remarquer John Patrick Bury, des voyageurs et des naturalistes ouvrent un second volet à la connaissance.[1] Enfin Strasbourg ne peut rester en dehors du phénomène de l'anglomanie précédant la Révolution.

Au VIe siècle, des moines écossais fondèrent à Strasbourg un établissement transformé ultérieurement en église collégiale par l'évêque Adeloch. Mille ans plus tard, en 1523, le curé de ce sanctuaire voué à St. Thomas a contracté mariage. La doctrine de Luther compte déjà de nombreux partisans. La plupart des institutions conventuelles va recevoir d'autres destinations, leurs revenus sont assignés à la santé publique ou à l'enseignement. Dans le ci-devant couvent des Carmes, l'ancien Chartreux Otto Brunfels (1488–1534) développe les sciences naturelles et prépare les *Herbarum vivae icones*.

C'est dans ce grand mouvement de la Réforme avec son particularisme strasbourgeois, qu'il faut rechercher avec Koszul et d'autres,[2] les débuts des relations culturelles avec l'Angleterre.

«In Strasburg that noble town
A city of most famous renown
Where the Gospel is freely preached» . . .

La satire aux vers médiocres, confiée à l'édition par William Barlow ou du moins par l'un des membres du «groupe des moines défroqués» s'étant réfugiés dans la vallée du Rhin, constitue selon Koszul le premier poème anglais édité à Strasbourg.[3]

Tandis que des pasteurs anglais, tels William Turner qui cultive la botanique et l'œnologie à Wissembourg, s'installent en Alsace,[4] la contre-réforme menace le protestantisme. Refusant d'accepter l' «intérim» imposé à la ville libre par Charles Quint en 1507, trois des représentants strasbourgeois les plus notoires vont émigrer dans le royaume d'Edouard VI, décidé à fonder l'anglicanisme. L'un d'eux, Martin Bucer (1491–1551) jouera un rôle de premier plan à Canterbury et surtout à Cambridge.

Déjà le cours de l'histoire change. Cinq ans après le décès de Bucer, la reine Marie Tudor fait déterrer son corps et le fait brûler publiquement. Devant l'intransigeante réaction de la nouvelle souveraine, ses sujets s'enfuient par centaines à Strasbourg.

Siècle de crise, le XVIe est aussi celui de l'humanisme. Moralistes et prédicateurs avaient donné le ton, qui sont trop nombreux pour être énumérés ici. En 1538 Jean Sturm (1507–89) obtient la transformation de la Haute-Ecole en Gymnase.[5] Ami intime de Vésale avec lequel il avait séjourné trois années durant à Paris, le nouveau recteur se souviendra de ses études de médecine.[6] L'année 1544, il fait venir auprès de lui Jean-Guinther d'Andernach, leur condisciple parisien. L'anatomiste-chirurgien enseigne le grec. Mais il est vraisemblable qu'il donnera ultérieurement des commentaires des Anciens. A la demande du Magistrat, il rédige un traité d'hydrothérapie et sur la peste. Inaugurés en 1545 par Sebald Hawenreuter (1508–89), les premiers cours de médecine n'ont pas un succès immédiat. Le but de l'enseignement au Gymnase était pourtant d'imposer aux étudiants des cours libres d'anatomie et des notions sur l'usage des parties aussi bien que des leçons de mathématiques, de physique ou de philosophie.

Mais c'est bien cette multivalence intellectuelle qui deviendra pour longtemps la caractéristique des maîtres strasbourgeois, autorisant leur permutation dans des chaires de lettres classiques ou de médecine théorique et pratique.

Sous l'autorité de Jean Sturm, l'établissement acquiert une réputation européenne, attirant des étudiants de toutes les nations. Le registre d'immatriculation de cette première période est malheureusement perdu. Une mise en condition doit y suppléer. La personnalité du recteur n'en est que plus intéressante, en particulier par les liens qui l'unissent à l'Angleterre. La correspondance avec la reine Elisabeth en est un des aspects.[7]

A Strasbourg même, Sturm compte des disciples et des amis anglais illustres, pour ne citer que John Hales,[8] Philip Sidney le familier de Henri Estienne et son frère Robert Sidney (1563–1626), les neveux du comte de Leicester. Sir Richard Moryson, ambassadeur à la cour de Charles Quint, décède à Strasbourg en 1556 après avoir été un fervent admirateur de Sleidan et de Sturm. De ce dernier, Moryson traduisit les œuvres et devint un propagandiste de Platon et d'Aristote, comme son secrétaire Roger Asham.[9]

Indissociable de cette grande concentration humaniste strasbourgeoise voulant réformer l'Eglise par la restauration des lettres, est le corollaire de l'imprimerie dont Jean Mentelin et Gutenberg sont les fondateurs. Les ouvrages médico-chirurgicaux sortis des officines de leurs successeurs sont classiquement connus. L'iconographie y joue un rôle capital. La prototypographie rhénane offre déjà sous le signe du temps, des traductions anglaises de la bible aussi bien que des traités de médecine.[10] Si Jean Fischart (né vers 1550) qui avait visité l'Angleterre au cours de sa vie errante fit imprimer chez son beau-frère Bernard Jobin une transposition vernaculaire de Gargantua,[11] il ne faut pas ignorer l'impression des deux premiers opuscules théologiques de Michel Servet à Haguenau.

Sebastian Brand (1457–1521) l'un des précurseurs de la Réforme, avait annoté une édition de Virgile, ornée de xylographies somptueuses. Mais il est surtout l'auteur de *Narrenschiff*[12] dont le succès fut immense. A partir des versions latines et françaises, Alexander Barclay invite dès 1509 en une adaptation anglaise ses compatriotes à s'embarquer dans *The Ship of Fools*. N'oublions pas que le successeur de William Caxton (1422–91) fut l'alsacien Wymherr de Worde ou Wörth.

Le 30 mai 1566, Sturm obtient de Maximilien II la transformation de la section supérieure du Gymnase en Académie habilitée à décerner les grades de bachelier et Maître-ès-Arts en théologie, philosophie, droit et médecine. L'empereur souhaite expressément l'assiduité des étudiants étrangers.

Arrivé à Strasbourg le 14 janvier 1537, Jean Sturm poursuit son œuvre jusqu'en 1581. Accablé à la fin de sa vie par l'ingratitude de ses concitoyens, il trouve encore la consolation dans les échanges épistolaires, voire les visites de ses admirateurs anglais en sa retraite de Nordheim.

Par un nouveau privilège, Ferdinand II érige l' «Academia Argentinensis» en Université, avec quatre Facultés, à partir du 5 février 1621. Peu propice aux échanges, la guerre de Trente Ans dure de 1618 à 1648, décime la moitié de la population. La «matricula studiosorum medicinae» nous livre cependant, pour cette période troublée, le nom d'un étudiant londonien, George Perkins, inscrit le 20 septembre 1626, sous le rectorat de Johann-Rudolf Saltzmann (1570–1657) docteur en médecine et professeur.[13] Assurant l'enseignement de l'anatomie entre le troisième et le quatrième de la dynastie des Sebiz, Jean Valentin Scheid (1637–1731), un successeur de Saltzmann, avait effectué auparavant un séjour en Angleterre.

De la permanence des liens religieux à cette époque, les faits archivés apportent encore le témoignage, moins de dix ans avant l'entrée des troupes de Louis XIV à Strasbourg. En effet l'année 1673 les luthériens de Londres demandent et obtiennent du Magistrat de la Ville un secours pour la construction d'une église.[14]

Si pour plus d'un siècle les registres d'imatriculation sont muets en ce qui nous concerne, et dans la méconnaissance ou nous sommes des noms des étudiants de l'Hôpital Royal Militaire, il nous faut désormais nous tourner vers la curiosité des voyageurs, des naturalistes.[15] La notoriété de l'un d'eux comble avec intensité le vide apparent.

C'est à la date du 27 juillet 1663 que John Ray (1628–1707) ancien Fellow of Trinity College de Cambridge, arrive de Heidelberg à Strasbourg, en compagnie de deux ou trois amis anglais.[16] Une heureuse fortune voulut qu'il y rencontrât un autodidacte dont il assurera la gloire.

Issu d'une famille de pêcheurs, ce Leonhard Baldner fut baptisé à Strasbourg le 11 janvier 1612. Il est successivement préposé au péage fluvial, en même temps aubergiste en 1650, puis garde forestier et maître des eaux et forêts. Assesseur au Grand Conseil à la fin de sa vie, il est un notable de la cité.

Voué dès l'enfance à l'observation de la nature, il ne connaît que le «Livre des animaux» de Conrad Gesner (1516–65) parmi les rares ouvrages parus jusque là.[17] Mais il ne s'appuie pas sur le texte de l'auteur suisse quand il se décide à rédiger, sans souci de système, ses propres constatations. La capture d'un certain nombre d'oiseaux étrangers à la faune locale l'a d'abord incité à en demander le dessin à un artiste. Ainsi naît au bout de vingt années de labeur, ce trésor zoologique du XVIIe siècle dédié aux amateurs de la pêche et de la chasse.

De fait il ne s'agit pas d'un travail destiné à la publication. Baldner confiait au scribe et au peintre les éléments du manuscrit, dont on ne connait, présentement, que trois exemplaires illustrés.

Le plus complet et aussi le plus parfait à ce qu'il semble fut détruit dans la nuit du 24 août 1870 lors de l'incendie de la Bibliothèque publique de Strasbourg.[18] En même temps disparut une copie moins riche. L'exemplaire brûlé était personnel à l'auteur qui en fit don, le 2 janvier 1687 à son plus jeune fils André. Agé de douze ans à cette époque, ce dernier exécuta lui-même une copie encore conservée à la Bibliothèque municipale de Strasbourg.[19] Les figures rehaussées de gouache et fixées sont d'une facture évidemment assez naïve.[20]

Un autre manuscrit illustré se trouve à la Bibliothèque de Cassel.

Mais il est plus essentiel de confronter le manuscrit de Strasbourg avec le volume in 4° oblong du British Museum.[21] Le frontispice, daté du 31 décembre 1653 représente une vue de la ville signée des initiales de l'artiste Jean-Georges Walther (1604–79) spécialisé en ornithologie. Un peu plus restreint que les autres, ce manuscrit de Londres a été étudié avec soin par l'alsacien Ferdinand Reiber en 1886.[22]

De manière plus générale, le plan d'ensemble de l'ouvrage de Baldner comporte une préface suivie de trois parties traitant des oiseaux; des poissons (avec les écrevisses) et des autres animaux aquatiques (quadrupèdes, insectes, vers, etc.). Même s'il arrive à Baldner d'interférer sciemment entre les espèces et les genres, son mérite est immense d'avoir coordonné seul les éléments de son travail d'observation. La perspicacité du pêcheur est significative, quand, à l'encontre de Gesner, il affirme que les carpes naissent des œufs et non de la vase. Des notions sommaires d'anatomie s'accompagnent des indications sur la nourriture même en captivité, sur les appâts, le gîte, le frai, la date et le mode de la récolte, le poids, la réglementation de la chasse et de la pêche. Au gastronome s'adressent des indications culinaires, le changement de couleur après la friture, et aussi la concordance avec les prescriptions écclésiastiques du carême, les interdits de la loi juive.

Il est hors de propos ici, de commenter les notions zoologiques après les travaux de Reiber, List, Seelig, Escherich et Lauterborn.[23]

Ray confirme l'acquisition des «figures de tous les oiseaux vivant près du Rhin, dessinés très artistement et avec une scrupuleuse exactitude, et réunies en un volume par Léonard Baldner, chasseur et pêcheur strasbourgeois qui avait tué tous ces spécimens, les fit peindre et les décrivit dans sa langue».[24]

La description, «in Germanico Idiomate», n'était assurément pas intelligible aux naturalistes anglais. Et ce ne fut sans doute pas chose facile à Frederick Slare (1647–1727), de traduire ce texte allemand, émaillé de locutions alsaciennes aujourd'hui précieuses pour le linguiste.[25]

C'est ainsi que l'iconographie et les textes de Baldner entrent dans la zoologie scientifique, avec la parution de l'*Ornithologie* et de l'*Ichtyologie* de Francis Willoughby (1635–72) peu après son décès, par les soins de son ami Ray en 1676. En 1686[26] John Jacob Scheuchzer (1672–1733) mentionne le manuscrit de Londres dans sa *Bibliographia scriptorum historiae naturalis*.[27] Quand le montpelliérain Antoine Gouan (1733–1821) fait paraître à Strasbourg en 1770 son *Historia Piscium*, il cite les divers auteurs qui ont décrit les poissons de leur contrée, mais Baldner lui est inconnu.[28] La méthodologie a cependant fait de grands progrès avec Linné, Berg, Catesby, Commerson.

A la fin du XVIIIe siècle, Jean Hermann (1738–1800), le naturaliste strasbourgeois surnommé «le Linné du Rhin», est décidé à publier le travail de son compatriote alsacien avec le concours de son fils Johann-Friedrich. Mais une mauvaise chance s'acharne sur ce projet, quand Joh.-Fr. Hermann fils succombe au typhus en 1793. La citation des noms de Willoughby et de Ray ainsi que plusieurs emprunts à Baldner sont le seul hommage transmis par Jean Hermann dans les *Observationes zoologicae*, posthumes.[29]

Après l'hydrographie, la topographie des environs immédiats de la ville nous apporte quelques renseignements intéressants. Le sol est encore particulièrement riche surtout à l'ouest. Le chroniqueur Jean-Frédéric Hermann, frère du naturaliste, revendique pour le XVIe siècle une curieuse raison de l'augmentation de la fertilité par la qualité «supérieure» des engrais provenant «des habitudes et de l'aisance d'une très grande partie des habitants qui ne fait pas maigre».

De fait, les cultivateurs anglais étaient très friands de la semence des oignons de Strasbourg, dont la culture était conditionnée par un règlement spécial.

Dans l'économie locale, le tabac jouait un rôle primordial. Une tradition encore vivante a conservé le nom du lieu où la plante aurait été cultivée pour la première fois, l'année 1620. C'est un négociant du nom de Robert Königsmann qu'en aurait rapporté d'Angleterre des graines et l'établissement fut nommé par la suite «Cour d'Angleterre».[31] Plus assurée est l'origine anglaise de l'introduction du maïs en Alsace. Connus depuis le Moyen-Age en Grande-Bretagne, les vins d'Alsace continuent à être très estimés.

Au vrai, pour les voyageurs anglais, qui à la seconde moitié du siècle des Lumières se conforment à la tendance générale en s'appliquant à étudier des choses de l'agriculture, l'Alsace apparaît comme un pays béni. Né terrien, Arthur Young (1741–1820) découvre, le 20 juillet 1789 «l'une des plaines les plus riches et les mieux cultivées que l'on puisse voir». Passionné par la méthode expérimentale et par les applications de la chimie agricole dont il avait entretenu Lavoisier en 1787, Young n'estime guère le «physiocratical rubbish». Il remet ses lettres de recommandations à Jean Hermann, professeur de botanique médicale et de chimie à l'Université. Celui-ci le renseigne sur un certain nombre de questions et lui fait sans doute visiter ses collections zoologiques encore existantes.[32]

Cette rencontre entre Young et Hermann nous induit à nous tourner vers la faculté de Médecine strasbourgeoise.

Grâce à la transcription de Knod, les registres d'immatriculation pour le XVIIIe siècle sont d'accès facile.[33] Et la déception est d'autant plus grande – même si l'on devait admettre des lacunes dans la transcription – qu'on ne trouve qu'un seul étudiant en médecine d'origine irlandaise. Il s'agit de Daniel O'Reilly «from Ireland, Carrickmakron from the county Managhan», inscrit le 15 décembre 1786 sous le rectorat de Joh. Laur. Blessig Phil. P.P.O.[34] Un chirurgien au patronyme français, Jack Desfontaines «Londoniensis eques, ocularius medicus» avait pris ses inscriptions dans sa catégorie le 17 mai 1740.[35]

Les investigations n'en sont pas moins instructives pour ce dernier tiers du siècle. D'après la «matricula didascalorum», l'enseignement de l'anglais est à ce moment fort actif. Quatre professeurs de langue sont inscrits de 1778 à 1789.[36] Leur activité s'éclaire pleinement par la remarque de Thomas Lauth, constatant qu'à cette époque «aucun homme instruit n'a droit à ce qualificatif, s'il ne pratique vraiment six ou sept langues modernes».[37]

Au vrai, l'anglomanie est à son apogée. Séjournant à Paris en 1785, la baronne d'Oberkirch en note les immenses progrès et le peu de conséquences de l'esprit national, qui cherche à effacer modes et usages pour adopter les idées nouvelles.[38] A Strasbourg, par le départ inopiné de Rousseau, l'Ecosse avait ravi à Jacques-Reinbold

Spielmann (1722–83), très célèbre professeur de chimie, de botanique et de matière médicale à la Faculté, un compagnon pour les excursions botaniques dans les Vosges et au Citoyen de Genève repos et santé. Mais dans l'étude des simples, Spielmann recommande particulièrement les images des plantes figurant dans le *Curious Herbal* d'Elisabeth Blackwell qu'il souhaite «voir entre les mains de tous». Les principaux ouvrages traitant de matière médicale des auteurs anglais lui sont connus.[39] Un recensement des ouvrages de sa bibliothèque riche de plus de 5.000 volumes, permet de dénombrer environ 235 livres imprimés en Angleterre, soit 4,60 pour cent de la collection.

A la vérité l'attirance de la médecine britannique reçoit sa pleine justification, par la réputation des maîtres, par l'organisation hospitalière et par la richesse des cabinets de collection.[40]

De fait, trois parmi les étudiants strasbourgeois qui atteindront à la notoriété, vont chercher à perfectionner en Angleterre l'enseignement reçu et pourront illustrer cette polarité.

Appartenant par sa mère à une lignée de théologiens protestants, Jean-Georges Roederer (1726–63) avait commencé sa médecine en 1744. Une large aisance matérielle lui permit de séjourner d'abord à Paris pendant un an. Agé de vingt-deux ans, il se rend alors à Londres et devient l'élève de Hunter en anatomie et de Lobb en médecine. Avec assiduité, il fréquente le cabinet du chevalier Hans Sloane, ainsi que les autres collections dont celles des machines de physique, les bibliothèques, le jardin des plantes médicinales de la capitale britannique. Richard Mead lui donne des lettres d'introduction pour l'Université d'Oxford. Initié à l'Art des accouchements en l'Ecole strasbourgeoise de Fried, il avait assisté à Paris aux leçons de Grégoire.

A Londres il suit deux cours chez Smellie, le second en 1752, après avoir pris entretemps le grade de docteur de Strasbourg. Une formation aussi étendue lui vaut la nomination par le roi d'Angleterre George II de la maison de Hanovre, à la chaire d'obstétrique, de gynécologie et de pédiatrie de Goettingue le 18 octobre 1751. Accumulant les charges honorifiques et les distinctions académiques, il est nommé médecin de sa Majesté britannique dans l'électorat du Hanovre. En sa qualité de Protecteur de l'Université, il devient le représentant direct du roi qui est recteur perpétuel.

Il succombe à une fièvre malgine au cours d'une halte à Strasbourg au retour d'un voyage à Paris, âgé de trente sept ans à peine.[41]

Orphelin à l'âge de sept ans, Jean-Michel Roederer (1740–98) reçut après ses humanités, une solide instruction en philosophie, lettres classiques et langues anciennes. Puis il assiste aux leçons de physique expérimentale de Grauel avant d'étudier la théologie protestante. Alors seulement il entreprend des études de médecine.

La soutenance d'une thèse *de valvula intestini coli* le libère de ses obligations et lui permet de poursuivre ses études en dehors de Strasbourg. En Août 1768 il se rend à Paris et y reste huit mois durant. Vers la mi-avril 1769, un bateau le mène de Dieppe à Brighton. Après une marche de trois jours, il atteint Londres. Il faut désormais écouter la relation personnelle qu'il donne de son séjour: «Là, pour autant que le trimestre déjà avancé le permet, je n'ai rien négligé de toutes les possibilités qui m'étaient offertes en cette saison pour perfectionner mes connaissances médicales.

Dans les hôpitaux correspondant à l'étendue de la cité, célèbres pour leur architecture et leur propreté que ce soit St. Bartholomew, Thomas, George, celui de Londres, du Middlesex ou d'autres, je me suis intéressé aussi bien aux consultations qu'au traitement des maladies surtout chirurgicales, dispensés avec beaucoup d'humanité par les médecins et les chirurgiens; au nombre de ces interventions et à part certaines plus communes j'eus la bonne fortune d'observer l'incision de la vessie par la méthode d'Hawkins pour l'extraction de la pierre ainsi que l'ouverture du crâne au moyen du trépan manuel des Anciens préféré habituellement par les chirurgiens Anglais pour l'aisance et la rapidité de sa rotation. En outre, j'ai pu observer des variolisations pratiquées adroitement chez un grand nombre d'enfants, selon la méthode de Dimsdal avec un grand succès, tant à l'hospice des nouveaux-nés, qu'à l'hôpital, uniquement grâce à la bienfaisance privée. Enfin, je n'ai jamais retiré autant de profit d'aucune leçon même de l'enseignement et de la bienveillance des hommes les plus illustres, supérieur à celui de Pringle, des frères Hunter, de Hewson, de Huck, de Turton.» Au mois de juillet, J. M. Roederer quitte enfin Londres pour la Belgique, il s'embarque en compagnie d'un ami alsacien déjà célèbre, l'helléniste et orientaliste, Joh. Schweighaeuser (1742–1830).[42] Second, puis premier obstétricien, il recevra la chaire d'anatomie et de chirurgie en 1784, lorsque Jean-Frédéric Lobstein l'Ainé (1736–84), prendra celle de pathologie.

Thomas Lauth (1758–1826) son successeur avait été formé par l'apprentissage de sept langues anciennes et modernes. Après son doctorat obtenu en 1781, il se rend d'abord à Paris, puis à Londres. Là, son ancien condisciple et ami, J. G. Schultz, lui facilite l'accès des sept hôpitaux principaux de la capitale: le Bartholomew Hospital où Pott dirige le service de chirurgie, le Westminster Hospital dans lequel exercent Watson et Justamond; le London Hospital dont Blizard est le chirurgien et enfin les institutions de Saint Thomas, Guy's, Middlesex et Saint-George. Avec F. F. Simmons, il se lie d'amitié et peut se familiariser sous sa conduite avec l'hospitalisation des aliénés à Saint-Luc. Elève de William Hunter peu avant la disparition de celui-ci, il visite ses collections anatomiques et celle de son collaborateur Cruickshanks. De Lowdher, il peut admirer les admirables préparations obstétricales. Et naturellement, il ne peut manquer la fréquentation du cabinet de John Hunter, avec les pièces de Watson. Parmi les célébrités du temps, le chirurgien Sheldon avait fait ces voyages en aerostat. Lauth fréquente aussi les expériences d'électrisation faites par Gray et par Birch. Chez le baronnet J. Banks, il rencontre l'ichtyologiste Broussonet ainsi que Scarpa qui devient son correspondant. De retour à Strasbourg, après avoir visité la Belgique, la Hollande et l'Allemagne, il reçoit la chaire d'anatomie, après la démission de Roederer en 1785. Dix ans plus tard il se verra maintenu dans ses fonctions comme Hermann, à la réouverture de l'Ecole de Santé, bientôt organisée en Faculté par décret impérial.[43]

Les liens se consolident par les échanges épistolaires. Et aussi dans les agrégations aux Sociétés Savantes. En 1788, Hermann qui correspondait avec Banks, Smith, Wonefe, fut associé à la Société Linnéenne de Londres. Parmi les membres d'honneur non-résidents de la Medical Society, «instituted of the Anatomical theatre, Great Queen Street, Lincoln's Inn Field» on trouve Thomas Lauth.[44]

A Strasbourg même, l'Université luthérienne a reçu son plus vif éclat de l'historiographe du Roi Jean-Daniel Schoepflin (1694–1775). En Angleterre, il avait lui-même étudié l'aspect politique du pays au lendemain de la mort de George 1er. Fondateur de l'Ecole politique et de diplomatie, il attire depuis 1750 un auditoire européen à ses cours privés et publics. Son élève Guillaume Koch (1737–1813) continue à alimenter le rayonnement qui séduit l'élite intellectuelle. Des vingt-trois Britanniques de distinction, la «matricula Serenissimorum et illustrissimorum» restitue de 1784 à 1790, les noms de George Henry Vansittard, Esquire de Londres; Francis Drake, capitaine au service du roi d'Angleterre; Thomas Mahon, gentilhomme Irlandais; Stephen Mahon et John Sulivan Wood, officiers anglais; Robert Meade, gentilhomme irlandais; Rowland Hill, Esq., du Shropshire.[45]

Mais déjà le temps est arrivé où Arthur Young doit assister avec stupeur au sac de l'Hôtel-de-Ville.[46] Et un autre voyageur anglais moins connu n'emporte plus, en 1793, qu'un souvenir médiocre de l'Université. «La plus grande ignorance dans toutes les branches et dans les sciences règne ici en même temps que la licence des moeurs . . . première vertu de la liberté» doit-il constater avec quelque excès.[47]

Notes et Bibliographie

1 BURY, JOHN PATRICK, 'Quelques voyageurs anglais en Alsace, 1660–1860', *Annuaire de la Soc. hist., litt. et scientifique du Club Vosgien*, Nelle série, vol. III, Strasbourg, Imp. Als., 1935, pp. 151–62.

2 Voir en particulier: CHRISMAN, MIRIAM USHER, *Strasbourg and the Reform. A study in the process of Change*, New-Haven and London, Yale University Press, 1967, in-8°, xii + 351 pp.

3 KOSZUL, ANDRÉ, 'Les relations entre l'Alsace et l'Angleterre au XVIe siècle', *Revue de Litt. comparée*, 1929, **9**, 5–24.

4 Réfugié à Wasselonne (Bas-Rhin), le célèbre théologien Edmond Grindel, futur evêque de Canterbury "avait acquis une si bonne connaissance de l'allemand, qu'il put bientôt prêcher dans cette langue", in FUCHS, F. J., *Les débuts du culte protestant a Wasselonne 1524–1575, d'après les rapports d'inspection éclésiastique* Soc. d'Hist. et d'Archéol. de Saverne et environs, cahier 58/59, pp. 41–45 (p. 42).

5 Originaire de Schleiden, près de Cologne, Jean Sturm fut appelé à Strasbourg par son homonyme, le stettmeistre Jacques Sturm von Sturmeck, qui prit une part très active dans l'humanisme alsacien.

6 Voir à ce propos: 'WICKERSHEIMER, ERNEST, Jean Sturm, ami Strasbourgeois d'André Vésale', *CR. XIXe Congrès Int. Histoire de la Médecine*, Bâle, 1964, pp. 25–32 (Karger, Basel/New York, 1966).

7 Correspondance de Jean Sturm. Lettres à Elisabeth d'Angleterre. 13 février 1561, 1 mai 1569, 16 novembre 1573, 24 février 1575, s.d. 1576, s.d. 1581, 4 septembre 1577. Arch. municip. Strasbourg, no. 163.

8 ROTT, JEAN ET FAERBER, ROBERT, 'Un Anglais à Strasbourg au milieu du XVIe siècle, John Hales,' *Etudes anglaises*, 1968, XXI, **4**, 381–89.

9 KOSZUL, ANDRÉ, 'Argentoratensis Britannica. Les Sidney et Strasbourg', *Bult. Fac. Lettres de Strasbourg*, 1938, **17**, no. 2, 37–44 et 1947–48, **26**, no 1, 232–47.

10 Cf. DUMAÎTRE, PAULE, *Communication XXVe Congrès Int. hist. Méd.*, Londres, 1972.

11 Rabelais, François, Von Thaten und Rhaten der Helden und Herren Grandgoschier, Gorgellantua und Pantagruel . . . in einem teutschen Model vergossen durch Huldrich Elloposcleron [Jean Fischart] [Strasbourg, Bernard Jobin], 1594, in-8°, ill.

12 BRAND, SEBASTIAN, *Das Narrenschiff*, Bâle, Bergmann de Olpe, 1494.

13 KNOD, GUSTAV C., *Die alten Matrikeln der Universität Strassburg, 1621 bis 1793*, 3 vols., in-8°, Strassburg, K. J. Trübner, 1897, tome II, p. 9.

14 Arch. Municip. Strasbourg, St. Thomas – Ordres religieux – no. 96, Carton 54, 16.

15 BURNET, GILBERT, *Travels, or a collection of letters to the Hon. Robert Boyle, Esq.; containing an account of what seem'd most remarkable in travelling thro' Switzerland, Italy, some parts of Germany, etc., in the years 1685 and 1686*, a new edition, London, 1737; BREVAL, J. D., *Remarks on several parts of Europe: relating chiefly to the history, antiquities and geography of those countries through which the author has travel'd; as France, the Low Countries, Germany, Lorrain, Alsatia, Savoy, Tirol, Switzerland, Italy and Spain*, London, 1726.

16 RAY, JOHN, *Observations Topographical, Moral and Physiological made in a journey through part of the Low Countries. Germany, Italy and France with a catalogue of Plants not native of England found spontaneously growing in those parts and their virtues*, London, 1673; *Travels through the*

Low Countries, Germany, Italy and France. With curious observations natural, topographical, moral, physiological, etc., also a Catalogue of Plants, found spontaneously growing in those Parts, and their virtues, 2nd ed., London, 1738.

17 GESNER, CONRAD, *Historiae animalium de quadrupedibus viviparis & oviparis, de Avium, Piscium, Aquatilium & Serpentum natura, Libri quinque. Tiguri, Froschoverus, 1551, 1555, 1558 and 1587*, in-fol., 4 vols. fig.

18 Recht natürliche Beschreibung und Abmalung der Wasservögel, Fischen, Vierfüssigen Thieren, Insecten und Gewürmb, so bey Strassburg in den Wassern seynt, die ich selber geschossen und die Fisch gefangen. auch alles in meiner Handt gehabt. Leonhard Baldner, Fischer und Hagmeister, in Strassburg gefertigt wotden im Jahr Christi 1666. Des copies sans figures existent: (1°) à la B.N.U. de Strasbourg sous les cotes 757 Als. 113 et 758 Als. 114; (2°) à la Bibliothèque Municipale de Strasbourg, cote MS.

19 Wahrhafte Beschreibung und nach dem Leben Contrafaitung, aller derjenigen Vögel, so sich allhier zu Strassburg, Inn- und bey der Statt, in den 4. Schiffreichen Wassern, nehren und auffhalten. Mit sonderbarem fleiss und Unkosten zusamen gebracht, durch mich Leonhardt Baldner, Dieser Statt wolbestelten Hagmeister. Geschen in dem Jahr Christi 1666. Bibl. municip. Strasbourg, MS. 655, in-fol. oblong, 114 fols., 126 figs. Le mot 'Hagmeister' est rayé.

20 La tendance actuelle est de considérer ce manuscrit comme l'œuvre autographe de Baldner père. Une liste intercalaire rédigée et signée 'Länhard baldner d[er] Elter' précise que le père a abattu lui-même tous les oiseaux entre 1646 et 1680. Seuls les poissons et écrevisses et les oiseaux sont représentés.

21 British Museum, cote MSS. 20789. Le manuscrit ne contient que 45 poissons, 57 oiseaux et 54 mammifères et insectes. Je remercie très sincèrement le Conservateur du British Museum d'avoir bien voulu mettre une copie du manuscrit à ma disposition.

22 REIBER, FERDINAND, *L'Histoire Naturelle des eaux strasbourgeoises de léonard Baldner (1666) Colmar*, Vve C. Decker, 1887, in-8°, pp. 1–114. *Extr. Bull. Soc. hist. nat.*, Colmar, 1886–88.

23 REIBER, F., op. cit., pp. 7–8, met en exergue son mérite d'avoir reconnu que '*l'Ammocoetus branchialis* n'est que la forme première du poisson *Petromyzon planeri*' fait non reconnu par Cuvier et Valenciennes (en réalité Cyclostome du genre Lampreta).
ESCHERICH, K., Leonhard Baldners, *Vogel. Fisch. und Tierbuch*, a.d. Jahre 1666, Münden, 1904.
LIST, WILLY, *Die Naturgeschichte der Leonhard Baldner*, Fischer zu Strasburg [Str. 1884].
SEELIG, FRIED, Wilh. L. Baldner's *Vogel-Fisch – und Thierburch 1666*, Eine bibliographisch-fischereigeschichtliche Studie [München, 1885].
LAUTERBORN, ROBERT, Leonhard Baldner, *Das Vogel – Fisch – und Thierbuch aus dem Jahr 1666*, Herausgegeben, mit einer Einleitung u. erläuternden Anmerkungen versehen von Robert Lauterborn, Ludwigshafen am Rhein, A. Lauterborn, 1903, in-8°, lxvi+177 pp.

24 *Ornithologia* (voir infra no. 26), Praefatio ad lectorem, p. 4.

25 *De historia piscium Libri quatuor* (voir infra no. 26), Praefatio, p. 2.

26 WILLUGHBY, FRANCIS, *Ornithologiae libri tres . . . Recognovit Joannes Raius*, Londini, J. Martyn, 1676, in-fol., 307 pp., 77 pl., atlas; *Ichtiographia*, Londini, Soc. Regalis, 1685, in-fol.; *De historia piscium Libri quatunor et Librum etiam primum et secondum integros adjecit Joannes Raius*, Oxonii, e theatro Sheldoniano, 1686, in-fol., 343 pp., av. un apendice de 30 pp. par Jean Nieuhof et un atlas de 12 pl.

27 SCHEUCHZER, JOHN JACOBUS, *Bibliotheca Scriptorum Historiae Naturali omnium Terrae Regionum inserviendum. Hist. Nat. Helvetiae prodromus. Accessit Jacob Le Long . . . de Scriptoribus Historiae naturalis Galliae*, Tiguri, Henr. Bodmer, 1716, in-8°, 241 pp., p. 19.
LELONG, JACQUES, *RP. Bibliothèque historique de la France. Nouv. éd. rev. corrigée et augm. par Fevret de Fontette*, A Paris, J. Th. Herrissant, 1768, 5 vols., in fol. tome I, Liv. I, Sect. VI, §I, no. 3547, p. 204:
'MS. Description des Oiseaux, Poissons & Insectes trouvés aux environs de Strasbourg; par Léonard Baldner: en Allemand, avec figures.
Baldner, Pêcheur de Strasbourg, homme intelligent, a fait dans le cours de 20 ans ce Recueil d'Animaux des environs de Strasbourg. Son Ouvrage, achevé en 1666, & écrit de sa propre main, est aujourd'hui dans la bibliothèque de M. Spielmann, Professeur de Médecine à Strasbourg, qui l'a reçu des Parents de Baldner, Bourgeois de Strasbourg. Le Chevalier François Willughby a fait usage des Observations de Baldner dans son Ornythologie (*Ornithologiae libri tres in quibus aves hactenus cognitae omnes accurate describuntur; ex recensione Joannis Raii: Londoni, 1676 & 1686*, in-fol.) & dans l'Ouvrage qu'il a donné sur les Poissons sous ce titre, *De Historia piscium libri quatuor, & recensione Raii, Oxon*, 1686, in-fol.]

28 GOUAN, ANTOINE, *Historia Piscium/Histoire des Poissons*, A Strasbourg chez Armand König, 1770, in-4°, xviii+252 pp., 4 pl. gr.

29 HERMANN, JOHANN, *Observationes zoologicae . . . Opus posthumus*, ed. Friedr. Ludwig Hammer, Argentorati et Parisiis, Armand König, an XII, 1804, in-4°, viii+332 pp., portrait (Fr. L. Hammer (1762–1837) était le gendre de Hermann).

30 Ce Robert Königsmann, en transformant son patronyme de Kingman, avait acquis le droit de bourgeoisie à Strasbourg (A.M.S. 1618, fol. 204). Un de ses parents, Philippe Königsman, avait présenté, le 7 aout 1596, une supplique au Magistrat pour jouer en compagnie de onze comédiens anglais des comédies et tragédies. L'autorisation fut accordée pour quinze jours (A.M.S. Protocolle des XXI, fol. 238). Voir à ce propos: Crüger, Englische Komödianten in Strassburg vor dem Ende des Dreissigjährigen Krieges, Strassburger Post, 28 decembre 1886 *et seq.*

31 HERMANN, JEAN-FRÉDÉRIC, *Notices historiques, statistiques et littéraires sur la ville de Strasbourg*, 2 vols., Strasbourg, chez F. G. Levrault, 1817, tome I, pp. 265–66.

32 YOUNG, ARTHUR, *Travels in France during the years 1787, 1788 and 1789*, edited by Constantia Maxwell, Cambridge University Press, 1950, in-8°, li+428 pp. (pp. 180–83). La première publication des 'Travels' in-4° eut lieu en 1792, à Bury St. Edmonds près de Bradfield. Une traduction française fut aussitôt donnée par F. Soulès (3 vols, Paris, 1793, Nouvelle édition en 1794) et une autre par Lesage en 1860. Plus recommandable est la traduction récente par Henri Sée (3 vols., in-8°, Paris, Armand Colin, 1931, cf. tome I, pp. 242–44).

33 KNOD, G., voir supra, note 13.

34 Ibid. tome I, p. 183 et tome II, p. 119. Matr. stud. med. 1785–87.

35 Ibid. Matr. didasc. atque servorum 1737. 41 tome I, p. 215.

36 L'un d'eux, William Taylor, d'Exmouth (Devon) habita chez le célèbre graveur Jean-Martin Weiss. Hendrix Nelson, de Londres, fut logé 'at the Blue Cloud on the Parade' (actuelle rue de la Nuée Bleue). Joseph Gosse, de Bristol, enseigna même la littérature anglaise.

37 LAUTH, THOMAS, *Vita Joaannis Hermann . . . Argentorati, Levrault, An X–1800*, in-8°, 64 pp. (p. 7, 'Doctus vero nostris temporibus nemo appellari sane potest, quin sex vel septem lingues vulgari usu tenre queat').

38 OBERKIRCH, BARONNE HENRIETTE-LOUISE D', *Mémoires sur la cour de Louis XVI et la société française avant 1789* (Nelle ed.), Mercure de France, 1970, in-8°, 56 pp., chap. XXX, p. 339.

39 Dans la bibliographie, il mentionne Georges Berkeley, Black, Digby, Dover et la Pharmacopée d'Edimbourg, Fall, Fordyce, Thomas Fuller, Huxham, William Lewis, la Pharmacopée de Londres de 1632, David Macbride, le 'Mechanical account of Poisons' (1702) de Richard Mead, Clephane, les 'Obs. on the diseases of the Army' de John Pringle, Stoughton, Thomas Sydenham, Daniel Turner, les 'Obs. on the nature' (1765) de Robert Whytt.

40 *Catalogus Librorum nuper mortalis Jacobi Reinboldi Spielmann . . . publice auctionis Lege divendendorum mense januarii A. MDCCLXXXV*, Argentorati, J. Heiz, 1784, in-12°, 303 pp.

41 LOUIS ANTOINE, *Eloge de Roederer. Eloges lus dans les séances publiques de l'Académie Royale de Chirurgie de 1750 à 1792*, Publ. par E. Fréd. Dubois d'Amiens, Paris, J.-B. Baillière et fils, 1859, in-8°, lxxvi+456 pp. Pp. 59–74 (Cet éloge fut le premier prononcé par Louis en qualité de Secrétaire perpétuel de l'Acad. de Chir., en séance publique du 18 avril 1765).

42 *Programma invitatorium ad Orationem inauguralem qua vir experientissimus Johannes Michael Roederer munus professoris anatomiae et chirurgiae ordinarii die XXVII aprilis A.R.S. MDCCLXXIV hora X ritu solenni auspicabitur*, Argentorati, J. H. Heitz, 1784, 7 pp.

43 VETTER, JEAN-MARIE, Thomas Lauth et l'individualisation de l'anatomie pathologique à Strasbourg. Thèse méd. Strasbourg, no. 140, 1968. Dact., 65 pp.

44 *Laws and Regulations of the Medical Society . . . dec. 19, 1779*, London, 1784, in-8°, 30 pp. (p. 4)

45 KNOD, G., op. cit. *Matr. Seren. et illustr.* (*1784–1787*), I, pp. 50–53.

46 YOUNG, A., op. cit. éd. C. Maxwell, pp. 182–83.

47 [Piaggino]. 'Reise eines Engländers durch einen Theil von Elsass und Nieder-Schwaben, in *Briefen verfasst und von seinem teutschen Freunde L.A.F.V.B. herausgegeben*, Amsterdam u. Stockholm, 1793, in-12°, 143 pp.

D. Wrotnowska
Paris (*France*)

Pasteur et la 'Royal Society of London'

Il aurait été fort émouvant de présenter, à l'occasion de ce Congrès, les rapports d'amitié que Ptaseur entretint avec la Grande Bretagne et ses savants. Il aurait fallu évoquer notamment Sir Joseph Lister qui, dès avant les chirurgiens français, appliqua à son art la doctrine pastorienne, le Dr. John Tyndall, défendant les principes de Pasteur contre ceux du Dr. Henry Charlton Bastian . . . et bien d'autres.

Le temps imparti ne le permettant pas il sera traité seulement des relations de Pasteur avec la Société Royale de Londres, grâce, notamment, à des documents inédits qu'avait bien voulu nous communiquer son bibliothécaire d'alors, M. L. Kaye.

Pasteur avait élaboré ses travaux sur la dissymétrie moléculaire, premier anneau de la chaine qui le conduira à la prophylaxie de la rage, alors qu'il était professeur de chimie à l'Université de Strasbourg,[1] de 1849 à 1854. Il en déduisit les premières conséquences à Lille[2] où, à 31 ans, il fut nommé, le 2 décembre 1854, doyen et professeur de chimie de la nouvelle Faculté des Sciences, dépendant de l'Académie de Douai. Malgré la charge accablante de l'organisation et de l'administration de cette nouvelle faculté, il sut se réserver des loisirs afin de continuer ses recherches dont l'éclat commençait à rayonner dans le monde.

La vénérable Société Royale de Londres s'intéresse aux travaux du savant. Elle avait été fondée en 1645 pour le développement de «toutes connaissances ayant pour objet d'appliquer la science [. . . et de] la rendre utile en même temps qu'attrayante».

Lors de sa séance du ler décembre 1856, le Conseil de la Société Royale[3] décide d'attribuer la Médaille Rumford à Pasteur. Le Président, Lord Wrottesley, dans un magistral exposé, retraça l'enchainement des découvertes de Pasteur qui sut voir des facettes droites ou gauches d'où leur influence divergente. «Ces patientes et laborieuses recherches pour la poursuite de la vérité, continue-t-il, sont maintenant récompensées par une découverte imprévue et brillante».

Le 7 novembre 1856, William Sharpey, secrétaire de la Société, annonce à Pasteur cette décision par une lettre connue par sa traduction[4]: «Le Président et le conseil de la Société Royale me chargent de vous informer qu'ils vous ont conféré la médaille Rumford de 1856, pour votre découverte de la nature de l'acide racémique et de ses rapports avec la lumière polarisée et pour les recherches auxquelles cette découverte vous a conduit.

«Les médailles dont la Société dispose, sont décernées publiquement par le président à la séance anniversaire de la Société, laquelle aura lieu, cette année, le lundi 1er décembre à quatre heures de l'après-midi. Ce serait avec un vif plaisir que la Société vous verrait lui faire l'honneur d'assister à cette séance pour recevoir la médaille Rumford de la main du président».

Le Secrétaire donne alors l'historique de ce prix: «La médaille Rumford a été créée par le comte de Rumford en 1796,[5] pour être affectée à la récompense des découvertes importantes ou des inventions utiles sur la chaleur ou sur la lumière. Le fondateur a de plus avisé à ce qu'une récompense en argent fut jointe à la médaille et remise en même temps.

«La somme qui vous revient s'élève à (mille cinq cents francs environ). Dans le cas où vous ne pourriez venir à Londres, je vous prierais de vouloir bien autoriser quelqu'un ici à la toucher pour vous.»

Pasteur, le 10 novembre, communique cette traduction au recteur de l'Académie de Douai, Guillemin[6]: «Je m'empresse de vous faire part de la traduction d'une lettre que je viens de recevoir de M. le secrétaire de la Société Royale de Londres par laquelle il m'informe d'une distinction très flatteuse pour l'Université et votre Académie. La Société Royale me confère la médaille du comte de Rumford [. . .].

«Je suis invité à me rendre à Londres, le ler décembre à cette occasion.»

Le lendemain, c'est au Président de la Société que s'adresse Pasteur[7]: [. . .] «Je suis, Monsieur le Président, profondément touché de l'honneur dont la Société Royale m'a jugé digne. Cette heureuse nouvelle m'a comblé de joie. Veuillez en agréer, Monsieur le Président, et en transmettre à la Société, l'expression de ma très vive reconnaissance.»

«Je désirerais pouvoir me rendre à Londres le jour de la séance annuelle de la Société; mais j'en serai forcément empêché par mes fonctions universitaires qu'il me serait impossible d'interrompre.»

Le 15 novembre 1856, le recteur Guillemin, à la séance de rentrée des Facultés à Douai[8] s'adressera, en ces termes, à ses professeurs: «Vos travaux sont connus, appréciés à l'étranger, hier même, j'apprenais que la Société Royale de Londres vient de décerner au savant doyen de la Faculté des sciences de Lille la Médaille Rumford pour ses belles découvertes en chimie [. . .].»

Au début de décembre, Pasteur reçut la somme annoncée, ce dont se réjouit Madame Pasteur «le meilleur collaborateur de son mari», a-t-on pu écrire. S'adressant à son beau-père, Jean-Joseph Pasteur, l'ancien soldat de Napoléon et tanneur, Madame Pasteur note, en s'identifiant à son mari[9]: «*Nous* avons reçu ces jours derniers le prix de la Société Royale de Londres. On *nous* a envoyé 1.750 francs sur un banquier de Lille, en *nous* annonçant que la médaille *nous* serait remise par une personne qui s'en chargerait en venant en France. Cette bonne aubaine *nous* met au niveau de nos affaires, au-dessus même.» Elle pense pouvoir ainsi acquérir un jardin, contigu à celui de la tannerie paternelle d'Arbois, aux bords de la Cuisance.

Pasteur ne put se rendre à Londres. Le 12 août 1857, il adresse la lettre suivante à O'Neil Nesbitt, professeur d'anglais au lycée de Lille, depuis le 2 septembre 1855[10]: «J'apprends que vous vous rendez à Londres prochainement. Seriez-vous assez bon pour aller de ma part demander au Secrétariat de la Société Royale de Londres, la Médaille Rumford qui m'a été décernée au mois de décembre 1856. Vous obligeriez beaucoup votre tout dévoué collègue.» La lettre porte, dans le bas, une annotation, datée du 26 août, signée d'O'Neil Nesbitt: «Reçu les deux médailles.»

Pasteur en avait conservé un exemplaire, en argent, qu'il plaça, avec quatre de ses premières médailles, dans un cadre que, plus tard, à l'Institut Pasteur, il fixa auprès de son lit, dans son appartement, transformé aujourd'hui en musée.[11]

De Lille, Pasteur présente sa candidature à l'Académie des Sciences, où, cependant, il ne sera élu qu'en 1862.[12] Dans ce but, il a, pour la première fois, recours à un savant anglais, membre de la Société Royale, le minéralogiste William Miller[13]: «Dans une affaire pendante et qui doit décider de mon avenir, on me conteste mes titres cristallographiques et l'importance de mes recherches sur les relations qui peuvent exister entre les propriétés physiques des minéraux et leur constitution moléculaire interne.

«Cette circonstance me fait penser que mes travaux n'ont pas été appréciés en France comme ils doivent l'être et je viens m'adresser à l'un des savants de l'Europe les plus compétents en pareille matière pour lui demander son opinion, et en quelle estime il tient mes travaux sous le point de vue que j'ai ci-dessus indiqué.»[14]

A Lille, en août 1857, Pasteur publiait son mémoire sur la *Fermentation appelée lactique*, démontrant qu'il s'agissait là d'un phénomène vital. Il ouvrait la voie à ses études sur les maladies infectieuses.[15] Cette année même, Pasteur est nommé administrateur de l'Ecole Normale Supérieure de Paris et Directeur des Etudes scientifiques. Là, il établira l'origine microbienne des fermentations organiques, puis le principe des générations non spontanées et la spécificité, d'où les cultures pures. Ensuite il étudiera les maladies des vins,[16] puis celles des vers à soie (la pébrine et la flâcherie) mettant au point le procédé de grainage.[17]

Le 12 mai 1869, Pasteur est informé que la Société Royale l'a admis au nombre de ses membres étrangers. Il remercie la Secrétaire de la Société[18]: «Occupé dans le midi de la France à des études sur les maladies qui déciment les vers à soie, j'ai reçu hier seulement, la lettre par laquelle vous m'informez que je viens d'être nommé, Membre de la Société Royale de Londres.

«Je suis extrêmement flatté de cet honneur que je considère comme l'un des plus grands parmi ceux qui m'ont encouragé dans ma carrière scientifique.

«Je vous prie d'être auprès de l'illustre Société que vous représentez dans cette circonstance, l'organe de mes sentiments de profonde gratitude.»

En septembre 1871, Pasteur, qui avait commencé à Clermont-Ferrand[16] des études sur la bière, se rendit à Londres pour visiter les grands brasseries «dont l'étendue est vraiment effrayante.»[20] Ne restant que peu de temps, il ne put faire d'expériences d'essai de la méthode qu'il préconisait. Il se borna à observer la fabrication anglaise et enseigna aux brasseurs anglais à utiliser le microscope pour l'étude des levures. Il se félicita de l'accueil reçu et sans doute siégea-t-il à une séance de la Société Royale. En 1873, Pasteur présenta à l'Académie des Sciences son procédé pour rendre la bière inaltérable.

Le 8 novembre 1874, il reçoit du Président de la Société Royale, Sir Joseph Hooker l'annonce d'un nouvel hommage[21]: «Le Conseil de la Société Royale vient de voter que la Médaille Copley vous soit décernée pour vos recherches sur la Fermentation et sur la Pébrine.

«En vous faisant part de cette résolution qui établit combien la Société apprécie hautement vos importantes recherches, je ne puis me passer de vous exprimer la satisfaction personnelle que j'en éprouve comme Président de la Société.»

En effet la Société Royale avait, dans sa séance du 3 novembre 1874,[22] décidé cet hommage. Le Président avait exposé les travaux de Pasteur sur la Fermentation

«Maintes et maintes habiles investigations, disait-il, ont été faites dans le même sens, elles soulevaient de telles difficultés que Dumas,[23] lui-même, recommandait à Pasteur de ne pas prodiguer son temps en travaillant sur un sujet sans espoir. Cependant pour le biologiste les recherches de Pasteur sont d'un grand intérêt et d'une grande importance.» Par la suite, Pasteur put prouver que la maladie des vers à soie était due à un parasite.

Dès le 7 novembre, Pasteur en informa son Maître vénéré, le grand chimiste Jean-Baptiste Dumas[24]: «Je veux que vous en soyez le premier informé par le souvenir que je conserverai toujours avec la plus vive gratitude du constant intérêt que vous m'avez témoigné dès mes premiers pas dans la carrière des sciences.»

Le lendemain, 8 novembre 1874, Pasteur remercia le Président de la Société[25]: «Profondément touché de cette marque d'estime, la plus haute que des travaux scientifiques puissent recevoir; j'ai l'honneur de vous prier, Monsieur le Président, d'adresser au Conseil de la Société l'expression de ma profonde gratitude [. . .].»

Cette médaille fut créée, au XVIIe siècle, par Sir Godfrey Copley,[26] membre de la Société Royale. Un exemplaire, en or, fut conservé par Pasteur dans le cadre auprès de la médaille Rumford.[27]

Pour la première fois, en 1880, Pasteur exposa à l'Académie des Sciences son principe des virus-vaccins (le choléra des poules).[28] Ce qu'il développera au Congrès international de Médecine de Londres, le 8 août 1881[29]: *Vaccination relative au choléra des poules et au sang de rate.* «J'ai donné, dira-t-il, à l'expression de vaccination une extension que la science, je l'espère, conservera comme un hommage au mérite et aux immenses service rendus par un des plus grands hommes de l'Angleterre, votre Jenner.» Pasteur fut ému des hommages chaleureux reçus à cette occasion.

En avril 1884, Pasteur se rendra une troisième fois en Grande Bretagne pour représenter l'Académie des Sciences au Tricentenaire de l'Université d'Edimbourg. Ses discours furent «couverts de bravos et de hourrahs, qu'il faut avoir entendus pour s'en faire une idée.»[30]

Comprenant la nécessité d'avoir auprès de lui un médecin pour pratiquer les inoculations, Pasteur s'attacha le Dr. Emile Roux qui, depuis lors, participa à toutes les expériences de son Maître. Dès 1888, suivant la méthode pastorienne, le Dr. Roux fait paraître un article intitulé[31]: *Contribution à l'étude de la diphtérie*, prélude à sa découverte du sérum diphtérique et de la sérothérapie.

Le Dr. Roux avait effectivement secondé Pasteur lors des recherches sur la prophylaxie de la rage, dont l'application souleva bien des contradictions. Dès le 12 avril 1886, en vue de vérifier l'efficacité de la méthode pastorienne, avait été nommée, par la Chambre des Communes, une Commission de la rage, présidée par Sir James Paget; Victor Horsley[32] étant secrétaire et parmi les membres: Sir Joseph Lister, les Drs. Henry Roscoe[33] et George Fleming.[34] La méthode que cette commission a suivie «peut servir de modèle».[35] Le Dr. Victor Horsley fit divers voyages en France pour étudier dans le détail les expériences de Pasteur, les répétant dans son laboratoire.[36] Un rapport[37] qui était «l'expression d'une confiance entière et unanime»[38] fut déposé en juin 1887. Il affirmait. «Les animaux peuvent être protégés contre la rage par l'inoculation de substances tirées des moelles épinières selon la méthode de M. Pasteur» et, plus loin, «après des études détaillées [. . .] de tous ces faits découle la certitude, pensons-nous, que les inoculations pratiquées par M. Pasteur chez des personnes mordues par des animaux enragés ont évité l'apparition de l'hydrophobie

[. . .]». Pasteur put dire[39]: «dans une carrière scientifique déjà longue, je n'ai jamais éprouvé une joie semblable à celle que j'ai ressentie à la lecture de ce Rapport». Il sera d'un grand poids pour confondre les détracteurs. On comprit alors que l'immunisation est une des lois de la nature et ce fut pour Pasteur l'apothéose.

S'affirmera alors l'amitié du savant et de l'instigateur de cette Commission, Sir James Paget dont Pasteur, en 1881, avait dit[40]: «Sa personne a comme un rayonnement de bonté émanant d'une flamme intérieure qu'il sait traduire, quand il le veut, avec toute la puissance des grands orateurs anglais.»

A la suite de ce succès, en 1889, Sir James Paget proposa à Pasteur, de présenter ses travaux dans une conférence à la Société Royale. Pasteur lui répondit, le 21 janvier[41]: «J'exprime au Conseil une très vive gratitude. Mais hélas! je suis personnellement impropre à remplir la tâche à laquelle vous avez la bonté de me convier.» Pasteur, le 23 octobre 1887, avait été frappé d'un second ictus et il lui était resté un «embarras de paroles très sensible». «J'offre, continuait-il, au Conseil de la Société Royale de désigner mon élève et mon ami, M. le Dr. Roux, pour faire cette année la conférence «Brownienne». Quant à moi, voulant remercier aussi dignement qu'il me sera possible MM. les membres du Conseil de la Société Royale [. . .] j'accompagnerais le Dr. Roux à Londres et me ferais un devoir et une joie d'assister à sa conférence, de l'intérêt de laquelle je réponds.» Quelques jours après il proposa le titre: «*Les vaccinations préventives, d'après les travaux du laboratoire de M. Pasteur* [. . .] *M. Pasteur étant empêché par l'état de sa santé, M. le Dr. Roux, chef de service à son laboratoire, fera la lecture.*»

A ce sujet sont conservées deux lettres de Pasteur à Michael Foster, secrétaire de la Société.[42] L'une du 10 mars 1889: «Je m'empresse de vous accuser réception de votre dépêche du 7 mars, renfermant le libellé de la décision du Conseil de la Société Royale, dont j'ai informé aussitôt M. le docteur Roux, chef de service à l'Institut Pasteur.

«M. le Dr. Roux se conformera aux indications de votre dépêche et se tiendra prêt à faire sa lecture le jour qui lui sera désigné ultérieurement par M. le Président du Conseil de la Société Royale – ce jour étant choisi du 20 au 31 mai.

«Si ma santé me le permet, je serai heureux d'être présent à la conférence du Dr. Roux et je remercie très cordialement M. le Président du Conseil de la Société de m'en exprimer obligeamment le désir.»

Puis le 24 mars, il écrit: «Je m'empresse de vous accuser réception de votre lettre que j'ai communiquée tout de suite au Docteur Roux en le priant de me donner par écrit une réponse adressée à M. le Président de la Royale Société. Cette réponse, je la joins à ces quelques lignes en vous priant d'agréer la nouvelle assurance de mes sentiments distingués et en vous réitérant mon désir d'accompagner M. Roux à Londres, si ma santé me le permet. Je me sens bien éprouvé maintenant par les premiers jours du printemps.» En effet, Pasteur dut renoncer à ce voyage.

Lors de cette conférence, le 25 mai 1889,[43] le Dr. Roux exposa les découvertes faites depuis le discours de Pasteur au Congrès de 1881. Il rappela que, le premier, Pasteur avait recherché, lors de ses études sur le choléra des poules, l'action des produits élaborés par les microbes. Le Dr. Roux conclut: «Les microbes sont surtout dangereux par les produits toxiques qu'ils fabriquent. [. . .] Dans les maladies infectieuses, la mort survient donc par intoxication. [. . .] L'immunité que nous ne savions donner jusqu'ici qu'au prix de l'introduction d'un virus vivant dans le corps peut donc être conférée par l'introduction d'un corps chimique dans les tissus» et, dans une vision de l'avenir, il ajouta: «Lorsque nous connaîtrons bien les substances toxiques que forment les microbes pathogènes nous pourrons peut-être leur trouver des contre poisons paralysant leur action au sein même du tissu.» En hommage à son Maître, il réclama «la reconnaissance de tous pour celui qui, par ses études sur les virus atténués et les vaccinations préventives, a permis d'aborder avec succès ce problème de l'immunité resté jusqu'ici impénétrable».

Cette reconnaissance, Pasteur l'avait reportée sur Jenner, en révélant au Congrès de 1881[44]: «Quel bonheur pour moi de glorifier ce nom immortel sur le sol même de la noble et hospitalière cité de Londres.»

Je suis heureuse d'avoir pu, ici même, me faire l'écho de ces paroles.

References

VALLERY-RADOT, R., *La Vie de Pasteur*, Paris, 1900, 702 pp., *passim*.
PASTEUR, *Oeuvres*, réunies par Pasteur Vallery-Radot, Paris, Masson, 1922–39, 7 vols., *passim*.
PASTEUR, *Correspondance*, réunie et annotée par Pasteur Vallery-Radot, Paris, Flammarion, 1940–51, 4 vols., *passim*.

1 WROTNOWSKA, D., 'Pasteur à Strasbourg. Ses difficultés administratives et financières', in *Histoire de la Médecine*, 7 juillet 1955; 'Pasteur, professeur à Strasbourg (1849–1854), in *92° Congrès des Sociétés Savantes, Strasbourg-Colmar, 1967. Comptes-rendus section des sciences*, Paris, Histoire des Sciences, 1969, **1**, 139–44.

2 WROTNOWSKA, D., *Pasteur, doyen de la nouvelle Faculté des sciences de Lille, 1854–1857*, sous presse.

3 *Proceedings of the Royal Society of London*, 1 decembre 1856, 1857, **8**, 254–57. Président de 1854 à 1858, John, Lord Wrottesley (1798–1867), Astronome.

4 Conservées aux Archives départementales du Nord, T182, 86; WROTNOWSKA, D., *Pasteur à Lille*, cit. William Sharpey, secrétaire du 30 novembre 1853 au 30 novembre 1872.

5 Rumford, Sir Benjamin Thompson, comte de (1785–1814), physicien et chimiste.

6 Arch. dép. Nord. T182, 86. J.-L. Guillemin, Recteur de l'Académie d'Ille-et-Vilaine, fut nommé recteur à Douai, le 22 août 1854. Il est l'auteur d'une histoire ancienne de l'Orient.

7 Conservée dans les précieuses archives de la Société Royale de Londres. MSS. Mc 6–309. Lettre autographe.

8 Archives Nationales, F17, 13204.

9 *Correspondance*, 1940, **1**, 411, cit.

10 Archives Roy. Soc., MSS. Mc. 6–293.

11 Musée Pasteur, inventaire, no. 538 (diamètre, 8 cm). WROTNOWSKA, D., 'Musée Pasteur' in *Bulletin de l'Association des Anciens élèves de l'Institut Pasteur*, 1960, **5**, 147–49.

12 WROTNOWSKA, D., 'Candidatures de Pasteur à l'Académie des Sciences', in *Histoire de la médecine*, no. spécial, 1958, 23 pp.

13 Miller, William Hollowes (1801–80), élu à la Société Royale en 1838.

14 *Correspondance*, cit., **1**, 419.

15 Choléra des poules, charbon des bovins, rouget du porc, péripneumonie des bovidés et FRANK, R., WROTNOWSKA, D., *Correspondance de Pasteur et Thuillier, concernant les vaccinations contre le charbon et le rouget du porc*, Birmingham, Les Presses Universitaires d'Alabama, Préface du Professeur Pasteur Vallery-Radot [1969], 240 pp., ill., bilingue; WROTNOWSKA, D., 'Recherches de Pasteur sur le rouget du porc', *Congrès des Sociétés savantes, Nice, 1965. Acte du Congrès*, 1966, **3**, 147–59.

16 PASTEUR, *Etudes sur le vin. Ses maladies, causes qui les provoquent, procédés nouveaux pour le conserver et le vieillir*, Paris, 1866, 264 pp. *Centenaire de l'ouvrage Etudes sur le vin. . . .* Paris, Office international de la vigne et du vin, Paris, 1966, 48 pp., ill. (P. Bréchot, Pasteur et le vin, T. Castelli, Etudes microbiologiques, A. Merine, La Pasteurisation, D. Wrotnowska, Genèse de l'ouvrage.)

17 PASTEUR, *Etudes sur la maladie des vers à soie, moyen pratique assuré de la combattre et d'en prévenir le retour*, Paris, 1870, 2 tomes en 1 vol., planches. D. Wrotnowska, Pasteur et l'Italie, *21e Congrès international d'Histoire de la Médecine, Sienne, 1968*, Rome, 1969, pp. 389–403; WROTNOWSKA, D., *Pasteur et Jeanjean à St-Hippolyte du Fort*, Congrès de la Société Américaine d'Histoire de la Médecine, avril 1970, à Birmingham (Alabama), à publier.

18 Archives de la Roy. Soc. MSS. Mc. 8.366. De la main de Mme. Pasteur. Le savant avait été frappé d'un ictus, le 19 octobre 1867. Secrétaire William Sharpey.

19 PASTEUR, *Etudes sur la bière, ses maladies, causes qui les provoquent, procédé pour la rendre inaltérable, avec une théorie nouvelle de la fermentation*, Paris, 1876. WROTNOWSKA, D., 'Pasteur et ses disciples en Auvergne', *88e Congrès des Sociétés Savantes; Clermont-Ferrand, avril 1963*, L964, 149–69, ill.; 'Une amitié de savants; Pasteur et Jacobsen', *Histoire des sciences médicales*, 1970, **3–4**, 131–42.

20 Notamment la brasserie Whitbread.

21 Archives de la Roy. Soc. MSS. MM 5–63; Sir Joseph Dalton Hooker (1817–1911), Botaniste.

22 *Proceedings of the Roy. Soc.*, 'séance du 3 novembre 1874', 1875, **23**, 68–70.

23 Dumas, Jean-Baptiste (1800–84), chimiste, biologiste et homme d'Etat.

24 *Correspondance*, cit., **2**, 592.

25 Archives de la Roy. Soc. MSS. MM 5–63 (minute autographe).

26 Copley, Sir Godfrey (mort en 1709), avait été élu à la Société Royale, en 1691.

27 Musée Pasteur, Inventaire, no. 539.

28 PASTEUR, 'Sur les maladies virulentes et en particulier sur la maladie appelée vulgairement choléra des poules', in *Comptes Rendus hebdomadaires des séances de l'Adadémie des Sciences*, **90**, (1880, 9, II), 239–48.

29 PASTEUR, 'Vaccination in relation to chicken-cholera and splenic fever', *Congrès international de Médecine de Londres*, 8 août 1881, in *Transactions of the International Medical Congress*, seventh session held in London, 2 to 9 August 1881, London, 1881, pp. 85–90.

30 *Correspondance*, cit., **3**, 416.

31 ROUX, E. et YERSIN, A., 'Contribution à l'étude de la diphtérie', in *Annales de l'Institut Pasteur*, 1887, **1**, 629–61.

32 Horsley, Victor, Président de la Société Royale, il eut avec Pasteur une nombreuse correspondance; *Correspondance*, cit., **4**, 2i lettres publiées.

33 Roscoe, Sir Henry, Membre du Parlement.

34 Fleming, George, Président du Collège vétérinaire.

35 BROUARDEL, 'discussion avec Peter', in *Bull. Académie de Médecine*, 2e série, **17**, 1887, 12, VIII, 37–68.

36 'Abstract Report of Mr. Horsley's Experiments', reproduit in *Nature*, 1887, **36**, 1er appendice, pp. 235–36 et 2e appendice, pp. 236–37.

37 Report of the Committee of inquiry into M. Pasteur's treatment of hydrophobia (to the local Government Board), reproduit in *Nature*, 1887, 7, VIII, **36**, 232–37.

38 PASTEUR, 'Note accompagnant la présentation du Rapport de la Commission anglaise de la rage', *Comptes Rendus hebdomadaires des séances de l'Académie des Sciences*, 1887, **105**, 6–7.

39 PASTEUR, 'Sur le traitement préventif de la rage après morsure', in *Bull. de l'Académie de Médecine*, 1889, 5, VII, **18**, 2e série, 6–7.

40 PASTEUR, 'Vaccination in relation to chicken . . .', cit.

41 *Correspondance*, cit., **4**, 283–85.

42 Archives de la Roy. Soc. MSS. Mc 15. 22 et MSS. Mc 16 30. Lettres autographes. Michael Foster, Secrétaire de 1881 à 1903.

43 Dr. E. Roux, Les inoculations préventives, Croonian Lecture, delivered 23 May 1889, in *Proceedings of the Royal Society*, 1890, **44**, 154–72; Sir George Gabriel Stokes, Bart, 1819–1903.

44 PASTEUR, 'Vaccination in relation to chicken . . .', cit.

S. Selwyn
London (Great Britain)

The origins of medical microbiology in Britain and abroad

Some of the principal fallacies in the history of medicine relate to bacteriology. The two most notable errors commonly made are to regard the science as having originated in the last quarter of the nineteenth century, and to ascribe it almost exclusively to French and German work. The current textbooks of microbiology possess in common with the standard works in medical history, a surprisingly short memory concerning bacteriology. Charles Singer had perhaps the least excuse for this partial amnesia when we consider his splendid studies of such pioneers in theoretical bacteriology as Fracastorius[1] and our own Benjamin Marten.[2] Yet in Singer's invaluable *Short History of Medicine* published in 1928 we read 'though but fifty years old, the science of bacteriology has itself undergone repeated subdivisions'. The student of the history of medicine thus receives authority for the popular view that bacteriology was born around the year 1880. The early work especially in Britain, has been comparatively neglected even by the few specialist writers.

Most medical historians, when seeking the origins of bacteriology, have erred in excessively limiting their field of enquiry. Viewing the subject from our modern vantage point, they have sought out early work on identifiable micro-organisms. They have, therefore, not usually neglected Leeuwenhoek – especially after the researches of Dobell[3] – nor have they ignored such eighteenth- and early nineteenth-century figures as Müller, Ehrenberg and Dujardin, who are of negligible medical importance. They have even paid commendable attention to the work of Redi and Spallanzani in the marathon battle against spontaneous generation. They have largely ignored, however, the vital but inextricably ramifying contributions to the development of bacteriology from such diverse fields as optics, parasitology, epidemiology, philosophical speculation and chemistry.

The historian of this vast and diffuse subject has one prime duty. He must try to bring order to the chaos that threatens to engulf him. His task entails unearthing the hidden roots of his science up to the level where 'the Birth of Bacteriology' is clearly visible – even to the writers of textbooks. He will find reassuring evidence of organic evolution, regions of hibernation and suspended animation, sudden germinations, violent mutations, lytic cycles and orgiastic cross-fertilizations.

It is convenient to consider our subject from three viewpoints: the central zone of studies into the biology of small organisms; the periphery of early immunology and work on fermentation, putrefaction, 'antiseptics' and spontaneous generation; and finally the nebulous realms of speculation and theorizing on infection, which float over the entire field.

EARLY PARASITOLOGY

At the centre, the relevant biological work began with an interest in small animal parasites that require magnifying glasses for their proper study. The larger intestinal worms had, of course, been observed from the earliest times, but were generally thought to have originated spontaneously in the host by a form of internal corruption. A more open-minded attitude was applied to the ectoparasites, for after all lice and fleas could be seen to change hosts on occasion.

While lice were for long accepted as normal features of human ecology – with possibly even a protective value (according to such authorities as Linnaeus) scabies created some confusion. It was usually regarded as a specially annoying consequence of louse infestation; and even when some early observers reported finding tiny animals in the lesions, these were thought to be young lice. This confusion was completely dispelled by the work of the first British microbiologist, Thomas Moffett, who, in 1589, produced a splendid description of the scabies mite.[4] This work, following, as it did, the first scientific observations on the liver fluke published by Fitzherbert[5] in 1523, established the traditional excellence of British parasitology which culminated in the nineteenth century with the researches of Erasmus Wilson, Cobbold, Manson, Ross, Bruce and others. Moffett at the outset showed that scabies was due to the burrowing habits of a minute parasite which differed from pediculi not only in its dermatozootic habitat but also in its anatomy, as viewed through a simple lens.

Despite Moffett's conclusive work, Bonanni one hundred years later depicted crab lice as the cause of scabies[6]; and even Linnaeus in his first great biological system named the parasite *Pedic. scabiei*, which he classified with the wingless insects.[7] However, the main disappointment one feels about scabies is to find that little or no attention was subsequently paid to its philosophical implications. After all it was, for more than 200 years following the death of Moffett, the only disease known to be due to a micro-organism, and one, moreover, that could be eliminated with specific 'antiseptic' treatment.

EARLY MICROSCOPY

The lens that was used to such advantage by Moffett probably owed much to the thirteenth-century studies of Grosseteste, Roger Bacon and others in England.[8] But the useful limits of a low-powered magnifying glass had already been reached by Moffett, in 1589, even though valuable work was yet to be done with a hand lens by Tyson in 1683 (on the relatively large segments of tapeworms and on nematodes).[9] However, by 1610 the first primitive compound microscopes had made their appearance. They seem to have been developed as modifications of the great sixteenth-century invention, the compound telescope, of which Leonard Digges' instrument of 1550 was one of the first bilenticular types.[10] Cornelius Drebbel, who spent much of his time in England, is one of the contenders for the disputed title of inventor of the microscope.[11]

Certainly all but two or three of the leading microscopists during the first hundred years were British. These pioneers, including Mundy, Charleton, Power, Grew and

Hooke, were mainly interested in the finer details of larger plants, insects and inanimate objects. Robert Hooke, however, in his *Micrographia* of 1665 introduced the earliest illustrations of a protozoan and a microscopic fungus, and described spore formation for the first time. Moreover, Hooke first described not only the dead 'cells' or cork, but also living cells, 'for in several of those vegetables, whilst green, I have with my microscope, plainly enough discovered these Cells or Pores filled with juices, and by degrees sweating them out'.[12] In the same year, another book published in London deserves mention. It was written by Marchmont Needham,[13] and contains a remarkably detailed account of the Germ Theory. However, the experiments described were modelled on those of Kircher[14] and deal only with microscopic 'vermicules', which were apparently true worms rather than bacteria, protozoa or microscopical fungi. In fact, the main advance made on the practical side of our subject before Leeuwenhoek's work was Hooke's innovation (inspired by Sir Christopher Wren) of accurate highly detailed engravings of microscopical objects.

The serious aberrations of seventeenth-century compound microscopes were all too obvious to Hooke who wrote that if a very small glass ball 'be fixt with a little soft wax against a small needle hole, prick'd through a thin plate of brass, lead, pewter or any other metal, and an object plac'd very near, be look'd at through it, it will both magnify and make some objects more distinct than any of the great microscopes'.[15] But few indeed could tolerate the strenuous discipline of the simple microscope. The great exception was, of course, Leeuwenhoek, who, ten years later, began his astonishing work with this instrument. His indebtedness to the Royal Society is very clear, but has not been sufficiently recognized. For a period of fifty years the Royal Society encouraged Leeuwenhoek in his extraordinarily painstaking and solitary labours, patiently receiving, translating, discussing and publishing his meandering observations. If bacteriology (and protozoology) was born out of Leeuwenhoek's work, the infant's foster mother was undoubtedly the Royal Society in London.

THE BIRTH OF BACTERIOLOGY

Immediately after London had received Leeuwenhoek's first reports of those animalcules that we now identify as true bacteria, Hooke extended the field of enquiry to deal with the bacteria that grow in wheat and other infusions. However, for almost twenty years after this burst of activity, there seems to have been no further bacteriological work, apart from an occasional observation by Leeuwenhoek mentioned in his published letters. Between 1693 and 1697, however, valuable studies on protozoa and bacteria were made by Sir Edmund King, the Reverend John Harris and Stephen Gray.[16] But even more impressive were the investigations of 'a Gentleman in the County' which were published by the Royal Society in 1703.[17] These ranged over the entire field of microbiology and were splendidly illustrated. The figures contrast strikingly with the very poor drawings which accompanied Leeuwenhoek's letters (but, as he was – by his own statement – without skill as a draughtsman, he commissioned the illustrations from others).

The next 140 years saw no discoveries in practical microbiology that were of any direct medical interest – though the position was rather different on the speculative side and in relation to the peripheral subjects such as fermentation and the spontaneous generation controversies. The only microbiological investigations carried out during this extremely long and barren period were exercises in arranging and classifying the multitudes of different 'infusoria' and 'animalcula', most of which had been discovered earlier. Thus, even before Leeuwenhoek's death in 1723, at the advanced age of ninety, a Frenchman, Louis Joblot, had issued a detailed work on protozoa. Many of Joblot's observations seem to have been copied from Leeuwenhoek – without acknowledgement. In contrast, Henry Baker did much to further Leeuwenhoek's memory.[18] Useful classifications were made in 1752 by John Hill,[19] and later by Müller and others. There was also the occasional piece of imaginative research, such as that of John Ellis in 1769 on the multiplication of protozoa.[20] But until the 1840s the landscape was indeed bleak in investigative bacteriology, even more than in protozoology.

Microscopy itself had advanced very little during this period. Even though Hall in 1733 and Dolland in 1758 had independently invented achromatic lenses these could not readily be applied to the microscope. Practical microscopy did not improve noticeably until 1830, when Joseph Jackson Lister solved the problem of spherical aberration.[21]

In 1842 the improved microscope produced its first fruits (in medical bacteriology) with the work of John Goodsir in Edinburgh.[22] His important pioneer work in cellular pathology was later recognized by Virchow, who dedicated his great book on this subject to Goodsir. However, it is the discovery of the *Sarcina ventriculi* by Goodsir that requires our attention here. This remarkable organism which occurs in packets of four cocci was found by Goodsir in the stomach contents of a patient who seems to have had gastric carcinoma. This work is important because Goodsir discovered a bacterium which he named, described fully and depicted adequately in association with a human disease. He then speculated reasonably (but incorrectly as it turned out) on a possible causal relationship between bacterium and disease. The name and description remain valid today – the earliest example of this in bacteriology. With his observations, Goodsir began an interesting relationship between the *Micrococcaceae* and Scotland. Almost forty years after the work on Sarcina – the first member to be discovered – Ogston in Aberdeen described, named and cultured the staphylococcus for the first time, distinguishing it from streptococci, and demonstrating pathogenic and commensal varieties.[23] Rather more than half a century later in 1937, Cruickshank finally demonstrated the complete correlation between coagulase production and pathogenicity in staphylococci, thus giving medical bacteriologists their first example of an *in vitro* indicator of disease-producing ability.

After 1842, there was, at last, increasing activity in bacteriology. Interest was stimulated by discoveries of non-bacterial pathogens including the first systemic mycoses in 1844 by Hughes Bennett in Edinburgh.[24]

The exciting work in mycology led to over-enthusiasm for a fungal theory of disease. After the arrival of asiatic cholera in Britain claims were inevitably advanced that fungi were responsible. Between 1846 and 1849 even the great epidemiologist William Budd, who carried out masterly research on typhoid, was led seriously astray on the fungi. Cowdell in 1848 was another notable exponent of the fungal origin of cholera.[25] The disproof of these ideas produced a set-back for the emerging Germ Theory that lasted a further twenty years.

In the meantime, Pouchet saw, in 1849, large number of 'vibrios' in choleraic stools but did not comment on their possible role in cholera.[26] Indeed, he remained a firm believer in spontaneous generation. Hassall, writing in 1855, seems to have been the first to suggest – albeit cautiously – a significant role for the 'vibriones' he found in the intestines of cholera victims and in their contaminated surroundings.[27] These vibriones provided physical reality for the specific animate contagion of cholera which John Snow had cogently postulated from 1849 onwards. Snow, a Yorkshireman and a former student at Westminster Hospital, convinced himself (and gradually most of his unbiased contemporaries) of the water-borne route of infection in cholera. Snow then compared the biological agent of cholera to the eggs of parasitic worms transmitted by water.[28]

The combined work of Hassall and Snow in London had, by 1855, produced a complete and accurate aetiology for cholera, but the world waited a further thirty years before crediting Koch with the great discovery (even though Koch's own 'postulates' could not be fully applied to the vibrios he belatedly demonstrated).

When by 1860, Davaine and others had discovered the anthrax bacillus in animals, the stage was indeed set for the advent of modern medical bacteriology. Although there is no danger of Pasteur's role in the subsequent events being overlooked, the valuable researches of British contemporaries – who were precursors of Koch – such as Andrew Smart, Burdon Sanderson and Joseph Lister (in his bacteriological capacity) have been sadly neglected. It is easy also to forget the importance of so apparently unrelated an event as the discovery by William Perkin in 1856, of the aniline dyes – which form the basis of the major bacteriological stains and of antimicrobial chemotherapy.

FERMENTATIONS AND PUTREFACTIONS

Turning towards the periphery of our subject, the benefits of fermentation and the unpleasantness of putrefaction had been taken for granted since at least the beginning of history, but the relevance of these processes to infection was appreciated only relatively recently. Possibly the earliest and certainly the most influential statements in this context were the rather cryptic remarks of Francis Bacon, Thomas Willis and Robert Boyle in the seventeenth century. Thus, Bacon in his *Novum Organum* of 1620 – one of the works that qualify him for the title 'Father of Experimental Philosophy' recommends that 'The different kinds of Putrefaction from which Animalcules are generated should be noted'.

This rather tenuous pronouncement and the similar dictum in Bacon's *Natural History*, 'That it is of excellent use to enquire into the means of preventing or staying putrefaction; which makes a great part of physic and surgery' proved so potent that well over 100 years later they formed the basis of Sir John Pringle's researches into 'Septic and Antiseptic Substances' as well as, later his celebrated *Observations on the Diseases of the Army* published in 1752.[29]

Unfortunately only passing mention can be made of the crucial work in 1748 of John Needham who stimulated Spallanzani's famous researches into 'spontaneous generation' – a heresy that was not finally overthrown until the work of Pasteur and John Tyndall over a century later. Similarly the immunological achievements of Edward Jenner and his predecessors Francis Home and Benjamin Jesty cannot be dealt with here. Nor can we consider further such isolated phenomena as the theoretical works of Benjamin Marten and Richard Bradley in 1720, or William Henry's remarkable experiments on heat disinfection in 1831 when active smallpox vaccine was the test system, or Joseph Lister's discovery of penicillin in 1871. I hope, however, that I have been able to show that medical microbiology has a respectably long history of 400 years and that the British contributions have been by no means inconsiderable throughout these centuries.

References

1 SINGER, C. and SINGER, DOROTHEA, 'The scientific position of Girolamo Fracastoro with special reference to the source, character, and influence of his theory of infection', *Ann. Med. Hist.*, 1917, **1**, 1–34.

2 SINGER, C., 'Benjamin Marten a neglected predecessor of Louis Pasteur', *Janus (Haarlem)*, 1911, **6**, 81–98.

3 DOBELL, C., *Antony Van Leeuwenhoek and his 'little animals'*, London, Bale, 1932.

4 MOFFETT, T. (1589) posthum. ed. *Insectorum sive Minimorum Animalium Theatrum*, London, Cotes, 1634.

5 [FITZHERBERT, SIR ANTHONY], *A newe Tracte or Treatyse moost profytable for all Husbandemen*, [London, 1532.]

6 BONANNI, P., *Observationes circa Viventia, quae in Rebus non Viventibus reperiuntur, Cum, Micrographia curiosa . . .*, Rome, 1691.

7 LINNAEUS, C., *Systema Naturae*, Leiden, Haak, 1735.

8 CROMBIE, A. C., *Robert Grosseteste and the Origins of Experimental Science 1100–1700*, Oxford, Clarendon Press, 1953.

9 TYSON, E., 'Lumbricus latus, or a discourse . . . of the joynted worms, wherein a great many mistakes of former writers concerning it, are remarked; . . . and the whole urged, as a difficulty against the doctrine of, univocal generation', *Phil. Trans. R. Soc. Lond.*, 1683, **13**, 113–44.

10 (DIGGES, L., 1550), cited by J. Needham and G. D. Lu in *Historical Aspects of Microscopy*, Cambridge, 1967.

11 (DREBBEL, C., *c.* 1610), cited by S. Bradbury in *The Evolution of the Microscope*, Oxford, Pergamon, 1967, pp. 21–22.

12 HOOKE, R., *Micrographia: or some Physiological Descriptions of Minute Bodies made by Magnifying Glasses. With Observations and Inquiries Therupon*, London, 1665 (licensed and printed, 1664), Preface, pp. 116, 125–28, 213–17.

13 (NEEDHAM, M.), *Medela Medicinae. A Plea for the free Profession, and a Renovation of the Art of Physick, . . . Tending to the Rescue of Mankind from the Tyranny of Diseases; and of Physicians themselves, from the PEDANTISM of old AUTHORS and present DICTATORS*, London, Lownds, 1665 (licensed, 1664).

14 KIRCHER, A., *Scrutinium physico-medicum contagiosae Luis, quae Pestis dicitur, quo origo, causae, signa, prognostica Pestis . . .*, Rome, 1658.

15 HOOKE, R., loc. cit., Preface.

16 *Phil. Trans. R. Soc. Lond.*, 1693, **17**, 861–65; 1696, **19**, 254–59, 280–87, 353–56; 1697, 539–42.

17 (ANONYMOUS), 'An extract of some letters sent to Sir C. H. relating to some microscopical observations', *Phil. Trans. R. Soc. Lond.*, 1703, **23**, 1357–72 (observations dated 1702).

18 BAKER, H., 'An account of Mr. Leeuwenhoek's microscopes', *Phil. Trans. R. Soc. Lond.*, 1740, **41**, 503–19.

19 HILL, J., *An History of Animals containing Descriptions of the Birds, Beasts, and Insects of the Several Parts of the World and including Accounts of the Several Classes of Animalcules visible only by the Assistance of Microscopes*, London, 1752, p. 1 et seq.

20 ELLIS, J., 'Observations on a particular manner of increase in the animalcula of vegetable infusions . . .', *Phil. Trans. R. Soc. Lond.*, 1769, **59**, 138–52.

21 LISTER, J. J., 'On some properties in achromatic object-glasses applicable to the improvement of the microscope', *Phil. Trans. R. Soc. Lond.*, 1830, **120**, 187–200 (read at Royal Society, 1829).

22 GOODSIR, J., 'History of a case in which a fluid periodically ejected from the stomach contained vegetable organisms of an undescribed form', *Edinb. med. surg. J.*, 1842, **57**, 430–33.

23 OGSTON, A., 'Ueber abscesse', *Arch. klin. Chir.*, 1880, **25**, 588–600; 'Report upon micro-organisms in surgical diseases', *Br. med. J.*, 1881, **i**, 369–74 and 453; 'Micrococcus poisoning', *J. Anat. Physiol.*, 1882, **16**, 526–67; ibid., 1883, **17**, 24–58.

24 BENNETT, J. H., 'On the parasitic vegetable structures found growing in living animals', *Trans. Roy. Soc. Edinb.*, 1844, **15**, 277–94.

25 COWDELL, C., *A Disquisition on Pestilential Cholera, Being an Attempt to Explain its Phenomena, Nature, Cause, Preventions, and Treatment, by Reference to an Extrinsic Fungous Origin*, London, Highley, 1848.
26 POUCHET, F.-A., 'Infusoires dans les dejections des choleriques', *C. r. hebd. Séanc. Acad. Sci., Paris*, 1849, **28**, 555–6.
27 HASSALL, A. H., 'Report on the microscopical examination of the blood and excretions of cholera patients', in Appendix to *Report of Committee for Scientific Inquiries in Relation to the Cholera Epidemic of 1854*, pp. 289–307.
28 SNOW, J., *On the Mode of Communication of Cholera*, 2nd ed., London, Churchill, 1855, pp. 15, 113.
29 SELWYN, S., 'Sir John Pringle: hospital reformer, moral philosopher and pioneer of antiseptics', *Med. Hist.*, 1966, **10**, 266–74.

E. Hickel
Braunschweig (West Germany)

British and continental nineteenth-century pharmacopoeias compared

Pharmacopoeias are usually considered by laymen as nothing but official drug-standards, which may have their significance for pharmacists and for the pharmaceutical industry. Professionals of the health professions, however, tend to look at the pharmacopoeia as a symbol of the intellectual capacity of their profession, and more than once they elevated the pharmacopoeia to a kind of National Monument. This may be understood by considering the fact that the development of pharmacopoeias took place on a purely national level until recent times; however, in judging and evaluating critically the problems and achievements of a pharmacopoeia, this way of thinking cannot be effective. Both the critic and the historian run the risk of taking for granted the particular conditions of their own pharmacopoeia – that is, the particular development of Public Health in their country – and to regard these as generally valid. Only by comparison with foreign pharmacopoeias and their conditions can the historian form a standard by which the characteristics of his own pharmacopoeia may be assessed.

Applied to the British pharmacopoeia this would mean that the British observer should abandon the idea that nineteenth-century pharmacopoeias were compiled exclusively by the medical profession and published by their organizations. For, on the Continent, e.g. in France and Germany, pharmacists and scientists were – in co-operation with the government – the main authors of the pharmacopoeias, and the government appeared as the guarantor for the validity of the pharmacopoeia by making it a legal code.

These fundamental differences necessarily must become manifest in the very different characters of the British and the Continental official pharmacopoeias. The latter, being legal codes, made every pharmacist liable to: (1) keep in his shop every drug mentioned in the pharmacopoeia (this list of drugs was the so-called 'series medicaminum'); (2) to prepare the compounds according to the pharmacopoeia-processes only: the formula of the pharmacopoeia had to be interpreted literally, even if the pharmacist knew a much better variation; (3) to apply the test- and assay-processes for drugs in every case where they were given in the pharmacopoeia; in particular, every pharmacist was obliged to meet all technical requirements which were necessary in order to perform such tests and assays.

In all these regards, the British druggists and chemists could take the pharmacopoeia more lightly. The public, on the other hand, in consequence of this freedom did not enjoy the same protection as on the continent. The greater liberality in

Great Britain may be considered as advantageous in so far as it permitted pharmacists to be more progressive than on the Continent in introducing new methods of drug-testing and assaying, because it was not necessary to take into consideration the facilities of every country pharmacist.

The London Pharmacopoeia of 1836 seems to prove – at first glance – the role of pace-maker in introducing new methods for drug-assay, for it listed gravimetric assays for a number of medicinal salts which were not to be found in the Prussian and in the French pharmacopoeias for a number of years. At the time, however, this progress was on paper only, for two reasons: on the one hand, the assay methods were not at all practicable as described in the London Pharmacopoeia; and on the other hand, there were at that time in England only a very small number of professional people who were able to put these methods – even if described correctly – into practice.

Here, it becomes obvious that there was in this regard a shortcoming in British public health in the nineteenth century, from which the effectiveness of pharmacopoeias and drug standardization suffered for several decades: even for a long time after the year 1841 (foundation of the Pharmaceutical Society) there was a marked lack of qualified authors as well as competent users of the pharmacopoeias. This was in contrast to continental pharmacy, where pharmacopoeias more than once fell behind the professional and technical level of the long-established and well-educated profession of pharmacy (this was true particularly in France); and where, on the other hand, pharmacopoeias could derive profit from the fact that at a much earlier time than in Britain highly competent public pharmacists entered the pharmacopoeia committees and took care that the practical requirements of the pharmacist's shop were considered sufficiently (which was true for instance in Prussia).

Not before the passing of the Pharmacy Act of 1852 can we expect to find similar conditions in Great Britain. In the course of the next twelve years the new profession of pharmacy succeeded (not least under the influence of the School of Pharmacy in London) in producing a sufficient number of competent pharmacists so that the British Pharmacopoeias of 1864 and 1867, presumably under their influence, became the most progressive pharmacopoeias in Europe (although the profession as a body was not mentioned in the pharmacopoeia itself). Nevertheless, it took at least another twenty years until the educational level of pharmacists was raised sufficiently to enable all of them to profit by the pharmacopoeia. For the first time in Europe the British Pharmacopoeias of the 1860s introduced the rather ambitious methods of volumetric analysis which had a special tradition in Britain since the time of Ure, which was later to dominate in foreign pharmacopoeias. The following editions of 1885 and 1898 maintained the outstanding position by introducing alkaloidal estimations (even if to a certain extent defective ones) in 1885, and a new system of impurity tests in 1898.

It surely is to be regretted that so far there have been no historical investigations into the pharmaceutical personalities who contributed to these epoch-making innovations in Great Britain, and that for example there are few details known of the life and the achievements of a person like John Attfield. As far as I am concerned, in the course of my researches on nineteenth-century pharmacy, I met with a number of names of public as well as industrial pharmacists who presumably contributed to the pharmacopoeia editions of 1867, 1885 and 1898 (e.g. Umney,

Bird, Walter Hills, Lucas, Barnard S. Procter). It would certainly be a rewarding task to elucidate the contributions of these people by investigation of archive material; this probably would tell us more about the 'professional standing' of nineteenth-century British pharmacists than most of the published intentions of the Pharmaceutical Society, and it would help us to understand the process of professionalization in British pharmacy.

For references and for more details see Erika Hickel, *Arzneimittelstandardisierung in den Pharmakopöen des 19. Jahrhunderts in Deutschland, Frankreich, Großbritannien und den Vereinigten Staaten von Amerika*, Stuttgart, 1973.

W. Kaiser
Halle/S (East Germany)

Über einige hallisch-englische Wissenschaftsbeziehungen des 18. Jahrhunderts

Als die Universität Halle im Jahre 1694 feierlich eröffnet wird und der zu diesem Zeitpunkt schon weithin bekannte Friedrich Hoffmann (1660–1742) das Amt des Professor primarius an der Medizinischen Fakultät übernimmt, ist damit ein Freund und Verehrer des 3 Jahre zuvor verstorbenen Robert Boyle (1626–91) zum Ordinarius an der neuen und bald in ganz Europa rennomierten Hochschule avanciert. Hoffmann hatte 1684 persönlich in England geweilt und dem Unterricht des berühmten Chemikers beigewohnt.

Zur gleichen Zeit lehrt mit Paul Hermann (1646–95) ein Sohn der Saalestadt als Ordinarius für Botanik an der niederländischen Universität Leiden. Auch er unterhält nach seinen England-Reisen von 1682 und 1683 enge Beziehungen zu den dort wirkenden Fachvertretern: neben John Watts, Henry Compton und Robert Morison hatte er Leonard Plukenet (1642–1706) aufgesucht, den ,,Queen's Botanist" und Vorsteher der Gärten von Hampton Court. Mit John Ray (1628–1705), dem Begründer der Systematik als eigenständigem biologischem Fachgebiet, steht er im beständigen Erfahrungsaustausch.

Denkt man schließlich daran, daß in der Gründungsphase der Universität Halle gleichenorts der Wundarzt Georg Händel (1622–97) wirkt, dessen Sohn Georg Friedrich die Beziehungen zwischen Halle und England außerhalb der Ars medica sinnfällig verdeutlicht, so sind damit einige Fakten aufgezeigt, die eine Analyse dieser Epoche unter dem generellen Aspekt der Wissenschaftskontakte sinnvoll erscheinen lassen.

Friedrich Hoffmann ist nicht der einzige bedeutende deutsche Arzt und Naturwissenschaftler, der sich auf die Schule eines Robert Boyle berufen kann. Die mit dem Namen des Hallensers verbundene Geschichte der Ätherdarstellung bezieht außerdem die in England tätigen Chemiker und Pharmazeuten Ambrosius Gottfried Hanckwitz und S. August Froben ein, die beide Mitglieder der Royal Society sind und von denen Hanckwitz wohl als erster Äther und Phosphorsäure in größerem Maßstab fabriziert. Schüler britischer Lehrer ist auch der deutsche Apotheker Caspar Neumann (1683–1737), der 1711 nach England geht und 1727 in Halle den Doktorgrad verliehen erhält.

Während der frühen Amtszeit von Friedrich Hoffmann sind die Medizinstudenten Henry Plumptre aus Nottingham und Thomas Kennedy aus Schottland in den Universitätsmatrikeln nachweisbar; beide legen 1705 ihre Inauguraldissertation vor. Plumptre fungiert später auf einer Professur in Cambridge; seine hallesche

Doktorarbeit über das Sal Carolinum ist 1714 in Dresden in deutschsprachiger Ausgabe verlegt worden. 1730 findet sich der aus London gebürtige Simon Adolphus (gente Iudaeus) unter den promovierten Absolventen; er kehrt allerdings nicht nach England zurück, sondern wird im niederrheinischen Kleve ansässig.

Ist die Zahl englischer Hörer relativ klein, so gehen umso mehr Studenten vo» Deutschland nach England. Für den um eine umfassende Ausbildung bemühten Mediziner versteht es sich von selbst, daß er nach Möglichkeit in Halle bei Friedrich Hoffmann und Georg Ernst Stahl (1659–1734) sowie in Leiden bei Hermann Boerhaave (1668–1738) Kollegs belegt, im Anschluß aber nach England reist, um die Vorlesungen eines Isaac Newton (1643–1727) zu hören und die botanischen Institutionen des Inselstaates aufzusuchen. Dieser Studiengang ist insbesondere für die aus den Ländern der Habsburgischen Krone nach Halle anreisenden Absolventen, die sich in der Heimat dem massiven Druck der Rekatholisierungskampagne ausgesetzt sehen, geradezu typisch. Dabei mag hinzukommen, daß ein 1692 durch Benjamin Woodroffe begründetes Kolleg (Gloucester Hall) diesem Personenkreis seine besondere Aufmerksamkeit widmete und dadurch ein Pendant zu Halle darstellte, wo in einem Pietismus spezifischer Prägung die Gedanken der Frühaufklärung bereits fest eingewurzelt waren. Repräsentanten dieses dreigeteilten Ausbildungsganges sind z.B. die Siebenbürger Mediziner Andreas Ajtai (1672–1733) und Franz Pariz Papai (geb. 1689): beide sind 1714 in Halle und 1715 in Leiden, absolvieren aber auch einen Teil ihres Studiums in England. Ebenso bemühen sich zahlreiche deutsche Mediziner um eine Fortbildung durch profilierte englische Fachvertreter. Bezeichnend ist der Werdegang von Johann Zacharias Platner (1694–1747), der 1717 in Halle promoviert wird und später als Ordinarius für Chirurgie in Leipzig amtiert. Platner rechnet sich zu den Schülern Hoffmanns, aber auch zu denen des jetzt im französischen Exil lehrenden Thomas Woolhouse (1650–1730), der am 14. Juni 1726 in die Academia Naturae Curiosorum berufen wird. Diese 1652 in Schweinfurt begründete und wissenschaftlich hochangesehene deutsche Gesellschaft baut damals in zunehmendem Maße ihre Kontakte zur Royal Society aus, wo Hans Sloane (1660–1753) ab 1727 die Präsidialfunktion innehat. Ein Jahr darauf kommt Johann Jakob Dillenius (1687–1747) als Professor der Botanik von Gießen nach Oxford; auch er ist seit dem 24. Juni 1713 Mitglied der Leopoldina. Carl von Linné (1707–78) sucht hier den Begründer der wissenschaftlichen Erforschung der Moose auf seiner England-Reise von 1736 auf.

Die Beziehungen zwischen der Academia Naturae Curiosorum und der Royal Society intensivieren sich noch mehr, als Andreas Elias Büchner (1701–69) das Amt des Akademiepräsidenten übernimmt (1735) und mit dem Wechsel vom Erfurter auf das hallesche Ordinariat (1745) das Sekretariat der Sozietät an die neue Wirkungsstätte verlagert. Unter seiner Leitungsära gelangen 6 in England tätige Wissenschaftler zur Rezeption: am 14. Mai 1737 der in London praktizierende Arzt John Henry Hampe (1697–1777), der bei seiner Berufung als Archiater der Prinzessin von Wales fungiert. Es folgen am 18. Juni 1739 der in Dublin lehrende Jakob Macdonald, am 16. Oktober 1749 der als Sekretär der Royal Society amtierende Cromwell Mortimer, am 8. September 1753 der in London tätige Emanuel Mendes da Costa, am 12. August 1761 der ebenfalls in London praktizierende Arzt John Hill und am 12. August 1762 Karl Morton vom Londoner Medizinalkollegium, gleichzeitig der Kustos der königlichen Manuskripte und des britischen Museums.

Der Name von Cromwell Mortimer (gest. 1752) erinnert nochmals an die Geschichte der Ätherdarstellung: dieser hatte nach dem Tode von Froben in den *Philos. Transact.* (Nr. 461) dessen bislang geheim gehaltene Rezeptur bekanntgegeben und eine Arbeitsvorschrift mitgeteilt, die Froben noch selbst im Februar 1740 der Royal Society vorlegen konnte. An gleicher Stelle teilt Mortimer die Geschichte der Äther-Veröffentlichungen und einiges über Frobens mystische Konzeptionen zu Ursprung und Natur dieses „Spiritus aetheri" mit.

Andreas Elias Büchner setzt es auch durch, daß dem Londoner Pharmazeuten William Watson (1715–87) im Jahre 1754 das Ehrendoktorat der Medizinischen Fakultät Halle verliehen wird, eine damals höchst seltene Auszeichnung. Einer von Büchners Hörern des Jahres 1758 ist der aus Berlin gebürtige Peter Simon Pallas (1741–1811), später bekannt als Begründer der paläarktischen Wirbeltierkunde. Auch Pallas hält sich noch an die Dreiteilung des Studiums an deutschen, niederländischen und englischen Universitäten: 1758 weilt er in Halle, 1760 in Leiden, 1761/62 in England. Zu seinen Lehrern der Botanik zählt er im erhalten gebliebenen Curriculum vitae drei Persönlichkeiten, deren Namen uns auch in der „Liste der Offiziere der Armee Floras" von Linné begegnen: Peter Collinson (Mercator Londinensis), Philipp Miller (Hortulanus Chelseensis) und Humphrey Sibthorp (Professor Oxoniensis). Außerdem beruft sich Pallas auf den Unterricht bei James Persons (1705–70), bei dem bereits erwähnten Leopoldina-Mitglied Emanuel Mendes da Costa und schließlich auch bei Karl Daniel Solander (1736–82), der an der ersten Cookschen Weltumseglung (1768–71) teilnimmt. Letzteres Ereignis lenkt die Aufmerksamkeit des Nachbetrachters auf die beiden Forster und damit auf zwei Persönlichkeiten, die erneut eine Wechselbeziehung zwischen England und Halle symbolisieren. Während Johann Reinhold Forster (1729–98) auf Vermittlung seines Sohnes 1777 von England aus als Ordinarius für Botanik nach Halle kommt, geht Georg Forster (1754–94), der im gleichen Jahr das Buch „A voyage round the world" über die zweite Cooksche Reise edierte, nach Kassel und Wilna, bevor er in Mainz in die Ereignisse der französischen Revolution verwickelt wird. In der Zwischenzeit legt er in Halle eine medizinische Doktorarbeit vor, die sich auf Forschungsresultate der Schiffsreise bezieht; die Leopoldina beruft ihn am 18. Juli 1780 in ihre Reihen. Ebenfalls 1777 wird der damals 22 Jahre alte Philipp Friedrich Theodor Meckel (1755–1803) zum Ordinarius für Anatomie, Chirurgie und Geburtshilfe in Halle bestellt, der sich gerade als Gast bei William Hunter in London aufhält. Es heißt, die frühe Berufung sei deswegen erfolgt weil die Gefahr bestanden habe, der begabte Anatom werde in England bleiben. Meckel hat wohl noch etwas geschwankt, ob er der Vokation folgen solle; er trifft erst 1779 in Halle ein.

Die Kontakte zwischen den britischen Gesellschaften und der Leopoldina halten auch im ausgehenden 18. Jahrhundert an. Am 26. März 1783 wird mit dem in London lehrenden Richard Kirwan (1735–1812) der Mitbegründer der Affinitätslehre in die Academia Naturae Curiosorum berufen, am 4. November 1789 der Botaniker Joseph Banks (1740–1820), ebenfalls ein Teilnehmer der ersten Cookschen Expedition. Am 14. Oktober 1793 folgt mit William Herschel (1738–1822) der Hofastronom Georgs III., am 6. Oktober 1794 mit Johann Latham (gest. 1837) ein Dartforder Arzt und Gynäkologe, am 10. Oktober 1797 mit Jakob Edward Smith (1759–1828) der Präsident der Linnéschen Gesellschaft zu London.

Abschließend sei noch einmal auf Friedrich Hoffmann verwiesen, mit dem diese kurze Studie begann. In dem von W. Lewis (gest. 1781) edierten ,,New Dispensatory" erscheint seine Äthermedikation als offizielles Arzneimittel; sein ,,Spiritus aetheris vitriolici compositus" ist im Londoner Arzneibuch von 1788 enthalten und bis auf unsere Zeit als ,,Hoffmanns anodyne" in Gebrauch geblieben, wogegen sich auf dem Festland eine nunmehr weinölfreie Präparation als ,,Hoffmannstropfen" durchsetzt.

Zahlreiche weitere Wissenschaftskontakte – erwähnt sei nur die Informationsreise des halleschen Chirurgen Carl Heinrich Dzondi (1770–1835) – bedürfen noch einer ausführlichen Analyse. Die vorliegende Abhandlung will im Sinne einer ersten Mitteilung verstanden sein, der eine ausführliche Darstellung folgen soll.

J. Kenéz
Budapest (Hungary)

Addison und die Nebennierenforschung auf dem Kontinent

Einleitend einige Worte über die Themenwahl. Seit Ende des zweiten Weltkrieges erscheinen immerwieder Monografien und Lehrbücher über die innere Sekretion, die weder im Text noch in ihrer geschichtlichen Einleitung die fundamentalen Versuche von A. Biedl (1869–1933) erwähnen und selbst seine Monografie über die Innere Sekretion, die jahrzentelang als das Standardwerk der inneren Sekretion gegolten hat und selbst in der Gegenwart nach Verstreichen von 60 Jahren noch immer eine unerschöpfliche Fundgrube von Daten und kritisch gesichtetem Material darstellt, wird nicht gebührend gewürdigt, ja unter den Standardwerken der inneren Sekretion nicht einmal angeführt.

Vor 3 Jahren, also anlässlich der loo-sten Wiederkehr seines Geburtstages, sind nur 2 Arbeiten erschienen. Eine von H. Prof. Kaiser, dem Vorsitzenden der medizinhistorischen Gesellschaft in der DDR, zusammen mit einem ungarischen Endokrinologen und die andere von mir.

Da unter den Themen des XXIII. Kongresses die Relationen der englischen Medizin zur Medizin im Ausland figurierte, habe ich mich entschlossen, die grundlegenden Versuche auf dem Gebiete der Nebennierenforschung vor diesem Forum zu erörtern, da einerseits die Befruchtung der Forschung durch einen englischen Mediziner Thomas Addison (1793–1860) am eindeutigsten ist und meines Erachtens die Versuche von Biedl die bedeutendsten eben auf diesem Gebiet sind.

In welchem Werk begegnen wir zum erstenmal dem anatomischen Begriff: Nebenniere?

Der wahrscheinlich in San Severino geborene Bartholomeus Eustachius Sanctoseverinatus (1524–74), der grosse Rennaissance Gelehrte und Leibarzt des Papstes war der erste der sie im Jahre 1564 beschrieb in seiner in Venedig erschienenen Opusculae Anatomicae. Im VI. Kapitel nannte er diese Organe *Glandulae quae renis incumbunt.* Das Werk gelang in Privatbesitz und ist 150 Jahre praktisch unbekannt geblieben. Später hat sie ebenfalls ein römischer Anatom, Giovanni Lancisi (1654–1720) mit seinen eigenen Notizen publiziert, da die Originalkommentare verschollen sind.

Eingehend beschäftigte sich auch mit diesem Organ beim Menschen der dänische, in Paris wirkende Anatom: Jacobus Benignus Winslow (1669–1764) in seinem Werk: *Exposition anatomique de la structure du corps humain.*

Weitere erwähnungswerte anatomische Arbeiten: Johann Friedrich Meckel (1781–1833) erhielt von Cuvier (1769–1832) zum Studium das grosse Tiermaterial des zoologischen Gartens in Paris und beschrieb die Nebennieren von vielen Tieren und auch von Menschen (*Abhandlungen aus der menschlichen und vergleichenden Anatomie und Physiologie*, Halle, 1806). Er beabsichtigte auch Tierversuche anzustellen, blieb jedoch nur bei der Absicht. Auf Alexander Ecker (1816–87) geht die Feststellung zurück, dass es sich um Drüsengewebe und zwar um eine Blutdrüse handelt (*Der feinere Bau der Nebennieren*, Braunschweig, 1846). Hinsichtlich der histologischen Struktur stammen wichtige Feststellungen von Rudolf Albert Koelliker (1817–1903), *Handbuch der Gewebelehre des Menschen*, Leipzig, 1852.

ÜBER DIE FUNKTION LAGEN JEDOCH MEHRERE JAHRHUNDERTE HINDURCH NUR UNFRUCHTBARE HYPOTHESEN VOR

In der Erforschung der Physiologie und der Klinik der Nebenniere bedeutet das Jahr 1855 einen Wendepunkt. Was bis dahin zutage gefördert wurde, bildet nur den geschichtlichen Unterbau für das grosse und später erbaute verzweigte wissenschaftliche Gebäude. Die makroskopisch-anatomischen und zum Grossteil auch die mikroskopischen Gesichtspunkte waren so gut wie abgeschlossen, es harrte vorerst die Physiologie ihrer Lösung.

Die Untersuchungen über die Funktion und die Physiologie dieses Organs wurde in bestimmtere Bahnen gelenkt als Thomas Addison, Arzt im Guy's Hospital in der Südwestlondoner Aerztegesellschaft einen Vortrag hielt, in dem er über 3 Fälle mit einer eigentümlichen Form der Anämie berichtete. Bei den Kranken bestand eine bronzene Verfärbung der Haut und sichtbarer Schleimhäute und die Sektion ergab eine völlige Zerstörung der Nebennieren. Bei 2 Fällen bestanden ausser der Destruktion der Nebennieren keinerlei sonstige Veränderungen.

Gedruckt erschien der Vortrag in der Londoner *Medical Gazette*, 1949, Nr 8. Addison stellt die Frage: könne es sich um eine zufällige Koinzidenz handeln?

Diese Frage hatte Addison selbst beantwortet in seiner im Jahre 1855 erschienenen Monografie. (On the constitutional and local effects of disease of the suprarenal capsules. Highley Verlag.). In dieser Monografie beschrieb er 11 autoptisch kontrollierte Fälle und nannte die Krankheit, die durch Anämie, Adynamie, und bronzerne Verfärbung der Haut und Schleimhäute charakterisiert war, Melasma suprarenale. Die Originalausgabe war mit 11 Bildern geschmückt. Französisch hatte Lasègue noch imselben Jahr in einer französischen Zeitschrift die Entdeckung von Addison besprochen, die deutsche Übersetzung erschien erst im Jahre 1912.

(Aus der Sicht der Gegenwart kann bemängelt werden, dass die Nebennieren histologisch nicht bearbeitet worden sind.)

Virchow (1821–1902) hatte den Zusammenhang nicht anerkannt. (Göschen, *Deutsche Klinik*, Bd. 9, 1857–59.)

Beim Erscheinen des Werkes von Addison schreiben wir das Datum 1855 und in Frankreich wirken zurzeit die Grössen der Physiologie und das Tierexperiment gehört zu den alltäglichen physiologischen Untersuchungsmethoden. Imselben Jahr prägt Claude Bernard (1813–78) den Ausdruck *Innere Sekretion* und er verstand darunter, dass gewisse Organe ihre Sekrete nicht durch Ausführungsgänge entlehren, sondern direkt an die Blutbahn abgeben. Er hat den Ausdruck für die Glykogenabgabe der Leber gebraucht, die zwar heute nicht mehr als innersekretorische Tätigkeit angesehen wird, der Ausdruck existiert jedoch noch in der Gegenwart.

Wie gesagt in Frankreich wo die Tierversuche in hohem Masse gehandhabt wurden begann kurz nach Erscheinen des Werkes von Addison die Prüfung der Funktion der Nebenniere im Tierversuch. Einer der Grössen der Physiologie im XIX Jahrhundert, der durch seine Selbstversuche unsterblich gewordene Ir-Franzose Charles Edouard Brown-Séquard (1818–94) hat den Reigen begonnen. Um einen Einblick in die Funktion der Nebennieren zu gewinnen, wollte er die Ausfallserscheinungen, die nach Extirpation der Nebennieren auftreten, beobachten.

Die Tierversuche boten aber dazu keine Gelegenheit, da die Tiere kurz nach Entfernung beider Nebennieren ausnahmslos unter Symptomen von allgemeiner Schwäche, Convulsionen, Delirien und Koma zugrunde gingen, nach einseitiger Epinephrektomie jedoch zum Grossteil am Leben blieben. Die Beschreibung seiner Beobachtungen trug er in der l'Academie de Science in Paris am 25/VIII und am 8/IX vor. Der Text im Autoreferat erschien in dem *Compt. Rend. de l'Acad. de la Science*, Paris, 1856, tome 43, nr. 8, S. 422 und 542.

Der Titel des ersten Vortrages: Recherches expérimentales sur la physiologie et pathologie des capsules surrenales. Sein weiterer Vortrag trug den Titel: Recherches expérimentales sur la physiologie des capsules surrenales. Er beruft sich auf die Feststellungen von Addison und zitiert auch einige anatomische Arbeiten.

Er führte seine Versuche an folgenden Tieren durch:

NN. Entfernung bilat. 5 Hunde, 44 Kaninchen, 2 Katzen und 5 Meerschweinchen.
NN. Entfernung unilat. 2 Hunde, 16 Kaninchen, 2 Katzen und 5 Meerschweinchen.

Seine Schlussfolgerungen lauteten: (1) La mort dépend surtout de l'absence des capsules surrenales c'est á dire de l'absence de leurs fonctions. (2) *Les fonctions des capsules surrenales sont essentiels à la vie.*

Er stellt die Frage: weshalb wurde dieses Organ bisher von den Physiologen und Klinikern negligiert? und beantwortet zugleich die Frage, es dünkt ihm, dass der Grund in der Winzigkeit des Organs zu suchen war.

Die Veröffentlichungen von Brown-Séquard hatten einen grossen Widerhall gehabt. Es erhoben sich die Forscher, die Brown-Séquard Behauptungen zu widerlegen versuchten. Der bekannteste unter ihnen war ein Mitarbeiter des anatomischen Institutes, späterer Leiter des anatomischen Lehrstuhls im Museum St. Hilaire, Louis Pierre Gratiolet (1815–65) der seine Versuche an Ratten durchführte und die Tiere überlebten. (Notes sur les effets, qui suivent l'ablation des capsules surrenales. *Compt. Rend. d l'Acad. Sci.* tome XLIII, 468.) Er stellte die Hypothese auf, dass die Tiere von Brown-Séquard an Sepsis bzw. an Operationsshock zugrunde gingen. Erwiderung von Brown-Séquard: es waren bei der Sektion weder Blutungen noch Hinweise auf eine Sepsis zu finden. Er liess jedoch die Möglichkeit offen, dass die Nebenniere bei den pigmentlosen Tieren nicht unbedingt lebensnotwendig ist.

In den darauffolgenden Jahren erschienen jedoch Arbeiten en masse, die den Standpunkt von Gratiolet zu unterstützen schienen, und das Interesse um die Nebennierenphysiologie flaute ab. Eine Arbeit aus dem Jahre 1889 erwies sich später als sehr wichtig.

H. Stilling, Privatdozent in Strassburg, veröffentlichte eine Arbeit: Über die kompensatorische Hypertrophie der Nebennieren (*Virch. Arch.* 1889, pp. 118, 569). Er stellte nach Entfernung einer Nebenniere beim Kaninchen die Hypertrophie der anderen fest. Er beobachtete ausserdem, dass die früher makroskopisch unsichtbaren, zerstreuten, winzig kleinen Nebennieren nach der unilateralen Epinephrektomie derart hypertrophierten, dass sie makroskopisch zur Sicht kamen. Bei der mikroskopischen Untersuchung zeigte es sich, dass diese neugebildeten, akzessorischen Nebennebennieren eine der Rinde entsprechende Struktur aufwiesen.

Es bestanden also diametral entgegengesetzte Meinungen und den Widerspruch, der wie sich herausstellte nur ein scheinbarer war, klärte ein junger Forscher aus dem Wiener Institut für experimentelle Pathologie: Artur Biedl. Er stammte aus Ungarn und sein Chef, Salomon Stricker (1834–98) war ebenfalls aus dem damaligen Ungarn gebürtig. Zur Klärung der Widersprüche nahm er einen bestechend einfachen, jedoch beweiskräftigen Modellversuch vor. Er entfernte die Nebennieren bei den Versuchstieren aus ihrer ursprünglichen Stätte und implantierte sie unter die Haut.

Die Tiere überlebten. In einer zweiten Sitzung hat er durch einen oberflächlichen Hautschnitt, die vorher eingepflanzten Organe entfernt und die Tiere gingen nach diesem sicher nicht traumatisierenden Eingriff ein. Brown-Séquard hat also Recht gehabt und seine Gegner begingen mehrere methodische Fehler. Einerseits haben sie an Tieren z.B. Ratten, die über ein ausgedehntes akzessorisches System von Nebennebennieren verfügen, gearbeitet, andererseits haben sie ihre getöteten Tiere nicht mit genügender Sorgfalt seziert und so entgingen ihnen die winzigen Restchen, die jedoch zum Weiterleben ausreichten. Diese Ansicht vertraten auch Abelous J. E. und P. Langlois: Note sur les fonctions des capsules surrenales chéz la grenouille. (*Compt. Rend. Soc. Biol.*, 1891, **43**, 292.)

Sie fanden, dass bei Fröschen und auch bei Meerschweinchen und Hunden die Entfernung einer Nebenniere keine wesentlichen Folgen hat. Erst Entfernung einer Nebenniere und eines Grossteils der anderen führt zumeist zum Tode. Werden jedoch grössere Teile einer Nebenniere zurückgelassen so trat der Tod-wenn überhaupt-erst nach längerer Zeit ein. Sie versuchten auch Extrakte herzustellen und konnten eine gewisse lebensverlängernde Wirkung bei ihren beiderseits epinephrektomierten Tieren beobachten.

Biedls Urteil über Brown-Séquard: wenn auch einige Tiere an postoperativem Shock oder an Sepsis zugrunde gingen, ist es sicherlich sein Verdienst den einzuschlagenden Weg vorgezeichnet zu haben. Nach der Klärung der Frage über die Lebenswichtigkeit der Nebenniere lautete die zweite zu beantwortende Frage: Welcher Anteil der Nebenniere ist aus der Sicht der Lebensnotwendigkeit entscheidend? Rinde oder Mark?

Biedls Versuche zeigten, dass ad conservandam vitae 1/8 der Nebennierensubstanz genüge, vorausgesetzt, dass es aus Rindegewebe besteht. Nach Entfernung einer Nebenniere und der Marksubstanz des Paarlings können die Tiere mit dem zurückbleibenden grösserem oder kleinerem Rindenrest ohne krankhafte Störung weiterleben. Bei Abtragung der Rindensubstanz gelingt es nicht die Tiere am Leben zu erhalten. Der bekannte Histologe A. Kohn (1867–1959) hat diese Beobachtungen insofern ergänzt, dass er nachwies, dass die Tiere zum Überleben keine Marksubstanz benötigen, da sie stets über genügendes chromaffines Gewebe verfügen-ausserhalb der Nebenniere und erst wenn es gelänge diese radikal zu entfernen, könnten schlüssige Beweise hinsichtlich der Funktion der Marksubstanz geliefert werden. Die Schlussfolgerungen von Kohn bestätigten die immer stärker betonte These von Biedl, dass die Rinde und nicht das Mark der lebenswichtige Anteil der Nebenniere ist.

Und dann kam eine Entdeckung, die trotz ihrer Grossartigkeit, die endgültige Klärung obiger Frage nachteilig beeinflusste. G. Oliver (1841–1915) und sein Mitarbeiter hielten am 10/II, 1894 einen Vortrag in der Londoner Physiologischen Gesellschaft. Sie berichteten, dass es ihnen gelang aus der Nebenniere eine blutdruckerhöhende Substanz zu isolieren. (The physiological effects of extracts of the suprarenal capsules', *J. of Physiol.*, 1895, **18**, 230.) Fast gleichzeitig-jedenfalls unabhängig von den englischen Forschern-berichteten polnische Forscher (N. Czybulsky, 1854–1919, und Mitarb. in Krakau) diese Stadt gehörte damals zur Donaumonarchie, dass es ihnen auch gelang eine blutdruckerhöhende Substanz zu isolieren (*Archiv. Akad. Wiss. Krakau*, 1895).

Die klinischen Erfolge waren mit dem Extrakt derart spectaculaire-was den Blutdruck und die Vasokonstriktion betrifft-dass man das Nebenierenproblem als gelöst angesehen hat. Bei der Anwendung von Addison Kranken kamen jedoch grosse Enttäuschungen, da weder mit dem Extrakt noch später mit der kristallinen Substanz die Kranken am Leben zu erhalten waren.

Es tauchte also wieder die Frage auf, war es nicht die Schuld der grossen Erfolge des Adrenalins, das Forschungsinteresse an der Nebennierenrinde in den Hintergrund zu drängen?

Und jetzt kamen die entscheidenden Tierversuche von Biedl!

F. Leydig (1821–1908, *Handbuch der vergleichenden Anatomie*, Bd 1, Tübingen, 1864) und F. M. Balfour (1851–82, *Monograph on the developement of the Elasmobranch Fishes*, London, 1878) wiesen nach, dass bei den Knorpel- und Knochenfischen vorkommende Interrenalkörper ihrem Baue nach der Nebennierenrinde der Säuger homolog sind (sie werden nach ihrem Erstbeschreiber H. F. Stannius, 1808–83, Anatom in Rostock, Stannius' sche Körper genannt).

Die paarigen, den sympathischen Grenzstrangganglien segmental anliegenden Suprarenalkörper dagegen sind als Homologe der Marksubstanz der Nebenniere der höchsten Vertebraten zu betrachten.

Im Jahre 1899 widmet sich Biedl während eines Studienaufenthaltes in der Stazione Zoologica Napoli und später in Triest der Untersuchung des Interrenalgewebes der Selachier (Knorpelfische) und konnte ihre vitale Bedeutung erweisen und sprach den Satz aus: „die Ausrottung des Interrenalgewebes allein mit der Fortdauer des Lebens unvereinbar ist und unter Erscheinungen zum Tode führt, welche den nach der Nebennierenextirpation zu beobachtenden an die Seite zu stellen sind.“

Die Entfernung der Adrenalorgane hatte die Lebenserwartung der Fische nicht grundlegend beeinträchtigt. Er wies zugleich nach, dass Extrakte dieser Adrenalorgane alle für das Adrenalin bis dahin bekannte physiologische Wirkungen zu entfalten vermögen. Bei der Registrierung des Blutdruckes bei den Torpedofischen und Rajas hat er ebenfalls beobachtet, dass in den Kiemenarterien dieselbe Wirkung zustande kommt wie nach der Verabfolgung von Adrenalin.

Nach Entfernung des Interrenalgewebes traten Pigmentveränderungen auf, und die Muskelschwäche zeigte weitgehende Parallelität mit der nach Rindenausfall bei Säugetieren.

Dieser als interrenopriver bezeichnete Symptomenkomplex konnte durch Adrenalin nicht behoben werden. Einige weitere Daten aus dieser Arbeit: 12 Squaliden hat er operiert. Davon überlebten d.h. sie starben erst nach 3 Wochen 10, kurz nach der Operation gingen 2 Fische ein. Die Sektion zeigte, dass nur bei den 2 unmittelbar Verstorbenen die Extirpation eine totale war, bei den übrigen blieben Restchen zurück. Bei den Rajiden gelang die Operation viel besser. Aus 32 Rajiden gelang es bei 27 total die Interrenalkörper zu extirpieren. Die Tiere zeigten eine ganz hochgradige Muskelschwäche.

Die Angaben von Biedl wurden auch bezweifelt.

Der bekannte englische Physiologe Swale Vincent hat diese Versuche bei den Teleostiern, bei einer Aalart wiederholt und die Tiere überlebten. Er beschrieb auch, dass die Extrakte der Stannius' schen Körperchen keine Adrenalin-Wirkung inne haben.

('The effects of extirpation of the suprarenal bodies of the Eel', *Proceedings Royal Society*, 1898, 62.)

Die Widersprüche wurden von dem berühmten italienischen Anatomen in Bologna Ercole Giacomini (1864–?) in befriedigender Weise geklärt. Er zeigte nämlich, dass bei den Teleostiern ausser den Stannius' schen Körperchen noch ein vorderes kraniales Interrenalsystem in Form einzelner Körperchen am vorderen Rande der Kopfniere ein konstantes Vorkommnis darstellt, also die Entfernung der Stannius' schen Körperchen für die Frage der Lebenswichtigkeit derselben keine Beweiskraft besitzen kann. Darüber berichtete er am 24/V, 1908 in Bologna. ('Il sistema interrenale e il sistema cromaffine nella anguilla, adulte, nelle cieche e nel leptocefali', *Bolletin Acad. di Sci.*, Bologna, 1908.)

Nach der Veröffentlichung von Giacomini glaubte Biedl seine Ergebnisse einem internationalen Forum vorlegen zu können. Auf der VIII internationalen Tagung, der Zoologen in Graz, vom 15, bis zum 20, August 1910, hielt er zwei Vorträge. I. Die funktionelle Bedeutung des Interrenalorganes der Selachier. II. Über das Adrenalgewebe bei Wirbellosen. In seinem Buche hat er auch ausführlich über seine Versuche berichtet und glaubte, dass seine Versuche den Streit über die Lebenswichtigkeit der Rinde eindeutig zu Gunsten der Rinde entschieden haben. Vincent hielt noch einige Jahre seine Zweifeln aufrecht, als aber B. Kisch (1890–1966) die Versuche in Neapel wiederholte und die Angaben von Biedl vollinhaltlich bestätigte, war auch Vincent überzeugt und in der *Festschrift der Endokrinologie* (1929, **5**, 335) die im Jahre 1929 anlässlich des 60 -sten Geburtstages von Biedl veröffentlicht wurde hatte er seine frühere Ansicht einer Revision unterzogen, umsomehr als damals schon die ersten Veröffentlichungen erschienen, die darüber berichteten, dass es gelang Nebennierenrindenextrakte herzustellen, mit denen die epinephrektomierten Tiere am Leben zu erhalten waren. (J. M. Rogoff und G. N. Stewart: 'The influence of adrenal extracts in the survival period of adrenalectomised animals', *Science*, 1927, **66**, 327.) Obige Autoren bestätigten auch die Angaben von Biedl über die Lebenswichtigkeit der Rinde.

Um den wirksamen Extrakt herzustellen hatte auch Biedl zahlreiche erfolglose Versuche angestellt. Er hatte jedoch erlebt, dass mit den wirksamen Nebennierenrindenextrakten auf der Mayo Klinik Addisonkranke mit Erfolg behandelt wurden.

Ich glaube, es wäre angebracht heutzutage, wo das Prednisolan zu unseren wirksamsten therapeutischen Mitteln gehört, auch des Pioniers dieser Forschungsrichtung zu gedenken, da die Versuche von Biedl sicherlich die Herstellung desselben um einige Jahre beschleunigt hat.

H. Kindt
Freiburg i.Br. (*West Germany*)

Henry Maudsley (1835–1918) und sein Beitrag zur Kinderpsychiatrie

Wenn wir heute über Henry Maudsley und seinen um 1870 geleisteten Beitrag zur Kinderpsychiatrie sprechen, so hat das nicht nur eine historische sondern auch eine unmittelbare und aktuelle klinische Bedeutung.

Die Kinderpsychiatrie wird erst heute in angemessener Weise als eigenständige akademische Disziplin akzeptiert. Ihrer Herkunft und Ausgrenzung aus der Fachkompetenz der Psychiatrie und Pädiatrie wird in den üblichen historischen Darstellungen lediglich mit wenigen übergreifenden Worten gedacht (Kanner, 1947; Shirley, 1963; Tramer, 1942–64). Die Anfänge und Schwerpunkte kinderpsychiatrischer Ansätze werden dabei mit großer Selbstverständlichkeit in das XX. Jahrhundert verlegt, lediglich einige, meist entwicklungspsychologische Hinweise, werden in das XIX. Jahrhundert zurückgeführt (Höhn, 1959). Erst in jüngster Zeit konnte begonnen werden, auf der Basis gründlicher historischer Studien zum Umgang mit dem kranken Kind auch die Entwicklung der Probleme des geistig behinderten Kindes zu erforschen. Dabei zeigte sich, daß das geisteskranke Kind gerade die Psychiater des XIX. Jahrhunderts zu Überlegungen zwang, die an Aktualität der Grundproblematik nichts eingebüßt haben. Von außerordentlicher Wirkungskraft erweist sich dabei der gedankliche Ansatz von Henry Maudsley, der als Gerichtsmediziner und Physician am Londoner West-End-Hospital zwischen 1860 und 1880 wichtige Arbeiten zu diesem Thema vorlegte.

Die allgemeine psychiatrische Betrachtungsweise auch kindlicher psychischer Störungen um die Zeit Maudsleys läßt sich in wenigen Sätzen zusammenfassen: „Auf der Grundlage der vorwiegend naturwissenschaftlich-physiologischen aber auch psychologisch-philosophischen Ausrichtung der Psychiatrie formieren sich in der zweiten Hälfte des XIX. Jahrhunderts fundiertere Vorstellungen über die Geisteskrankheiten vornehmlich als Gehirnkrankheiten (Griesinger). Die Überlegungen, welche Teile der Seele, des Bewußtseins, der Vernunft, des Verstandes oder des Willens erkranken können, münden in breit angelegte Systematisierungsversuche einer wissenschaftlich begründeten Psychopathologie."

Kindliche pathologische Lebens- und Verhaltensäußerungen werden zunächst in einer absoluten Gleichsinnigkeit der Phänomene zum Erwachsenenalter gesehen, wozu sich erste Ansätze nicht nur im Bereich der Psychiatrie, sondern auch innerhalb der Pädiatrie finden lassen. Die am frühesten beachtete Form kindlicher Geistesstörung, der Idiotismus, stellt dabei ein wichtiges Kriterium für die vergleichende Beurteilung und Akzeptation auch anderer kinderpsychiatrischer Erkrankungen dar, die zunächst rein deskriptiv und ohne weitergehende differential-diagnostische Erwägungen über Ätiologie und Pathogenese in die pädiatrische und psychiatrische Fachliteratur Eingang finden.

Gezieltere und definiertere Überlegungen zur Genese auch kindlicher Geisteskrankheiten werden 1857 in der von Benedict Augustin Morel (1809–73) niedergelegten Degenerations-lehre formuliert – ein Konzept, auf das Maudsley unmittelbar aufzubauen scheint, wenn er schreibt: ,,. . . das Irrsein . . . ist nur eine Stufe, die nach abwärts zum sterilen Idiotismus führt . . .'' und etwas später: ,,. . . Diese durch Generationen sich fortsetzende Degeneration ist eine retrograde Bewegung, entgegengesetzt jener progressiven Spezialisierung und stets zunehmenden Vielseitigkeit der Beziehung zur Außenwelt, die . . . als charakteristisch für die fortschreitende Entwicklung bezeichnet wurde'' (H. Maudsley, *Physiologie und Pathologie der Seele übersetzt von R. Böhm*, 1870, pp. 225, 226). Er resümiert hierzu weiterhin: ,,Die Fähigkeit zur Entwicklung schließt die Fähigkeit zur Entartung in sich'' (loc. cit. p. 215).

Wir haben es jedoch bei Henry Maudsley nicht nur mit einem Anhänger und Verteidiger der hereditären Prädisposition der Geisteskrankheiten und deren degenerativen Verlauf zu tun. Auf dem Hintergrund einer umfassenden eigenen Kenntnis nicht nur medizinisch-naturwissenschaftlicher sondern auch kulturanthropologischer und philosophischer Theorien gelingt es ihm, wichtige und originelle weiterführende Denkansätze zu entwerfen.

In gleicher Weise wie für Maudsley im Irrsinn des Erwachsenenalters ,,kein Zufall herrscht'' (loc. cit. p. 205) hält er auch die kindlichen Geistesstörungen für abhängig von physiologischen Bedingungen des jeweiligen Lebensalters und von diesen sogar in ihrer Phänomenologie geprägt. Damit ist er in der Lage – und darin liegt das Besondere an Maudsleys Betrachtungsweise – neben entwicklungsbedingten, ätiologischen Faktoren dennoch eine Ganzheitsbetrachtung des Kindes zu versuchen. Danach besitzt jeder zeitspezifische Abschnitt des Kindesalters sein eigenes und eigenständiges Kranksein – dies ist ein Gedanke, der in der Zeit Maudsleys durchaus nicht selbstverständlich – da er eine deutliche Abhebung von der Erwachsenenpathologie impliziert.

Um das Gesagte zu vertiefen, müssen wir einige Gedanken aus Maudsleys Konzept der sich aus dem Rückenmark bis zum Gehirn ausbildenden und zur Vollkommenheit aufbauenden Seele aufgreifen. Das Rückenmark bedeutet für Maudsley dabei lediglich den Sitz der ,,Reflex-action'' – ein Begriff, für den unter anderem von Thomas Willis (1621–75), Marshall Hall (1790–1857), Johannes Müller (1801–58) und Eduard Pflüger (1829–1910) ein empirisch faßbares Korrelat gesucht wurde. Dabei steht eine neurologie-historische begriffsgeschichtliche Abgrenzung zwischen ,,Reflex-action'' und Reflextätigkeit bzw.-bewegung noch aus.

Auf der Grundlage dieses so verstandenen Rückenmarks sind die ersten Bewegungen des Kindes als reine Reflexe auf empfangene Eindrücke aufzufassen. Eine Störung der ,,Reflexaction'' kann sich folglich als ,,Irrsein der Reflexzentren'' in motorischer Unruhe manifestieren. Stufenweise entwickeln sich dann in den ersten Lebensjahren ein ,,Sensorium commune'' – unter welchem Terminus alle gemeinsamen Zentren für Sinnesempfindungen zusammengefaßt wurden, ein ,,Intellectorium commune'' als Zentrum der Verarbeitung von Eindrücken in Vorstellungen und Ideen und ein ,,Motorium commune'', als Gebiet der ,,Actuation'' (loc. cit. p. 174) in dem die Fähigkeit zu bestimmten koordinierten Bewegungen enthalten ist.

Von diesen Begriffen hat das „Sensorium commune" als Zentrum der Sinnesempfindungen eine lange Tradition und ist vielfältig in philosophischen, psychologischen und staatstheoretischen Bereichen verankert, währenddessen die anderen, dem „Sensorium commune" bewußt angeglichenen Begriffe von Maudsley nach seinen Angaben neu eingeführt werden und von ihm als Stationen der Seelenentwicklung verstanden werden.

Bei dieser Auseinandersetzung um das Übergreifen von motorischen in sensorische Phänomene fällt auf, daß Maudsley auch auf Erasmus Darwin (1731–1802) zurückgreift, dessen Beobachtungen aus der *Zoonomia* er für die Erklärung seines Sympathiebegriffes heranzieht. So führt Erasmus Darwin unter anderem aus: „. . . daß eine Art Delirium nichts Anderes ist als Convulsionen der Sinne und daß unsere Vorstellungen die Bewegungen dieser Organe sind . . ." (*Zoonomia*, I, 25–26), Überlegungen, die Maudsley in dem Konzept einer Entwicklungsphysiologie der Seele verarbeitet hat. Wie die motorischen-sensomotorischen und sensorischen Lebensäußerungen fließend in die intellektuellen Fähigkeiten wie Verstehen, Einbildung und Phantasie übergehen, stehen auch die physiologischen Nervenzentren in vor- wie auch in rückläufiger Beziehung zueinander und ermöglichen dem Individiuum ein evolutiv-fortschreitendes aber auch ein regressiv-krankhaftes Verhalten. Gesundheit einerseits als fortschreitende Entwicklung oder Irrsinn andererseits als rückschreitende, „retrograde Metamorphose", auch dies ist ein ätiologischer Denkansatz, der für die Mitte des XIX. Jahrhunderts sicher ungewöhnlich ist. Maudsley dürfte einer der ersten ernstzunehmenden Psychiater sein, der hierbei auch die Entwicklungsgedanken Charles Darwins übernommen und in sein eigenes Konzept eingebaut hat.

Das Kindesalter selbst mit der naturgemäß vorgegebenen „Vermischung krankhafter Zustände" ist für Maudsley nun untrüglicher Beweis seiner aufgestellten Theorien: Auch die Entwicklungsstadien des Irreseins und dessen Phänomene sind – wie oben bereits angeführt – gleichermaßen zum spezifischen Zeitpunkt der jeweils vorhandenen physiologischen Bedingungen wie aber ganz besonders unter dem Aspekt der Ganzheitsbetrachtung des Kindesalters zu sehen. Diese Gedanken werden allerdings von Maudsley nur theoretisch diskutiert und finden nur bedingt Eingang in seine kinderpsychiatrische nosographische Systematisierung. Gleichwohl muß gesagt werden, daß sie für heutige Vorstellungen eine noch immer richtungsweisende Relevanz besitzen. Er stellt sieben ätiologisch begründete Gruppen auf, unter denen sich nach seiner Ansicht kindliches Irresein manifestiert und die allein wegen ihrer präzise dargestellten Phänomenologie auch unser heutiges Interesse beanspruchen können. Es sind dies

1. Monomanie = partielles Irresein im Vorstellen.
2. Chorea-artiges Delirium.
3. Kataleptisches Irresein.
4. Epileptisches Irresein.
5. Manie.
6. Melancholie.
7. Affektives oder Moralisches Irresein.

Zur Erläuterung der eingangs betonten auch aktuellen klinischen Wichtigkeit sei das affektive Irresein kurz herausgegriffen. Aus diesem Krankheitsbild lassen sich zwei wesentliche Aspekte besonders deutlich herausarbeiten – nämlich Maudsleys Verhältnis zum Unbewußten und sein Konzept einer infantilen Triebsstruktur.

Wenn Maudsley Überlegungen wie diese trifft, daß das „Selbstbewußtsein in seinen Aussagen nicht zuverlässig ist", sondern „. . . von einem großen und wichtigen Teil der Seelentätigkeit gar keinen Bericht erstattet . . ." oder er anmerkt, „daß jeder, der sorgfältig auf seine Träume Acht gibt", findet, „daß viele von den scheinbar unbekannten Dingen, mit denen seine Seele im Traum beschäftigt ist und welche ihm als neue unbekannte Vorstellungen erscheinen, sich auf . . . unbewußte Assimilation des Tages zurückführen" lassen, so fällt es nicht schwer zu sehen, wie diese Gedanken Charcots und Freuds Konzept des Unbewußten zumindestens parallelisieren.

Der zweite Aspekt, der von Maudsley im Sinne einer kindlichen Triebstruktur herausgearbeitete Instinktbergriff zeigt diesen wirkungsgeschichtlichen Ansatz noch deutlicher: „Mit dem Instinkt der Appropriation, vermöge dessen assimiliert wird, was dem Ich zuträglich ist, ist als notwendige Kehrseite ein destruktiver, abstoßender Instinkt oder Trieb verbunden, der alles, was dem Ich nicht angenehm ist, zurückweist, ausstößt oder vernichtet. . . ."

Maudsley kann also von „Heuchelei" sprechen, wenn es um die ihm fragwürdige Möglichkeit einer Reinheit und Unschuld der kindlichen Seele geht, weil er die destruktiven Triebe oder Leidenschaften in gleicher Weise in die Seelenentwicklung eingebaut sieht wie die Entwicklung von Selbsterhaltungstrieb, Affekten und Emotionen, deren krankhafte Störung dann allerdings zur pathologischen Äußerung des Affektiven- oder Instinktiven Irreseins führt.

Diese wenigen Äußerungen, die den weitverzweigten Gedankengängen Maudsleys nur unvollkommen gerecht werden können, sollten lediglich auf die Notwendigkeit hinweisen, sich nicht nur für die historische Analyse, sondern vor allem im Hinblick auf die saubere Abgrenzung heutiger kinderpsychiatrischer Begriffe mit dem gesamten Hintergrund der Problematik zu befassen. Henry Maudsley nimmt hierbei einen bisher kaum beachteten, für die Genese heutiger Vorstellungen aber umso wichtigeren Platz ein.

E.-H. Lochmann
Hannover (West Germany)

Die Kontakte zwischen Ulrich Friedrich Hausmann und Wilhelm Herschel sowie dessen Familie

Ulrich Friedrich Hausmann leitete von 1820–47 als Direktor die Thierarzneischule in Hannover. Er war der Sohn eines Landwirtes und wurde am 10. September 1776 im Fürstentum Lippe geboren, das heute zum Regierungsbezirk Detmold im Bundesland Nordrhein-Westfalen der Bundesrepublik Deutschland gehört. 1794 trat er als Scholar in die damalige hannoversche Thierarzneischule, die heutige Tierärztliche Hochschule Hannover ein, die er drei Jahre später mit einem überdurchschnittlichen Zeugnis als Tierarzt verließ. Anschließend erweiterte und vertiefte er seine Kenntnisse an der Thierarzneischule in Berlin und studierte außerdem an der dortigen Universität Physik und Chemie. Auch in Berlin erhielt er beim Abgang 1798 gute Zeugnisse, die sicherlich mit den Ausschlag gaben, daß er im selben Jahr die Stelle des Hoftierarztes am Hofe Karl Augusts in Weimar erhielt. Weimar, heute Kreisstadt in Thüringen in der Deutschen Demokratischen Republik, war damals Hauptstadt des Herzogtums Sachsen-Weimar-Eisenach. Der Herzog hatte bekanntlich 1775 Johann Wolfgang v. Goethe zu sich berufen; dieser war übrigens auch an den Belangen der Tiermedizin interessiert und er rief 1816 in Jena ein tierärztliches Institut ins Leben, das heute noch besteht, allerdings nur bis 1843 Tierärzte ausbildete. Von Weimar aus bewarb sich Hausmann um die frei gewordene Stelle des zweiten Lehrers an der Thierarzneischule in Hannover, die er Ende 1802 antrat, nachdem er während eines halbjährigen Urlaubs in Göttingen Physiologie, Chemie, Physik, Botanik und Logik gehört hatte. 1820 folgte seine Ernennung zum Direktor der hannoverschen Anstalt als Nachfolger des 1819 verstorbenen August Conrad Havemann. Ende 1846 wurde er krankheitshalber von allen dienstlichen Verpflichtungen entbunden und er verstarb am 25. Januar 1847.

Obwohl Hausmann also über 44 Jahre die Stelle eines Lehrers und später des Direktors an der Thierarzneischule in Hannover inne hatte, wirkte er doch nur etwa 32 1/2 Jahre wirklich dort. 1803 nämlich, als sich die Franzosen Hannover näherten, mußte er die hannoverschen Marstallpferde nach England begleiten. Er tat in London mit dem Charakter eines Stalloffiziers als Marstallpferdearzt Dienst. Man scheint ihn und seine Arbeit geschätzt zu haben, denn bereits nach einem Jahr wurde sein Gehalt verdreieinhalbfacht. Erst nachdem Hannover wieder frei von französischer Besatzung war, kehrte er im Herbst 1814 nach dort zurück.

In Hausmanns Nachlaß befinden sich auch schriftliche Quellen zu einem betimmten, im Zusammenhang mit seinem Englandaufenthalt stehenden Erlebniskomplex, über den hier berichtet werden soll. Anlaß dazu gibt auch, daß sich im

August 1972 zwei in der Wissenschaftsgeschichte bedeutsame, Hausmann zumindest indirekt berührende Ereignisse zum 150. bzw. 200. Male gejährt haben.

Am 25. August 1822 verstarb in Slough unweit von London der königliche Hofastronom Friedrich Wilhelm Herschel. Genau 50 Jahre vorher, im August 1772 hatte er seine nachmalige Assistentin, seine Schwester Karoline Lucretia aus ihrer gemeinsamen Geburtsstadt Hannover nach England geholt. Beide sind bekanntlich während 50-jähriger gemeinsamer astronomischer Arbeit zu Weltruhm gelangt.

Wieso aber haben diese beiden Daten Bedeutung für Hausmann, außer daß der eine in Hannover wirkte und die anderen dort geboren worden waren?

Hausmann hat die Familie Herschel in England kennengelernt. Das ist an und für sich noch nicht von großem Belang, denn die Bekanntschaft des angesehenen Wissenschaftlers Herschel suchten zahlreiche Menschen. Hausmann war aber nicht nur bekannt, sondern befreundet mit den Herschels. Das geht aus recht persönlichen, leider nur zum Teil datierten Briefen im Hausmann-Nachlaß hervor, die Wilhelm Herschel, seine Schwester Karoline, sein Sohn John Frederick William und die Nichte seiner Frau Sophia Baldwin an Hausmann geschrieben haben.

Wilhelm Herschel spricht in drei Briefen einerseits von Linsen, Spiegeln, Zinn (offenbar für die Herstellung von Spiegeln), Werkzeug und irgendeinem Modell, was auf die Beteiligung Hausmanns an astronomischen Forschungen hinweist. Andererseits bittet er Hausmann um tierärztliche Hilfe für eines seiner Pferde. – Auch Karolines Briefe, so u.a. ihre Nachrichten über die gesundheitliche Wiederherstellung Wilhelms und ihre Frage nach dem Wohlergehen einer gemeinsamen Bekannten, lassen die freundschaftliche Verbundenheit erkennen. – John spricht zweimal, offenbar zu verschiedenen Zeiten, sehr herzliche Einladungen aus. – In einem Brief aus dem Jahre 1815 versichert Miss Baldwin, daß die Familie Herschel sich gern Hausmanns erinnert, seinen Weggang von England bedauert und sich über ein Wiedersehen ganz besonders freuen würde. Auch alles weitere in diesem dreiseitigen Brief ist das Geplauder mit einem guten Freund.

Weiterhin weisen astronomische Notizen, Berechnungen, Tabellen, Skizzen usw. in Hausmanns Nachlaß auf seine enge Verbundenheit mit den Herschels hin.

Neben dem Nachlaß geben auch die 1877 von Mary Cornwallis Herschel herausgegebenen Tagebücher und Briefe Karoline Herschels manchen Hinweis, indem Hausmann mehrmals in der Art erwähnt wird, wie man von einem lieben, alten Freund spricht. Allerdings finden sich in dem Buch Bemerkungen über ihn erst nach Karolines Rückkehr nach Hannover am 28. Oktober 1822.

Gleich in ihrem ersten Brief vom 30. Oktober 1822 aus Hannover an ihre Schwägerin schreibt sie „. . . Mr. Hausmann machte mir gestern seinen Besuch . . .“. Dann findet sich z.B. bei den Tagebucheintragungen aus dem Jahre 1838 die Bemerkung „31. Januar. Dr. Hausmann brachte mir einige Journale und sprach eine Stunde lang mit mir über alte Zeiten, was er immer tut, der gute Mann!“ Unter dem 24. Oktober 1838 lesen wir „Dr. Hausmann . . . nahm den Kasten mit dem Spiegel zu meinem Kometensucher mit . . . Ich bin froh, daß mein armer Sucher nun in guten Händen ist!“ In einem Brief vom 5. April 1840 an ihre Nichte, die Frau ihres Neffen John, teilt sie dieser offensichtlich erleichtert und einer Sorge enthoben mit „Mein Kometensucher . . . befindet sich jetzt im Besitz des guten, ehrlichen Dr. Hausmann . . .“

Um diese, ihren Kometensucher betreffenden Bemerkungen in ihrer Bedeutung richtig ermessen zu können, muß man wissen, daß sie dieses Instrument Newtonscher Bauart 1783 von ihrem Bruder Wilhelm für eigene Beobachtungen bekam. Sie entdeckte damit selbständig u.a. acht Kometen, davon fünf neu, und fand 14 Nebelflecke. Nicht zuletzt durch diese Entdeckungen begründete sie ihren hochgeachteten Platz in den Annalen der Astronomie. Man kann es leicht nachempfinden, daß ihr das Gerät sehr ans Herz gewachsen war, weshalb es in Hannover einen Ehrenplatz in ihrem Wohnzimmer fand. Sie war besorgt darum, daß es nach ihrem Tode in unrechte Hände käme und der Umstand, daß sie es Hausmann anvertraute, spricht für sich selbst. Sie konnte allerdings damals nicht ahnen, daß er noch vor ihr verstarb, fast genau ein Jahr. Der Sucher aber blieb in seiner Familie. Auch Karolines sehr geliebter Neffe John, ebenfalls Wissenschaftler, u.a. Astronom, hieß die Entscheidung seiner Tante über den Verbleib des Gerätes gut, schreibt er doch am 10. August 1840 an sie „Die Telescope sind jetzt, wie ich hoffe, in passender Weise untergebracht. Dr. Hausmann hat den Kometensucher, den er zu schätzen wissen wird, . . .“.

Erstaunlich ist es, daß diese Kontakte Herschel – Hausmann nicht oder nur vereinzelt bekannt sind, obwohl darüber schon publiziert worden ist. Einerseits existiert eine die Kontakte etwas ausführlicher behandelnde Veröffentlichung von Häpke aus dem Jahre 1910 und kurze Bermerkungen dazu stammen von Froehner (1953). Andererseits erwähnt Buttmann in seiner Herschel-Biographie (1961) Hausmann überhaupt nicht und er teilte auch persönlich mit, daß ihm bei seinem Quellenstudium der Name Hausmann nie begegnet sei. Auch eine Rückfrage bei Mrs. E. D. Shorland, einer Ururenkelin Wilhelm Herschels,[1] blieb erfolglos; sie konnte keine Erwähnung Hausmanns finden.

Diese Umstände ließen es nicht nur gerechtfertigt, sondern notwendig erscheinen, die freundschaftlichen Beziehungen zwischen dem Astronomen Wilhelm Herschel und seiner Familie einerseits sowie dem Tierarzt Ulrich Friedrich Hausmann andererseits vor dem Vergessenwerden zu bewahren, zumal dies gerade 1972 und in London möglich war.

ZUSAMMENFASSUNG

Der von 1802–47 als Lehrer und ab 1820 als Direktor an der damaligen Thierarzneischule in Hannover, der heutigen Tierärztlichen Hochschule Hannover wirkende Ulrich Friedrich Hausmann weilte von 1803–14 als Begleiter der wegen der französischen Besetzung Hannovers evakuierten hannoverschen Marstallpferde in London. Dort machte er die Bekanntschaft des Astronomen Wilhelm Herschel und seiner Familie, die sich zur Freundschaft entwickelte und auch nach seiner Rückkehr nach Hannover bestehen blieb. Er hat sich in England an astronomischen Untersuchungen beteiligt und Karoline Herschel anvertraute ihm in hohem Alter ihren Kometensucher, der ihr sehr viel bedeutete, damit das Instrument nach ihrem Tode nicht in unrechte Hände geriete.

Schrifttum

BUTTMANN, GÜNTHER (1961), *Wilhelm Herschel – Leben und Werk* (Große Naturforscher. 24), Wissenschaftliche Verlagsgesellschaft, Stuttgart; (1972), persönliche Mitteilung vom 30 März.

[1] Für die Überlassung der Anschrift gilt Herrn Günther Buttmann mein aufrichtiger Dank.

HÄPKE, L. (1909/10), 'Karoline Herschel und ihr Kometensucher', *Himmel und Erde*, **22**, 156–64.
HERSCHEL, MARY CORNWALLIS (Frau John Herschel) (Hrsg.) (1877), *Caroline Herschel's Memoiren und Briefwechsel (1750–1848)*, Aus dem Englischen von A. Scheibe, Verlag Hertz, Berlin.
FROEHNER, REINHARD (1953), in *Die Tierärztliche Hochschule in Hannover 1778–1953*, Verlag Schaper, Hannover, S. 84.
SHORLAND, E. D. (1972), persönliche Mitteilung vom 16 Mai.

G. Risse
Madison, Wis. (U.S.A.)

Scottish medicine on the Continent: John Brown's medical system in Germany 1796–1806

During the last quarter of the eighteenth century medicine was beginning to experience a deep crisis of confidence. Medical theory was gradually losing its credibility since the previous simplistic and mechanical models of physiopathology were forfeiting their appeal in the face of new biological observations and discoveries. The concept of a self-propelled human machine was being supplanted by that of an organism governed by a supreme director.

Thus, there was a considerable turnover of medical systems on the Continent, from Boerhaave's to Hoffmann's, and Stahl's to Gaub's. Their individual obsolescence created confusion but the earlier goal of arriving at a rational explanation of disease production and subsequent cure remained.

Beginning in the 1750s and largely as a result of Albrecht von Haller's experimental conclusions, a new pathogenesis emerged. Instead of stressing humoral changes in hydrodynamic terms, the newer medical systems focused their attention on the disturbances of those vital motions occurring primarily in the neuromuscular structures of the body.

Undoubtedly Haller's irritability and sensibility did not appear to respond to mechanical principles and also acted independently of the mind. A gap seemed to exist between the explanations of voluntary movements of the skeletal muscles and the physical properties inherent in the body's own constitutive elements. Such a hiatus was filled by postulating the existence of a series of harmonious and unconscious motions necessary for the survival of the organism.

The cause for these phenomena was largely unknown and increasingly ascribed to one chief vital force or power responsible for physiology, pathogenesis and healing.

Hence, the stage was set for the appearance of a novel medical system which could draw its fundamental principles from such a vital power and, in that framework, present a series of logical explanations of disease formation. Moreover, the system was expected to provide – in the early eighteenth-century rationalist tradition – clear guidelines for the practitioner based directly on the main theoretical postulates.

These expectations were fulfilled in 1780 with the publication, in Latin, of a work called *Elementa Medicinae*. Its author was a hitherto obscure disciple of William Cullen, named John Brown. Originally a theology student, Brown had already begun his medical studies in 1759 under Cullen's patronage, although his many-sided interests slowed his progress considerably.

In 1770, an unexpected event had occurred in Brown's life which, by his own admission, profoundly changed his medical views and ultimately his entire career.

According to his own testimony, Brown suffered a series of severe attacks of gouty arthritis in spite of the antiphlogistic regime prescribed by Cullen. Frustrated and impatient by his confinement as well as dissatisfied with the ineffective treatment, Brown abandoned the earlier food restrictions and returned to his meat and alcohol. Unfortunately for Brown's judgment the change in treatment apparently coincided with the onset of an intercritical period common in gout, and he remained symptom-free for several years in spite of gross dietary and alcoholic indiscretions.

Brown's apparent cure led to deep disagreements with his teacher, William Cullen, and the formulation of a new medical system which to some extent simplified the propositions advanced by Cullen himself. This system reflected Brown's inadequate clinical knowledge, his own experience with gout and a vehement desire to provide medicine with a more exacting theory and precision for the administration of drugs.

Brown accepted one fundamental principle in his system which he called 'excitability'. The name vaguely designated a bodily capacity of perceiving external or internal impressions and the ability to respond to these stimuli. For Brown, 'excitability' was the ultimate cause of life and, in his words, like Newton's gravity, incapable of further definition. In his scheme the impact of the various stimulating influences on the 'excitability' was supposed to generate the necessary vital actions to preserve and maintain the organism: life 'excitement'.

A corollary of Brown's framework was the idea that life could not be viewed as a spontaneous or independent phenomenon. Rather, vitality was the result of constant environmental and internal agents acting on the 'excitability'. Food, poisons, climate, contagion, emotions and thoughts all 'consumed' specific quantities of 'excitability' in order to generate well-defined amounts of 'excitement'. Since the differences among these factors were solely seen in quantitative terms, Brown declared that the entire physiology, pathogenesis and therapeutics could be subjected to mathematical analysis.

Health was defined by Brown as an optimum balance between adequate stimuli and the proper amount of vital activity needed to keep the body in good working order. The equilibrium was always precarious and could easily be tilted to produce so-called 'asthenic' diseases – if the stimulation decreased – or 'sthenic' illnesses – when excessive influences conveyed upon the organism. From his writings it is clear that Brown based his entire physiopathology on a simple imbalance between the body's 'excitability' and the stimulating agents. He therefore paid little attention to symptoms, disease classifications and pathological anatomy which for him were only secondary manifestations of disturbed 'excitability'.

For Brown the basic issue in medicine was the need for certainty and precision, both in medical theory as well as in practice. He strongly believed that the establishment of some fundamental principles of vitality – his 'excitability' and 'excitement' – would contribute to an understanding of the underlying causes of disease formation. Since Brown wanted infallibility and exactness in medicine, he attempted to subject his 'excitability' – for him the Newtonian medical principle – to mathematical computation. He thus adopted a purely hypothetical and arbitrary scale on which both 'excitability' and 'excitement' were each divided into eighty degrees.

In Brown's view, the physician virtually became a bedside mathematician who when called, took an inventory of the stimulants which had affected the patient prior to his illness with the help of a comprehensive medical history. Once in possession of this information, the Brownian practitioner could promptly diagnose the exact degree of 'excitability' and decide on a plan of cure aimed at restoring the healthy balance.

Hence, there was only one form of treatment in Brown's system: the administration of stimulants to adjust the disturbed 'excitability'. Brown was vehemently opposed to the so-called antiphlogistic method of cure with its copious bleedings, vomitings and purgings. By contrast, he used dietary manipulations and a few drugs, notably opium, for the restoration of his 'excitability'. The emphasis was on gradual and precise dosages as well as the use of therapeutic trials. Such a simple and exact medical practice appeared impressive on paper but was nearly impossible to carry out at the bedside in the face of insufficient clinical and pharmacological knowledge. Brown, however, remained confident in his therapeutical procedure, basing his conclusions largely on the handling of his own gout. Over the years he had developed a keen insight into his exact needs for opium, to which he had become addicted, in order to quell the gouty pains. Under such circumstances, Brown seems to have been proud of his own therapeutic precision.

Brown's system of medicine found few adherents in Britain because it was difficult, if not impossible, to implement clinically. His personal vituperation of William Cullen and blanket indictment of the entire Edinburgh medical establishment cast Brown in the role of an ignorant challenger, morally despicable because of his alcoholism and drug addiction.

In France, Brownianism encountered early opposition from the leaders of the Paris School, because of their negative attitude toward medical systems and stress on clinical medicine. Thus French medicine was spared from the acrimonious controversies which arose in German and Italian medical circles following the introduction of the Brownian system.

Brown's departure from Scotland and subsequent death in London, in 1788, did not extinguish the interest in that peculiar living quality frequently called irritability. Perhaps as a result of the controversies between the adherents of Cullen and Brown, the works of Haller and Fontana received wide attention in Edinburgh's medical circles.

Among those visiting the centre of Western medicine in 1789 was a Swiss physician, Christoph Girtanner (1760–1800), who acquired a manuscript of Brown's medical lectures. Shortly after his return to the Continent, Girtanner published a paper in France dealing with irritability as the highest principle in nature.

Regrettably, however, the Swiss author used most of Brown's ideas to fashion his own medical system without acknowledging his Scottish source. Girtanner proposed to transform the healing art into a mathematically correct science along Brownian lines, although he added some chemical speculations of his own, declaring that the newly discovered oxygen was the principle of irritability. Conversely, all interactions between stimuli and irritable fibres were thought to occur because of their chemical affinity.

Girtanner's work was immediately translated into English and German, and his piracy unmasked. An English medical student then travelling through Göttingen, who had studied at Edinburgh, clearly recognized Brown's system in its new chemical garb and accused Girtanner of plagiarism. The spirited controversy was vented in the most prominent German medical journals thereby attracting considerable attention to Girtanner's sources.

In Germany, the ensuing curiosity about the original Brownian theories was temporarily satisfied in 1794 with a reprint of Brown's original Latin text. This was followed in 1795 by a veritable flood of translations from Italian sources as well as German commentaries and abridgments.

In the meantime the battle continued to rage in Germany between those who claimed that Haller's properties were expressions of one single 'Lebenskraft' or vital force and the new adherents of Galvani's animal electricity. The latter group sought to interpret the body's vitality in terms of electrical phenomena.

Amidst such theoretical disputes, the very ambiguity and scope of Brown's 'excitability' seemed to satisfy, at least temporarily, both the vitalists and Galvanists. The recent promulgation of Fontana's laws of irritability gave Brownianism a truly modern look. At the same time, simple and seemingly logical formulations continued to please those physicians interested in a coherent synthesis of medical knowledge.

One such practitioner was the German Melchior A. Weikard (1743–1803), whose extremely fertile pen and pungent writing truly introduced Brown's medical system among the German physicians. Weikard carried out his vigorous promotion of Brownianism between 1795 and 1798 in the face of mounting hostility from leaders of the medical profession because of his insulting diatribes. Paradoxically, Weikard's shock treatment alienated many of his colleagues while others were prompted into a fierce rejection of the ideas he so zealously attempted to propound.

Nevertheless, Brownianism could hardly have made such a great impact in Germany without this climate of scandal and controversy created by Weikard's own defective personality. He provided a crucial impetus and challenge with his summaries of Brown's original ideas and the numerous German translations of Italian sources on Brown. The net result of Weikard's activity was an unexpected and rather remarkable resurrection of a defunct medical system almost twenty years after its inception in Edinburgh, where originally it had been conceived merely as a local alternative to William Cullen's ideas.

If the theoretically inclined physicians derived satisfaction from the Brownian system, the German clinicians who attempted to apply it at the bedside were sceptical. The majority of practitioners were unsure regarding the diagnostic criteria, the dosages of the drugs employed and the evaluation of therapeutical results. Under those circumstances two physicians with excellent medical credentials – Johann P. Frank (1745–1821), and his son, Joseph Frank (1771–1842) – came to the rescue of clinical Brownianism. They both established useful and limited applications of Brown's ideas and laid the groundwork for better diagnosis and treatment along Brownian lines. By 1797 and largely through the efforts of both Franks, Brownianism became a viable method of cure in opposition to the evacuation procedures favoured by the physicians still adhering to humoural theories or those too weak to break their old therapeutic habits.

At the theoretical level a new movement got under way in 1798 to establish a true 'science' of medicine. Largely stimulated by Kantian epistemology, the German approach centred on the search and discovery of the ultimate causes of life, health and disease. Thus Kantian philosophy began to significantly influence the character and course of German medicine, and Brown's principle of 'excitability' was chosen to become a pure Kantian *a priori* concept.

The result of such philosophical efforts was the establishment of a 'pure science' of medicine, the ultimate and apodictically certain system of medical knowledge. The attempt was led by Andreas Röschlaub (1768–1835), professor of medicine at the University of Bamberg, and resulted in the establishment of a modified Brownian theory called the 'Erregungstheorie'. The new system postulated that life was an expression of the general forces operating in nature, and Röschlaub proposed thirty different laws dealing with 'excitability' and its possible variations. Together these rules made up a complete and 'scientific' medical system of apodictic certainty, a national scheme in which vitality could be properly defined.

These lofty theoretical efforts engaged only a minority of 'philosophical' physicians who still believed that medical certitude could only be achieved through a solution of the hitherto hidden nature of life. Their heavy reliance on philosophy – especially Kant's critical thought – made their enterprise seem highly respectable.

The majority of more clinically oriented healers were, however, more concerned with the establishment of a medical practice which could be based on the principles of Brown and Röschlaub. The previous routine of excessive and often indiscriminate bleedings and purgings lost favour. More meticulous medical histories, improved dietary instructions and a judicious, gradual administration of certain drugs were adopted in many places.

If the practice of medicine gained significantly through the efforts of those physicians who attempted to make Brownianism a clinical success, it did so without slavish adherence to the philosophically deduced laws. A significant shift from the older evacuation procedures only occurred as many practitioners used those Brownian propositions which were found to be useful at the bedside. As Brown's theory subsequently fell victim to newer philosophical formulations, this change in the therapeutic approach became one of the more lasting contributions made by Brown and his adherents to the practice of medicine.

In Germany, the final chapter in the history of the Brownian medical system took place during the first decade of the nineteenth century. At that time, Brownianism became largely dependent on the biological formulations of the philosopher Friedrich W. J. von Schelling (1775–1854). Schelling's writings on 'Naturphilosophie', published between 1797 and 1799, became extremely popular in Germany, and satisfied numerous intellectuals anxious for an overall scientific synthesis which would systematically order and contain the baffling new discoveries of chemistry, electricity and biology.

Many physicians were therefore attracted to this philosophy of nature which purported to unveil the intimate structure of nature by allowing glimpses of the ultimate origins of life.

Schelling's comprehensive efforts to project into nature a series of laws discovered through philosophical reflexion was much bolder and greater in scope than the previous Kantian attempt to establish a 'science' of medicine. Since he largely used Röschlaub's modified Brownianism to express the new order, most philosophically oriented German physicians avidly adopted Schelling's ideas, convinced that 'Naturphilosophie' would greatly improve their chances for an understanding of the real essence of vitality.

Gradually, however, from 1801 to 1805, Schelling began to displace the Brownian 'excitability' from the central explanation of life until he eliminated the concept altogether. The shift brought to a conclusion the persistent efforts of Schelling's friend and follower, the physician Andreas Röschlaub, who had vainly attempted to harmonize his 'Erregungstheorie' with the changing concepts of the 'Naturphilosophie'. For all purposes Schelling's new attitude sounded the death knell for Brownianism as a medical system in Germany.

Röschlaub failed in his theoretical efforts because he had welded the rather simple Brownian scheme to a highly abstract idealist philosophy. The changeover from the Kantian garb to Schelling's philosophy of nature exceedingly complicated Brownianism, totally divorcing the speculative and philosophical theory from its clinical application on the patient. While the theory dissolved under the impact of newer medical systems based on Schelling's ideas, Brownian practice lingered on as one modality of therapy among others which had to justify its viability on clinical grounds rather than through some philosophical speculation.

Thus ended one of the most confusing periods of German medicine, marred by bitter personal controversies and characterized by an impressive flood of argumentative publications. Bothered by the impressive cleavage between medical theory and practice, dazzled by the discoveries of animal electricity and organic chemistry, the German physicians had set out to achieve medical certainty. They did so by adopting a foreign system which offered an apparent solution to their problems. Thus, an impressive array of well-known medical figures worked on the task of securing the Brownian theory with the help of Kant's and Schelling's philosophies, while others sought to establish a viable practice according to Brownian principles.

In a sense, Brown's Scottish medical system was unsuccessful in Germany. Heralded as *the* final dogma for a rational practice of medicine, it collapsed under the brunt of new biological discoveries and philosophical speculations thereby dashing the hopes of many German physicians for a static and monolithic system of medicine. Yet, the story of Brown's failure is another chapter in the gradual and often tortuous road towards medical enlightenment. The spirited controversies, endless polemics and resulting disappointments gradually sharpened the practitioner's powers of understanding and streamlined his methods of inquiry. The more critical and discerning attitudes that developed among subsequent physicians made the growth of modern medicine a reality.

Selected Bibliography

BROWN, JOHN, *Johann Browns Grundsätze der Arzeneylehre*, trans. M. A. Weikard, Frankfurt a.M., Andreae, 1795.

BROWN, WILLIAM CULLEN, *The Works of Dr. John Brown*, 3 vols., London, J. Johnson, 1804.

CULLEN, WILLIAM, *First Lines of the Practice of Physic*, new enl. ed. 4 vols., Edinburgh, C. Elliot, 1784.

FRANK, JOSEPH, *Erläuterungen der Brownischen Arzneilehre*, Heilbronn, Class, 1797.

FRANK, JOSEPH, *Heilart in der klinischen Lehranstalt zu Pavia*, foreword by Johann P. Frank, Vienna, Camesina, 1797.

GIRTANNER, CHRISTOPH, *Ausführliche Darstellung des Brownschen Systems der praktischen Heilkunde, nebst einer vollständigen Literatur und einer Kritik desselben*, 2 vols., Göttingen, J. G. Rosenbusch, 1797–98.

HUFELAND, CHRISTOPH W., *Bemerkungen ueber die Brownsche Praxis*, Tübingen, Cotta, 1799.

ROESCHLAUB, ANDREAS, *Von dem Einflusse der Brownschen Theorie auf die praktische Heilkunde*, Würzburg, Kölische Buchhandlung, 1798.

SCHELLING, FRIEDRICH W. J. VON., *Erster Entwurf eines Systems der Naturphilosophie*, Jena and Leipzig, Gabler, 1799.

WEIKARD, MELCHOIR A., *Entwurf einer einfachern Arzneykunst oder Erläuterung und Bestätigung der Brownischen Arzneylehre*, Frankfurt a.M., Andreae, 1795.

C. Martínez Durán
Guatemala City (*Guatemala*)

L'influence de la médecine britannique dans les thèses de Licence et de Doctorat des étudiants de médecine de l'Université de San Carlos de Guatemala au XVIIIe siècle et au commencement du XIXe

Dans cette brève étude, nous voudrions démontrer que, malgré l'isolement dans lequel se trouvait notre Université au XVIIIe siècle, la médecine moderne de cette époque a pénétré suffisamment dans la pensée des universitaires et que, bien que ces derniers n'aient pas abandonné totalement la médecine d'Hippocrate, de Galien, et d'Avicenne enseignée dans toutes les universités du monde, ils ont incorporé dans leurs études Descartes, Locke, Boerhaave, Santorio, Baglivus, Van Swieten, Heister, Helmontio, Solano (espagnol), Piquerius, Astruc, Corsinus, et les britanniques Macbryde, Cullen, Harvey et tout particulièrement, Thomas Sydenham, presque toujours présent dans les sujets de leurs thèses médicales: De Rebus naturalibus, de Rebus non naturalibus, de Rebus Praeter Naturam, de Febribus, de Locis Affectis, de Methodo Medendi, de Sanguine missione, de purgatione, de pulsibus, de Ex Chirurgica, de Medicam, de Ex Physica, de Ex Generatione, etc.

Dans ces considérations trop brèves, nous ne pouvons pas nous étendre dans les détails mais nous voulons seulement détacher les points concrets dans les sujets des thèses qui concernent la médecine britannique, en choisissant quelques exemples importants.

Dans les thèses de Manuel Vasquéz de Molina, en juin 1735, nous lisons dans «de Febribus» que malgré la théorie de Galien qui traite de l'échauffement inhabituel du corps humain provoqué par les quatre humeurs, Willisio ou Willis (célèbre médecin anglais) affirmait avec raison que la fièvre vient de la fermentation du sang et non de l'échauffement.

Le célèbre médecin vénézuelien et guatémaltèque Narciso Esparragosa y Gallardo, dans sa thèse (janvier 1789) «De Rebus Praeter Naturam» citait Sydenham (*Dissert. Ep.* p. 413) au sujet des femmes hystériques. La maladie dépend d'esprits animaux qui se manifestent sous forme de spasmes et d'excitations douloureuses.

Dans «De Methodo Medendi» (Sydenham, sec. 2, p. 68) le Dr. Esparragosa affirme que ce qui compte surtout dans les maladies c'est de mettre immédiatement en action les moyens de guérir sans se perdre dans d'autres considérations et d'agir sans délai en se conformant à la nature. Notre art complète la nature.

Il y a dans cette thèse un point important au sujet de la quinine originaire du Pérou qui «peut guérir de nombreuses fièvres sans danger même chez les malades très affaiblis». Il est très important aussi de remarquer dans la thèse de José Luís Franco (mars 1798) le postulat de Boerhaave dans «De non naturalibus»: il y a trois principes pour rester en bonne santé: maintenir la santé présente, prévoir les maladies contagieuses cachées dans l'atmosphère et faire tout son possible pour obtenir la longévité des hommes.

Mariano Antonio de Larrave cite dans presque toutes les propositions de sa thèse (juillet 1798) Cullen, Macbryde et Harvey.

Dans «De anatome et chirurgia» il affirme, selon Cullen que la thérapeutique de l'acide carbonique est la plus indiquée pour les tumeurs cancéreuses.

Reprenant la doctrine de Cullen, il insiste sur tous les problèmes de l'excitation et de la stimulation et dans sa proposition «De pulsibus» il en établit l'importance pour le diagnostic des maladies.

Dans «De Generatione», le Dr. Larrave s'en tient aux idées d'Harvey au sujet du développement de l'oeuf.

Dans la période de 1800 à 1820 toutes les thèses maintiennent dans leurs propositions les doctrines physiques de Cullen et les indications thérapeutiques et chirurgicales de Macbryde.

Pour conclure, je considère comme très important que nous nous souvenions du grand maître de la Médecine Moderne Thomas Sydenham qui a toujours signalé dans la pathologie la nécessité de l'observation clinique rigoureuse avant de se perdre dans des hypothèses incertaines ou dans des systèmes philosophiques. Sydenham, avec une clarté prévoyante, n'a-t-il pas assuré que les maladies aigües sont biologiques et que les maladies chroniques sont humaines étant de véritables biographies des hommes.

J. Honti
Budapest (Hungary)

Richard Bright, Edward Brown, and John Paget's travels in Hungary

Along the past centuries quite a number of notable British physicians and natural scientists have visited Hungary. They have given an account of their travelling experiences in books, describing the natural and economic geography of the country and telling about the life, folk-costumes and customs of the population. Among the physician-travellers perhaps the three most famous are: Richard Bright, Edward Brown and John Paget. They attained to the highest rank in medicine and did their best in getting remote Hungary acquainted and loved by the society of their age.

Richard Bright (1789–1858) was a medical student and he became a member of George Stuart Mackenzie's expedition to Iceland. Mackenzie published an account about the experiences of his expedition and Richard Bright wrote the botanical and zoological chapters. In 1827 he published his most significant work *Reports of Medical Cases*, . . ., which meant a milestone in the history of medical science concerning the pathology of kidneys. He established a renal department at Guy's Hospital, London, in 1842. To the memory of his work a group of renal diseases is called Bright's disease all over the world.

In 1814 Richard Bright was a young doctor when he started visiting some Dutch, Belgian and German universities and hospitals. While in Berlin he got news of the Vienna Congress approaching its end. He hurried to Vienna to be present at the closing celebrations. After his arrival it turned out that the Napoleonic War had not been finished yet, consequently he decided to continue his travel to Hungary. In March 1815 he arrived in Budapest starting from Vienna and travelling through Pozsony and the Hungarian Highland (north Hungary). Then he returned to Vienna and this time, equipped with letters of recommendation from Hungarian lords staying in Vienna, in April 1815 he made his close acquaintance of Hungary travelling around Transdanubia. His experiences were recorded in his voluminous 762-page diary which was published in Edinburgh and London in 1818 under the title *Travels in Lower Hungary*.

When he arrived in Budapest the spring fair was just beginning. He gives a lively picture of the everyday life in the streets, and of the social and economic situations. He delivers an account about the theatre life, and Hungarian language and literature. He highly appreciated the Hungarian arts, visited the National Museum, the University Library, the Observatory on the Gellért Hill and the University itself. About the latter he says: 'The University, . . . has been of considerable advantage to Pesth, both by increasing the concourse of people, and by diffusing more generally a literary taste and spirit amongst the inhabitants.' He describes in detail the Pest university of medicine, makes the following statement: 'The examinations . . . are strict, and include a clinical trial of the candidate's proficiency.' Then he writes: 'Professor Kitaibel accompanied me one day to the Clinical Hospital, which forms an appendage to the University. It is small, but excellently calculated both for the benefit of the patients, and for the instruction of the pupils. It consists of several small wards, each containing six beds only', and then he gives a detailed description of the clinic and the educational system prevailing there. He highly praises what he saw and tells: 'I was much pleased with the order and regularity with which this hospital is conducted; and am not sure, that more celebrated institutions might not gather hints from the proceedings of this distant and almost unknown medical school.'

In the botanical garden he was accompanied by Professor Paul Kitaibel, who is characterized by him like this: 'Professor Kitaibel, . . . is well known by his writings in the scientific world.'

He describes the Pest festival, the hot-baths of Buda, speaks about the police and fire brigade of Pest, all in much detail. He writes about the Hungarian handicraft and his account of the capital is finished by a short story of the town.

Along his journey in April 1815 he visited the estate of Duke Eszterházy, the Lake of Balaton, and he was the guest of Count Festetich in Keszthely, where he studied the organization and function of Georgicon, the internationally famous agricultural High School of the time. He climbed the surrounding hills, namely Badacsony, Szigliget, etc., which are world-wide well-known Hungarian wine-growing districts and he fulfilled some geological observations, compared the hills with those volcanic groups which he saw some years earlier in Iceland. He studied the geography of Lake Balaton in his book, and this description was long mentioned among the best. From Keszthely he travelled to Croatia and then through Pécs, Mohács and Szekszárd again he arrived in Budapest, but this time he stayed in the capital for only a short period. He was the guest of the Brunszvik family in Martonvásár, the same family which gave well-known hospitality to Beethoven only fifteen years earlier. Via Székesfehérvár, Veszprém, Sümeg and Graz he travelled to Vienna. Returning home he delivered a special account about his observations in Badacsony, Szigliget, etc., to the British Geological Association and this lecture was published in the Association's journal.

He gathered together substantial material about Hungarian literature which he was going to publish in a separate work. Later he was so deeply involved in the practice of medicine that he could not afford the time to publish his material on Hungarian literary life.

Edward Brown lived and visited Hungary much earlier than Richard Bright. Brown was born in Norwich in 1644. He attended the famous Trinity College in Cambridge, where he graduated as B.M. He continued his medical studies in Oxford and attained to M.D. Later he became a member of the Royal Society. In his youth he made some journeys in Europe, among them in the autumn of 1669 he started from Vienna, and through Hungary – along the Danube – he travelled south to the Balkans and turned back to Vienna through Bulgaria. During his journeys he made close observations of the natural phenomena and of the outstanding historical events, as well as about everything which was closely connected to his profession. He drew sketches, some of which are preserved in the British Museum. He studied the ancient Greek monuments and he tried in his imagination to copy Hippocrates. Later he became the family doctor of the King, a member of the College of Physicians and he lived at Salisbury Court in Fleet Street. He was elected to be the physician to St. Bartholomew's Hospital, London, and later he was first the bursar, then the president of the College of Physicians.

Edward Brown published a 144-page book in 1673 under the title: *A Brief Account of Some Travels in Hungaria, etc.* In this book he gave an account of his travels in Hungary. He describes the situation of the country which was under Turkish occupation at that time. He made observations about the country's copper-, silver-, mercury- and gold-mines, and about the baths of Buda. Further he writes that the thermal baths of Buda are esteemed as the most magnificent ones of Europe, not only on account of the abundance of fountains and their hot water, but on account of the ornamental buildings as well. He visited eight baths and he gave detailed descriptions of them. He paid a visit to the Turkish convent where he was welcomed by the Turkish General Gülbaba. He writes about the Hungarian bread and wine: 'where I travelled, I met with so good and well tasted Bread, that with Wine, it was to me a Feast; and with Water a sufficient Repast. Grapes they have very delicious and large; . . . Wines also of a generous and noble sort, the Wines of Tokay are highly esteemed.' His experiences in Hungary made a great impression on him, as he often refers to Hungary in his essays containing the description of his journeys in other countries. His references were used for comparisons.

His book is illustrated with pictures, e.g. Hungarian man, Hungarian landscape, etc. In connexion with the latter he puts down: 'in this country many families, and the inhabitants of diverse little towns, live all under ground.' Richard Bright, who had known Edward Brown's book and the above-mentioned picture, quotes this part of Brown's book and tells that such houses caved into the ground could be seen by him only in the surroundings of Martonvásár.

In recent years significant data have come to light by the publication of the Royal Society's Oldenburg correspondence, which yields new and important facts in connexion with Edward Brown's journeys in Hungary. Two outstanding representatives of the history of science, Rupert and Marie Boas Hall, published this correspondence in 1968 and the fifth volume discloses six letters, among others, between Oldenburg (secretary of the Royal Society) and Edward Brown who was travelling in Hungary at that time. Edward Brown was travelling in Eastern Europe and in Hungary on the commission of the Royal Society. We can conclude from the data of the correspondence that Edward Brown visited Hungary twice: first in spring 1669 to the Highlands (North Hungary), second in summer 1669, when he followed the Danube along the middle of the country.

The book written by Edward Brown about Hungary achieved publication in foreign languages as well, among them German, French, Dutch and English. Published many times, it was an outstanding travel book of the age.

Travellers from later periods knew Edward Brown's works well. Richard Bright in several parts of his diary refers to Edward Brown's book and it seems that Bright in choosing his travelling direction accepted Edward Brown's experiences gathered some 150 years ago.

The third traveller John Paget visited Hungary somewhat later than Richard Bright. He was born in Thorpe Satchville, Leicestershire in 1808. He finished his medical studies with outstanding results at Edinburgh University. He went to Paris to study the hospital work there and he was awarded the first prize for his essay on cholera. Later he was in Italy for a study-tour and here he made the acquaintance of the niece of Baron Nicholas Wesselényi (an esteemed Hungarian liberation fighter and humanist of the age). John Paget married a Hungarian girl and since that time he was closely connected to Hungary. He travelled to and fro in Hungary and Transylvania in 1835–36. He published his two-volume book about his travels under the title: *Hungary and Transylvania; with remarks on their condition, social, political and economical*, which attained to some English and German editions. Some chapter titles from his book include: Buda-Pest, Füred and the Balaton, Country Life and Peasantry, The Puszta, Winter Journey across the Puszta, The Carnival in Pest.

John Paget settled down in Transylvania, had a castle built in the English style, and was deeply engaged in agriculture, having big estates there. He participated in the Hungarian war of independence in 1848–49 and devotedly fought with sword and pen for the independence and development of his adopted country. He was the correspondent of the English press and the events of the war were announced by him. He was one of the aides of General Bem, the legendary hero of Polish origin. After the defeat in the war of independence he and his wife found refuge in England, where he prepared for the reception of Kossuth, the great Hungarian freedom-fighter. He tried to get support in England for the continuation of the Hungarian war of independence. Later he returned to his castle in Transylvania where he found everything destroyed. His knowledge of the Hungarian language was perfect, and he could write some Hungarian articles in professional magazines about agriculture, and viticulture. He established an English club in Kolozsvár and bestowed a two-thousand-volume library upon it. He died in Transylvania in 1892. It is worthwhile to know that his descendants participated in the progressive public life.

These English physician-travellers and their work and travels are well known in Hungary. In recent years their affairs were often the topic of different articles published in Hungarian magazines, and a book has been edited, which contains some translations with quotations from Bright's diary of travels. A relief was erected in Keszthely at the entrance of the Festetich Castle in memory of Bright. A relief can be found in Balatonfüred and Thorpe Setchville in memory of Paget. Hungarian cultural organizations offered a relief to Guy's Hospital, London, to be placed on the wall in memory of Bright. I am deeply honoured to present you with the experiences and works of the three famous English physicians who travelled in our country and did their best in establishing the highly appreciated and traditional English-Hungarian friendship.

T. J. S. Patterson
Oxford (Great Britain)

The transmission of Indian surgical techniques to Europe at the end of the eighteenth century

The operation to reconstruct a nose has always been regarded as the hallmark of that branch of surgery which has come to be known as plastic surgery. In Europe in the fifteenth and sixteenth centuries the nose was made by transferring a flap of skin from the upper arm, a technique which was brought to perfection by Gaspare Tagliacozza, Professor of Surgery in Bologna. After his death in 1599, the whole subject incurred the displeasure of the Church, and was not revived for two hundred years, although the principle of this 'Italian' method is sound, and still used today. Reconstruction of the nose by a flap of skin from the forehead, however, had been practised in India many centuries before Tagliacozza, although the information about this did not reach Europe until the end of the eighteenth century. The first account of this 'Indian' method appeared in a letter to the *Gentleman's Magazine* for October 1794, over the initials 'B.L.'. This gave a detailed description of an operation, which had been witnessed near Poonah by two of the medical gentlemen of the Bombay presidency. Cowasjee, a bullock-driver with the English army in the war of 1792, had had his nose and one of his hands cut off when he was taken prisoner by Tippoo, and in this state he became a pensioner of the East India Company. His nose was reconstructed from a flap of the skin of the forehead, by a man of the Brickmaker caste, who had been brought to Poonah at the instigation of Sir Charles Malet, the British Resident. The letter added that 'this operation is not uncommon in India, and has been practised from time immemorial'.

It is, perhaps, surprising that news of this had not reached Europe earlier. Eduard Zeis of Dresden, who collated all the references to the literature of plastic surgery up to 1863, made some caustic remarks about this failure to transmit such important information. In a section headed 'On the lack of information about the Art of making noses in India' he says: 'When you think that the English have already lived for a couple of hundred years in India, it is astonishing that, if rhinoplasty has really been practised there from time immemorial, the news did not reach Europe earlier than 1794. It is also remarkable that, in all this time, no English doctor living on the spot has investigated the history of this Art in India . . . again, there is no record whether, after the operation on Cowasjee, a similar operation has ever been carried out by an Indian surgeon.' Brett, in a textbook of surgery published in Calcutta in 1840, could have given part of the answer to this: 'A tribe of Koomhars or Potters who reside at Kot-Kangra in the hills north of the Suttledge, have long been famed for their dexterity in this operation, and numbers of mutilated individuals resort to them; but from the cases I have witnessed I had no reason to admire their performances.' He then gives a detailed account of his own technique, based on the same method. However, he was writing at a time when the technique of rhinoplasty was well established in Europe, and Zeis' rebuke would seem to have been justified when applied to the earlier surgeons in India. No record has yet been found of the involvement of Europeans in Hindoo surgery in the eighteenth century, apart from the Cowasjee episode, and fleeting references to a 'Mr. Lucas', who is thought to have been the first European in India to carry out such an operation.

Lucas' name is first mentioned in a leading article in the *Bombay Courier* of Saturday, 4 April 1795, in which the editor laments that most Europeans have applied themselves rather to the speculative than to the practical parts of the knowledge of India – ignoring, in particular, the Hindoo art of making noses. 'We have seen a Letter from Mr. Lucas, an ingenious Surgeon of Madras, describing very particularly the operation of putting on Noses, which in one case he himself performed with success. This differs but little from the Indian method practised by the Koomas, a cast of Hindoos. . . .' Lucas is also referred to by Carpue in 1816 in the first account in English of the technique of reconstructing the nose by a flap of skin from the forehead in the Indian method: 'I am obligingly informed by Major Heitland, of the Indian service, that in India, several years ago, in the time of Hyder Ali, Mr. Lucas, an English surgeon, was, in several instances, successful in the operation, which he copied from the Hindoo practitioners.'

If this information was correct, Lucas must have been operating before Hyder Ali (father of Tippoo) died on 7 December 1782. From a study of the official lists it seems probable that this 'Mr. Lucas' was Colley Lyon Lucas (1730–97), although his name is incorrectly given in the original List of the Medical Officers of the Indian Army for the Madras Presidency as *Colley*, L. Lucas. Carpue's 'Major Heitland' can be identified as William P. Heatland who served in the Infantry in the Madras Presidency from 1782 until he retired as a Major on 26 August 1807 (Patterson, 1971). Colley Lyon Lucas, born 1730, was appointed to the Army Medical Department in 1761, and went to Madras in 1762, where he was continuously employed until his death in 1797. He was a well-known Freemason, and a member of the Medical Board in Madras. He had a distinguished military career, becoming Surgeon-General to the Madras Army. In 1794 he joined the Honourable East India Company Service as 'full' Surgeon, with the equivalent rank of Colonel. Here, then, is a distinguished surgeon of Madras, whose career would fit with the little that we know of 'Mr. Lucas'. He would have been active in the time of Hyder Ali, and there would have been ample opportunity for Carpue's 'Major Heatland' to make his acquaintance, as they both served in the Madras Presidency.

Since the letter to the *Gentleman's Magazine* was signed 'B.L.', it has been suggested that this must have emanated from Lucas. However, this letter starts with the words: 'A friend has transmitted to me, from the East Indies, the following very curious, and, in Europe, I believe, unknown chirurgical operation, which has long been practised in India with success: namely, affixing a new nose on a man's face.' Thus, 'B.L.' could not have been the same person as 'Mr. Lucas' of Madras (Freshwater, 1972). The surgical details which are given in this letter are very similar to those in the *Bombay Courier* a year later; in some cases the wording is identical.

The latter, however, has a fuller account, and includes more technical medical terms. No document has yet been found to confirm this report that Lucas successfully carried out the operation of rhinoplasty himself, although there would certainly have been no lack of a suitable opportunity. Surgeons in India writing a little after this time comment on the frequency of nasal mutilation and on the consequent experience of reconstruction, which was far greater than that of their contemporaries in Europe.

The copper-plate print of the Cowasjee episode was engraved by James Wales, and was published in Bombay at the end of March 1794. The subscription-book for this has been found among the Malet papers in the India Office Library (Sir Charles Warre Malet was the Resident in Poonah at the time of the operation on Cowasjee, and he was also Wales' father-in-law). The list of subscribers does not contain Lucas' name. The name of the Company's ship is given – *Earl Fitzwilliam* – by which copies of the print could be sent to England. By this means it would have been in time to appear in the *Gentleman's Magazine* in October of the same year.

This news, and the demonstration of the practicability of the technique by Carpue in England and von Graefe in Germany, led to the widespread revival of interest in reconstructive operations which laid the foundations of the modern specialty of plastic surgery.

References

BRETT, F. H., *Surgical Diseases*, Calcutta, 1840, p. 453.
CARPUE, J. C., *An Account of Two Successful Operations for restoring a Lost Nose*, London, 1816, p. 40.
FRESHWATER, M. F., *Plastic and Reconstructive Surgery*, 1972, **49**, 78.
Gentleman's Magazine, 1794, p. 891.
PATTERSON, T. J. S., *Plastic and Reconstructive Surgery*, 1971, **48**, 68.
ZEIS, EDUARD, *Die Literatur und Geschichte der plastischen Chirurgie*, Leipzig, 1863–64, p. 213.

K. K. Roy
Calcutta (India)

Early relations between the British and Indian medical systems

India had its initial contact with the British medical system when the first fleet of the East India Company under the command of Captain (later Sir James) Lancaster set out for the East in December 1600 with four ships. Each ship carried 'Surgeons Two and a Barber'. These 'Surgeons Two and a Barber' were the pioneers who brought English or modern medical science to India. They constituted the origin of what subsequently developed into the Indian Medical Service under British rule.

The Indian Medical Service dates back to 1612 when it was started by the East India Company under John Woodall as the first Surgeon General. Under him medical officers (mainly civilian) were recruited. Subsequently when the Company found it necessary to maintain a regular body of troops in India, they commenced employing military surgeons from 1745 onwards. It was not until 1764 that these surgeons were organized into a regular establishment of the Company's Armies. Thus the Bengal Medical Service was formed in 1764, the Madras Medical Service in 1767 and the Bombay Medical Service in 1779 for the three Presidency Armies of Bengal, Madras and Bombay. The heads of the Presidency Medical Services were called the Head Surgeons and they controlled the civil and military needs. Alongside these Presidency Medical Services, the Company began to employ the services of Vaidyas and Hakeems for their native troops and local personnel. These Vaidyas and Hakeems were in no way subordinate to the Head Surgeons and mostly functioned independently.

During the eighteenth century, there were far too many obstacles for these Indian Medical Services personnel such as non-availability of British medicines and surgical appliances, which had to be imported in large quantities to replenish the stock in India as the Company's activities began to spread in the interior of the country. It cannot, however, be denied that the earnestness evinced by early British doctors to make life in India 'sweet and wholesome' for the British settlers was the motive that led to reasonably healthy towns springing into existence on 'sodden swamps, masses of Jungles, fetid ponds and jheels'. Calcutta soon became a leading centre in the Orient for advanced medical treatment and study, with Ayurvedic and Unani medical systems running side by side for the native populace.

The East India Company rightly felt at that time that protective medical measures were very necessary as, more than the mutinies, wars and sniping by terrorists, it was the climate and epidemics which took the largest toll of British lives in India. This was indeed true taking into consideration the fact that while the Battle of

Plassey in 1757 had cost Robert Clive's 1,096-strong army 'only seven killed and thirteen wounded', the great sickness of 1762, took a toll of 800 British lives in Bengal alone.

But for this, the British had none but themselves to blame, as Dr J. R. Martin, who is credited with preparing the earliest medical topography of India points out 'that the British of all European nations who have planted distant settlements, have invariably shown least regard to the proper selection of localities for the sites of their colonial cities'. Till this time the British doctors in India had shown no interest in any of the local medical systems, Ayurvedic or Unani.

Till the end of the eighteenth century, life in India was considered by the British as 'unhealthy'. Diseases rife, very frequent and mostly fatal in epidemic form were as dreadful as cholera, smallpox, typhus, malaria, bacillary dysentery, hepatitis, etc., but many of these had not been accorded nomenclatures as such. The rainy season when the epidemics raged was called 'the season of death'. Even more dreadful than the killer monsoon, perhaps were remedies prescribed by British doctors who were grappling with unforeseen symptoms of the then virtually unknown tropical diseases.

It is on record that at first 'the remedies reckoned effectual' for cholera known since 1698 as 'Indian Mordechi' (mort de chien) were either 'applying a red hot iron across the ankles and taking "Kanji" [a herb] water with pepper' or 'after giving brandy and laudanum [opium mixed in alcohol], placing the patient in a hot bath and bleeding him white through the arms [not a drop of water to be drunk by the patient]'. Though later 'emetics, opiate, hartshorn [for its abundant ammonia] and water' used to be prescribed. A phenomenon observed in an early British army camp in India led to the permission for drinking water being accorded to cholera patients. When a cholera epidemic was raging there, those patients who 'disobeying the ban against water and got it by stealth' were found to have 'rapidly recovered'.

The treatment of dysentery was even more fantastic. According to Dr. Goodeve, who made an extensive research into the early state of medical treatment in British India. 'As the strength must be supported in dysentery, patients were allowed pillaos, curries, grilled fowl, and peppered chicken broth, "ad libitum" with a glass or two of medicines or a little brandy and water and dessert of ripe fruit.'

These incidents show that when wholly British methods of treatment would produce no effect, Indian Doctors (Vaidyas and Hakeems) with their hot and cold remedies for hot and cold diseases and their 'Mantras' and 'philtres' were sometimes called in by these British doctors and settlers. The reason for such consultations with Indian doctors was largely due to the influence the Christian missionaries had on the British settlers, since they were the ones who had more contact with the natives and were beginning to place reliance on these Indian doctors. Most of the missionaries were in remote places away from the Presidency towns and therefore quite out of reach of British doctors. In their times of sickness, Indian doctors were often called in, with the result that the Christian missionaries had slowly begun to trust such Vaidyas and Hakeems. A few missionaries had gone even further. They had read some of the Ayurvedic and Unani texts and had begun to have faith in these systems of medicine.

But while these Indian doctors mostly treated their patients free of charge, medical practice in eighteenth-century India proved a veritable gold mine for British doctors. 'The Medical gentlemen then made their visits in palanquins and received one gold mohur from each patient for every common attendance; extras were enormous.' Medicines were expensive too, the first apothecary's shop in Calcutta opened in Fort William in 1780 charged 'Rs. 3 for an ounce of Bark. Rs. 2 for a Blister and Rs. 1 for a Bolus'. Obviously the British doctors could not have cared a whit for Rs. 50 per mensem which the East India Company used to pay them as salary.

This by and large reflects the early relations which Ayurveda had with the British or modern medical science. The Unani system was at the time still under the patronage of various Muslim nawabs of different principalities all over the country, but the Ayurvedic system had no such royal patronage. It flourished wherever the Hindus were living in a majority. Dr. Buchanan, as reported by Montgomery in his book *The History, Antiquities, Topography and Statistics of Eastern India* (1807) notes:

> Besides the professors of medicine, about 700 families of Brahmins, almost all of Sakadwipa, practise the art and are the only Hindu physicians who possess anything like science, except three of the medical tribes of Bengal who have settled at Patna (Bihar). The traditional system of training of Kavirajas (Vaidyas) which had lasted for many centuries in Bengal was exclusively on a residential tutorial system. The Vaidyas learnt the medical science mainly from books and also through oral instructions from their masters or gurus, who were adept in the science. The knowledge imparted was mostly voluntary and free of cost too. Similar practices still exist in Tols.

The propagation of the Unani system also continued along the same pattern as that of Kavirajas in Madrassa (schools) with the only difference that Unani knowledge was directly imparted to the students by Hakeems at whose places the students usually resided. As the Unani system was then accorded official patronage by both the Mughal Kings at Delhi and the Nawabs of Bengal, the East India Company in order to win over the Muslims opened the Calcutta Madrassa and started Unani medical system classes. No such help was given to the Hindus who followed the Ayurvedic system. It was not until 1811 that the East India Company made an effort to help the restoration of indigenous learning in medical science under its own management and control. The Court of Directors pointed out the richness of Sanskrit, in that it contained many an excellent treatise on ethics, medical plants and drugs, astronomy and mathematics. The Court also advocated that necessary steps should be taken 'to induce people to adopt modern improvement in science'. In pursuance of the Court's directions, instruction in Ayurvedi began to be imparted in the Sanskrit College in 1812.

Alongside this introduction of Ayurvedic teaching, the British medical system firmly transplanted itself with the opening of a chemist's shop in Calcutta by Mr. Bathgate, a young Scot who was a trained pharmacist and came to India with the Company. Bathgate soon became the most familiar source of supply of British and European medicines to the citizens of Calcutta. Ten years later, in 1821, the firm of Stainstreet was started by Surgeon J. Robinson and Dr. James Williams as a small apothecary's shop. A few years later Dr. John Smith and Dr. Thomas Dawson Stainstreet bought this concern and renamed it as Smith Stainstreet & Co. Both these firms still exist in Calcutta though under Indian management. There was, however, no commercial shop at the time to sell Ayurvedic or Unani medicines which were only available from the Kavirajas and Hakeems who used to make medicines themselves by purchasing herbs and plants from wandering ascetics.

In 1824 the General Committee of the Sanskrit College decided to impart knowledge of medical science, both British and Indian, to the students. This was the first time that British medicine was being taught in India regularly. Dr. Tytler began his lecture on medicine according to British methods and trained Indian Kavirajas were appointed to teach Charaka, Sushruta, Bhavaprakasa, etc. to Ayurvedic students. The classes were well attended. The famous Indian scholar of the time, Pt. Madhusudan Gupta, was a student of this class and learned medical science according to both the systems. Later on he became a Professor of the Native Medical Institution at Calcutta and was entrusted with the teaching of British medicine as well. He was probably the first Indian Professor of Medicine whose students handled bones and dissected animals. It is on record that gunfire from the ramparts of Fort William greeted the achievement of British medical teachers headed by Dr. Tytler when they successfully prevailed upon Pt. Gupta to overcome his inhibitions against the dissection of a corpse. Alongside Dr. Tytler, Dr. James Grant, the Apothecary General began his lectures on Anatomy and Physiology, Diagnosis and Surgery in 1831 (see *Minutes of Evidence of the House of Commons on the Affairs of the East India Company*, 1832).

Credit is mainly due to Lord William Bentinck, the then Governor General of India, for initiating higher medical education in India. He improved upon Warren Hastings's efforts and was deeply interested like him in Ayurveda and wanted it to develop alongside the British system. In 1833, he appointed a Committee for improving the Native Medical Institute of Calcutta and the education imparted there. The members of this Committee were Surgeon John Grant, Apothecary General and lecturer at the Native Medical Institute, J. C. C. Sutherland, Secretary to the Education Committee and a noted Sanskrit Scholar, C. E. Trevelyan, Deputy Secretary, Political Department, Assistant Surgeon Spens of the Bodyguard, Assistant Surgeon M. J. Bramley, Assistant Marine Surgeon and Babu Ram Komal Sen. The deliberations of the Committee known as the Grant Committee have had a most profound effect on the future course of British and Indian medical systems. After more than a year of meetings and deliberations, the Grant Committee submitted a lengthy report and made several recommendations for the improvement of the Native Medical Institution, Calcutta. It is interesting to note from this report that on one point the members of the Committee were divided, namely, whether the medium of instruction should be an Indian vernacular or English. Rev. Dr. Duff, a leading missionary of the time, and his party had succeeded in influencing the Grant Committee members for adopting English as the medium of instruction against Dr. Tytler's group who maintained until the very last that both the systems of medicine could be taught through the medium of any Indian vernacular. Dr. Tytler tried to win over the Committee members by trying to impress upon them the fact that ever since 1824, he and his staff at the Medical School were teaching the students in Sanskrit and Bengali medium. Dr. Grant himself was of the opinion that it will be extremely difficult to translate new medical terms and phrases into the Indian vernacular languages and efforts made in translating British medical books into Indian languages would be quite useless owing to a very wide and diverse variety of Indian languages being read and spoken all over the country. He also rejected the arguments put forward by Babu Ram Komal Sen in favour of adopting Sanskrit as a medium of instruction on the grounds that the Muslims and growing number of

Indian Christians will object to it. According to the famous minutes of 2 February 1835, Lord Macaulay won a definite victory for the anglicists over the orientalists. The result was that the Native Medical Institution at Calcutta was abolished and a new Medical College of Bengal was sanctioned days after the Grant Committee report was accepted. The old order had changed, yielding place to new. Dr. M. J. Bramley, an Assistant Marine Surgeon and a member of the Grant Committee, was made the Superintendent of the new College with Dr. H. H. Goodeve as his assistant. Pt. Madhusudan Gupta was transferred to the New College and had two assistants assigned to him. The Unani and the Ayurvedic systems of Indian medicine were thus shelved permanently in favour of the British system. No students were allowed to continue Ayurvedic classes at the Bengal Medical College under orders of Dr. Bramley and surprisingly no leading Indian citizens of the day like Dwarkanath Tagore and Raja Rammohun Roy raised their voices at this step.

It must be pointed out at this stage that no member of the Grant Committee, much less Lord Macaulay or even the Governor General, Lord William Bentinck were against teaching the Ayurvedic system alongside the British system. There decidedly was a difference of opinion as to the medium of instruction, but no mention was ever made that only the British medical system be taught in English, and the Ayurvedic and Unani systems be brushed aside. Dr. Bramley's decision was therefore not the official endorsement of the Grant Committee. In all fairness to the Grant Committee it must be stated that they really wanted Ayurvedic and Unani systems to be taught in English alongside the British or the modern system. But this is not what happened.

We must now take up the question as to why did not Pt. Madhusudan Gupta, the Indian professor both at the Native Medical Institute and the new Bengal Medical College, take pains to seek clarification in the Grant Committee report about the brushing aside of the Indian medical system. There is also no record of his ever taking up the matter with Dr. Bramley the Superintendent. It, however, transpires from several Bengali publications of the time that Pt. Madhusudan Gupta was himself undecided at that time. He realized that without a radical reform of the Ayurvedic medical system, there was no point in simply switching over the medium of instruction from Sanskrit to English. The Ayurvedic system had virtually made no progress from the time the Muslims began to rule India and as such the science was nearly two thousand years old. On the other hand if British medical science was taught to his countrymen, it would consequently promote a more liberal and an enlightened system of medical instruction, embracing Anatomy, Physiology, Diagnosis, Surgery, and other useful branches of medical science which may be accomplished with the sum proposed to be spent by the Governor General, by employing a few doctors of talent and learning like Bramley and Goodeve, who were educated in England. He wanted the new Medical College furnished with the necessary books, instruments and other apparatus and desired with all his heart that Indians by the study of modern medicine might throw off superstition bred of ignorance and take to the path of enlightenment as was being done in the countries of Europe where modern medical science was working wonders. The consciousness of a broader medical education had dawned at last.

Pt. Madhusudan Gupta was thus not merely any occidentalized oriental, no Hindu polished into the doubtful semblance of an Englishman, as some of the educated

Indians of his times were trying to be. If we follow the right line of his thinking, we find that he tried to lead the way from the orientalism of the past, not to, but through British medical science, towards developing the science of medicine which is neither British nor Indian, but something vastly larger and nobler than both. He preserved continuity throughout, by virtue of his having studied both the British and the Indian systems of medicine which in reality applied the motive force of his progressive thought. He thus brought a period of renaissance to the Indian medical system and has in a way been responsible for the introduction of modern medicine in India.

When Lord William Bentinck found that the leading Indians of the day have reconciled themselves to adoption of the British medical system in favour of the Indian, he made his next move and directed Sir Frederick Adams the then Madras Governor, to start a medical school there on the same lines as the earlier one at Calcutta. A medical school was thus established there in 1835 with Surgeon William Mortimer and Assistant Surgeon George Harding. Here also Indians knowing the Ayurvedic system were recruited to teach students British medical science after undergoing thorough training.

Likewise the Bombay Governor, Sir Robert Grant, first organized the Medical and Physical Society of Bombay in 1837 where British doctors and surgeons used to lecture members on various aspects of modern British medicine and when sufficient members got interested in the modern medical system, the Grant Medical College was established with Dr. Charles Moorhead as the Principal and John Peet and H. Giraud as Professors in 1845.

We thus see that by 1845 the British system of medicine had come to stay in India and many educated Indians of affluent means had come to realize by that time that the East India Company genuinely desired an all-round improvement of the British native population and the introduction of a modern medical system as an essential part of it.

A year earlier than the opening of the Grant Medical College at Bombay, four Indian students of the Bengal Medical College, Calcutta, Gopal Chandra Seal, Dwarkanath Basu, Surjee Kumar Chakravarty and Bholanath Basu had sailed for England by the ss. *Bentinck* on 8 March 1844 for higher medical studies under the dual patronage of Dr. H. H. Goodeve and Dwarkanath Tagore, grandfather of Rabindranath Tagore, the well-known poet.

By this time and quite unfortunately, as in any other systems of our activity, the development of Indian medical science came to a standstill. It got arrested. People who were practising it were content with merely repeating what had been handed down to them, but were not making any progress due to lack of support by the then Government with the result that Ayurveda fell on evil days. It must, however, be admitted that the British rulers of India at the time, including the doctors and settlers, were sincerely interested in training suitable Indian personnel in British medicine. In addition they hired trained Indian doctors in medical research work which they did in India such as: (1) Lewis's work on trypanosomes; (2) Vandyke Carter's work on spirillum of relapsing fever, leprosy and mycetoma infections; (3) Ronald Ross's great discovery of the transmission of malaria by the anopheles mosquitoes in 1898; (4) James Esdaile's work on mesmerism. He demonstrated the possibilities of performing major surgical operations painlessly under anaesthesia caused by mesmerism; (5) Haffkine's work on plague in Bombay and his success in manufacturing plague vaccine as a prophylactic.

Soon Indian doctors of modern medicine also came of age such as Dr. Amulyacharan Bose of the Bengal Chemical and Pharmaceutical Works, Dr. K. N. Brahmachari, Sir Nilratan Sircar, Sir Nusserwanji Choksey, Dr. R. Rao, Dr. Surveyor and others.

In the evolution of early Indo-British relations in the history of medicine, we can thus trace a number of stages: an early state in which the two systems functioned independently without influencing each other: a stage in which the importance of a study of Ayurvedic and Unani systems had been sufficiently impressed on the British doctors by Christian missionaries, a stage in which British doctors and surgeons realized that Ayurveda and Unani medical systems were founded on proper scientific fundamentals and were not just 'native magic' a stage in which anatomy and physiology of the human being drew attention by Kavirajas and Hakeems and finally a stage in which British medical system came to stay in India.

References

Bengal Herald, May 1829.
Bengal Hurkaru, February–December 1835.
Bengali Spectator, February–December 1835.
BHATIA, S. L., *History of Medicine with Special Reference to India.*
BHATIA, S. L., *The Medical Heritage of India.*
Calcutta Journal, February–December 1835.
CRAWFORD, D. G., *History of the Indian Medical Service*, London, Thacker, 1914.
MCDONALD, DONALD, *Surgeons Two and a Barber. History of the Indian Medical Service 1600–1947*, London, Heinemann, 1950.
DUTTA, UDAY CHAND, NIDAN, 1882.
India Gazette, February–May 1835.
KASHIKAR, C. G., *Indian Medicine.*
Minutes of Evidence of the House of Commons on the Affairs of the East India Company, 1832.
MOORHEAD, CHARLES, *Report of the Grant Medical College*, Bombay, 1845–46.
MONTGOMERY, *The History, Antiquities, Topography and Statistics of Eastern India*, 1807.
MUKHOPADHYAYA, GIRINDRANATH, *History of Indian Medicine*, Calcutta, 1923.
ROY, P. C., *History of Chemistry in Ancient and Medieval India.*
Samachar Chandrika, February–May 1835.
Samachar Darpan, Serampore, February–May 1835.
Sambad Kaumaudi, February–May 1835.
SANYAL and DUTTA, *Ban-glar Samajik Ithias.*

M. Nadjmabadi
Tehran (Iran)

Les relations médicales entre la Grande Bretagne et l'Iran et les médecins anglais serviteurs de la médecine contemporaine de l'Iran

Il y a près de deux siècles que les relations médicales entre la Grande Bretagne et l'Iran sont établies, quoiqu'on compte quelques médecins anglais qui étaient en Iran à des dates plus reculées.

Après l'an 1818 (= 1234 de l'Hégire) quand le premier étudiant persan, diplomé de la Faculté de Médecine d'Oxford était de retour à Iran, ces relations médicales entre les deux pays ont pris un nouvel aspect.

Il faut noter qu'un nombre de médecins anglais étaient venus en Iran sous le titre de médecins de l'Ambassade Britannique ou comme médecins de la Cour Impériale, ainsi que médecins du bureau de Telegraphe Indo-Europe. Parmi ces médecins figure le Dr. Briggs qui était assistant chirurgien et après chirurgien de l'ambassade de la Grande Bretagne à Téhéran (1799 = 1214 de l'Hég.) et le Dr. Andrew Jukes qui exerçait la chirurgie à Bombay et arriva à Téhéran en l'an 1808 = 1223 de l'Hég.). Il est mort à Isfahan en l'an 1821 (= 1237 de l'Hég.). Après lui un autre chirurgien, le Dr. Campbell vint à Téhéran; il exerçait aussi la chirurgie. Il est mort en mars 1818 (= 1234 de l'Hég.). Après le Dr. Campbell, Dr. John McNiel était nommé comme médecin de la compagnie d'Inde Orientale. Né en 1795 (= 1213 de l'Hég.), diplomé de la Faculté de Médecine d'Edinbourg, il devint médecin de l'ambassade de la Grande Bretagne en Iran. Pendant son séjour en Iran il a pu transmettre la connaissance de la médecine européenne au roi de Perse (Fath-Ali-Chah), qu'il visitait chaque jour à la Cour Impériale.

Un autre médecin anglais, Dr. John Cormick, était le médecin privé du Prince Héritier (Abbas Mirza fils du Fath Ali-Chah). Dr. McNiel devint le médecin de Mohammad Chah (fils d'Abbas Mirza). Dr. McNiel vécut longtemps en Iran et jouait un rôle bien important dans les courants diplomatiques.

Après les guerres entre l'Iran et la Russie Tsarique de 1803–13 (= 1218–28 de l'Hég.), Abbas Mirza envoyait un nombre d'étudiants en Angleterre. Parmi ces étudiants un jeune iranien nommé Mirza Baba Afchar, était le premier médecin qui a introduit la médecine européenne en Iran. Il a étudié la médecine à Londres et après à Oxford. Le Dr. Afchar retourna en Iran en 1818 (= 1234 de l'Hég.) et devint médecin du Prince Héritier Abbas Mirza. Dr. Afchar a fait un deuxième voyage en Grande Bretagne comme surveillant d'un groupe d'étudiants persans. Il devint médecin privé et chef des médecins du successeur d'Abbas Mirza, Mohammad Chah, jusqu'à 1838 (= 1254 de l'Hég.). Donc le Dr. Afchar, diplomé de la Faculté de Médecine d'Oxford, était le premier Médecin persan de l'école médicale anglaise.

Il faut noter que le Dr. John Cormick, fils du Dr. Richard Cormick, était le médecin particulier d'Abbas Mirza, et a écrit un livre sur la vaccination antivariolique traduit en persan par un médecin nommé Mohammad fils d'Abdos-Sabour en dix chapitres et une préface. Le livre était imprimé en 1829 (= 1245 de l'Hég.) à Tabriz, centre de la grande province nordouest de l'Iran (Azarbaidjan). Ce fut le premier livre médical imprimé en Iran. Dr. John Cormick est mort en Iran en 1833 (= 1249 de l'Hég.).

En l'an 1824 (= 1240 de l'Hég.) un autre chirurgien anglais, accompagné du Colonel MacDonald, vint en Iran. Il exerçait la chirurgie d'abord à Shiraz, chef-lieu de Fars, la grande province du Sud de l'Iran, et après à Téhéran comme chirurgien de l'Ambassade de la Grande Bretagne. Après lui un autre chirurgien, le Dr. Riach, était nommé comme chirurgien (1826 = 1242 de l'Hég.) à Buchihr, port situé à l'ouest du Golfe Persique, ensuite à Tabriz (Tauris); ce dernier avait en même temps une carrière diplomatique.

Après la mort du Colonel MacDonald (1830 = 1246 de l'Hég.) à Tabriz, le capitaine Campbell lui succéda et le Dr. McNiel fut son médecin et assistant. Le Dr. McNiel avait établi une collaboration médicale bien sincère avec le Dr. Afchar, ainsi qu'avec d'autres médecins persans. Il a pris de sévères mesures médicales et hygiéniques pendant les épidémies en Iran.

Outre les médecins mentionés ci-dessus, on doit signaler dans l'histoire médicale de la Perse d'autres médecins comme le Dr. Griffith, le Dr. Clarck (les deux médecins consultants de Mohammad Shah), ainsi que le Dr. Bell, un autre chirurgien à Tabriz. Un autre chirurgien de l'Ambassade de la Grande Bretagne nommé Dr. Dixon exerçait la chirurgie pendant à peu près quarante ans en Iran et a rendu beaucoup de services aux Iraniens.

A noter qu'après deux voyages du Dr. Afchar en Angleterre et quelques autres visites d'étudiants qui ont pris le chemin de ce pays, l'introduction de la médecine européenne, était établie en Iran.

Après l'inauguration de l'Université de Téhéran (= Darol-Founoune) grâce aux efforts du grande ministre Iranien Mirza Taghi Khan Amir Kabir en 1851 (= 1268 de l'Hég.) et l'arrivée des professeurs en Iran pour enseigner dans cette Université la Séction médicale (= la classe médicale) s'est établie à Darol-Founoune. Les professeurs de l'Université de Téhéran venaient de l'Empire Autriche-Hongrie et enseignait la chirurgie, l'anatomie et la pharmacologie. Parmi eux le Dr. Edouard Jacob Polak enseignait l'anatomie et la chirurgie et le Dr. Focatti la pharmacologie. Leurs leçons étaient purement conformées aux méthodes européennes. Peu à peu les étudiants iraniens se sont habitués à apprendre la médecine d'après la méthode occidentale.

Disons quelques mots à propos des hôpitaux, dispensaires fondés par les médecins anglais: le premier hôpital fondé par la mission religieuse anglaise en Iran était à Isfahan (centre de l'Iran). Cet hôpital était établi par le Dr. Robert Bruce au sud de la ville d'Isfahan dans une petite ville (ou quartier) nommée Djulfa qui avait des habitants arméniens. Le Dr. Bruce a rendu beaucoup de services aux habitants d'Isfahan, ainsi qu'à la province d'Isfahan. En l'an 1885 (= 1303 de l'Hég.) un autre médecin anglais nommé Dr. E. F. Hoernle de la mission religieuse a construit un nouvel hôpital. Dr. Scully était le médecin de la légation de la Grande Bretagne en Iran en 1896. C' était pendant ce temps que le roi de la Perse Nassredin Chah fut tué dans une petite ville située près de Téhéran. Sir M. Durand, le ministre plénipotentiaire de la Reine de la Grande Bretagne, l'a envoyé pour examiner le cadavre du Chah. Il a informé le ministre britannique que la balle était introduite entre le 5e et 6e côte gauche de la poitrine et qu'elle avait pénétré le coeur. Cet évnement a eu lieu pendant que le Marquis de Salisbury était le ministre des affaires étrangères britannique.

Parmi les médecins et chirurgiens qui ont travaillé dans l'hôpital, d'Isfahan, les Dr. Donald et W. Carr jouissaient d'une réputation considérable à Isfahan et dans tout l'Iran. Ils ont laissé de bons souvenirs dans notre pays. Les vieux médecins iraniens les connaissent par leurs travaux médicaux et humanitaires. Le Dr. Donald a fondé quelques dispensaires dans la province d'Isfahan, ainsi qu'un département pour la gynécologie et obstétrique sous la direction du Dr. Emanelina Stuart. Outre le Dr. Carr quelques autres médecins et chirurgiens ont rendu de grands services médicaux à Isfahan; le plus renommé parmi eux était le Dr. Schafter. A l'état actuel, le Dr. Eric B. Wild est le directeur responsable de l'hôpital, et je le remercie ainsi que mon confrère Dr. M. Filsouf pour les renseignements qu'ils m'ont donnés concernant cet hôpital. Malheureusement en 13 Juin 1972 un chirurgien de cet hôpital, le Dr. Ian Thomas, est mort par un accident d'auto. Outre les médecins et chirurgiens mentionnés, douze autres ont travaillé à l'hôpital d'Isfahan en collaboration avec ceux de l'Iran. Ainsi à Téhéran, la capitale du pays, des confrères anglais avaient établi une bonne collaboration avec leurs confrères persans. A noter que les médecins et chirurgiens anglais ont fondé des hôpitaux et dispensaires dans quelques villes de l'Iran comme à Isfahan, Kerman (ville du sud-est du pays), Kermanchah (ville de l'ouest du pays), Recht (ville du nord du pays), Hamadan (ville de l'ouest du pays), Meched (ville de l'est du pays), Yezd (ville de centre du pays).

Parmi les médecins anglais celui qui a proposé pour la première fois d'établir une quarantaine aux bouches du Golfe Persique était le Dr. Colville.

J'ouvre une paranthèse pour dire qu'il existait dans notre pays, un «conseil sanitaire gouvernemental» que «L'administration de la Santé Publique» et après «le ministère de la santé publique» remplacèrent plus tard. Ce conseil se composait de membres persans et non persans, parmi eux un médecin anglais, et un de ses devoirs était l'empêchement de l'entrée des maladies épidémiques. Il y a à peu près soixante ans que ce conseil n'existe plus en Iran et que le ministère de la Santé Publique lui a succédé, donc ce sont les médecins persans qui s'occupent des sujets hygiéniques, quarantaines, etc. Les anciens médecins anglais étaient employés comme médecins des quarantaines des bouches du Golfe Persique, à cause des intérêts commerciaux et diplomatiques de la Grande Bretagne et du voisinage du pays avec l'Inde.

Le statut de conseil sanitaire était codifié en 1904 (= 1322 de l'Hég.) et le gouvernement persan a pris des mesures actives pour que les quarantaines des ports du golfe persique soient surveillées par les médecins persans et peu à peu les confrères anglais n'avaient pas occasion d'intervenir sur ce sujet.

J'ajoute qu'avant la première guerre mondiale (1914–18) la majorité des médecins persans diplômés des Facultés d'Europe étaient sortis des facultés de médecine françaises, et aussi que l'enseignement médical en Iran était conforme à la méthode française et avec les livres médicaux français. Donc la deuxième langue pour les médecins persans était le français. Après la première guerre mondiale, entre les deux guerres, et après la deuxième guerre, des étudiants et médecins ont pris le chemin de la Grande Bretagne, l'Amérique du Nord et l'Allemagne. La conséquence était que la langue anglaise succéda à celle française.

Permettez moi de dire quelques mots à propos de deux médecins anglais qui ont travaillé longtemps en Iran et ont laissé de bons souvenirs dans notre pays.

(1) Dr. Antony Richard Neligan, M.D., London, D.T.M., H. Il est né à Tralee et mort le 8 decembre 1948 à Birmingham). Fils du Dr. J. W. Neligan, il étudia à Barts. Décoré de la medaille d'or de Matthews Duncan et plusieurs autres, il devint Bachelier ès Sciences (M.B.) en 1903 et trois ans après docteur en médecine de l'Université de Londres.

Il était médecin de l'ambassade de la Grande Bretagne en Iran de 1906–26. Ensuite il fut nommé membre du conseil sanitaire (de l'Hygiène) de l'Iran, où il a rendu de bons services; Pendant son séjour en Iran, il a travaillé aussi pour diffuser la vaccination antivariolique dans le pays. Il était en même temps chef du service médical à l'hôpital gouvernemental à Téhéran, où il collaborait avec le Dr. Scott, le chirurgien anglais, chef de la section chirurgicale de l'hôpital, ainsi qu'avec d'autres médecins persans.

Dr. Neligan avait des relations amicales et professionnelles avec les médecins persans, l'Institut Pasteur, etc.

Il avait un grand enthousiasme pour le sport et était pendant des années sous-directeur de «l'association du progrès du Football» en Iran, dont j'étais à ce temps secrétaire. Donc, je le connais de près et je peux dire qu'il était un sportsman correct et aimable.

Il avait sa clinique privée à l'ambassade de la Grande Bretagne, où quelques étudiants travaillaient avec lui.

Dr. Neligan retourna en 1926 en Angleterre et fut successivement directeur de la clinique pour les soins du rhumatisme de la Croix Rouge (à Londres), chef des Bains Royaux à Brighton, membre de l'Association Internationale de l'Hydrologie, membre du comité international pour la lutte contre le rhumatisme, membre de l'Association Médicale Royale de la Grande Bretagne. Il a écrit un article à propos de l'état hygiénique et sanitaire et la vaccination antivariologique en Iran dans le *Lancet* (1926); il a aussi préparé une brochure comme guide pour les voyageurs qui venaient en Iran.

Son fils, le jeune Dr. Neligan, est un pédiatre. Je l'ai vu en 1951 à Newcastle.

(2) Dr. Cyril L. Elgood, M.A., M.D., F.R.C.P. Le Dr. Elgood était un des médecins anglais qui avaient une réputation considérable parmi les milieux médicaux et scientifiques de Téhéran. Il était pendant dix ans médecin de l'Ambassade Britannique en Iran, ayant sous ses soins en même temps des malades persans et a fait des voyages dans tout l'Iran. Aussi bien que médecin pratiquant, le Dr. Elgood était un écrivain et historien qui avait de bonnes relations scientifiques, avec les médecins iraniens et avec toutes les institutions médicales du pays, surtout avec l'Institut Pasteur de l'Iran.

Il a laissé deux œuvres médicales pendant de son séjour en Iran: (*a*) *Medical History of Persia and the Eastern Caliphate*, Cambridge, 1951. (*b*) *Safavid surgery*, Pergamon Press, 1966. Dans la préparation de toutes les deux œuvres historiques et médicales, il avait été aidé par des confrères persans.

Il se rendit en Angleterre après sa retraite. J'étais en correspondence avec lui et je lui avais envoyé mon livre «Histoire de la Médecine en Iran avant l'Islam»; il m'envoya des îles des Seychelles, dans l'Océan Indien à l'ouest de Bombay, son œuvre sur *La chirurgie au temps des Safavides.* Il vint en Iran en 1964 et m'écrit une lettre pour me voir, mais malheureusement j'étais en Europe. A son retour aux Seychelles, il avait toujours la bonne volonté de m'écrire des lettres. Cette correspondence a duré jusqu'à mars 1970. Au mois d'Avril 1970, j'ai reçu une lettre de son épouse m'informant que mon éminent confrère est mort le 29 Mars 1970 aux Seychelles. Je crois franchement que les deux œuvres du Dr. Elgood sont des documents historiques d'importance pour l'histoire de la Médecine en Iran.

Après le Dr. Elgood un autre chirurgien anglais, le Dr. Davies, était le médecin de l'Ambassade Britannique; il a fondé un hôpital privé pour les anglais à Téhéran.

C'était grosso modo quelques mots a propos des relations médicales entre la Grande Bretagne et l'Iran, ainsi que les services des médecins anglais en Iran.

V. Busacchi
Bologna (Italy)

L'università di Bologna e l'Inghilterra

I rapporti culturali tra lo Studio di Bologna e l'Inghilterra sono sempre stati intensi, ma non così cospicui come con la Spagna o la Germania. Ho avuto occasione di interessarmi varie volte di questi rapporti che ci conducono a ricordare nomi come quelli di George Scharpes[1] di Marcello Malpighi,[2] di Polidoro Virgilio,[3] ed anche di Harvey,[4] per rammentarne solo alcuni dei principali.

Un letterato italiano, Arturo Farinelli[5] ha esaminato accuratamente i rapporti fra i due paesi nel secolo della rinascita fino a Shakespeare (1564–1616) il massimo poeta inglese morto quando Harvey iniziava le *Lectures on the whole of anatomy* (1616–26).

Lewis Einstein in un suo volume del 1902 *The italian Renaissance in England* ha messo in evidenza quanto questi rapporti siano stati profondi nel tempo e particolarmente nel periodo da lui preso in considerazione. E così noi possiamo ritrovare con soddisfazione e anche con tenerezza fra le memorie dei nostri popoli atteggiamenti dell'animo, gusti, curiosità, interessi culturali che ci riportano addietro di secoli.

I primi rapporti sicuri fra l'Università di Bologna e l'Inghilterra risalgono al Secolo XII e riguardano il diritto. Infatti nel 1140 Teobaldo, Arcivescovo di Canterbury, chiamò in Inghilterra Vacario che nell'antica Cronaca di Normandia è considerato lombardo. Questo dottore bolognese, scolaro di Irnerio, fondò in Oxford una scuola di diritto che gli procurò una grande fama. Passò poi al servizio di Ruggero, Arcivescovo di York. Nel 1198 era ancora vivente.

Lo studio del diritto romano indusse molti inglesi, anche dotti a venire in Italia a perfezionarsi a Bologna. Fra questi merita di essere particolarmente ricordato Tommaso Becket o Tommaso di Canterbury (1118–70) poi martire, innalzato agli onori degli altari e già sulla fine del secolo XII festeggiato da numerosi inglesi suoi connazionali accorsi a Bologna e onorato colla erezione di un altare nella Chiesa di S. Salvatore.

Sembra poi che un inglese, Pietro Blesense, poco dopo il 1150, dopo avere appreso le leggi, le professasse a Bologna.

Tutti coloro che finora ho ricordato hanno però insegnato leggi. Per quei lontani tempi infatti si affermava che Bologna era una città europea che eccelleva nelle leggi, Parigi nelle scienze, Orleans nelle lettere e Montpellier nella medicina. Galfrido di Vinosalvo (lat. *Galfridus de Vino Salvo*) inglese, che visitò Roma e fu in relazione con Innocenzo III lasciò scritto:

In morbis sanat medica virtute Salernum aegros; in causis Bononia legibus ornat nudos; Parisius dispensat in artibus illos panes, unde cibat robusto: Aurelianis educat in cunis auctorum lacte tenellos.[6]

Nessuna nazione, nel secolo XII, ebbe un concorso di studiosi di legge a Bologna maggiore di quella inglese. Ma non mancarono nemmeno i nomi di coloro che insegnarono medicina.

Fra questi debbo anzitutto ricordare Nicolaus de Fernham o de Fuly che fece parte di quel gruppo di persone che nel 1229 *Oxonium Parisiis concessit* per i contrasti sorti in quella Università come Bulaeus espone nella sua storia della Università di Parigi.[7]

Il Sarti e Fattorini,[8] si trovano incerti sul modo di classificare l'insegnamento impartito da questo inglese che insegnò inizialmente filosofia a Parigi e poi medicina a Bologna dedicandosi completamente alla teologia acquistandosi grande fama.

Ma noi qui lo considereremo particolarmente come medico in quanto insegnò questa disciplina a Bologna, e secondo quanto dice il suo coetaneo ed amico Matteo da Parigi non molto dopo il 1230.[9]

Fu poi creato Vescovo e per lui avvenne il fatto singolare che il Re e la Regina d'Inghilterra non solo lo assunsero come Consigliere familiare ma anche come guida spirituale e medico dei loro corpi.

Nel secolo XIII troviamo altri dati di notevole interesse: per esempio nel 1265 viene ricordato Enrico d'Inghilterra (*Enricus de Anglia*) come Rettore degli scolari ultramontani.[10]

Sempre nel 1265 da un atto che proviene dal Convento di S. Francesco in Bologna abbiamo notizia della Nazione degli Inglesi che era evidentemente incorporata nella Nazione germanica: in seguito a contrasti fra gli scolari sulla elezione del Rettore di questa Università che comprendeva anche gli inglesi viene redatto un atto notarile che vede anche come testimoni Alessandro de Orfort e Henrico de Ludela inglesi.[11]

E, sul finire di questo secolo, il 31 maggio 1293 come risulta da un testamento dell'Archivio di S. Francesco in Bologna Dominus Franciscus dottore di leggi, figlio del dottore di leggi Accursio lascia fra i suoi lasciti testamentarii, due donazioni per ospedali di Londra;

Item hospitali posito in Anglia in Londonijs, quasi in introitu civitatis quando venitur de Francia et itur in Anglia, quinque libras bononenorum.

Item Hospitali sive Domus, que vocatur Sanctus Thomas de Acri, posito in Anglia in civitate Londonijs in contrata que dicitur Guazapa Quinquaginta libras bononenorum.[12]

Attraverso i documenti relativi allo Studio di Bologna si possono trarre altri elementi per fissare i secolari rapporti con l'Inghilterra.

Durante il rinascimento si deve ricordare Polidoro Virgilio. Nacque verso l'anno 1474. Nei suoi scritti si professa sempre urbinate anche dopo aver assunto la cittadinanza inglese. Si fece ecclesiastico e dopo avere studiato a Padova e completato la sua cultura a Bologna restò per breve tempo in questa città dedicandosi alle belle lettere. Divenne in seguito segretario del Duca di Urbino Guidobaldo I. In questo ufficio dimostrò notevole abilità tanto che il Papa Alessandro VI lo creò collettore apostolico e lo inviò in Inghilterra ai primi del secolo per raccogliere l'obolo di S. Pietro. Tale tassa, detta in Inghilterra 'Romescot' era stata istituita attorno all'VIII secolo e fu soppressa nel 1532. Serviva in gran parte al mantenimento di un Ospizio per pellegrini inglesi in Roma.

A questo suo incarico certamente non fu estranea l'indicazione del Cardinale

Adriano Castellesi, valente latinista, suo parente, che in lui aveva intuito un ottimo umanista ed una persona atta a propagare il gusto della latinità fra i dotti inglesi.

La missione di Polidoro Virgilio ebbe buon esito. Enrico VII (+21 aprile 1509) lo volle alla sua corte e lo tenne in grande considerazione. La medesima considerazione ebbe per lui Enrico VIII. Nel 1507 ebbe l'Arcidiaconato di Wells. Nell'ottobre 1510 assunse la cittadinanza inglese. Ebbe durante il suo soggiorno vicissitudini varie e notevoli amarezze. Fu anche rinchiuso per oltre sei mesi nella torre di Londra da cui fu liberato per l'intervento di Leone X (II)e dell'Università di Oxford.

Nel 1538 lasciò l'Inghilterra e per qualche tempo ritornò in Italia. Sul finire del 1551, essendo la sua salute malferma chiese ed ottenne il permesso di tornare in Italia ad Urbino e qui venne a morte nel 1555.

Questa la vita e questa l'opera di Polidoro Virgilio che abbiamo voluto considerare da un punto di vista particolare. Non è senza significato che questo umanista italiano proprio in questi ultimi tempi venga di nuovo studiato e per così dire riscoperto. John F. Fulton, l'insigne fisiologo e storico della medicina nord americano, poco più di una decina di anni or sono definiva Polidoro Virgilio il primo storico della medicina dopo l'avvento della tipografia, e non bisogna dimenticare che nel *De inventoribus rerum* ci ha dato anche una storia della stampa, e il primo autorevole storico dell'Inghilterra.[13,14]

Poco dopo la sua partenza e precisamente con un viaggio durato dal febbraio al dicembre 1552 un altro grande italiano, un medico, Girolamo Gardano (1501–76), si recava in Inghilterra e raggiungeva la Scozia per visitare John Hamilton, Arcivescovo di S. Andrea a Edimburgo, fratello di James Hamilton, Reggente durante la minore età di Maria Stuarda.[15] Riuscì a guarirlo da una forte forma asmatica.

L'elenco dei laureati[16] ci fornisce elementi che dimostrano come gli studenti di medicina nel 1400 e nel 1500 si siano venuti diradando in quanto troviamo soltanto tre inglesi che si laureano in medicina e cioè:

D. Nicolaus Calvoodley Anglicus in utraque censura (cioè in medicina e filosofia) il 16 febbraio 1602; *D. Benedictus* (*de*) *Mondforte Anglicus in medicina* (24 gennaio 1617); *D. Johannus Cademanus Anglus in medicina* (24 luglio 1636).

Sono numerosi, come risulta dai Rotuli dei lettori, gli insegnamenti nella Università di Bologna. Dovrò fare un arido elenco di nomi, ma in questo caso anche i nomi hanno la loro importanza.

Così per l'anno 1486–87 troviamo il *D. M. Gulielmus Balce de Scotia artistarum et medicorum dignissimus Rector ad lecturam Medicine diebus festis*; nel 1584–85 *D. M. Gualterus Ricardi de Laciis de Anglia, dominorum scolarium artistarum et medicorum dignissimus Rector* ha la *lecturam medicine diebus festis.*

Nel 1601 il nobile inglese Nicolaus Calvoodley insegnò logica.

Sono anche numerosi nel 1600 gli scozzesi.

Lo scozzese Dempster (*Thomas Deppster baro*(*a*) *Muresk*) nato a Cliftbog nel Aberdeenshire nel 1579 e morto a Bologna nel 1625 insegnò nella Università degli artisti dal 1619–20 al 1624–25 umane lettere. Questa cattedra era considerata come prestigio *eminente.* Il Dempster seppe congiungere nel suo sapere veramente enciclopedico, come ebbe a scrivere il Calcaterra, poesia e naturalismo, filosofia e diritto, mitologia e geografia, filosofia e storia, ricerche glottologiche e osservazioni anatomiche, antiquaria e modernità; creando una nuova unità di sapere.

Fra i suoi scritti ha ancora valore storico il *De Etruria regali* con cui tentò di chiarire le origini degli etruschi ed il loro linguaggio. L'opera fu pubblicata postuma a Firenze nel 1723–24. Può essere considerato per questa opera il vero iniziatore degli studi di etruscologia per la accurata raccolta di materiali storici e archeologici.

Scrisse anche un *Antiquitatum Romanorum corpus absolutissimum* (Parigi, 1613) che ebbe varie edizioni.

Mente eclettica, lasciò una storia naturale, come supplemento a quella dell'Aldrovandi di cui aveva avuto l'incarico di sovrintendere alla stampa delle opere e persino una *anatomia partium corporis humani.*

Nel 1634 l'irlandese Giorgio Scharpes (latinamente *Sciarpius*) fu chiamato da Montpellier a Bologna e insegnò teorica della medicina dal 1634–35 al 1636–37. Insegnò con tanto onore che i reggitori dello Studio dopo la sua morte (1638) per i suoi meriti straordinarii e per aiutare la sua famiglia chiamarono suo figlio Claudio, allora giovanissimo dottore a insegnare logica, considerata allora una delle prime materie di insegnamento. Era il primo gradino per ulteriori avanzamenti. E poichè anche questi morì dopo breve tempo, per i suoi meriti e a ricordo di quelli del padre fu concesso alla famiglia lontana un quarto dello onorario.[17]

La cattedra di Teoria della medicina straordinaria restò senza titolare fino all'anno accademico 1642–53.

In precedenza *Scottus Constantius* (ciè Costanzo scozzese) aveva insegnato dal 1626–27 al 1641–42 e poi, dal 1646–47 al 1651–52 prima logica, poi teorica della medicina straordinaria e in seguito contemporaneamente pratica della medicina ordinaria e anatomia.

Nel 1562–63 venne costruito in Bologna il nuovo edificio delle scuole, l'Archiginnasio, che racchiudeva nel vasto e centrale edificio le aule dei legisti e degli artisti. L'edificio si venne arricchendo nel tempo di stemmi ed iscrizioni. Vi si trovano alcuni nomi di inglesi e anche di italiani che furono consiglieri della Nazione inglese.[18]

Penso valga la pena di ricordare alcuni di questi nomi:
Anglorum D. Jo. Baptista Scaynus Salodiensis.
Angliae D. Jacobus Franciscus Viscardus Novars. (Da Cravegna frazione di Crodo (Novara). Lo stemma appartiene a Consigliere artista del 1601).
Jo. Baptista Thadeus.
Anglensium D. . . . ac Cavalerius Bergomensis.

Nel 1600, nella solenne processione che che si svolse per accogliere il genovese Domenico Spinola, eletto Rettore generale dello studio si trova, come rappresentante della nazione inglese nello studio *D. Jo. Settonus Scotiensis.*
Nell'aula II dei legisti si trova: *Anglorum D. Cuno baro de. . . .*

Ma chi maggiormente ha contribuito a sottolineare i rapporti scientifici fra l'Italia e in particolare Bologna e l'Inghilterra è stato Marcello Malpighi (1628–94) nato a Crevalcore presso Bologna, maestro a Bologna di Anton Maria Valsalva (1666–1723) e attraverso l'allievo di Giambattista Morgagni (1682–1771).[19]

Il 2 ottobre 1667 Enrico Oldenburg, segretario della Royal Society of Medicine gli inviò una lettera chiedendogli notizie scientifiche e ragguagli dei suoi studii. La corrispondenza coll'Oldemburg divenne poi notevole e frequente e costituisce un elemento interessante per conoscere la vita del Malpighi.

I rapporti del Malpighi con la grande Società inglese furono di notevole importanza per la ulteriore attività del Maestro e gli italiani hanno certamente un debito di riconoscenza verso la grande Istituzione sempre viva e rinnovantesi nel tempo. Nel 1669 Egli spedisce alla Società la sua opera sul baco da seta con disegni autografi. Il 26 marzo 1669 il Segretario Oldenburg gli comunica la sua cooptazione a socio. E' interessante leggere la corrispondenza in latino, allora ancora lingua universale dei dotti, con la Royal Society.

Il Malpighi seguitò a mandare i suoi scritti alla Società: il *De formatione pulli in ovo*, prima opera embriologica con intendimenti scientifico sperimentali e sopratutto l'*Anatome plantarum* che giunse contemporaneamente a quella di Nehemias Grew nel 1671.

La Royal Society conserva un ritratto del Malpighi che le fu donato dallo stesso nel 1680 su richiesta del Consiglio direttivo. Questo risulta da una lettera a Hooke con la quale il Malpighi accompagna una cassettina contenente, come risulta dall'elenco in calce, *effigies mea* e alcuni libri. E nell'aprile del 1682 il Malpighi ringrazia per la sede onorifica in cui la Società si è degnata di porre il suo ritratto. Il quadro fu collocato inizialmente vicino al ritratto di Newton, in seguito a quello di Harvey.[20]

A dimostrare la universalità della scienza l'Università di Bologna conserva anche nella biblioteca dell'istituto matematico un busto marmoreo di Isaac Newton, fondatore della moderna fisica matematica e della astronomia fisica (1642–1727).

Nel museo dell'Aldrovandi si trova un busto in gesso di Richard Owen (1804–92), zoologo, anatomico, e paleontologo, oppositore delle teorie evoluzionistiche e del Darwin in particolare.

E posso concludere questi cenni sommarii sui rapporti fra la più antica Università ed un grande Paese ricordando che questa e le sue Facoltà, dopo l'unità d'Italia, hanno inviato discorsi e lettere in latino a università, società scientifiche e studiosi di tutto il mondo.[21] Ricordo quelli inviati in Gran Bretagna:

Università di Exeter (1956).

Università di Glasgow per il 450° anniversario della fondazione (1901) e 500° anniversario della fondazione (1950).

Università di Kingston a Hull per la sua fondazione (1955).

Reale Società di Scienze naturali di Londra per il 350° anniversario della fondazione (1912).

Università di Londra in occasione della assunzione da parte di S. Maestà la Regina Madre dell'ufficio di Cancelliere (1955).

Al Presidente del quinto Congresso di Gastroenterologia, Londra (1956).

Alla Università di Southampton (1953).

Il Preside della Facoltà di Giurisprudenza a William Galbraith Miller, dell'Università di Edimburgo (1903).

E finisco leggendo il messaggio che l'Università di Bologna inviò nel 1928 al Royal College of Physicians di Londra in occasione della celebrazione del III centenario dell'opera di Harvey:

La Regia Università di Bologna e la sua Facoltà di medicina hanno già risposto con grato e lieto consenso all'illustre Reale Collegio dei Medici di Londra, che le invitava alla celebrazione del III centenario dalla pubblicazione di quell'esercitazione anatomica di Guglielmo Harvey sul movimento del cuore, che, dissipate tenebre secolari, aperse un campo immenso alla ricerca scientifica.

Abbiamo dunque mandato il Professor Mariano Luigi Patrizi, ordinario di

Fisiologia, che offrirà al genio inglese i lauri d'Italia e ricorderà la fausta coincidenza dell'anno 1628: allora spuntò tra noi l'astro di Marcello Malpighi, il quale, osservando tra l'altro la circolazione del sangue nei vasi capillari, gettò nuova luce sulla grande scoperta di Guglielmo Harvey, come se illuminasse giorno con giorno e assicurasse una gloria ormai senza fine e senza limiti alla scienza sperimentale.

7 maggio 1928.

Bibliografia e Note

1 BUSACCHI, V., *L'écossais George Scharpes lecteur à Montpellier et à Bologne*, Scalpel, 1963, **3**, no. 11 del 16.

2 *Celebrazioni Malpighiane. Discorsi e scritti*, Contiene scritti del Card. Lercaro, Prof. F. Battaglia, Prof. G. Sotgiu, Prof. V. Busacchi, Prof. G. Gentili, Dott. P. Gelmetti, Prof. L. Münster, Dott. M. Fanti. A cura della Università, Azzoguidi, Bologna, 1966.

3 BUSACCHI, V., *Polidoro Virgilio da Urbino, storico della medicina e della scienza*, Atti I Convegno Marca firmana storia della medicina, Fermo, 1955.

4 BUSACCHI, V., 'Harvey in Italia', *Arch. di Pat. e Clin. medica*, 1964, **41**, 48.

5 FARINELLI, A., *Inghilterra e Italia nel secolo della Rinascenza fino a Shakespeare*, Sta in. Divagazioni erudite, Bocca, Torino, 1925.

6 FARAL, E., Les arts poétiques du XIIe et XIIIe siècle, Paris, 1923.

7 BULAEUS, cit. Da Sarti e Fattorini: vedi nota 8.

8 SARTI, M. e FATTORINI, M., *De claris Archigymnasii bononiensis professoribus a saeculo XI usque ad saeculum XIV*, Bononiae, 1888–96, tomo I, p. 535.

9 MATTEO DI PARIGI, *Chronica maiora*, Londra, 1687–80.

10 L'atto, che proviene dal Convento di S. Francesco è pubblicato in *Acta Nationis germanicae Universitatis bononiensis ex archetipys tabularii Malvezziani*, iussu instituti germanici savignyani ediderunt Ernestus Friedlander et Carolus Malagola, Berolini, Typis et impensis Georgii Reineri, 1887, pp. 347–48.

11 Vedi testo a nota 10.

12 Riportato dal Sarti e Fattorini (loc. cit.), vol. 2°, pp. 70 e 71.

13 FULTON, F. J., 'Polydor Vergil, his chapters on the History of Physick and his Anglica historia', *Bull. Hist. Med.*; Suppl. no. 3, 1944, pp. 65–88.

14 BELLONI, L., *Polidoro Virgilio*, Castalia, 1951.

15 CARDANO, G., *Autobiografia*, cap. XXIX.

16 BRONZINO, G., *Notizia Doctorum sive catalogus doctorum qui in Collegiis Philosophiae et medicinae Bononiae laureati fuereunt ab anno 1480 usqua ad annum 1800*, Giuffré, Milano, 1962.

17 BUSACCHI, V., loc. cit.

18 FORNI, G. G. e PIGHI, G. B., *Gli stemmi e le iscrizioni minori dello Archiginnasio*, Bologna, Tip. Compositori, 1964.

19 Oltre al volume citato alla nota 2 vedere anche; *Notizie edite ed inedite della vita e delle opere di Marcello Malpighi e di Lorenzo Bellini raccolte da Gaetano Atti*, Bologna, 1847.

20 FOSTER, M. A., *Malpighi e la Società reale di Londra*, con appendice documentaria. Sta in: Marcello Malpighi e l'opera sua; scritti raccolti e ordinati a cura di U. Pizzoli, Vallardi, Milano, 1897.

21 *Acta Universitatis bononiensis*. Orationes et epistulae ab MCCCLXXIII ad MCMLIX, Bologna, Tip. Luigi Parma, 1959. Accanto al testo latino è riportata la traduzione italiana a cura di G. B. Pighi.

U. Ceccarelli
Lucca (Italy)

A physician from Lucca at the court of the king of England during the middle ages

I do not want to repeat the subject so learnedly discussed by Professor Coturri (see pp. 754–55), therefore I shall not mention Pancio da Controne and other medieval physicians from Lucca who could reach and become a part of the highest and most representative social circles of England. One of these doctors, for example, was Magister Agostino de Agostini, highly esteemed by Henry VIII. On the contrary, I am going to dedicate this paper to a very important physician from Lucca, Davino Nigarelli, King Henry IV's physician, who lived during the fourteenth century. I think he is worthy of consideration and study even if he is not well known to the historians of medicine. Also Magister Davino, following the example of other doctors from his town, came to the court of the king of England, not only in a spirit of adventure or greed for profit, but, above all, for his own professional value and ability, already known beyond the Alps. From the thirteenth century, when the first universities flourished, these doctors followed the way paved and made easier by the indefatigable and intelligent work of the great Tuscan merchants, who had been able to create a very active web of relations and interests, spreading through it, from finance to culture, from political relations to social questions. No wonder that in the huge Filze collection of the notorial archives of the Republic of Lucca, I personally carried out careful researches about this famous doctor.

Being the chief physician of Paolo Guinigi, the founder of one of the greatest medieval 'Signorie', he treated also his wife Ilaria del Carretto. He was also the chief physician of Henry IV. Davino Nigarelli, Dino's son, was born in Lucca at the beginning of 1350. This was a very bad period for his town, because, thereafter 'Signoria of Castruccio Castracani', the small Tuscan state, politically and economically exhausted, was, for over half a century, subdued and ruled by various imperial delegates, by the Scaligeri, the Florentines and by 'the hated tyrants' from Pisa.

In 1369, however, when Magister Davino was nearly twenty and devoted himself to the study of medicine, the Republic of Lucca again succeeded in getting its freedom, which was to last, except for the 'Guinigeo' period, until the early nineteenth century, that is to the Napoleonic period.

As a matter of fact, on 6 June 1369, Emperor Charles IV granted the state of Lucca the foundation of a 'University Studium', for the teaching of canon and civil law, notorial studies, logic, philosophy, and even medicine. A few years later, a bull of Pope Urbano IV confirmed such privileges. The teaching of medicine, however, was not carried out, even if some attempts were made to invite 'Maestri pro tempore a legere medicinam volentibus audire'. Therefore Davino Nigarelli had to leave Lucca and go to the famous University of Bologna, which attracted students from every country of the world.

Here Magister Davino graduated in medicine, after having spent also a year in the University in Padua. Then he returned to Lucca where he practised his profession with such devotion and skill as to be appointed the family doctor of the 'Guinigi', who were distinguished for their cleverness in public and private affairs. They had their best representative in 'Paolo di Francesco'. It was during this period that Magister Davino was personally called as a court physician at Windsor by Henry IV, King of England, and made up his mind to leave for this distant land. This happened at the beginning of the fifteenth century.

In a few years, from his fiftieth to his sixtieth year, Magister Davino gained such a remarkable reputation and trust that the king himself wanted to introduce him to the highest personages of the English court. Among the several acquaintances he made, we must remember his sincere and lasting friendship with John Gower, who, as a poet, played an important role in the development of the English language, in a period when Norman French was the dominant language. He was so highly appreciated by the king as to get from him many precious English books scrupulously preserved in his royal library such as the *Scripta Super Libro Rectoricorum* by the Franciscan English Friar William Ockam, and the *Liber Continens Scriptis Super I II III Partes* by the English theologian, Walter Burley. Such books enriched his considerable library, made up, above all, of medical texts, later on inherited by his son Matteo who was a physician too.

During the regency of Henry V, Duke of Aquitaine and Lancaster, in the years 1410–12, Henry IV was seriously ill for a long time and, relieved of royal engagements, could, as a patient, strike up a closer friendship with his chief physician (according to some authors King Henry IV was afflicted by leprosy). He was even allowed to dedicate to the king himself his collection of valuable prescriptions collected in his *Liber In Papiro Particularum Receptarum Compilatarum Ab Ipso Magistro Lucense Davino*. We are, however, given a further proof of the friendly and highly esteemed relations between these two men, by a letter of King Henry IV to Paolo Guinigi, 'Signore of Lucca', when after twelve years' stay in England (from 1400–12), Nigarelli became very homesick for his native land. In his letter, the king apologized for being compelled to keep the 'Maestro' in his country, because he highly appreciated him for his merits and his sharing of sentiments concerning Catholicism, but above all, because of Nigarelli's presence at the court, Henry IV felt tranquil about his weak health. The letter reads:

Henricus, Dei gratia Rex Angliae et Francae et Dominus Hiberiae, strenuo et spectabili Viro Paulo De Guiniziis, Domino Civitatis Lucanae, amico nostro sicere dilecto cum interni amoris affectionem salutem.

Amice sincere, dilecte habentes in confidentia magna ea quae nostris nituntur beneplacitis vobis etiam complacentiam allectura et dilectioni vestrae significamus quod veniente super regnum nostrum Angliae dilecto nobis Magistro Davino de Nigarelli phisico subdito et cognato vestro, vobis quoque de ipsius scientia virtutibus et meritis intimato, ipsum penes nos in domum nostram recepimus, ubi tam laudabilia tamque fructuosa reperimus eius obsequia, quod praesentiam suam nobiscum et circa personam nostram desideranter appetimus, ipsumque propterea penes nos in praesenti duximus cum vestri licentia retinendum.

Datum sub signeto nostro apud castrum novum de Windesore mensis octobris Die XIII.

This precious letter together with other papers, represents additional proof of the brave spirit of the noble and intelligent citizens from the Republic of Lucca, who beyond the Channel, could bring great prestige to our country.

Bibliography

Archivio de' Notari, Ser. Domenico Lupardi, no. 290, Reg. I, Arch. Stato Lucca.

Archivio de' Notari, Ser. D. Lupardi, no. 291, Reg. I, Archivio di Stato di Lucca.

BONGI, S., *Inventario Arch. Stato di Lucca*, vol. III.

Carteggio di Paolo Guinigi, Codice 113, Biblioteca Govern. Lucca.

Carteggio di Paolo Guinigi, Filza, no. 12, Biblioteca Govern. Lucca.

DEL CARLO, T., *Storia popolare di Lucca*, Lucca, 1880.

LAZZARESCHI, E., *Le ricchezze di due medici lucchesi nella Rinascenza*, Siena, 1915.

LAZZARESCHI, E., *Lucca nella storia, arte ed industria*, Pescia, 1941.

MANCINI, A., *Storia di Lucca*, Florence, 1949.

GAIRDNER, S., *House of Lancaster and York*, 1874.

FLEMMING, S. H., *England under the Lancastrians*, 1927.

ROSSI, M. M., *Storia d'inghilterra*, Florence, 1953.

WYLIE, S. H., *History of England under Henry IV.*, 1884–1898.

G. Pezzi
Rome (Italy)

L'Italia ed i rapporti medici coll'Inghilterra durante il periodo romantico

Fra i periodi storici che maggiormente s'impongono all'attenzione di quanti vogliano indagare le origini e l'affermarsi della moderna concezione medica, nessuno è più interessante e suggestivo di quello compreso fra gli ultimi decenni del XVIII° secolo e la prima metà del XIX°: il periodo, cioè, contrassegnato dal nascere e fiorire del 'romanticismo'. Il termine romanticismo fu coniato, come è noto, per indicare un fenomeno per il quale le arti in genere e la letteratura in ispecie subirono un particolare mutamento, un rivolgimento di indirizzo. Ma, come il termine 'umanesimo' fu originariamente usato per indicare principalmente quel rinnovamento spirituale e letterario che si iniziò col Petrarca ed il Boccaccio, con i cosidetti 'studia humanitatis', e poi fu esteso ad ogni espressione artistico – culturale, così anche il termine 'romanticismo' venne a comprendere un campo ben più vasto di quello a cui si riferiva inizialmente. Ed è appunto per la molteplicità e complessività degli influssi, che il romanticismo esercitò sull'evoluzione del pensiero non soltanto speculativo ma anche scientifico, morale, sociale, politico, così come per la varietà di atteggiamenti e di espressioni ch'esso assunse attraverso il procedere del tempo e, anche, in armonia con le tradizioni nazionali dei vari popoli, che riesce impossibile darne una precisa definizione. Quello che appare certo é che il bisogno di rinnovamento che diede origine al romanticismo, scaturì dall'evoluzione generale degli spiriti in Europa; evoluzione che é contrassegnata dal sentimento dell'illimitata potenza creatrice dello spirito, del valore assoluto della coscienza o, meglio, dall'autocoscienza e, quindi, dall'esigenza di affermare il proprio io, il mondo interiore individuale.

E' noto come il movimento romantico abbia avuto inizio nel campo letterario: 'romantici' chiamarono sé stessi, nella seconda metà del XVIII° secolo, alcuni scrittori e studiosi germanici che, alla pedissequa imitazione dei classici, e in particolare dei classici francesi del 'secolo d'oro', volevano contrapporre un'arte autonoma e nazionale.

In Germania sorse, nel 1797, la prima scuola romantica, che, dalle pagine della rivista *Athenaum* contemporaneamente fondata, proclamò i suoi principi e ideali: concezione della poesia come voce della natura, come effusione del sentimento, della passione, dell'istinto al di fuori ed al di là di ogni modello, di ogni precettistica.

Nel 1798, cioé solo un anno dopo la costituzione della scuola romantica tedesca, il programma pubblicato da Wordsworth e Coleridge in aggiunta alle *Lyrical Ballads* segnò la nascita del romanticismo inglese, il quale appare per certi aspetti il più affine a quello germanico. Lo spirito inglese, del resto, come per temperare l'innato senso realistico, aveva sempre nutrito una viva predilezione per la leggenda, la fiaba, l'avventura, il mondo della cavalleria, predilezione testimoniata dalla grande poesia di Shakespeare e Spencer via via fino al romanzo gotico del XVIII° secolo. Certo si é che il periodo romantico é uno dei più fulgidi della letteratura inglese e si fregia di nomi consacrati all'immortalità: Byron, Shelley, Keats, per non parlare degli stessi Wordsworth e Coleridge, e di Southey, Moore, Bulwey, Tennyson, Elisabeth Barret, Robert Browning, Walter Scott.

E in Italia? Forse in nessun altro paese come in Italia esisteva un clima spirituale ed estetico remoto che, per certi rispetti, pareva aver precorso il romanticismo. I romantici guardavano infatti a Dante e all'Ariosto come a degli antesignani, mentre é innegabile che la filosofia del Rinascimento, dagli inizi al Bruno e al Campanella, aveva segnato l'alba del nuovo pensiero e che dell'evoluzione di questo pensiero, della formazione d'una coscienza nuova s'era fatto mirabile, acutissimo indagatore e interprete il Vico.

Come sistema di concezioni e dottrine letterarie il romanticismo comparve primamente fra noi con l'opuscolo sul *Cacciatore feroce* e sull'*Eleonora* di G. A. Bürger, lettera semiseria di Crisostomo, composto e pubblicato dal Berchet nel 1816. In esso l'autore afferma che la poesia deve esser libera espressione del sentimento e precisamente di quei sentimenti ed affetti che trovano eco nelle anime moderne.

Ma chi conferì sostanza vitale e potenza di suggestione al romanticismo italiano fu il Manzoni. E ciò non soltanto per gli inni sacri e le odi civili e patriottiche, e per l'*Adelchi* e il *Conte di Carmagnola*, che, come ben osserva il Gabetti, per la libertà della struttura interna, per la lirica del tono, per la religiosità profonda dell'ispirazione, per il colore poetico furono le prime tragedie romantiche di reale rilievo nella letteratura dei paesi latini, ma anche e soprattutto per *I Promessi Sposi*, in cui dalla ispirazione profondamente cristiana derivò vigore alla nuova spiritualità e alle nuove concezioni sociali.

L'esigenza di rinnovamento che, come abbiam sopra detto, impronta di sé il pensiero romantico, si manifesta vigorosamente anche nel campo scientifico, e in particolare in quello della medicina. In questo, tuttavia, diverse e talora contrastanti appaiono le forme in cui tale esigenza s'esprime sì che qualche studioso é giunto a parlare di crisi del pensiero medico in questo periodo; noi preferiremmo dire che si tratta d'un travaglio interiore, d'un'ansiosa ricerca del vero, quale sempre caratterizza ogni passo sulla via del progresso.

Esaminiamo per primi i 'sistemi', che costituiscono uno degli aspetti tipici della medicina di questo periodo e nei quali é più evidente l'influsso della corrente filosofica romantica. Sono teorie o, piuttosto, speculazioni scientifiche che riguardano specialmente il campo della patologia e dell'eziopatogenesi e che, mentre tendono a obliterare le vestigia dello scolasticismo galenico, voglion anche annullare il residuo influsso dei principi cui s'eran ispirate le due grandi scuole del secolo precedente, la iatromeccanica e la iatrochimica, fondate rispettivamente da Gian Alfonso Borelli e da Giovanni Battista Von Helmont.

Tralasciando di parlare della medicina sistematica nei diversi paesi, in specie in Germania ed in Francia, in questo breve lavoro intendiamo ricordare l'influsso che le nuove teorie ebbero in Inghilterra ed in Italia.

In Inghilterra, la medicina sistematica ha il suo primo insigne assertore in William Cullen di Edimburgo, eccellente clinico e acuto indagatore. Il suo sistema segna un sensibile progresso rispetto a quello dell'Hoffmann, da cui pur aveva attinto concetti fondamentali: in esso, infatti, riceve pieno e più esatto risalto l'importanza della funzione del sistema nervoso nell'equilibrio dell'organismo. Quando il sistema nervoso é turbato da stimoli e traumi esterni, si verifica negli organi o un'eccitazione abnorme, uno 'spasmo', o una 'atonia'. Nella terapia, il Cullen, mentre prescrive come benefico l'uso dei tonici del sistema nervoso, quali la china e la canfora e di sedativi, denuncia il gran pericolo rappresentato dal troppo frequente e largo impiego dei lassativi e degli evacuanti.

Ma il più noto dei medici sistematici inglesi fu John Brown, scolaro del Cullen, creatore del sistema che ebbe, nell'evolversi della pratica medica di questo periodo, una diffusione enorme e che fu appunto chiamato 'brownianismo'. Esso s'impernia su un solo fondamentale principio: é l'azione degli stimoli che, eccitando gli organi, dà la vita. Tutti gli agenti esterni ed interni sono degli eccitanti: la vita e la salute sono determinate dalla loro influenza più o meno intensa o, meglio, dalla giusta proporzione tra gli stimoli e l'eccitabilità degli organi. Questa dottrina era una reazione plausibile contro gli 'animisti' ed i 'meccanicisti'. Ma il Brown che, nel suo *Elementa Medicinae*, propugnava con grande ardore questo sistema, non chiariva, sorvolava anzi, sull'essenziale, e cioé sullo studio dei fenomeni di azione e reazione incessanti che sono la manifestazione stessa della vita.

In Italia la medicina sistematica non trovò un'atmosfera propizia ad una rigogliosa fioritura e ciò é da attribuirsi prevalentemente al fatto che presso di noi eran più vivi e operanti che altrove le grandi tradizioni rinascimentali e il prestigio di quel metodo sperimentale che aveva già dato così mirabili risultati nel XVII° secolo. Nessun sistema è legato al nome di medici italiani; dei celebri sistematici stranieri uno solo conseguì, tuttavia, notorietà e favore nell'ambiente medico italiano: il Brown, la cui opera, *Compendio di medicina* fu tradotta e pubblicata da Giovanni Rasori, professore all'Università di Pavia, il quale aveva concepito un'entusiastica ammirazione per le teorie del sistematico inglese.

Il Rasori nato a Parma nel 1766 aveva ottenuto a 19 anni, il titolo di 'Dottore' con una brillante tesi che richiamò l'attenzione del duca di Parma, Don Ferdinando di Borbone, il quale volle inviare il giovane a viaggiare in Italia ed all'Estero. Il Rasori fu, infatti, prima a Firenze ove strinse amicizia col Fontana, poi a Pavia ove conobbe il Volta, lo Spallanzani e lo Scarpa; indi si recò a Londra ed infine a Edimburgo, ove rimase alcuni mesi ed ove poté apprendere direttamente le teorie dei due sistematici inglesi, William Cullen e John Brown, interessandosi però, in particolar modo, al pensiero ed agli insegnamenti del Brown.

I rapporti medici fra il Rasori e la scuola del Brown durarono per lungo tempo, anche perché il Rasori, dotato di una geniale potenza di volgarizzazione, circondato da allievi numerosi e fedeli aveva potuto allargare e far conoscere in Italia le teorie del medico inglese. Delle due fondamentali opere del Brown: *Compendio di medicina e farmacologia* e *Elementi di medicina* il Rasori pubblicò, nel settembre del 1792, la traduzione della prima; gli *Elementi di medicina* furono pubblicati, nei primi mesi dello stesso anno, da Antonio Moscati, che aveva avuto l'opera da Giovanni Locatelli, professore di clinica medica nell'Ospedale Maggiore di Milano. Il Locatelli aveva fatto numerosi viaggi in Inghilterra allo scopo di ben conoscere le dottrine dei due sistematici inglesi. Sostennero le teorie del Brown e del Rasori numerosi studiosi e illustri professori universitari: Siro Borda, insegnante nell'Università di Pavia, Luigi

Valeriano Brera, professore nell'Università di Padova, Giuseppe Mocini, Giuseppe Matteo Menegazzi, Luigi Emiliani, professore a Modena, e infine, Giacomo Tommasini, professore a Bologna.

Il Mocini pubblicò sul *Giornale di Medicina* (maggio 1793) numerosi scritti e lettere elogiative inviate al Brown; Giuseppe Matteo Menegazzi nel 1800, pubblicò in difesa delle teorie del Brown, il suo libretto: *Adversaria medica in doctrinam Brunonis*; opera che ebbe ampia diffusione in Inghilterra; Luigi Emiliani diede alle stampe in Bologna, nel 1795, alcuni scritti divulgativi sul brownianismo ed infine molti lavori del Tommasini apparvero su *La Gazzetta di Parma* fin dal 1787. Ma il Rasori ed il Brown ebbero in Italia anche altri sostenitori: Giovanni Bondioli, professore di materia medica a Padova, alcuni scritti del quale, tradotti in lingua inglese, ebbero ampia diffusione in Inghilterra; Antonio Fanzago che nel 1820 scrisse delle virtù controstimolanti della digitale, Giuseppe Ambrì di Parma, amico del Tommasini, autore di varie memorie pubblicate sul giornale della Società Medico-chirurgica parmense, alcune delle quali furono ben conosciute in Inghilterra. Altri ammiratori del Cullen, del Brown, del Rasori e delle loro scuole furono Giuseppe Della Valle, Antonio Caimari, Francesco Chiaverini di Napoli, Giovanni Zecchinelli, Francesco Vasani, il Giannini, il Guani, il Gelmetti, il Gandini che fece numerosi viaggi in Inghilterra, il Rubini ed infine Carlo Botta, seguace appassionato del brownianismo; il Botta, infatti pubblicò a Grenoble, in lingua francese, nel 1789, una *Apologia della dottrina del Brown*.

Tutti questi studiosi furono i principali artefici dei rapporti medici intercorsi fra l'Italia e l'Inghilterra durante il periodo romantico.

Ma già numerose ed autorevoli voci cominciarono a criticare ed a contrastare prima il Cullen, per i principi teorici esposti sulla sua, pur mirabile opera, 'Materia Medica', e poi il Brown, il Rasori ed i rasoriani. Primo fra tutti Luigi Rosa, maestro di Maurizio Bufalini; Nicolò Olivari allievo del Borsieri e del Frank, insegnante di Clinica Medica a Genova, il quale scrisse un piccolo, ma interessantissimo libro, tradotto anche in inglese e in tedesco, contro le teorie del Brown, nel quale esaltava la medicina ippocratica. Bassiano Carminati pubblicò a Pavia, nel 1787, il suo *Adversaria in principia theoriae Brunonianae*, con quale attaccava la teoria sulla irritabilità, sostenuto, in questa forte polemica, da Francesco Villa di Lodi, da Francesco Agliati, da Gaetano Strambio e da Ignazio del Monte. Ma fra tutti gli oppositori alle nuove teorie eccelsero – come é noto – i tre autorevolissimi maestri: Francesco Vacca Berlinghieri, Maurizio Bufalini e Domenico Cotugno. Ma già i nuovi sistemi cominciavano a declinare; lo stesso Rasori cominciò a poco a poco ad abbandonarli ed anche il Tommasini finì col riconoscere i tratti più discutibili di tali sistemi, come ben chiaramente si rileva dal suo libro *Della nuova dottrina medica italiana*, pubblicato nel 1817. A tale declino molto contribuì lo stesso Brown, il quale, di carattere intollerante e violento, nel suo 'Elementi di medicina' aveva attaccato lo stesso Cullen, suo maestro e protettore, tanto che allontanato dalla facoltà medica, dovette lasciare Edimburgo e trasferirsi a Londra, ove visse in miseria; disordinato, irreligioso, intemperante, ricoperto di debiti, venne anche arrestato; stava, tuttavia, per esser chiamato a Berlino, allorquando, colpito da apoplessia, moriva a 58 anni, nel 1788. Anche il Cullen, pochi anni dopo, chiudeva la sua vita terrena e ben può dirsi che, con la sua fine, vennero a cadere molti di quei legami di sincera amicizia che, per lungo tempo, avevano unito studiosi inglesi ed italiani durante questo periodo tanto interessante per l'evoluzione della letteratura e delle scienze. I sistemi andarono poi rapidamente declinando poiché si andò formando, così in Italia come in Inghilterra e negli altri paesi, una scuola di clinici che fondavano l'arte medica sull'esperimento ma, soprattutto sull'osservazione attenta del malato. Era questa la via verso la quale la medicina si era ora indirizzata, la via maestra che avrebbe condotto, ben presto, alle più alte conquiste del sapere.

Z. Ohya
Kyoto (Japan)

Rapports entre la médecine anglaise et celle japonaise au point de vue médico-historique

Keiki, le dernier Shôgoun, se soumit au décret, tandis que ceux de ses tenants qui refusèrent de suivre son exemple furent défaits d'abord à Fushimi, près de Kyoto (17 janvier 1868), puis à Ouyeno, faubourg de Yedo (4 juillet 1868) ensuite dans le district d'Aizou (6 novembre 1868) et définitivement à Hakodate (27 juin 1869), où certains d'entre eux avaient essayé de fonder une république indépendante. William Willis, après l'achèvement de ses études à la Faculté d'Edinburgh, débarquait au Japon en 1861, en qualité de chirurgien attaché à la légation anglaise, alors âgé de 25 ans. Il participait à la guerre civile de Fushimi et traitait nombre de blessés dans l'Hôpital du clan Satsouma de Kyoto. L'Hôpital militaire provisionel de Yokohama était fondé en 17 avril 1868; Willis était élu le chef. En 20 août 1868, il allait à la guerre d'Aizou et il pratiquait 16 cas d'amputation avec grand succès. En septembre 1868, l'Hôpital militaire de Yokohama déménageait à Tokyo et devenait le Dai-Byôin (L'Hôpital grand); Willis était nommé le directeur, il enseignait la chirurgie anglaise: l'anesthésie générale par l'inhalation du chloroforme, l'antiseptique par la solution du permanganate de potassium et la technique de l'amputation. Ishigouro Chûchokou, Ikeda Kensai et Sasaki Tôyô furent les éminents parmi ses élèves. Il contribuait grandement au développement de la chirurgie japonaise. En 1870, Sagara Kôan et Iwasa Jun décidaient en faveur du système allemand au lieu de celui anglais pour l'éducation médicale japonaise. Donc, Willis donnait sa démission comme directeur de Dai Byôin (Le grand Hôpital). En 12 décembre 1869, l'Académie provinciale de Kagoshima était fondée à Kagoshima. Willis était élu le professeur par la recommandation de Saigô Takamori, l'homme influent. Takagi Kenkan, Saneyoshi Yasouzoumi et Mitamoura Tadakouni furent les premiers élèves. Après le long séjour d'une dizaine d'années à Kagoshima, il rentrait dans son pays natal en 1881. Ultérieurement, il ouvrait l'Hôpital à Bangkok, la capitale de Thaïland en 1885. Il mourut en février 1894 à Bangkok. En septembre 1867 l'Hôpital de femmes publiques était fondé à la rue Yoshihara de Yokohama; Newton, le médecin militaire anglais était élu le chef, il pratiquait les injections sous-cutanées de la solution du sublimé. Ensuite, il fondait l'Hôpital de syphilis de Nagasaki en 1870. Okouyama Tora-aki, le médecin de la Marine de guerre, compilait le dictionnaire des termes techniques de médecine anglo-japonaise en 1872. C'est le premier dictionnaire de ce genre au Japon. Hobson, le médecin anglais résidant à Canton en Chine, laissait trois ouvrages médicaux écrits en caractères chinois; Hirose Genshû traduisait un des ouvrages, nouveau manuel de gynéco-puériculture, en 1874. Palm, le médecin et missionnaire anglais, allait à Niigata où il faisait le compte rendu sur la fièvre fluviale du Japon en 1875. William Anderson, le médecin anglais était élu le professeur d'Académie de médecine de la Marine de guerre en 1873. Ensuite, Yoshida Kenzô, Takagi Kenkan, Saneyoshi Yasouzoumi, Tozouka Kankai et Souzouki Shigemichi étaient envoyés à Anleterre pour y étudier la médecine anglaise en 1875, ils étaient nommés les professeurs de l'Académie de la médecine de la Marine de guerre. La méthode antiseptique de Joseph Lister était introduite au Japon par Sato Sousoumou en 1875. John Hill, le médecin anglais, était nommé le chef de l'Hôpital de syphilis de Yokohama en 1877.

Agnes Vetch, l'infirmière anglaise, enseignait sur les soins des malades à l'école des infirmières de la Faculté de Tokyo en 1887. Takagi Kenkan et Saneyoshi Yasouzoumi enseignaient sur la médecine anglaise à l'Académie privée de la médecine de Jikei de Tokyo en 1891. Saneyoshi Yasouzoumi, le médecin inspecteur général de la Marine de guerre, était élu le «honorary fellow» de la Faculté d'Edimbourg en 1905.

S. Kottek
Strasbourg (*France*)

Médecins juifs en Angleterre du XIIe au XVIe siècle

I. XIIe–XIIIe SIÈCLES

Cecil Roth leur consacre un chapitre de son livre «Essays and portraits of Anglo-Jewish History». D'autre part, dans une petite plaquette intitulée «The intellectual activities of medieval English Jewry», il donne une liste de 18 noms dont il a pu retrouver la trace. Il s'élève contre l'assertion de Neubauer affirmant que les Juifs anglais au Moyen-Age n'avaient aucune notion de médecine et faisaient appel en cas de besoin à des médecins chrétiens.

Nous reproduisons ici cette liste

1.	Un médecin (?) de Lynn	1190
2.	Joseph le Médecin	1190
3.	Isaac Medicus (Londres)	1192
4.	X, père de Joseph (Londres)	avant 1192
5.	Ursellus (= Josué) Medicus (York)	1208
6.	Deodonatus Medicus (York)	1208
7.	Magister Benedict (Norwich)	1234
8.	Isaac le Médecin (Norwich)	avant 1266
9.	Salle le Mire (Norwich)	1266
10.	Salomon le Médecin (Norwich) id. au précédent?	1264
11.	Samson le Cyrurgeon (Londres)	1273
12.	'Hak (Isaak) le Mire (Londres)	1274
13.	Jacob Medicus ou Le Mire (York)	1275
14.	Magister Simon le Mire (Bedford)	1275
15.	Leo le Mire (Bristol)	1278
16.	Elias le Mire (Londres)	1280
17.	Magister Elias de Londres	1284
18.	Bateman fils de Deulecresse (Norwich)	1290

A propos de *Salomon le Médecin*, de Norwich, il faut signaler que ce médecin possédait dans cette ville, exactement dans Saddlegate Street, un herbier ou un jardin de plantes médicinales (vers 1266). Selon Ch. Singer, ceci peut-être considéré comme le premier jardin-des-plantes privé connu dans l'Angleterre du Moyen-Age.

Mais le nom qui ressort nettement dans cette liste est celui de *Magister Elias*, fils de Magister Moïse de Londres, plus connu en hébreu sous le nom de Rabbi Elija Mena'hem de Londres (1220?–84).

Son père, Rabbi Moïse de Londres, était un talmudiste et grammairien connu, de la lignée des grands Massorètes.

Magister Elias, fut une personnalité réellement marquante, aux multiples facettes. A la fois talmudiste éminent ayant composé des commentaires appréciés sur certains traités du Talmud, mais aussi homme d'affaires dont les transactions s'étendaient sur tout le pays. Enfin, médecin de valeur internationale. En effet, il fut appelé en consultation en 1280, aux Pays-Bas par Jean d'Avesnes, comte de Hainault, neveu du Comte de Flandres. Après bien des démarches, il fut autorisé à se rendre en Flandres avec un assistant. Le patient guérit. Les lettres échangées à cette occasion existent toujours et de nombreux documents jettent une lumière assez vive sur ce personnage exceptionnel.

En ce qui concerne la présence de médecins juifs dans l'Oxford médiéval, Cecil Roth la met en doute (cf. *The Jews of Medieval Oxford*, p. 149, n. 3). Il cite l'opinion du Rev. C. W. Boase, que nous rapportons: «a medical school which we find established in the twelfth century can hardly have been other than jewish». De même, H. S. Wellcome (*Oxford Medical lore*, 1904), pense que le premier professeur de médecine à l'Université, qui s'appelait Stokes, enseigna probablement à l'école de médecine juive. Mais ceci semble rester dans le domaine des probabilités, car on manque de documents sur cette époque. Ce qui est sûr, c'est qu'une communauté israélite existait à Oxford au XIIIe siècle. Le propre frère de Magister Elias de Londres (Magister Jacob fils de Moïse) y habitait.

En conclusion, il y eut en Angleterre au Moyen Age, et jusqu'en 1290 (date de l'expulsion de tous les Juifs du pays) une présence de médecins juifs dont la liste publiée ne donne sans doute qu'une faible idée. Cependant il n'y eut pas de figure très marquante, à part Magister Elias de Londres.

II. XIVe–XVe SIÈCLES

Dans la période intermédiaire, que Hyamson appelle the «Middle Period» (1290–1550), on dit communément qu'il n'y avait pratiquement pas de juifs en Angleterre. En fait, il y eut constamment des individualités juives bien qu'aucune communauté organisée n'ait existé jusqu'au règne de Charles 1er. On dit qu'à Oxford, un petit noyau se maintint longtemps après 1290. En 1310, une délégation de 6 juifs, dont l'un était médecin, vint en Angleterre pour essayer de négocier le retour des juifs dans le pays, apparemment sans succès.

Vers la fin de sa vie, le Roi Henry IV, étant tombé malade et ayant été traité sans succès par ses médecins, appela à son chevet le médecin juif Elias Sabot (Elija de Sabatto) de Bologne. Celui-ci arriva en Angleterre en 1410, muni d'un sauf-conduit avec licence de se déplacer et de s'établir dans tout le pays. Ce médecin, appelé encore Elija Beer (Fonte) Ben Shabbetai, fut médecin de cour du Pape Martin V (1417–31) puis d'Eugene IV (1431–47). Il fut fait officiellement citoyen de Rome en 1405 par une lettre patente qui a été conservée jusqu'à ce jour. Il prêta le serment d'allégeance sur les Saintes Ecritures, et put alors porter ses armes et fut dispensé de porter l'insigne des Juifs. Tout ceci a été rapporté pour souligner la notoriété de ce médecin.

Hyamson cite par ailleurs un autre médecin, David di Nigarellis de Lucca, dont l'adhérence au Judaïsme n'est que suspectée. En tout cas il ne se déclara jamais comme tel, car il fut naturalisé Anglais avec tous les droits qui en découlent.

Enfin, en 1409 un médecin du sud de la France, Maistre Sampson de Mierbeawe judeus reçut le droit de se déplacer, de pratiquer son art et de se fixer dans tout le Royaume pour une durée d'un an. Il avait été appelé par Sir Richard Wittington, le fameux Lord-Maire, au chevet de sa femme Alice.

Cependant, c'est au XVIe siècle que nous allons trouver des figures marquantes de médecins juifs qui furent, contrairement aux précédents, profondément enracinés en Angleterre.

III. XVIe SIÈCLE

Il est bien connu que les Juifs furent expulsés d'Espagne en 1492, puis du Portugal en 1497. Ceux qui restèrent sur place subirent une conversion forcée, et ces «Nouveaux Chrétiens», appelés par le peuple Marranos furent en butte à la suspicion d'abord, puis aux persécutions de l'Inquisition. Il y eut dès lors une émigration continue, principalement en direction de la Hollande (Amsterdam) et de l'Italie, où ils étaient bien accueillis, mais aussi dans d'autres pays d'Europe, dont l'Angleterre. Cette petite communauté juive d'Angleterre comprenait un nombre relativement important de médecins. Les recherches de Lucien Wolf, Cecil Roth et Harry Friedenwald ont permis de mieux les connaître. Cependant la petite communauté crypto-juive fut dispersée en 1542 à la suite d'une dénonciation et de l'intervention des autorités espagnoles.

Parmi les médecins marranes de la période précoce de colonisation, on cite Maître Diogo (env. 1535), Maître Antonio (env. 1540), Emanuel Fernandes et surtout Dionysius Rodriguez. Ce dernier avait été médecin de la Reine du Portugal et s'était ensuite enfui à Londres avec ses 3 fils; par la suite il s'établit à Anvers en 1538. Il mourut à Ferrare en 1541. Son fils Manuel Brudo, pratiqua quelque temps avec succès la médecine en Angleterre, et sa clientèle comprenait des personnalités telles que Sir Thomas Audley, lord Chancellor et Sir William Sidney, lord Chamberlain. Il publia un ouvrage *De ratione victus in singulis febribus* qui connut au moins 4 éditions, la première en 1544. Cet ouvrage est divisé en 3 livres, le deuxième et le troisième sont dédiés «ad Anglos».

Il faut noter ici que le grand médecin juif portugais Amatus Lusitanus a rencontré aussi bien Dionysius que son fils Manuel Brudo, et qu'il les cite dans ses œuvres. Il parle notamment d'une controverse qui opposa Dionysius au médecin français Brissot à propos du diagnostic de la pleurésie: chacun d'eux devait publier une «apologia» sur ce sujet.

Hyamson cite par ailleurs un médecin nommé Ferdinando Lopes, qui vécut à Londres (St. Helens) vers 1550, et qui fut arrêté, jugé et expulsé du pays pour une cause mal précisée. (*The Jews in England*, pp. 124 et 136).

Amatus Lusitanus cite aussi «notre ami Petrus Fernandus qui exerça la médecine avec beaucoup de succès parmi les Anglais à Londres, et qui maintenant prospère à Venise».

Enfin, citons encore Antonio Brandão (ou Brandan) qui était le propre neveu d'Amatus et exerça la médecine à Bristol.

Dans cette même ville de Bristol on trouve à la tête de la Communauté juive, un médecin, le docteur Henrique Nuñez, qui s'y installe avec sa famille, en 1545. Toutefois, en 1555, il émigra en France, sans doute à la suite de la réaction contre la réforme au temps de la «bloody» Queen Mary.

Cependant, un peu plus tard, sous le règne d'Elizabeth, et après la victoire du Protestantisme en Angleterre, la communauté marrane connaît un nouveau développement. A cette époque, deux noms de médecins surgissent nettement du lot: Rodrigo Lopez et Hector Nunez.

Rodrigo Lopez, né au Portugal en 1525, arriva à Londres en 1559, selon certains en temps que prisonnier de Sir Francis Drake. On a très peu de renseignements sur ses origines, sa formation, sa vie privée. On sait qu'il fut le premier médecin-résident au St. Bartholomew's Hospital, de 1567 à 1575, où il eut pour collègue, entre autres, le chirurgien William Clowes qui le cita dans un de ses ouvrages, élogieusement. Voici ses paroles: «he showed himself to be both careful and very skilful, not only in his counsil in dieting, purging and bleeding, but also his direction of Arceus' apozema . . .».

Vers 1586, il fut nommé médecin de la Reine, après avoit été employé par le Comte de Leicester et avoir été lié avec Walsingham et le Comte d'Essex. Il eut cependant le tort de se mêler de politique, ce qui entraîna sa perte. En octobre 1593, il fut arrêté et accusé d'avoir voulu empoisonner la Reine sur l'instigation du Roi d'Espagne. Après un long procès, il fut exécuté à Tyburn le 7 juin 1594. Il y eut à ce moment une petite vague d'antisémitisme en Angleterre, ce qui entraîna le déclin de la communauté marrane. A ce moment, la pièce de théâtre en vogue à Londres était le «Juif de Malte» de Marlowe, et Shakespeare faisait jouer peu après son «Marchand de Venise».

Hector Nuñez (parfois appelé «Docteur Hectour») né à Evora au Portugal, ayant fait ses études à Coïmbra, arriva en Angleterre vers 1550. L. Wolf retrouve sa trace dès 1549, à la paroisse de St.-Olafe, Hart Street. Il fut admis au Collège Royal des Médecins et à celui des Chirurgiens dès 1554. Par ailleurs, il fut également un grand brasseur d'affaires et ses nombreux correspondants étrangers lui font jouer un certain rôle politique. Il fut naturalisé Anglais en 1568. Ce fut Nuñez qui le premier annonça l'arrivée de la Grande Armada à Lisbonne, sur le chemin du retour. Il fut lié aux ministres Burleigh et Walsingham. Il semble avoir pratiqué le judaïsme en secret, car on a pu montrer qu'il fut membre de la Synagogue clandestine d'Anvers, sous le nom de Francisco Pessoa. Il mourut en septembre 1591 et fut enterré à Stepney Churchyard, à côté de sa belle-sœur Grace Freire.

A la fin du XVIe siècle, la petite colonie marrane d'Angleterre connait un déclin dont nous avons brièvement rappelé les causes. Le XVIIe siècle verra les efforts de Manassé ben Israël pour le revivifier et ses démélés avec Cromwell. Mais nous limitons notre étude au XVIe siècle. Si l'on ne retient de cette période que les noms de Dionysius Rodriguez et de son fils Manuel Brudo, de Rodrigo Lopez et de Hector Nuñez, on aura du moins en mémoire des figures attachantes de médecins juifs ou crypto-juifs ayant pleinement participé à la vie de leur patrie d'adoption: l'Angleterre.

Bibliographie

ADLER, M., *Jews of Medieval England*, London, 1939.
FINESTEIN, I., *A short History of Anglo Jewry*, 1957.
FRIEDENWALD, H., *Jews and Medicine*, Baltimore, 1944.
GOLDSCHMIDT, S., *Die Geschichte der Juden in England im XI. und XII. Jht M.G.W.J.*, Berlin, 1885–86.
HENRIQUES, H. S. Q., *The Jews and the English Law*, Oxford, 1908.

HYAMSON, A. M., *History of the Jews in England*, 2nd ed. (1928), London.
JACOBS, J., *The Jews of Angevin England*, London, 1893.
JACOBS, J. et WOLF, L., *Bibliotheca Anglo-Judaica*, London, 1888.
PICCIOTTO, J., *Sketches of Anglo-Jewish History*, London, 1875.
ROTH, C., *A History of the Jews in England*, Oxford, 1941.
ROTH, C., *The Jews of Medieval Oxford*, Oxford, 1951.
ROTH, C., *Essays and Portraits in Anglo-Jewish History*, 1962.
STOKES, H. P., *Studies in Anglo-Jewish History*, London, 1913.
TOVEY, D'B., *Anglia Judaica*, Oxford, 1738.
WOLF, L., *Essays in Jewish History*, London, 1934; 'Jewish Physicians at the England Court', *Brit. Med. J.*, 1907, **2**, 151–52.

N.B. Une bibliographie détaillée à propos de Rodrigo Lopez sera donnée dans un travail ultérieur.

P. Boeynaems
Antwerp (Belgium)

Irish doctors in the southern Netherlands

The continuous religious troubles in Ireland in the sixteenth, seventeenth and eighteenth centuries caused many Irish to leave their home-country and seek refuge abroad. This emigration was at its height in the midst of the seventeenth century after Oliver Cromwell had disembarked on the island and started his campaign to suppress a new rebellion.

It is not surprising that many emigrants sailed to the Low Countries, i.e. the Netherlands, particularly in the south. Many reasons may be considered for this choice. In contrast to the northern part of the Low Countries, which had turned to Protestantism, the south remained a stronghold of Catholicism. Moreover it stood under the rule of Spain, which was at war with England, and it is possible that the emigrant Irish hoped that the king of Spain would help them in their fight for freedom of their country in the future. Indeed many of them joined the Spanish army which had its own Irish Brigade. For the same reason there was an Irish Brigade in later years in the service of France. There was no country in Europe at that time with which the Irish were more connected than with the southern part of the Netherlands. Most of the Irish refugees, however, never returned to their home-country and integrated themselves with the native population of the country of their adoption.

I tried to collect the names of Irish medical practitioners who stayed in the southern Netherlands in the course of the seventeenth and eighteenth centuries and to find out what were their medical activities. As far as I could trace, most of them received their medical degree, which was a degree of Licentiate in Medicine, at the University of Louvain. I did not find a graduation at any other university. Louvain was a centre of attraction for the Irish. Not less than three flourishing Irish colleges were established in that town, and as one author said 'The Irish colleges of Louvain remain a proud and lasting monument of the learning and zeal of the Irish Nation'. After their graduation in medicine the Irish doctors began to practise in the big centres, including the towns of Antwerp, Bruges, Brussels and Mons. Because of their poor knowledge of the Dutch native language, they avoided practice in the country places.

Was their medical career a successful one? No information could be found so far as to their private practice. But on the other hand there is evidence that some of these Irish doctors enjoyed the esteem of the local authorities and their colleagues. While some of them received appointments by the town councils such as 'médecin pensionnaire' or posts in hospitals, others were chosen by their colleagues as chairmen of the local medical societies.

Here follows the list of the Irish doctors who practised medicine in the seventeenth and eighteenth centuries in the southern Netherlands so far as they can be traced, together with some biographical and bibliographical information.

Dolphin, Henry. Born in Ireland and studied medicine at the university of Louvain where on 16 May 1704 he received his degree of licentiate in medicine. He settled at Bruges and was elected in that city as chairman of the Society of St. Luke in 1717 and in 1723.[1]

Downing, Joannes Mattheus. A medical student at Louvain. Preparatory to his degree of Medicinae Licentiatus, he submitted in 1777 to the authorities of the medical faculty, together with three other fellow students, a *Repetitio de praecipuis morbis contagiosis*, Lovanii. 4°, 12 pp. The title-page of this leaflet mentions as Downing's place of origin *Talloniensi Hiberno*.[2]

Mac Grath, Raymond. A medical officer in the Austrian army. By will he bequeathed in 1780, for the benefit of students of his kinship, 9,402 florins to the Collegium Pastorale Hibernorum at Louvain.[3]

Meagher, Jean. Received his degree at Louvain on 2 March 1712. He practised medicine at Brussels where he was entered on the list of the doctors of the Collegium Medicum Bruxellense on 17 November 1747 with the mention: Irishman.[4]

Meagher, Jacques. Probably a son of the preceding. He took his degree at Louvain on 10 June 1749 and was entered on the list of the doctors of the Collegium Medicum Bruxellense on 17 July 1751.[5]

Magher [*sic*], Thomas. He took his degree on 9 March 1758 and was entered on the list of the Collegium Medicum Bruxellense without a date of admission.[6]

O'Dwyer, John. Born in Cashel in the year 1620, studied medicine at Louvain where he received the degree of licentiate in medicine and settled in the town of Mons. For a long time he was a military doctor in the Spanish army. After leaving the military service he was appointed 'médecin pensionnaire' by the magistrate of his town of adoption. O'Dwyer is the author of: *Querela Medica, seu, Planctus Medicinae Modernae Status*. 1686, 8°. In this book, which he dedicated to his colleague and fellow countryman doctor Edm. Trohy of Antwerp, O'Dwyer protests against the abuses in medicine, the incompetence of some practitioners and the credulity of patients.[7]

O'Sullivan, Jeremias. Born in the county of Kerry in 1697, O'Sullivan studied medicine at Louvain where he received his degree of licentiate in medicine on 29 November 1724. After his graduation he went to Ostend and afterwards settled at Bruges, in which town he was appointed physician at the St. John's hospital. From 1746 till 1765, he was chairman of the Society of St. Luke in Bruges. On account of a report made by O'Sullivan the Magistrate of Bruges in 1751 published an order prohibiting the sale of mussels which were declared harmful to public health.[8] O'Sullivan died in Bruges on 17 November 1769 at the age of 72 and was buried in the church of the Holy Redeemer.[9]

de Trohy, Edmond. Licentiate in medicine. After having been admitted as a citizen of the town of Antwerp on 15 October 1666 he practised medicine there and was appointed sworn physician by the magistrate. In 1678 he was one of the four sworn physicians who addressed an attestation to the council of the town declaring that the reigning sickness was not contagious.[10]

Tully, Florent Guillaume. Born in Ireland, and came to Dunkirk where he was appointed as 'médecin pensionnaire' and became an alderman of the town. He died there in 1768 or 1769. Tully is the author of: *Essai sur les maladies de Dunkerque*, Dunkerque, 1759.[11]

Verron, Andrew. He came from Dublin and received his medical degree at Louvain on 6 June 1663. He practised medicine at Brussels where he was entered on the list of the doctors of the Collegium Medicum Bruxellense on 21 October 1663.[12]

References

1 DE MEYER, *Suite aux Analectes médicaux*, Bruges, [n.d.], p. 213.
2 This leaflet was in my possession but was unfortunately destroyed during the last war.
3 O'FLANDRES, *Erin*, Nieupoort, 1922, p. 414.
4 BROECKX, C., *Histoire du Collegium Medicum Bruxellense*, Anvers, 1862, p. 458.
5 Ibid. p. 459.
6 Ibid. p. 459.
7 ELOY, N. F. J., *Dictionnaire Historique de la Médecine*, Mons, 1778, vol. III, p. 414.
8 DE MEYER, *Analectes médicaux*, Bruges, 1851, p. 239.
9 DE MEYER, *Suite aux Analectes médicaux*, Bruges, [n.d.], pp. 217–18.
10 VAN SCHEVENSTEEN, A. F. C., 'Naamlijsten van Antwerpsche Geneesheren etc.', in: *Antwerpsch Archievenblad*, 1922, nr. 2, pp. 12, 37; Idem., *Documents pour servir a l'étude des maladies pestilentielles dans le marquisat d'Anvers*, Brussels, 1932, vol. II, p. 359.
11 FAIDHERBE, A., *Les Médecins et les Chirurgiens de Flandre avant 1789*, Lille, 1892, p. 331.
12 BROECKX, C., op. cit., p. 455.

G. T. Haneveld
Utrecht (The Netherlands)

The Schroeder Van der Kolk museum collection

Jacobus Ludovicus Conradus Schroeder Van Der Kolk (1797–1862) was appointed to the chair of anatomy, morbid anatomy and physiology at the university of Utrecht in 1827. He published many articles on (comparative) anatomical, physiological and medical subjects. His book on *The Minute Structures and Functions of the Spinal Cord and on the Treatment of Epilepsy* (1859) and his handbook *The Pathology and Therapeutics of Mental Diseases* (1863) were translated into German and English (1870).

For his studies on tuberculosis, the fine structures of the placenta – he was the first to describe the Langhanslayer in the chorionic villi – the diagnosis of sputum, he made use of a beautiful achromatic British microscope bought from the royal optician Dollond, which is still in perfect working order in Utrecht. He was one of the first to propagate the need for microscopic examination of the excision margins in excised tumours. The latter half of his life was devoted to the care of the insane, which earned him the name 'Father of Dutch psychiatry'.

During his lifetime he worked at perfecting a private collection which expanded to 770 pathological preparations, including nearly 400 skeletons and skulls and 337 anatomical and ethnological preparations. After his death in 1862 this collection was offered for sale for £1,000. The whereabouts of this collection were unknown until in 1970, when by pure chance, Henry Acland, Regius professor at Oxford, was found to have purchased part of the collection for the Oxford Museum. Part went to Dr. Humphrey in Cambridge.

The Van Der Kolk collection served as the nucleus of the medical collection of the Oxford Museum together with two smaller collections from Christ Church, made by Dr. Kidd.

Over 200 of the original specimens – dried bone preparations and wet specimens – could be retraced in the William Dun School of Pathology and in the Radcliffe Infirmary, thanks to Dr. Robb-Smith and the late Dr. French. Even more valuable was the rediscovery of the complete handwritten catalogue stating all clinical details, post-mortem findings, correspondence, references to publications, and fifteen doctors' theses, etc.

The Dutch Schroeder Van Der Kolk collection, now in Oxford, is a typical early nineteenth-century collection showing the beginning of modern pathology and the infancy of pathological histology.

G. A. Lindeboom
Amsterdam (The Netherlands)

Boerhaave's influence on British medicine

INTRODUCTION

Leyden University was founded by William the Silent in 1575 as a reward for the courageous behaviour of the citizens during the siege by the Spaniards. From the very beginning English students came to Leyden to matriculate in various faculties. In fact, the first student to be inscribed in the Faculty of Medicine, in 1581, was an Englishman, John James.[1]

When a century later, in 1673, the Test Act closed the Universities of Oxford and Cambridge to students being non-members of the Church of England, the English Roman Catholics and Protestant dissenters had to go elsewhere for a university education. Besides, facilities for an all-round medical education in England remained unsatisfactory for a long time. Still in 1714, the year in which Boerhaave was vice-chancellor of Leyden University, an English writer published a plea for greater facilities for medical education in his country.[2] Hence, many medical students from Oxford and Cambridge went to Holland to complete their studies; most of them graduated at Leyden or Utrecht, or at a French University. Innes Smith, in his *English-speaking Students at the University of Leyden* listed some two thousand English students who matriculated at Leyden University in the first three hundred years of its existence.

BRITISH STUDENTS AND GRADUATES

Boerhaave taught medicine at Leyden from 1701 till his death in 1738 – first as a reader (lector) and since 1709 as professor. During this period of thirty-seven years he lectured on medicine, but on other subjects too. He was appointed first as professor of botany and medicine, gave bedside teaching from 1714 and was also professor of chemistry from 1718 till 1729 when he resigned from his professorships of botany and chemistry.

When, in the beginning of his academic career, Govert Bidloo (1649–1702), physician-in-ordinary to King William neglected the teaching of anatomy, and Jacobus Le Mort (1650–1718) that of chemistry, English students requested Boerhaave to deliver private lectures in these sciences. The Leyden professors were entitled to give such lectures for which the students had to pay; to Boerhaave they paid 30 Dutch guilders for a course of one hour daily (four days a week) during the academic year. Boerhaave lectured privately until the year of his death on theoretical and on practical medicine. His cheerfulness, his eloquence and his excellent teaching qualities attracted many students to his lecture-room, who flocked there from all over Europe.

BRITISH STUDENTS AND GRADUANDS

Boerhaave's audience was international: about half of his students were foreigners, of which a large proportion were British. During the period of Boerhaave's professorship, that is – between 1709 and 1738 – the total number of students at Leyden enrolled in the Faculty of Medicine amounted to 1,919; of these 659 were English-speaking: 340 came from England, 205 from Scotland, 107 from Ireland and a few from 'the British colonies beyond the sea'.[3] Thus more than a third of Boerhaave's students came from Great Britain.

These figures corresponded well with the class lists of Boerhaave's last courses on theoretical and practical medicine (1737) which by chance have been preserved. In one of these lists 97 students signed; among the 60 foreigners 23 were Englishmen, 5 Scotsmen and 3 Irishmen; again the British made up about a third of the total.

Usually the British students completed their medical studies in a period of about two years; but some graduated after a much shorter time. As already stated others went to France to graduate at some French University (Rheims, Angers, etc.), but a considerable number graduated at Leyden.

For his degree the candidate had to write and to defend a thesis publicly. Such a thesis, usually of 20–30 pages, was printed by the university printers, who since 1628 had been the Elseviers. Boerhaave taught more disciplines than the other professors, and hence not only promoted more students yearly than they did, but also proportionally more foreigners. Of the 178 students who were promoted by him, 102 were foreigners. Among these were 43 English-speaking students, made up of 31 Englishmen, 5 Scotsmen, 5 Irishmen and 2 English–Americans.

Recently Underwood[4] established that, in the first half of the eighteenth century, excluding the men educated only at Oxford or Cambridge, of 130 Fellows or Licentiates of the Royal College of Physicians of London, no less than 75 were educated in Holland. It may be assumed that the greater part of these men had enjoyed the teaching of Boerhaave.

All these figures demonstrate two things: first that, apparently, in the early eighteenth century Leyden exerted a great attraction for foreign medical students as their number surpassed that of the native Dutchmen; and secondly, that among the foreign students of medicine the English-speaking proportionally formed the majority. There can be little doubt that, apart from the excellent facilities of the Faculty, which had at its disposal a rich botanic garden, a chemical laboratory, an anatomical department, a hospital and a well-stocked library, Boerhaave's enthusiastic teaching and his cheerful and charming personality were the main attraction. 'In the hospital he was at his best and nowhere else could the students get such instruction.'[5]

The British students who crossed the sea to Holland, also provided a means of communication between Boerhaave and British scientists. Some of them came to Leyden and called on Boerhaave with a recommendation from Sir Hans Sloane (1660–1753) or from Richard Mead (1673–1754). After their graduation, such students would not fail to take leave of their beloved professor. When such an opportunity presented itself, Boerhaave used to give the young doctor a good testimonial. Often, too, he would ask the young man to be the bearer of a gift to one of Boerhaave's friends, such as a copy of an oration he just had delivered or of a book that he had recently published, or even some plants for the Chelsea Garden.[6] In this way Boerhaave preserved the bonds with his British friends, most of whom he had never met.

Further, once Boerhaave's former pupils were established in practice, they enjoyed the unwritten privilege of consulting their famous professor by letter in difficult cases. British students were particularly in the habit of doing so, perhaps when their treatment of distinguished or aristocratic patients was not entirely successful. They would describe in detail the symptoms and signs of such an illness as well as the drugs they had prescribed without success. In such a letter the writer would often send Boerhaave a fee in the form of a bill of exchange. Boerhaave, despite the fact that he was overburdened and without the benefit of a secretary, never failed to answer within a few days. He would express his opinion on the case and give some sound general advice such as on diet, on riding or bathing. He always added some prescriptions and often ended with good wishes for the recovery of the patient – be it a noble lady with habitual abortion, the most illustrious Admiral of England with a skin disorder, the Earl of Berkeley[7] with, perhaps, gouty attacks, a gentleman with asthmatic bronchitis, or a patient with symptoms of any disease.

BOERHAAVE'S MEDICAL BOOKS IN ENGLAND

Very soon after his appointment as professor of medicine and botany in 1709, Boerhaave began to achieve international fame. This was largely due to his two medical textbooks, written during the eight years of his lectureship, which had just been published. Written in Latin, which was still the language of science, they soon found their way beyond the borders of his own country and made his name widely known abroad.

The first of these books, the *Institutes of Medicine* (1708) dealt with theoretical medicine and offered, in fact, a comprehensive and consistent system of medical knowledge. The other, *Aphorisms concerning the Knowledge and Cure of Diseases* (1709), covered the practice of medicine in 1479, and aphorisms on the diagnosis and treatment of diseases. Though both the *Institutes* and the *Aphorisms* were primarily written as a basis for his own teaching (*in usus annuae exercitionis domesticos; in usum doctrinae domesticae*) they were soon welcomed as very useful textbooks by other teachers at foreign universities. They went through several editions prepared by the author himself – the *editio Leydensis* was authoritative – but they were also reprinted surreptitiously in France, Italy and Germany. Moreover, translations into modern languages began to appear within a few years. In Britain plagiarized editions, adaptations and translations began to appear from the year of 1714 for the *Institutes*, and from 1715 for the *Aphorisms*.[8]

The course of lectures on the *Institutes*, which Boerhaave delivered in 1710 and in which he gave an extensive introduction to the study of medicine, was worked up by some English pupils into the spurious book entitled *A Method of studying Physick* (London, 1719). Though Burton attributes 'many blunders and absurdities' to this work, it seems to give a very good idea of Boerhaave's teaching, and in any case it was very successful. It was reprinted, adapted, and also translated into Latin, and ultimately corrected by no less a man than Haller.[9]

Finally, when Haller, after the death of his Master, edited the *Institutes* together with the lectures Boerhaave had delivered on them, this six-volume work also appeared in English and was reprinted nine times. In this way the essence of the Leyden medical teaching became extensively available in Britain for all those who were interested in a systematic exposition of the theory and practice of medicine.[10]

But it was not his books but his lectures that made the deepest impression on Boerhaave's own pupils, and this statement is especially true of his clinical demonstrations in the old St. Caecilia Hospital.

Until 1637 medical education at Leyden University, as in all other medical schools on this side of the Alps, did not include clinical instruction. Bedside teaching to classes of students was initiated at Padua about the middle of the sixteenth century. In Western Europe clinical teaching was given for the first time in Holland in 1637, at Utrecht and at Leyden. However, at Utrecht it was not continued for long, and even at Leyden, where two of the professors had to give it in turn for a period of three months, the Curators had to take special action in order to keep it going. Again and again it was neglected. Such a period occurred after the death of Govert Bidloo, who had been physician to William III of England, in the year of 1714, when Boerhaave was Rector Magnificus of the University. It was perhaps at his own request that bedside teaching was now entrusted to Boerhaave, and for nearly a quarter of a century he gave it enthusiastically to larger and larger classes. Many of the students who passed through the gateway of that hospital were to become leading physicians in their own countries in later years.

BOERHAAVE AND EDINBURGH

Boerhaave must have appreciated very greatly his election in 1730 as a Fellow of the Royal Society, on the proposal of its Secretary, Cromwell Mortimer, who had been one of his own pupils. In view of the high esteem in which Boerhaave was held in Britain and his eminence in science and in medicine, his election came rather late in his career.[11] However, the prosperous development of the young Medical School at Edinburgh must have given him even greater satisfaction. First of all – Boerhaave was a teacher, a devoted, enthusiastic and indefatigable teacher. With unceasing efforts he endeavoured to raise the standard of medical education. His shining example must have inspired the four young men, John Rutherford, John Innes, Andrew St. Clair and Andrew Plummer, who started at Edinburgh in 1724 on their own initiative courses in medical subjects. From this beginning a complete Medical Faculty developed within a few years, and this Faculty, modelled on the Leyden pattern, became the foremost in Great Britain during the whole of the eighteenth century. Boerhaave's textbooks were used there and the spirit of Boerhaave dominated all the teaching. His authority remained unshaken for decades. William Cullen (1710–90), remembering his medical education at Edinburgh, wrote: 'I learned the system of Boerhaave; and except it maybe the names of some ancient writers, of Sydenham, and a few other practical authors, I heard of no other names or writers on physic; and I was taught to think the system of Boerhaave to be very perfect, complete and sufficient.'

After his appointment as professor of the theory of medicine at Edinburgh in 1766 Cullen took the liberty of differing from Boerhaave on some points, but he immediately met with severe criticism as 'a whimsical innovator'. He was requested to 'avoid differing from Dr. Boerhaave' as such behaviour 'was likely to hurt himself [myself] and the University'.[12]

CONCLUSION

We owe to one of Boerhaave's English pupils, William Burton, the first biography, a carefully written *Account of the Life and Writings of Herman Boerhaave.* In the Preface of his book he justifies his undertaking, saying that it seemed 'strange, that four years should elapse from the death of Dr. Boerhaave, e'er any *separate* Piece on his Life and Writings appear'd in the language of *that people*, from whom, during a length of time, he received singular encouragement, whilst they in return have been proportionally benefited by his skill, and precepts'.[13]

Perhaps the debt of British medicine to Boerhaave has been best expressed by Charles Singer, who summed up his appreciation of Boerhaave in two statements. First: 'Through his pupils he is the real founder of the Edinburgh Medical School, and through it of the best medical teaching in the English-speaking countries of the world' in the eighteenth century.[14] And secondly: 'Taking one thing with another, considering his influence as a teacher, his clinical acumen, his power of inspiring younger workers, his wide learning, his balanced vision, his eagerness for new knowledge, his sanity, his humanity, his generosity, and his prophetic power, Boerhaave must be regarded as the greatest physician of modern times. To him the debt of British medicine, and through it of British well-being, is quite incalculable.'[14]

References

1 John James matriculated on 21 September 1578, and in 1581 he was the second man to graduate in medicine.

2 BELLERS, J., *An Essay Towards the Improvement of Physick*, London, 1714, pp. 7, 14.

3 KROON, J. E., 'Boerhaave as Professor-Promotor', *Janus*, 1918, **23**, 291–311.

4 UNDERWOOD, E. ASHWORTH, 'English-speaking medical students at Leyden', *Nature, Lond.*, 1969, **221**, 810–14.

5 COMRIE, J. D., 'Boerhaave and the Early Medical School at Edinburgh', in *Memorialia Herman Boerhaave Optimi medici*, Haarlem, Bohn, 1939, p. 33.

6 LINDEBOOM, G. A., *Boerhaave's Correspondence*, Leiden, Brill, 1962, vol. 1, p. 191.

7 Ibid. pp. 225, 227.

8 LINDEBOOM, G. A., *Bibliographia Boerhaaviana*, Leiden, 1959, pp. 33, 38, 46.

9 BURTON, W., *An Account of the Life and Writings of Herman Boerhaave*, London, 1743, p. 225.

10 The genealogy of the Latin edition, entitled *Methodus discendi artem medicam* and *Methodus discendi medicinam* is not quite clear. Haller gave the book the name *Methodus studii medici* (*Bibliogr. Boerh.*, pp. 36–37, 98–103).

11 For the possible reasons see G. A. Lindeboom, *Herman Boerhaave. The Man and His Work*, London, Methuen, 1968, pp.170–71.

12 THOMPSON, JOHN, *An Account of the Life, Lectures and Writings of William Cullen*, 2 vols., Edinburgh, London, 1859, vol. I, pp. 118–19; quoted by L. E. King, *The Medical World of the Eighteenth Century*, Chicago, 1958, pp. 59–60.

13 BURTON, W., loc. cit., p. 11.

14 SINGER, CHARLES, *A Short History of Medicine*, Oxford, 1928, pp. 140, 142. E. A. Underwood, in his revised and greatly enlarged second edition of this work (Oxford, 1967, pp. 149–50), allowed these sentences to stand unaltered as expressing also his own view.

G. S. Rousseau
Los Angeles, California (U.S.A.)

Mandeville and Europe: medicine and philosophy

Bernard Mandeville, born about 1670 in Holland and died in 1733 in London, remains one of the least well-known figures of European intellectual history. Almost nothing of substance is known about his life except that he studied medicine in Leyden in the 1680s, later settled for unknown reasons in London where he never acquired practice or reputation, and was known in distilling circles only. A lack of extant documents and the further unlikelihood that any will ever come to light, cast permanent gloom on the possibility of knowing the man firsthand.[1] Whatever reputation he thus far possesses rests upon a single iconoclastic work *The Fable of the Bees*, published in 1714, a large Hobbesian tome attempting to prove systematically that 'private vice is public good' and that the whole social order rests upon this rudimentary but quintessential principle. Fourteen other published works are attributed to Mandeville, all relatively brief and inconsequential except one, *A Treatise of Hypochondriack and Hysterick Passions*, first published in 1711.[2] This work amounting to 280 quarto pages is almost as long as *The Fable of the Bees* but has gone unnoticed and unappreciated for two and a half centuries except for a brief word of praise from Dr. Johnson,[3] and while its contents are not nearly so radical its obscurity among medical historians remains somewhat mysterious.[4] No one, it seems, has actually bothered to read it.

The *Treatise* is cast in the form of three dialogues between a physician Philopirio and his patient Misomedon; Misomedon's wife Polytheca, their daughter, and a druggist named Pharmaenio also enter into the dialogue as minor figures, but the first two, physician and patient, are the main characters. Misomedon suffers from the hyp,[5] as do his wife and daughter, but he is also manic-depressive and undergoing male menopause; Philopirio, the model of a competent physician and Mandeville's mouthpiece,[6] attempts to cure all three. By the conclusion Philopirio has prescribed such an extensive programme of remedies that Misomedon, who promises to follow his advice, is kept too busy to contemplate his aches and pains. Philopirio doubtlessly espouses Mandeville's own beliefs, but since absolutely nothing is known about Mandeville as a physician, one cannot get anywhere by taking this line as a strategy for explication and interpretation. The Misomedon family, on the other hand, are *hypochondriaci*, all suffering from the conventional symptoms: fits, flutters, flushes, indigestion, heart pain, headaches, sore eyes, and of course wild flights of the imagination and bizarre dreams.

So far nothing indicates that the *Treatise* deserves more attention than dozens of other similar works written throughout the seventeenth and eighteenth centuries in England and on the Continent: and even Mandeville's flair for language, his quick wit and biting satire, cannot compensate, one might well argue, for a lack of new material on the matter. After all, both hypochondriasis and hysteria were prevalent, popular diseases and by 1700 enough ink had been spilled about both to render still another book on the subject gratuitous – *liber non grata*. Ever since the Renaissance and probably before then, physicians, surgeons, barbers, apothecaries, empirics, quacks, nurses, and even handmaidens had prescribed for this curiously nebulous ailment which few understood and even fewer could cure; by 1700 one became afflicted with it almost as one faces rain and slush in winter – with the sure knowledge that both are unpleasant and that do what one may they will again return. At least from the time of Burton's prescriptions in the *Anatomy* to the giant moneymaking cures of the eighteenth century, every pill and potion, powder and water, had failed.[7] Why then, one might ask, bother with a single treatise about the hyp? Merely because it was written by the heterodox Mandeville? Surely this answer will not suffice as a valid reason for considering the work important or even of mild interest to the history of medicine.

Other reasons exist, not all of them immediately apparent on a first reading. For example, from the Renaissance to the nineteenth century the literature of hypochondria, especially in England, is an impoverished literature.[8] Few, if any, works contain the substance of Burton's and most are like Sir John Hill's treatise of 1766, a paltry and hastily written handbook of sixty pages professing to be a *vade mecum* for the patient but in fact a parade of the author's own penchant for spleenwort, root of valerian, bardana, and other ineffective herbs he was then growing in his lucrative garden at Bayswater.[9] Mandeville's treatise rises far above such works by taking its subject more seriously and by investigating the relation of melancholy to non-medical aspects of culture generally. In both areas Mandeville was ahead of his time, and if his argument is not put forward with the same brilliant originality one discovers in *The Fable*, also a dialogue, this can be held against him to a degree only since he was politically radical and medically conservative. For the purposes of clarity and brevity I have summed up his achievement, at least as it appears to me, in ten distinct categories:[10]

1. DEFINITION

Mandeville believes that the *condition*, hardly a single disease, encompasses so many different symptoms and courses of treatment that it is meta-definitional. He therefore indicates at considerable length why hypochondria or hysteria cannot be reduced to a *single* disease, and he never hazards definitions that would be painfully simple-minded and clinically reductionistic to knowledgeable men; but unlike most other writers, he is nevertheless acutely sensitive to the definitional problem, one not altogether dissimilar from that attached to neurosis in this century.[11] So many medical authors of his period still adhered to the old conception of hyp as a *single* ailment, pasteurized, homogenized, and packaged, as it were, into one person that Mandeville's treatise stands out solitary. Just why the hyp evolved into the English malady *par excellence* is another matter[12]; what counts here is Mandeville's grasp of it as a complex system of behavioural conditions arising from a large number of different sources, not merely the usual ones, solitude, sedentary life, too much reading, and so forth.

2. CURABILITY VERSUS INCURABILITY

Something of a paradox exists here: the title-page advertises the *Treatise* as one 'in which the Symptoms, Causes, and Cures of those [hypochondriacal] Diseases are set forth after a Method intirely new', as if to suggest that cure exists, and yet Philopirio makes it perfectly clear that no real cure exists at all.[13] Whatever the name given to the cluster of conditions or constellation of diseases designated by the term hypochondriasis Mandeville believes that most, if not all, cases are virtually hopeless. The phrase 'incurable' is actually used (p. 200) and there can be no doubt about Mandeville's drift: although Philopirio prescribes extensive lists of drugs and activities, especially exercise, for his melancholic patients and is optimistic to the extent of feigning cheerfulness, he does so with a knowledge of their incurability. This inner sense of ultimate incurability is rare in seventeenth- and eighteenth-century treatises and anticipates later theory.[14] Mandeville sees some hope for partial cure through strengthening of the doctor–patient relationship, an attachment not often commented upon in medical treatises at the turn of the eighteenth century.[15] Here one sniffs the seeds of the complicated process called 'transference' in modern psychiatry, a subtle and elusive concept that theoreticians today are just beginning to comprehend, especially in the realm of child psychiatry.

3. 'A PRIORI' AND 'A POSTERIORI' REASONING

Observation and empiricism are the sole worthy guides in the treatment of disease according to Mandeville, and for this reason Philopirio must evaluate each hypochondriacal case on its own terms as a medically unique phenomenon. Mandeville entertains no preconceived notion whatsoever about the form a particular case may take, his wisdom deriving largely from definitional sophistication but also from experience in treating patients for several decades. While there is nothing unusual about the presence of *a posteriori* reasoning in medical treatises of the eighteenth century, it is a rare work that espouses it at the beginning of the period over *a priori* reasoning *both in theory and in practice*. In a survey of medical treatises written in England from 1700 to 1800, I discovered that the former type of reasoning overtakes the latter in both realms, theory and practice, after 1740 and does not really establish itself until the 1770s.[16]

4. NECESSARY AND ADEQUATE CONDITIONS

Mandeville disqualifies *necessary* conditions on definitional grounds and replaces them with *adequate* conditions; in other words four or five symptoms are sufficient to indicate the presence of the condition but no specific four or five are necessary.[17] The distinction between these conditions is subtle and not commonly found in the literature of melancholy until the mid-nineteenth century, certainly not as a guiding methodological principle.

5. THE 'PROCATARCTIC CAUSE'

Mandeville believes that the hyp, unlike most other diseases, is not occasioned by bodily disturbances but by external, non-bodily conditions; thus his insistence on the physician's discovery of a procatarctic, or external, cause. Stated in less antiquated terms, Mandeville would consider it unlikely that a young or middle-aged woman who manifested all the typical signs of hypochondria could be dying from hypoglycaemia; her hypoglycaemia could be the bodily manifestation of an external procatarctic agent, usually some disturbance in her environment, but the origin of the entire condition could not be hypoglycaemia. In distinguishing internal and external agents, and, beyond that, secondary bodily manifestations, Mandeville's work is important in the history of the psychosomatic theory of medicine. Nowhere in the writings of Cheyne, Robinson, or Highmore, for example, is a 'procatarctic cause' so clearly delineated nor does it determine so clearly the author's argument.[18]

6. RELATION OF THE 'PROCATARCTIC CAUSE' AND THE PHYSIOLOGICAL ASPECTS OF HYPOCHONDRIASIS

Although the condition usually originates in external sources, it naturally manifests itself later in the body, and Mandeville spends much time demolishing theories that incorrectly account for the role of the stomach, spleen, brain, and animal spirits in its mechanical phases. Space here does not permit a detailed analysis of Mandeville's grasp of the functions of these organs, but while he is not truly original he distinguishes well between superior and inferior anatomists and relies on the best ones for his purposes. For example, he recognizes the valuable contribution that Willis's brain theory makes to diagnosis and treatment of the hyp and he discards lesser theorists whom time has proved inconsequential. Furthermore, he believes that the animal spirits play a smaller role once the condition is actually underway than do his contemporaries, and he assigns a greater role to the brain – as if to suggest that throughout its course the illness is more psychological than physiological.[19]

7. THE TREATISE AS A DOCUMENT IN THE HISTORY OF MEDICINE

Obviously it is impossible to rate documents according to any yardstick of measurement other than extremely concrete ones. Nevertheless some works are clearly more important than others for a great variety of reasons including direct and indirect influence. While Mandeville's *Treatise* was not influential either as a direct source or an indirect system of medical thinking it is one of the lengthiest treatments ever given to the hyp; and if it cannot hope to assume the importance of Burton's *Anatomy of Melancholy* or Cheyne's *English Malady*, it will nevertheless fascinate students of Mandeville's thinking in general as well as historians of psychiatry. But most of all it must engross historians of medicine whose range is far and wide because of the variety of subjects it treats, for example rationalism and empiricism, estimates of seventeenth-century medicine in the eyes of a practising eighteenth-century physician, the quarrel of the Ancients and the Moderns, the decline of Galenism, the role of book learning in actual treatment, theories of venereal disease, the relative merits of the medical schools of Europe, controversies over the chemical nature and mechanical operations of the animal spirits, the anatomical function of the stomach in digestion and of the brain in thinking, and many others – these will arrest at least the passing interest of medical historians. Moreover, this work represents philosophical medicine at its best,[20] always centred on its avowed topic but perpetually aware of the larger implications, historically and medically, of its subject matter.

8. THE TREATISE AS A LITERARY DOCUMENT

Literary critics are just beginning to appreciate Mandeville's satirical gifts, especially his penchant for irony and rhetorical inversion.[21] These talents abound in the *Treatise*, itself a satire of bad doctors, bad patients, and false medical reasoning, addressed primarily to an audience of patients rather than doctors; in addition it is logically organized and well written. Too little, however, has been written about the dialogue tradition in English literature to assign it an unequivocal role,[22] but one can fairly say that dialogue here admirably serves the author's purposes: through Philopirio Mandeville is able to speak autobiographically (a liberty he does not even take in the *Fable*), and his three other characters allow him to demonstrate important varieties of the hyp plus such qualities as Misomedon's pedantic learning in, yet amateur knowledge of, medicine. Because the treatise is ostensibly medical in content it cannot hope to interest such a wide audience as can the *Fable*; but if literary historians could somehow transcend their feelings that the history of medicine is entirely a technical and specialized subject remote from their (the literary men's) domain, they would discover here a document every bit as polished and tightly organized, especially in its well-wrought preface, as *The Fable*.

9. THE TREATISE AS A SOCIOLOGICAL DOCUMENT

Statistically speaking at least half the *Treatise* is devoted to subjects other than hypochondriasis, to the quarrel between physicians and apothecaries, to the true duties of different types of medical men, to the role of hypotheses in medical theory, and to such seemingly remote topics – remote, that is, from the hyp – as diet and exercise. In considering all these subjects Mandeville demonstrates more than a usual grasp of the social dimensions of illness, a deep sense that medicine, even in its abstractest theories about the aetiology and pathology of disease, remains firmly tied down to social processes – to economics, politics, education, and even to language. Among all these diverse social topics Mandeville devotes the greatest space to two matters, the quarrels between the physicians and the apothecaries, and the role of the physician in society-at-large.

Regarding the first, Mandeville sums up the arguments on both sides and maintains throughout an objective, almost dispassionate, stance: while he himself probably continued to practise medicine as a physician throughout his life, he understands the grievances of the apothecaries.[23] Here it is not an adjudication in favour of one side or another that matters but rather Mandeville's acute understanding that the dispute had greater social ramifications than his contemporaries imagined – that it was the symptom of a deep malaise, *au fond* economic but also signifying the emergence of professional groups within a single vocation.[24] By devoting so much attention to the dispute he underscored its social relevance, especially the role of pride within a professional group and the psychological way in which group jealousies manifest themselves professionally.

Regarding the second, the physician's role, I have discovered no other work written in English in the eighteenth century, with the exception of Smollett's inimitable satires,[25] which grasps so well as Mandeville's the overarching role of a physician, his strengths and weaknesses, frailties and foibles, potentials and limitations. It is indeed no exaggeration to say that Mandeville, writing almost 300 years ago, has prophetically anticipated the medical problems facing such a nation as the U.S.A., for example, in which present-day discussions about socialized medicine evolve around the physician's conception of himself as an economic creature, a social creature, an ethical and, of course, a professional creature diagnosing and curing illness.[26] Mandeville's originality on this subject includes the radical notion that a doctor is nothing more than the sum of what his society imagines him to be; if he is imagined as the Godhead, omniscient and infallible, he, the physician, will attempt to fulfil this imagined posture even though he knows that such a stance engages him in pretension and outright dishonesty. For precisely this reason Misomedon is made to conceive of Philopirio in impossibly grandiose terms missing no opportunity to display his (Misomedon's) learning in medicine; and also for this reason Philopirio is portrayed as humbler and less dishonest than many practising hyp physicians of his time. Eighteenth-century medical writers adhere, whether they are aware of it or not, to a typology of the physician and Mandeville stands on the side of those who would melodramatically diminish his profits, radically alter his role, and therefore hopefully enlarge his true medical calling within the community.[27]

10. MEDICINE, A SCIENCE OR AN ART?

Finally, the treatise must be viewed as one more link in the long chain of seventeenth- and eighteenth-century debates about the status of medicine as a science or an art.[28] Mandeville's unequivocal insistence *on experience* as the essential attribute of every good physician leaves no doubt about his opinion of the matter: if book learning and school training are worthwhile, experience alone teaches the doctor to cure, i.e. to fathom the secrets of Nature. Medical treatment therefore requires more skill than knowledge, and is at bottom an art. Here, again, the prophetic Mandeville anticipates a future debate, one that hardly died in his own epoch but that continued to gather momentum in the next two centuries, in fact one that remains far from a satisfactory solution in 1972.

References

1 The available sources are very few; there are less than a dozen letters revealing almost nothing, no diaries, journals, or commonplace books, and no biography other than the brief life in the *Dictionary of National Biography* and in F. B. Kaye's introduction to his scholarly edition of *The Fable of the Bees* (Oxford, Clarendon Press, 1924, 2 vols.). The legend that Mandeville's commonplace book is extant and housed in the library of the Earl of Macclesfield in Oxfordshire has now been disproved by G. S. Rousseau in 'Mandeville and the First Earl of Macclesfield', *Notes and Queries*, 1971, **216**, 335. If Mandeville's biographical statements in the *Treatise* are true, this adds considerably to our meagre knowledge about him. See below, n. 6.

2 In London by Dryden Leach, 'in Elliot's Court, in the Little-Old-Baily, and W. Taylor, at the Ship in Pater-Noster-Row'. Although Dryden Leach was a well-known London printer (see Plomer, *Dictionary of the Printers and Booksellers . . . in England 1726–1775*, Oxford, Oxford

University Press, 1932, p. 151), nothing is known about the circumstances of publication of Mandeville's *Treatise*. According to records in the Stationers' Hall it was entered against the name of 'B. de Mandeville Feb. 27 1710/11', his only work listed there.

3 BOSWELL, JAMES, *The Life of Samuel Johnson, LL.D.*, London, 1791, 2 vols., vol. 2, p. 107.

4 Both in conventional medical histories and works solely devoted to the history of hypochondriasis. Here one could compile a long list of important secondary works that omit it.

5 Abbreviated form of hypochondriasis used in the eighteenth century in common parlance and throughout this paper.

6 No reason exists to disbelieve Mandeville's statement in the preface, p. xi: 'In these Dialogues, I have done the same as *Seneca* did in his *Octavia*, and brought my self upon the Stage; with this difference, that he kept his own Name, and I changed mine for that of Philopirio, a Lover of Experience, which I shall always profess to be; Wherefore I desire my Reader to take whatever is spoke by the Person I name last, as said by my self.' Even the author's vigorous irony and calculated rhetoric of understatement should not lead us to distrust this important remark. Nor should his disclosures about his father's medical practice in Holland and the social standing of his family be discredited, a significant utterance because so little is known about Mandeville's family background: 'The two Populous Cities there meant, are *Amsterdam* and *Rotterdam*; in the latter of which, the Physician mention'd in the same Place, lived in Repute above Thirty Years, and for the greatest part of that time in Request among the better sort of People than any other; as no body can be ignorant of, that lived there before the Year 92, and knew any thing at all' (p. xii). If Mandeville's statement about his own career as a physician is true, then we perhaps ought to revise our conception of his medical practice: 'Mine [my thesis] was *de Chylosi vitiata*, which I defended at Leyden in the Year 1691, Dr. *William Senguerdus*, Professor of the Aristotelian Philosophy, being then *Rector Magnificus*. My reason of telling you this, which otherwise might seem impertinent, is because I have often thought it very remarkable, that I always had a particular Eye upon, and have been led, as it were, by instinct to what afterwards appear'd to be the cause of the Hysteric and Hypochondriack Passions, even at a time, when I had no thought of singling out these Distempers for my particular Study, and was only design'd for general Practice, as other Physicians are' (p. 121).

7 In the sense that only incidental, fortuitous cure was obtained; obviously the problem is somewhat circular: one cannot cure a condition that one knows little about.

8 On several counts: (1) as well-written literature; (2) insofar as it deals with its ostensible subject of discourse; (3) regarding originality and the relationship of intuition and execution of such intuition; (4) in the degree to which it plundered and plagiarized from other authors; and most important, (5) in taking itself far too seriously to permit truly spontaneous flashes. Some sense of this literature may be found in Ilza Veith, *Hysteria, The History of a Disease* (Chicago, University of Chicago Press, 1964); John Sena's recent bibliographical survey of works on melancholy 1600–1800; and Lawrence Babb, *The Elizabethan Malady: A Study in Melancholia in English Literature from 1580 to 1642* (East Lansing, Michigan State College, 1951).

9 ROUSSEAU, G. S., *Sir John Hill: The Life of a London Literary Quack*, 1973, in press, chap. vi, 'Hill's Herbal Remedies'.

10 Obviously there are others, for example Mandeville's indebtedness to other writers, but extensive revision of these sections has persuaded me that these categories are the most important.

11 Every psychiatrist or historian of twentieth-century psychological jargon will agree with this observation, that a distinction must be drawn. The term neurotic poses vast definitional problems as soon as it is brought, as it were, into the realm of society: for example, society considers it 'neurotic' to be a 'neurotic compulsive worker', yet the question is begged whether that so-called neurotic condition is any more neurotic than equally irrational modes of mass behaviour, such as the cigarette smoking condoned by much of society. How then does one adequately define neurotic? Similar difficulties exist for the term hypochondriacal or melancholic at the turn of the eighteenth century, a term which by then had become so various in its meanings that Mandeville saw the urgent need for a discrimination of 'hyps', or barring that, the meaninglessness of the term altogether. See *Treatise*, pp. 210 ff.

12 Some reasons have been offered by Cecil A. Moore in *Backgrounds of English Literature, 1700–1760*, Minneapolis, University of Minnesota Press, 1953.

13 See his final programme of remedies beginning on p. 255 of the *Treatise*. Misomedon is to be kept so busy taking purges and vomits that he will literally not have the time to realize he has not been cured.

14 This intuitive sense of the incurability of major diseases is almost non-existent among Mandeville's contemporaries. While numerous medical authors admit to having no certain remedy for a particular disease, almost all express the certainty of being on the verge of the discovery of one; and it was precisely this certainty in cure that caused physicians of the mid- and late eighteenth century to criticize earlier ones. Mandeville's extraordinary trust in 'experience' over

'reason' taught him that the hyp frequently cannot be cured at all, and engendered in him a type of medical scepticism about cure in general.

15 Many passages make this point perfectly clear, as, for example, *Treatise*, preface, p. iv.

16 ROUSSEAU, G. S., ' "Sowing the Wind and Reaping the Rain": Rationalism and Empiricism in Eighteenth-Century Medicine', in *Studies in Change and Revolution: Aspects of English Intellectual History 1640–1800*, ed. P. J. Korshin, London, Scolar Press, 1972, pp. 129–59. The matter is of course more complicated than this and involves the whole history of critical thinking in medicine, not merely the somewhat artificial division into 'reason' and 'experience'; and because Mandeville favoured experience over reason, his hero, as stated in the preface (pp. iv–v), is Baglivi. Like Baglivi, he, too, distinguished sharply between theory and practice, diminishing greatly the value of reason in practice, as seen throughout Philopirio's prescriptions. In the realm of theory, Philopirio's briefest and clearest statement is made on p. 269 of the *Treatise*: 'The reason you [Misomedon] give may be good for ought I know: Being made *a Posteriori*, it cannot mislead us, yet it is far from being satisfactory to me.' Throughout the study of the role of reason and experience in medical writing, I have benefited from the work of Dr. Lester King.

17 See, for example, p. 80. Here, again, experience alone is a worthy guide.

18 To prove this rigorously one would naturally have to read many treatises about a single disease and then show the absence of a procatarctic cause; this I have undertaken for the hyp and find Mandeville's work fairly singular. See my introduction to the Augustan Reprint Society Edition of John Hill's *Hypochondriasis: A Practical Treatise 1766*, Los Angeles, California, 1969, pp. i–xiii. Also influencing Mandeville's theory of a procatarctic cause is his intuitive sense of the hyp as forming part of a realm of non-physiological conditions having somatic consequences. While he does not carry his ideas very far, he does intimate time and again that medicine must explore this nebulous region of illness. Mandeville, in any case, is not a systematic thinker in medicine (in the sense that Linnaeus was in botany) but he does have a considerable 'medical intuition' that guides him well.

19 See, for example, *Treatise*, p. 277, in which Philopirio forbids the use of redundant medicines 'in all Distempers, but more especially those [like the hyp], in which the Fancy has so great a share, and the least trifle is of moment.' These and other similar remarks reveal the large role of 'Fancy' in the aetiology of the condition.

20 A type of medical writing that did not really get under way until the 1760s and which flourishes in the writings of Drs. Robert Whytt, William Cullen and John Brown.

21 PRICE, MARTIN, *To the Palace of Wisdom: Studies in Energy and Order*, New York, Doubleday, 1962, pp. 122–37; Robert Hopkins, 'The Cant of Social Compromise: Some Observations on Mandeville's Satire', in *Mandeville Tercentenary Essays*, ed. Irwin Primer, *in press*. Other essays in this opulent volume also are devoted to Mandeville's style.

22 Standard works say little about the eighteenth century altogether, leaving out such important works as Hume's *Dialogues of Natural Religion* and Mandeville's *Fable of the Bees*. In the case of the *Treatise*, the dialogue form draws attention to the doctor-patient relationship, which Mandeville considers therapeutic and beneficial to cure, if incorporating a strong sense of trust.

23 See *Treatise*, pp. 215–20, 260 ff. The quarrel had flared up during the 1690s and again at the turn of the eighteenth century, but Mandeville's lengthy descriptions do more than state the case for each side: they present the strengths and weaknesses with detached, almost dispassionate understanding.

24 The organization of various medical groups with different professional aims at the turn of the eighteenth century has not received attention except in passing. See, for example, Sir George N. Clark's *A History of the Royal College of Physicians*, Oxford, The Clarendon Press, 1964–66, 2 vols. A sociology of medicine, taking account of these professional developments, is badly needed.

25 Especially in *Humphry Clinker* and *Peregrine Pickle*. Smollett's vision is essentially negative, concentrating the thrust of its energetic attack on all those abominable qualities physicians seemed to have acquired since the Restoration: pride, smugness, pretence, obsession with lucre, heartless disconcern if they cured or killed. In some deep ways Mandeville and Smollett are not so far apart: they were both physicians, both practised, and both intuitively aware of the foibles of medical men.

26 Here, again, Mandeville's medical intuition, as I have been calling it, has proved right. At a recent meeting in April 1972 in Washington, D.C., young doctors were told by senior medical officers of the medical profession that they should make all the money they expected to make in the next seven or eight years, for by 1980 American doctors would be earning just about the same as other workers – i.e. socialized medicine. This is, of course, not the case at present, when doctors are probably the very highest paid members of any profession.

27 The typology is complex and changed from decade to decade; for example, the 'pedantic Canting Physician', as one medical author calls it, remained a stock image throughout the century, while the 'lucre-seeking mongrels', described by another, faded in and out. I have attempted to survey

the typology of doctors throughout the century in *Doctors and Medicine in the Novels of Tobias Smollett*, Princeton University Ph.D. Dissertation, 1966, chap. i.

28 The standard histories of medicine (Garrison, Castiglione, Singer, etc.) say very little about this debate; to find anything substantial about it the student must look in periodical literature, articles. In any case, almost nothing to my knowledge has been written about the debate in the eighteenth century; and while it is not usually of prime concern to that century, say to the extent that whole works are devoted to the question, it does play a role as a *topos* in a great deal of medical writing.

R. E. Wright-St. Clair
Hamilton (New Zealand)

The Edinburgh influence on New Zealand medicine

New Zealand became a British colony in 1840. Before the town of Auckland was established as the capital in 1841 the area was inhabited by Maoris and two white men, one of whom was John Logan Campbell, M.D., M.R.C.S. Edinburgh. He had been the first person to graduate M.D. *in absentia* from Edinburgh and the Senatus Academicus had to establish a special procedure for him to do so because he was on the point of emigrating to the colonies. When the Colonial Government officers arrived to establish the new capital Campbell set up a trading establishment. He did not practise medicine but he was a very successful merchant. Later he entered local politics and became a Member of Parliament, Superintendent of Auckland Province (a sort of provincial governor) and Mayor of the city. He is remembered today as Auckland's greatest benefactor, the giver of parks and endowments which have created much of the character of Auckland.

The primitive society of the new colony had only a limited use for doctors. The population consisted of the indigenous Maoris who, although they had been afflicted with white man's bacteria, were on the whole suspicious of white man's medicine, and immigrant Europeans, mostly of British stock, who had come through the rigours of five or six months under sail across stormy seas. Those who were not determined did not set out on the voyage and those who were not hardy did not survive it, so that the colonists were a selected group. Those who had money used it to buy land and stock it, and although the land eventually gave them a good return its value was in capital accretion rather than in quick profits. The working-class immigrants had mostly used their life savings for the voyage out and spent their new lives saving again; if they succeeded they too put their money into land. So there was little affluence in the colony.

A young, healthy, impecunious, hard-working people imbued with Victorian fatalism towards child mortality gave little employment to doctors, and a population thinly scattered over the country in small settlements separated by mountainous and heavily forested terrain was not conducive to easy practice. The immigrant doctor, however, had his sound classical education and usually a little money behind him. In the colonial community with no aristocracy of birth to form its ruling class and where the landed gentry were too busy with their sheep to form a leisured class, the doctor became a natural leader and many of them proved to be very able politicians.

Andrew Sinclair, M.D. Edinburgh, was Colonial Secretary, the chief administrator before representative government. Isaac Earl Featherston, M.D. Edinburgh, was a member of the first Parliament and first Superintendent of Wellington Province. J. A. R. Menzies, M.R.C.S. Edinburgh, was a Member of Parliament and first Superintendent of Southland. Ralph Richardson, M.D. Edinburgh, was a Nelson settler who became a member of the first Parliament. Sir David Monro, M.D. Edinburgh, son of Professor Alexander Monro *tertius*, was a leader of the Nelson settlement, a member of the first Parliament and the second Speaker of the House of Representatives.

There is thus no doubt about the influence of Edinburgh medicine on New Zealand politics which were shaping the character of the colony. For a few early years New Zealand was divided into two provinces. The southern province, called New Munster, introduced medical registration several years before the United Kingdom. The proposal was no doubt based on Thomas Wakley's unsuccessful bills in 1846 and 1847 in the House of Commons. David Monro, one of the Edinburgh doctors mentioned above, was a member of the Legislative Council of the province and although he was not the originator of the scheme for medical registration he gave it powerful support and assisted materially in assuring its passage through the council. This scheme came into effect in 1850.

When representative government was introduced in 1853 the Province of New Munster was abolished and its medical registration died with it. The colony was then divided into six provinces with a central Parliament. In Wellington, formerly part of New Munster, the Provincial Council tried to continue medical registration but was frustrated by the Superintendent, Isaac Featherston, another Edinburgh doctor, who was opposed to registration. After an abortive attempt in the central Parliament in 1860, led by Drs. Menzies and Monro, registration eventually came in for the whole colony in 1867. The first president of the registering board was Sir James Hector, M.D. Edinburgh, F.R.S. Hector was a geologist who did not practise medicine. He is remembered in Canada as the discoverer of the Kicking Horse Pass and in New Zealand as the great doyen of science in the late nineteenth century.

The country round Otago harbour in the South Island of New Zealand was settled in 1848 by a group of immigrants belonging to the Free Church of Scotland. The principal town of the settlement was named 'Dunedin', the old and poetic name for Edinburgh. This new Edinburgh carried to the antipodes many of the traditions of the Scottish metropolis: the street names were all there, the Scottish love of education was there, what more natural than that a university and medical school should be established? Dunedin had a population of less than 15,000 when the University of Otago was founded in 1869, but after all Edinburgh had been little larger when its university was established in the sixteenth century.

The University of Otago was established as a teaching and degree-giving institution on the Scottish model but after several years of wrangling it gave up its right to grant degrees in favour of the University of New Zealand, an examining body on the original London model. This arrangement lasted for ninety years. Medicine was one of the subjects included in the Provincial Act incorporating Otago University but for a start there was no medical school. One of the first four professors appointed was an Edinburgh medical graduate, Duncan Macgregor, M.B., C.M., but his appointment was as Professor of Mental and Moral Philosophy for he had had a brilliant career in classics and philosophy before taking up medicine.

Although Macgregor was never a member of the staff of Dunedin Hospital he took charge of the first case treated in New Zealand on the antiseptic principles which he had learned from Lister in Edinburgh. It was a case of a compound comminuted fracture of the forearm which occurred in 1872. The patient did well and the new method was thereafter adopted in Dunedin. Macgregor was a charismatic teacher of commanding stature who was to have a profound influence on the future of medical practice in the colony. He served for twenty years as Inspector-General of Hospitals, in which capacity he laid many of the foundations of the present public hospital system of New Zealand. He also introduced state registration of nurses in 1902 and of midwives in 1904.

A medical school was ever close to the heart of Dunedin citizens with memories of Edinburgh, and in 1874 the first steps were taken to bring this school into being. James Gow Black, Professor of Natural Science, was an Edinburgh graduate. He was not a medical man but he held the first D.Sc. in chemistry ever granted in Edinburgh and his old University was prepared to grant recognition to his lectures in chemistry as part of a medical course. The post of Professor of Anatomy and Physiology was advertised at a salary of £600 with class fees. One of the eighteen applicants was D. J. Cunningham of Edinburgh, later famous as Professor of Anatomy there.

The appointee to this first medical chair in New Zealand was Millen Coughtrey, M.B., C.M. Edinburgh, who had worked as a demonstrator in Anatomy under that great Edinburgh teacher, Sir William Turner. A two-year course was proposed with students going to the United Kingdom to complete their training. The project was a failure and Professor Coughtrey resigned. Coughtrey was a competent practitioner who put unusual stress for that period on preventive medicine. He remained in practice in Dunedin and was the founder of the New Zealand Medical Association which became the New Zealand Branch of the British Medical Association and is now the Medical Association of New Zealand. Coughtrey should not perhaps be blamed for the failure of the medical school scheme which may well have been premature when the total European population of New Zealand at the time was 342,000 with 47,000 Maoris.

The University of Otago was certainly not discouraged by Coughtrey's resignation and decided to carry on with its medical course. Cunningham was approached for the anatomy chair but he was not available. When the post was advertised there were, surprisingly, twenty-five applicants. John Halliday Scott, M.D. Edinburgh, was appointed: he was aged twenty-five and was demonstrator in anatomy at Edinburgh. 'This was a most fortunate appointment for the young struggling school. The university and medical school secured a first-rate person of the highest personal character and with qualities academic and administrative which secured the future success of the medical school.' Professor Scott came to a primitive university and a non-existent medical school. With Scottish thoroughness he set quietly about establishing a school on the model that he knew from Edinburgh.

Although the Dunedin course was recognized in Glasgow, Dublin and London as well as in Edinburgh, it was to Edinburgh that nearly all the New Zealand students went to complete the course or to do the full course and their success was phenomenal. Many of them won prizes and gained distinction in Edinburgh. At least two of them served in the office of President of the Royal Medical Society.

Despite the success of New Zealand students in Edinburgh after the two-year course in Dunedin it was clear to Professor Scott that the truncated school should be completed. This was achieved in 1885 and the first graduate was capped in 1887. This was W. L. Christie who subsequently became Lord Mayor of Bristol. The qualifying degree was M.B., Ch.B., a style which Edinburgh did not adopt until after 1893. Even later many New Zealanders continued to go to mother Edinburgh to take the medical course. Until the establishment of the Auckland medical school, which will graduate its first students next year, Otago remained the sole medical school in the country.

Among subsequent Dunedin professors who were Edinburgh graduates six names stand out most prominently: Sir Louis Barnett, John Malcolm, Sydney Champtaloup, Murray Drennan, Frank Fitchett and Sir Gordon Bell. Sir Louis Barnett was one of the early students at Otago who graduated in Edinburgh. He returned to Dunedin where he became Professor of Surgery. He taught surgery to such leaders of the profession as Sir Archibald MacIndoe, Sir Arthur Porritt and Sir Douglas Robb: he was the first surgeon in New Zealand to wear rubber gloves and a mask while operating; he pioneered research into hydatid disease; he was founder and first President of the Royal Australasian College of Surgeons. John Malcolm was a Highland Scot who worked as assistant to Schafer in Edinburgh before being appointed Professor of Physiology at Otago in 1905, a post which he occupied for almost forty years. When Malcolm retired he had taught physiology to almost every member of the profession in New Zealand. I am just old enough to have learned my physiology from Malcolm who had learned it from William Rutherford and Edward Schafer in Edinburgh.

Sydney Champtaloup was a New Zealander who graduated in Edinburgh and then took the new chair of bacteriology and public health at Dunedin. He developed the new department with great vigour and ability. Although he died at a regrettably early age he had taught and strongly influenced his successor, Sir Charles Hercus, a powerful and long-serving Dean of the school. It was also through Champtaloup's influence that his fellow student from Edinburgh, Murray Drennan, came to Dunedin as Professor of Pathology. One of Drennan's important innovations was a teaching method he had learned from J. L. Smith, his former chief in Edinburgh, consisting of teaching Pathology on a disease basis rather than an organ basis and always closely related to clinical findings. Drennan and Hercus embarked on an active research programme on colloid goitre which was endemic in New Zealand. They proved that the fault was iodine lack in the soil and this has subsequently been remedied by iodized salt with virtual disappearance of the previously common simple goitres. Drennan subsequently returned to Edinburgh where he succeeded Smith in the chair of pathology.

Frank Fitchett and Sir Gordon Bell were both New Zealanders who graduated in Edinburgh. Fitchett became Professor of Clinical Medicine; he was an incomparable teacher and a great exponent of the art of clinical examination. He is remembered as a tremendous 'character', sharply intolerant of fools and the source of many entertaining anecdotes. Gordon Bell succeeded Sir Louis Barnett in the chair of surgery and taught sound clinical practice in surgery for almost thirty years. These two New Zealand-born Edinburgh graduates between them occupied the chair of surgery for nearly sixty years and dominated surgical teaching and practice in the Antipodes.

Of course there were members of the faculty who did not come from Edinburgh. Sir Lindo Ferguson, Scott's successor as Dean, was Scottish born but was educated and graduated in Dublin; he brought to Dunedin the earthy wisdom of the Irish school. Daniel Colquhoun, the first Professor of Medicine, was a Scot who graduated in London; he brought the dignity and urbanity of a London physician with a good touch of the gold-headed cane about him – a valuable influence among rough-and-ready colonials. Frank Ogston, the first Professor of Medical Jurisprudence and Public Health, was an Aberdonian and a member of a leading medical family in that city. Percy Gowland, Professor of Anatomy for thirty years, was from Manchester and brought a salty Lancashire tongue to Dunedin.

New Zealand medicine was therefore a hybrid. Like many other aspects of life in a new country it was of mixed descent with a strong overlay of colonial pragmatism; but the dominant strain was Edinburgh and that is the likeness that has remained.

In my own hospital, Waikato Hospital, Hamilton, established eighty-five years ago, the first Medical Superintendent was a Glasgow graduate, but the second was an Edinburgh graduate who held the post for a record twenty-one years and really put the hospital on an efficient basis. Of the seven Superintendents who have served since then, all but one were New Zealand graduates and of these three had Edinburgh higher qualifications.

One notable New Zealander who qualified in Edinburgh was Sir Truby King. He graduated M.B., C.M. and then took the new B.Sc in Public Health. King was an eccentric but in New Zealand he became a great reformer in the fields of psychological medicine, nutrition and infant feeding. He made considerable improvements in the mental hospital system and founded the Plunket Society which is still a powerful influence in promoting good child care.

From the foundation of the Otago medical school until Sir Gordon Bell retired in 1952, one or more of the teachers from Edinburgh mentioned in this paper taught every doctor who graduated in New Zealand. In 1939, just before the outbreak of war, there were 1,559 names on the New Zealand medical register. On these, 277 (18 per cent) were Edinburgh graduates or held Edinburgh higher qualifications and 982 (63 per cent) were New Zealand graduates. The former figure is almost certainly an understatement because higher qualifications were not always registered. Nowadays more New Zealanders go to London than to Edinburgh for postgraduate study; still, many of their teachers in London come from the Scottish metropolis anyway.

The clinical teaching tradition which began in Padua in the sixteenth century spread from there to Leyden and from there to Edinburgh where it reached its greatest flowering in the eighteenth century. The Edinburgh medicine which was transplanted to New Zealand was that of the later nineteenth century, a time when Edinburgh was no longer the capital of the world of medicine. Nevertheless, the Edinburgh of James Syme, Joseph Lister, James Young Simpson, Robert Christison and John Hughes Bennett was not a city that could be medically ignored; it was a font of new ideas in surgery, midwifery, anaesthesia and physiology and these new ideas took ready root in the new colony giving New Zealand medicine a heady exciting quality that was to last for its first few decades until colonial life, and with it its medicine, set into its own pattern, indigenous yet moulded by its antecedents in the Old World.

Bibliography

CAMPBELL, J. L., *Poenamu*, 2nd ed., Christchurch, Whitcombe & Tombs, 1952.
COMRIE, J. D., *History of Scottish Medicine*, London, Wellcome, 1932.
FULTON, R. V., 'Medical Practice in Otago and Southland in the Early Days', *Otago Daily Times*, Dunedin, 1922.
HERCUS, SIR CHARLES and BELL, SIR GORDON, *The Otago Medical School under the First Three Deans*, Edinburgh, Livingstone, 1964.
JONES, D. W. CARMALT, *Annals of the University of Otago Medical School*, Wellington, Reed, 1945.
Minutes, Senatus Academicus, University of Edinburgh, 1839.
MORRELL, W. P., *The University of Otago: A Centennial History*, Dunedin, Otago University Press, 1969.
WRIGHT-ST CLAIR, R. E., 'Medical men in early New Zealand politics', *N.Z. med. J.*, 1955, **54**, 551–55.
WRIGHT-ST CLAIR, R. E., 'The beginning of medical registration in New Zealand' *N.Z. med. J.*, 1955, **54**, 693–97.

E. Coturri
Florence (Italy)

Maestro Pancio da Controne, physician of King Edward II, King Edward III and Queen Isabel

We know for certain from many official acts, that the physician Maestro Pancio da Controne, so named from his native country, near Bagni di Lucca, 'a famous corner of Tuscany', as the English writer Whipple wrote at the beginning of our century,[1] lived at St. James's Court. He was the physician of King Edward II and King Edward III, as well as Queen Isabel, wife of the former and mother of the latter.

The most ancient act concerning Maestro Pancio da Controne is that dated 11 November 1317 and this is an order, from King Edward II to the Chancellor of the Exchequer, for the payment of £25 a year to Maestro Pancio da Controne, physician, 'so long as he shall remain in the Realm, the King's leek and clerk'.[2]

At that time Maestro Pancio had probably been in England only a short time, because the acts dated 11 November 1317 and 14 August 1318,[3] show a remarkable uncertainty in the writing of his name, an uncertainty which does not appear later when his name became well known at the English court.

In fact, Maestro Pancio's reputation reached an important goal in a short time: he became consultant physician to the Queen and accumulated a lot of money, acquiring great fame in his profession. Maestro Pancio took advantage of this situation for his own commercial affairs and for helping his friends and countrymen. He even succeeded in obtaining, from the king, the pardon of an emigrant from the city of Lucca who, during a fight, had killed an English nobleman.[4]

Maestro Pancio was still alive on 11 December 1340, when 'in aegritudinis lecto recumbens', he dictated a codicil to his will drawn up two years before in London in St. Agostino's sacristy, by the notary Uguccio Sensi de Ficullis of the Diocese of Orvieto.[5] From that time we know nothing more about him.

His good name, no doubt, developed and grew in consequence of the successful treatments given to the king, the queen and some dignitaries of the Court, but Maestro Pancio was, at the same time, a man of science. This is demonstrated, at least, by Maestro Pancio's wish expressed in his previous will, to establish in Bologna, where perhaps he had studied, a college for students from Lucca who had gone there in order to attend that famous university. And if the college was not established it was not Pancio's fault.

Neither did he neglect his own studies. Gentile da Foligno, Alderotti's famous pupil and Master of Medicine at Perugia, in the 'Quaestio undecima' of his treatise *De febribus* debating 'utrum febris sit passio cordis sive verum subiectum febris sit cor', thoroughly examines and then confutes Pancio da Lucca's opinion that the heat of fever depended on a passion of the liver. And moreover, Code XXV, 4 of the Malatestiana Library in Cesena, coming from 'ex libris bonae memoriae Magistri Johannis physici de Arimino', contains in the papers 74–76 verso, a 'Quaestio magistri Pancii de Luca' still unpublished. Also this 'quaestio', refers to the pathogenesis of the fever, but the problem examined here is if the fever presupposed a corruption of the blood, namely, if the fever is 'ex sanguine putrescente' or 'ex sanguine manente in propria norma'. The title of 'quaestio' is formulated in the following way: 'Quaestio proposita fit utrum ex sanguine manente in propria forma sanguinis possit fieri febris'. It would seem that Gentile da Foligno in his confutation had referred to another 'quaestio', so that we may deduce that the contributions to the subject of the fever brought by Maestro Pancio had been more than one.

Our Maestro Pancio da Controne, so, takes part, by full right, both in the history of the Court, of English trade, and the history of medicine.

The present work could be continued with research on other Italian physicians in service at St. James's Court during that time. From the documents of the Public Record Office – from which we have obtained information on Pancio – we notice that a certain John Paladyn, in the year 1363,[6] was physician at the English Court and he was probably an Italian from Lucca like Pancio. Then we have evidence of a certain Peter de Florence who was physician, in the year 1368, at the English Court with the salary of £40 a year,[7] and finally an act dated 18 February 1413 reports, namely, the 'Nauralisation of David de Nigerellis de Luca, K's Physician'.[8]

As you can see the subject may still be considered open, and it might perhaps be connected with the arrival in Italy, later, of Englishmen such as Caius, Harvey, etc.

References

1 WHIPPLE, E. E., *A Famous Corner of Tuscany*, London, 1928.
2 *Cal. Pat. Rolls*, III, p. 57.
3 Ibid. p. 199.
4 Ibid. p. 132.
5 Archiv. di Stato in Lucca, Opera di S. Croce, n. 15.
6 MANCINI, A., *Catruccio in Inghilterra*, Florence, 1934, p. 159.
7 Ibid.
8 Ibid.

E. Herman
Lodz (Poland)

The connexions between Polish and British neurology in historical perspective

Before discussing the problem of the relations between Polish and British neurology, it might be worthwhile to reflect on the circumstances which led to the creation of an opportune background for such relations. The first circumstance was created by Polish political exiles who had emigrated to Great Britain which became their adoptive country. The second circumstance was the attraction of English medical centres where the Polish neurologists endeavoured to supplement their knowledge. The third circumstance arose from the intellectual relationship between the leading Polish neurologists and distinguished British neurologists.

As regards the first circumstance, it found its reflection in World War II when many doctors found themselves in Great Britain by reason of their participation in the military operations. The friendly attitude of the Englishmen towards the Poles led to the creation of the Polish School of Medicine in Edinburgh. Dr. Jakub Rothfeld-Rostowski, professor of the Lwów University, lectured in this school on neurology in 1941–49. His name is well known to the British neurologists for the syndromes which he described, namely gelolepsia – the loss of muscular tonus during laughter, and orgasmolepsia – the loss of muscular tonus during orgasm, and for the Balduzzi-Rothfeld sign. Within eight years 228 physicians graduated from the Polish School of Medicine in Edinburgh, and among them the neurosurgeons H. Masłowski, B. Sedzimir, and H. Urich, professor of neuropathology in London.

But the mutual relations between Polish and English physicians originated far in the past, for instance in the second half of the nineteenth century, when Joseph Lister (1827–1912), the founder of antiseptic surgery, won over to his side many Polish physicians, and even earlier in the first half of the sixteenth century, at the reformation period, when some Scottish and Englishmen settled in Poland. I shall mention here Marcin Foxius, a Scot who was professor of medicine at the Jagiellonian University in Cracow, or Bernard O'Connor who was physician in ordinary of the king Jan III and later professor of anatomy and physiology in Oxford and Cambridge, and the author of a two-volume work entitled *The History of Poland*.

In 1830–31, during a Polish uprising, Andrew Buchanan, later professor and a co-founder of the *Glasgow Medical Journal*, fought against the epidemic of cholera in Poland.

As regards the second circumstance – the education of Polish physicians in English medical centres – it must be admitted that at that time Polish neurologists kept in closer touch with French and German neurology. Nevertheless we can cite a number of instances of the migration of Polish physicians to English medical centres. For example, Edward Sawicki, head of the Lwów hospital, wrote in his report of his scientific journey around England about the experiments of the Scottish neurologist Sir David Ferrier (1843–1928), professor of neuropathology at King's College, London, the author of the works entitled *The Functions of the Brain* (1876) and *Cerebral Localisation* (1878): 'In Germany Ferrier was even suspected of plagiarism, while in England he proved that his discovery was genuine.' Another example may be Kazimierz Funk (1884–1971) who isolated a crystalline substance free from protein, fat and sugar and containing no phosphorus which cured beriberi. In 1910 Funk worked at the Lister Institute in London with Martin as its director. He was instigated in his scientific research by Eijkman (1858–1930) who, together with Sir Frederick Gowland Hopkins (1891–1947), the famous English biochemist, was awarded in 1929 a Nobel Prize in physiology and medicine for his pioneer work on vitamins. In 1911 Funk published in the *Lancet* his article entitled 'Experiments on the causation of beriberi', and in 1912 another article in the *Journal of State Medicine* entitled 'The etiology of deficiency diseases'.

Perhaps it would be also advisable to mention here the name of a Pole, David Keilin who, while working in Cambridge at the Molteno Institute and doing research work on myohematin, isolated cytochrome which plays a highly important role in biochemical processes of the muscles. I also mention the name of Dr. Józef Handelsman, later professor of psychiatry at the Warsaw University, who worked with Sir Victor Horsley (1857–1916) and published with him a work on experiments on the hypophysis.

The third circumstance concerns the union of thought of the leading Polish neurologists and of the British neurologists.

Adolf Beck (1863–1942), professor of physiology at Lwów University, a co-worker of Napoleon Cybulski (1854–1919), professor of physiology at the Jagiellonian University in Cracow – did research work on the localization in the brain and in the spinal cord with the use of electrical phenomenona (1891) which later gave rise to the foundation of electroencephalography. Beck's publications called forth a response on the part of the English research workers Gotch, Horsley and Caton whose experiments were different and unknown to Beck.

Oliver together with Schafer confirmed the results of the experiments of the Cracow scientists – a physiologist Napoleon Cybulski and a histologist Władysław Szymonowicz – on physiology of the adrenal cortex (epinephrines according to the nomenclature of the Polish research workers).

In 1685 Thomas Willis described myasthenia – a disease thoroughly defined in 1891 by Samuel Goldflam (1852–1932), and entitled Erb-Goldflam disease.

In 1927 Spiller published in *Brain* a description of subcortical epilepsy which in 1924 was defined by a Polish neurologist Sterling as extrapyramidal epilepsy, and in 1925 by Wimmer as striatal epilepsy.

Henry Charlton Bastian, an English neurologist (1837–1915), became famous for the description of a law called the Bastian law – the abolition of the tendon reflexes of the lower extremities in a complete transverse lesion in the spinal cord. Flatau, a Warsaw neurologist, together with a German neurologist Gad performed experiments on dogs which gave him good reason for criticizing Bastian-Bruns law. He prepared in 1894 an atlas of the human brain, published also in the English language, and he is also the author of the Flatau law about an excentric arrangement of the long fibres of the spinal cord.

Wood, a Scottish physician, published in 1829 in the *Edinburgh Medico-chirurgical Transactions* an article entitled 'Observations on neuroma', and later a Polish neurologist Orzechowski coined a name 'neurinomatosis centralis' and brought Bourneville's disease into relationship with Recklinghausen's disease (neurinomatosis multiplex).

Natalia Zand (1883–1941), a Warsaw neurologist, working on the observations of Sherrington on decerebration rigidity, demonstrated in her experimental studies the significance of bulbar olives in the muscular tonus.

Adam Opalski, professor of neurology at Warsaw University, revealed gigantic glial cells, called Opalski's cells, which are characteristic of Wilson's disease.

Eugeniusz Brzezicki, professor of psychiatry at the Cracow Medical Academy, investigated angio- and glioplastic properties of the basal ganglia of the brain, characteristic of Wilson's disease.

Jan Mazurkiewicz (1871–1947), professor of psychiatry at the Warsaw University, became a exponent of the modern theory of Jackson (1834–1911) by writing an article entitled 'Evolution and dissolution of the cortico-psychic activity'.

Łucja Frey (1889–1943) described in 1923 an auriculotemporal syndrome called Frey's syndrome in the English encyclopaedia which had already been described in 1897 by Parkes Weber in the *Clinical Society's Transactions*.

L. K. Glinski (1870–1918), an anatomopathologist of the Jagiellonian University in Cracow, described in 1911 cachexia hypophyseopriva – three years earlier than a neurologist research worker M. Simmonds. This fact was emphasized for the first time by J. D. Robertson.

The above examples constitute a sufficient explanation of the basis of the third circumstance under consideration – the intellectual relationship between the Polish and the British neurologists.

These short illustrations show the existing bonds between Polish and British neurology.

M. Lyskanowski
Warsaw (Poland)

Recognition of the English 'no-restraint-system' in the Warsaw medical milieu of the nineteenth century

Towards the close of the eighteenth century, as a result of partition, Poland was divided among Austria, Russia and Prussia. Each of the invading states tried to absorb the occupied territories by introducing its own legislation and bureaucracy.

Polish physicians who at that time were engaged in treating mentally ill patients worked in very hard conditions, without proper financial provisions, training facilities, or appropriate official and legal rights. Despite so difficult a situation, they worked out a number of instructions and regulations aimed at protecting the interests of the mentally diseased. Undoubtedly, they showed a humane, highly thoughtful attitude towards the mentally sick in the period under discussion, nevertheless they could not change the general situation. Adolf Rothe (1832–1903), one of the most outstanding Polish psychiatrists of the nineteenth century wrote in the columns of *Tygodnik Lekarski* (Medical Weekly) in 1864: 'The number of our hospitals destined entirely for the mentally diseased is so small, in relation to the number of the sick, that very often there is no room for them at all.'[1]

Soon after that, in 1865, the Chief Tutelar Council (Rada Główna Opiekuńcza), an institution responsible for hospitals, decided to construct a modern mental hospital outside the city of Warsaw.[2] In 1866, Count Berg, the Emperor's governor, ordered the recall from Petersburg of an eminent psychiatrist of Polish origin Proffessor Jan Balinski (1827–1902), and asked for his advice and instructions regarding the construction of the new hospital. Professor Baliński arrived, and suggested that the hospital should be divided into two parts: for female and male patients, each of them having five wards: for calm, turbulent, severely ill, incontinent patients, and violent patients. Besides, he suggested the establishment of wards for epileptics. He also proposed to introduce belts for those excited.

In 1868, Adolf Rothe, together with an architect, Turnell, was sent abroad to get acquainted with the furnishings of modern mental hospitals. Subsequently, they wrote a memorandum which, together with the plan for the construction of a new hospital for 400 beds, was handed to the emperor's authorities in Warsaw. The authorities accepted the memorandum and decided that a detailed plan of the hospital should be made. Rothe and Turnell estimated the cost of the construction at one million roubles and worked out the plan for the hospital, based upon the pavilion system. Five years later, i.e. in 1874, Petersburg answered, that the cost was too high and so the ministry rejected the plan.

However, at the time when Adolf Rothe and Turnell were working on the above plan, in the columns of the contemporary polish medical press there broke out a discussion on modern ways of attending the mentally diseased. Undoubtedly, Rothe's declaration published in *Tygodnik Lekarski* in 1864, as well as the feasible perspectives of founding the new hospital in the vicinity of Warsaw contributed to the discussion.

The floor was taken by the following physicians: Stanisław Chomętowski (1838–81), Stanisław Markiewicz (1839–1911), Zygmunt Dobieszewski (1836–81) and, a number of times, Adolf Rothe.

In December 1868, *Pamiętnik Towarzystwa Lekarskiego Warszawskiego* 'Warsaw Medical Society Memorials', published an article by Stanisław Chomętowski: 'On treating the mentally diseased without using any restraining means'. The author wrote:

> The total abandonment of the restraining means, i.e. the so called No-Restraint-System, was introduced for the first time in England, in 1837, by Dr. Charlesworth and Dr. Gardiner Hill, to the hospital in Lincoln and, two years later, it was disseminated and improved by Dr. Conolly in the large hospital in Hanwell. This system, according to its advocates, consists in the influence of sane people upon the minds of the sick, by evoking in the latter pleasant impressions and by averting from them all unpleasant effects. This kind of treatment deserves to be called moral: it rejects any thought of restraining the sick, or, worse still, inflicting any penalty on them. A sick person who acts improperly should be made to understand that their behaviour annoys those whose favour and friendship they desire.[3]

In his reasoning, Chometowski, quoted a statement by Conolly:

> Together with the introduction of No-Restraint, dreadful images of prison, punishment or cruel death disappear from the hospitals. When the sick are treated severely, their fear and excitement are increased; kind treatment, in favourable conditions, considerably hastens the recovery. Every sick person is carefully examined after an attack so that in future it would be possible to remove the cause of the excitement and thus once and for ever prevent him from such attack.

It should be stressed that Dr. Chomętowski, who was so much in favour of the 'No-Restraint-System', with pride and satisfaction pointed out the achievements of Warsaw mental hospitals: 'However, in the large mental hospital in Hanwell, according to Dr. Sankey's latest lectures, families and friends were allowed to visit the sick formerly twice a week and now four times a week, while in Warsaw mental hospitals they are allowed to do it every day, although the "No-Restraint-System" has not been introduced here.'

In 1879, the question of the 'No-Restraint-System' was again discussed in the columns of the press. This time, the discussion was a result of the book by Alfons Erlicki (1846–1902) published in Warsaw, entitled: *Clinical Lectures on Mental Diseases.* Erlicki was an assistant to a famous Russian psychiatrist of Polish origin, Jan Lucjan Mierzejewski (1839–1908) from Petersburg. In his manual, Erlicki, being an advocate of the strait jacket, approached critically the 'No-Restraint-System'. He thought that the advocates of this system locked the excited sick: 'in separate rooms, for a long period of time and do not pay attention to the fact that such measure is more restraining than a strait jacket, and the more humiliating if there is a secret hole in the door to the room in which the sick has been locked and through it the sick is spied like a criminal or a wild animal.'[4]

The isolated opinion of Dr. Erlicki did not sum up the discussion on the 'No-

Restraint-System'. It was the statement by Dr. Adolf Rothe pronounced the same year that may be considered its summing up: 'The idea of total abandonment of restraining measures', wrote Rothe in his *Contribution to Practical Psychiatry*, 'was introduced by Conolly in the Hanwell Hospital in 1839. Indeed, it is a long step forward and a beautiful idea, treating the mentally diseased without mechanical restraining measures'. Further on we read: 'And so, a new epoch has come about in treating mental diseases: the so called "No-Restraint".'[5]

Along with the discussion of the specialists, a campaign was led for the construction of the new hospital. It was decided that it would be situated in Tworki near Warsaw. The corner-stone for its construction was laid only in 1888 (i.e. when the Polish community had collected among themselves 500,000 roubles),[6] and it was opened on 15 November 1891. It was undoubtedly a great achievement of the enthusiasts of modern treatment of the mentally diseased, nevertheless it was a drop in the ocean. No wonder that in the same year in the magazine *Health* (Zdrowie) there appeared an article: 'The fate of mentally diseased in the Congress Kingdom of Poland', in which an anonymous author stated: 'Whoever should think that together with the completion of the hospital in Tworki the question of the mentally diseased in the Congress Kingdom of Poland has been solved would be mistaken. . . . Although with the opening of the hospital in Tworki we shall have a little better proportion than that in the Empire, it will still be far from the norm . . . despite the completion of the Tworki Hospital, not even half of the mentally diseased who require medical attendance will get it. . . .'[7]

The above article, similar to the previously quoted one by Adolf Rothe, was very harsh; it was directed against the contemporary authorities who did anything to improve the bad situation. Against this background, the more outstanding are the merits of the Polish physicians treating the mentally diseased, who – despite such difficult working conditions – tried to treat their patients in the most humane way. They knew the modern trends and methods of medical treatment applied abroad, they also knew well the English 'No-Restraint-System'. Being characterized by great culture and humanitarianism it conformed to the spirit of Polish psychiatry as well as to the activity and proceedings of Polish psychiatrists of the contemporary period.

References

1 ROTHE, ADOLF, 'Krótki rys historii psychiatrii', *Tygodnik Lekarski*, 1864, nr. 1, p. 47.

2 BUCELSKI, STANISŁAW, 'Dzieje budowy zakładu dla obłąkanych w Królestwie Polskim oraz stan obecny szpitala w Tworkach', *Pamiętnik Towarzystwa Lekarskiergo Warszawskiego*, Warsaw, 1905, **101**, 581.

3 CHOMĘTOWSKI, STANISŁAW, 'O leczeniu obłąkanych bez użycia środków krępujących (No-Restraint-System)', *Pamiętnik Towarzystwa Lekarskiego Warszawskiego*, Warsaw, 1868, **6**, 283.

4 ERLICKI, ALFONS, *Wykłady kliniczne o chorobach umysłowych*, Warsaw, 1897, p. 198.

5 ROTHE, ADOLF, 'Przyczynek do psychiatrii praktycznej', *Pamiętnik Towarzystwa Lekarskiego Warszawskiego*, Warsaw, 1879, **75**, 90–91.

6 BILIKIEWICZ, TADEUSZ, *Jan Gallus. Psychiatria Polska na tle dziejowym*, PZWL, Warsaw, 1962, p. 139.

7 *Los obłąkanych w Królestwie Polskim (artykuł wstępny) Zdrowie*, tom VII, 1891, nr. 68.

S. Szpilczynski
Wroclaw (Poland)

Bernard O'Connor from Ireland: aulic physician to the Polish King Jan III Sobieski. A contribution to the development of medical thinking at the turn of the seventeenth century

The traditions of cultural links between Poland and England, in the field of medicine, can be traced back to the remote past; their development fluctuated during the course of history, depending on circumstances which brought closer or drove apart both countries. The seventeenth century is to be regarded as that of rapprochement, as shown, among others, by the presence of British physicians at Polish courts. To name but a few there was an outstanding physician John Jonston[1] (1603–75), whose father was a Scot and whose mother was of Polish origin; he stayed at the court of Rafal Leszczynski in the first half of the century; his brilliant works in the field of natural sciences and medicine made him famous throughout the world. In 1661–68 the physician-in-ordinary at the court of King Jan Kazimierz and his wife Marie Louise was William Davidson,[2] also of Scottish origin. By the end of the seventeenth century it was the Irishman Bernard O'Connor,[3] personal physician to King Jan III Sobieski, who became famous. His views, as precursors of concepts postulated in the eighteenth century, hardly found any repercussions in the literature; nor could I find any pertinent mention in D. Guthrie's *History of Medicine*. That is why I welcome this opportunity to shed some light on this interesting personality.

Bernard O'Connor (1666–98) came from the county of Kerry in Ireland. He studied medicine from 1686 in Montpellier, then in Rheims, where he received his medical degree. For some time he stayed in Paris; then he visited Germany, Italy and Austria. In Vienna he met Poles and travelled with them through Moravia and Silesia to Cracow and next to Warsaw (1693). As a result of the intervention of the Venetian deputy – Hieronim Alberti de Conti – he was admitted to the court of King Jan III Sobieski, in the capacity of personal physician. While holding this post (for a period of one year) he was concerned with collecting records concerning the history of Poland. O'Connor probably feared that the king would soon die, as he was suffering from gout and, being corpulent, tended to develop oedema; frequent catarrhal affections of the upper respiratory tract were also among his complaints. The king took a fancy to O'Connor, did him many favours but at the same time put his talent to many acid tests, from which he used to emerge victorious. In the king's Court O'Connor did not enjoy benevolence and popularity, this fact was accounted for by several circumstances. One of them was that the practitioner stressed the importance of anatomy in medicine whereas the Polish society at that time adhered to the false notion that taking up anatomy and surgery was unbecoming for the highly educated physician, who was thought to be equal to the philosopher. Such activities were regarded as the duty of quacks, and this attitude lead to dereliction which was abolished only by the Kollontaj's reform (1793). Another circumstance which interfered, to some degree, with O'Connor's popularity was his bold prophecy concerning the prompt death of the king's sister, Radziwillow's wife, who was an exceptionally talented woman; she wrote Latin, and described, among others, her journey to Egypt. This said prevision roused in the king's court a feeling of anxiety and resentment towards O'Connor. To make matters worse the prediction came true, and also the diagnosis made by O'Connor (liver abscess) was confirmed by post-mortem examination; the additional finding was the presence of stones in the gall and urinary bladder. The loss of his sister did not affect the king's attitude to O'Connor; it is even likely to have enhanced the king's respect for his knowledge, but this was not enough to suppress the unfavourable atmosphere of his milieu. The last straw to complete his unpopularity was his bold utterance at the session initiated by the king, with participation of bishops and high clergy; when asked by the king which parts of the human body harbour the soul, when does it enter and leave the body, O'Connor bravely revealed his views which considerably departed from those postulated by the Christian philosophy.

With no prospects for winning popularity and credit with Polish society, and considering the poor health of the protector himself, O'Connor took the opportunity when the king was about to send his only daughter, the wife of the Bavarian elector, to Brussels, to persuade the king, again by mediation of the Venetian deputy, to allow him to join her court. So he left Poland and after two months he reached his destination. On the way he visited many places where the king's daughter was given a solemn welcome. In Brussels the medical care about the twenty-three-year-old daughter of King Jan III was taken over by the court physician of the Bavarian elector and O'Connor, delivered of his duties, went to Oxford and then to Cambridge where he lectured on anatomy and published his papers including *Oeconomia animalis, De principiis medicinae et fermentatione*. They earned him the fellowship of the Royal Society and the College of Physicians. Some of his dissertations such as *Evangelium Medici, sive medicinam mysticam de suspensis naturae legibus, sive de miraculis* (London, 1697, Amsterdam, 1699, Jena, 1707) postulating that the miracles described in the gospel are easily explainable in a natural way, were an alarming sign for the Church; as a result, their propagation was prohibited. Soon O'Connor's brilliant career was cut short through his sudden death.

Among the works immediately connected with Poland and Poles is *The History of Poland* published in London, 1698 by D. Brown and A. Ropert; vol. I, pp. i–xvi, 1–352, vol. II, pp. 1–236, 1–124. A German edition *Beschreibung des Königsreichs Polen* appeared in Leipzig in 1700. Individual chapters are presented in the form of letters to persons of quality. In the *History of Poland* O'Connor undertook as he put it 'Giving an Account of the Antient and Present State of that Kingdom, Historical, Geographical, Physical, Political and Ecclesiastical; Its Origin and Extent, with a Description of its Towns and Province; the Succesion and remarkable Actions of all its King, and of the Great Dukes of Lithunia; the Election, Power, and Coronation of the King, the Senate, or House of Lords; the Diet and form of Governement; the Privileges of the Gentry, their Religion, Learning, Language, Customs, Habits, Manners, Riches, Trade, and Military Affairs, together with the State of Physick and Natural Knowledge, as also an Account of the Teutonic Order, and of the Duke of Curland, his Family and Territories, with Sculptures, and a new Map after the best Geographers.'

In preparing the *History of Poland* O'Connor consulted the memoirs of outstanding writers from their travels and took advantage of his own observations.

He depicted[4] in detail sanitary and hygienic conditions in Poland. O'Connor was convinced that compared to the neighbouring countries like Sweden, Russia and Germany, Poland was a healthier nation and explained this fact by circumstances such as the diet consisting of fresh meat, proper beverages, the way of living with no beds to sleep in and no bedclothes to cover the body; love for hunting, physical fitness and a bright disposition were among other characteristics of Poles, as observed by O'Connor.

As to hygienic conditions in Polish houses Connor states that each of them possesses a washbasin, separate for men and women, to wash their hands and face in cold water, which, in his opinion, accounts for the rarity of scabies in children; the incidence of malformations and disabilities seems to be lower, as compared with that in children of other countries.

In Poland, physicians were few, mostly French, Italian and German. As a rule, Poles are not attracted by medical studies.

In practice, the medicine in Poland left much to wish for; physicians were not familiar with the latest achievements, this being particularly true for anatomy and chemistry; they knew little about materia medica and mostly used Galenics, and what is worse, of the poorest sort. Polish physicians would use the same drugs as their English colleagues, i.e. mercury, iron, antimony, quinine, sal volatile, spiritus vitalis, etc.; they were brought to Warsaw either by themselves or through mediation of German pharmacists, without knowing the exact mode of their administration. When meeting to discuss a case they showed, as a rule, little concern for the causes of the disease, endorsing indiscriminately the authority of a writer (professor), regardless of given circumstances.

According to O'Connor, the number of physicians living at that time in Warsaw amounted to ten, but many pseudophysicians practised medicine too. He described one of them as he saw him at his home; he lived six miles from Warsaw and concerned himself particularly with venereal diseases; his charge for the therapy was never more than two talars; the treatment lasted eight days. For the first four days patients were bathed in water containing concoction of three or four medicinal herbs (helleboraster, capillus veneris, maiden hair, nieswurzel) and to quench their thirst they were given a mixture of the same components. The next four days were spent in a sweating bath, treated with the same herbs; they were lying on special plank beds so as to expose the whole body to the action of hot air with resulting profuse sweating, their thirst being quenched with the concoction as given in the first four days of the therapy. O'Connor states that the management of syphilis was efficient, as judged by accounts of trustworthy patients.

Cases of venereal diseases would be fairly frequent, the preferred treatment consisting more in procedures stimulating profuse sweating than in salivation produced by mercury ointment, as was the case in England. O'Connor probably ignored Wojciech Oczko,[5] who early in the sixteenth century called attention to the danger of intoxication with mercurotherapy, which might have caused abandonment of this method in favour of sweat-inducing procedures in the seventeenth century.

O'Connor observed in Poland cases of erysipelas treated successfully with white chalk powder. Infrequent in this country was scurvy and malignant fever; generally, there were fewer diseases in Poland as compared with other countries; wounds and leg ulcers were regarded as untreatable.

In the *History of Poland* more space is devoted to the disease called plica polonica; the physician of King Jan III, a Jew, treated it by excision; plica was formed by intertwisted, felted hairs, occasionally overnight; sometimes, hair reaching to the shoulders underwent complete stiffening. Cutting off a plica resulted in headaches lumbar pain, vomiting, twisting and stiffening of limbs, with appearance of white spots on the nails and skin eruption. As a rule, early ablation of plica was contraindicated for fear of impending blindness. Plica had no characteristics of venereal, rheumatic disease or of arthritis; it was never accompanied by caries of bones; only exceptionally was it associated with ulcers of the mouth. Some, according to O'Connor, regarded plica as a hereditary, others, as a contagious disease that could be transmitted from people to animals. In Lithuania the incidence of the disease was higher, whereas it was not seen in Tartars and in Moscow.

Dealing with diseases O'Connor also quoted a case of cancer of the tongue concerning a laywer; moreover, he described a case of a child with mental disorders; this child would be fed, in the postnatal period by a female bear; he included a copperplate with a picture of a bear feeding a human baby together with bear cubs.

The *History of Poland* also contains descriptions of curative waters, e.g. in Jawor, Szkło where sulphur water of crystalline transparence was found; it was recommended for general invigoration of the patient, in scrophulosis of children and to combat ulcers.

Among peculiarities described by O'Connor a mention is deserved of a practising woman; she possessed knowledge of Latin and used to speak this language; she was the owner of a gallery of petrified bodies. In the pertinent description O'Connor refers to Dr. Bernitz, the physician of King Jan Kazimierz. He also mentions some charlatans, among others, those who treated wounds caused by glass with cauterization.

O'Connor's review of the sanitary conditions in Poland is mingled with descriptions of curiosities: he reports on a fish of huge dimensions (4 elbows and 8 feet long, 5 feet wide), and about people (probably alchemists) whose occupation was to dissolve silver.

In the *History of Poland*, the letter IV (vol. I) 'to Right Honorable Wiliam of Yarmouth'[6] is of special interest, as it depicts the terminal stage of the disease of King Jan III. Included, is the text of the letter he received from the Plock bishop Zaleski, asking for advice on the king's severe condition. The text reads as follows:

> His Majesty's Feet, Legs and Thighs, as likewise the lower Part of his Belly, have been considerably swell'd for a good while. These Swellings have daily encreas'd since they began this Summer, notwithstanding the most effectual Remedies, both inward and outward, which have been made use of to prevent their Progress, and to discuss them, when these Tumors are press'd with one's Finger, they do not pit, for they are almost as hard as Iron, and as heavy as Lead. When His Majesty walks, he imagine he has a great Weight ty'd to his Legs. The Hardness of these Tumours cannot be sustened. Nevertheless, when the swollen Parts are rubb'd a little with a hot Cloth, they seem immediately to be reduced and eas'd; but soon after they return to their former condition. The Colour of the Swellings is not pale, but reddish, something inclining to Purple.

A week later he learned about the king's death. The pertinent account is as follows:

A Week after I receiv'd this Letter news came that this Prince was dead, as I could not but reasonably expect he would be, labouring under so rare and dangerous a Disease being a Dropsy turn'd into Schirrus, or into hard and insensible Tumor. Cases of this nature my Lord, are very seldom seen. I have spoken lately with some old Practionners in Physick that had never met with any; for my part I have never observ'd any Disease like it, and I was at first surpris'd that the King's Legs that us'd to pit an Inch deep when I was at his Court, should become so very hard and so heavy afterwards. But considering that in our Mass of Blood there is, even naturally, a great deal of earthy Parts or Dreggs, and that these lees may, by way of Sediment, fall into the Legs, and that their Weight and Quality can hinder them from ascending to the Heart with the circulating Fluids. I rather admir'd why Cases of this nature do not more frequently happen, particularly in old and Plethoric People, as the King was. These hard Swelling of his Legs hinder'd the Blood to circulate downward, and to drove up all Humors to the Head; which opressing and overflowing the Brain, caus'd an Apoplexy of which he died the 17th of June, fifteen days after the date of my Letter, in the Year 1696, in the sixty sixth Year of his Age, and the 22d of his Reign. He was oldest King then in Christendom.

Then he enumerates the merits of the king.

The above-quoted description of the disease of King Jan III is an interesting contribution to his medical history, with the direct and indirect reasons of his death. This problem was already dealt with in detail by W. Ziembicki in his paper entitled 'Health and ill-health of Jan III Sobieski'.[7] The author believed that Jan III Sobieski's death was due to uraemia preceded by chronic renal disease.

The copy of the *History of Poland* belonging to the Ossolineum (Library of the Polish Academy of Sciences in Wroclaw, sign. XVII 5997 III/1–2) volume I is catalogued under the title 'A Compendious Plan the Body of Physics'.[8] The title is followed by the text of a letter by a gentleman from Cambridge to O'Connor, with 'Dr. O'Connor's Answer, containing a Plan of his *Corpus Rationale Medicum* or of his new and compendious Method Chymical and Anatomical, for understanding the *Oeconomia Animalis*, the Nature of Disease, and the *Materia Medica*.' This answer goes as follows:

Sir,

Whatever you are pleased to say in Commendation of me or my Book, I must wholly attribute to your Civility, and will return no other Compliment to you for it, but that I shall endeavour to deserve your good Opinion. I am extreamly oblig'd to your Correspondent in Oxon for the advantagious Character he gives of me; and I assure you that I have not met with better Discipline, nor with Persons more universally learned in any University of Europe.

As for the Method or Scheme I observed at Oxford to lead the Proficientia in Physick, and other ingenious Gentleman there into the Knowledge of the Fabrick, natural Functions, and Distempers of the Human Body, as likewise into the Knowledge of the Materia Medica to cure the same Diseases, it is follow.

I consider'd Man, in the first place, as a Being compounded of Spirit and Matter, but seeing it is only the last of these Parts wherein our Faculty is concern'd. I took a stricter of most other Animals. But to have any accurate Knowledge of Man, we must not only have a distinct Account of his constituent Parts, but likewise of all the external Bodies which any way affect him, or contribute to his Preservation. Since therefore he cannot live without Earth to tread upon, Air to breath, Animals and Vegetables to feed upon, Sun and Stars to afford him Warmth and Light, etc. we must by consequence examine the System and Elements of the World, and particulary as they concur to the Preservation or Destruction of Man. We must be very well acquainted with the nature of Vegetables, and Minerals, before we can give any tolerable Account of the Generation, Nourishement, Health, Diseases, or Death of Man; before we can discover the admirable Fabrick and Contexture, the Mechanick and Hydraulical Actions, Chemical Preparations, the various Operations of Medicine and an infinite number of other surprising Phenomena in the Human Body.

The best Method therefore, I presume, is to proceed Analytically from the previous Examination of all the known Parts of the great World, to particular Enquiries into the Microcosm. Now the first step to this Method, is a good Insight by Chymical Experiments into the Nature, more especially the Figuration and Qualities of the Principles of mixt Bodies, and chiefly of the Blood. For the want of such a Discovery (which is not impossible) has hitherto been a great Obstruction to the Improvement of Natural Phylosophy, and the Practice of Physick. It is plain to me, that a Man void of all Prejudice, and who considers that all the Operations of Bodies are perform'd by natural Causes without Miracles, may be easily convinc'd that the Causes of Diseases, and the true use of Applications to cure them, can be render'd very intelligible; so that vulgar Axiom, that ther's no certainty in Physick, will be found most erroneous.

I don't Sir, pretend to have discover'd this just Method, which I hold necessary to lead us into the abstruse Secrets of Nature, but I would fain hope that the following Scheme, which is that I observ'd at Oxford, may approach it in some degree, which Method, tho it may be call'd altogether new, may perhaps be a just Model for others to imitate hereafter in the true Theory and Practice of Physick which rightly consider'd are one and same thing.

In the first, above, part of O'Connor's answer his views are those postulated by Paracelsus and his adherents from the sixteenth century and by neo-paracelsists, iatrochemists in the next century; they assume a dependence of microcosmos on macrocosmos, as well as analytical methods and chemical experiments to explain phenomena of life without resorting to supernatural forces (miracles). O'Connor, however, while being an iatrochemist did not reject the 'hydraulic' mechanism, as proposed by iatrophysicists of the seventeenth century for interpretation of the human body.

The next part of O'Connor's answer deals with 'A new Plan of Animal Oeconomy demonstrated in the Spring Anno 1695, at London the Winter following, and at Cambridge in the Year 1696' and concerns as follows:[9]

1. Of the Elements, Fabrick, and System of the World, with the mutual Cohesion, Influence, and Dependance of its Parts.
2. Of the Elements of Terrestrial Bodies, where (after various Chymical Experiments) are consider'd the Nature, Properties, Figures, and Effects of the four Chymical Principles, Earth, Water, Salt and Sulphur, and their main mutual Action, Fermentation; as also the Production of Animals, Vegetables and Minerals.
3. Of the Structure of the Human Body, and its division into fluid and solid Parts; where a particular and new Account is given of the Nature and Contexture of the solid Parts, being all made of Vascular Fibres, and demonstrated to the Eye by Dissection.
4. Of the fluid Parts of the Human Body; of the Nature, Principles, Fermentation, and Circulation of the Blood; of Nutrition, of the Temperaments, of the Humours contain'd in the Blood, of the seat and Nature of Fevers, where likewise of Youth, old Age, and Death.
5. Of the Reparation of the Blood, of the Cycle, Lactaeus Vessels, Chyliferous Duct, of Appetite, Mastication, Digestion, and the Ferment, of the Stomach; of the Precipitation or Separation of the Excrements from the Chyle, where of the Structure of the Oesophagus or Gullet, of that of the Stomach, and all the Intestines, of the

Peristaltic and Antiperistaltic Motions of the Guts, of the Glands, of the Mesentery, of the Lympha, and the Lymphatic Vessels.

6. Of the Structure, Motion, and Use of the Heart, where of the various Kinds of Pulses, of the Polypus in the Heart, Palpitation, and Swooning; likewise a new Hypothesis of the Motion of the Heart, and of Sanguinication.

7. Of the Contexture of the Windpipe, or Trachea Arteria, and the Lungs, where of the Cause and Use of Respiration; a new Account of the Nature of the Air, Nitre, and the Unvoluntariness of Respiration, of the Hiccough.

8. Of the Praecordia . . .

9. Of the numerous Ramifications of the Vena Porta . . .

10. Of the Ramifications of both the Aortas . . .

11. Of the Brain and Cerebellum; a new Account of the Animal Spirits, their Generation, Motion, and Use; of Perception, Sleeping, Waking, and the Influence of the Soul upon the Body, whereof Sensation, and the five Senses.

12. Of the Eye, Tears, Nosal and Aqueous Ducts . . .

13. Of the Fabrick of the Nose . . .

14. Of the Tongue, Palat . . .

15. Of the Larynx . . .

16. Of Feeling, the cuticula, Skin, Hairs, miliary Glands, the mucous and reticular Bodies; of Fat, Transpiration, Sweet, the Iter, Cutaneous Diseases, Palsy, the Plica Polonica.

17. Of the Ear, Aquaeduct, Hearing . . .

18. Of the Structure, Use and Number of the Nerves . . .

19. Of the Structure and various Figures of the Muscles, the vascular Fibres, where Muscular, Natural, and free Motion are explain'd, as likewise stretching and gaping, leaping, swimming, and flying, with Convulsive, Tonic, Systaltic, Epileptic, and Hysteric Motions of Vapour and Rheumatism.

20. Of the Liver, Gall, and Pancreas, where the Secretion . . .

21. Of the Nature and Difference of all the Glands or Strainers of the Body; a new Account of the various Filtrations of the excrementious and recrementious Humours, as Lympha, Spittle, Gall, Urine, Seed, etc. Of Obstructions and Dropsies.

22. Of the Structure and Use of the Spleen and what Melancholy . . .

23. Of the Reins or Kidneys . . .

24. Of the Structure and Use of the Bones, Marrow, Ligaments . . .

25. Of the Parts of Generation in Man . . .

26. Of the Parts of Generation in the Woman of the Eggs and Ovarium; of Generation, Conception, going with Child, Flowers, Birth, Monsters, Floodings, false Conceptions, Whites etc.

27. Of the Posture and Nourishment of the Embryo . . .

28. Some Consideration of the Union of the Soul and Body, where the Laws and Effects of that Union are inquired into.

The 'Plan of animal oeconomy' constitutes an overall programme of medical knowledge. The characteristic elements of his approach are contained in the last part of his 'Answer'; it reads:[10]

You see, Sir, that after having examin'd the different Parts of the World, and the Elements of Bodies by Chemistry, I have divided the Human Body into solid and fluid Parts. Before I consider'd by way of Chemistry, to be acquainted with all the Humours, and specially with the Principles and Motions of the Blood, which is the Primum mobile of the whole Machine; for which purpose it is fit to know how by Digestion the Meat becomes Chyle, the Chyle becomes Blood, how the Blood becomes Flesh and Bone, and consequently how it must be continually repaired by Aliment; how the Heart is put in Motion to communicate the Fame to the Blood; how the Blood expelled by the Heart, after . . .

Man, as I said before, is made of two Substances, Soul and Body. The Soul preserves the Body by Reason, and governs its voluntary Motion. The Body furnishes the Soul with Ideas of Corporal Beings. The Life of Man is the Correspondence between Soul and Body; but the Life of the Body is the natural Motion of the Blood and Spirits, the Cessation of which Motion is Death. The solid Parts of the Body have no Motion (or Life) of their own, but such as they borrow from the Blood and Spirits. The Blood and Spirits have none neither, but such as they are allowed by the general Laws of Nature, establish'd by a Supreme Being. To maintain this mutual Correspondence and Dependance between Soul and Body, all the Organs, Springs and Humours of the Body, must be in their due Disposition; for the Death of the Body is properly the loss of this Disposition, and not the Separation of the Soul, as is commonly believ'd; for the Body is dead before the Soul is gone out of it; and the going out of the Soul is but the Cessation of its Correspondence with the Body for want of Motion in the latter. This Disposition is disordered or ruined by Diseases, all which Diseases have their first Seat in the Blood, from whence they are communicated to the solid Parts; and the solid Parts being affected, they reciprocally infect the Blood. But tho the Blood was never infected, and Man never sick, yet he should die of course, by the Relaxation and Attrition of his solid Parts from the long and continual Circulation of the Humours through them, which we call Old Age.

As to what relates to the *Materia Medica*, or the Account I have given of the Virtus and due Application of inward Medicines in the Practice of Physick I should likewise give you a Series of the different Subjects I treated of, as I have in my Plan of the Animal Oeconomy; but finding it too tendious, and needless, I will only mention in general, that all inward Diseases have their first Seat in the Mass of Blood, that they are causes by a Ferment or Matter hot in it, which deriv'd its Origin from some outward Causes. That there are no Specific Medicines for any Part of the Body, as for the Head, Heart, Liver, Stomach, Spleen, but that they must all operate upon the whole Mass of Blood; that consequently outward Applications cannot avail much for inward Distempers, that the Medicines must be carried in a convenient Vehicle through the Blood to the place where the Distemper lies, and that then they either carry its Cause out of the Body by Evacuation or change the Nature of it within by altering the Mass of Blood.

I may therefore reasonably divide all the Materia Medica described by so many voluminous Authors, only into two Classes of Medicines. Evacuating and Alterating. I did not so much talk of those Remedies that evacuate only from some Parts of the Body, as Bleeding, Clysters, Leeches, Issues, Blisters, Setons, Gargles, Snush, and the like, for they can hardly ever cure any inward Disease; but of such as evacuate the Morbific Matter from the whole Mass of Blood by the five general ways, Stool, Vomit, Urine, Sweat and Salivation; where, without recurring to occult or precarious Qualities, I reduce to the Principles of Chemistry and Reason, the Nature and Operations of Purgative, Emetics, Diuretics, Diaphoretics, of Antimony and Mercury, of Veneral and other Diseases, as likewise the Nature and Usefulness of Bath, and other mineral Waters.

I have likewise examin'd and endeavour'd to explain the Nature and different Effects of Alterating Medicaments, which operate in the Mass of Blood without any Evacuation, such as sweeten the Blood when fewer, that thin it when gross and thick that hasten its too slow Circulation, that stop its too rapid Motion as in Fevers; that cool the Blood, that heat it, and raise the Spirits, as Cordials; that calm the Spirits, as Narcotics; that strengthen the Tone of the Parts, as Styptics, and Astringents; that open Obstructions, as Aperitives. Here therefore I had Occasion to consider the Virtues and Operations of Steel, Opium, Jesuits Powder, of Alcalious and Acid Medicines, and of the whole Tribe of other alternating Remedies.

The above somewhat shortened 'answer' by O'Connor, along with a new plan of animal economy, constitutes an interesting source for studies on medical thinking at the turn of the seventeenth century. It may be envisaged as a synthesis of ancient views (Hippocrates, Aristotle, Galen) related to philosophy of nature, cosmology (notion of elements, their coexistence and interactions, concept of the movement, parts of the body with their properties etc.), with new ideas initiated in the sixteenth century by Paracelsus and his adherents, enriched in the seventeenth century by the iatrochemical trend in medicine. O'Connor did not reject, however, some achievements of another main concept reigning in the medicine of the seventeenth century, i.e. iatrophysics (iatromechanics). He was also familiar with ideas postulated by outstanding representatives of natural sciences, outside the circle of iatrochemists and iatrophysicists such as William Harvey, Marcello Malpighi, etc., as well as with new elements of materialistic philosophy (René Descartes). Thus, selecting various concepts of the human organism, in health and disease, he assumed a system which he referred to as a 'new' approach to animal economy. The term 'new' is repeated in O'Connor's 'answer', with regard to the title 'New Plan' under Nos. 3, 6, 7, 11, 21. What accounts for O'Connor's 'newness' or originality, when assumed it was neither nominal nor of the kind as exemplified by *Totius medicinae idea nova* (1671) by de le Boë (1614–72)? Like the aforementioned author O'Connor did not share the iatrogenic views of van Helmont (1577–1644); he dismissed his metaphysicodynamic system and developed one based on *a priori* assumptions and deductions, with rather indiscriminate extrapolation of chemical processes in nature to the human organism; he accepted a notion of fermentation processes in the body fluids according to the theory of acrimonies (bases and salts), fashionable in the seventeenth century, but, in contradiction to de le Boë, he dismissed personification of vital force, as preached by Paracelsus and J. B. van Helmont, and replaced it by the notion of 'soul', which at that time was gaining ground in England with the increasing popularity of Descartes' philosophy; he rejected also the notion of de le Boë – *Spiritus animales et volatiles* – superseded by his concept of 'spirit' (*Spiritus*), harboured by the human body in health. In O'Connor's opinion it has an existence of its own and does not leave the body at the moment of death. In this respect O'Connor is to be regarded as one of the first to discern what is nowadays referred to as 'clinical death'.

In the light of philosophy, O'Connor started from the deistic point of view; he admitted God as a source of all things, but simultaneously refused to attribute to Him the governing power of the world, interpreting the phenomena of life in a mechanical way, thus departing from the pure chemistry of the seventeenth century. The materialistic tendencies of O'Connor are stressed, among others, by his notion of megalomany of humans who find their species to be superior, as compared with animals; in the eighteenth century this idea culminated in utopic searches for separate zoologic classification of people. Unlike representatives of extreme materialism, O'Connor did not militate against teleology and was not a believer in extreme mechanistic theories, as represented in the eighteenth century by La Mettrie (1709–51) author of *L'homme machine* (1748). During O'Connor's life medicine in Europe was under the influence of mechano-materialistic theories of moderate nature, as postulated by Giovanni Alfonso Borelli (*De motu animalium*, 1690), or by Giorgio Baglivi (1668–1706) who interpreted the human body according to hydraulic laws (the organism would consist of innumerable tubes with the heart as a pump).

As far as embriologic problems are concerned O'Connor must have known the dissertation of G. Sperlinger, *Tractatus physicus de formatione hominis* (1661). O'Connor was also familiar with the analytical method as proposed by Robert Boyle (1626–92) and with the experimental one advocated by van Helmont in chemistry. In 'New Plan' he quoted under paragraph 7 the view of J. Mayow (1641–79) and of

R. Hooke (1635–1703), for whom the respiration was related to the presence in the air of the so-called 'Nitrate', a compound which they also thought to be indispensable for combustion; in this respect they were predecessors of Lavoisier who discovered oxygen in the air.

Unlike chemiatrists of the seventeenth century, O'Connor showed a predilection for anatomy, which may be gathered from paragraph 6 of the 'New Plan' containing a mention about that W. Harvey's discovery and from paragraph 21 suggesting that he did not ignore the merits of Malpighi.

From the above consideration it can be readily concluded that O'Connor was abreast of latest achievements in the field of natural and medical sciences of which he took advantage in his 'New Plan' by integrating theoretical and practical knowedge to coin one system. Against the picture of medicine in the baroque era O'Connor emerges as a type of scientist with moderate mechano-materialistic tendencies under the auspices of iatrophysicists and chemiatrists with vitalistic concepts about phenomena of life in health and disease. In practice he had much in common with neo-paracelsists searching for efficient treatment in experiments designed to find out the essential property of the drug – *Virtus*. In his physics as explanation of natural phenomena his approach to the latter is a somewhat pantheistic one. The emphasis he laid on the necessity of anatomic knowledge is related to traditional notions about phenomena of life, as since Galen's era anatomy was closely linked with physiology, or physiology was still an animated anatomy. By the end of the seventeenth century O'Connor could hardly depart from this narrow concept, abandoned only at the turn of the eighteenth century. Thus, the 'New Plan' by O'Connor could not play a major role, though it harboured a great deal of elements paving the way to modern medicine.

In conclusion I find it hard to understand from the historical point of view why O'Connor's contribution to the development of medical thinking has fallen into oblivion.

References

1 BILIKIEWICZ, T., *Jan Jonston*, Warsaw, 1931, pp. 1–233.

2 KOŚMIŃSKI, S., *Słownik Lekarzów polskich* [Medical Dictionary], Warsaw, 1888, p. 85.

3 KESTNER, C. W., *Med. Gelehrten Lexicon*, Jena, 1740, pp. 213–14; JÖCHER, C. G., *Allg. Gelehrten Lexicon*, Leipzig, 1750, col. I, p. 2050; GASIOROWSKI, L., *Zbiór wiadomości do historii sztuki lekarskiej w Polsce* [Collections new to the Polish history of medicine], Poznan, 1853, vol. II, p. 297; KOŚMIŃSKI, S., op. cit., p. 74: PODGÓRSKA-KLAWE, Z., 'Bernard O'Connor lekarz nadworny Jana Sobieskiego, autor dzieła The history of Poland' [B. O'Connor aulic physician of John Sobieski author of the History of Poland], *Archiwum Historii Medycyny, Warszawa*, 1966, **29**, 133–39.

4 *History of Poland*, vol. I, p. 190 ff.

5 OCZKO, W., [Albertus Occius] (1537–1626), author of *Przymiot* [Syphilis], Cracow, 1581, pp. 1–664.

6 *History of Poland*, vol. I, pp. 153–211.

7 ZIEMBICKI, W., 'Zdrowie i niezdrowie [Health and ill health] Jana Sobieskiego', *Archiwum Historii i Filozofii Medycyny*, Poznań, 1930, **10**, 193–225, **11**, 26–46.

8 O'CONNOR, B., *A new Plan . . .*, p. 289–99.

9 Ibid. pp. 293–96.

10 Ibid. pp. 297–99.

J. Caria Mendes
Lisbon (Portugal)

John Hunter, his travels in Portugal, and his probable influence on Portuguese medicine

During the campaign of 1762–63 between Portugal and Spain (War of the Spanish Succession), some British troops arrived at Lisbon from Belle Isle to help their old ally. The British troops were estimated as ten thousand men of infantry and artillery. The Portuguese–English Army was under the general command of the Count of Lippe.

As a military surgeon of the British troops, John Hunter, aged thirty-six, arrived at Lisbon probably on 6 June 1762. He accompanied all the movements of the troops from Lisbon to the Portuguese border through the valley of the River Tagus. In Santarem he worked in the military hospital. One attack of the Spanish Army obliged the Count of Lippe to defend the Mondego valley and, with a tremendous sweep of nearly forty kilometres per day, the troops moved quickly to Coimbra. Afterwards, the Army came back south again and John Hunter arrived in Abrantes, a town and a fortress on the Tagus valley where the headquarters of the Count of Lippe was situated.

John Hunter was ordered to go to Portalegre, a small town near the border, to be the director of the military hospital there. He stayed there nearly three months, until December, when he came back to Lisbon and we think he embarked to England in the beginning of February 1763. The Peace of Paris was signed in November.

There are some letters of John Hunter concerning his travels in Portugal at the Library of the Royal College of Surgeons, London, some of them already published. They are very interesting documents.

Very probably, not only John Hunter but all the staff of the military service of the Army have had some influence on the evolution of medicine in Portugal. We try to see it through the following facts and dates:

1762–63, Portuguese–Spanish War.

On 1772, nine years after, the University of Coimbra, that had been until this time under a very strong medieval influence, was reformed.

Manuel Constancio, a military surgeon of the Portuguese Army, born near Abrantes, instituted great improvements on the studies and practices of Medicine in Lisbon. He was an anatomist and professor of the Royal Hospital of Lisbon. He very probably knew John Hunter personally.

Under the influence of Manuel Constancio some Portuguese postgraduate medical students of the next generation came to London and Edinburgh on scholarships. It was this generation, immediately after the Napoleonic Wars and Wellington, that developed a liberal, social, political and cultural movement in Portugal, under a strong British influence. They founded the Society of Medicine of Lisbon (1822), one of the oldest societies in Europe conserving the same name and rules, and in 1825, the Royal Medical School of Lisbon and Oporto. On Portalegre, the small town where John Hunter stayed longer, a very characteristic regional hospital was built, very probably concerned with the military hospital of 1762–63. It is a hospital nowadays.

C. Bart and E. Bart-Racoveanu
Bucharest (Romania)

Works of English physicians in the Batthyaneum Library

Libraries containing countless treasures, as well as museums displaying valuable collections and historic milestones can be found even in the most remote areas of a country. Generally these are known only to the specialist and scholar.

That is the case of 'Batthyaneum', a library at Alba Iulia (the old Apulum), a small town in the middle of Transylvania, a region of Romania. The Library was founded by the bishop, the Earl J. Batthyany (1741–95). Although a clergyman he was a personality holding wide humanistic views. All his life he gathered manuscripts, incunabula and books concerning not only theology but all fields of science. Two years before his death he founded a public library in Alba Iulia, where he was primate of the catholic church of Transylvania.

It goes without saying that the Batthyaneum Library can be compared neither with the library of the British Museum nor with that of the Wellcome Institute of the History of Medicine, nevertheless it can be looked upon as one of the richest and most interesting libraries of south-east Europe. It houses a fine collection of 1,300 manuscripts, 600 incunabula and about 100,000 printed books.

As regards English medical science as a whole, i.e. works written in English as well as translations from English authors, there are to be found four manuscripts, four incunabula, and around 150 books by English authors, published after 1500.

If, comparatively, English medical science is represented by a smaller number of authors than that of authors of German or Italian origin, still it surpasses the number of Spanish, Hungarian or Armenian authors. This can be explained by the fact that the founder lived for a while in Rome, then within the boundaries of the former Hapsburg Empire, acquiring also the library of Carindal Migrazzi of Vienna.

Here are some of the English Medical Collections that can be found in the library:

(A) Manuscripts all belonging to the fourteenth century: 'De proprietatibus rerum . . .' by Bartholomeus Anglicus, 'Magisterium de arte alchemicae' by Michaele Scotus, 'Rosarius' by Johannes Dastinus Anglicus, 'Speculum astronomiae' or 'astrologiae' by Rogerus Bacon.

(B) The Incunabula (chronologically) are: 'Auctoritatis Aristotelis' by the Venerable Bede, Coloniae, 1447, apud J. Guldenschaefium; 'Repertorium, sive tabula generalis auctoritatium Aristotelis cum commento' also by the Venerable Bede, Nurenbergae, 1490, apud P. Wagnerium; 'Cursus librorum philosophiae naturalis secundum viam doctoris subtilis Scoti', published by an unknown, Basilae, 1494, apud Furterum; 'Liber physionomiae in multis secretis mulierum' by M. Scotus printed in Venetiae, the year of publication is not mentioned, but it is considered by Denis as an incunabulum.

Manuscripts and incunabula concerning medical sciences, as might be expected, are rather scarce. Alchemy and astrology are the fields mostly dealt with. It should also be noted that the manuscripts as well as the incunabula above mentioned are the works of clergymen and not of physicians. But one has to bear in mind that in Europe as well as in England, during the Middle Ages, only clergymen specialized in the medical sciences. This fact was stressed also by C. H. Talbot in his work, *Medicine in Medieval England*, London, 1967. And if these clergymen were highly influenced by Aristotle or Pliny, as concerns medical sciences they opposed the Arabic influence and therefore we are not faced with a process of erosion of antiquity as has been upheld by some authors.

(C) Now, let us consider the works of English authors written after 1500. We are neither going to list here the names of all these authors nor their works. We shall attempt to give some general information only. Mentioning manuscripts and incunabula all written by priests, it may be supposed that Batthyany showed a special leaning towards collecting only these kinds of works. However, looking through the collections of the library one can see that he was fairly impartial.

In the Batthyaneum Library one can find the complete book collection of such authors as Sydenham, Willis, Robert Morton, or some works by James Primrose, Johnstone, W. Colle, while John Caius is represented in the library by his *De mendendis methode* (1544), Thomas Browne by his *Religio Medici* (1452) alongside with B. O'Connor's *Evangelium Medici* (1699) or Gideon Harvey's *Ars curandi morbes ex expectatione*, bound together with *De vanitatibus dolis et mendaciis medicorum* (1695), as well as many other authors. Works written in English as John Armstrong's *Preserving Health*, Bellinger's *Nutrition of the Foetus*, James Keill's *Animal Oeconomy*, W. Read's *The Whole Practice of Chirurgery*, as well as many others are also represented. Besides it should be noted that the works of many English authors such as R. Bacon, Ch. Bell, F. Home, R. Lower, William Musgrave, W. Prout, C. Wintringham, translated into French or German are also to be found in the Library. This is a token of the appreciation these authors enjoyed in such a medical centre as Vienna.

We should like to mention also English authors, physicians or laymen who are represented in the Library by one or several works. Among these may be quoted Ray's famous *Historia Plantarum . . .* (London, 1693), Parkinson's *Paradise of Flowers* (London, 1655), Helsham's *Physica experimentalis* (1769) as well as Fr. Bacon's work in no less than four editions. The great esteem enjoyed by Bacon's work can be seen also from the fact that, as in his London (1638) edition was lacking the chapter *Historia Vitis et Mortis*, this one had been replaced by a handwritten copy.

Also to be found there are English works of value concerning other fields of science such as: *Flos historiarum terrae Orientis* by John Haythonus (manuscript, 1307), *Physica Experimentalis* by Helhalmus (ex Londonensi anglica, editione in latinum, translata Vindobone, 1769) and *Historia naturalis de quadrupedibus libri*, by John Johnstonus (1657) and many others. But of course we are not going to deal with these.

Before closing we should like to add a few words that might be of interest to the bibliophile.

The Batthyaneum Library contains other treasures including illustrated copies in all fields of interest, rare collections, or editio princeps, or even unique copies, illuminated manuscripts, in folio volumes with marginal notes. Among these can be mentioned the 'Codex Aureus', a manuscript of the ninth century, the gospel according to St. Mark, 'Naturalis imago diversiorum conchyliorum coloribus ad vivum depictorum' a manuscript unique in the world as it concerns the contents and its presentation.

All these increase the interest for this library – that is why scholars will travel long distances personally to examine an original item.

J. C. Bercus
Bucharest (Romania)

The activity of the English doctor J. B. Mawr in Bucharest

Together with many foreign doctors coming from abroad and professing medicine in Wallachia in the second half of the nineteenth century, the name of the English doctor John Barker Mawr is recorded as having played an important role in the medical and cultural life of the country.[1]

J. B. Mawr was born in London in 1815, studied medicine there and got a doctor's degree in 1840. He came to Romania to accompany Ion C. Brătianu, the important Romanian statesman, and settled in Bucharest.[2] He was granted the right for a free practice of medicine in 1859.[3]

Eager to make for himself a name in the medical life of Romania, Dr. J. B. Mawr addressed a memorial, on the 12–24 September 1858, to the Minister of the Home Department (Prince Constantin Ghica), proposing the nomination of an Inspector General for public sanitation in Bucharest. His proposal was made because of the conditions he noted in Bucharest, and to the 'hearty welcome' of the Prince Alexandru Ghica.

'I consider the nomination of an Inspector general of public sanitation a very important matter' appears in Mawr's memorial. 'My observations have convinced me that the diseases and mortality are more frequent here than in other countries . . . and their causes are far too little studied; as for hygiene it is completely misunderstood and badly observed that is why it is necessary to take the most definite steps required by science and experience in order to avoid epidemics and epizoty in order to maintain hospitals, charity establishments, barracks, monastries, schools, towns and villages in the best conditions'.[4] Mawr's project went on mentioning a series of measures to be taken, such as: to remove dirt, to drain stagnant ponds, analyse drinking water, to clean away from the streets and markets 'everything that could work up and bring about diseases; consequently, at least half of the diseases in this country would be lessened'.

On 13 September, Mawr's memorial – translated – was sent off to the Health Committee which, in its turn, delivered it to the Medical Council. Having studied it, the Medical Council showed in its answer of 20 September that there were still many things to be done as regards the improvement of public health, where the lack of hygienic conditions was not caused by disregard of science but 'it had been – up to now – due to some causes independent of the field of medical men's activity'. As far back as three years, the Council had minutely elaborated a work meant to take the steps demanded for public health, but the 'political and economical state of the country had not allowed to put into practice all the measures suggested, such as street sewerage and pavement, drainage of moorlands with standing waters etc., although part of it has already been put into work'. In its answer, the Council mentioned once more the tasks of the veterinary surgeons, and of the doctors belonging to the Commissions charged with inspecting public markets. Even the anterior provisions of Art. 47 of the Organic Regulations stipulated a series of prerogatives which the Medical Council, the chemists in the Capital, and district doctors are today charged with.

As a conclusion the signatories to the answer given by the Medical Council (Dr. N. Gusi, president, Dr. C. Bacaloglu, Dr. I. Barsch, Dr. C. Leib, Dr. G. Athanasovici, members, and G. Polizu, secretary) 'are of the opinion that the setting up of a General Medical Inspector for Public Health is unnecessary. It is desirable only that the future circumstances of the country should permit the exact execution with all the necessary vigour of the public health measures which already exist and those which are added to them day by day corresponding to the development and civilization of the country'.[5]

In February 1859, Dr. Mawr was appointed 'Secondary Doctor' to the Brâncovenesc Hospital, together with the 'Primary Doctor', Emanoil Triandafilidis, as well as a physician to the 'Domnita Bălașa' Asylum, both in Bucharest. He worked in those appointments until 1876 when he asked for his retirement.

On 22 August 1863, The Scientific Medical Society from Bucharest held an extraordinary meeting in the building of the Colțea Hospital, and among the new members admitted to the Society was also to be found Mawr. He seemed not to have actively participated in the debates of this Society, although on 8 October 1864, he was chosen together with Dr. N. Turuescu, Dr. Gh. Athanasovici, Dr. L. Fialla and Dr. G. Kiriazi to draw up a report on the fees of medical consultations.[6] He was a member of the Royal College of Surgeons and Physicians in London, and as a correspondent of the English medical newspaper the *Lancet* he published a number of notes and reports in which he related aspects of medical life.

During the 1877–78 War of Independence of Romania, Dr. J. B. Mawr maintained thirty beds in a hospital for the wounded by the aid of a contribution received from England.[7]

On retiring, Mawr published his work *The Art of Caring for little children. A Guide for young mothers for the upbringing of children*, Bucharest, 1883.

'Doctor Mor' or 'The Englishman' as he was called, enjoyed a great reputation in the hospital, in the medical life of Bucharest especially as a paediatrician. He died in Bucharest in 1892.

References

1 Among the foreign doctors who had come to Wallachia in that time, we should mention M. Mingarelli (Italian); D. Lamberty, G. Papadopulo-Kiriazi, T. Vaias, D. Ziteseos, Em. Triandafilidis (Greek); P. Protici, G. Athanasovici, P. Beron (Bulgarian); N. J. Russel, P. Alexandrof (Russian); J. Koperniki (Polish); L. Fialla, J. Oroszhegyi (Hungarian); J. N. Meyer (Austrian); J. G. Andreas Grunau (German); C. Davila, A. Lebiez (French), etc.

2 The doctor J. B. Mawr lived on Serafim Street nr. 3 and Fortuna nr. 5.

3 The *Journal of the Medical Council of the Principality of Wallachia* from 28 June 1858, signed by the doctors: N. Gusi, C. Leib, I. Barasch. See address of the Medical Council and of the Pharmaceutical College nr. 82 from 9 and 17 July 1858, as well as Th. St. Buc., Fond D.G.S.S. dossier nr. 22/1858.

4 Arh. St. Buc., Fond. D.G.S.S., dossier 105/1858, fol. 4.
5 Idem, fols. 3 and 6; *Official Bulletin*, nr. 6 from 19 January 1858, p. 23. See G. Barbu, *The Art of Healing in the Bucharest of the Past*, Bucharest, 1967, pp. 126, 127 and 163.
6 *Official Gazette*, nr. 25/5 September 1863, pp. 194–95; V. Gomoiu, *From the History of Medicine and of the Medical Teaching in Romania*, Bucharest, 1923, pp. 564, 573; Idem, *Catalogue of Physicians, Pharmacists, Veterinary Surgeons . . .*, Brăila, 1938, p. 273; Idem, *An Addition to the Report*, vol. I, Bucharest, 1941, p. 104; *The Annual of Sanitary Service*, 1964, pp. 21–26.
7 GOMOIU, V. and PLĂTĂREANU, V., *The Centenary of the Hospital Brăncovenesc*, Bucharest, 1927, p. 95.

B. Dutescu and I. C. Pop
Bucharest (*Romania*)

Exposé sur les relations médicales entre la Grande Bretagne et la Roumanie dans le domaine de l'histoire de la médecine

Nous ressentons un grand plaisir en présentant à la tribune de ce Congrès international quelques informations concernant les relations scientifiques dans le domaine de l'histoire de la médecine entre la Roumanie et la Grande Bretagne.

Notre communication présente les relations que l'éminent et érudit chirurgien roumain le Dr. Victor Gomoiu (Président de la Société Internationale de l'Histoire de la Médecine entre 1936–70) a eu avec les savants de Grande Bretagne.

Nous précisions, dès le début, que nos informations ne peuvent pas être complètes, car le musée d'histoire de la médecine créé et organisé par Victor Gomoiu, ainsi que sa bibliothèque personnelle, ont été partiellement détruits pendant la guerre. Parmi les documents sauvés nous avons retrouvé un cahier contenant les adresses de plusieurs personnalités scientifiques de divers pays. Nous citons celles provenant de la Grande Bretagne: le Professeur A. Crombie de Oxford, le Professeur Charles Singer de Londres, le Professeur Geoffrey R. Edwards de Londres (ancien secrétaire de la Société Royale des médecins de Londres), le Professeur I. E. Mours de Glasgow, le Professeur Sir Arthur S. MacNalty de Londres (ancien président de la Société de l'Histoire de la Médecine) le Professeur Rollestone de Londres, le Dr. A. V. Hill de Londres (ancien président de la Société Royale des médecins de Londres) le Dr. I. Connie de Edimburg, le Dr. Norman de Londres, le Dr. A. E. Williams de Londres et le Dr. Peter I. Johnston – Saints de Londres. Nous allons nous occuper seulement de ceux pour lesquels nous avons trouvé des dates et une partie de leur correspondance avec le Dr. V. Gomoiu.

La personnalité de Victor Gomoiu est bien connue, de même que son rôle dans le mouvement scientifique international dans le domaine de l'histoire de la médecine. En 1970 Editura Medicală a publié la monographie signée par un de nous 'Victor Gomoiu 1882–1960' qui présente la vie et l'œuvre de cette dynamique personnalité médicale.

Un de ces plus grands mérits est celui d'avoir beaucoup travaillé pour que les Sociétés scientifiques nationales d'histoire de la médecine se connaîssent mieux, collaborent plus fructueusement et soient plus actives dans la grande famille de la Société Internationale de l'histoire de la médecine. Pour ses mérites dans l'assistence médicale et dans l'activité scientifique, l'état Roumain et d'autres états et sociétés savantes ont conféré à Victor Gomoiu plusieurs titres de grand honneur.

Pour le zèle qu'il avait prouvé pendant la première querre mondiale quand il a été chirurgien, le Gouvernement de la République Française lui a accordé la Légion d'honneur (Chevalier). Il a été élu membre des plus prestigieuses sociétés d'histoire de la médecine; la société française (1926); les sociétés: hellène (1932), belge (1935), allemande (1936), anglaise (1939), etc.

Voilà pourquoi nous considérons très intéressant de présenter à l'occasion de ce Congrès et comme un pieux hommage porté à nos prédécesseurs, les liaisons scientifiques permanentes qui ont existé entre eux, assurant une meilleure connaissance des gens, la promotion de la science, de la collaboration et la bonne entente.

Le Professeur Gomoiu avait connu le Professeur Ch. Singer en 1927 à l'occasion du VIe Congrès International qui a eu lieu à Leyde. Les rapports des deux savants ont été peu fréquents jusqu'en 1932 (les félicitations à l'occasion des Fêtes de l'An et des rencontres à l'occasion des Congrès qui ont suivi). Pendant la période des préparatifs pour le IXe Congrès International de Bucarest (1932) leur amitié s'est affermie; l'échange de lettres et d'idées entre les deux hommes est devenu plus vif. Le Professeur Ch. Singer fut designé comme représentant de l'Université de Londres au Congrès de Bucarest. Mais, à la veille de l'ouverture du Congrès on a annoncé officiellement que le Professeur Ch. Singer ne pouvait pas participer, étant retenu par d'autres charges. Les regrets du Professeur Ch. Singer sont presentés dans la lettre qu'il a envoyée au Dr. V. Gomoiu qu'il appelle «Mon cher collègue et ami» et où il exprimait son regret de ne pas pouvoir connaître la Roumanie.

En échange, ce fut le Dr. John Davy Rollestone – ancien secretaire général du Congrès International de l'histoire de la Médecine de Londres (1922) et auteur d'un important travail sur les maladies infectieuses aiguës et de nombreux articles sur l'histoire de la médecine, la pédiatrie et les maladies infectieuses qui prit part au Congrès de Bucarest de 1932.

Vieux membre de la Société internationale de l'histoire de la médecine, le Dr. J. D. Rollestone a participé presque à tous les congrès internationaux de la Société.

Il avait connu le Dr. Gomoiu à l'occasion du VIIe Congrès de Oslo et il l'avait revu à Rome à l'occasion du VIIIe Congrès. Le IXe Congrès de Bucarest a affermi l'amitié des deux savants, qui est restée sincère et durable.

Les lettres qu'il ont échangés à l'epoque nous permettent de connaître les rapports d'amitié et de considération qui existaient entre eux.

La séance du Congrès du 13 septembre 1932, ayant comme thème «La défence de l'Europe contre la peste» a été présidée par le Professeur Dr. I. Cantacuzino et le Dr. Rollestone; à la tribune du Congrès le Professeur Rollestone a présenté l'étude *Cancer and Medieval medicine*. A l'occasion de ce Congrès sur la recommendation du Dr. V. Gomoiu, le Dr. J. D. Rollestone a été honoré avec la décoration «Le mérite culturel» – Ie classe, qui à l'époque était le plus haute distinction roumaine pour les gens de lettres.

En 1936, une lettre adressée par le Dr. J. D. Rollestone au Dr. V. Gomoiu confirme qu'il avait reçu les livres et les objets qu'on lui avait envoyé à Londres.

Nous n'avons pas pu retrouver le titre des livres et, de même, nous ne connaissons pas quelles dates, objets (pièces) ou photos de pièces chirurgicales anciennes trouvées sur le territoire de notre pays avaient été envoyées au Professeur Rollestone par le Dr. Gomoiu.

Nous n'avons trouvé qu'un reçu postale avec quelques mots de V. Gomoiu qui certifient l'expédition de ce qu'on lui avait demandé. Il s'agit, sans doute, de pièces chirurgicales trouvées sur le territoire de la Dacie et datant du temps de l'occupation romaine.

Un autre participant au IXe Congrès de la Société Internationale de la médecine qui a visité notre pays en 1932 en tant que représentant du «Wellcome Historical Medical Museum» et du Ministère de l'instruction publique a été le Capitaine P. Johnson-Saint.

Après le Congrès, a son retour en Angleterre, le délégué du «Wellcome Historical Medical Museum» écrivait au Dr. Gomoiu avec beaucoup de chaleur:

> Au moment de mon retour à Londres du Congrès à Bucarest, j'estime que c'est mon premier devoir de vous écrire pour vous remercier en votre qualité de Président du Conseil de la Société roumaine de l'histoire de la médecine des amabilités et du bon accueil que l'on m'a temoignés pendant mon séjour à Bucarest comme délégué officiel de la Grande Bretagne.
>
> Je suis sûr que tous ceux qui assistaient au Congrès seront de mon avis, que l'assemblée a eu un succès complet autant qu'agréable pour tout le monde, grace en grande partie aux efforts amicaux de madame Gomoiu et de vous-même, mon cher confrère. . . .

Voila seulement quelques aspects des nombreuses liaisons d'amitié qui ont existé entre la Société roumaine d'histoire de la médecine et le Dr. Victor Gomoiu et d'éminents savants, médecins et historiens de Grande Bretagne. Ce sont de vifs exemples qui incitent au développement future de ces relations.

Nous sommes contents de constater qu'une importante délégation d'éminentes personnalités de l'histoire de la médecine anglaise, sous la direction du Dr. F. N. L. Poynter, a participé au XXIIe Congrès International de Bucarest en 1970 et que de même ici, à Londres, se trouvent les représentants des plus importants médecins-historiens roumains.

V. C. Ionescu and C. Angelescu
Bucharest (Romania)

L'insuline de Banting et Best (1922) et la pancréine de Paulesco (1921)

Dans l'un des derniers numéros du périodique belge *A.B.D.* (Association Belge du Diabète), le Professeur Bastanie (Bruxelles), en faisant l'historique de la découverte de l'insuline par Banting et Best, évoque après la description des travaux canadiens, qu'à l'autre bout du monde, un auteur roumain – Paulesco – professeur de physiologie à la Faculté de Médecine de Bucarest, effectuait lui aussi des recherches similaires, *avec les mêmes résultats*. . . . En 1921, dans une revue belge de Frédericq de Liège et Héger de Bruxelles, Paulesco publiait un article merveilleux, intitulé modestement: «Recherches sur le rôle du pancréas dans l'assimilation nutritive.» En effet, Paulesco obtenait *les mêmes résultats*, mais il les obtenait . . . *huit mois avant les canadiens.*

Le Professeur Bastanie décrit les canadiens «comme étant deux jeunes gens, l'un chirurgien, âgé de 30 ans, formé par l'expérience de la guerre, l'autre étudiant en médecine».

Qui était Paulesco, dont Sir Edward Sharpey Shafer, dans son traité *The Endocrine Organs*, London, 1926, p. 344, en parlant de la sécrétion interne du pancréas, précisait: «La même année que Paulesco *publiait* ses premières expériences, J. C. Banting et C. H. Best commençaient leurs expériences à ce sujet.»

Et sur l'autre continent, les savants brasiliens Alfredo Sordelli et Juan Lewis, dans leur livre *L'insuline*, Buenos-Aires, 1924, mentionnaient: «Paulesco mérite une mention spéciale dans ce chapitre et même nous pourrions dire dans l'ensemble du problème de l'insuline, car en 1921 il a préparé un extrait aqueux de pancréas très actif . . . qui lui a permis d'obtenir *les mêmes résultats* que ceux publiés sept mois plus tard par les canadiens.»

N. C. Paulesco est né à Bucarest en 1869. Ayant une culture générale exceptionelle, parlant parfaitement le latin, le grec et le français, il part à Paris en 1888 et s'inscrit à la Faculté de Médecine. En 1892, il occupe par concours la place d'externe à l'Hôpital Hôtel-Dieu, dans le service du Professeur Lancereaux. Ici il se fait remarquer par son intélligence éclatante et par une exceptionnelle activité dans le service. En 1894, l'illustre clinicien Lancereaux, appréciant l'originalité et la profondeur de sa pensée, prend le jeune externe roumain comme Interne à l'Hôpital Notre Dame du Perpétuel Secours, où il était Médecin Chef. En 1897, Paulesco obtient le titre de *Docteur en Médecine et Chirurgie* de la Faculté de Médecine de Paris avec la mention «Extrêmement Bien». Il est nommé la même année Médecin

Adjoint de l'hôpital où il travaillait. En 1899, il obtient le titre de *Docteur ès Sciences Naturelles* à la Sorbonne et en 1901 celui de *Docteur de l'Université de Paris.*

De simple élève, Paulesco devient le collaborateur du Professeur Lancereaux. Des articles et des études de spécialité de la plus grande importance se succèdent à courts intervalles.

En 1902, l'Etat français lui accorde «les Palmes Académiques», en le nommant «Officier d'Académie».

On lui offre une belle situation à l'hôpital où il travaillait, pour qu'il s'établisse en France.

Une chair lui est offerte à l'Université de Friburg (Suisse).

Le 16 octobre 1897, avec l'apparition du *Journal de Médecine Interne*, publié sous la direction scientifique de Lancereaux, Paulesco est nommé secrétaire de rédaction, charge qu'il détient jusqu'en 1900, quand il est appelé comme Professeur de Physiologie à la Faculté de Médecine de Bucarest.

Le premier travail monumental de Paulesco est le *Traité de Médecine*, en collaboration avec Lancereaux. Le grand clinicien et président de l'Académie de Médecine de Paris, le considère comme le plus digne à le seconder dans l'accomplissement de cet important ouvrage.

En 1908, Paulesco publie L'*Hypophyse du cerveau*, une magistrale étude sur l'hypophyse, dans laquelle il décrit pour la première fois une nouvelle voie d'accès pour son extirpation. Cette étude a eu un grand retentissement dans le monde entier et le grand neuro-chirurgien américain Cushing, qui lui a adopté la méthode dans la chirurgie sur l'homme, déclarait que «c'était de beaucoup la plus importante contribution dans ce domaine».

Il écrit en 1913 un ouvrage sur le *Traitement de la Fièvre.*

En 1921 il publie en français un *Traité de Physiologie* en trois volumes, le résumé de son cours proféssé à la Faculté de Médecine de Bucarest et que le grand physiologiste Maurice Arthus de Lausanne salue de la sorte: «Mon traité a besoin d'un chapitre de physiologie pathologique et de pharmacodynamique, afin que l'étudiant soit préparé à aborder la clinique; le vôtre est complet.»

Mais son génie scientifique atteint l'apogée en 1921 quand, après des années d'études et de recherches sérieuses, commencées du temps où il se trouvait encore à Paris, il publie dans les Comptes Rendus de la Société de Biologie de Paris et dans les Archives Internationales de Physiologie de Liège, son célèbre ouvrage intitulé «modestement» comme le disait Bastanie, *Recherches sur le rôle du pancréas dans l'assimilation nutritive*, dans lequel il décrit l'insuline nommée par lui Pancréine.

Le traitement du diabète était dès lors découvert. Il est vrai, dans un petit coin de l'Europe assez peu connu alors, dans un petit pays appauvri par la guerre et par l'occupation ennemie de 1916–18, et se trouvant dans une grande crise économique à cause des transformations politiques, enfin par un modeste homme de science qui, comme il déclarait plus tard, était convaincu que la date des publications scientifiques le mettait à l'abri de toute iniquité ultérieure. Il brévète son invention en avril 1922, mais le pays ne possède pas d'industrie pharmaceutique ni les fonds nécessaires pour la créer. La pancréine ne peut donc pas être diffusée.

Banting et Best de Toronto, qui ont pris connaissance de cet ouvrage et qui commettent l'imprudence de la signaler dans la bibliographie de leur premier article, répètent les expériences de Paulesco et, *huit mois plus tard*, ils obtiennent l'extrait aqueux de pancréas à caractères hypoglycémiants. Ils annoncent bruyamment leur résultat, ils *dénaturent* ceux de Paulesco, et ils s'associent un biochimiste de grande classe, Collip, qui sépare à partir de cet extrait le principe actif, dénomé par eux «Insuline». Enfin, ils font tout de suite appel aux services d'Elli Lilly Comp., qui, avec ses vastes possibilités, dans un temps record, inonde le monde entier avec le précieux médicament anti-diabétique. Les canadiens reçoivent les honneurs, et Paulesco reste désabusé; ses travaux seront bientôt complètement oubliés.

Cinquante ans passent et le Professeur Ian Murray de Glasgow, membre fondateur de la Fédération Internationale du Diabète et Membre du Conseil de Direction de l'Association Britannique du Diabète, chercheur passionné et homme de science correct, dans une minutieuse étude d'histoire de la médecine rétablit la vérité concernant la priorité de la découverte de l'insuline par Paulesco (Paulesco and the Isolation of Insulin by Ian Murray, *Journal of the History of Medicine and Allied Sciences*, no. 2, April 1971).

Des personnalités scientifiques de grande valeur reconnaissent de même aujourd'hui Paulesco comme découvreur de l'insuline: Professeur Eric Marin de Genève, Professeur Rolf Luft de Suède, Dr. Rodrigues Minon d'Espagne, Professeur R. Korec de Tchekoslovaquie, Professeur I. Magyar d'Hongrie etc., etc., remettent Paulesco dans ses droits de découvreur de l'insuline.

L'activité scientifique de Paulesco prend fin avec une autre étude de valeur mondiale, en démonstrant l'inexactitude des lois uréo-sécrétoires d'Ambard. Les lois d'Ambard et sa Constante uréo-sécrétoire *sont erronées*. Et cette constante qui a fait tant de bruit pendant toute une époque, a été définitivement éliminée de la science par les recherches expérimentales de Paulesco.

«Ces distingués chercheurs de laboratoire (Paulesco et collaborateurs), écrivait F. Cathelin dans les Travaux annuels d'Urologie 1926, apportent la confirmation expérimentale des idées que je défends seul en France depuis plus de dix ans, que les lois d'Ambard sont erronées.»

Paulesco est mort en juillet 1931.

Nous avons cru utile la publication succinte de ces dates pour donner la possibilité a ceux qui connaissent le palmarès de l'équipe de Toronto, publié avec beaucoup de détails dans la presse mondiale, de connaître aussi la modeste activité scientifique du Professeur N. C. Paulesco, le vrai découvreur de l'insuline.

M. G. Marinescu and I. Popescu-Sibiu
Bucharest (Romania)

The scientific relations of Prof. Dr. Gh. Marinescu with scientists in the U.S.A. and Canada

Professor Marinescu's relations with the scientific centres in the U.S.A. and in Canada are reflected in the content of about seventy letters sent from fourteen localities (most of them – thirty-eight – from New York), signed by over thirty scientific personalities and conserved in the archives of the Professor G. Marinescu Memorial Museum in Bucharest. These relations have expanded in all the fields of research where – neurology having its deep implications – the Romanian scientist has made a precious contribution. They represent an exchange of experience both through his collaboration to numerous reviews and through his membership of some scientific North American speciality societies.

These relations started in 1913. Using a polyomyelitic virus sent by Professor Flexner (Rockefeller Institute, New York), by means of his experiments on apes, Professor Marinescu thoroughly described the localization process of the virus in the nervous system. In 1932, Flexner wrote a letter in which he particularly expressed his appreciation of the work about 'Encephalomyelitis' sent to him by Professor Marinescu.

Professor E. V. Coudry, from the same Institute, praises Professor Marinescu's initiative in the researches concerning the part played by oxidases in the neuro-histologic phenomena, expressing at the same time his satisfaction of the fact that the Romanian scientist agrees with the conclusions he himself arrived at when studying the intramuscular inclusions of the rabies virus.

In 1926, Professor Emile S. Jeliffe, general secretary of the editorial board of the *Review for Neurology and Psychiatry* in New York, considers the researches made by Professor Marinescu in the field of epidemic encephalitis (carried out in London in 1917) as a precious contribution to the work of Van Economo on this subject. Two years later he published two papers in this American review and in 1932, when his work about the *Tonus of the Striated Muscles* (published in French in Bucharest, prefaced by Sherrington and dedicated to Pierre Marie) came out, he wrote to his Romanian colleague: 'with admiration for your stimulating researches which considerably contributed to the progress of neurology'.

In 1929, Professor Richter, the famous neurologist from Cornell University, New York, expressed his thanks for the interesting photos (neurochemistry and physiology) and reproduced them in the university's *Review of Neurology*. 'Through the precious researches you have carried out, you have reinforced Claude Bernard's law'. The neurologist Professor Berhard Sachs from New York stressed in a letter the value of the original articles 'The amaurotic idiocy' and 'The development of the cerebellar cortex'; he expressed his wish to meet him at the Neurology Congress in Berne (1931), where they actually met.

In the field of biochemistry, Professor Marinescu exchanged works with Dr. Bertrand M. Brickner, concerning the sclerogenous character of lipasia and the possibility of inactivating it by an early treatment with hydrochloric quinine.

In 1932, Professor Armando Ferraro, the director of the Institute and Hospital for Psychiatry from New York, thanked Professor Marinescu for the oxidase preparations which he sent and wrote to him: 'I wish I could come to Bucharest as an old and great admirer of your monumental work which contributes to the progress of neurology, to know you personally in order to cooperate in the field of intracellular chemism'.

The same year, Sir Clifford N. Beers informed him of his election as a member of the International Society for Mental Hygiene from New York. Professor O'Brien from the Rockefeller Institute, expressed his admiration for his pupil O. Sager whom he met when he was a scholar of this institute, as well as his wish to come to Bucharest in order to have the honour of making his acquaintance and start a collaboration. In other letters from New York signed by Dr. F. Tilha (1931) from the Institute for Neurology, Sir Alsop Riley (1931), Dr. Abner Volt (1935), we find the same concern for the exchange of experience and works in the above-mentioned fields. The same year, Dr. Ralph C. Gerhard wrote about a scientific interest for genetics and its problems which he discussed at a congress with Dr. Bagdasar.

The last six letters from New York (1937–38), signed by Dr. Gersberg from the Medical Association of Spanish Language, referred to the elaboration of the programme for a scientific session, asking Professor Marinescu to write an article for the *Blue Book* issued by this association.

As early as 1925, the first letter from Washington written by Dr. E. Folkner, director of the *Review of the American Association for Medical Researches*, informed Professor Marinescu that he had been elected a member of this association and collaborator to the review. One year later, Professor R. C. Cook from the American Association for Genetics and the *Review for Genetics*, requested his collaboration, especially concerning the laws of heredity, informing him that he had often been quoted in works of psychopedagogy or of a social character, and also that he had been elected a member of this association and collaborator of the review.

In 1929, Dr. Frankwood Willie, the president of the first American Congress for Mental Hygiene (5 May 1930), invited Professor Marinescu to this Congress in order to start at the same time a collaboration with the American Association for Geriatrics in Washington. A month after Professor Marinescu's death, a letter (20 July 1938) came from Professor Welling Othmar Solnieky, dean of the Faculty of Medicine of Georgetown University, in which he asked for a photograph in order to 'honour us by entering in our collection of the famous research workers of the world'.

The first letter (in the archives of the Museum), dated from 1921, is signed by the professor for physiology, Dr. E. M. Child from the Faculty of Medicine of Chicago University, requesting his scientific collaboration. Four years later, the Chicago department of the Society 'Science Extension' suggested the creation in Romania of a department of this society, as had been done in several European countries, in order to achieve a systematic organization of the exchange of experience among all the research centres in the world.

Shortly after this, Professor Max Thorek, one of the greatest surgeons of the time, asked him, because of the admiration he had for his work, to review some of his papers and give him his opinion.

Professor Parkval Beck, of the same Faculty, read the work Professor Marinescu had published together with Dr. Goldstein about the myoblasts of a tumour, asked him to send the microphotographs for his collection, as such a tumour is extremely rare.

The echo of Professor Marinescu's work made its way also to California since 1927, when his first two articles to appear in this part of the world were published in the *Review for Endocrinology* issued by Dr. Achard from Los Angeles: 'About senility and the endocrine glands' and 'Old age, rejuvenation from the endocrinologic point of view'. The same year, while Professor Marinescu was in Cordoba, a letter came from Dr. L. Pomery (from Los Angeles), informing him of the scientific interest he found in the method of titrating ethylic and methylic alcohol in live organisms and in cadavers, he asked him to send the original works he published about this method.

A particular interest was also aroused in Philadelphia whence Dr. Friedrich Rand from Pennsylvania University and the Union of the American Societies for Biology suggested a collaboration and asked for extracts of the problems of biology and pharmacology tests which the Romanian scientist wrote about.

In the same spirit, the Gladwyne Laboratory for Biochemistry from Philadelphia wanted to know the technique of the researches carried out by Professor Marinescu concerning Charcot's disease and the colloidal chemism of the nervous system, new discoveries which were considered as very promising on the grounds of the original conception of Professor Marinescu. Finally, Professor S. I. Sperling from the same town wrote to thank him for the interesting work about the *Epidemy of Polyomyelitis in Romania* (1928), published in our country.

From Boston, Dr. Loring T. Swain from the A. Brigham Hospital (1931–35) wrote, thanking Marinescu for the works which he received and particularly appreciated, and in 1937, Dr. A. Meyersohn asked the Romanian scientist to give his opinion about a recent classification of neurosis made by neurologists and psychoanalysts.

Finally, from Baltimore, Professor Warren H. Leirs, and Dr. R. M. Perdue from Kansas (who met Marinescu in Italy in 1926), expressed the same regard when suggesting a scientific collaboration.

A few days before his death, Professor S. C. Aunoy wrote from New Orleans informing him that, much to his regret, he could not take part to the congress about 'Rabies', but he sent his paper.

From Canada, two letters attest of a brief scientific relation. One is dated 1928 and comes from Ontario University, concerning biochemistry; the other, dated 1932, comes from Professor A. Barbeau from the Montreal University, asking for Professor Marinescu's work 'About old age', which he considers of real value.

This high scientific world-wide regard for the work of the Romanian scientist never stopped asserting itself, as the value of his discoveries had a lasting, far from ephemeral character; they have been confirmed by the evolution of contemporary science.

Effectively, the actual value of his work has been stressed on the occasion of the centenary of his birth (1963) which was celebrated in the great scientific centres of the world under the care of the World Council for Peace. Recalling only the scientific relations of Professor Marinescu's work with the North American scientific centres, we will mention part of a letter written by Professor Houston Merritt from the Columbia University in New York at the centenary celebrations: 'I would have liked to be present to the honour of the commemoration of one of the world's leading neurologists. He has not only been the founder of Romanian neurology: his work has had a considerable influence on the development of neurology in the world'.

Finally, we will quote a fragment of the report which Professor Murray Barr, the holder of the Chair for Microscopic Anatomy of Ontario University, published in 1951 in the review *Science* about the two volumes *La cellule nerveuse*, a work issued in Paris in 1909. 'Some branches of science – writes Murray Barr – are based on such new conceptions and methods that older literature presents but little interest. This does not happen with neuro-anatomy. It is not admissible that an up-to-date research worker studying in this field, should not know this meticulous and brilliant work carried out in Europe half a century ago . . .'.

M. M. Grecu
Cluj (Romania)

Old medical works by English authors in some Romanian libraries

The development of the Romanian medical culture presents endeavours and fundamental achievements in the field of medical studies, outstanding personalities, and scientific works through which the Romanian Medical School integrated itself into the great torrent of world medicine.

The contribution of the Romanian Medical School to world medicine is already known, but we all know that it has not developed completely isolated, as a mountain flower on a peak. The direct and indirect influences of some other schools or their representatives whose books reached us, or the Romanian physicians who studied in other European centres, made these links turn to good account and brought about the achievements well known in our days.

In the present paper I shall deal with only one aspect of the documentation problem, that is medical books of English origin, their presence in our state and private libraries, books that in the seventeenth and eighteenth centuries made possible the links, more difficult at that time, between our medical world and the English one, having in mind the considerable distance, the limited possibilities of communication and the strong French and German influence on our culture, generally speaking.

Romanian being a Romance language, and as the majority of the old medieval works were published in Latin, they were easily accessible to our scientists so that it is not at all surprising that an appreciable number of books written by English physicians (in English too) reached us, constituting precious documentary material. To these are added non-medical books of the natural sciences, physics, chemistry, mathematics (e.g. the famous physics by John Wallis – an English mathematician – professor at Oxford (1616–1703), a book that was found in the bookcase of the Romanian humanist Constantin Cantacuzino).

Let us discuss the problem of how these books came to us. A part of them were brought by those who had studied in the western universities, others were brought by those who had travelled through Europe, another part reached us by trade; a number of books by English authors became known especially in Transylvania – through German translations.

One of the libraries in Transylvania that contains an appreciable number of old books is the Library of Brukenthal Museum in Sibiu, where, by thorough research work I have found the books of some English physicians and scientists such as: Thomas Sydenham, Nicholas Culpeper, Francis Fuller, Robert Boyle, John Fothergill, etc. To these are added those existing in the Library of the History of Medicine Department in Cluj, books by William Cullen, Thomas Willis, James Currie, John Howard, etc. These works are only a part of those that circulated in the intellectual circles of our country. I am going to refer to some of them.

I. One of the first works of a British man of culture that entered our libraries is that written by Robert Boyle (1626–91), the son of the Earl of Cork, who devoted his wealth and talent to science. His work to be found in the library of Brukenthal Museum is entitled: *Medicina hydrostatica sive hydrostatica materiae medicae applicata*, which appeared in Geneva in 1693. The work appears with others in the third volume of the *Opera Varia* and has seventy pages.

II. William Cullen (1710–90) born at Hamilton, in Lanarkshire, was the son of a lawyer. Studied at Glasgow Faculty, became apprentice to a surgeon in Glasgow, later to an apothecary in London. He went to the West Indies as ship's surgeon. Settled then, in his native town where he practised medicine. Later on we see Cullen at Glasgow conducting a large practice and lecturing with the approval of the authorities not only on his favourite subject – chemistry, but also botany, materia medica and practice of physic. He may indeed be regarded as the founder of the Glasgow School of Medicine (the opinion of D. Guthrie). In 1751, at forty-one years of age, he became Professor of Medicine in Glasgow, until 1755. His lectures were the first to be given in the vernacular instead of Latin. In Edinburgh he delivered lectures on clinical medicine in the Royal Infirmary. In 1766 he added the Chair of Physiology which had become vacant by the death of Robert Whytt. Cullen is the author of a successful book: *First Lines of the Practice of Physic* (London, 1777) in which he underlines the importance of the nervous system in different diseases and attempts a classification of the diseases. His books to be found in the History of Medicine Department Library in Cluj are:

1. *Synopsis nosologia methodicae*, Tomus primus, 2nd edition, Venice, 1792, in 8^0 Johan Anton Pezzana tip. ed.

2. *Abhandlung über die Materia Medica* (trans. into German by Samuel Hohnemann), vol. I, Leipzig, 1790; vol. II (pharmacology), Leipzig, 1790.

III. Nicholas Culpeper (1616–54), studied at Cambridge (known as an astrologer too) distinguished himself due to his extraordinary medical zeal. He was an extremely prolific author.

His work *Medicaments for the Poor or Physick for the Common People* (in two books), written while he was a student, 'contains excellent remedies for most Common Diseases incident to mans body, made of such things as are common to be had in almost every country in the world, and are made with little Art and small charge. First written in Latin by that famous and learned Doctor John Prevotius, Philosopher and public Professor of Physick in Padua. Translated into English with additions by Nicolas Culpeper student in Physick and Astrology' (London, 1670), the book is to be found in the Library of Brukenthal Museum in Sibiu. In his moving preface Culpeper speaks about the two absolutely necessary qualities of a physician: '*Skill to cure* the sick and *great charity to the Poor*, without which there can hardly be so much sense of anothers misery that can invite one carefully to lend his utmost help'.

IV. James Currie (1756–1805) a Scot who practised in Liverpool, took up the idea inaugurated by Sanctorius, and while treating typhoid fever with cold baths checked his results by thermometry. So he was one of those who introduced the thermometer into clinical practice.

One of his works can be found in the History of Medicine Department Library in Cluj and it is written in German: *Wirkungen des kalten und warmen Wassers als eines Heilmittels im Fieber und in andern Krankheiten* (Preface by Brandis, 1st vol., Leipzig, 1801, and 2nd vol., Leipzig, 1807).

V. John Fothergill (1712–80) born on 8 March in Yorkshire, distinguished himself while still a student in several fields. He took his doctor's degree in 1736 in Edinburgh. His study trips included Holland, Germany, France. Settling in London he soon acquired a large practice and popularity. His work: *An Account of the Sore Throat Attended with Ulcer*, 1748, brought him fame. He was greatly interested in botany and in the introduction of new plants into England. To this end, in 1762 he planted a large botanical garden of five acres at Upton in Essex. He brought exotic plants there, especially medical ones. He extended the use of quinine (Peruvian bark), advised the use of (conium) hemlock for neuralgia, introduced the astringent gum known as *kino*, and revived the use of antimony. He popularized the use of coffee and promoted the cultivation of the plant in the West Indies. One of his most interesting papers deals with the *History and Use of Coffee*. Another important one was his account of *Weather and Disease* as well as *Rules for the Preservation of Health*, London, 1762. The work we have got in the Library of the Brukenthal Museum is a German translation entitled: *Sämtliche medizinische und philosophische Schriften . . . aus dem Lateinischen und Englischen übersetzt*, Alternberg, 1785.

VI. Another English physician and author whose work we have is Thomas Fowler, born on 22 January 1736 in York. He studied pharmacy and practised it for fifteen years. In 1774 he went to Edinburgh for medical studies. After four years he took his degree with the dissertation on the treatment of smallpox by the help of mercury. He settled in Stafford and took the leadership of a hospital. In 1791 he returned to York where he treated with great success asthma convulsium and became the chief physician of Quaker-Hospital, where he worked until his death. To his name is connected the preparation of the medicament: *Solutio arsenicalis Fowlery* used even today in therapy. His work represented in the Library of the History of Medicine Department in Cluj is a translation in German: *Bemerküngen über die Kur des hitzigen und chronischen Rheumatismus durch Aderlassen Schwitzmittel und Blasenflaster* (1795).

VII. Another representative of the seventeenth century is Francis Fuller. He was maître-ès-arts at St. John's College at Cambridge. The book we have was mistakenly attributed to Thomas Fuller by Albrecht Haller. However, this misconception was finally corrected. So Francis is the author of *Medicina Gimnastica or a Treatise Concerning the Power of Exercise with Animal Oeconomy, and the Great Necessity of it in the Cure of Several Distempers*, a book that is in the Library of the Brukenthal Museum in Sibiu. The book was printed in 1705 by John Matthews for Robert Knaplock, at the Angel and Crown in St. Paul's Church Yard, London, 1705.

VIII. Thomas Fuller (1654–1734) physician from Kent, wrote a series of pharmacopoeias among which is *Pharmacopoeia extemporanea* (13th ed., Lausanne, 1737), a book that we have, and which came out in nineteen editions. This book is to be found in the History of Medicine Department Library in Cluj.

IX. John Howard (1726–1810), a surgeon of great merit, and pupil of Percivall

Pott, was famous for his endeavour to reform the prisons and hospitals in England and other countries of Europe. He travelled much to this end. By his works Howard contributed to the reformation of these institutions. His work translated in German: *Nachrichten von den vorzüglichsten Krankenhäusern in Europe* (Leipzig, I. Göschen, 1791, XVI, pp. 616, 5 plans) is to be found both in the Brukenthal Museum Library and in the History of Medicine Department Library in Cluj.

X. Richard Mead – an important English practitioner, born at Stepney, London, on 11 August 1673. Followed his father, a presbyterian priest, who took refuge in Holland. He studied at Leyden, then in Padua. Here, in 1696, he got the title of doctor in medicine and philosophy. He stayed for a time in Naples and Rome. Later he came back to London where he became the private physician of the Prince of Wales, the future King George II. He was vice-president of the Royal Society. He died in February 1754. Mead was a protector of science and art. At his initiative a hospital was created.

His work, that we have in the History of Medicine Department Library in Cluj, is entitled: *Mechanica expositio venenorum* (Amsterdam et Denuo Neapoli in 1739) to which it is also attached a work by Herman Boerhaave: *De mercurio experimenta,* that appeared in *Philosophical Transactions* in 1738.

XI. By far the greatest clinical physician of the seventeenth century was Thomas Sydenham (1624–89) born in Wynford-Eagle, Dorset, well-named 'the English Hippocrates'. The studies he began in 1642 at Magdalen College, were continued after an interruption at Montpellier. In 1663 he got the right to practise and settled in Westminster. In 1676 at Cambridge he received the title of doctor in medicine. His best known works are *Medical Observations* and *A Treatise of the Gout*. He was one of the first physicians to prescribe iron for anaemia. He contributed to the development of symptomatology.

He used opium as a remedy in the form of a tincture to which were added saffron, cloves and cinnamon. *Sydenham's laudanum*, as it was called, remained a popular remedy for many years. Among his works of a practical application is also the one we have in Brukenthal Museum Library: *Tractatus de Podagra et hydrope* (Lugdunum Batavorum Johannes Prius, 1684), as well as the following ones that are to be found in the History of Medicine Department Library in Cluj:

1. *Médecine pratique de Sydenham*, Nouvelle édition, Avignon–Paris, an VII (1799), trans. by Professor A. F. Jault.
2. *Medizinische Werke*, Wien, 1786–87; I–II vol.
3. *Opera Medica*, Venice, 1735 and 1762.
4. *Opera Universa*, Leyden, 1726 and 1754.

XII. Another representative of the seventeenth-century medical English world is the Irishman Edmundo (Dermutius) de Meara, who studied medicine at Oxford. He is represented in the History of Medicine Department Library in Cluj by a volume containing two of his works: the first is a polemical work entitled: *Examen-diabribae Thomae Willisii* (Amsterdam, 1667) and *Pathologia haereditaria generalis sive de morbis haereditariis* (Amsterdam, 1666). The latter may interest those that study the history of medical ideas regarding the hereditary diseases.

XIII. Richard Morton (1635–98) famous English physician, Sydenham's rival, was born in a small town in Suffolk. Initially he was a theologian in Oxford, later he studied medicine. In 1670 he graduated in medicine at Oxford and moved to London where he became a member of the College of Physicians and doctor of the prince of Orange. He is so well known due to his works on tuberculosis and infectious diseases:

1. *Phthisiologia seu exercitationes de phthisis libri III*, London, 1689; English version in London, 1694, 1720.
2. *Pyretologia seu exercitationes de morbis universalibus acutis*, London, 1692, 1693.
3. *Pyretologia s. de febribus inflammatoriis universalibus*, London, 1694.

A complete edition of his works appeared in Geneva 1696, and in Amsterdam, 1696, 1699.

The book we have in the Library of Brukenthal Museum is the English translation of his first work: *Phthysiologia or a Treatise of Consumption* (it contains three books: (1) Of Original Consumptions from the Whole Habit of the Body; (2) Of an Original Consumption of the Lungs; (3) Of Symptomatical Consumptions or Such as are the Effects of Some Other Distempers).

The Library of the History of Medicine Department in Cluj has some old British pharmacopoeias in Latin and German; e.g. (1) *Pharmacopoeia Pauperum in usum Nosocomii Regii Edinburgensis*, Edinburgh, 1759; (2) *Pharmacopoeia Colegii Regalis Medicorum Londonensis*, Londini, Joseph Johnson et Rotherdami, C. R. Hake, 1788, xxiv+156 pp.; (3) *Pharmacopoeia Colegii Regii Medicorum Edinburgensis*, 2nd editionis Novisimae exemplar recusa. In usum Prelectionum Academicarum, Bremae et Lipsiae Imp. Georgii Ludovicii Foersteri MDCCLVIII (1758), xii+146 pp. and index.

In listing these old medical works, which have contributed to the training of our medical students for centuries, I wanted to illustrate the assertion made at the beginning of my paper, that the human natural desire for knowledge, determined man to search, to collaborate directly or indirectly with his fellow men; and that in the field of the Romanian–English medical relations, at least for a period of time, these relations were covered by books, some of which I have just mentioned. The list of these books is far from being complete, because there are other libraries in Romania that possess a great number of old books and among them a good deal of English medical ones, but I considered it interesting to research this, and to offer this material to those interested.

H. Goerke
Munich (Germany)

Johan Henrik Engelhart (1759–1832), Wegbereiter der Neuralpathologie in Schweden

Im Jahre 1776 erschien in Edinburgh das Buch von William Cullen (1712–90), das den Titel *First Lines of the Practice of Physic* trug und die Grundzüge eines medizinischen Systems enthielt, das als Neuralpathologie nachhaltigen Einfluß auf das ärztliche Denken in England, dem europäischen Kontinent und in Nordamerika gewann. Die Einfachheit der von Cullen vertretenen Lehre, die herausgehobene Bedeutung des Nervensystems für die Funktion des gesunden Organismus und für Störungen bei Krankheiten ermöglichte es jedem Arzt seine therapeutischen Entscheidungen verhältnismäßig leicht zu treffen. Cullen hat sich selbst zu den Ansichten des Hallenser Klinikers Friedrich Hoffmann bekannt, dessen „Nervenfluidum" und bipolare Konzeption von „Spasmus" und „Atonie" Anknüpfungspunkte für seine pathogenetischen Vorstellungen gewesen sind. Cullens Schüler John Brown (1735–88) hat außerhalb Englands mit seinen 1780 in erster Auflage erschienenen *Elementa medicinae* viel Zustimmung gefunden. Seine an Hallers Irritabilitätslehre anschließenden Anschauungen von der *Sthenie und Asthenie* fanden besonders in Deutschland und Italien viele Anhänger. Neuralpathologische Lehren sind im 20. Jahrhundert erneut in Erscheinung getreten und haben wiederum die begeisterte Zustimmung der Ärzte gefunden. Die Gründe dafür unterscheiden sich nicht so sehr von denen, die man für die Lehren Cullens und Browns vorgebracht hat. Verbunden ist diese moderne Neuralpathologie mit den Namen Gustav Ricker und Alexej Dimitrijewitsch Speranski.[1]

Für die Rezeption neuralpathologischer Lehren in Skandinavien, insbesondere in Schweden hat Johan Henrik Engelhart (1759–1832) eine wichtige Rolle gespielt. Als Sohn des Stadtchirurgen Dietrich Engelhart in Göteborg geboren, kam er mit 17 Jahren als Student an die südschwedische Universität Lund, wurde dort 1778 Magister der Philosophie und erhielt zwei Jahre später die medizinische Doktorwürde. Im Jahre 1780 trat er eine mehrjährige Auslandsreise an, die ihn nach England, Holland und Frankreich führte. Die engen Verbindungen seiner Vaterstadt Göteborg zu England waren sicher ausschlaggebend für sein erstes Reiseziel und sein langes Verbleiben in England und Schottland. Engelhart blieb zuerst drei Jahre in Edinburgh und kam in engen persönlichen Kontakt mit William Cullen und Alexander Monro (1733–1817) Secundus, der selbst auf einer Studienreise zum Kontinent Berlin und Leiden aufgesucht hatte, sowie anderen bedeutenden Ärzten der Edinburgher Schule. Neben Monro, der den Lehrstuhl für Anatomie und Chirurgie bekleidete, und Cullen, der seit 1773 den Lehrstuhl für praktische Medizin innehatte, hat auch der Arzt Joseph Black (1778–99), dem 1766 der Lehrstuhl für Chemie übertragen worden war, einen erheblichen Einfluß auf Engelhart ausgeübt. Im September 1783 reiste Engelhart weiter nach London,[2] wo er sich 8 Monate aufhielt, in Krankenhäusern arbeitete und Vorlesungen hörte. Seine Reise ging dann weiter nach Paris. Dort blieb Engelhart einundeinhalbes Jahr und reiste schließlich im September 1785 über Holland, Norddeutschland und Dänemark zurück nach Schweden. Nach fast 6-jähriger Abwesenheit traf er am 6. März 1786 in Göteborg ein. Zwei Jahre später wurde Engelhart Professor für praktische Medizin an der Universität Lund. Aus seinem weiteren Lebenslauf sei hier nur noch berichtet, daß er sich später mehr und mehr der Theologie zuwandte und schließlich als Arzt und Geistlicher gleichzeitig tätig war. Nachdem er 1815 die Pfarramtsweihe erhalten hatte, gab er ein Jahr später seine Professur auf und wurde Pfarrer einer großen Gemeinde in Mittelschweden. Auch in dieser Stellung, die er 17 Jahre lang bis zum Tode ausgeübt hat, gab er die ärztliche Tätigkeit nicht auf. Während seiner Zeit als Professor der Medizin in Lund trat Engelhart erfolgreich für die medizinische Ausbildung von Theologiestudenten ein.[3] Aus seinem Lebenslauf verdient noch die Tatsache der Erwähnung, daß er es gewesen ist, der während seines Aufenthaltes in London 1783 für den Nachlaßverwalter Linnés die Verbindung zu James Edward Smith hergestellt hat, der den wissenschaftlichen Nachlaß Linnés erwarb, der sich heute im Besitz der Linnean Society in London befindet.[4]

In welchem Ausmaß Engelhart von den ärztlichen Systemen, mit denen er in Edinburgh und London in Berührung gekommen war, der Neuralpathologie Cullens und Browns, beeinflußt worden ist, wie er diese selbst mit den Auffassungen anderer und eigenen Erfahrungen vermischt weitergegeben hat, dafür gibt es relativ weniges dennoch ausreichendes Material. Unter seinen Veröffentlichungen[5] findet man die ersten Hinweise, wobei man lediglich die unter seinem Präsidium abgehaltenen Disputationen auszuwerten braucht. In zwei verschiedenen Disputationen haben Nic. Fr. Freese (1805) und Car. Joh. Furst (1812) das Thema *Doctrina Brunonis de Opportunitate Expositio critica*, vier seiner Schüler (Pehr Brantström, 1806; Thure G. Rothstein, 1809; Jac. Berggren, 1812 und Jan. Trobeck), *Aphorismi de Viribus et Usu Opii* und Joh. Magnus Allgulin 1810 *De Asthenia directa ab indirecta distinguenda* abgehandelt. Allein die Themenwahl bestätigt die Verbindung zur Neuralpathologie.

Der als letzter genannte Johann Magnus Allgulin hat am 12 März 1805[6] eine handschriftliche Ausarbeitung seiner Kollegaufzeichnungen unter dem Titel *Föreläsningar af Medicinae Pract. Professorn Konungens Förste Lif-Medicus Med. et Philos. Doctorn Herr John. Hind. Engelhart* abgeschlossen, zu der auch ein „zweiter Teil" gehört. Der erste Teil hat einen Umfang von 319 Seiten im Folioformat, der zweite umfaßt 214 Seiten. Sie bietet einen ausgezeichneten Einblick sowohl in die Unterrichtsmethodik als auch in die medizinischen Anschauungen Engelharts und ist darüber hinaus ein schönes Beispiel für die Universitätsmedizin um die Wende zum 19. Jahrhundert.

Die Einteilung des im ersten Teil vorgelegten Vorlesungsstoffes ist in fünf Kapiteln erfolgt mit folgenden Überschriften[7]: (1) Allgemeines über Fieber, (2) Entzündungsfieber, (3) Fieberhafte Exantheme, (4) Hämorrhagien, (5) Flüsse (Profluviae). Über *Asthenie, Shenie und Hypersthenie* finden wir schon auf S. 6 die ersten Bemerkungen, so z.B. daß die antisthenische Behandlungsmethode der antiphlogistischen der alten

Ärzte entspricht und bei sthenischen Krankheiten Anwendung findet. Im Abschnitt über *Intermittente Fieber* wird in sthenische, asthenische und symptomatische eingeteilt und darauf hingewiesen, daß Brown das Vorkommen von sthenischen intermittenten Fiebern abgelehnt habe.[8] Bei der Besprechung der Fiebermittel empfiehlt Engelhart übrigens die Chinarinde als besonders wirksam und wendet sich unter Berufung auf Werlhof und van Swieten gegen die Behauptung, ihre Anwendung sei mit Gefahren verbunden. Auf S. 60 bezieht er sich bei Besprechung der ,,kontinuierlichen Fieber" direkt auf Cullen und gibt dessen Definition dieser Krankheitsgruppe an. In gleicher Weise begegnen uns die Zitate dieses von Engelhart besonders geschätzten Lehrers in fast allen Abschnitten des Manuskripts. Cullen ist eindeutig der mit Abstand am häufigsten und auch ausführlichsten zitierte Autor. Immer wieder heißt es: ,,Cullen definiert . . .", ,,Cullen nimmt an . . .", ,,Cullen behauptet . . .", ,,Cullen sagt . . .". Seine ausführlichen lateinischen Krankheitsbeschreibungen werden fast bei jedem Krankheitsbegriff wiedergegeben. In einigen Fällen findet man jedoch auch kritische Anmerkungen zu dem, was von Cullen mitgeteilt wurde. So heißt es auf S. 133 bezüglich der von diesem angegebenen Einteilung der Angina in 5 verschiedenen Formen: ,,Diese Einteilung ist nicht ganz richtig". Bei der Erörterung der Ursache des Podagra ist Engelhart auch auf die Ablehnung und die Begründung dafür eingegangen, die Cullen zu der Theorie von Stahl gegeben hat und dabei hat er auch Cullens eigene Ansichten eingehend dargestellt. Im Vergleich zu der Häufigkeit, mit der auf Cullen Bezug genommen wird, kommen andere Autoren selten zu Wort und es verbleibt dann auch fast immer bei der Nennung des Namens. Bei allen ätiologischen Erörterungen werden stets die Begriffe Sthenie und Asthenie verwendet.

Der zweite Teil des Manuskripts lehnt sich in der Gliederung an das System von Sauvage[9] an, auf den auch mehrfach verwiesen wird, gelegentlich unter Erwähnung abweichender Ansichten Cullens. Bei der Besprechung der ,,Apoplexia" heißt es (S. 1) ,,Cullen nimmt fälchliseherweise an, daß es davon 9 Arten gibt, eigentlich gibt es nur drei", die er dann als ,,Apoplexia sanguinea", ,,Apoplexia serosa" und ,,Apoplexia nervosa" beschreibt (S. 3). Neben Cullen werden an englischen Autoren genannt außer Brown und Monro auch Willis, Lind, Sydenham, Widders, Hamilton, Hull und auch einfach nur ,,ein englischer Arzt".

So sehr dieses Vorlesungsmanuskript dazu verlocken muß, es noch weiter und hinsichtlich anderer Autoren sowie der eigenen Ansichten und persönlichen Beobachtungen Engelharts zu analysieren, so genügt es doch in diesem Zusammenhang sich auf vorstehende Erhebungen zu beschränken.

Daraus geht hervor, daß Engelhart, der gerade nach diesem Manuskript seiner Vorlesung ein außergewöhnlich guter Lehrer gewesen sein muß, von den neuralpathologischen Vorstellungen, die er in Schottland und England selbst kennengelernt hatte, nicht nur wesentliche Teile übernommen, sondern sie auch im Unterricht eindrucksvoll vertreten hat. Dadurch wird seine Rolle als Vermittler der Neuralpathologie im Sinne Cullens und auch Browns und zugleich seine Bedeutung für die Beziehungen zwischen der englischen und der schwedischen Medizin eindeutig nachgewiesen.

Anmerkungen

1 Vgl. RATH, GERNOT, Neurol. Pathology, *Bull. Hist. Med.*, 1959, **33**, 526–41.

2 Vgl. RIEPPEL, F. W., *Die Blütezeit der Medizinschule von Edinburgh*, Basel, Ciba-Zschr., 1948, **10**, H. 113; S. 4181–188., Magn. Laur. Ståhl, *Biographiske underrättelser om professorer vid kongl. universitetet i Lund.* Christianstad, 1834, S. 287 f., Martin Weibull u. Elof Tegner, *Lunds universitets historia 1668–1868*, bd. 2; Lund, 1868; S. 147 f.

3 Vgl. GOERKE, HEINZ, 'Medizinische Ausbildung von Theologiestudenten an der Universität Lund von 1813 bis 1840', in *Medizingeschichte in unserer Zeit*, Festgabe f. Edith Heischkel u. Walter Artelt z. 65. Geb. Tag. Stuttgart, 1971, S. 352–58.

4 FRIES, TH(ORE) M(AGNUS), *Linné Lefnadsteckning*, bd 2, S. 417 f.

5 GABR. MARKLIN, *Catalogus Disputationum*, Tabl. 2, Uppsala, 1820, Martin Weibull u. Elof Tegner a.a.O.

6 Handschr. Abt. Univ. Bibl. Lund, MS. nr. 373. Das Manuskript in schwedischer Sprache ist durchweg z.T. sogar innerhalb einzelner Worte in einer Mischung von deutscher und lateinischer Schrift geschrieben. Die Datierung bereitet etwas Schwierigkeiten. Der erste Teil des MS. ist mit dem Datum 12 März 1805 versehen. wobei die '5' jedoch von anderer Hand korrigiert ist, der zweite Teil trägt die Jahreszahl 1801. Da Johann Magnur Allgulin (1784–1819) erst 1804 sein Studium in Lund aufgenommen hat, 1908 Dr. phil. und 1813 Dr. med. wurde, spricht viel gegen 1801 als Jahr der Niederschrift des 2. Teils des Manuskripts (vgl. *Svenska Läkaresällskapet 1808–1908*, Porträtt och biografier, Stockholm [1909], S. 48.)

7 Dieses und die folgenden Zitate sind Übersetzungen des schwedischen Originaltextes.

8 Vgl. *John Browns System der Heilkunde*, 3, Aufl. Hrsg. v. C. H. Pfaff, Wien, 1807; S. 378–89.

9 Francois Boissier Sauvages de Lacroix (1706–67), seit 1734 Prof. der Medizin in Montpellier. Sein nosologisches Krankheitssystem veröffentlicht als *Pathologia methodica, seu de cognoscendis morbis*, Amsterdam, 1752.

W. Kock
Stockholm (Sweden)

Sweden's medical contacts with England during the eighteenth and nineteenth centuries

The Serafimer Hospital in Stockholm was Sweden's first national hospital. It came into existence in 1752 as a joint establishment for Sweden and Finland and had eight beds. In connexion with its 200th anniversary, an exhibition was arranged. This included a map, showing the journeys which the hospital's first senior physician and senior surgeon made in Europe in the 1740s for the purposes of study. This map covered not only Denmark, Germany, Holland, Switzerland, Italy and France, but also England, which was represented primarily by London and Oxford. This map was for long of great interest to young Swedish doctors, who for years to come were more or less compelled to conclude their studies with a long sojourn abroad, after they had learnt all they could in Sweden, which was then still a very isolated country.

Even in Sweden, the foundation of the Royal Society in 1662 seems to have stimulated great interest in studies at seats of learning in England. However, it is perhaps even more noteworthy that the Royal Society itself showed interest at an early stage in establishing links with Sweden. In this connexion the names of Urban Hiärne and Olof Rudbeck appear early on. Urban Hiärne was the first Swedish doctor to have the great honour of being elected to the Royal Society. He was introduced in 1669 by Jakob Barkman Lejonberg, the Swedish Resident Minister, who had himself been elected a member in 1667, Hiärne was a frequent guest of the Society during his stay in London in 1669–70. He then proceeded to Paris for three years of study. In 1712 Hiärne was to dedicate his book *Acta et tentamina chymica* to the Royal Society. However, the English scientists were primarily interested in Olof Rudbeck, who from 1668 onwards received several offers of co-operation but made no response until 1681, when he sent an apologetic letter and a present of two volumes of his *Atlantica.* He became a member of the Royal Society in 1682.

Among the other Swedish doctors who had contacts with England at this time, I may mention the Scot, Jacob Robertson à Struan, who was physician-in-ordinary to Gustav Adolf II and Queen Christina, Petrus Kirstenius, Otto Sperling, Herman Fuchs, the barber-surgeon, and Johan Svensson Rothman, who studied medicine and chemistry in England for a few years at the end of the seventeenth century and is said to have lectured on chemistry at Oxford. One also encounters the names of Andreas Drossander, who obtained some of his physics equipment in England, Lars Roberg, Johan von Hoorn, Olaus Rudbeck the younger, Magnus Bromelius, Johan

Martin Ziervogel, Gustaf Lohreman, who regarded England as one of the leading countries, along with Germany, France and Holland, in which 'knowledge could be gained', and Magnus Detterberg. England was not perhaps the most important destination for Swedish doctors travelling abroad to study, but it had come to the fore as one of the more important. In the first two decades of the eighteenth century, there were not many Swedish doctors who were in a position to travel abroad to study, partly, of course, as a result of the difficult political and social conditions in Sweden during Charles XII's campaigns.

However, Magnus Gabriel Block, who regarded Italy as his second fatherland but who later became a district medical officer in the Swedish province of Östergötland and was ennobled under the name of von Block, came to London in 1702 and sent reports back to Urban Hiärne. Like several other Swedish doctors, he made the acquaintance of Sir Hans Sloane. Nils Boy, a Swede of Scottish descent who later became the Stockholm City Medical Officer and was one of the founders of the Serafimer Hospital, visited London and Oxford in 1706. He took home with him, amongst other things, his observations of the importance of drinking spa waters to cure diseases, a practice which became very popular in fashionable circles in the Swedish capital.

Several Swedish doctors made their way to England during the 1720s and 1730s. We meet with the names of Carl Alstrin, Peter Petersen (ennobled under the name of von Heidenstam), Evald Ribe, Urban Hiärne's son Christian Henrik Hiärne, and Gustaf Zimmerman, who later became the Stockholm City Medical Officer. Gustaf Harmens, who later became a professor of medicine and physics, spent seven months in England in 1726, visiting London, Oxford and Cambridge. Harmens was one of the comparatively few Swedish doctors of the period who could speak English.

Here I shall pass over, as being too well known, the visit which Carl von Linné (Linnaeus) paid to England in 1736; it was brief and was mainly in consequence of his interest in the natural sciences. However, I may point out that his stay in England was later of great significance for many Swedish doctors. In a letter written in 1771, he declared that 'the English have furthered the cause of natural science more than the French or indeed all the other peoples put together'. Linnaeus did not understand English and carried on his extensive correspondence with the English scientists in Latin (although he is not regarded as having been particularly fluent in Latin either).

In his doctoral thesis entitled *Svenska studieresor till England under frihetstiden* (Swedish Students in England during the Period of Liberty),[1] Sven Rydberg makes particular mention of the visits to England at this time of three Swedish doctors – Herman Schützer (he was later ennobled under the name of Schützercrantz), who, together with a French surgeon, studied operations for the stone under Drs. W. Cheselden and S. Sharp, Olof Acrel, who later became the senior surgeon at the Serafimer Hospital and was ennobled under the name of af Acrel, and Abraham Bäck, who became the senior physician at the Serafimer Hospital. I shall discuss here the journeys abroad made by the last two.

Between 1740 and 1745, Olof Acrel (1717–1806) was engaged in a journey of extreme variety, which even involved a period of confinement as a prisoner of war

[1] The period between the death of Charles XII in 1718 and the *coup d'état* by Gustaf III in 1772 is called the 'Period of Liberty' in Sweden.

during the War of the Austrian Succession, in which he served as a surgeon in the French Army. He left Sweden as an apprentice surgeon in 1740 and spent some time in Denmark, Germany, Switzerland, northern Italy and France (Paris and Rouen). He arrived in Rouen in the spring of 1743 and there studied operations for stone in the bladder under Le Cat for a couple of weeks on his way to England. He travelled to England via Dieppe, together with a friend and fellow student from Switzerland. After landing at Bristol, Acrel had a hazardous journey to London, where he visited several hospitals and famous collections. However, he concentrated his studies on St. Thomas's Hospital, where the famous Dr. Cheselden was a surgeon, and on Guy's Hospital, where his instructor was Dr. S. Sharp. However, when the War of the Austrian Succession broke out, he hastened back to the Continent. In 1745, he returned to Sweden, where he quickly took his medical examinations and in 1752 was appointed senior surgeon at the then newly opened Serafimer Hospital. He is regarded as the father of Swedish surgery.

One of the great names in Swedish medicine during the 'Period of Liberty' was that of Abraham Bäck (1713–95), who, as senior physician at Serafimer Hospital, was Acrel's colleague. Like Acrel, Bäck pursued his studies abroad during the period 1741–45, when he stayed mostly in Holland and France. However, he spent three months in England in the autumn of 1742. Like Linnaeus, he devoted himself primarily to the study of botany. Naturally he was particularly attracted to Sir Hans Sloane's museum collections in Chelsea and to the garden which Sloane had presented to the Society of Apothecaries in 1722. The collections consisted of a library (which occupied many rooms), living and pressed plants, living, stuffed and preserved animals, mineral specimens, antiquities, coins, etc. Bäck was so fascinated that he planned to enter Sloane's service but after mature consideration he did not proceed with his application. His interest in botany was later to be of some importance in connexion with the garden at the Serafimer Hospital, for 'immediately in 1753 a sort of botanical garden was projected there'. Bäck also collected and presented some seeds for this garden, the purpose of which was twofold – to provide the hospital dispensary with various essential medicinal plants and to enable botanical instruction to be given in the garden.

However, Bäck also found time for medical studies during his stay in London. Together with a French surgeon, Pierre Guérin, he studied operations for the stone carried out by Cheselden and Sharp. He was able to attend a ceremonial meeting of the College of Physicians, although he does not seem to have derived much benefit from it on account of language difficulties – in spite of the fact that he had practised his English at his lodgings with 'a young and beautiful but honest girl' and her girl friends, who were by no means tongue-tied. He had the privilege of meeting Dr. Richard Mead, perhaps the most famous doctor in England at that time, whose large income allowed him to be an art collector on a large scale. Naturally, Bäck also often attended the meetings of the Royal Society. He spent a week in Oxford, the sights of which, including the Bodleian Library and several of the colleges, he described in detail. However, he found that the academic ceremonies were mostly 'scholastic fussiness and pedantry'. He also visited Harwich, Canterbury, Dover and Greenwich with its hospital for 'infirm seamen'.

His programme also included literature and English drama and he took home a large quantity of literature. As Rydberg has pointed out, Bäck was later active as a translator; in 1769 he translated Thomas Dimsdale's book *The Present Method of Inoculating for the Small-pox* into Swedish. It was natural that his good friend Linnaeus should write the preface to the Swedish edition.

The middle and later years of the eighteenth century saw several Swedish doctors in England. I may mention Carl Diedrik Engelhart, a Gothenburg doctor, Johan Gustaf Siefvert, a regimental medical officer, Samuel Aurivillius, who later became a professor, Johan Bergstral, David Schulz von Schulzenheim, who later became the first Swedish professor of obstetrics, Pehr Bierchén (ennobled under the name of af Bjerkén), Evald Ribe the younger (ennobled under the name of Ribben), Jacob Gabriel Rothman and Henrik Gahn, who later became a naval doctor. I shall discuss here the visits paid by only four of these men.

David Schulz (he took the name of von Schulzenheim when he was ennobled) was born in 1732 and died in 1823. At the age of twenty-five he was already a doctor of medicine and in 1755 he left Sweden for England to learn inoculation against small-pox at the request of the Health Commission, to which Bäck had put forward his name (despite protests from Linnaeus, who feared that he lacked experience). As a result of Lady Mary Wortley Montagu's propaganda, England had become the leading country in the field of inoculation, although doctors in Sweden had learned something of it at an early stage also through the information sent by Emanuel Timoni to Charles XII, Samuel Skragge, his physician-in-ordinary, and Melchior Neumann, his surgeon-in-ordinary.

Schulz now visited 'small-pox hospitals' and 'inoculating houses', where he gained experience in exchange for high fees. The results of inoculation in the cases he saw were very favourable; in all the ninety-seven cases he followed up, the outcomes were successful. Naturally he met, besides a number of barber-surgeons, several famous English doctors, including William Smellie the obstetrician (obstetrics was a subject which particularly interested Schulz), Peter Shaw, a physician-in-ordinary to George II, Matthew Maty, Edward Archer and Sir John Pringle. On his return to Sweden, Schulz published in 1756 a book entitled *Berättelse om koppors ympande*, which came out in London two years later under the title of *An Account of Inoculation* (it was probably translated by Archer, who was the superintendent of the Smallpox Hospital in London). During his stay in London until the turn of the year in 1755, Schulz, like Bäck, devoted himself to his literary interests, together with like-minded medical colleagues.

Of course, surgeons as well as doctors left Sweden in order to travel and increase their professional knowledge. When in 1756 the Swedish Riksdag (Parliament) decided to establish a fund to support the Health Collegium, Salomon Schützer, the director-general of the Surgical Society promptly applied to the King-in-Council for the grant of three or four scholarships from this fund. As a result, 1,000 silver riksdalers were allotted each year for 'the travelling expenses of two young surgeons and scholarships for two years'. These scholarships were primarily intended to create a corps of surgeons with experience of surgery on active service in wartime. If we examine the correspondence between these scholarship holders and their counsellors in Sweden, who supervised their charges with great zeal, we shall find that two of them made their way to England (one even to the U.S.A.), although the majority studied at seats of learning on the Continent.

Pehr Bierchén was born in 1731 and died in 1774. He was ennobled under the name of af Bjerkén. At the beginning of 1758 he arrived in England bearing letters of recommendation from Schulz von Schulzenheim. He spent eighteen months there and visited Oxford and Cambridge. He was clearly very well received and in a letter to Abraham Bäck he wrote: 'No country in the world can match England in its public charitable institutions'. He did most of his studying in London, especially at the London Hospital. As Hjelt has pointed out, one of the reasons for Bierchén's long stay in England was his negotiations on behalf of the Swedish Government (although at his own suggestion) with Richard Guy, the surgeon, about the purchase of the latter's secret remedy for curing cancer. He bought Guy's remedy for some £4,000 and this remedy led to his having great success as a doctor after his return to Stockholm. It was later transferred to David Schulz von Schulzenheim and Henric Gahn, but otherwise the secret was never revealed.

Among the other surgeons who visited England in this period were Carl Henrik Deneke and Daniel Theel. Deneke later became a regimental surgeon. In the summer of 1766 Daniel Theel was a diligent student at Guy's Hospital and St. Thomas's Hospital, where he learned how to operate for the stone, in which field he later became the leading surgeon in Sweden.

Johan Gabriel Rothman (1721–72) was something of an adventurer but was favoured by Linnaeus and Nils Rosén von Rosenstein, at any rate to begin with, and was even offered the post of Professor of Anatomy at Stockholm. He spent too much time abroad and for this reason was even deprived of the assistant professorship at Uppsala which he had in fact received but had never taken up. He lived in London in the 1750s and married an Englishwoman. After a hasty visit to Sweden, he is said to have returned to London in 1762. He devoted himself to his literary and social interests. In the paper which he published in 1756, entitled 'Skäl och Ordsaker Til Swenska Folkets Utflyttning' (The Reasons for and the Causes of the Emigration of the Swedish People) (his answer to a question in a competition set by the Royal Swedish Academy of Science), he analysed Swedish society. He praised England especially for its educational system and its medical services and stated that there were a hundred times as many doctors in England as in Sweden.

Henric Gahn (1747–1816) became a physician to the Swedish Admiralty after his travels abroad. When he arrived in England at the end of August 1771, he had the advantage of having had the ground well prepared for him by his maternal uncle, David Schulz von Schulzenheim, and, of course, also by his teacher, Linnaeus. These years in England were to be the most instructive and enjoyable period of his life and he came to reckon England as 'his second homeland'.

Captain Cook had recently completed his first voyage round the world, which at that time was the talk of London. Daniel Solander, Gahn's fellow countryman, offered him a post as a collector on the new expedition which King George III had ordered. However, he refused the offer and instead went on with his medical studies, which went smoothly with the help of such men as Schulzenheim's friends, Sir John Pringle and Dr. John Fothergill, who were at that time the leading doctors in private practice in London. Gahn attended the lectures given by Sir John Pringle and William Hunter and practised at St. Thomas's Hospital, which was also an emergency hospital with 500 beds. He met many of the famous men of the period, such as Samuel Johnson and Benjamin Franklin. He faithfully attended the meetings of the Royal Society (although a contemporary observer described them as 'often so trifling that they were scarcely worth sitting through'). He was also in touch with 'the Corporation of Surgeons' (who, according to another traveller, were 'all fat and corpulent and do talk of nothing but eating and drinking'). Gahn does not seem to have shared the view expressed in these malicious comments, although it was well known that the Royal Society was not going through one of its more brilliant periods at that particular time.

Gahn travelled far more widely in England than the majority of other Swedish doctors at that period. Together with – and at the expense of – Carl Anders von Plommenfelt, he made a journey through England, Wales and Scotland to study mining and trade. But the pair found it difficult to agree and Gahn longed to continue his medical studies in Edinburgh, which was then a flourishing medical centre, with 300 students. He attended the lectures of William Cullen, Alexander Monro *secundus*, Thomas Young, Francis Home and others. He followed Young's teaching with particular care, as he was regarded as the leading specialist in obstetrics and paediatrics in Great Britain. Before he ended his visit to England in 1773, Gahn made a thorough study of the medical service in the Royal Navy. Among the men he met during his stay in England was the famous James Lind.

By the beginning of the nineteenth century there were already lively interchanges between Sweden and England in the fields of medicine and natural history. The blockade instituted by Gustaf Adolf IV and his government for political reasons gave rise to difficulties in importing scientific literature into Sweden. The first real medical association in Stockholm was a little society formed in 1798 under the name of 'The Society'. Its actual founder was Christopher Carlander, who spent much of his income on the purchase of books and ordered most of his literature from England, the most important country in Europe in the field of medicine at that time. Through agents, he procured literature both for himself and for his friends in Gothenburg, Stockholm and elsewhere. 'The Society' was short lived but provided the model for the Swedish Society of Medical Sciences, which was founded in 1807 and was also partly a 'reading society'.

Swedish doctors' journeys abroad to study naturally increased greatly in the nineteenth century, but Swedish surgeons' journeys for this purpose increased still more, judging from the study trips undertaken by the senior physicians and senior surgeons at the Serafimer Hospital. I have chosen two examples of surgeons who made these trips, one from the beginning and the other from the later half of the nineteenth century.

In his autobiography, Carl Johan Ekströmer (1793–1860) writes as follows of his stay in London: 'With reference to my stay in London, which was undoubtedly the most interesting and instructive part of my travels abroad, I have, however, less to say than about any other period of them; this was because the period of 7–8 months which I spent in this capital of the world did not, on the whole, offer any variety but consisted of an unbroken series of studies and visits to hospitals. Throughout my travels up to then I almost invariably enjoyed the goodwill and friendship of my teachers and my contemporaries among the doctors whom I visited and got to know, but this was the case to an even greater extent in England.'

Bearing letters of introduction from Berzelius and others, Ekströmer went to see Sir Astley Cooper, 'the most famous surgeon of his time in England and perhaps in Europe'. He was received by him 'from the very first with almost paternal kindness and was also introduced to all that was excellent in London in the spheres of medicine and surgery'. Among his teachers he also mentions Travers and Green at St. Thomas's, Abernethy and W. Lawrence at St. Bartholomew's, and Sir Everard Home and B. Brodie at St. George's Hospital. He had the pleasure of becoming a member of a club consisting of seven London surgeons, who met every Monday at the house of one of the members to dine and to discuss scientific problems. He also had the honour of becoming a member of the 'Medico-Chirurgical Society', in which, many years later, he was to be elected an honorary member in the place of Dupuytren, a distinction which he considered to be 'the most precious of the many which, quite beyond my merits, have fallen to my lot'. His good relations with the English surgeons were later also to benefit many young Swedish surgeons, as had happened 100 years before, with regard to the Swedish doctors and natural scientists with letters of introduction from Linnaeus.

Unfortunately, Ekströmer's funds were insufficient to enable him to visit Edinburgh and Dublin. 'My stay in London was expensive; not, however, on account of the actual cost of living, for I paid in all £2 a week for board and lodging, but books, clothes, instruments, etc. accounted for large sums'.

There was also John Berg (1851–1931), who was later to be the teacher of an entire generation of Swedish hospital doctors, in his capacity as Professor of Surgery at Karolinska Institute and as senior surgeon at Serafimer Hospital. In June 1879 Berg was twenty-eight years of age and had recently graduated as licentiate of medicine. He was ready to begin his grand tour abroad, which lasted until 1880. At this time, when antisepsis was slowly but steadily gaining ground in England, it was, of course, England in particular that primarily attracted him. He arrived in London in August 1879 and had the good fortune to find accommodation in a small boarding-house in Harley Street, where he associated with the highly educated officials on the staff of the Swedish–Norwegian Legation. He visited several of the famous hospitals and certain special hospitals, such as orthopaedic, urological and proctological clinics, representing specialities which were not to come to the fore in Sweden for many years. Despite the distances, which made it impossible to visit more than one hospital per day, Berg was able to see eight to ten major operations at a stretch. However, Lister was away and therefore Berg decided to leave London and return there the following summer. He made his way to Vienna. This young surgeon, who had been warmly welcomed by his colleagues in London, now found himself a student harassed by courses and lectures. On his return to London after his stay on the Continent, which naturally also included a sojourn in Paris, he was able in July to meet Sir Joseph Lister, who from his little ward of thirty beds dictated laws for the world of surgery. Berg describes his impressions of Lister, the first time he heard him lecture, as follows: 'He is entirely straightforward and unaffected in his manner and in his lectures, which are sometimes interrupted by an incompletely suppressed stammer. Curiously enough, he spoke today about the entire theory on which he based his dressing of wounds. The other members of the audience had certainly heard it more than once and he himself has spoken of it more than a hundred times. Perhaps it was a gesture of courtesy to the guest from Scandinavia, which he visited in the autumn of 1879 and of which he said that he had very pleasant memories.'

Lister's methods had been successfully simplified in many quarters on the Continent, but Lister himself adhered strictly to all his instructions about sprays and bandages: '. . . at the same time he operated in his usual long frock-coat and only rolled up his sleeves, removed his cuffs and quickly dipped his hands in a 5% solution of carbolic acid, before he took up the knife. In this connexion he seemed to me to be a typical example of stubborn English conservatism and subjectivism. But then he was in everything a pattern of an English gentleman.'

Berg himself later wrote an account of Lister's method, which he added as an appendix to his interesting description of his travels.

The letters of recommendation which Berg had from his future father-in-law, Professor Carl Gustaf Santesson, who was regarded in his time as the leading surgeon in Scandinavia, opened many doors for him in London. He was able to meet Sir James Paget, Sir Henry Thompson, Professor John Erichsen and a large number of younger surgeons and he also had time for a number of agreeable amusements. He rounded off his stay in Great Britain with a visit to Dr. George Murray Humphry, the Professor of Anatomy at Cambridge, and spent a few days in Edinburgh and Glasgow, where he described the very highly respected surgeon, William McEwen, as a 'refreshing acquaintance'. After his eleven-month study trip, he was soon back in Stockholm and was able, as time went by, to put into practice the experience he had gained – especially that acquired during his successful visit to England – to the benefit of Swedish surgery.

By way of conclusion, I may recall that the contacts with England in the field of medicine also included contacts in the history of medicine, even during what may perhaps be called the period of its establishment as a science in Sweden. In 1907, on the initiative of Vilhelm Djurberg (1865–1933) in particular, the Medical History Section of the Swedish Society of Medical Sciences was founded as the second (after that of obstetrics and gynaecology) of the now more than fifty sections. Its first international contact would seem to have been in 1909, when Mr. Henry Wellcome in London requested the Section to help him by lending objects illustrating the history of medicine in Sweden in connexion with the plans to arrange a medico-historical exhibition at the International Medical Congress held in London in 1913. Having received a government grant of 500 kronor, Djurberg visited this exhibition in August 1913 and lectured on it to the Section the same year.

We all know the magnificent results which have followed from Henry Wellcome's interest in the history of medicine. The lively contacts which in recent years have linked the Stockholm Museum of Medical History with the Wellcome Institute for the History of Medicine and its director are a constant stimulus to us in our own work.

References

EKSTRÖMER, CARL JOHAN, *Kirurgminnen från Karl Johanstiden* (ed. W. Kock), Stockholm, 1964.

GRAPE, ANDERS, *Ihreska handskriftssamlingen i Uppsala universitets bibliotek*, vol. I, Uppsala, 1949.

HJELT, OTTO E. A., *Svenska och finska medicinalverkets historia 1663–1812*, vols. I–III, Helsingfors 1891–1893.

KOCK, WOLFRAM, 'Berömda svenska läkares utländska studieresor i gångna tider', *Sv. Läk. tidn.*, 1953, **50**, 1821–39 (also in *Föreningen medicinhistoriska museets vänners årsskrift*, 1953).

Idem, 'John Bergs utlandsresa 1879–80. Ett bidrag till kirurgiens historia', *Lychnos*, 1953, pp. 203–34.

Idem, 'Karl XII i Balkanländerna – några medicinhistoriska notiser', *Nord. med. hist. årsbok*, 1970, 144–51.

Idem, *Kungl. Serafimerlasarettet 1752–1952*, Jönköping, 1952.

Idem, *Medicinhistoriens grunddrag*, Halmstad, 1955.

Idem, *Olof af Acrel*, Stockholm, 1967.
Idem, 'Som Chirurgiska societetens resestipendiat i 1700-talets Europa', *Sv. Läk. tidn.*, 1941, **38**, 2502–33.
Idem, 'Svenska Läkaresällskapets medicinsk-historiska sektion genom 50 år', *Sv. Läk. sällsk. handl.*, 1957, **77**, 1–20 (also in *Med. hist. årsbok*, 1958).
LENNMALM, FRITHIOF, *Svenska Läkaresällskapets historia 1808–1908*, Stockholm, 1908.
RYDBERG, SVEN, *Svenska studieresor till England under frihetstiden*, Uppsala, 1951.
SELLING, OLOF H., 'Henric Gahn (1747–1816)', *Nord. med. hist. årsbok*, 1968, pp. 136–46.
UGGLA, ARVID HJ., 'De tidigaste förbindelserna mellan Royal Society och Sverige', *Lychnos*, 1940, pp. 302–24.

B. N. Sehsuvaroglu
Istanbul (Turkey)

British physicians in the service of the Ottoman Empire

The Ottoman Empire, which was spread over parts of three continents and whose European borders reached the Danube and the centre of Hungary, was at first a closed social unit. For this reason its relationship with its European neighbours was very limited. With the passage of time, it was inevitable that more close political, economic and cultural relationships had to be developed; and these relationships were established at a fast rate starting from the seventeenth century.

For long centuries Ottoman medicine had an islamic, eastern and classical character and only after the seventeenth century was co-operation with the western medical world begun. At first this co-operation started with nations located on the continent like Italy, Austria and France and later with England.

The medical relationship with England reached its peak in the nineteenth century. During the first half of the century, establishment of the Ottoman Quarantine Administration (1831–40), the Crimean War (1853–56) and Turkish–Russian War (1877–78) were important factors in this development. The Ottoman Quarantine Administration was temporarily established in 1831 and permanently in 1838, by the efforts of some Ottoman statesmen, especially the Foreign Minister Mustafa Reşit Pasha, and it became an international organization in 1840.

The personal effort of some British physicians, like Dr. McGuffog, physician to the Ambassador of England to Turkey, must also be mentioned. Dr. McGuffog, during his long stay in Turkey, learned to speak Turkish and helped in maintaining contact between the Sultan and the ambassadors. He was the trusted interpreter between Sultan Mahmut II (1809–39) and the British Ambassador Sir Stratford Canning (1786–1880) in 1832. Dr. McGuffog was also among the founders of the first Turkish medical society (Imperial Medical Society of Turkey).

Our research on the History of the Turkish Quarantine Administration starting in 1947 has enabled us to locate many of the names of physicians who worked there. There are many British subjects who were active in the organization and among the most famous are:

Cleman (M.D.). He worked in Turkey for a number of years at the beginning of the twentieth century.

Dickson (M.D.). He stayed in Turkey for a long period and he was therefore awarded both with the Osmanî and Mecidî orders of the third degree.

Both of these physicians represented England for a long time at the Turkish Council of the Quarantine Administration.

McCarty, J. W. (M.D.). He came to Istanbul while teaching in the Vienna School of Medicine and was also a member of the Vienna Medical Society. He worked as a palace physician during the reign of Sultan Mahmut II and was also a member of Council of the Quarantine Administration. He treated Sultan Mahmut II just before he died and later served again as a palace physician to Sultan Abdülmecit (1839–61).[1]

The Crimean War started in 1853 between Russia and Turkey, then one year later some European nations joined. Among them, England entered the war on the Turkish side. The following medical staff are those that went to Turkey with the British forces.[2]

Anderson, David (M.D.) (1821–54). Graduated from Edinburgh Medical School, was one of the British Army Surgeons of second class. Died at Military Hospital of Scutari, 4 November 1854.

Anderson, William Abbot (M.D.) (1822–55). He was a British Army Surgeon and worked with the British forces in Crimea. He was one of the physicians that attended Miss Florence Nightingale when she became ill in Crimea.

Dr. Anderson died on transport *Columbus* in Balaclava Harbour, 3 January 1855.

Blackwood (M.D.). After the battle of Inkerman, he came to Turkey together with his wife Lady Alice Blackwood and worked at Scutari Barracks Hospital.

Butler (M.D.). He stayed in Turkey for a long time and took part in the Crimean and Turkish–Russian War of 1877–78.

Cumming (M.D.). He worked as a member of the Medical Commission of the Scutari Barracks Hospital.

Dwight (M.D.). No information can be found about his life.

Forrest (M.D.). After the recall of Dr. Menzies, the former head of the Scutari Barracks Hospital, he was appointed as the chief physician. He was discouraged after working a few weeks, therefore he resigned and returned to England.

Hall, John (M.D.). He was the chief physician of the British Army in Crimea.

Lawson (M.D.). After Dr. Forrest he was appointed the chief physician of the Scutari Barracks Hospital. He had a notorious reputation, like Dr. Menzies, of being very harsh with the sick and wounded soldiers.

Mapleton (M.D.). He was the chief physician of the British Army in Turkey and was also the founder of Scutari Barracks Hospital.

McGregor, James (M.D.). He was a first-class British Army surgeon and was also the chief physician of the Scutari Barracks Hospital. He died in the winter of 1855, during a typhus epidemic, together with five other British physicians.

Menzies (M.D.). He was the first chief physician of the Scutari Barracks Hospital. He was dismissed from his post by the inspection team that inspected the hospital in the spring of 1855 for being very harsh to the sick and the wounded and also because of his rough and selfish attitude towards other people.

Meyer (M.D.). He came to Turkey together with the second group of nurses under the leadership of Lady Mary Stanley.

O'Conner, Nicholas (M.D.) (1814–56). He was a first-class British Army surgeon, and he died during the Crimean War at Balaclava, 7 June 1856.

Sutherland (M.D.). He worked for the British Forces in the Crimea. He was also one of the physicians that took care of Miss F. Nightingale when she was ill there.

Sandwith, Humphrey (M.D.). He was a British physician who worked at Kars front during the Crimean War. He is the author of the book *The Siege of Kars* which was published in London in 1856. Later a Turkish general, Sait Pasha of Eğin (1830–95) translated this work into Turkish. Sandwith is also the author of another work, *The Hekrimbaşi.*

Tice, John Charles Graham (M.D.) (1810–62). British Army surgeon of the first class.

I would like to mention the names of the British nurses, the real assistants of physicians, who contributed much to the emergence of the modern nursing, while staying in Turkey during the Crimean War.

Barnes, Miss Sophia. She came to Turkey with Florence Nightingale's group. She died in 1855 while working in the Scutari Barracks Hospital. She is buried in Haydarpaşa English Cemetery. Her tomb is still very well kept.

Blackwood, Lady Alice. During the Crimean War, after the Battle of Inkerman, she came to Turkey together with her husband Dr. Blackwood, travelling at their own expense.

Bracebridge, Mrs. Charles. She came to Turkey together with her husband Mr. Charles Bracebridge, the uncle of Miss F. Nightingale. She worked in the Scutari Barracks Hospital and roomed with Miss Nightingale in one of the towers of the Scutari Barracks. Died 31 January 1874.

Goodman, Miss Margaret. She came to Turkey with the Nightingale group and worked in the Selimiye Barracks Hospital.

Moore, Mrs. Charlotte. She was the widow of Colonel Moore. She came to Turkey with the Nightingale group and worked in the Scutari Barracks Hospital. She died in 1855 and was buried in the Haydarpaşa English Cemetery. Her tomb is still very well kept.

Nightingale, Florence (1820–1910). The founder of the modern nursing.

Roberts, Mrs. She came to Turkey with the Nightingale group and worked in the Scutari Barracks Hospital.

Stanley, Lady Mary. After Miss Nightingale's group, she organized a second group and came to Turkey. She worked in the Kuleli Barracks Hospital.

Stewart, Mrs. Show. Coming from noble descent, she studied nursing in Germany, later worked in many different London hospitals. She came to Turkey with the Mary Stanley group, and worked mostly in the Crimea.

After the Crimean War, foreign physicians together with the British physicians founded the first Turkish medical society (Imperial Medical Society of Turkey) on 1 March 1856. Among the founders of this society the following were the British members:

McCarthy (M.D.). Physician to the palace and a founding member of the society.

McGuffog (M.D.). Physician to the British Ambassador and a founding member of the society.

Meredith (M.D.). A founding member of the society.

Millingen, Jules (M.D.). A founding member of the society.

Foreign medical institutions, like the English, French and Austrian hospitals which later continued their activities in Istanbul, were the souvenirs of the Crimean War.

The Turkish–Russian War of 1877–78 which started right after the coronation of Abdülhamit II (1876–1909) caught Turkey unprepared, even though this war created major trouble for the Russians. Tsar Nicholas II had to call for volunteers from all over Europe and only Romanian troups responded to his call. 50,000 Romanian soldiers played an important role in the final outcome of the war. During this time Turkey, through its embassies in Europe advertised for foreign medical personnel. English physicians and surgeons who came to Turkey during the war and those that were already in Turkey at that time are listed below:

Beresford (M.D.). No information has been found about his life.

Black, Surgeon. Worked in Vidin; in his youth he was a brilliant surgeon. In his later years, due to alcohol, he lost much of his skill.

Busch (M.D.). No information has been found about his life.

Butler (M.D.). Also took part in the Crimean war.

Buckle (M.D.). Was captured by the Russian forces at the Erzurum front in 1877.

Casson (M.D.). Was captured by the Russian forces at the Erzurum front in 1877.

Denniston, James, Surgeon. A graduate of Glasgow Medical School.

Featherstonbough, Charles. Surgeon. Worked in Erzurum.

Foley (M.D.). No information has been found about his life.

Forbes, Litton (M.D.). From the British Red Cross. Worked in Nish Military Hospital.

Gethardth (M.D.). No information has been found about his life.

Geoffery (M.D.). From Edinburgh Medical School.

George, Fritz (M.D.). He was Colonel in the British Army.

Gill (M.D.). After working for a long time in Turkey, he went back to England to become a well-known physician at Welshpool.

Guppy (M.D.). Worked in Erzurum and died from typhoid fever in 1878.

Hurvey (M.D.). No information has been found about his life.

James (M.D.). He was a captain in the British Army.

Keen, Howard. Surgeon. Worked in Nish Military Hospital.

Kronberg (M.D.). No information has been found about his life.

Kustler (M.D.). He was an Australian.

Leslie, Armond (M.D.). From the British Red Cross. Worked in Nish Army Hospital as a surgeon. Later went to Egypt and was killed there.

Leslie, Ralph (M.D.). No information has been found about his life.

Moore, Bond (M.D.). From Stafford House Medical Committee. Worked under Osman Pasha in Plevne.

Mackeller (M.D.). No information has been found about his life.

Morisot (M.D.). A captain in the British Army.

Pinkerton, John (M.D.). From Edinburgh. Died from typhus at Erzurum in 1878.

Rockl (M.D.). No information has been found about his life.

Ryan, Charles (M.D.). An Australian. Worked in Plevne and in Erzurum. Later published his memoirs in 1897.

Roy (M.D.). Worked in Erzurum in 1878. He was sent by the British Red Cross.

Stoker, George (M.D.). A physician from Harley Street. Worked under Osman Pasha in Plevne.

Stephenson (M.D.). From Edinburgh Medical School.

Strewen (M.D.). No information has been found about his life.

Stanley (M.D.). No information has been found about his life.

Temple (M.D.). Worked for Ottomans for many years.

Weniberger (M.D.). An Australian.

Waldemann (M.D.). No information has been found about his life.

Woods (M.D.). From Northern Ireland.

This communication is an opportunity to pay our respects to the memory of those who served Turkey faithfully and devotedly in the past.

References

1 MCCARTHY, J. W., and CARATHEODORY, C., *Relation officielle de la Maladie et de la Mort du Sultan Mahmud II*, Paris, 1841.

2 HAMLIN, C., *My Life and Times*, Boston and Chicago, 1893.

WOODHAM-SMITH, CECIL, *Florence Nightingale, 1820–1910*, London, Constable, 1950.

Bibliography

HAMLIN, C., *My Life and Times*, 5th ed., Boston and Chicago, 1893.

RYAN, CHARLES S., *Under the Red Crescent, Adventures of a British Surgeon with the Turkish Army at Plevne and Erzurum, 1877–1878*, London, 1897.

SANDWITH, HUMPHREY, *The Siege of Kars*, London, 1856.

SLADE, ADOLPHUS, *Turkey and the Crimean War: A Narrative of Historical Events*, London, 1867.

ŞEHSUVAROĞLU, BEDI N., *Histoire de la Quarantaine en Turquie*, İst. Üniv. Tip Fak. Mec. no. 3, 1957, no. 4, 1958, no. 1, 1958, no. 1, 1959.

ŞEHSUVAROĞLU, BEDI, *Kirim Harbi'nde İstanbul Hastaneleri*, Hayat-Tarih Dergisi, no. 10, İstanbul, 1965.

Wellcome Institute of the History of Medicine's Archives.

POOLE, STANLEY LANE, *Life of Lord Stratford de Redcliffe*, London, 1888.

Mareshal Ferid Pasha's unpublished memoirs (1849–71), in B. N. Sehsuvaroglu's private archives.

C. R. Burns
Galveston, Texas (U.S.A.)

Reciprocity in the development of Anglo-American medical ethics, 1765–1865

From the beginnings of recorded human history, ideals *and* ideas about values have been associated with the personal and professional activities of medical practitioners. The professional values can be classified best under the following four headings: (1) the education of medical practitioners, (2) consultations with other practitioners, (3) transactions between physicians and patients, and (4) relationships between medical practitioners and communities. During the one hundred years encompassed by this study, Anglo-American physicians experienced value changes within all four of these categories of interpersonal relationships. These changes are well illustrated by the ideals of three British physicians: John Gregory (1724–73), Thomas Percival (1740–1804), and Michael Ryan (1800–41).[1]

After joining the Edinburgh faculty as professor of medicine in 1765, Gregory gave several introductory lectures about the qualifications and duties of physicians. He published six of them in 1772. His ideals primarily involved the education of a physician and the nature of medical science. He strongly believed that a formal education in particular subjects constituted the ethical basis for medical practice. Education, science, and ethics were inseparable. Even when dealing with the public, Gregory's scientific emphasis continued. He was less concerned about what physicians should do for the community than about what laymen *qua* scientists could do for medicine. Somewhat randomly he exhorted his students to attend to the professional decorums that underlay interactions of practitioners and transactions between practitioners and patients. A more detailed analysis of these latter two groups of professional ideals was made by Thomas Percival, a Manchester physician who had carefully studied Gregory's book.

After a decade of private practice, Percival was appointed physician to the Manchester Infirmary. As hospitals became more exclusively concerned with the care of the sick during the eighteenth century, they provided a new arena for the struggles of British physicians, surgeons, and apothecaries. After verbal and emotional conflicts persisted among the physicians and surgeons of the Manchester hospital, Percival was asked – in 1792 – to draft a code of rules to regulate and govern practitioners at that hospital.

Since he had no vested interest in the principal London guilds, Percival could view the nexus of traditional relationships as an outsider, so to speak. He realized that the moral statutes of the various colleges of practitioners exerted little significant influence in hospital practice. But, by altering and expanding these statutes, particularly those of the Royal College of Physicians of London, and by using the highest moral sentiments of the age in dealing with the practical problems of hospital practice, Percival cleverly adapted guild regulations to the hospital setting. These rules were accepted by the trustees two years later, and they eventually became the first chapter of a book on medical ethics. After adding three chapters – one about private practice, one about relationships with apothecaries, and one about the legal duties of practitioners, Percival published his *Medical Ethics* in 1803.

There were major differences between the ideals of Gregory and the precepts of Percival. In view of Gregory's thorough discussion, Percival probably thought it superfluous to devote much attention to educational and scientific ideals. Besides, Percival did not believe that an 'academical' education was absolutely necessary for a medical practitioner even though he himself was a scholar and an ardent proponent of the experimental philosophy.

Gregory had offered a few standards about interactions of practitioners and about patient care. In appreciating the centrality of consultation in both private and hospital practice, Percival offered many precepts about transactions between physicians, surgeons, and apothecaries. In contrast to the guild statutes, though, Percival emphasized that all matters of consultative decorum should be judged in terms of better patient care. For example, in rural areas, apothecaries usually knew considerably more about the patient than anyone else. Thus, consultation and co-operation between physician, surgeon, and apothecary were desirable not only for professional improvement, but also for a more judicious decision about the care of the patient. In fact, ideals about the conduct of practitioners towards patients were pre-eminent in Percival's code.

There was a third major difference between Gregory's values and those of Percival. Gregory had urged laymen to devote their attention to basic problems of health and disease, but he had not discussed the social obligations of medical practitioners. Percival not only attended to public health obligations, but he also recognized the ethical significance of legal requirements. In return for exemptions from military service and jury duty, for example, physicians were required to meet certain demands of society, including testimony at judicial proceedings requiring medical evidence. This recognition of the impact of laws on professional ethics was a unique contribution by Percival. When applied to medicine, 'jurisprudence' meant primarily forensic medicine to the majority of British physicians who practised in the eighteenth and nineteenth centuries. 'Jurisprudence' signified moral injunctions to a few, including Percival and Michael Ryan.

A medical graduate of Edinburgh and a member of the College of Physicians in Edinburgh and in London, Ryan was editor of the *London Medical and Surgical Journal* in the 1830s. In 1831, he published a manual of medical jurisprudence, and, five years later, he issued an enlarged edition. The three sections of Ryan's compendium dealt respectively with medical ethics, laws in Britain relating to medicine, and forensic medicine.

Written primarily as a text for students, Ryan wished to prepare a 'concise and comprehensive compendium of the moral and legal duties of a medical man'. In the section on moral duties, Ryan essayed a history of medical ethics – probably the first in the English language. He did not analyse basic problems of professional values, as had Gregory and Percival.

Nevertheless, Ryan is singularly significant because he attempted to correlate medical ethics, health legislation, and forensic medicine. He realized that any society could incorporate its values about professional behaviour into civil statutes and, consequently, impose both moral and legal obligations on professional persons. Moreover, practitioners could not satisfactorily discharge professional obligations without understanding community expectations embodied in laws, and a satisfactory fulfilment of certain community obligations involved a special knowledge of law as well as medicine. Thus, Ryan sustained Percival's emphasis on the moral import of laws as well as his understanding of the forensic responsibilities of practitioners.

Various editions of Gregory's monograph, Percival's code, and Ryan's manual appeared between 1770 and 1850. In using these, British and American physicians began to deal with problems of medical ethics in a more thoughtful and organized fashion.

Physicians in the United States who considered problems of medical ethics were well acquainted with the writings of these three men. Benjamin Rush had read Percival's *Medical Ethics*, but, above all else, Rush had been profoundly influenced by his teacher, Gregory. As a professor in Philadelphia, Rush gave at least seven lectures about particular aspects of medical ethics. For example, in 1789 and again in 1801, Rush lectured about the immorality of scientific falsehoods in medicine. Medicine would be vastly improved if the scientific causes that retarded medical progress were removed. Rush repeated some of the causes that Gregory had listed in 1772, and he added some of his own.[2]

After Gregory's lectures were reprinted at Philadelphia in 1817, his influence became even greater. Hugh Hodge, in an oration to the Philadelphia Medical Society, reiterated Gregory's suggestions about the importance of certain subjects in medical education. Hodge had also studied Percival's book, and an abridgement of the same was published at Philadelphia in 1823. In that same year, the New York State Medical Society adopted its first code of medical ethics. However, it was not the first American code.

A few rules of professional ethics had been included in the by-laws adopted by some of the medical societies established in the United States before 1800. During the first half of the nineteenth century, these norms were frequently separated from the main group of by-laws and incorporated into codes of ethics, etiquette, or police. The first code was adopted by the Boston Medical Association in March of 1808. Known as the *Boston Medical Police*, this code had been prepared by a committee of doctors who claimed that they used the writings of Gregory, Percival, and Rush. Actually, all of the precepts in the *Boston Medical Police* could be found in the second chapter of Percival's *Medical Ethics*, the chapter that discussed such situations in private practice as consultations, arbitration of differences, interferences with another's practice, fees, and seniority among practitioners. Furthermore, the Boston physicians did not explain their reasons for ignoring Percival's precepts about hospital practice, apothecaries, and laws. Although there were few apothecary-practitioners in the United States at this time, there were hospitals, druggists, and medically-related laws. In spite of these exclusions, or, perhaps because of them, the *Boston Medical Police* became *the* model for codes of medical ethics adopted between 1817 and 1842 by at least thirteen societies in eleven states, New York not included.

The New York physicians did not simply imitate the Boston code. They included the forensic obligations so important to Percival. On the other hand, they championed Gregory's ideal about the social arrangement of medical practitioners. Percival had desired that a rigid distinction be maintained between physicians, surgeons, and apothecaries whereas Gregory had challenged British practitioners to learn and practise all branches of medicine. In agreeing with Gregory, the New York physicians expressed the sentiments of other American practitioners who saw no value in supporting the British hierarchy of social distinctions.[3]

The code of the New York State Medical Society exerted obvious influence on those who prepared a code for the Medico-Chirurgical Society of Baltimore in 1832.[4] The committee of Baltimore physicians also used the code of the Connecticut Medical Society (based on the *Boston Medical Police*) and the writings of Percival, Gregory, Rush and Ryan. In that same year, R. E. Griffith of Philadelphia, had issued an American edition of Ryan's *Manual of Medical Jurisprudence*. To the fifth chapter of this edition, Griffith added a synopsis of Rush's list of duties for patients. This synopsis became part of the fifth section of the code adopted in Baltimore and part of the first chapter of the code adopted by the American Medical Association fifteen years later.

Rush had offered his ideals about the obligations of patients in another lecture to students in 1808. According to Rush, patients should select only those physicians who have received a regular medical education. Moreover, patients should select only those doctors who have regular habits of life and are not devoted to company or pleasure at the theatre, turf, or chase. Patients should send for the doctor in the morning but be ready to receive him at any time of the day. They should communicate the history of their complaints fully but not relate the tedious or unimportant details. They should promptly obey the doctor's prescriptions. They should express appropriate gratitude and pay their fees promptly. Thus, the Baltimore doctors added a new dimension to American medical ethics by codifying the ideas of Rush regarding the responsibilities of patients toward their physicians.

With the momentum generated by local and state societies and their codes, it is not surprising that one of the earliest resolutions passed by the delegates to the first national medical convention in the United States involved the creation of a code of medical ethics. The committee who drafted this code reported that 'a great number of codes of ethics adopted by different societies in the United States,' were 'all based on that by Dr. Percival'.[5] In preparing their code, the committee attempted to preserve the words of Percival, although a 'few of the sections were in the words of the late Dr. Rush', and 'one or two sentences' were from other writers. On the afternoon of 6 May 1847, the committee's report was adopted as the first code of medical ethics for the American Medical Association.

Between 1765 and 1847, therefore, interested Americans unquestionably studied and utilized the British heritage bequeathed by Gregory, Percival and Ryan.[6] This heritage was essential to the beginnings of American medical ethics. In fashioning their ideals, American physicians borrowed many, but not all of the values offered by the British doctors. Furthermore, there was a major paradox in the transmission of professional values from Great Britain to the United States. Americans had rejected the British arrangements of medical practitioners and had grouped together in local, state, and national societies. In preparing codes of ethics for these societies, though, the Americans adopted many ideals about professional conduct that Gregory and Percival had offered to improve relationships between members of the British guilds. Nevertheless, with the adoption of the national code in 1847, American values and ideals returned to influence British doctors.[7]

The AMA code was divided into three chapters. The first dealt with the duties of physicians to their patients and, vice-versa, the duties of patients to their physicians. The latter section was exclusively Benjamin Rush. The former included summaries of the comments about patient care scattered throughout Percival. Chapter 2 reviewed the obligations that physicians had toward each other. It included all of the aforementioned precepts about consultations, interferences, and disagreements. Chapter 3 included the obligations of the profession to the public and, conversely, the obligations of the public to the profession. The latter were generalizations based on the requisites of Rush. The former preserved the concerns of Percival and Ryan by obligating American doctors to attend to matters of public health and forensic medicine.[8]

In 1849, a third edition of Percival's *Medical Ethics* was published in London, but the momentum of American influences was strikingly increasing in Great Britain. In an essay that appeared in the *London Medical Gazette*, W. B. Kesteven quoted several clauses from the AMA code.[9] The London publishing firm of John Churchill reprinted the AMA code and some essays on the duties of physicians written by a Boston physician, John Ware.

The most important American author, though, was a private practitioner in Connecticut, Worthington Hooker. In 1849, Hooker published a monograph with the following title: *Physician and the Patient or, a Practical View of the Mutual Duties, Relations, and Interests of the Medical Profession and the Community*. With this book, Hooker became the only American physician to write an extensive interpretation of the AMA code, and he was also the only nineteenth-century American physician to write a comprehensive monograph on the subject of medical ethics.

In 1850, an edition of Hooker's book was published in London. The editor, Edward Bentley, understood the historical significance of Hooker's book. 'It has been the subject of common remark', said Bentley in his preface, 'that no work upon the mutual duties, relations, and interests of the medical profession and the community has hitherto appeared in England, and considering the many able men capable of performing this task and whose opinions and experiences in such matters would carry weight and add importance to this interesting subject, it certainly is a matter of surprise . . .'. It is difficult to say which was more surprising to Bentley: the fact that no British physician between 1803 and 1850 had written a monograph on medical ethics, or the fact that a Norwich, Connecticut, practitioner had written one that so forcefully illustrated the dimension of mutuality or reciprocity in physician-patient relations. Although calling Hooker 'William' instead of Worthington on the title page of his London edition, Bentley could not change the fact that an American doctor had made a significant contribution to Anglo-American medical ethics.

Hooker believed that physicians had profound obligations to develop the highest of professional skills, especially those involved in clinical observation and evaluation. He also expected the public to correct their errors about professional skills and to learn how to distinguish between good and bad practices. Furthermore, physicians must understand and adhere to all of the rules of professional decorum, and the public must also understand these rules and appreciate the consequences of interfering with the activities of competent practitioners. With these and other analyses of the mutual obligations of physician and patient – of the medical profession and the community – Hooker championed the ingenuity of the AMA code and brilliantly depicted a feature of professional ethics that was not emphasized by Gregory, Percival, or Ryan.

The American novelty was widespread codification culminating in the AMA code of 1847. This code was voluntarily adopted by many state societies during the ensuing eight years. In 1855, the AMA resolved that all state and local societies had to adopt the code if they wished to send delegates to its annual convention. But compulsory acceptance did not guarantee higher standards or uniform enforcement. In 1857, one critic of codification observed that professional conflicts and abuses were as evident in England where there were no codes as they were in America with codes. Hooker might have retorted that the goods of professional life were more recognizable in the United States with codes than in Great Britain without codes. No American claimed that codes guaranteed medical righteousness. Codes simply provided physicians with some knowledge of the difference between right and wrong professional conduct. Without some ideals and some means of institutionalizing them, there would be little chance to alter professional evils anywhere.

Spurred by the AMA code, the British Medical Association attempted to develop a code of ethics. Prior to 1858, at least two committees faltered. At the Edinburgh meeting in July of 1858, a thirty-four-member committee was established with Charles Hastings as chairman and T. Herbert Barker and Alexander Henry as secretary. At the meeting in 1859, Barker was granted additional time to prepare his report. It had not materialized by 1865.[10]

The American efforts afforded British doctors a mirror by which they could judge the relevant and less relevant parts of their own professional values. Perhaps the British practitioners understood the problems of enforcement and compromised professional freedom inherent in codes. Whatever the reasons, Great Britain did not have a nationally accepted set of ethical guidelines by 1865.

In summary, the international exchange of professional ideals was not exclusively from Great Britain to the United States between 1765 and 1865. Primarily one-way before 1830, the influences began to shift afterwards. By the middle of the nineteenth century, British practitioners were well aware of developments in the United States, including the adoption of the AMA code in 1847 and the publication of Worthington Hooker's *Physician and Patient* in 1849. After 1850, practitioners in both countries recognized the challenge of a principle of mutual obligations between practitioners and patients and they reciprocally influenced each other as they created and changed their professional values.

References

1 KING, LESTER S., *The Medical World of the 18th Century*, Chicago, 1958, pp. 244–60; FORBES, ROBERT, 'Medical ethics in Great Britain', *Wld med. J.*, 1954, **1**, 297–99.

2 RUSH, BENJAMIN, *Sixteen Introductory Lectures*, Philadelphia, 1811, pp. 141–65.

3 *A System of Medical Ethics, Published by the Order of the State Medical Society of New York*, New York, 1823.

4 Medico-Chirurgical Society of Baltimore, *The System of Medical Ethics Adopted by the Society, Being the Report of the Committee on Ethics*, Baltimore, 1832.

5 *Proceedings of the National Medical Conventions, Held in New York, May, 1846, and in Philadelphia, May, 1847*, Philadelphia, 1847, p. 92.

6 Between 1832 and 1847, the writings of Gregory and Percival had been cited by several other American physicians. In 1834, sections from Percival's books were published in an issue of the *United States Medical and Surgical Journal*. In 1836, Gregory's lectures and Percival's book were recommended to candidates for licensure examination by the Massachusetts Medical Society. Robley Dunglison, in 1837, recommended that medical students carefully study the books on medical ethics written by Gregory and Percival. In an address to a group of Lexington doctors in 1839, Thomas Mitchell referred to Percival.

7 Influences from the United States began to be visible in the 1830s. When Michael Ryan revised his book on medical jurisprudence in 1836, he transformed chapter 5 into a section entitled 'American Medical Ethics'. This chapter was actually a reprint of the talk that had been given to the Philadelphia Medical Society in 1826 by John Godman. Ryan had not prepared a history of 'American medical ethics' nor had he mentioned the synopsis of Rush's essay on the duties of patients that Griffith had added to the Philadelphia edition of Ryan's book. But Ryan had acknowledged the existence of an 'American' medical ethics.

8 Thomas Percival's grandson, James Haywood, visiting Philadelphia in December of 1848, expressed his appreciation to one of the members of the AMA committee for their use of Percival's moral precepts. 'In England', said Haywood, 'I believe that my grandfather's Medical Ethics are generally looked upon as a standard work on that subject, and it is gratifying that you have honored him with a similar confidence on this side of the Atlantic.' Letter to Isaac Hays from James Haywood, 3 December 1848; located in Isaac Hays' Papers, Library American Philosophical Society, Philadelphia, Pennsylvania.

9 KESTEVEN, W. B., 'Thoughts on medical ethics', *Lond. med. Gaz.*, 1849, **9**, 408–14.

10 *Br. med. J.*, 1858, pp. 657–58; ibid., 1859, p. 631.

E. T. Carlson
New York (U.S.A.)

The impact of British medicine on Benjamin Rush[1]

On the wall of his bedroom Benjamin Rush (1745–1813) proudly hung the sword of his great-great-grandfather John – a symbol of his reverence for his British forebears and his pride in their revolutionary spirit. The 'Old Trooper' as Rush fondly called him, had fought with Oliver Cromwell and had, according to family legend, won high respect in his command of a 'troop of horse'. Later, John Rush had turned Quaker and in an atmosphere of intolerance of the Restoration period, welcomed an opportunity to emigrate. In 1683 he settled in William Penn's new colony with his children and grandchildren. It was to this strong-minded man that Benjamin ascribed the source of 'a large portion of my republican temper and principles'.

But the revolutionary spirit that guided Benjamin Rush's life had more contemporary roots. While a medical student at the University of Edinburgh (1766–68) he became friends with a British classmate, John Bostock, who likewise cherished a Cromwellian ancestor. The progressive spirit that Bostock inherited still burned within him and rekindled in Rush what would become a lifetime of political self-questioning. His initial doubts on the validity of hereditary rights for the monarchy matured into strong support for the republican way of life. His first major step toward realization of this ideal came on 4 July 1776 when he fixed his name among the fifty-six signers of the Declaration of Independence. For the remainder of his life Rush would be involved in numerous political, educational, and medical reform movements that touched virtually every area of society in his time.[2]

While at Edinburgh, Rush studied under Dr. William Cullen, a man whom Rush found attractive for the brilliance of his mind, yet disturbing because of his profound religious scepticism. Nor was Rush to be taken by the Deism of another acquaintance, David Hume. Rush shared the rationalistic orientation so prevalent in the late eighteenth century but he had no use for overt Deists. Baptized in the Episcopal church of his father, he was raised in this faith till the age of five when John Rush died. Thereafter, his mother brought him up in the Presbyterian church of Gilbert Tennet, an evangelical leader in the Great Awakening.

The Great Awakening was essentially a reform movement among the different groups of the Church of England. It was brought to America by George Whitefield (whom Rush often visited while in London) and spread rapidly through the churches of North America. The New Side Presbyterians supported the doctrine of 'irresistible grace', a belief embraced by Rush which enabled him later to accept the principle of universal salvation. Opposed to the older and more severe Calvanism, New Side-ism was an optimistic movement that initiated many important social changes in America. Rush believed strongly that man was created to do God's work on earth and New Side-ism offered him a viable structure in which to affect man's turning toward God. Man could work toward perfection but could not achieve it, for he was a fallen angel whose ultimate salvation lay in God's hands. God was perfection; His world demonstrated this by its integral unity. It was belief in this integral unity, this same organization and striving toward perfection that motivated Rush in the construction of his medical theories.[3]

Rush finished his religious education at the New Side College of New Jersey (now Princeton University) and started his medical apprenticeship under Dr. John Redman of Philadelphia. Redman had received his degree from Leyden after training at Edinburgh and London. It was Redman who introduced Rush to the great physicians Sydenham and Boerhaave. Rush's enthusiasm for Sydenham never ceased, though it was greatly modified as Rush himself matured. Rush named his farm after Thomas Sydenham and late in his life, he produced the first American edition of his works.[4] But, as we have seen, Rush met his greatest medical hero several years later when he went to Edinburgh and heard the stimulating lectures of William Cullen. Returning to Philadelphia to establish his practice, Rush incurred the emnity of the largely-Boerhaavian physicians there by vigorously promulgating the Cullenian system. It would be many years before Rush would break away from his master and feel free to develop his own theory. A combination of factors made this possible: Cullen's death in 1790, Rush's own intellectual development, but most importantly, his appointment in 1791 as Professor of the Institutes of Medicine at the University of Pennsylvania.

Rush was honoured to follow in the tradition of Cullen who also had been Professor of Chemistry and who had just taken over the chair of Institutes before Rush's arrival at Edinburgh. His new position forced Rush to analyse and compare current theories of medicine for presentation to his students. His own theories were developed by the time of the 1793 yellow fever epidemic in Philadelphia, and completed by 1795.[5] Rush took this challenge seriously, and spent a great deal of time preparing his lectures. He found the works of David Hartley particularly useful for this task. His library suggests that Rush first used Joseph Priestley's 1775 condensation of Hartley before obtaining the 1791 complete edition.[6]

Hartley's natural theology had a strong appeal to Rush.[7] Hartley was one of a long line of English physico-theologians who sought not only to worship God through the beauty and intricacy of His wordly creation, but to keep secure God's position of supremacy against the threat of a growing number of philosophers who found motion and matter, but not God, in the world. In so doing, he followed the eighteenth-century genius, Isaac Newton, in his suggestion that the natural phenomenon of nature be derived from 'mechanical principles' which would clarify God's handiwork. Hartley followed Newton further, into the new area of moral philosophy and its outgrowth, psychology. Like Locke before him, Hartley believed the individual started with an empty brain capable of responding to sensory impressions. These impulses caused vibrations in a Newtonian-like ether located in the branches of the nervous system, which were ultimately transmitted to the brain where first they produced simple, and then complex ideas from which the several faculties emerged. Man himself could not initiate motions; that ultimately belonged to God – as Rush also believed. This fitted well with what Rush had learned from William Cullen, who had stressed the capacity of the solids of the body and especially of the nervous system to respond to stimuli with either sensation or motion. Life, then, was 'a forced state'.

But Rush, in his eagerness to become his own system builder, did two things: first, following the thought of another of Cullen's students, John Brown, he simplified Cullen's theory by focusing on the body's capacity to respond. He called this capacity 'excitability' and the response itself, 'excitement'. Both could vary in degree and in regularity. Second, Rush believed that the amount of energy or excitability not only varied but could be distributed and transmitted throughout the body. Rush made the arterial system the main vehicle of transmission and not the nervous system. Disease, then, resulted from a disturbed motion in the arteries; and reflecting the unitary hand of God, there could be, therefore, but one disease.

Rush also applied his theory to psychiatry. 'The cause of madness is seated primarily in the blood vessels of the brain, and . . . it depends upon the same kind of morbid and irregular actions that constitute other arterial diseases. There is nothing specific in these actions. They are part of the unity of disease, particularly of fever; of which madness is a chronic form, affecting the part of the brain which is the seat of the mind.'[8] The shape of the mental illness that followed this disturbance was determined by which of the faculties of the mind were affected.

At this juncture Rush diverged from Hartley. They both believed that this is not an 'ideal disease' but a physical illness – that somehow the mind was physically dependent on the brain. How mind and body interacted they were both unable to say, and ended by falling back on a form of psychophysical parallelism. Hartley followed Locke, and built his faculties on association guided by the reactions of pain and pleasure. Rush agreed to a certain point. He could concur that this was so for the intellectual faculties, but in regard to those that determined man's moral behaviour he became acutely uncertain. Rush who has never been known for his philosophical acumen, showed his inconsistency and limitations at this point in postulating an innate moral faculty which automatically knows right from wrong.

Nonetheless, these faculties were clinically useful to Rush. Nine in number, they included three intellectual faculties (understanding, imagination, and memory), three miscellaneous (the will, passions, and the principle of faith), and the three moral faculties (the moral sense, conscience, and the sense of Deity). There is no evidence that his selection came from any one person or source. Several of them were traditional; Hartley spoke of at least five, and the Scottish philosophers whom Rush often mentions had many more. These faculties acted in concert in all human actions, certain of them exerting greater force, according to the needs of specific situations. If one or several of them fell victim to disordered action, what Rush called 'derangement' followed.[9]

Intellectual derangement was of three types and, although in all three the understanding was most easily disturbed, disruptions of the memory and of the imagination usually accompanied it. The first type was delirium, in which the brain, through a sympathetic response via the blood vessels, is disturbed by a derangement elsewhere in the body. The second type was phrenitis, the result of an acute inflammation of the brain. The third type, madness, was a chronic form of inflammation which could be either partial or general.

Partial intellectual derangement was represented by the traditional categories of hypochondriasis and melancholia. In his discussions thereof, Rush cited a number of English physicians: Joseph Mason Cox, John Ferriar, William Heberden, and Thomas Perceval, for example.

General intellectual derangement was most clearly manifested in mania, both acute and chronic. Rush was influenced in his thinking on the acute form of mania by the three major figures of English psychiatry of his time: Thomas Arnold, Alexander Crichton, and John Haslam. In his discussion of the treatment of this condition, he cited Erasmus Darwin and mentioned a letter from the Reverend Francis Willis, Sr., who had treated the English monarch, George III.

Derangement of the imagination received little or no attention from Rush, but he devoted an extensive chapter to disorder of the memory, reflecting the influence of such diverse scientists as Isaac Newton, Joseph Priestley, and John Pringle.

In the *Diseases of the Mind*, Rush devoted a separate chapter to each of his three miscellaneous faculties. Under disorders of faith, or the believing faculty, he obviously relished presenting the example of Dr. George Berkley and his followers, but he marshalled no English authorities for his discussion of disorders of the will. His chapter on the passions is profusely illustrated. John Gregory's *A Father's Legacy to His Daughters* was used in his discussion of love; on anger, he advocated John Arbuthnot's diet of milk and vegetables to temper this destructive passion; and he quotes John Hunter's personal use of opium to reduce fearfulness.

In his presentations on the moral faculties, Rush was careful to avoid any indication that the sense of Deity, a faculty he adapted from Lord Kames, could become disordered. The moral faculty proper, or moral sense, was a concept developed from several sources, but primarily from James Beattie, the minor Scottish poet and philosopher. Rush was far in advance of his time in suggesting that the moral sense could be disordered. This idea would not achieve wide acceptance until the mid-nineteenth century, when it was popularized by James Cowles Prichard as moral insanity.[10]

The above brief account naturally does not exhaust the range of British influences on Rush. Not mentioned are the many literary allusions – to Milton and Pope, to Boswell and Johnson (whom Rush had met in London), to Sterne, and to his two favourite authors, Shakespeare and the contemporary poet, William Cowper. These appear throughout all his writings. Rush was widely read in British sources – religious, philosophical, literary and medical – and they all helped to shape his psychiatric thought.

Although he saw himself as a revolutionary, history has judged Rush to be more moderate than extremist. His espousal of a republican form of government over a hereditary monarch constituted his most radical departure. In his medical thought, the 'Father of American Psychiatry' held closely to what he had learned from his forebears, teachers, and contemporaries of the English scene.

References

1 The author wishes to acknowledge the assistance of Beatrice T. Heveran and the support in part of N.I.H. grant LM00919 from the National Library of Medicine.

2 CORNER, GEORGE W. (ed.), *The Autobiography of Benjamin Rush*, Princeton, N.J., for the American Philosophical Society by the Princeton University Press, 1948, pp. 22–25, 46. See also David Freeman Hawke's, *Benjamin Rush: Revolutionary Gadfly*, Indianapolis, Ind., Bobbs-Merrill Company, 1971, p. 6.

3 HEIMERT, ALAN, *Religion and the American Mind: From the Great Awakening to the Revolution*, Cambridge, Mass., Harvard University Press, 1966. Very useful is Donald J. D'Elia's 'The Republican Theology of Benjamin Rush', *Pennsylvania History*, 1966, **33**, 187–203.

4 RUSH, BENJAMIN (ed.), *The Works of Thomas Sydenham, M.D.*, Philadelphia, Penn., Benjamin and Thomas Kite, 1809. A second edition was published by E. Kimber in Philadelphia in 1815.

5 CARLSON, ERIC T. and SIMPSON, MERIBETH M., 'The definition of mental illness: Benjamin Rush (1745–1813)', *Amer. J. Psychiat.*, 1964, **121**, 209–14.

6 Benjamin Rush's personal copies are at the Library Company of Philadelphia. Joseph Priestley's *Hartley's Theory of the Human Mind, on the Principle of the Association of Ideas*, London, J. Johnson 1775, is more heavily annotated than David Hartley's *Observations on Man, his Frame, his Duty and his Expectations*, London, J. Johnson, 1791, 3 vols.

7 D'ELIA, DONALD J., 'Benjamin Rush, David Hartley, and the revolutionary uses of psychology', *Proc. Amer. Phil. Soc.*, 1970, **114**, 109–18.

8 RUSH, BENJAMIN, *Medical Inquiries and Observations upon the Diseases of the Mind*, Philadelphia, Penn., Kimber and Richardson, 1812, pp. 17–18.

9 RUSH, BENJAMIN, 'Lectures on the Mind'. This manuscript is at the College of Physicians of Philadelphia and was used through the courtesy of W. B. McDaniel, 2nd.

10 CARLSON, ERIC T. and SIMPSON, MERIBETH M., 'Benjamin Rush's medical use of the moral faculty', *Bull. Hist. Med.*, 1965, **39**, 22–33.

J. B. Eklund and A. B. Davis
Washington D.C. (U.S.A.)

Some thoughts on the influence of British medicine on American medicine in the eighteenth century

Demonstrating the influence of British medicine on its colonies may be the most venerable tradition in the history of medicine in America. Even before the first American medical school was dedicated, John Morgan was totting up his debt to his Edinburgh professors.[1] Subsequent reviews of American medicine throughout the nineteenth century acknowledged Britain's role[2] and no less a person than William Welch on no less an occasion than the seventieth birthday of Sir William Osler in 1919 chose it as his subject.[3] Throughout this century, distinguished historians of medicine have commented on the relationship between the medicine of the two countries, though, curiously, they seldom mention each other's work.[4] Our purpose here is not to condemn, or even to contradict these earlier efforts. Rather, it is to review both their achievements and their methodology, and to suggest directions for additional research.

Arguing for something as tenuous as intellectual influence between two cultures, however similar, surely offers some of the most intriguing problems in historiography. The most ponderable approach is to demonstrate a transfer of matter, as it were. That is, to note the immigration to America of British medical men who later achieved a prominent practice; thus such names as William Douglas, John Kearsley Sr., William Shippen Sr., Cadwalader Colden and those three refugees from the '45, Peter Middleton, Lionel Chalmers and Hugh Mercer, can be seen in many articles on the subject.

Of course, non-living matter may be transferred as well, and thus the late Professor Sigerist noted the use of a number of publications – continental as well as British – which were used in teaching native American medical students at home.[5] And although the actual importation of British masonry had to wait until the nineteenth and twentieth century (capped, of course, by London Bridge itself), more than one colonial rejoiced in the architectural similarities between the Philadelphia Hospital and Edinburgh's impressive Royal Infirmary.[6]

But hospitals are not the only institutions for export. Writers on British influence have justly focused their attention on the similarities between Edinburgh's Medical School and the Medical Department of the College of Philadelphia. For a medical faculty to be connected to a university or college was usual enough in England with its long educational traditions, but the College of Philadelphia began a trend which, though interrupted by the era fondly known as 'The Rise of the Common Man', has continued to the present day. Completely reversing the English custom of small private hospital schools, Edinburgh and Philadelphia consciously gave an academic cast to medicine which, though scientifically premature, kept alive both the enlightenment's optimism for the future of man on earth, and the medical profession's dream of a draw, if not a win, with disease.[7] But if the goal set by the intellect could not be reached, the philosophical approach could be borne in mind, and the knowledge of the form that the solution would have to take radiated out from college to medical society to the club and thence to town, village and hamlet.[8]

But curricula, courses and texts are dull stuff without the men who invented, taught and used them, and thus few discussions of British influence omit a description, however brief, of the brilliant Edinburgh Faculty. The names, specialities, educational backgrounds of and occasional anecdotes about the first great (though not the first) medical faculty in Edinburgh – the two Monros, Innes, Sinclair, Rutherford and Plummer – have been, and will be, fondly retold by all authors who have come under eighteenth-century Edinburgh's intellectual spell.[9] Such later additions to the faculty as Robert Whytt, Charles Alston, and the biting critical intellect of William Cullen not only paved the way for the scientific achievements of Joseph Black but also stimulated the thought of American physicians from John Moultrie to Benjamin Rush and beyond.[10] Snippets from the journals of various foreign students suggest that life was not always the daily round of two to five classes, along with service at the apothecary shop and the infirmary.[11]

Although sometimes it seems that Edinburgh was the only city to which American medical students resorted, such was not the case as we all know. London got its share, particularly in surgery, which the anatomical brilliance of the Monros had kept from full fruition in Edinburgh. Starting with William Cheselden, there was a long line of exciting surgeons who drew not only American students, but graduates of Edinburgh as well. One thinks immediately of the skill of Percivall Pott, John Pringle and the Hunters. There, too, were several physicians such as Fothergill and, later, John Coakley Lettsom who served *in loco parentis* to Americans who arrived with the proper credentials. These might be from former students or, best of all certainly, from Benjamin Franklin, who himself served as friend and protector during his long sojourns in England.[12]

Most of all, medical historians have been intrigued with the students themselves. Starting with Moultrie, who graduated with an M.D. from Edinburgh University in 1749, there has been great concern with tracing out the student experiences and subsequent careers of Americans who studied in Britain. Because of his political prestige and as the author of a medical system which aroused respect and controversy abroad as well as at home, Benjamin Rush has surely received the lion's share of historical attention. Similarly, the other lights of Philadelphia – John Morgan and William Shippen Jr. – have been understandably celebrated in their role as the founding fathers of the Medical School in Philadelphia. In interest, they are closely followed by such later members of that faculty as Adam Kuhn, Caspar Wister and William Syng Physick. Since medical education in New York followed so closely on Philadelphia's heels, there has been similar interest in Samuel Bard and Peter Middleton, not to mention another medical man who, with Wistar, was one of the first important American chemists: Samuel Latham Mitchell. The earlier generation, too, has been the subject of much research. One thinks immediately of John Kearsley Sr., William Shippen Sr., John Bard, John Redman, William Douglas and

Cadwalader Colden.[13] In addition to those works which address themselves directly to the problems of 'influence' there are, of course, sections of articles with different intent and of books on various subjects which discuss the problems in passing. The number of these is so large that few bibliographic efforts would be more useful than a general survey of the relevant existing literature.

Now it seems to us that these are all reasonable approaches, and their execution in various combinations by various authors are, for the most part, admirable efforts. Indeed, we are happy to be able to report that those who are interested in this area can look forward to some interesting reading. In particular, two related areas – public health and medical practices during epidemics – have received a good bit of competent attention and will not be dealt with here.[14]

But admirable though the existing literature may be, one is left vaguely dissatisfied and, indeed, somewhat empty. Nowhere does a very clear picture emerge of the actual practice of those who studied abroad or, for that matter, those who did not. Specifically, we do not gain a feeling for the way in which their learning experience abroad translated itself into their modes of practice at home or even into the teaching of medicine in America.

Happily, in the latter case a start has been made. For example, Dr. Bell, in his superb study of the life of John Morgan, has pointed out that Morgan's lectures on materica media and chemistry were for the most part just synopses of Cullen.[15] Perhaps we may hope for similar detailed comparison between student notes known to exist from Edinburgh and Philadelphia, New York and Harvard.

The relationship between British *thought* and American *practice* is even more difficult, largely because we know so little about the 'average' practitioner, even 'average' in the sense of being university-educated but less famous than, say, a founder of the medical school in Philadelphia or a signer of the constitution. It is an historiographic fact of life that we almost always know more about the atypical, whether it is a person or an object, for the atypical is (almost by definition) valued more than the typical. Even, here, however, close study will continue to prove rewarding. Thus, for example, detailed comparison between Benjamin Rush's analysis of Dr. Hugh Martin's cancer remedy and the standard methods of chemical identification as taught by Cullen and Black suggests that though Rush did a workmanlike job, it was hardly as remarkable as some have thought.[16]

Most disturbing, perhaps, is the allegation, either explicit or implied, that individual practice was virtually helpless in the face of disease. Often this takes the more subtle form of repeatedly pointing out that public health during this period was more *effective* than private practice. By present-day standards, this is certainly true, but this seems to us to distort, rather than help, the attempts at historical analysis. A more cogent question, it seems to us, is to ask how the practitioner himself viewed his medical choices. Certainly in sheer number, they were impressive. Few can fault contemporary treatises on the practice of medicine or, for that matter, the pharmacopoeias, for not being sufficiently ponderous in terms of weight or tone. Indeed, Sydenham, Boerhaave, Salmon, Cullen and Brown – together or singly – can make up many a long evening's reading even now, as many of you can attest. Surely there is enough in any one of these authors to give the eighteenth-century practitioner a feeling that something by way of a cure might turn up if he just looked long enough and tried enough of the suggestions.

In fact, we doubt very much that, even though an individual's 'normal' practice lacked the drama of fighting an epidemic or the success of public health measures, the eighteenth-century practitioner saw his work as anything other than useful and even, on occasion, exciting. And with good reason. One need not depend on such sources as David Ramsay's ebullient review of the century's progress in medicine to convince oneself of this. As one might expect, reading the case reports of a master like Cullen will do as well. Even though one can argue with hindsight that the various procedures and medicines applied did no 'real' good, or even harm, the number of accounts which end with the words 'Dismissed, cur'd' would hardly lead to a pessimistic outlook on the medical practices of that time.[17]

But one need not limit the search to the best. A glance at the confident comments on medicines and the detailed observations on morbidity in the commonplace book of the relatively commonplace American practitioner, Elizur Hale of Glastonbury, Connecticut (fl. 1750–80) shows a richness of thought in a local man which seldom emerges in existing studies.[18] Even the dry day-books of Timothy Horton of West Springfield, Massachusetts, suggest a wide variety of responses to disease.[19] Painful as it might be, the task of counting and correlating the incidences of prescriptions for emetic powder and cholic pills vs. bitters and anodynes in such sources would tell us something useful about even the most empiric practice. While we shall probably need more casebooks, wastebooks, student notebooks etc. than we shall ever get, such material is slowly becoming available and its analysis will eventually allow useful comparisons with contemporary British practice.

In the last analysis, however, the most profound influence of British medicine on American practice – or at least the university variety – had the curious effect of limiting that very influence. The spirit of doubt and enquiry which characterized the best of British medical thinking in both Edinburgh and London allowed the American physician to strike out on his own; it allowed the American environment and experience, as reflected in American social and intellectual practices, to mould and attenuate British and continental ideas to fit American situations.

The most important vehicle for this expression of medical independence was the theory that a strong factor in the nature of disease was 'climate'. The term was meant in its broadest sense to include institutional and political as well as the natural environment. Discussions on the impact of climate on disease had engaged medical writers since antiquity, and received special attention in the eighteenth century by both British and Continental physicians and philosophers.[20] Not unexpectedly, the theory was transmitted to America where Thomas Bond[21] (1712–84), Peter Middleton[22] (d. 1781), Samuel Bard[23] (1742–1816) and Lionel Chalmers[24] (1715–77) among others believed that every climate and society gives rise to diseases peculiar to itself. In the later, post-revolutionary period, Rush and Charles Caldwell (1772–1853) both strongly urged that both the political climate and a physical climate which was causally tied to American methods of cultivation had an effect on disease problems.

Influenced by the work of the Americans John Mitchell (1690?–1768?), John Lining (1708–60) and William Currie (1754–1828), Rush and, later, Caldwell based their theories of fever on climatic conditions.[25] Caldwell's interest in the causes of variations in animals had led him to translate the 'climatist' Blumenbach's *Elements of Physiology* in 1795. Unlike European authors, who argued that America's climate led to overall weakness and greater susceptibility to disease, Caldwell saw America as part of a bold and gigantic hemisphere in which nature was at her best. But along with the great diversity and wealth of creatures America spawned, there were more virulent diseases which were difficult to control.[26] The proof that diseases were more powerful in America than in Europe was that to cure them one needed to apply stronger treatments such as greater bloodletting and to administer more potent drugs.[27] It appeared that the warmer temperatures – especially in the South – produced putrefaction throughout the countryside with its consequent evolution of 'Marsh miasmas' or gases that became the predisposing causes of a variety of fevers.[28] Such fevers included intermittent, remittent, malignant, cholera, dysentery and inflammation. Caldwell, following ancient theory, assumed that if the land would be properly cleared of rotting vegetation, these diseases would diminish or disappear. Other causes including rich and improper diet, contaminated water and insufficient clothing contributed to the type and severity of disease. All seemed to depend on the stage of civilization in America. Political events also were 'influential in modifying the constitutions, temperaments [and] diseases of the inhabitants. The general cheerfulness and the national diathesis [bodily constitution which predisposes to a disease or class of diseases] is such as to invite and suffer inflammatory diseases of an exalted grade.'[29]

Finally, perhaps it is not amiss to remind ourselves that, however great the influence of British medicine on its American counterpart, and however closely attuned America's medicine may have been to its own cultural factors, influence between cultures is invariably a reciprocal process. Thus America's effect on British medicine should, as in the case of smallpox, continue to prove an interesting area of study. As Lawrence Cremin recently pointed out, '. . . the very existence of the New World stirred the imagination of the Old, requiring it to rethink many of its time-honored beliefs. From More to Locke, philosophers located their utopias in America; and a steady flow of information concerning the realities of the colonial world . . . worked a transforming influence on [British] political, religious and scientific ideas.'[30]

References

1 MORGAN, JOHN, *A Discourse Upon the Institution of Medical Schools*, Philadelphia, 1765, pp. 29–31.

2 DINGLEY, AMASA, *An Oration on the Improvement of Medicine*, New York, 1794, pp. 15–33; RAMSAY, DAVID, *A Review of the Improvements, Progress and State of Medicine in the Eighteenth Century*, Charleston, 1801, *passim*; BECK, JOHN B., *An Historical Sketch of the State of Medicine in the American Colonies*, Albuquerque, Horn & Wallace, 1966, a reprint of the original of 1850, p. 23. Predictably, as America matured, there was less and less emphasis on Britain's role in the development of American medicine during the colonial period. Beck barely acknowledges it at all.

3 WELCH, WILLIAM H., 'Influence of English medicine upon American medicine in its formative period', in *Contributions . . . dedicated to Sir William Osler Bart, M.D., F.R.S. in Honor of his Seventieth Birthday*, 2 vols., New York, 1919, vol. 2, pp. 811–17.

4 See, for example, MILLER, GENEVIEVE, 'European influences in Colonial medicine', *Ciba Symp.*, 1947, 8, 514 ff.; MERCER, SIR WALTER, 'The contributions of Edinburgh to early American medicine', *J. R. Coll. Surg.*, 1962, 7, 180–92; MALLOCH, ARCHIBALD, *Medical Interchange Between the British Isles and America Before 1801*, London, 1946.

5 SIGERIST, HENRY E., 'Boerhaave's influence upon American Medicine', *Nederland. Tijd. Geneesk.*, 1938, 82, 4822–28.

6 KRAUS, MICHAEL, 'American and European medicine in the eighteenth century', *Bull. Hist. Med.*, 1940, 8, 689 ff.

7 GAY, PETER, *The Enlightenment, an Interpretation*, 2 vols., New York, Alfred A. Knopf, vol. 2, pp. 3–55.

8 WELCH, WILLIAM, op. cit. p. 813; PACKARD, FRANCIS R., 'How London and Edinburgh influenced medicine in Philadelphia in the eighteenth century', *Trans. Coll. Phys., Phil.*, 1931, **53**, 164; SIGERIST, op. cit., pp. 4825–26; SHRYOCK, RICHARD H., 'Pennsylvania and Edinburgh', *Penna Gaz.*, 1939, **37**, 272; KRAUS, op. cit., pp. 682 ff.

9 Including the present authors. See our 'Joseph Black matriculates: medicine and magnesia alba', *J. Hist. Med.*, 1972, **27**, 396–417.

10 See, for example, WELCH, op. cit., pp. 814–15; WILSON, J. GORDON, 'The influence of Edinburgh on American medicine in the eighteenth century', *Proc. Inst. Med. Chicago*, 1929, **7**, 132–34; PACKARD, op. cit., pp. 158–62; MILLER, op. cit., pp. 517–21.

11 See, for example, COZENS-HARDY, BASIL (ed.), *The Diary of Silas Neville*, London, Oxford University Press, 1950, pp. 136–56; a fascinating letter by a French student at Edinburgh has been published by Genevieve Miller, op. cit., pp. 519–21.

12 PACKARD, op. cit., p. 164, and especially KRAUS, op. cit., pp. 680–81, 684 ff.

13 Here the list of authors is almost as long as the list of subjects. A useful, though by no means exhaustive, catalogue of students by geographical area can be found in MERCER, op. cit., *passim*. Although the list is too long to be all-inclusive, see, for example, WELCH, op. cit., pp. 811–13, 814–16; WILSON, op. cit., pp. 134–38; PACKARD, op. cit., pp. 162–80; SIGERIST, op. cit., pp. 4824, 4826 ff.; and MILLER, op. cit., pp. 517 ff.

14 Works which come most readily to mind, are John Blake's *Public Health in the Town of Boston*, Cambridge, Harvard University Press, 1959, John Duffy's *Epidemics in Colonial America*, Louisiana State University Press, 1953, and, of course, Richard H. Shryock's *Medicine and Society in America, 1660–1860*, New York University Press, 1960.

15 BELL, WHITFIELD, *John Morgan, Continental Doctor*, Philadelphia, University of Pennsylvania Press, 1965, pp. 134–35.

16 RUSH, BENJAMIN, *Medical Inquiries and Observations*, Philadelphia, 1789, pp. 188–94; BLACK, JOSEPH, 'Elements of the Theory and Practise of Chemistry', National Library of Scotland, MS. 3533, pp. 176–82; cf. HINDLE, BROOK, *The Pursuit of Science in Revolutionary America*, Chapel Hill, University of North Carolina Press, 1956, pp. 297–98.

17 Casebook of William Cullen, National Library of Medicine, MS. B 15.

18 HALE, ELIZUR, Medical Commonplacebook, 1746–1783, National Library of Medicine, MS. fB 118.

19 HORTON, TIMOTHY, Daybooks (9 vols.), 1780–1833, National Library of Medicine, MS. fB 23.

20 For a compilation of ancient authors see ALBINUS, B. S., *De sede et causa Aethiopium*, Leyden, 1737. For eighteenth-century writers see HALLER, ALBRECHT VON, *Element. physiologiae corporis humani*, Lausanne, 1757–63, vol. 5. James Cassedy discusses the British and American interest in climate and disease, indicating how this marked the beginning of experimental medicine with the gathering of meteorological observations. 'Meteorology and medicine in Colonial America. Beginnings of the experimental approach', *J. Hist. Med.*, 1969, **24**, 193–204. The interplay between eighteenth-century European and American writers on climate and the development of organisms is analysed by Gilbert Chinard, 'Eighteenth-century theories on America as a human habitat', *Proc. Amer. phil. Soc.*, 1947, **91**, 27–57. See also BOORSTIN, DANIEL J., *The Lost World of Thomas Jefferson*, Boston, 1966, chap. 2.

21 In his 'Introductory Lecture to a Course of Clinical Observations in the Pennsylvania Hospital', of 1766 Bond commented: '. . . every Climate produces Diseases peculiar to itself, which require experience to understand and cure; and even the Diseases of the several Seasons in the Same Country, are found to differ so much some years, from what they were in others, . . .'. BRIDENBAUGH, CARL, 'Dr. Thomas Bond's essay on the utility of clinical lectures', *J. Hist. Med.*, 1947, **2**, 12. On Bond see THOMSON, ELIZABETH, 'Thomas Bond, 1713–84: First professor of clinical medicine in the American Colonies', *J. med. Educ.*, 1958, **33**, 614–24.

22 *A Medical Discourse . . .*, New York, 1769. Middleton spoke to the difficulties 'that young practitioners must be under to accommodate what they witnessed in America and compare it with foreign observations as they represented it in their medical texts', p. 68.

23 *A Discourse Upon the Duties of a Physician*, New York, 1769. Bard wrote: 'Every country has its particulair Diseases; the Varieties of Climate, Exposure, Soil, Situation, Trades, Arts, Manufacturing and even the Character of a People, all pave the Way to new complaints, and vary the Appearance of those, with which we are already acquainted;' p. 16.

24 *An Account of the Weather and Diseases of South Carolina*, London, 1776. Chalmers' intention was to discuss the temperament of the people of South Carolina, 'For it greatly concerns those, who undertake the cure of diseases in any country, to know somewhat of the constitutions of its inhabitants . . .', p. 39. In an *Essay on Fevers* (London, 1768), he claimed, 'In some countries bleeding may perhaps be more necessary in inflammatory fevers than I have generally found in South Carolina', p. 53.

25 An excellent account of Rush's actions during the yellow fever epidemic of 1793 appears in POWELL, JOHN H., *Bring Out Your Dead*, Philadelphia, 1949. Rush's own account was pub-

lished in his *Medical Inquiries and Observations*, 4 vols. in 2 reprinted by Arno Press and New York Times, 1972, vol. 2. A good summary of Mitchell's scientific interests appears in Raymond Phineas Stearns, *Science in the British Colonies of America*, Urbana, University of Illinois Press, 1970, pp. 539–59. The nature of the epidemic has been challenged by several historians: DUFFY, JOHN, *Epidemics in Colonial America*, Baton Rouge, 1953, p. 151; JARCHO, SAUL, 'John Mitchell, Benjamin Rush and yellow fever', *Bull. Hist. Med.*, 1957, **31**, 132–36. JONES, GORDON W., 'Dr. John Mitchell's yellow fever epidemic', *Va. Mag. Hist. and Biog.*, 1962, **70**, 43–48. While Mitchell appears to have been incorrect in his diagnosis he does deserve more study for the variety and extent of his scientific and medical thought.

26 CALDWELL, CHARLES, *An Oration on the Causes of the difference . . . between the Endemic Diseases of the United States of America and those of Countries of Europe*, Philadelphia, 1802.

27 Ibid., pp. 14–15.

28 Ibid., p. 26. Another who commented on the relationship between cultivation of the land and its effect on the climate and on disease is Amasa Dingley, op. cit., p. 7.

29 Ibid., p. 31.

30 CREMIN, LAWRENCE A., *American Education in the Colonial Experience 1607–1783*, New York, 1970, p. 24.

S. J. Reiser
Boston, Massachusetts (U.S.A.)

Aspects of role of the stethoscope in the introduction of auscultation to Great Britain and the United States

The stethoscope, invented by Laennec in 1816 and introduced to the world in his 1819 treatise on auscultation, was the symbol of the new age of physical diagnosis. It was the first instrument of diagnosis ever used on a large scale in medicine. It stood for a new perception of disease in which cause was circumscribed in the anatomical lesion; a new physical relation of doctor with patient; a new search for signs of disease in the interior recesses of the body, and a forsaking of older disease signs discerned on the body's outer surface or from the questioning of patients. It exerted significant psychological effects on Laennec, and the patients and physicians who observed or employed it. As the mediating agent of auscultation the problems and advantages surrounding its use determined in large part the reception of the technique.

Through comments on the stethoscope, one is able to form a picture of the effect of the notion and act of physical diagnosis on the patient, to whom the experience of being actively examined by doctors was new. Some were apprehensive: reports appeared of adults who refused examination with the instrument,[1] and some children did not permit its steady application.[2] Doctors learning the procedure compounded the problem by setting the instrument upon the chest of patients with excessive force or asking them to make frequent changes in posture. Medical students in Edinburgh at one time were denied permission to practise with the stethoscope on patients because, as novices, they were apt particularly to make such mistakes.[3] Some patients associated the stethoscope with surgical instruments and became alarmed that an operation would be performed. Physicians hence were cautioned against its unnecessary display.[4] Such assertions were challenged, one physician claiming as early as 1828, that he never attended a patient who refused to be ausculted.[5] Nonetheless, the act of auscultation fostered a new physical association between patient and doctor which required significant psychological adjustment on both sides.

The idea of anatomization of the living body through auscultation affected patients profoundly. Internal illness of the chest could no longer be concealed – the patient was autopsied while alive. The omnipotence of this method became personified for the public in the stethoscope, as the following English newspaper account illustrates:

A wonderful instrument called the stethoscope, invented a few months ago, for the purpose of ascertaining the different stages of pulmonary affections, is now completely in vogue in Paris. . . . It is quite a fashion, if a person complains of a cough, to have recourse to the miraculous tube, which, however, cannot effect a cure; but should you unfortunately perceive in the countenance of the Doctor, that he fancies certain symptoms exist, it is very likely that a nervous person might become seriously indisposed and convert the supposition into reality.[6]

Expression of concern over disclosures of the disease within the body are contained in a poem 'To the Stethoscope' which appeared in *Blackwood's Edinburgh Magazine* of 1847. The editor introducing it wrote that the instrument was well known to physicians and that to most families it had proved 'an object of horror and the saddest remembrance'. So often was it connected with predicting the loss of close relatives, it was a device upon which 'the hopes and fears, and one may also say the destinies of mankind, so largely hang'. Thus, the stethoscope was thought an admirable subject for poetic exposition.[7]

Stethoscope! thou simple tube,
   Clarion of the yawning tomb,
Unto me thou seem's to be
   A very trump of doom.

. . .

Wielding thee, the grave physician,
   By the trembling patient stands,
Like some deftly skilled musician;
   Strange! the trumpet in his hands.
Whilst the sufferer's eyeball glistens
   Full of hope and full of fear,
Quietly he bends and listens
   With his quick, accustomed ear –
Waiteth until thou shalt tell
   Tidings of the war within:
In the battle and the strike,
Is it death, or is it life,
   The fought-for prize shall win?
Then thou whisperest in his ear
   Words which only he can hear –
Words of woe, and words of cheer.
   Jubilates thou hast sounded,
   Wild exulting songs of gladness;
Misereres have abounded
   Of unutterable sadness.
Sometimes may thy tones impart,
   Comfort to the sad at heart;
Oftener, when thy lips have spoken,
Eyes have wept, and hearts have broken.[8]

Because the impoverished state of therapy meant that many diagnoses carried with them a death warrant, the accuracy of the stethoscope was feared. However, the enigmatic character of the instrument, which heard sounds silent to the patient, combined with its accurate forecasts, produced a rapid public veneration and acceptance. Indeed, beginning in the late 1820s, public sentiment in favour of the stethoscope grew to the extent that the practitioner forsaking the instrument placed his reputation in jeopardy. Dr. J. P. Kay wrote in 1828 that objection to the stethoscope would be 'suicidal' to professional standing.[9] A doctor signing himself 'One of the New School' declared that physicians undervaluing the stethoscope were 'unworthy of public patronage'. There is one comfort however still in store – we now know who the physicians are that duly appreciate this inestimable discovery, and who are really deserving of the public's support. Doubtless they will receive it, for a John Bull is attached to the good things in life. . . . The pages of *The Lancet* are widely read, and ere long the names of those physicians who 'close their ears to the voice of the charmer,' will be as regularly shown up, as in times past, and in the columns of John Bull, were those of the clergy, who persisted in praying for Queen Caroline.

It has been declared by Dr. Kay of Manchester, that by-and-by, 'it will be dangerous, positively *suicidal* to the professional reputation, to object to the stethoscope.' Dr. Kay will excuse me, but the time is already arrived.[10]

Such sentiment encouraged doctors of the time who could not distinguish a wheeze from a murmur to carry the stethoscope for purposes of public display. This charade produced caustic comments from the auscultors. A stethoscopist claimed to see one of these pretenders,

the other day put on a look of great wisdom – applying the wrong end of the stethoscope to his ear – hold the other end about two inches from the patient's chest – and sagely remark, that he heard, very distinctly, the respiratory murmur! This respiratory murmur was no other than the murmur of a hackney coach, passing over a piece of newly macadamized street, opposite to the patient's house![11]

Physicians of high repute in the 1830s publicly sneered at what they referred to as the quackery of the stethoscope and prophesied its existence would be short-lived. Their predictions failing, they resorted to carrying the instrument about under the pretext of being a learned auscultor. The pretenders were described as knowing as much about the use of the stethoscope 'as a state trumpeter in one of our city pageantries, knows of the use of the instrument of music which he idly carries as a part of the show,'[12] or as deriving as much benefit from applying the stethoscope 'to the seat of honor as to the chest'.[13]

Physicians in this period found that patients denigrated those relying solely on words to arrive at diagnoses.

[The public] will no longer tolerate the mere symptomatic doctor of the last century. Something more than an acquaintance with a Latin and Greek Vocabulary, some other badge of professional knowledge besides the wig and gold-headed cane, is now required from the medical graduates for public confidence. We would venture a small wager that so much abused, insignificant-looking little instrument, the stethoscope, would prove assured passport in the hands of a young medical aspirant for public employment, and a more certain means of obtaining public confidence as a physician, than the gold-headed cane of Sydenham, Meade, or of any other of the medical sages of former times.[14]

In the 1840s the stethoscope continued to be used by practitioners unable to gain diagnostic information from it but forced by public sentiment to carry it. Accusations continued to be made that some set the instrument to the chest 'not because they themselves can thereby derive any real benefit, but because it is the fashion, and gives the appearance of accuracy and profundity'.[15] The *Lancet*, in 1842, condemned the physician who used his stethoscope in examination 'all the while looking thoroughly wise, yet remaining with a mind uninformed, and an ear unimpressed by a single idea derived from his hypocritical performance.'[16]

These events demonstrate the effect of public pressure on professional behaviour in medicine. They clarify the role that a technological instrument can exert in favour of an intellectual innovation such as auscultation.

The stethoscope was the focus of comment and debate not only by patients and physicians who were opposed to or disquieted about the acceptance of auscultation in general, but also by the auscultors themselves. Although Laennec had striven mightily to wed the performance of auscultation to the stethoscope, only several years after his treatise appeared arguments were raised which asserted the instrument held no superiority over the unaided ear and was in many circumstances inferior to it. Laennec noted the competition in the second (1826) edition of his treatise: 'Since the publication of my researches, some physicians have attempted to repeat them by immediate auscultation; and there is one or two of these who seems to give this method the preference.'[17]

There were three medical circumstances favouring use of the unaided ear over the stethoscope. First, it was generally agreed that learning to auscult was more difficult with the stethoscope than with the naked ear, the former requiring more practice, attention and time.[18] Reflecting on his observations at the Paris hospitals between 1825 and 1826, Dr. Charles Williams said that in mastering auscultation 'the management of the stethoscope was a stumbling block to not a few',[19] and for this reason, the French often discarded it. He illustrated the problem with an anecdote about the visit of Sir Charles Scudamore to Laennec's hospital in 1826 to take lessons from the master. Laennec was untiring in his efforts to teach Sir Charles but in vain, for the English doctor claimed he could hear nothing through it. Critical investigation revealed that because the tragus of Sir Charles' ear was uncommonly large the pressure of the stethoscope pushing it had caused blockage of the auditory canal. By slightly hollowing the flat end of the stethoscope, 'Sir Charles's ear was thus opened. He returned to London rejoicing: and shortly after, published a pamphlet in favour of auscultation.'[20] Though the advocates of the stethoscope acknowledged these difficulties, they insisted the slight additional trouble of learning to use the instrument would be repaid by the greater distinctness and certainty of its indications. They sarcastically asserted that auscultation with the naked ear (immediate auscultation) because more easily learned than that with the stethoscope (mediate auscultation) would always have advocates among those who preferred ease to exactness. Wrote one in 1837: 'It is, beyond doubt, more difficult to learn mediate auscultation than immediate; just as it is easier to whistle than to play the flute.'[21]

The inconvenience of carrying the stethoscope was the second factor and was cited by Laennec as a main source of opposition to the instrument.[22] Andral had predicted that because the ear was more readily available than the stethoscope, the former was more likely to be used in auscultation.[23] To make matters worse, Laennec's original stethoscope, as described by Jacob Bigelow, was 'large and clumsy'.[24] Although the dimensions of the stethoscope were modified and the instrument made more portable,[25] the physicians of this period resented the inconvenience of transporting their medical apparatus.

A third factor favouring immediate auscultation was the time saved for the physician, owing to the greater rapidity with which it could be applied when large areas implicated by disease had to be investigated.[26]

On the other side, most auscultors agreed with Laennec that the stethoscope was indispensable not only in unclean cases and when treating females, but also in examining portions of the body such as the axilla, the neck, or the malformed chest wall, where the application of the ear was physically impracticable.[27]

Laennec had asserted categorically that 'the repugnance which everyone must feel to apply the ear to the chest of a patient that is dirty or whose chest is bathed in perspiration, must always prevent the habitual or frequent use of this method [immediate auscultation]'.[28] Most auscultators substantiated Laennec's statement, noting that application of the ear also placed the nose and face in contact with the unclean patient.[29] Wrote Williams: 'To apply it [the ear] to the chest of a patient labouring under an infectious disorder, is neither pleasant or safe.'[30] This problem was joined to the issue of delicacy. In relating the circumstances leading to his notion to construct a stethoscope, Laennec had observed that the sex and young age of the female whom he had to examine induced him to auscult through a rolled quire of paper rather than place his ear directly on her chest. He asserted that to auscult over the mammae of females with the naked ear was inadmissible for 'reasons of decorum'.[31] In this matter too, there was general agreement that the stethoscope had the advantage over the naked ear. For example, Williams remarked: 'to apply it [the ear] to the person of a young female, whether pleasant or no, would certainly not be proper.'[32]

Touch and manipulation of the body can be threats to human dignity. The patient, unaccustomed to physical familiarity as part of his relation to the physician, was prone to feel controlled and object-like with auscultation. Physicians were also clearly disturbed by the intimate physical contact imposed upon them by the procedure of auscultation. The stethoscope allowed them to disengage from direct physical contact and increase the distance between the patient and the examiner. It thereby served a critical psychological function.

Apart from the relative advantages granted to the two methods, auscultors disagreed over their comparative accuracy in a number of circumstances. Laennec insisted on the superiority of the stethoscope in locating small lesions.[33] He and others argued it circumscribed, augmented, and transmitted sounds better and thereby marked their limits more precisely.[34] The dissentors from this proposition asserted that the well-practised ear could localize lesions with a precision equal to that of the stethoscope. Commented Andral: 'Neither can I agree with him [Laennec] that the stethoscope is better than the ear for distinguishing the sounds of the part under consideration from those proceeding from the adjacent parts. I have never found any difference in this respect between the two methods of auscultation.'[35]

A second point at issue involved the relative physical inconvenience of each technique for the physician. The assertion was made that placing and keeping the stethoscope in good contact with the patient's body required considerable skill. In some postures the patient assumed in bed it was thought impossible even for experts to hold the stethoscope with sufficient firmness to keep it in the proper place. The application of the ear was said to demand less constrained positioning than the application of the stethoscope.[36] The advocates of the instrument disagreed. Williams wrote: 'Unless your neck be pretty long and flexible, you will find this easy method [immediate auscultation] after all more irksome and fatiguing than the mediate method.'[37] Laennec too had noted that the posture one was forced to assume when practising immediate auscultation caused blood to rush to the head and consequently made the hearing dull.[38] He and other auscultors claimed also that placing the naked ear to the chest engendered more extraneous sounds than when the stethoscope was applied.[39] As Hughes declared:

The rustling of the clothes of the patient, in consequence of a larger surface being covered by the side of the head than by the end of the stethoscope, is more likely to interfere with the sounds proceeding from the chest. The hair of the auscultor himself, by the motion of the patient's body, frequently gives rise to sound nearly resembling those arising from disease. These may be incorrectly supposed to proceed from the chest and may thus become a source of error.[40]

Andral categorically denied both assertions. He stated the stethoscope occasioned no fewer adventitious sounds than the naked ear when the former was set upon the patient.[41]

The advocates of immediate auscultation also challenged Laennec's belief that certain pathognomonic sounds of disease were only transmittable through the stethoscope. A good example of such a sign was the phenomenon of pectoriloquism that consisted of the direct transmission of the voice from the chest to the ear through the stethoscope. Laennec found this sign to exist in all patients who had excavations in the lung caused by tuberculosis. He believed pectoriloquism was a pathognomic sign of tuberculosis which could be trusted diagnostically in the absence of all other symptoms or signs of the disease.[42] Laennec said that the unique sound of the transmitted voice heard through the stethoscope was changed into simple resonance when the naked ear was used to detect it, thereby losing the value of a sign of great significance in diagnosis.[43] However, it was argued by Andral that though pectoriloquism was sometimes more distinct and perfect under the stethoscope, it could be distinguished quite well with the naked ear.[44]

Finally, it was a moot point whether use of the stethoscope or naked ear was of greater benefit to the physician's reputation and abilities in the eyes of the patient. On the one hand, a physician arguing for the use of immediate auscultation wrote in 1825: 'But certainly the application of the stethoscope carries with it an *appearance* of quackery, which it is desirable to avoid, at least among the higher ranks of society, who are apt to canvass a medical man's actions, as well as words.'[45]

The similarity between auscultation with the stethoscope and surgery was marked. Both used instruments and were manual in character. These qualities had caused physicians to disdain surgery. Physicians saw their art primarily in terms of the intellectual synthesis of symptoms and associated the surgeon who used tools and manually laboured on the body with tradesmen of a distinctly lower class. As one practitioner explained:

Physicians, almost from the days of Linacre, have reprobated that branch of medicine which is denominated 'surgery', as the '*instrumental*' branch of the science – the chirurgical, the manipulating department, – and affecting to despise all mechanical contrivances, the M.D.'s, both Dubs and Regulars, have rejected every species of chirurgical instrument, from the lancet down to that dextrous finger of Sir Astley Cooper which forced its way to the aorta of a suffering being who ended his existence in Guy's hospital.[46]

In one of the earliest English reviews of Laennec's treatise, a critic remarked that two large volumes devoted to the diagnosis of diseases of the chest, using signs perceived by one sense through an instrument, led him to suspect a little charlatanism was at hand.[47] This fear that an adverse collegial image would be created by using the stethoscope was commented upon by John Forbes in the preface to his 1821 translation of Laennec. He said that one of the primary barriers to its application was the 'ludicrous' picture presented by the image of the grave physicians listening to a patient's chest through a long tube as if 'the disease inside were a living thing that could communicate its condition' to the engrossed practitioner.[48]

Auscultation with the ear also was held to cause no pain to the patients[49] and no anxiety to youngsters[50] as did the stethoscope. On the other hand, as I have pointed out, for many patients the stethoscope symbolized the diagnostic accuracy attributed to auscultation, thereby seeming to give therapeutic advantage to physicians using it. It personified and represented the content of the new technique and the set of perceptive and personal relations that came with it.

By the 1840s, the medical literature in the United Kingdom and the United States reflected the belief that Laennec had exaggerated the advantages of mediate over immediate auscultation. A critic of the stethoscope wrote that it 'possesses no magical properties; it is merely a conductor of sound, and a good auscultator and pathologist who has never seen one in his life could hear as much on his first attempt as the man who had never ausculted without it'.[51] In both the United Kingdom and the United States, some auscultors exclusively used one or the other method,[52] while others argued that neither be solely adopted but used alternatively depending upon the medical circumstances.[53] Though the stethoscope had lost some of its popularity it had inspired discussion, study and use of auscultation and thereby performed a central role in fostering acceptance of the technique by the medical profession and society.

It is important to appreciate the significance of the psychological effect it exerted upon Laennec. The mediative qualities he believed the stethoscope to uniquely possess encouraged him in the pursuit of the phenomena of auscultation. It seemed to delineate and clarify internal sounds in ways not possible by using merely unaided senses. Laennec believed ordinary sensory powers needed augmentation to discern the hidden lesions beneath the skin. The stethoscope represented the first major effort in medicine to convince doctors that man's natural faculties were no longer adequate to diagnose disease. Only by their technological expansion could the senses attain the acuity to detect the disease processes within. The use of Laennec's stethoscope represents a shift from the doctor's personality, intellect, and unaided senses as his primary diagnostic instruments, to his instrumental extensions.

References

1 Review of Forbes' 1827 translation of Laennec, *Mthly J. for. Med.*, 1828, **1**, 193.

2 WILLIAMS, CHARLES J. B., *Lectures on the Physiology and Diseases of the Chest, including the principles of physical and general diagnosis*, Philadelphia, Haswell, Barrington & Haswell, 1839, p. 78; also BARTH, M. and ROGER, HENRY, *A Practical Treatise on Auscultation*, trans. Patrick Newbigging, Lexington, Ky., Scrugham & Dunlap, 1847, p. 8.

3 LAENNEC, R. T. H., *A Treatise on Diseases of the Chest, and on Mediate Auscultation*, trans. from the 3rd French ed. by John Forbes; additional notes by Professor Andral, trans. by John D. Fisher from the 4th French ed., New York, Samuel S. & William Wood, 1838, p. 31. See also COMINS, NICHOLAS P., Letter to the editor, *Lancet*, 1828–29, **ii**, 685; and HUGHES, H. M., *A Clinical Introduction to the Practice of Auscultation*, Philadelphia, Lea & Blanchard, 1846, pp. 97–98.

4 HUGHES, op. cit., pp. 27–28.

5 See ref. 1 above.

6 *The Times*, 19 December 1824, as quoted by George Rosen, 'A note on the reception of the stethoscope in England', *Bull. Hist. Med.*, 1939, **7**, 93–94. It is interesting that though physicians were aware of the stethoscope in 1820, the popular press four years later reports it just recently discovered.

Another example of the sensitive qualities the stethoscope was thought to possess is found in a short limerick appearing in the *Lancet*, 1829, **i**, 96, entitled 'Auscultation extraordinary':

Quoth Rod'rick, 'I'll a place contrive
So dark and safe, no man alive
Shall to our private meeting grope:'
'Egad,' cries Johnny, 'that won't do,
If there's no crack to listen through,
They'll take "reports" by Stethoscope.

7 'To the stethoscope', *Blackwood's Edinb. Mag.*, 1847, **61**, 361.
8 Ibid. The remainder told of its role in predicting the death of a patient.
9 KAY, J. P., letter to the editor, *Lancet*, 1827–28, **i**, 757.
10 One of the New School, letter to the editor, *Lond. med. Gaz.*, 1828, **2**, 408–9.
11 Review of Stokes' *A Treatise on the Diagnosis and Treatment of Diseases of the Chest*, Part I . . ., *Med. chir. Rev.*, 1838, **8**, 33.
12 Review of Kennedy's *Observations on Obstetric Auscultation . . ., Dubl. J. med. chem. Sci.*, 1834, **5**, 90.
13 See ref. 11.
14 Review of Duncan's *Empyema and Pneumo-thorax*, *Med. chir. Rev.*, 1828, **8**, 131–32.
15 Review of Maillot's *A Practical Treatise on Percussion . . ., Mthly J. med. Sci.* (*Edinb.*), 1847–48, **8**, 189.
16 'Auscultation', *Lancet*, 1843–84, **i**, 268.
17 LAENNEC, R. T. H., *A Treatise on the Diseases of the Chest and on Mediate Auscultation*, trans. John Forbes from the 2nd French ed., London, T. & G. Underwood, 1827, pp. 23–24.
18 See, LAENNEC, 1838 translation, p. 3. See also WILLIAMS, CHARLES J. B., *A Rational Exposition of the Physical signs of the Diseases of the Lungs and Pleura . . .*, London, 1828, p. 51; and HUGHES, op. cit., p. 97.
19 WILLIAMS, C. J. B., *Memoirs of Life and Work*, London, Smith, Elder, 1884, p. 48.
20 Ibid. See also, *Memoir of James Jackson, Jr., written by his father . . .*, Boston, Hilliard, Gray, 1836, pp. 109–14.
21 Review of Stokes, Meriadec, Laennec and Andral, *Br. for. med. Rev.*, 1837, **4**, 295. See also, WILLIAMS, *Lectures on the Physiology and Diseases of the Chest . . .*, p. 77.
22 LAENNEC, 1827 translation, p. 24. Piorry had mentioned this as a problem in the use of his plenimeter, *supra*, p. 69.
23 LAENNEC, 1838 translation, p. 32.
24 BIGELOW, JACOB, 'Brief rules for exploration of the chest, in diseases of the lungs and heart', *Boston med. surg. J.*, 1839, **20**, 373.
25 There were many changes in the form and size of the stethoscope during the period 1819–50. It assumed several shapes and was made smaller. The stethoscope Laennec described and recommended in his 1819 treatise was one foot long, one and a half inches wide, came apart in the middle for more convenient carrying, and was made of wood.
26 See, HUGHES, op. cit., pp. 97–98. See, BENNET, HENRY, 'Remarks on the comparative value of auscultation practised with and without the stethoscope', *Lancet*, 1843–44, **i**, 464. See also GERHARD, W. W., *Lectures on the Diagnosis, Pathology, and Treatment of the Diseases of the Chest*, Philadelphia, Haswell & Barrington, 1842, p. 26; and review of Phillipp, Gerhard, Cowan and Trier, *Br. for. med. Rev.*, 1837, **3**, 188.
27 See, LAENNEC, 1827 translation, p. 24; 1838 translation, p. 32; WILLIAMS, *Lectures on the Physiology and Diseases of the Chest . . .*, p. 78; BARTH and ROGERS, op. cit., pp. 7–8; and BENNET, op. cit., p. 464.
28 See ref. 17, pp. 4, 24.
29 WILLIAMS, op. cit., p. 78, See also BENNET, 'Remarks on the comparative value of auscultation practices with and without the stethoscope', *Lancet*, 1843–44, **i**, 464; HUGHES, op. cit., p. 99; and BARTH and ROGER, op. cit., p. 7.
30 WILLIAMS, op. cit. One of the few to disagree with this point was Andral who asserted: 'As to the offensive condition of the patient from lack of cleanliness, etc., a remedy is easily found in placing a handkerchief or a napkin over the surface to be examined' (Laennec, 1838 trans., p. 25).
31 LAENNEC, 1827 trans., p. 25; see also LAENNEC, 1821 trans., p. 284.
32 WILLIAMS, op. cit., p. 78. See also BARTH and ROGER, op. cit., pp. 7, 24, 204. Dr. John Burne in 1841 reported that he has met women who would not allow even the stethoscope to be applied on them by the doctor because of the proximity and exposure made necessary by the procedure. ('An account of a new Plesser and Plessimeter', *Lond. med. Gaz.*, 1840–41, **ii**, 468.)
33 LAENNEC, 1827 trans., p. 24.
34 One physician raised the question that if the stethoscope indeed circumscribed and magnified sounds, could not one be sure that, as in the case of the microscope or telescope, the sound was not somehow distorted? (CLUTTERBUCK, HENRY, 'Lectures on blood-letting', *Lond. med. Gaz.*, 1837–38, **ii**, 698). Furthermore, though Laennec and other auscultors observed that stethoscopes made of dissimilar materials transmitted sounds differently (LAENNEC, 1821 trans., pp. 284–85)

they never examined the perceptual consequences of the phenomenon. (See, LAENNEC, 1827 trans, pp. 24 and 284. See also, GERHARD, op. cit., p. 26; HUGHES, op. cit., p. 98; and Review of Stokes, Meriadec, Laennec and Andral, op. cit., p. 295.)

35 LAENNEC, 1838 trans., p. 32. See also BARTH and ROGER, op. cit., p. 8. The following argument to demonstrate the principles underlying the superiority of immediate versus mediate auscultation in locating lesions of the lungs was made by Dr. Henry Bennet in 1842. He claimed it was evident that the more intense the sounds, the more clearly they were perceived by the ear. Since the intensity of a sound depended in part on the number of distinct vibrations heard, it followed that the greater the number of vibrations perceived, the clearer would be the aural recognition of them. Because the ear directly applied to the chest detected a greater number of vibrations than the stethoscope, the sounds of the healthy or diseased body would be heard with greater distinctness with the former than with the latter. By comparing the clearly perceived sounds in normal and pathological areas, the differences existing between them could be accurately appreciated (BENNET, op. cit., pp. 463–64.)

However, in so far as the heart was concerned, even Dr. Bennet agreed that the stethoscope was superior to the naked ear. He wrote that 'if we wish to form an accurate diagnosis to ascertain which of the valves or regions of the heart is the seat of the disease, then the stethoscope becomes indispensable'. This was so because 'the respiratory murmur, not serving as a point of comparison, as is the case in auscultation of the lungs, interferes with the perception of the cardiac sounds. . . . The stethoscope only giving distinctly the sounds created underneath the area which it covers, enables us to exclude, to a certain extent, the respiratory murmur. . . . It also enables us to examine separately, and to compare the varied nature and intensity of the sounds in each of the regions we have mentioned, which are scarcely possible if the ear cover at the same time both the base and the apex of the heart. Thus it will be seen that the same principles which induce me to confine myself almost entirely to that instrument when examining the heart' (ibid., p. 465).

36 See, LAENNEC, 1838 translation, pp. 31–32; and BENNET, op. cit., p. 464.

37 WILLIAMS, op. cit., p. 78. See also LAENNEC, 1827 translation, p. 24.

38 LAENNEC, 1827 translation, p. 25.

39 Ibid., pp. 24–25. See also WILLIAMS, op. cit., p. 78.

40 HUGHES, op. cit., p. 98.

41 LAENNEC, 1838 translation, p. 31.

42 See, LAENNEC, 1821 translation, pp. 297–301.

43 LAENNEC, 1827 translation, p. 25.

44 LAENNEC, 1838 translation, p. 32.

45 Review of Forbes' *Original Cases . . .*, *Med. chir. Rev.*, 1825, **2**, 65.

46 TOWNSHEND, RICHARD, 'Tabular view of the principal signs furnished by auscultation and percussion . . .', *Lancet*, 1831–32, **ii**, 121–22. The identification of surgery with technology as it affected the adoption of instrumental aids to diagnosis by physicians is a subject requiring further study.

47 Review of LAENNEC's *On Mediate Auscultation . . .*, op. cit., p. 165.

48 LAENNEC, R. T. H., *A Treatise on the Diseases of the Chest*, trans. John Forbes in 1821 from the 1st French ed.; intro, by Paul Klemperer, New York, Hafner, 1962, p. xix. See also Review of Andral's *Clinique Médicale . . .*, *Med. chir. Rev.*, 1825, **3**, 493.

49 LAENNEC, 1838 translation, p. 31; and HUGHES, op. cit., pp. 97–98.

50 WILLIAMS, op. cit., p. 78; and BARTH, M. and ROGER, H., op. cit., p. 18.

51 BENNET, op. cit., p. 465.

52 See, WILLIAMS, op. cit., p. 77; HUGHES, op. cit., p. 97; GERHARD, op. cit., p. 26, and BIGELOW, op. cit., p. 373.

53 See, BARTH and ROGER, op. cit., p. 78; and HUGHES, op. cit., pp. 97, 114–15.

M. H. Saffron
New York (U.S.A.)

The influence of Dublin on American medicine

By the year 1670 England had gained undisputed control of the eastern seaboard of North America from Massachusetts to the Carolinas, and medical practice in the now unified colonies soon began to follow the pattern of the mother country very closely. Qualified physicians with degrees were rare, but these few studied the theories of Willis, Sydenham and Mead as closely as did their counterparts in the British Isles. The lack of medical schools and the serious shortage of trained medical men in the early eighteenth century led to the revival of an ancient form of education – the preceptorship – and many an excellent practitioner received all of his medical training while serving as an apprentice to some well-known physician.

As the eighteenth century progressed an increasing number of colonials began to find their way to the medical centres of Europe. Although Leyden managed to attract a few, and we hear of an isolated student at Rheims and Paris, the great majority of Americans were drawn to Edinburgh, then enjoying its period of greatest fame. The 'Edinburgh period' of American medicine has rightly received a great deal of attention. Such celebrities as William Shippen, Jr., John Morgan, Benjamin Rush and Samuel Bard received in the Scottish capital not only an excellent education but the inspiration to found at Philadelphia and New York the two earliest medical schools in North America. Before returning home many Edinburgh graduates stopped off at London to walk the hospitals for six months or longer.

I turn now to another centre of medical instruction in the British Isles – one which has received little attention as a source of influence on American medicine. Although I know of no eighteenth-century American who came to Dublin for the sole purpose of studying medicine, I hope to show that a trio of Irish physicians who were educated in Dublin or practised there before migrating to America were to exert considerable leadership in the medical life of their adopted country. It will be noted that I have more than a superficial interest in each of these men.

First in point of time was Samuel Clossy (1724–86). A native of Dublin, Clossy took his arts and medical degrees at Trinity where he found himself attracted first to natural philosophy and later to the rising science of morbid anatomy. While still an undergraduate in medicine he was accorded the unusual privilege of performing all the autopsies at the famous Steevens' Hospital. Clossy also spent several summers in London, attending the lectures of William Hunter and working in the dissecting rooms at St. George's Hospital. At Dublin he had found a kindred soul in George Cleghorn, a master anatomist who had spent many years as an army surgeon on the island of Minorca, studying the comparative anatomy of the Barbary ape and man, and eventually incorporating his observations in a printed volume which appeared in 1751. In 1762 while the French and Indian War was still being fought in America Clossy received news that a military hospital was to be erected in New York. Caring little for the actual practice of medicine Clossy saw in this project a rare opportunity to continue his anatomical studies unhampered by the usual restraints of authority. In the summer of 1763 he came to London to supervise the publication of his only printed work *Observations on Some of the Diseases of the Parts of the Human Body*. This is certainly one of the earliest attempts at a systematic review of pathology in the English language, antedating the better known and more comprehensive effort of Mathew Baillie by half a century. In a reprint of Clossy's book which I edited in 1967 the striking resemblance of his methodology in case presentation to the protocol of the modern clinico-pathologic conference was emphasized.

Arriving in New York in September 1763, Clossy was shocked to learn that because of the cessation of hostilities, plans for the hospital had been abandoned. He nevertheless decided to remain in the attractive town, and two months later wrote Cleghorn a glowing letter reporting a successful course in human anatomy, the first complete course on the cadaver to be given in New York. Clossy was undoubtedly the best-trained and most scientific physician to reach America in his day – a master of mathematics and physics, he was eagerly welcomed at the fledgling King's College (now Columbia) which had been founded a mere ten years earlier. Clossy was invited by the second president, Myles Cooper, to become Professor of Natural Philosophy, with the result that his second annual course in anatomy was given under the auspices of the College and within her walls, thus making Clossy the first professor of a medical subject in North America. After serving as a medical faculty of one for three years Clossy was joined by five other men in the opening of the medical department at King's (1767). I was fortunate enough to find and acquire Clossy's original manuscript, *The Uses of Anatomy* delivered at the opening ceremonies, 2 November 1767, and this I presented to Columbia, my alma mater, two hundred years later to the exact date and time of day. In this paper Clossy mentions the purchase of a copy of the *De Sedibus et Causis Morborum* of Morgagni, a man whom he worshipped as a demigod.

Clossy continued as Professor of Anatomy until 1776 when the outbreak of the Revolution interrupted his successful teaching career. During the conflict he lost his cherished library, anatomical preparations and manuscripts. Stunned by this reversal of fate and the ruin of his ambitions Clossy was forced to remain in New York while serving as a lowly surgeon's mate in the British army. When he returned to England (1780) he was an ill, thoroughly defeated man. In Dublin he was made an honorary member of the Royal College of Physicians, but when he died a few years later he was already a figure of the past, and relatively disregarded on both sides of the Atlantic. Had history not dealt him such cruel blows his important contributions to pathology and medical education would be much better known today.

The second physician of Irish extraction who made medical history in the United States was John Crawford (1746–1813), the son of a physician, and the older brother of Adrian Crawford, physician at St. Thomas's Hospital and a well-known figure in England for his writings on the subject of 'Animal Heat'. John had a most interesting and exciting career. Having studied medicine at Trinity he did not proceed directly to the M.D. degree (which he later obtained elsewhere), but enlisted in the British naval service, taking two trips to the East Indies before being assigned to a hospital in Barbadoes. Here and later at Demerara he performed many autopsies while studying the relationship of parasites to plants, and slowly began to formulate the theory of contagion by 'animaliculae' which was to occupy his thoughts for the remainder of his days. At the age of fifty (1796) he settled in Baltimore where he soon took a most active role in the medical and civic life of the rapidly growing community. He corresponded frequently – and on terms of equality – with Benjamin Rush, discussing among other matters a project for founding a dispensary in Baltimore. Finally receiving the necessary approval of the city fathers Crawford opened this pioneer institution in 1801. Just one summer earlier Crawford had received from Dr. John Ring of London a sample of Jenner's vaccine, which he used with apparent success at almost the same time that Benjamin Waterhouse was experimenting with the new method in Boston. Although the question of priority cannot be resolved it is quite possible that Crawford may indeed have been the second, if not the first, to perform vaccination against smallpox in the New World. In 1807 he adverts to the fact that 'the discovery of inoculation divested the cause of smallpox of a large portion of its destructive powers, and the innoculation of kine-pox has rendered it nearly harmless'. Crawford must have been a man of unusual vitality and social consciousness: among the institutions he helped to found were the Baltimore Public Library, the Bible Society, the Maryland Society for Promoting Useful Knowledge and the Maryland Penitentiary. Nevertheless, as a very positive person, brooking no opposition to his opinions or theories, he did not always find favour with the medical faculty of the town, then actively engaged with plans to found a medical school, nor indeed does his name appear as one of the fathers of that institution (1807). We now come to the principal area of disagreement between Crawford and the medical establishment, namely his theories about Quarantine and Contagion. As for the first Crawford rightly points to the failure of such measures as quarantine to prevent the spread of epidemic diseases, and to the futility of depending on them alone. But it was his theory of contagion which was considered anathema at the time. Unable to secure publication in any reputable medical journal Crawford went to the extreme of founding a weekly journal for the intelligent layman in 1804, and it was in *The Observer* (as it was later called) that he developed at length the remarkable doctrine for which he is justly famous. He shows his vast erudition by paying respect to his predecessors in the theory of a 'contagium animatum', namely, Kircher, van Swammerdam, Redi and Von Plenciz, noting also the negative opinions of such authorities as Boerhaave, van Swieten and Morgagni. He agrees with Von Plenciz that diseases cannot originate in a common cause, 'in every instance varying in nature and qualities as do the several seeds of vegetables from one another'. Crawford's prophetic vision of insects as vectors of 'animaliculae' so minute as to escape observation by the naked eye did not escape the vigilance of William Osler, who while in Baltimore had become familiar with Crawford's theory, and had been shown the remnants of his library. Osler writes: 'Thayer had copied for me for Sir Ronald Ross, Crawford's remarkable papers on "Quarantine" from the Baltimore "Observer" 1806–1807. Ross deposited the papers in the Library of the School of Tropical Medicine, Liverpool. Crawford suggests the importance of insects as transmitters of disease.'

Crawford's latter years were not free from the contentions and frustrations which seem to have characterized his entire career. In 1809 he recommended – unsuccessfully – that a full-time medical supervisor be appointed to the Board of Health, but this suggestion had to wait twenty years before being implemented; in the same year, however, his theory of contagion did receive an honourable presentation to the medical world when it was published in the *Baltimore Medical and Physical Recorder*. Rankled by his exclusion from the faculty of the medical school Crawford wrote to Rush outlining a plan for giving his own series of lectures on medicine. In 1811 there appeared *An Introduction to a Course of Lectures on the Cause, Seat and Cure of Diseases*, but the project never got off the ground, so to speak, and the Faculty of the medical school proceeded to mollify Crawford by appointing him 'Lecturer on Natural History' (1812). My own interest in Crawford is therefore twofold: he did have some connexion, albeit fragile, with the University of Maryland, my medical alma mater, but of greater importance is the fact that he was a devoted bibliophile, who like Grolier and Mead loved to share his books with others. After his death his daughter advertised: 'Those gentlemen who have been in the habit of borrowing books from the late Doctor Crawford are earnestly solicited to examine their libraries, and if any belonging to him should be found to return them to the subscriber without delay.' Fortunately a goodly portion of Crawford's library was sold after his death to the University of Maryland which now proudly displays about 400 items from this remarkable collection which may justly lay claim to be the oldest medical private library in continuous existence in the United States.

The third and final member of this Irish trio was another individual of abounding energy and magnetism, an unusual combination of idealism and pragmatism. William James MacNeven (1763–1814) was born in Galway, but studied medicine at Prague and in Vienna where a paternal uncle had become physician to Empress Maria Theresa. Following graduation he entered on a very successful practice in Dublin, but after a decade his revolutionary activities drove him first to Switzerland and then to France. A writer and poet of considerable charm he published in 1803 *A Ramble through Switzerland in the Summer and Autumn of 1802*. In 1805 he arrived in New York where he was befriended by the influential Dr. David Hosack, and soon developed a large practice. Appointed first to the chair of Midwifery at the College of Physicians and Surgeons, he was later, at the reorganization of the school (1811) made Professor of Chemistry, a position much more to his liking and competence. MacNeven is credited with founding the first chemical laboratory in New York City, and his studies on the minerals of several counties in New York and New Jersey are of considerable historic importance. He also studied the waters of a spa in Schooley's Mountains, comparing the virtues of this place with those of Cheltenham and Scarborough. His most ambitious work, *Exposition of the Atomic Theory of Chemistry and the Doctrine of Definite Proportions* (New York, 1819) was a spirited defence of Dalton's theory, which at the same time gave credit to such precursors as Higgins and Thomson. MacNeven also edited, with numerous emendations, the then influential textbook on chemistry of W. T. Brandes, and acted as co-editor for a brief period of the *New York Medical and Philosophical Journal and Review*. The honours which MacNeven received were numerous: he was elected to the American Philosophical Society and the Literary and Philosophical Society of New York; his monograph on the Daltonian theory was honoured by being reprinted in the *Annales de Chimie*. A brilliant teacher and lecturer who accompanied his talks by demonstrations and historical references, he may have been among the first in America to demonstrate the beneficial effects of the Galvanic current. As early as 1809 he was honoured by election as the first president of the Medical-Surgical Society of New York.

MacNeven held very high ideals about medical education, and poured his wrath on the 'village schools where they pretend to teach anatomy and surgery without subjects and the practice of physic without a patient', such as were then cropping up in New York State. In 1825 he delivered at the New York Athenaeum a series of lectures (later published) on *The Application of Chemistry to Agriculture*. In these he urged American young men of means to 'return to the farm', ending with a prophetic verse which bears repeating:

So with superior boon may your rich soil
Exuberant, nature's blessings pour
O'er every land, the naked nations clothe,
And be th' exhaustless granary of the world.

After having taught for twenty years MacNeven and a few colleagues withdrew from the College of Physicians and Surgeons, disturbed by the lowered standards for admission and the poor quality of the candidates for the degree. In 1827 the dissidents founded a new school, Rutgers Medical College, affiliated for the purpose of granting degrees with Rutgers College of New Brunswick, New Jersey. Unfortunately, authorization for this arrangement could not be obtained from the New York Board of Regents, and the entire venture continued for only a few years. Although this ended MacNeven's career as a teacher, he continued to interest himself in his practice and in the welfare of his immigrant compatriots, for whom his generosity was unbounded. Like Crawford, MacNeven was a man of great culture and wide reading, and the possessor of a fine library. A classical scholar, he knew German, French and Italian as well as Gaelic. More than twenty years after his death MacNeven, himself a Catholic, was accorded the exceptional honour of having a monument erected to his memory in the graveyard of Protestant St. Paul's Chapel, a firm indication of the gratitude felt for his efforts by many citizens of New York.

Finally, as lecturer in the History of Medicine at the present Rutgers Medical School, the College of Medicine and Dentistry of New Jersey, I am happy to claim some affinity to this humanist and physician who did so much for medicine and the sciences in his adopted country.

America has good reason to be proud of the remarkable contributions made by this unusually productive group of Irish-born medical men.

J. A. Shilinis
Moscow (U.S.S.R.)

On the history of the Russian-British connexions in general pathology

The establishment of the Russian–British medical connexions dates from the times of Peter the Great, Reformer of Russia. Robert Erskine was one of the first to promote these connexions. Born in Scotland, he took his medical degree at Oxford University, and became a Fellow of the Royal Society. R. Erskine came to Russia in 1706 and at first became Prince A. D. Menschikov's physician. From 1713 onwards he was physician-in-ordinary to Peter the Great who, on 30 April 1706 by a special charter signed in the town of Gdansk, gave R. Erskine the title of archiatre (senior physician) and President of the Medical Faculty of Russia. R. Erskine accompanied the Tzar in his journeys through Germany, Holland and France. Peter the Great appreciated Erskine's erudition so that he appointed him the chief of the Cabinet of Curiosities and the Library. Erskine died in the town of Olonez in December 1718 and was buried in Alexander Nevski Abbey in St. Petersburg.

Russian–British medical connexions continued in the second half of the eighteenth century. From 1776 to 1782 the Russian physician E. F. Zveraka was perfecting his knowledge in different European universities and on 24 May 1779 he obtained his medical degree at Edinburgh University. On returning to Russia Zveraka practised medicine, and in 1794 at the request of the famous general A. V. Suvorov was appointed professor of the Medico-Surgical School in the town of Elisavetgrad where he taught chemistry, botany, pathology and therapy.

From 1780 the Russian doctor D. J. Pisechkov studied for two years in London and one year at Edinburgh University. On 2 August 1784 he took his medical degree in Aberdeen for the thesis 'De novo methodo psoram sanandi'. In addition to medicine, Pisechkov studied agronomy abroad and received the title of professor of agriculture. In 1800 he translated into Russian and published with many corrections and additions *The Medical Pocket Book containing a short but plain account of the symptoms, causes and methods of cure of diseases incident to the human body* (London, 1781). The author of this book, Sir John Elliott (1736–86), born in Edinburgh, was formerly physician to the Prince of Wales.

Still more popular in Russia than Elliott's *Pocket Book* was *Domestic Medicine, or the Family Physician* by the Scottish physician William Buchan (1729–1805). The Russian Empress Catherine II rewarded W. Buchan for his book with a gold medal and a commendatory letter. The book was first published in England in 1769 and then passed through nineteen editions and was translated into all the main European languages. The Russian translation was made from the French edition with comments and explanations and published in five volumes twice – in 1790–92 and in 1809–13 under the title *Full and Universal Domestic Book on Medicine, written to preserve health by reliable means and also to cure diseases of all kinds. . . . This is a creation of W. Buchan who is the famest English physician of our century.* The translator of the book consulted outstanding Russian doctors, such as S. G. Zybelin, Skiadan, and Keresturi, and as a result made corrections and additions to adjust the handbook of medical advice to the Russian climate and mode of life.

This handbook was used not only by Russian doctors but also by educated people of Russia of that time. This is evident from *Family Chronicle* by S. T. Aksakov (1791–1859), an outstanding Russian author whose mother used Buchan's handbook to treat first her father and then her little son. Aksakov wrote that the results of the treatment were successful: 'My recovery was considered by the doctors themselves to be a miracle. . . . Buchan received the title of my saviour and my mother taught me in my childhood to pray for Buchan at my morning and evening prayers' (S. T. Aksakov, *Sobranie sochineniy* [collected works], Moscow, 1966, vol. 1, p. 271).

Except that handbook one more of Buchan's works was published in Russian. It was *On the Offices and Duties of a Mother* (1800), translated from French by Ivan Keppen and entitled in Russian *True keeper of the health of mothers and children* (Moscow, 1826). To this translation was added a paper *On the utility and method of smallpox inoculation* by E. O. Muchin, professor of Moscow University.

Thus Russian physicians of the early nineteenth century paid great attention to Buchan's works which summarized his vast medical experience. Meanwhile they knew very well and critically appreciated doctrines of Scottish physicians W. Cullen and John Brown on general pathology. Professor F. G. Politkovski of the Moscow University pointed out that a new period in the development of medicine, that is a transition from humoral to solid pathology, was connected with W. Cullen's name. F. G. Politkovski wrote about Cullen: 'He had argued and overthrown deeprooted prejudices of many physicians and thus had surpassed the renowned Boerhaave himself.'

In 1818 *Handbook on the knowledge of nosology and therapeutics* was published in Russian in St. Petersburg. The book was compiled from Cullen by the latter's disciple Josef Townsend and translated into Russian by A. Kreisty.

Professor J. V. Keir was Cullen's disciple in Edinburgh. Afterwards he was invited to Russia by J. V. Willie, Scottish by birth, who was the President of the Medico-Surgical Academy and Physician-in-ordinary to Alexander I. Keir lectured at the Moscow Medico-Surgical Academy on general pathology and therapeutics basing his teaching on the doctrines of W. Cullen and the German physician F. Hoffmann. Many of the Russian scientists of the late eighteenth and early nineteenth centuries creatively developed the principles of solid pathology, as Cullen did, and paid particular attention to the role of the nervous system. But their ideas on the 'nervous principle' in pathology were materialistic and not so one-sided and contradictory as those of Hoffmann and Cullen.

Especially critical was the attitude of Russian scientists to John Brown's system, based on the doctrines of H. Boerhaave, W. Cullen, and mostly on A. Haller's works on irritability and sensibility. J. Brown's medical ideas became known in Russia from a translation of Thomas Beddoes's book *The Elements of Medicine of John Brown* (London, 1795) first translated into German by Ch. Hirtanner (Copenhagen, 1796) and then into Russian by A. Archangelski under the title *Johann Brown's System of Medicine* (St. Petersburg, 1806–7). A course on general pathology was held only at the St. Petersburg Medico-Surgical Academy for a short period by professors I. A. Smelovski and K. F. Uden. Both of them, however, made additions to 'brownism' from the point of view of their own experience. But most Russian scientists did not share the universal passion for Brown's system. They considered it to be contradictory to experience and it omitted disease specificity, individualization of an ill person and the material principles of pathological phenomena.

Searching for the material substratum of disease was the reason for the vivid interest of Russian physicians in the first English book on morbid anatomy entitled *The Morbid Anatomy of some of the most important parts of the human body*, which was published in 1795 by John and William Hunter's disciple Matthew Baillie (1761–1823), a Scot, and Fellow of the Royal Society. This valuable book was translated into Russian by Ivan Kostomarov, professor of the Moscow Medico-Surgical Academy, who dedicated his work to J. V. Willie and published it under the title: '*The morbid anatomy of the most important parts of the human body chiefly situated in the four main cavities.* A composition by Mat. Baillie, Medicinae Doctor, Fellow of the Royal Societies of London and Edinburgh, Physician extraordinary to the King of England, Fellow of the Royal College of Physicians; translated from the 5th corrected edition with explanatory and complementary comments. To this has subjoined Ivan Kostomarov his own Treatise on the relation of morbid anatomy to other medical sciences, as well as on methods with the help of which it may be cognizable and perfected, with an addition of a short preliminary account of its history.' The translator had approached his task creatively, taking into consideration the drawbacks of the original text as well as the achievements of Russian science in physiology and functional pathology. For example, speaking on the relation of morbid anatomy to physiology and clinical evidence I. Kostomarov put a question: 'Is it enough when studying a disease to limit oneself with the changes in material parts without penetrating into the mechanism of their origin and development, and without trying to comprehend changes in vital functions which accompany them?' The answer to this question was: 'It seems the questions to be solved by physiology, which in this connexion may be rather called pathological, must necessarily occupy our mind in studying organic diseases, otherwise our science would be a dead one if it will limit itself but with a dead body' (pp. xxiii–xxiv).

I. Kostomarov formulated the tasks of morbid anatomy as follows: (1) to study the pathological changes of the structure of different organs in their regular connexion; (2) to study the mechanism of the origin and development of pathological changes from the point of view of physiology and patho-physiology; (3) to determine the connexion between organic and functional manifestation of disease, to draw clinico-anatomical parallels.

Thus I. Kostomarov made an essential contribution to M. Baillie's work by underlining the necessity of combination of patho-anatomical and functional study of disease. Vital power and fruitfulness of these ideas were proved by the whole subsequent development of medicine in Russia. Experimental research methods, achievements of physiology and clinical medicine favoured synthetic understanding of the general laws of the origin and pathogenesis of human disease. In the middle of the nineteenth century special chairs of general pathology parallel with the chairs of pathological anatomy were already established in Russian universities, and there appeared original scientific schools of general pathologists headed by such prominent scientists as V. V. Pashutin, A. B. Foght, I. I. Mechnikov, V. V. Podvysotski and others.

One of the outstanding representatives of Russian general pathology was Vladimir Georgiyevich Korenchevsky (1880–1959), founder of the International Gerontologic Association, named by some British and American authors (E. V. Cowdry and others) 'The Father of Gerontology' not only in Great Britain but in the whole world. It is of interest to find out the origins of Korenchevsky's creative work, which E. Cowdry characterized as 'a gift from Russia to humanity of far-reaching consequences'. V. G. Korenchevsky received his medical degree at the St. Petersburg Military Medical Academy where he attended the lectures of the great physiologist I. P. Pavlov and other representatives of scientific schools of I. M. Sechenov and S. P. Botkin. When still a student he occupied himself with experimental pharmacology and at the laboratory of Sechenov's disciple professor N. P. Kravkov he prepared a paper: *Comparative pharmacological study on the effect of poisons on unicellular organisms*. The idea of essential difference between the process of premature pathological ageing and that of a normal physiological one came to him in 1906 when he visited an asylum for the aged in Moscow. V. G. Korenchevsky's aim was to study these processes in order to discover the potential ability of an aged person and to contribute to the prevention of premature ageing. In 1907 Korenchevsky started his research work on digestive pathology at the Moscow university under the guidance of professor A. B. Foght, the founder of the Moscow scientific school of pathologists marked by clinico-experimental trends. The leading problem of the research work was the so-called 'reserve powers' and compensatory adaptation of an organism in pathologic conditions. The investigation included the pathology of cardio-vascular, endocrine, lymphatic and urinary systems.

While preparing his dissertation V. G. Korenchevsky used his scientific mission in Paris to visit I. I. Mechnikov's laboratory at the Pasteur Institute, where he carried out a number of experiments. He maintained his doctoral thesis: 'On the doctrine of gastrointestinal autointoxication' – at the Moscow University on 13 May 1909.

During March–August 1910 Korenchevsky worked under Pavlov's guidance at the physiological department of the St. Petersburg Institute of experimental medicine and also at the chair of physiology of the Military Medical Academy, where he fulfilled three experimental studies. From 1912 to 1919 V. G. Korenchevsky headed the chair of general and experimental pathology at the Petersburg Military Medical Academy which was famous for studies on the interchange of gases and the problem of hunger. Korenchevsky himself and his co-workers studied mainly the effect of sex and thyroid hormones on the somatic organs and their function.

Research work, carried out at the chair, dealt with gas and nitrogen interchange in castrated animals; connexion between thyroid and sex glands taking into account their effect on metabolism; the effect of sex gland emulsion – testicles and ovaries – on metabolism of normal and castrated animals as well as animals with simultaneous thyroidectomy and castration; gas and nitrogen interchange in animals with simultaneous castration and thyroidectomy. The result of the research work had proved that the achievements of endocrinology might be used to solve the problem of ageing.

The analysis of Korenchevsky's works carried out during the span of his life shows that he developed the ideas of the three Russian scientific schools of pathologists, those of I. I. Mechnikov, A. B. Foght, and V. V. Pashutin as well as the great Pavlov's physiological school. By all his subsequent work Korenchevsky propagated these ideas and favoured their use for the research work on the gerontologic problems all over the world.

Thus we see that Russian–British connexions in medicine dating from long ago were of a creative character and contributed greatly to the progress of medical science.

J. C. Sokolov
Moscow (U.S.S.R.)

On connexions between medieval Russian medicine and some countries of the east which were members of the British Commonwealth

One of the most interesting but not well enough elaborated aspects of the history of medicine is the study of the interaction and reciprocal enrichment of folk medicine of different countries, and the penetration into the true historical essence of certain ideas and basic theories, which are international in their character. This trend, once begun by P. M. Factorovitch, is being continued by his followers.

The connexions between medieval Russia, India and Pakistan were accomplished in several ways. In ancient times extensive trade and culture relations existed between Russia and the countries of Middle Asia and the East. One can draw such a conclusion on the basis of the records of the Arab author Ibn-Hardadbekh, who wrote that the Russians shipped out the goods by the Sea of Jurdasan (southwestern part of the Caspian Sea) and brought them in by camels to many large towns of the East. According to the works of Byzantine historians, several Russian merchants who lived in Constantinople were among the suite of grand duchess Olga during her christening in 957.

Of note is a well-known journey of Aphanasey Nikitin, a merchant from Tver who lived in India for a certain period of time. It took him six years (1466–72) to make his journey. A little later in September 1532 an Indian merchant, Hodja Husein, arrived in Moscow (V. Bartold, 1925).

Ancient manuscripts and books published both in Russia and on the territory of the Indostan subcontinent were another way of interconnexions. In the seventeenth century a library containing many books in the original tongues as well as translated ones existed under the jurisdiction of the Chemist's Office. In 1678 the post of a translator of foreign books from which 'the Russian people could become excellent physicians and chemists' was established at the above-mentioned Office.

Up to the nineteenth century there existed the opinion that the oldest medical manuscript in Russian was translated from Polish in 1588. This opinion has been expressed in the well-known works by Willhelm Richter in which he writes the following: 'The oldest medical manuscript known to me in Russian is translated from Polish. It is one of the books on folk medicine which were called Lechebnicks [a manual for treatment]. This book is of a small sheet in size, it is handwritten and is divided into two columns.' In this book one can find direct references to initial connexions between Russian and British medicine, for instance, at the beginning of the seventeenth century a wide assortment of drugs which were employed by Russian physicians was supplied by the drugs imported by the British chemist James French.

We cannot consider that the opinion of W. Richter regarding the above-mentioned book is correct, because one can name more than ten other manuals for treatment and other handwritten books which had been issued long before the one mentioned by W. Richter. These books are: *The Book of Enoch's Sacred Mysteries*, *Svyatoslav's Collections* (1073), *Explanatory Paleya* and others. When we study the list of drugs imported by James French we can draw the conclusion that many of them had been employed in medical practice since old times both in Russia and Middle Asia. Among them were such drugs as pomegranate, wormseed, sulphur, wormwood, filices roots, pepper and others. ('Ancient manuscripts', 'Galinovo na Ipokrata', 'Hartus Amoenus' and others.) We consider that the probable contacts between Russian medicine and that of the countries of the East are reflected in the works published long before.

And there are good grounds to prove this. As archaeological studies have shown, India and Pakistan are countries of highly developed ancient culture, with their particular flora and fauna. In one of the most ancient books about animals entitled *Physiologist*, which appeared in our country before the thirteenth century, many of the animals inhabiting the Indostan Peninsula are described.

As early as that time excellent methods of teaching medicine, high standards in the development of chemistry and materia medica, and perfect surgical techniques (plastic operations in particular), existed in India. We must also remember that it was in Jundishapoor where the well-known Medical Academy, which was the centre of the development of medicine in the East, was situated.

The coincidence of a number of points of view allows us to conclude that the relations between our countries might have existed at an even earlier period. A peculiar resemblance can be observed in the foodstuff classifications which are given in ancient Indian literature and those employed by tabibs in Middle Asia. All of them considered that curative substances of foodstuffs possessed such properties which could be classified as hot and cold, dry and moist. In the book *Hartus Amoenus* published in 1672 similar differentiation of these substances is given.

A wide assortment of curative substances which were used both on the territory of the Indostan subcontinent and in Russia is well known. The treatment based on resemblance had been employed there since time immemorial.

Many pieces of advice on how to preserve health and extend the life-span, which can be found in ancient Russian manuscripts are similar to those which were recommended by such Indian physicians as Katka, Ibn-Bekhtishu and others. The manual for treatment (Lechebnick), which was kept under the number 481 in the Library of the Moscow Patriarch, is particularly remarkable for the study of the contacts between medieval Russian medicine and that of the countries of the East. The third chapter of this book contains descriptions of the origin of the human body which greatly resemble those given both by the ancient Indian authors and Hippocrates (M. Lakhtin, *Ancient Medical Manuscripts*).

Almost identical considerations about the influence of climate on health can be found both in Sushruta's works and our doctors. In the ancient medical manuscripts 'Explanatory Paleya' and 'Galinovo na Ipokrata' which appeared in Russian in the fifteenth to sixteenth centuries one can find considerations about the particular significance of climate and seasons for men. The issue of Tolkovaya Paleya known to us dates as far as 1406, but we can assume that it was known in medieval Russia even earlier (V. Uspenskey, *Tolkovaya Paleya*, Kazan, 1876). It is possible to postulate that Hippocrates' works, who as is well known paid particular tribute to climate, were the source of such considerations. For he said: 'One who desires to study medical art properly must do the following: first of all he must take into consideration seasons'.

The descriptions of a number of surgical operations (for instance – lithotomy) given by Sushruta and Ibn-Sina are almost identical. Both of them were advocates of linked theories of the etiology of diseases (humoralpathologic); they shared the opinion about the role and the wide choice of curative substances, metals in particular, which were used by them in treatment.

Investigating the relationship between the States of the Indostan peninsula and the peoples that once inhabited Middle Asia our precursor Factorovitch wrote that in a number of towns (Samarkand, Bukhara, etc.) as well as in the Buddhist monasteries in India there were 'bekhars' in which the study of natural sciences was flourishing.

In Middle Asia, as well as in Ancient India colloid gold was employed for the treatment of cardio-vascular diseases during many centuries. The data about this 'drinking gold' appeared in Western Europe a little later. A striking resemblance in the methods of its preparation cannot but draw our attention: thin golden leaves were heated, then sunk into milk, oil or some other substance five to seven times to obtain a colloid solution.

The study of these works manifest the antiquity and original character of Russian medicine and natural sciences, their broad links with the countries of the East, which were able to borrow much from Russia. It is known that the town of Kiev, Russia, had a high standard of sanitary town planning and organization of public services. The case history of Svyatoslav Jaroslavich who underwent an operation for the incision of gland tumours in 1076 illustrates the high standard of medical development in Russia. The question arises why during the following years the scientists did not appreciate the achievements of that period and did not know about the above-mentioned works. The fact that the owners of such works were being persecuted by the ruling circles during a prolonged period of time is of great significance in this matter.

In 1676 during the reign of Tsar Fedor Alekseevitch, boyar Artamon Matveev was brought to trial. He was charged with custody of a certain notebook, in which the ways 'to treat different diseases are described and the prescriptions are given not in letters but in figures'. For this notebook Matveev was exiled to a monastery and deprived of all his property. Shortly after (1677) another case was investigated. Several serfs who were charged with copying prescriptions from Matveev's notebook were brought to trial. The decision of this trial reads as follows: 'Markusha Tarakanov for exorcism letters which he copied from lechebnick [manual for treatment] and then gave this lechebnick to a certain man, Mishka Stashevsky by name, for exorcism for trembling palsy must be whipped and exiled to Astrakhan and the lechebnick with the exorcism letters and the exorcism for trembling palsy themselves must be flogged.'

Many other facts illustrating the cruel persecution for copying, reading and custody of medical manuscripts in the seventeenth century can be cited. These facts vividly demonstrate a keen interest of the common people in the study of the human body, diseases and their treatment. They also manifest the fact that long before the translation from Polish (1587) of the lechebnick mentioned by Richter, the Russians already possessed a large storage of medical knowledge, derived not only from the lechebnicks which had appeared before but from the long-standing experience of fishermen, hunters, agrarians, tradesmen, soldiers and sorcerers.

The above facts show that medieval Russian medicine employed for its development many achievements and experience of physicians who lived in the countries of the East, which were included in the British Commonwealth. These achievements and those based on its own research have enabled our medicine to enrich world science with many discoveries.

I. V. Vengrova
Moscow (U.S.S.R.)

Some parallels in the history of public health in Russia and England

The problem of parallels in the history of the Russian and English public health is of great interest because the development of public health is closely connected with the mode of production of material values, with the capitalist mode of production in particular, and with the development of the working class movement. The development of capitalism in England and in Russia was one of the main premises of the origin of social hygiene. In both countries the working class movement had the determinative effect on the formation of progressive views of medical men and on their attitude to the professional and social medical activity.

Study of the history of public health proves how right was F. Engels when he stated that the same social system in different countries gave birth to similar social phenomena and this was clearly manifested in the effect of the capitalist system on the condition of the proletariat.

England was the first capitalist country. When Russia entered the path of capitalism in 1861 England had already become the classic capitalist country with all its contradictory consequences, that is concentration of large masses of population in industrial centres, endless prolongation of the working day, especially for women and children, destruction of family traditions, lack of houses, food and clothing and other social evils. The contradictions of the capitalist system were the main reason of the first mass revolutionary movement of the working class – chartism. Under the conditions of this movement and of the rise of social enthusiasm connected with it progressive-minded English doctors put forward the questions of preserving the health of the working population which had been thrown into quite new circumstances of life. These doctors had carried out numerous studies of labour and life conditions of different population groups such as factory and agricultural workers, working women and children, etc. The most successful in this connexion was the activity of a medical team headed by John Simon, an outstanding English medical officer of health.

Rapid development of capitalism in Russia after the abolition of serfdom, increase of industry and population of manufacturing towns had also drawn the attention of progressive-minded Russians including many physicians. The revolutionary situation in Russia in 1859–61, diffusing the ideas of Russian revolutionary democrats (A. I. Hertsen, V. G. Belinsky, N. A. Dobrolubov), and the atmosphere of social enthusiasm deeply influenced the development of a democratic trend in Russian medicine which was expressed by progressive Russian medical periodicals. This trend manifested itself in the aspirations of physicians to improve the welfare of the people. Medical care for the population was considered by progressive-minded Russian doctors to be one of the first tasks. These questions were raised in connexion with the hard living conditions of the working population. Physicians considered these conditions to be the cause of many social and sanitary evils in Russia.

Beginning with simple descriptions of labour conditions, most advanced periodicals came to demand the improvement of social, economic and sanitary conditions of the people. They suggested measures to prevent the spread of epidemic diseases, underlined the necessity to improve sanitary conditions of labour by law, and agitated for mass health education. The first of such periodicals was *Archives for Forensic Medicine and Social Hygiene*, especially in the period of 1865–70, when it was edited by S. P. Lovtsov (1823–76), a noble Russian patriot, who was a highly educated, social-minded, physician and contributed greatly to the development of social hygiene in Russia in the 1860s and 1870s.

The aim of the *Archives* was to inform Russian physicians about the best Russian and foreign works on forensic medicine and social hygiene, and encourage discussions on these questions. To this end besides original papers the magazine published reviews of works by native and foreign authors. Since 1868 in each copy of the magazine there was a special section 'On the sanitary condition of workers'. A large part of this material was foreign, English in particular. Very often it dealt with the results of public health work by English physicians in the 1830s to 1860s. Sometimes these data were published with the aim of using comparison with England to draw attention to social evils existing in Russia. This was one of the secret ways of putting forward urgent public health problems, because under the tsar it was not always possible to speak openly about serious public health evils and especially to analyse their social causes.

For instance, a big review of Simon's report, *Ninth Report of the Medical Officer of the Privy Council* (London, 1867), was published in the *Archives* in 1868. P. A. Khlebnikov, professor of Petersburg medico-surgical academy, the author of this review, writes: 'This book is a symposium of reports on the condition of people's health which are annually submitted to the English parliament by the Privy Council with the aim to improve people's health . . . the meaning of this book is strengthened by the fact that for the first time it deals with the results of the sanitary measures which has been designed recently by medical science and carried out on a wide scale to improve sanitary conditions of towns of Great Britain'. Professor Khlebnikov underlined that figures cited in this report proved clearly the benefit of these measures.

Control of cholera epidemics in Russia was one of the urgent public health problems at that time. It was widely discussed by medical men in the pages of medical periodicals. Russian scientists took an active part in the controversy about the mode of diffusion of cholera. This question drew great attention by scientists of different countries because the control of cholera was closely connected with problems of public health. Russian and English physicians as well had seen that cholera epidemics, when starting, spread mostly among the working population.

An interesting example of scientific collaboration of Russian and English physicians on the problem of cholera control is a booklet published by J. Simon entitled *Papers submitted by the Medical Officer relating to the Recent Diffusion of Cholera in Europe* (London, 1874). The booklet contains: Introductory Letter to the

President of the Local Government Board by J. Simon; Observations by Dr. Pelikan, Director of the Medical Department of the Russian Government, on Mr. J. Netten Radcliffe's Report (May 1872) on the Recent Diffusion of Cholera in Europe; Dr. Pelikan's Memorandum (1866) on the Measures for the Prevention of the Introduction of Cholera and Plague from Persia into Russia; Dr. Arkhangelsky's Account (1871) of the Great Cholera Epidemic of 1852–55 in Russia; Memorandum by Mr. J. Netten Radcliffe on Dr. Pelikan's Observations; Dr. Tholozan's Note on Cholera in North-East Persia, in the years 1867–69.

In spite of some differences of views on the mode of cholera diffusion Russian and English scientists were unanimous in the socio-hygienic appreciation of the meaning of cholera control. In the above-mentioned introductory letter J. Simon writes: 'I observe with particular pleasure and hopefulness the emphasis with which Dr. Pelikan applies this principle . . . with reference to the vast analogous interest which Continental Europe has in its own hygienic progress, I may observe that the facts which Dr. Pelikan brings to our knowledge seem to me singularly suggestive. Whether it has been by re-infection or by continuance of infection that Eastern Europe has been able to provide during so many years an habitual lodgment and breeding-place for Cholera, equally I would concur with our eminent Russian fellow-worker in urging that thorough investigation should be made of the local circumstances under which that sad susceptibility to the infection exists.'

Academician N. F. Gamaleya, a distinguished Russian scientist, microbiologist and epidemiologist, appreciates in his turn the achievements of Simon's team of physicians in the control of cholera. In his paper *Cholera and its Control* (1905) he wrote: 'At that time in England there appeared a pleiad of talented hygienists with John Simon as the head and they had succeeded not only in practical solution of the most important questions of the cholera epidemiology but had also laid the foundation of the modern public health'.

In the early 1870s Russian doctors were considering on the problem of the establishment of a system of sanitary reform in Russia. In this connexion a number of papers on the sanitary system in England were published in medical periodicals. Analysing the achievements of the Englishmen, Russian doctors made sharp social comments. For instance, I. E. Andreevsky, a progressive public man, professor of Petersburg University had quite correctly pointed out one of the main reasons for passing the Public Health Act in 1848. He wrote: 'Passing of this famous Public Health Act by the way was provoked by the general movement of workers in 1848. By passing this act the English government begins a new policy of solving the labour question, that is to meet by governmental action such workers' needs of which the latter are already fully aware and if these needs would not be met it might involve a social upheaval dangerous for the state' (*Zdorovje*, 1874, **4**, 74).

F. F. Erisman (1842–1915), a prominent Russian hygienist gave also an original explanation of the reasons for success of the public health system in England. In his paper 'System of public hygiene in Russia' (1876) he states that these achievements were promoted not so much by the proper work of the sanitary board but rather by socio-medical work of advanced social men and by publication of the reports submitted to Parliament.

A lot of data about English public health are included in Erisman's work 'Occupational hygiene or hygiene of mental and manual labour' (1877). In this work

Erisman repeatedly cites *The Capital* by K. Marx. Analysis of these parts of Erisman's book shows that he chooses those pages of *The Capital* where Marx discusses socio-hygienic questions of the working class condition and cites in his turn a lot of material from the reports of Simon's team. Data from Simon's reports, cited by Marx, were used by Erisman when discussing such problems as: the effect of the economic condition of the working class on its sanitary conditions and the effect of the industrial development on the death rate and on the growth of the population; children's death rate in industrial districts; working hours; participation of women and children in industry; living conditions of workers of different categories; food and clothes. It is seen from this enumeration how similar were the problems in which English and Russian doctors were interested.

F. F. Erisman himself points to this similarity. He writes in the above-mentioned book: 'The picture drawn by Dr. Ambleton (his evidences are included in a report of J. Hunter, one of the doctors of Simon's team) is very similar to that which we ourselves have seen in Prince Viazemsky's and Lord Pirogov's lodging houses and others in St. Petersburg and to the state of common lodging houses in Moscow and other Russian towns about what we learn from the press'.

Speaking about the parallels in the history of public health in Russia and England we must point out, however, that progressive-minded Russian doctors manifested a more profound social approach to the problems of public health. They underlined the direct connexion of these problems with the capitalist relations of production, with working-class movement. The most clear evidence of this we find in a paper 'On the condition of workers in Western Europe from a socio-hygienic point of view' published in the above-mentioned *Archives for Forensic Medicine and Social Hygiene* in 1870. It is stated in this paper that Marx's doctrine gives a singularly true approach to the discussion of socio-hygienic problems. The authors of the paper write: 'In order to realise how those ugly conditions which we are to encounter could have come to life it is quite enough for us to be aware of the essence of the relation between capital and labour . . . the readers will see that the facts we shall cite are inevitable logic consequences of the very essence of this relation between capital and labour, and that is why these facts are not exceptional but general phenomena characteristic of the condition of the working class as a whole, and not in a certain area or country but in any place where the relation between capital and labour is in existence, that is in all the civilized countries'.

Thus, the comparison of public health undertakings of Russian and English doctors allows us to speak about the similarity of their activity. Russian as well as English doctors put forward wide problems of the improvement of the conditions of working people and to this end they thoroughly studied the working-class conditions, organized epidemic control, designed new forms of public health systems, demanded the passing of new public health acts and so on. By this activity social-minded doctors in Russia and England were putting pressure upon governmental authorities, and brought public opinion to the necessity of care for the health of people. Objectively in their reports and works they gave the scientific ground to the demands of the working class.

It was hard labour, often without reward, persistence, initiative, self-sacrifice, devotion, and the struggle against the ruling classes that characterized the public health activity of Russian and English doctors.

V. Bazala
Zagreb (Yugoslavia)

Bemerkungen zu einigen englischen Reiseberichten über Kroatien

Die besten Verbindungen zwischen den verschiedenen Ländern werden hergestellt durch die Reisenden, die heimgekehrt ihre Reiseeindrücke und Erlebnisse aufschreiben und veröffentlichen.

Im Jahre 1511 erschien in London *This is the begynnynge and contynuance of the Pylgrymage of Sir Richard Guylforde*, wo sich eine Beschreibung von Dubrovnik (Ragusa) befindet. Die Stadt wird hier Arragonse genannt.

Der englische Geograph Richard Hakluyt (1553–1616) hat im Jahre 1589 die wichtigsten englischen Reisen, Schiffahrten und Entdeckungen von der frühesten Zeit bis zur Zeit der Königin Elisabeth I zusammengestellt (*The principal navigations, voyages, and discoveries of the English nation*, 1589; 2. Auflage 1589–1600).

Im Reisebericht Nr. 20 erwähnt er die Reise Roberts Ketenensis nach Dalmatien usw. (*The voyage of Robert Ketenensis . . . to Dalmatia, Greece and Asia*, Anno 1143.) Auf der Reise begleitete ihn Hermanus Dalmata, eine der größten Persönlichkeiten aus dem Gelehrtenkreis des 12. Jahrhunderts, Übersetzer und Abschreiber arabischer Werke in Latein, Angehöriger der philosophischen Schule in Chartres, der in Spanien (hauptsächlich in Toledo) und in Frankreich (hauptsächlich in Toulouse) tätig war. Man kann ihn für den ersten Gelehrten aus den kroatischen Ländern ansehen, der seine Rolle in der großen Welt spielte. Mit Petrus Kluniacense (nicht mit Robert de Retine, wie man öfters aber fälschlicherweise angibt) übersetzte er den Kur'an ins Latein, und selbst übersetzte er mehrere arabische Werke. Seine Übersetzung des Planisphaerium von Claudius Ptolomaeus war von größter Bedeutung für die westliche Welt und ihre Wissenschaft, denn die europäischen Gelehrten haben sich durch diese Übersetzung mit dem damaligen Hauptwerk der Astronomie bekannt gemacht. In seinem philosophischen Werk De essentiis befasst sich Hermanus mit den fünf physikalischen Begriffen (causa, motus, spatium, tempus und habitudo). Robert Ketenensis hat auf seiner Reise wohl keinen besseren Begleiter haben können.

Im Reisebericht Nr. 24 wurde *The famous voyage of Richard the first, King of England into Asia, for the recouering of Jerusalem. . . . Anno* 1190 beschrieben. Darin steht unter anderem, daß der englische König Richard I. Löwenherz von einem Sturm an die Küste von Histria (Istrien) geworfen wurde, was dennoch nicht der Wahrheit entspricht. Der König rettete sich in den gut gesicherten Hafen von Ragusa (Dubrovnik). Die Stadt hatte ihn herzlich empfangen und er schenkte ihr 100.000 Dukaten für den Bau der Kathedrale als Lösung eines Gelübdes für die glückliche Rettung aus dem Sturm.

Im Reisebericht Nr. 52 wird *The voyage of the John Lock to Jerusalem, Anno* 1553. und im Reisebricht Nr. 56 *The voyage of M. Henry Austel by Venice to Ragusa and thence over-land to Constantinople . . . Anno 1586* beschrieben. Der letztgenannte Reisebericht ist auch gesondert als Buch erschienen. Lock reiste entlang der kroatischen Adriaküste mit dem Schiff bis Dubrovnik und von hier bis Constantinople auf dem Karawanenweg durch die Mitte der Balkanhalbinsel.

Das Werk von Hakluyt hat Samuel Purchas fortgesetzt und seine Wallfahrt im Jahre 1613 beschrieben unter dem Titel *Hacluytus Posthumus, or Purchas his Pilgrims* (1613, 2. Aufl. 1619, 3. Aufl. 1625).

George Sandys' Reisebericht aus dem Jahre 1610 erschien in London im Jahre 1615 unter dem Titel *A Relation of a Journey begun A. Dom. 1610*, und Fynes Morysons *Itinerary* wurde im London im Jahre 1617 gedruckt.

William Lithgow gab einen ausführlichen Bericht über seine 19-jährige seltsame Reise und mühsame Irrfahrt in seinem Reisebericht *Total discourse of the Rare Adventures and Painefull Peregrinations of long nineteene yeares Travayles from Scotland to the most famous Kingdomes in Europa, Asia and Africa* (London, 1632).

Henry Blount gab im Jahre 1634 seinen Reisebericht *A Voyage into the Levant* heraus, der später noch mehrmals gedruckt wurde.

Alle diese Reiseberichte beschreiben ausführlich auch die kroatische Adriaküste und teilweise auch ihr Hinterland.

Der englische Diplomat Paul Rycaut (1628–1700) hält sich 6 Jahre in der Türkei und schrieb das bekannte Werk *The present state of the Ottoman Empire. Containing the maxims of the turkish politic, the most material points of the Mahometan religion, their sects and heresies, etc.* (London, 1668, 3. Aufl. 1670, 5. Aufl. 1682). Von diesen Werk bestehen auch eine französische Übersetzung von M. Briot aus dem Jahre 1672, eine deutsche Übersetzung aus dem Jahre 1671 und 1699, und eine russische aus dem Jahre 1741. Obzwar Rycaut selbst nicht Bosnien durchreiste, war er sehr gut über die Verhältniße in Bosnien benachrichtigt und zwar von den Besuchern, die ihm zuverlässige Berichte gebracht haben. Ganz besonders interessant sind seine Bemerkungen über Bogumilen, bosnische Patarenen.

Der englische Arzt Edward Browne (1642–1708) beschreibt in seinem Werk *A brief account of some travels in Hungaria . . .* (London, 1673, 2. Aufl. 1685) seine Beobachtungen auf der Reise über Süd-Europa und berichtet auch über die gesundheitlichen Verhältnisse in Kroatien. Über diesen Reisebericht schrieb ausführlich F. N. L. Poynter in der Neuburger Festschrift, Wien, 1941, S. 381.

Georg Wheler durchreiste mit dem französischen Arzt Jacques Spon im Jahre 1675 und 1676 Italien, Dalmatien, Griechenland und die Levante. Einen Reisebericht darüber schrieb Spon unter dem Titel *Voyage d'Italie, de Dalmatie, de Grèce, et du Levant* (Lyon, 1678), den anderen Wheler unter dem Titel *A Journey . . .* (London, 1682). Diese Berichte sind wichtig, weil die Reisenden zum erstenmal mehrere Pestlazarette in Dalmatien wie auch das Schwefelbad in Split (Spalato) und den Diocletian-Palast aus der damaligen Zeit beschrieben haben. Aus diesen Beschreibungen wissen wir wie dieser Palast damals ausgeschaut hat.

Der englische Architekt Robert Adam besuchte im Jahre 1757 Spalato in der Begleitung des französischen Baumeisters C. L. Clerisseau und des Italieners A. Zucchi und schrieb ein bedeutendes Werk über diese Stadt und den Diokletian-Palast. Inspiriert von diesem Prachtbau baute Adam an der Themse die prachtvolle

Adelphi Terrace, mit vielen großmächtigen Wölbungen, Hallen und Rundbögen, die an den erwähnten Palast erinnerten. Die Beschreibung Adams *Ruins of the Palace of Emperor Diocletian in Spalato in Dalmacia* (London, 1764) ist noch heute lesenswert.

In dem Werk *Travels in Hungary, with a short account of Vienna in the year 1793* (London, 1797) hat Robert Townson seine Reise über Österreich, Ungarn und teilweise über Kroatien beschrieben.

Der englische Kliniker und Pathologe Richard Bright (1789–1858) hielt sich mehrmals am Kontinent auf, besonders aber im Jahre 1814, anlässlich des Wiener Kongresses und in nachfolgenden Jahren. Heimgekehrt beschrieb er diese Reise in einem Buch von über 600 Seiten, das in Edinburgh erschienen ist unter dem Titel *Travels from Vienna through Lower Hungary with Some Remarks on the State of Vienna during the Congress in the Year 1814* (Edinburgh, 1818). Das Buch war illustriert mit eigenhändigen Zeichnungen, die über seine auserordentliche zeichnerische Fähigkeiten Zeugnis ablegen. Enthält gute Beschreiburg des nördlichen Teiles von Kroatien, auf mehr als 40 Seiten des Buches, wie folgt:

Im April 1815 fuhr er fort aus Wien und besuchte den Plattensee. Im Keszthely war er Gast des Grafen Festetics. Von hier, über Hidvég, Kiskomáron und Nagy Kanizsa erreichte er die Mur, die er mit einer Fähre überfuhr. Nachher besuchte er Vidovec und Prelog und erwähnt auch viele andere Dörfer, Siedlungen, Häuser, Leute und Volksbräuche dieser Gegend. Einige Tage verweilte er in der Stadt Čakovec, besuchte hier das Franziskaner-Kloster, die Burg der Grafen Zrinjski und andere Sehenswürdigkeiten. Es ist bekannt, daß er sich für die Gefängnisse interessierte und desswegen wundert uns nicht, daß er auch das Gefängnis in Čakovec beschreibt. Dadurch ist er ähnlich dem englischen Juristen John Howard (1726–90) der durch sein Week *State of Prisons* (1777) viel zur Reform der Gefängnisse beigetragen hat. Am Lande besuchte er die Schafsfarmen, interessierete sich über die Molkerei und die Milchverarbeitung, für die Mais – und Tabakzucht wie auch für den Weinbau. Ausführlich beobachtet und beschreibt er die Goldwäsche. Beim Dorf Paklenica besuchte er die Erdölquelle (heute bestehen viele solche in dem Mur-Drau-Zwischenland). Aufgrund eigener Beobachtung in Prelog bescheibt er auf mehren Seiten des Buches die Aufzucht der Seidenraupen. Er war auch im Nedelišće. Nachher besuchte er Varasdin, vormals Hauptstadt von Kroatien von wo er auch die schönste Zeichnung gemacht hat. Nach dem Besuch von Ludbreg und Koprivnica durchfuhr er die Drau und über Fünfkirchen erreichte er Buda.

Er reiste mit dem Postwagen und auf der Bauernfuhre. Mit der Bevölkerung in Kroatien verständigte er sich leicht mit Lateinisch und Deutsch. In Verbindung mit Kroatien beschreibt er die tausendjährige Geschichte des Staates und das Volk, die natürliche und wirtschaftliche Geographie, das Leben der Leute besonders der Bauern, ihre Art der Bekleidung, die Volksbräuche und trachtet immer ein treues Bild des Landes zu geben, was ihm aufgrund seines scharfen Blickes, Genauigkeit und Gründlichkeit im größtem Maße gelingt.

In seinen Abhandlungen *Dalmatia . . .* (Oxford, 1887) wie auch *Rambles in Istria, Dalmatia and Montenegro* (London, 1875) gibt T. G. Jackson viele wertvolle Angaben und erwähnt auch eine bekannte wie seltsame kroatische Persönlichkeit aus dem Ende des 16 und dem Beginn des 17 Jahrhunderts, den früheren Erzbischof von Spalato, Marc Anton de Dominis (1560–1624). Dieser hat nach dem Konflikt mit seinem Kapitol und der Römischen Kurie Spalato verlassen und ist geflüchtet nach Venedig. Hier machte er Bekanntschaft mit dem englischen Gesandten in Venedig Sir Henry Wotton und mit seinem Kaplan Bedell. Im Jahre 1616 begleitete er diese Herren nach London, wo der König James I. Dominis zum Decanus der Hofkapelle von Windsor ernannte. Es ist bekannt, daß Dominis hier das Werk *De Republica Ecclesiastica* gegen den Papst geschrieben hat, aber nachher kehrte er doch zurück zur römisch-katholischen Kirche und ersuchte Ablaß beim Papst. Deswegen kam er nach Rom aber hier wurde er der Inquisition übergeben und ins Gefängniß gesetzt wo er starb.

In seinem Vorwort zur 4. Auflage des Buches *Travels in the Slavonic provinces of Turkey-in-Europe* (London, 1877) der englischen Journalistinnen G. Muir Mackenzie und A. P. Irby, erklärt und bekennt sich der englische Politiker William Ewart Gladstone für die Befreiung Bosniens von der rohen türkischen Verwaltung.

Zum Schluß soll noch erwähnt werden Laurence Sterne (1713–68) der mit seinem exzentrischen *The Sentimental Journey* einen starken Einfluß auf viele Schriftsteller ausgeübt hat, unter diesen auch auf den kroatischen Schriftsteller Antun Nemčic, der unter diesem Einfluß seine erdichtete Reisebeschreibungen ,,Putositnice" geschrieben hat.

VII MEDICINE AND THE HUMANITIES